P9-DEC-074

Principles and **Practice** of **Ophthalmology**

SECTION EDITORS

Mark B. Abelson, M.D.
Daniel M. Albert, M.D., M.S.
Dimitri T. Azar, M.D.
George B. Bartley, M.D.
Leo T. Chylack, Jr., M.D.
Donald J. D'Amico, M.D.
Mohamad-Reza Dana, M.D., M.P.H.
Claes H. Dohlman, M.D.
Richard K. Dortzbach, M.D.
C. Stephen Foster, M.D.
Alec Garner, M.D.
Evangelos S. Gragoudas, M.D.
Eve Juliet Higginbotham, M.D.
Frederick A. Jakobiec, M.D., D.Sc.(Med.)
Joel A. Kraut, M.D.
A. Van C. Lanckton, J.D.
Simmons Lessell, M.D.
Leonard A. Levin, M.D., Ph.D.
C. Patricia McCabe, M.P.H., P.T.
Travis A. Meredith, M.D.
William F. Mieler, M.D.
Joan W. Miller, M.D.
Monte D. Mills, M.D.
Frances E. Nason, M.S.W.
Arthur H. Neufeld, Ph.D.
Deborah Pavan-Langston, M.D.
William J. Power, M.Ch.
Richard M. Robb, M.D.
Andrew P. Schachat, M.D.
Johanna M. Seddon, M.D., M.P.H.
J. Wayne Streilein, M.D.
Janey L. Wiggs, M.D.

Monte D. Mills, M.D.
Assistant Professor, Departments of Ophthalmology and Visual Sciences and Pediatrics, University of Wisconsin Medical School, Madison, Wisconsin

Martin C. Mihm, Jr., M.D.
Clinical Professor of Pathology, Harvard Medical School; Adjunct Professor of Pathology, Albany Medical College, Albany, New York; Adjunct Professor of Psychiatry, Vanderbilt University School of Medicine, Nashville, Tennessee; Senior Dermatopathologist, Associate Dermatologist, and Pathologist, Massachusetts General Hospital, Boston, Massachusetts

Jordi Monés, M.D.
Vitreoretinal Consultant de Institut Microcirurgia Ocular de Barcelona; Department of Ophthalmology, Hospital de la Creu Roja, Barcelona, Spain

Eric Mukai, M.D.
Resident in Medicine, Oregon Health Sciences University Hospital, Portland, Oregon

Shizuo Mukai, M.D.
Assistant Professor in Ophthalmology, Harvard Medical School; Associate Surgeon in Ophthalmology, Massachusetts Eye and Ear Infirmary, Boston, Massachusetts

Michael L. Murphy, M.D.
Assistant Professor, Department of Ophthalmology, Medical College of Wisconsin; The Eye Institute, Milwaukee, Wisconsin

Robert P. Murphy, M.D.
Co-Director, The Glaser-Murphy Retina Treatment Center, Chevy Chase, Maryland

Timothy G. Murray, M.D.
Associate Professor of Ophthalmology, Bascom Palmer Eye Institute, University of Miami, Miami, Florida

Timothy J. Murtha, M.D.
Instructor in Ophthalmology, Harvard Medical School; Senior Staff, Joslin Diabetes Center, Boston, Massachusetts

Frances E. Nason, M.S.W.
Adjunct Associate Professor, Simmons College School of Social Work, Boston; Private Practice (Psychotherapy), Chestnut Hill, Massachusetts

J. Daniel Nelson, M.D.
Professor of Ophthalmology, University of Minnesota Medical School—Minneapolis; Associate Medical Director, Surgical Specialties, HealthPartners, Minneapolis, Minnesota

Peter A. Netland, M.D., Ph.D.
Associate Professor of Ophthalmology, University of Tennessee, Memphis, College of Medicine; Surgeon in Ophthalmology, University of Tennessee Hospital, Memphis, Tennessee

Arthur H. Neufeld, Ph.D.
Bernard Becker Research Professor of Ophthalmology, Department of Ophthalmology and Visual Sciences, Washington University School of Medicine, St. Louis, Missouri

Eric A. Newman, Ph.D.
Professor, Department of Physiology, University of Minnesota Medical School—Minneapolis, Minneapolis, Minnesota

Nancy J. Newman, M.D.
Cyrus H. Stoner Professor of Ophthalmology, Associate Professor of Ophthalmology and Neurology, and Instructor in Neurosurgery, Emory University School of Medicine, Atlanta, Georgia; Lecturer in Ophthalmology, Harvard Medical School, Boston, Massachusetts; Director of Neuro-Ophthalmology, Emory Eye Center, Atlanta, Georgia

Eugene W. M. Ng, M.D.
Clinical Fellow, Wilmer Ophthalmological Institute, Johns Hopkins University School of Medicine, Johns Hopkins Hospital, Baltimore, Maryland

Quan Dong Nguyen, M.D.
Clinical Fellow, Retina Specialists of Boston, Boston, Massachusetts

Don H. Nicholson, M.D. (retired)

John H. Niffenegger, M.D.
Director, Retina, Vitreous, Macula, Eye Centers of Ohio, Canton, Ohio

Gary D. Novack, Ph.D.
President, PharmaLogic Development, Inc., San Rafael, California

Kenneth D. Novak, M.D.
Clinical Assistant Professor of Ophthalmology, University of Rochester School of Medicine and Dentistry, Rochester, New York

M. D. Oberlander, M.D.
Chief Resident, Department of Ophthalmology and Visual Science, University Hospital Clinics, Galveston, Texas

Joan M. O'Brien, M.D.
Director, Ocular Oncology Unit, University of California, San Francisco, School of Medicine, San Francisco, California

R. Joseph Olk, M.D., F.A.C.S.
Staff, The Retina Center of St. Louis, St. Louis, Missouri

Karl R. Olsen, M.D.
Clinical Assistant Professor of Ophthalmology, University of Pittsburgh School of Medicine; Active Staff, Department of Ophthalmology, Children's Hospital of Pittsburgh; Provisional Staff, Department of Ophthalmology, Allegheny General Hospital and St. Francis Central Hospital; Consulting Staff, Department of Ophthalmology, Department of Veterans Affairs Medical Center and Western Pennsylvania Hospital, Pittsburgh; Courtesy Staff, Department of Ophthalmology, Conemaugh Memorial Hospital, Johnstown, and Shadyside Hospital, Pittsburgh, Pennsylvania

E. Mitchel Opremcak, M.D.
Clinical Associate Professor of Ophthalmology, Ohio State University College of Medicine; The Retina Group, Columbus, Ohio

Dennis A. Orlock, C.R.A.
Director, ICG Reading Center, Manhattan Eye, Ear, and Throat Hospital, New York, New York,

Robert H. Osher, M.D.
Medical Director, Cincinnati Eye Institute, Cincinnati, Ohio

Randall R. Ozment, M.D.
Attending Surgeon, Fairview Park Hospital, Dublin, Georgia

Millicent L. Palmer, M.D.
Assistant Clinical Professor, University of Arizona College of Medicine; Chief, Ophthalmology, Kino Community Hospital, Tucson, Arizona

Susanna S. Park, M.D., Ph.D.
Assistant Professor of Ophthalmology, University of Texas Southwestern Medical Center at Dallas Southwestern Medical School, Dallas, Texas; Staff Ophthalmologist, Department of Ophthalmology, The Permanente Medical Group, Inc., Sacramento, California

Richard K. Parrish II, M.D.
Professor and Chairman, Department of Ophthalmology, University of Miami School of Medicine; Medical Director, Anne Bates Leach Eye Hospital, Miami, Florida

M. Andrews Parsons, M.B., Ch.B., F.R.C.Path.
Senior Lecturer in Ophthalmic Pathology and Director of Ophthalmic Sciences Unit, University of Sheffield; Honorary Consultant in Ophthalmic Pathology, Central Sheffield University Hospitals Trust, Sheffield, England, United Kingdom

Samir C. Patel, M.D.
Assistant Professor of Ophthalmology, University of Chicago Division of the Biological Sciences, Pritzker School of Medicine; Director, Vitreoretinal Service, University of Chicago Hospital/Clinics, Chicago, Illinois

Deborah Pavan-Langston, M.D., F.A.C.S.
Associate Professor of Ophthalmology, Harvard Medical School, Boston, Massachusetts

Mark A. Pavilack, M.D.
Instructor in Ophthalmology, Wills Eye Hospital, Philadelphia, Pennsylvania; Private Practice, Lancaster, Pennsylvania

John R. Perfect, M.D.
Professor of Medicine, Duke University School of Medicine, Durham, North Carolina

Henry D. Perry, M.D.
Clinical Associate Professor of Ophthalmology, Cornell University Medical College, New York; Chief, Corneal Service, North Shore University Hospital, Manhasset; Chief, Cornea and External Disease, Nassau County Medical Center, East Meadow, New York

Richard Pesavento, M.D.
Retina Specialist, Inland Eye Institute, Colton, California

Robert A. Petersen, M.D., Dr. Med.Sc.
Assistant Professor of Ophthalmology, Harvard Medical School; Senior Associate in Ophthalmology, Children's Hospital, Boston, Massachusetts

Joram Piatigorsky, Ph.D.
Chief, Laboratory of Molecular and Developmental Biology, National Eye Institute, Bethesda, Maryland

Eric A. Pierce, M.D., Ph.D.
Scheie Eye Institute, University of Pennsylvania School of Medicine, Philadelphia, Pennsylvania

Michael K. Pinnolis, M.D.
Clinical Assistant in Ophthalmology, Harvard Medical School; Associate Surgeon, Massachusetts Eye and Ear Infirmary, Boston, Massachusetts

Constantin J. Pournaras, M.D.
Chargé de Cours, University of Geneva, Geneva School of Medicine; Director of Outpatient and Ambulatory Patient Department, Medicine Adjoint, University Hospitals of Geneva, Department of Clinical Neurosciences, Division of Ophthalmology, Geneva, Switzerland

William J. Power, M.B.B.C.H., F.R.C.S., F.R.C.Ophth.
Royal Victoria Eye and Ear Hospital, Dublin, Ireland

Steven G. Pratt, M.D.
Head, Oculo-Plastics Service, University of California, San Diego, School of Medicine, San Diego; Surgeon, Scripps Memorial Hospital, La Jolla, California

Carol C. Prendergast, A.B.D.
Early Childhood Special Education, Columbia University Teachers College; Infant Development Specialist, New York University Medical Center, New York, New York

Ronald C. Pruett, M.D.
Associate Clinical Professor in Ophthalmology, Harvard Medical School; Surgeon in Ophthalmology, Massachusetts Eye and Ear Infirmary, Boston, Massachusetts

Amy Pruitt, M.D.
Assistant Professor of Neurology, University of Pennsylvania School of Medicine; Staff Neurologist, Hospital of the University of Pennsylvania, Philadelphia, Pennsylvania

James L. Rae, Ph.D.
Professor of Physiology and Biophysics and of Ophthalmology, Mayo Clinic, Department of Education Services, Rochester, Minnesota

Michael B. Raizman, M.D.
Assistant Professor of Ophthalmology, Tufts University School of Medicine; Ophthalmologist and Director, Cornea and Anterior Segment Service, New England Eye Center, New England Medical Center; Ophthalmic Consultants of Boston, Boston, Massachusetts

Gary A. Rankin, M.D.
Private Practice, Greensboro, North Carolina

Elio Raviola, M.D., Ph.D.
Professor of Neurobiology, Harvard Medical School, Boston, Massachusetts

Chittaranjan V. Reddy, M.D.
Vitreoretinal Surgeon, Retina Consultants of Central Illinois, Peoria, Illinois

Charles D. J. Regan, M.D.
Associate Professor of Ophthalmology, Emeritus, Harvard Medical School; Surgeon in Ophthalmology, Emeritus, Massachusetts Eye and Ear Infirmary, Boston, Massachusetts

Elias Reichel, M.D.
Assistant Professor of Ophthalmology, Vitreoretinal Diseases and Surgery; Tufts University School of Medicine; Director, Electroretinography Service, New England Eye Center, Boston, Massachusetts

Martin H. Reinke, M.D.
Private Practice, Minneapolis, Minnesota

Leon L. Remis, M.D.
Instructor in Ophthalmology, Harvard Medical School, Boston, Massachusetts; Courtesy Staff, Massachusetts Eye and Ear Infirmary, Boston, Massachusetts

Marsha B. Rich, B.S.N.
Case Manager, North Shore Rehabilitation Center, Danvers, Massachusetts

Thomas M. Richardson, M.D.
Assistant Clinical Professor of Ophthalmology, Harvard Medical School; Assistant Surgeon in Ophthalmology, Massachusetts Eye and Ear Infirmary, Boston, Massachusetts

Claudia U. Richter, M.D.
Clinical Assistant in Ophthalmology, Harvard Medical School; Assistant Surgeon in Ophthalmology, Massachusetts Eye and Ear Infirmary; Ophthalmic Consultants of Boston, Boston, Massachusetts

Klaus G. Riedel, M.D.
Clinical Professor, Ludwig-Maximilians University; Director, Eye Infirmary Herzog Carl Theodor, Munich, Germany

Joseph F. Rizzo III, M.D.
Associate Professor of Ophthalmology, Harvard Medical School; Staff, Massachusetts Eye and Ear Infirmary, Boston, Massachusetts

Richard M. Robb, M.D.
Associate Professor of Ophthalmology, Harvard Medical School; Ophthalmologist-in-Chief, Children's Hospital, Boston, Massachusetts

Alan L. Robin, M.D.
Professor, University of Maryland School of Medicine; Associate Professor, Wilmer Ophthalmological Institute, and School of Hygiene and Public Health, Johns Hopkins University; Chairman, Glaucoma Department, Greater Baltimore Medical Center, Baltimore, Maryland

Joseph R. Robinson, Ph.D.
Professor of Pharmacy and Ophthalmology, School of Pharmacy, University of Wisconsin, Madison, Wisconsin

Rebecca L. Rockhill, M.S.
Research Technician, Howard Hughes Medical Institute, Boston, Massachusetts

Edward J. Rockwood, M.D.
Staff, Glaucoma Department, Division of Ophthalmology, Cleveland Clinic Foundation, Cleveland, Ohio

I. Rand Rodgers, M.D.
Director, Ophthalmic Plastic and Reconstructive Surgical Service, North Shore University Hospital, Manhasset; Attending Physician, Department of Ophthalmology, Mount Sinai Medical Center, and Manhattan Eye, Ear and Throat Hospital, New York, New York

Merlyn M. Rodrigues, M.D., Ph.D.
Professor of Ophthalmology and Pathology, University of Maryland School of Medicine, Baltimore, Maryland

Shiyoung Roh, M.D.
Instructor, Department of Ophthalmology, Harvard Medical School, Boston; Staff Surgeon, Lahey Clinic, Burlington, Massachusetts

Dorothy J. Roof, Ph.D.
Assistant Professor of Ophthalmology, Harvard Medical School; Massachusetts Eye and Ear Infirmary, Boston, Massachusetts

Jack Rootman, M.D., F.R.C.S.C., Dipl.A.A.O.
Professor and Chairman, Department of Ophthalmology, and Professor, Department of Pathology, University of British Columbia Faculty of Medicine; Head, Department of Ophthalmology, Vancouver General Hospital; Chairman, Ocular and Orbital Tumor Group, British Columbia Cancer Agency, Vancouver, British Columbia, Canada

Steven J. Rose, M.D.
Clinical Assistant Professor of Ophthalmology, University of Rochester School of Medicine; Associate Attending in Ophthalmology, Strong Memorial Hospital, Rochester, New York

Robert C. Rosenquist, M.D.
Assistant Clinical Professor, Loma Linda University, Loma Linda, California

Perry Rosenthal, M.D.
Assistant Clinical Professor of Ophthalmology, Harvard Medical School, Boston, Massachusetts

Peter A. D. Rubin, M.D.
Assistant Professor of Ophthalmology, Harvard Medical School; Director, Ophthalmic Plastic, Orbital, and Cosmetic Eyelid Surgery, Massachusetts Eye and Ear Infirmary, Boston, Massachusetts

Shimon Rumelt, M.D.
Senior Ophthalmologist, Hadassah University Hospital, Jerusalem; Western Galilee–Nahariya Medical Center, Nahariya, Israel

Anil K. Rustgi, M.D.
T. Greer Miller Associate Professor of Medicine, University of Pennsylvania School of Medicine; Chief of Gastroenterology, Hospital of the University of Pennsylvania, Philadelphia, Pennsylvania

Mark S. Ruttum, M.D.
Professor of Ophthalmology, Medical College of Wisconsin; Director of Graduate Medical Education in Ophthalmology, Children's Hospital of Wisconsin, Milwaukee, Wisconsin

Allan R. Rutzen, M.D.
Assistant Professor of Ophthalmology, University of Maryland School of Medicine; Co-Director, Refractive Surgery, External Eye Disease and Uveitis Service, Maryland Center for Eye Care, Baltimore, Maryland

Edward T. Ryan, M.D., D.T.M.&H.
Instructor in Medicine, Harvard Medical School; Assistant in Medicine, Division of Infectious Diseases, Massachusetts General Hospital, Boston, Massachusetts

Alfredo A. Sadun, M.D., Ph.D.
Professor, Departments of Ophthalmology and Neurosurgery, University of Southern California School of Medicine; Director of Residency Program in Ophthalmology, Doheny Eye Institute, Los Angeles, California

José A. Sahel, M.D.
Professor of Ophthalmology and Director, Eye Pathology Laboratory, Louis Pasteur University; Head, Vitreoretinal and Oncology Unit, Ophthalmology Clinic, Hôpitaux Universitaires de Strasbourg, Strasbourg, France

Michael A. Sandberg, Ph.D.
Associate Professor of Ophthalmology, Harvard Medical School; Associate in Ophthalmology, Berman-Gund Laboratory for the Study of Retinal Degeneration, Massachusetts Eye and Ear Infirmary, Boston, Massachusetts

Guitelle H. Sandman
Department of Social Work and Discharge Planning, Massachusetts Eye and Ear Infirmary, Boston, Massachusetts

Maria A. Saornil, M.D., Ph.D.
Associate Professor of Ophthalmology, Medical School, University of Valladolid; Ocular Pathology and Oncology Unit, Instituto de Oftalmobiologia Aplicada, University of Valladolid, Valladolid, Spain

David A. Saperstein, M.D.
Assistant Professor, Department of Ophthalmology, Emory University School of Medicine, Atlanta, Georgia

Joseph W. Sassani, M.D.
Professor of Ophthalmology and Pathology, Pennsylvania State University College of Medicine; Penn State–Geisinger Health System, Hershey, Pennsylvania

Stephen J. Saxe, M.D.
Eye Care Specialists, Cape Girardeau, Missouri

Andrew P. Schachat, M.D.
Professor of Ophthalmology, Wilmer Ophthalmological Institute, Johns Hopkins University, Baltimore, Maryland

Oliver D. Schein, M.D., M.P.H.
Associate Professor, Department of Ophthalmology, Johns Hopkins University Medical School; Wilmer Ophthalmological Institute, Baltimore, Maryland

Wiley A. Schell, M.S.
Associate in Research, Department of Medicine, Duke University Medical Center, Durham, North Carolina

Gretchen Schneider, M.S.
Genetic Counselor, Children's Hospital, Boston, Massachusetts

Jan Schreiber, Ph.D.
President, MicroSolve Corp., Waltham, Massachusetts

Alison Schroeder, B.A.
Laboratory Manager, Erickson Laboratory, Department of Ophthalmology, Boston University School of Medicine, Boston, Massachusetts

Ronald A. Schuchard, Ph.D.
Associate Professor of Medicine and Physics, University of Missouri—Kansas City School of Medicine; Director of Research, Eye Foundation of Kansas City, Kansas City, Missouri

Joel S. Schuman, M.D.
Professor of Ophthalmology, Tufts University School of Medicine; Director, Glaucoma Service, and Director, Residency Training, New England Eye Center, New England Medical Center, Boston, Massachusetts

Kevin R. Scott, M.D.
Assistant Clinical Professor of Ophthalmology, Georgetown University School of Medicine; Center for Sight, Georgetown University Medical Center, Washington, District of Columbia; Attending Surgeon, Fairfax Hospital, Fairfax, Virginia

Marvin L. Sears, M.D.
Professor, Department of Ophthalmology and Visual Science, Yale School of Medicine, Yale–New Haven Hospital, New Haven, Connecticut

J. Sebag, M.D., F.A.C.S., F.R.C.Ophth.
Adjunct Associate Clinical Scientist, Schepens Eye Research Institute, Harvard Medical School, Boston, Massachusetts; Associate Clinical Professor of Ophthalmology, Doheny Eye Institute, University of Southern California School of Medicine, Los Angeles, California

Johanna M. Seddon, M.D., S.M.
Associate Professor of Ophthalmology, Harvard Medical School; Associate Professor of Epidemiology, Harvard School of Public Health; Director, Epidemiology Unit, Massachusetts Eye and Ear Infirmary, Boston, Massachusetts

Robert P. Selkin
Fellow, Corneal and Refractive Surgery Service, Massachusetts Eye and Ear Infirmary, Boston, Massachusetts

Richard D. Semba, M.D.
Associate Professor, Johns Hopkins University School of Medicine, Baltimore, Maryland

M. Bruce Shields, M.D.
Sears Professor and Chairman, Department of Ophthalmology and Visual Science, Yale University School of Medicine; Chief of Ophthalmology, Yale–New Haven Hospital, New Haven, Connecticut

Bradford J. Shingleton, M.D.
Assistant Clinical Professor in Ophthalmology, Harvard Medical School; Associate Surgeon in Ophthalmology, Massachusetts Eye and Ear Infirmary; Surgeon in Ophthalmology, Boston Eye Surgery and Laser Center; Ophthalmic Consultants of Boston, Boston, Massachusetts

S. Madeline Shipsey, M.S.W., Lic.C.S.W. (retired)
Formerly Director of Social Work, Social Service, Massachusetts Eye and Ear Infirmary, Boston, Massachusetts

Yichieh Shiuey, M.D.
Clinical Fellow, Cornea and Refractive Surgery, University of Utah, Salt Lake City, Utah

John W. Shore, M.D., F.A.C.S.
Associate Clinical Professor of Surgery, Uniformed Services University of the Health Sciences, F. Edward Hébert School of Medicine, Bethesda, Maryland; Staff Physician, Department of Surgery, Seton Medical Center; Texas Oculoplastic Consultants, Austin, Texas

Santiago Antonio B. Sibayan, M.D.
Fellow, Glaucoma Service, Massachusetts Eye and Ear Infirmary, Boston, Massachusetts

Richard J. Simmons, M.D.
Associate Clinical Professor, Harvard Medical School; Massachusetts Eye and Ear Infirmary, Boston, Massachusetts

Omah S. Singh, M.D., F.R.C.S.(C.)
Assistant Clinical Professor of Ophthalmology, Tufts University School of Medicine, Boston, Massachusetts

James W. Slack, M.D.
Assistant Professor of Ophthalmolgy, George Washington University School of Medicine and Health Sciences; Director of Cornea and External Disease Service and Attending Physician, George Washington University Medical Center, Washington, District of Columbia

Stephen G. Slade, M.D., F.A.C.S.
Clinical Faculty, Hermann Eye Center, University of Texas Medical School at Houston; National Medical Director, The Laser Center; Medical Director, The Laser Center of Houston, Houston, Texas

William E. Smiddy, M.D.
Associate Professor of Ophthalmology, Bascom Palmer Eye Institute, University of Miami School of Medicine, Miami, Florida

Lois E. H. Smith, M.D., Ph.D.
Assistant Professor of Ophthalmology, Harvard Medical School; Senior Associate in Ophthalmology, Children's Hospital, Boston, Massachusetts

Neal G. Snebold, M.D.
Clinical Assistant in Ophthalmology, Harvard Medical School; Assistant in Ophthalmology, Massachusetts Eye and Ear Infirmary, Boston, Massachusetts

Sandra J. Sofinski, M.D.
Instructor in Clinical Ophthalmology, University of Southern California School of Medicine; Attending Staff Ophthalmologist, John F. Kennedy Memorial Hospital, Indio, California

John A. Sorenson, M.D.
Assistant Clinical Professor of Ophthalmology, Columbia University College of Physicians and Surgeons; Attending Surgeon, Department of Ophthalmology, Manhattan Eye, Ear and Throat Hospital, New York, New York

Sarkas H. Soukasian, M.D.
Clinical Assistant Professor of Ophthalmology, Tufts University School of Medicine; Director, Cornea and External Diseases, Ocular Immunology and Uveitis, Lahey Clinic Medical Center, Burlington, Massachusetts

Richard F. Spaide, M.D.
Vitreous-Retina-Macula Consultants of New York, New York, New York

Janet R. Sparrow, Ph.D.
Associate Professor of Ophthalmic Research, Department of Ophthalmology, Columbia University College of Physicians and Surgeons, New York, New York

Charles S. Specht, M.S., M.D.
Staff Pathologist, Department of Ophthalmic Pathology, Armed Forces Institute of Pathology, Washington, District of Columbia

Tomy Starck, M.D.
Assistant Professor of Ophthalmology, University of Texas Medical School at San Antonio; Director, Refractive Surgery Service, University of Texas Health Science Center at San Antonio, San Antonio, Texas

Walter J. Stark, M.D.
Professor of Ophthalmology, The Johns Hopkins University School of Medicine; Director, Cornea Service, The Wilmer Eye Institute, The Johns Hopkins Hospital, Baltimore, Maryland

Christopher E. Starr, M.D.
Resident in Ophthalmology, Massachusetts Eye and Ear Infirmary, Boston, Massachusetts

Scott M. Steidl, M.D., D.M.A.
Assistant Professor in Ophthalmology, University of Maryland School of Medicine; Director, Retina Service, and Clinical Director of Ophthalmology, University of Maryland Medical Center, Baltimore, Maryland

Roger F. Steinert, M.D.
Assistant Clinical Professor, Harvard Medical School; Surgeon, Massachusetts Eye and Ear Infirmary and Boston Eye Surgery and Laser Center; Ophthalmic Consultants of Boston, Boston, Massachusetts

Leon Strauss, M.D., Ph.D.
Instructor, Johns Hopkins University School of Medicine; Wilmer Ophthalmological Institute, Baltimore, Maryland

Barbara W. Streeten, M.D.
Professor of Ophthalmology and Pathology and Director, Eye Pathology Laboratory, State University of New York Health Science Center at Syracuse, Syracuse, New York

J. Wayne Streilein, M.D.
Professor of Ophthalmology and Dermatology, Harvard Medical School; President and Director of Research, Schepens Eye Research Institute, Boston, Massachusetts

David A. Sullivan, M.S., Ph.D.
Associate Professor of Ophthalmology, Harvard Medical School; Senior Scientist, Schepens Eye Research Institute, Boston, Massachusetts

Francis C. Sutula, M.D.
Instructor, Harvard Medical School, Boston, Massachusetts

Paul P. Svitra, M.D.
Private Practice, New Hyde Park, New York

Jonathan H. Talamo, M.D.
Assistant Clinical Professor of Ophthalmology, Harvard Medical School; Associate Surgeon in Ophthalmology, Massachusetts Eye and Ear Infirmary; Medical Director, The Laser Eye Center of Boston, Cornea Consultants, Boston, Massachusetts

Richard R. Tamesis, M.D.
Associated Eye Specialists, Pasig City, Philippines

Kristin J. Tarbet, M.D.
Clinical Instructor, University of Wisconsin Medical School; Staff, Davis Duehr Dean Clinic, Madison, Wisconsin

John V. Thomas, M.D.
Clinical Instructor in Ophthalmology, Harvard Medical School; Clinical Assistant Professor of Ophthalmology, Tufts University School of Medicine; Clinical Assistant in Ophthalmology, Massachusetts Eye and Ear Infirmary, Boston, Massachusetts

Joseph M. Thomas, M.D.
Fellow, Department of Ophthalmology, Case Western Reserve University School of Medicine; Fellow, Department of Ophthalmology, University Hospitals of Cleveland; Private Practice, Cleveland, Ohio

David P. Tingey, M.D., F.R.C.S.(C).
Assistant Professor of Ophthalmology, University of Western Ontario Faculty of Medicine, London, Ontario, Canada

King W. To, M.D., M.M.S.
Associate Clinical Professor of Ophthalmology and Pathology, Brown University School of Medicine; Director of Residency Training, Department of Ophthalmology, and Director of Ophthalmic Pathology, Department of Pathology, Rhode Island Hospital, Providence, Rhode Island

Ikuko Toda, M.D.
Assistant Professor of Ophthalmology, Tokyo Dental College, Tokyo, Japan

Felipe I. Tolentino, M.D.
Associate Clinical Professor, Department of Ophthalmology, Harvard Medical School; Surgeon in Ophthalmology, Massachusetts Eye and Ear Infirmary, Boston, Massachusetts

Michael J. Tolentino, M.D.
Clinical Fellow, Retina Service, Scheie Eye Institute, University of Pennsylvania School of Medicine, Philadelphia, Pennsylvania

Trexler M. Topping, M.D.
Clinical Instructor and Associate Clinical Professor, Tufts University School of Medicine; Staff, New England Medical Center; Associate Surgeon in Ophthalmology, Massachusetts Eye and Ear Infirmary; Ophthalmic Consultants of Boston, Boston, Massachusetts

Paul E. Tornambe, M.D.
Consultant, Department of Defense, Balboa Naval Hospital, San Diego; Retina Consultant, Mericose Eye Institute, La Jolla, California

Christopher M. Tortora, M.D.
Medical Director, Hawaiian Eye Center, Wahiawa, Hawaii

Daniel J. Townsend, M.D.
Instructor, Harvard Medical School; Instructor, Tufts University School of Medicine; Assistant Surgeon, Ophthalmology, Massachusetts Eye and Ear Infirmary, Boston, Massachusetts

Theresa Tretter, M.D.
Resident in Ophthalmology, Manhattan Eye, Ear and Throat Hospital, New York, New York

S. D. Trocme, M.D.
Associate Professor and Vice Chairman, and Director, Corneal and Research Services, Department of Ophthalmology and Visual Sciences, University of Texas Medical School at Galveston, Galveston, Texas

Michele Trucksis, Ph.D., M.D.
Associate Professor of Medicine, Center for Vaccine Development, Division of Geographic Medicine, Department of Medicine, University of Maryland School of Medicine; Staff Physician, Veterans Administration Medical Center, Baltimore, Maryland

Ilknur Tugal-Tutkun, M.D.
Associate Professor of Ophthalmology and Ocular Immunology and Uveitis Services, Department of Ophthalmology, Istanbul University Faculty of Medicine, Istanbul, Turkey

Paulette Demers Turco, O.D.
Clinical Instructor, Department of Ophthalmology, Harvard Medical School; Adjunct Clinical Instructor of Rehabilitation Medicine, Boston University School of Medicine; Adjunct Faculty, Graduate School of Education, University of Massachusetts; Associate Director, Vision Rehabilitation Service, Department of Ophthalmology, Massachusetts Eye and Ear Infirmary, Boston, Massachusetts

Ira J. Udell, M.D.
Professor, Albert Einstein Medical College, New York, New York

Nurşen Ünlü, Ph.D.
Associate Professor, School of Pharmacy, University of Ankara, Ankara, Turkey

Paul F. Vinger, M.D.
Clinical Professor of Ophthalmology, Tufts University School of Medicine, Boston; Ophthalmologist, Lexington Eye Associates, Lexington, Massachusetts

Nicholas J. Volpe, M.D.
Assistant Professor of Ophthalmology and Neurology, University of Pennsylvania School of Medicine; Residency Program Director, Scheie Eye Institute, Philadelphia, Pennsylvania

Michael D. Wagoner, M.D.
Professor of Ophthalmology, University of Iowa, Iowa City, Iowa

Michael Wall, M.D.
Professor of Neurology and Ophthalmology, University of Iowa College of Medicine; Staff, University of Iowa Hospitals and Clinics and Veterans Administration Medical Center, Iowa City, Iowa

David S. Walton, M.D.
Associate Clinical Professor of Ophthalmology, Harvard Medical School; Surgeon, Massachusetts Eye and Ear Infirmary, Boston, Massachusetts

Martin Wand, M.D.
Associate Clinical Professor of Ophthalmology, University of Connecticut School of Medicine, Farmington; Senior Surgeon, Hartford Hospital, Hartford, Connecticut

Martin B. Wax, M.D.
Associate Professor, Department of Ophthalmology and Visual Sciences, Washington University School of Medicine, St. Louis, Missouri

David V. Weinberg, M.D.
Assistant Professor of Ophthalmology, and Director, Vitreoretinal Service, Department of Ophthalmology, Northwestern University Medical School, Chicago, Illinois

Mark J. Weiner, M.D.
Director, Eye Surgery Center, Northside Hospital–Cherokee, Canton, Georgia

Fran A. Weisse, B.A.
Manager, VISION Information Center, VISION Foundation, Inc., Watertown, Massachusetts

David J. Weissgold, M.D.
Assistant Professor of Ophthalmology, University of Vermont College of Medicine, Burlington, Vermont

John J. Weiter, M.D., Ph.D.
Associate Clinical Professor, Department of Ophthalmology, Harvard Medical School; Clinical Senior Scientist, Schepens Eye Research Institute, Boston, Massachusetts

Christopher T. Westfall, M.D.
Associate Professor of Ophthalmology, University of Arkansas College of Medicine; Chief of Ophthalmology Services, Arkansas Children's Hospital, Little Rock, Arkansas

Roy Whitaker, Jr., M.D.
Director of Glaucoma Service, Georgia Eye Institute, Memorial Medical Center, Savannah, Georgia

Scott M. Whitcup, M.D.
Clinical Director, National Eye Institute, Bethesda, Maryland

Valerie A. White, M.D., F.R.C.P.(C).
Assistant Professor, Departments of Pathology and Laboratory Medicine and of Ophthalmology, University of British Columbia Faculty of Medicine; Consultant Pathologist, Vancouver General Hospital, British Columbia Cancer Agency, and British Columbia Children's Hospital, Vancouver, British Columbia, Canada

William L. White, M.D.
Clinical Assistant Professor of Ophthalmology, University of Missouri—Kansas City School of Medicine; St. Joseph's Health Center, Kansas City, Missouri

Janey L. Wiggs, M.D., Ph.D.
Assistant Professor of Ophthalmology, Genetics, and Pediatrics, Tufts University Medical School and Tufts University Sackler School of Graduate Biomedical Sciences; Director, Molecular Genetics Laboratory, Department of Ophthalmology, New England Medical Center, Boston, Massachusetts

Jacob T. Wilensky, M.D.
Professor of Ophthalmology, University of Illinois College of Medicine at Chicago; Director, Glaucoma Service, University of Illinois Eye and Ear Infirmary, Chicago, Illinois

A. Sydney Williams, M.D.
Associate Clinical Professor, Department of Ophthalmology, University of California, San Francisco, School of Medicine, San Francisco, California

M. Roy Wilson, M.D., M.S.
Dean and Professor of Ophthalmology, Creighton University School of Medicine, Omaha, Nebraska

William J. Wirostko, M.D.
Fellow, Vitreoretinal Section, Medical College of Wisconsin, Milwaukee, Wisconsin

John J. Woog, M.D., F.A.C.S.
Associate Clinical Professor, Tufts University School of Medicine; Clinical Instructor, Harvard Medical School; Co-Director, Eye Plastics and Orbit Service, New England Medical Center; Associate Surgeon, Massachusetts Eye and Ear Infirmary, Boston, Massachusetts

Nimit Worakul, M.S.
School of Pharmacy, University of Wisconsin at Madison, Madison, Wisconsin

Shirley H. Wray, M.D., Ph.D., F.R.C.P.
Professor of Neurology, Harvard Medical School; Director, Unit for Neurovisual Disorders, Department of Neurology, Massachusetts General Hospital, Boston, Massachusetts

Jean Yang, M.D.
Clinical Assistant Professor of Ophthalmology, State University of New York Health Science Center at Brooklyn, Brooklyn, New York

Michael J. Yaremchuck, M.D., F.A.C.S.
Assistant Professor of Plastic Surgery, Harvard Medical School; Assistant Surgeon, Massachusetts General Hospital, Boston, Massachusetts

Lawrence A. Yannuzzi, M.D.
Professor of Clinical Ophthalmology, Columbia University College of Physicians and Surgeons; Vice-Chairman, Department of Ophthalmology, and Director of Retinal Services, Manhattan Eye, Ear and Throat Hospital, New York, New York

R. Patrick Yeatts, M.D.
Associate Professor of Ophthalmology and Otolaryngology and Director, Ophthalmic Plastic and Reconstructive Surgery, Bowman Gray School of Medicine of Wake Forest University, Winston-Salem, North Carolina

Sonia H. Yoo, M.D.
Instructor, Harvard Medical School; Staff, Massachusetts Eye and Ear Infirmary, Boston, Massachusetts

Timothy T. You, M.D.
Retina Specialist, Pacific Clean Vision Institute, Eugene, Oregon

Lucy H. Y. Young, M.D., Ph.D.
Associate Professor of Ophthalmology, Harvard Medical School; Associate Surgeon in Ophthalmology, Massachusetts Eye and Ear Infirmary, Boston, Massachusetts

Beatrice Y. J. T. Yue, Ph.D.
Professor of Ophthalmology, Department of Ophthalmology and Visual Sciences, University of Illinois College of Medicine at Chicago, Chicago, Illinois

Bruce M. Zagelbaum, M.D., F.A.C.S.
Assistant Professor, New York University School of Medicine, New York; North Shore University Hospital, Manhasset, New York

James D. Zieske, Ph.D.
Assistant Professor of Ophthalmology, Harvard Medical School; Senior Scientist, Schepens Eye Research Institute, Boston, Massachusetts

Lorenz E. Zimmerman, M.D.
Chairman Emeritus, Division of Ophthalmic Pathology, Armed Forces Institute of Pathology, Washington, District of Columbia

PREFACE TO THE SECOND EDITION

It was our vision when **Principles and Practice of Ophthalmology** was first conceived to create a comprehensive multivolume text of the highest level of accuracy, authority, scope, and style. We aspired to provide a definitive text that would gain a place in the professional lives of ophthalmologists in the 1990s and beyond, corresponding to what Duke-Elder's *Textbook and System* had achieved in the mid-20th century. Together with the publisher, editors, and chapter authors of this work, we were gratified by the widespread use and favorable reviews that the first edition received. In the year of its publication, 1994, **Principles and Practice of Ophthalmology** won first prize in medical sciences from the Association of American Publishers as the best new medical book. We believe that the first edition met its objectives.

Now, 6 years later, there is a large accumulation of new data and information pertaining to the treatment of eye disease. Areas with breakthroughs in new knowledge have included the genetics of inherited retinal disease; treatment of macular holes, retinitis, and endophthalmitis; genetics and therapy of glaucoma; treatment of retinoblastoma; diagnostic immunohistochemical staining; refractive surgery techniques; and cosmetic surgery. We requested the assistance of many of our former section editors and authors from the first edition, and we included new experts in various ophthalmic subspecialties, in order to provide an updated and improved second edition.

A major change in the text's format has been to move most of the chapters that appeared previously in the basic science volume to the appropriate clinical section. Many of these chapters have been revised and rewritten to make them more pertinent for the clinician. In other cases, chapters with limited use to the clinician have been dropped. Once the revised structure of the second edition was established, the two senior editors then divided the contents into separate areas of editorial responsibility. I worked extensively with the sections on Glaucoma, Lids, Orbit, Ophthalmic Pathology, Neuroophthalmology, Pediatric Ophthalmology, Ocular Oncology, and Trauma and also with Psychological, Social, and Legal Aspects. Included among the new section editors with whom I had the pleasure of working are Drs. Travis Meredith (Toxicology), Eve Higginbotham (Glaucoma), George Bartley (Lids and Orbit), Alec Garner (Pathology), Leonard Levin (Neuroophthalmology), Monte Mills (Pediatrics), Andrew Schachat (Oncology), and William Mieler (Trauma). Dr. Jakobiec had principal oversight for the sections on the Conjunctiva, Cornea and Sclera, Uveal Tract, Lens, Retina, Vitreous, Eye in Systemic Disease, and Optical Principles.

The goal of the team involved in producing the second edition of **Principles and Practice of Ophthalmology** has been to make this an even better text than the first edition. It is written with expertise, and I congratulate the section editors and chapter authors for their outstanding work. I am grateful to several other individuals who made this text a reality: Nancy Robinson and Susan Power, the Managing Editors; Lewis Reines, President of the W.B. Saunders Company; Richard Lampert, Senior Medical Editor; and Hazel Hacker, Senior Developmental Editor. The production staff at W.B. Saunders included Copy Editors Marjory Fraser, Judy Gandy, and Mimi McGinnis; and Production Managers Peter Faber, Linda Garber, Jeff Gunning, Shelley Hampton, Denise LeMelledo, Frank Polizzano, and Natalie Ware.

The second edition of this work provides a current and comprehensive overview of ophthalmology. I believe it will be a valuable source of information and guidance for ophthalmologists in the care of their patients.

Daniel M. Albert, M.D., M.S.
Madison, Wisconsin

PREFACE TO THE SECOND EDITION

In antiquity, the creation of a new text or codex (a scroll) often entailed, first, the rubbing off of the previous script from the underlying parchment or vellum (this layering of old and new texts is referred to as a palimpsest), in order to conserve these valuable and then exiguous materials. With the importation of paper from China (the first extant sheets there date from 100 to 105 AD) into Western Europe in the 14th century, and with the invention of the printing press by Gutenberg in the middle of the 15th century, a second edition did not obligate the immolation of the first. The earliest printed books documented before 1501 are called incunabula. In comparison with the past 500 years, what a distance we have traveled over the past 20 years with today's panoply of computerized manuscript preparation, printing, and CD-ROM technology!

We are delighted that the highly favorable reception of the first edition of the **Principles and Practice of Ophthalmology** encouraged us to write a second edition. This edition was conceived under a good karma: In 1994, the book won the accolade of being judged the best medical publication across all specialties by the Association of American Publishers. The six volumes were widely disseminated throughout the United States and abroad and were even translated into Italian. Mainly highly laudatory reviews in the foremost ophthalmic journals and incessant inquiries by trainees, basic scientists, and clinical ophthalmologists about when a second edition might appear confirmed our decision to proceed.

Major changes in the second edition consist of the following: the relocation of many chapters covering basic sciences, which now appear as early chapters in the clinical sections; the incorporation of the radiology and aging chapters into appropriate clinical sections; the addition of more than 500 new color illustrations; the introduction of more than 100 new chapters; the complete revision of all other retained chapters; and an emphasis on new entities, therapies, and the latest basic science developments that can have impact on patient care—for example, in the area of neoangiogenesis, about which there are three new chapters.

Numerous new section editors and authors and coauthors were selected; they turned in a virtuosic performance that revitalized and tightened up the textual, illustrative, and bibliographic compass of this endeavor. This impression is ratified by the reduction in total chapters from 434 to 422 between the first and second editions—a remarkable accomplishment at a moment in our global culture that is characterized by logorrhea on the one hand and by tabescent scholarship on the other. F. Scott Fitzgerald commented sententiously and somewhat autobiographically that in American literature, after successful first novels, there are no second acts (e.g., J. D. Salinger, J. Heller). In contradistinction, in medical publishing the second edition is frequently the best in the lifetime of a textbook, because enthusiasm remains high among the chief editors and the participating authors, who typically respond positively to the fillips of praise and constructive criticism engendered by the first edition.

With Daniel Albert's move to Madison, Wisconsin, he and I divided up the logistics attendant upon the preparation of the second edition. I decided to inveigle two colleagues at the Massachusetts Eye and Ear Infirmary, Drs. Dimitri Azar and Evangelos Gragoudas, to assist me as Associate Chief Editors. They assumed substantial editorial roles, including presiding over large chunks of the textbook as section editors, and provided me with spiritual succor and intellectual camaraderie. Ms. Susan Power, my devoted and loyal administrative manager at the Infirmary, served as managing editor for those portions of the textbook emanating from Boston. Her tenacity, intelligence, and attention to detail have been indispensable for the launching of the second edition. Mr. Richard Lampert, Senior Editor at W.B. Saunders, and Mrs. Hazel Hacker, Senior Developmental Editor, have been caryatids throughout the entire project: The former helped to negotiate the architecture of the enterprise, made us hew to deadlines, and cajoled the occasional dilatory contributor; the latter massaged the potentially polyglot manuscripts into a seamless style that is both readable and graceful.

Of the 73 individuals whom I cited at the end of my preface to the first edition as playing mentoring and supportive roles in the development of my career, I am sad to report that six have passed on: Drs. Henry Allen, Frederick Blodi, David Cogan, Thomas Duane, and Robert Ellsworth and Mr. William Renchard. Their loss impoverishes me personally and, more important, the larger universe of their families, friends, and acquaintances whose lives they enriched. I have no other mentors to add to this list because I have entered the earliest stages of encephalomalacia, but I am also at an enjoyable point in my trajectory in which I am trying to give back to my students, patients, and faculty the beautiful gifts of love, kindness, and knowledge that have been showered upon me by my many wonderful colleagues and associates.

I hope that I might be indulged two short philosophical riffs. In my first preface, I alluded to the phenomenon that a comprehensive textbook can be only a temporary approximation of the truth; from the moment that it appears, it undergoes an accelerating obsolescence. One might think that this would be a deterrent to subsequent editions, owing to the inescapable investment of the Herculean energies that are required; nonetheless, each new edition approaches truth asymptotically, rather than experiencing the Sisyphean tragedy of having the effort fall back to ground zero. This is a more optimistic position than that adopted by Democritus (*c.* 460–370 BC), an early Greek atomist, "In truth we know nothing, for truth lies in the depths" (fragment 117). When Jesus Christ was asked by Pontius Pilate, "What is truth?" (John 18:38), no answer was recorded, although Pilate, an enervated but by no means undiscerning pagan, said to the crowd assembled outside his palace: "I find in him no fault at all." Perhaps the essence of truth is ultimately inexpressible, even if knowable. When asked a similar question by Thomas, Jesus responded obliquely and without any designated omega-point: "I am the way, the truth, and the life" (John 14:6). Regardless of one's theological convictions, Jesus displayed wisdom in defining truth, from his top-down perspective of revelation, as a process that is surely ever-unfolding for us mortals. We must be fully cognizant that human knowledge cannot be "clearer than the truth"; otherwise, the former is self-serving advertising or propaganda. The French Jesuit philosopher and paleontologist Pierre Teilhard de Chardin (1888–1955) clairvoyantly portrayed humankind and the universe in terms of noögenesis and noösphere (the development of the mind and the infinite enlargement of the life of the mind); the dynamics of intellectual generativity have become the new Heraclitian flux, as witnessed by the emergence of cyberspace, cybertexts, the Internet, and the World Wide Web.

My second tangent has to do with a medical scientist's and physician's apparent fascination with disease. Without such a paraphilia, we could not sustain the intellectual and emotional capital investment that is necessary for success in our fields. The antidote to such morbid interest is supplied by the moral and ethical dimension of seeing each individual patient holistically. In fact, we are probably never more lovable or in need of kindness than when we are weak and vulnerable. We should revel trepidatiously in our ability to alchemize our most contrary and unseemly impulses into the beauty of knowledge and service. As the ancient Latin poet Terence (*c.* 186–159 BC) put it in his *Heauton Timoroumenos* (*The Self-Tormentor,* 163 BC)—"Homo sum: humani nil a me alienum puto" (I am a man: nothing human is alien to me).

FREDERICK A. JAKOBIEC, M.D., D.SC.(MED.)
BOSTON, MASSACHUSETTS

PREFACE TO THE FIRST EDITION

"INCIPIT." The medieval scribe would write this Latin word, meaning *so it begins,* to signal the start of the book he was transcribing. It was a dramatic word that conveyed promise of instruction and delight. In more modern times INCIPIT has been replaced by the PREFACE. It may be the first thing the reader sees, but it is, in fact, the last thing the author writes before the book goes to press. I appreciate the opportunity to make some personal comments regarding **Principles and Practice of Ophthalmology.**

One of the most exciting things about writing and editing a book in a learned field is that it puts the authors and editors in touch with those who have gone before. Each author shares with those who have labored in past years and in past centuries the tasks of assessing the knowledge that exists in his or her field, of determining what is important, and of trying to convey it to his or her peers. In the course of the work the author experiences the same anticipation, angst, and ennui of those who have gone before. He or she can well envision the various moments of triumph and despair that all authors and editors must feel as they organize, review, and revise the accumulating manuscripts and reassure, cajole, and make demands of their fellow editors, authors, and publisher.

This feeling of solidarity with early writers becomes even more profound when one is a collector and reviewer of books, and conversant with the history of one's field. In Ecclesiastes it is stated, "of the making of books, there is no end" (12:12). Indeed, there are more books than any other human artifact on earth. There is, however, a beginning to the "making of books" in any given field. The first ophthalmology book to be published was Benvenuto Grassi's *De Oculis* in Florence in 1474. Firmin Didot in his famous *Bibliographical Encyclopedia* wrote that Grassus, an Italian physician of the School of Solerno, lived in the 12th century and was the author of two books, the *Ferrara Quarto* (1474) and the *Venetian Folio* (1497). Eye care in the 15th century was in the hands of itinerant barber-surgeons and quacks, and a treatise by a learned physician was a remarkable occurrence. The next book on the eye to appear was an anonymous pamphlet written for the layperson in 1538 and entitled *Ein Newes Hochnutzliches Büchlin von Erkantnus der Kranckheyten der Augen.* Like **Principles and Practice of Ophthalmology,** the *Büchlin* stated its intention to provide highly useful knowledge of eye diseases, the anatomy of the eye, and various remedies. It was illustrated with a full-page woodcut of the anatomy of the eye (Fig. 1). At the conclusion of the book, the publisher, Vogtherr, promised to bring more and better information to light shortly, and indeed, the next year he published a small book by Leonhart Fuchs (1501–1566) entitled *Alle Kranckheyt der Augen.*

Fuchs, a fervent Hippocratist, was Professor first of Philosophy and then of Medicine at Ingolstadt, Physician of the Margrave Georg of Brandenburg, and finally Professor at Tübingen for 31 years. Like the earlier *Büchlin,* his work begins with an anatomic woodcut (Fig. 2) and then lists in tabular form various eye conditions, including strabismus, paralysis, amblyopia, and nictalops. The work uses a distinctly Greco-Roman terminology, presenting information on the parts of the eye and their affections, including conjunctivitis, ophthalmia, carcinoma, and "glaucoma." The book concludes with a remedy collection similar to that found in the *Büchlin.* Most significant in the association of Leonhart Fuchs with this book is the fact that a properly trained and well-recognized physican addressed the subject of ophthalmology.

Julius Hirschberg, the ophthalmic historian, noted that Fuch's *Alle Kranckheyt,* along with the anonymous *Büchlin,* apparently influenced Georg Bartisch in his writing of *Das Ist Augendienst.* This latter work, published in 1583, marked the founding of modern ophthalmology. Bartisch (1535–1606) was an itinerant barber-surgeon but nonetheless a thoughtful and skillful surgeon, whose many innovations included the first procedure for extirpation of the globe for ocular cancer. Bartisch proposed standards for the individual

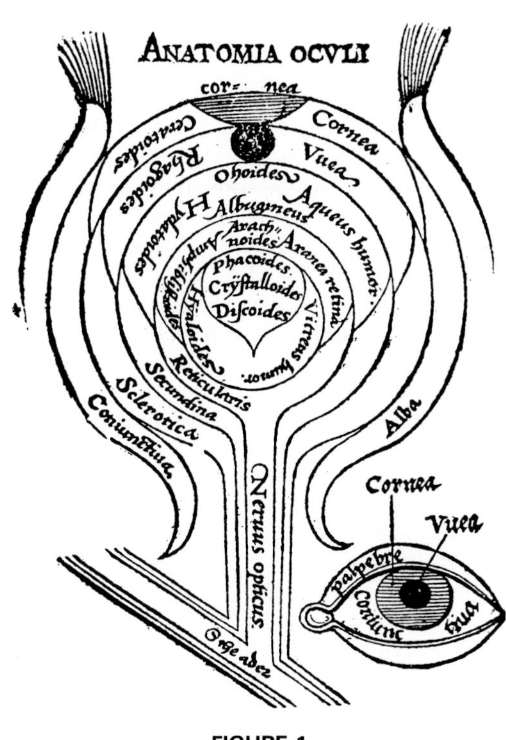

FIGURE 1

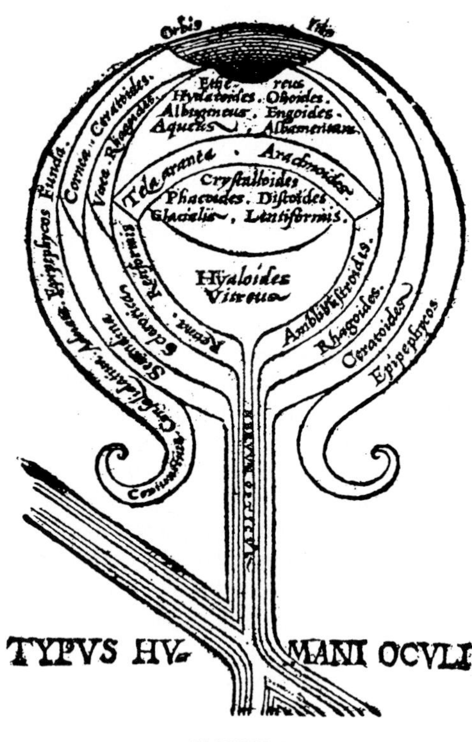

FIGURE 2

who practices eye surgery, noting that rigorous training and concentration of effort were needed to practice this specialty successfully.

By the late 16th century, eye surgery and the treatment of eye disease began to move into the realm of the more formally trained and respected surgeon. This is evidenced by Jacques Guillemeau's *Traité des Maladies de L'Oeil,* published in 1585. Guillemeau (1550–1612) was a pupil of the surgical giant Ambroise Paré, and his book was an epitome of the existing knowledge on the subject.

The transition from couching of cataracts to the modern method of treating cataracts by extraction of the lens, as introduced by Jacques Daviel in 1753, further defined the skill and training necessary for the care of the eyes. The initiation of ophthalmology as a separate specialty within the realm of medicine and surgery was signaled by the publication of George Joseph Beer's two-volume *Lehre von den Augenkrankheiten* in 1813–1817. Beer (1763–1821) founded the first eye hospital in 1786 in Vienna, and his students became famous ophthalmic surgeons and professors throughout Europe.

In England, it was not only the demands of cataract surgery but also the great pandemic of trachoma following the Napoleonic wars that led to the establishment of ophthalmology as a recognized specialty. Benjamin Travers (1783–1858) published the earliest treatise in English on diseases of the eye, *A Synopsis of the Diseases of the Eye,* in 1820. In the United States, acceptance of ophthalmology as a specialty had to await the description of the ophthalmoscope by Helmholtz in 1851, and the additional special skills that using the early primitive "Augenspiegel" required.

As the complexity of ophthalmology increased and as subspecialization began to develop in the 19th century, multiauthored books began to appear. This culminated in the appearance in 1874 of the first volume of the Graefe-Saemisch *Handbuch.* The final volume of this great collective work, of which Alfred Carl Graefe (1830–1899) and Edwin Theodor Saemisch (1833–1909) were editors, appeared in 1880. The definitive second edition, which for more than a quarter of a century remained the most comprehensive and authoritative work in the field, appeared in 15 volumes between 1899 and 1918. The great French counterpart to the Graefe-Saemisch *Handbuch* was the *Encyclopédie Française d'Ophtalmologie,* which appeared in nine volumes (1903–1910), edited by Octave Doin, and filled a similar role for the French-speaking ophthalmologist.

In 1896, the first of four volumes of Norris and Oliver's *System of Diseases of the Eye* was published in the United States. The senior editor, Dr. William Fisher Norris (1839–1901), was the first Clinical Professor of Diseases of the Eye at the University of Pennsylvania. Charles A. Oliver (1853–1911) was his student. Norris considered the *System* to be his monumental work. For each section he chose an outstanding authority in the field, having in the end more than 60 American, British, Dutch, French, and German ophthalmologists as contributors. Almost 6 years of combined labor on the part of the editors was needed for completion of the work. In 1913, Casey A. Wood (1856–1942) introduced the first of his 18 volumes of the *American Encyclopedia and Dictionary of Ophthalmology.* The final volume appeared in 1921. Drawn largely from the Graef-Saemisch *Handbuch* and the *Encyclopédie Française d'Ophtalmologie,* Wood's *Encyclopedia* provided information on the whole of ophthalmology through a strictly alphabetic sequence of subject headings.

The book from which the present work draws inspiration is Duke-Elder's *Textbook of Ophthalmology* (7 volumes; 1932) and particularly the second edition of this work entitled *System of Ophthalmology* (15 volumes, published between 1958 and 1976). The *System of Ophthalmology* was written by Sir Stewart Duke-Elder (1898–1978) in conjunction with his colleagues at the Institute of Ophthalmology in London. In 1976, when the last of his 15 volumes appeared, Duke-Elder wrote in the Preface:

> The writing of these two series, the *Textbook* and the *System,* has occupied all my available time for half a century. I cannot deny that its completion brings me relief on the recovery of my freedom, but at the same time it has left some sadness for I have enjoyed writing it. As Edward Gibbon said on having written the last line of *The Decline and Fall of the Roman Empire:* "A sober melancholy has spread over my mind by the idea that I have taken everlasting leave of an old and agreeable companion."

Duke-Elder adds a final line that I hope will be more àpropos to the present editors and contributors. "At the same time the prayer of Sir Francis Drake on the eve of the attack of the Spanish Armada is apposite: 'Give us to know that it is not the beginning but the continuing of the same until it is entirely finished which yieldeth the true glory.'" The void that developed as the Duke-Elder series became outdated has been partially filled by many fine books, notably Thomas Duane's excellent 5-volume *Clinical Ophthalmology.*

Inspiration to undertake a major work such as this is derived not only from the past books but also from teachers and role models. For me, this includes Francis Heed Adler,

Harold G. Scheie, William C. Frayer, David G. Cogan, Ludwig von Sallmann, Alan S. Rabson, Lorenz E. Zimmerman, Frederick C. Blodi, Claes H. Dohlman, and Matthew D. Davis.

Whereas the inspiration for the present text was derived from Duke-Elder's *Textbook* and *System* and from teachers and role models, learning how to write and organize a book came for me from Adler's *Textbook of Ophthalmology*, published by W.B. Saunders. This popular textbook for medical students and general practitioners was first produced by Dr. Sanford Gifford (1892–1945) in 1938. Francis Heed Adler (1895–1987), after writing the 6th edition, published in 1962, invited Harold G. Scheie (1909–1989), his successor as Chairman of Ophthalmology at the University of Pennsylvania, and myself to take over authorship. We completely rewrote this book and noted in the Preface to the 8th edition, published in 1969: "This book aims to provide the medical student and the practicing physician with a concise and profusely illustrated current text, organized in a convenient and useable manner, on the eye and its disorders. It is hoped that the beginning, or even practicing, ophthalmologist may find it of value."

In 1969 it was apparent that even for the intended audience, contributions by individuals expert in the subspecialties of ophthalmology were required. The book was published in Spanish and Chinese editions and was popular enough to warrant an updated 9th edition, which appeared in 1977. One of the high points of this work was interacting with John Dusseau, the Editor-in-Chief for the W.B. Saunders Company. As a 10th edition was contemplated, I became increasingly convinced that what was needed in current ophthalmology was a new, comprehensive, well-illustrated set of texts intended for the practicing ophthalmologist and written by outstanding authorities in the field. I envisioned a work that in one series of volumes would provide all of the basic clinical and scientific information required by practicing ophthalmologists in their everyday work. For more detailed or specialized information, this work should direct the practitioner to the pertinent journal articles or more specialized publications. As time progressed, a plan for this work took shape and received support from the W.B. Saunders Company.

Memories of the formative stages of the **Principles and Practice of Ophthalmology** remain vivid: Proposing the project to Frederick Jakobiec in the cafeteria of the Massachusetts Eye and Ear Infirmary in early 1989. Having dinner with Lewis Reines, President and Chief Executive Officer, and Richard Zorab, Senior Medical Editor, at the Four Seasons Hotel in May 1989, where we agreed upon the scope of the work. My excitement as I walked across the Public Garden and down Charles Street back to the Infirmary, contemplating the work we were to undertake. Finalizing the outline for the book in Henry Allen's well-stocked "faculty lounge" in a dormitory at Colby College during the Lancaster Course. Meeting with members of the Harvard Faculty in the somber setting of the rare book room to recruit the Section Editors. Persuading Nancy Robinson, my able assistant since 1969, to take on the job of Managing Editor. The receipt of our first manuscript from Dr. David Cogan.

We considered making this work a departmental undertaking, utilizing the faculty and alumni of various Harvard programs. However, the broad scope of the series required recruitment of outstanding authors from many institutions. Once the Section Editors were in place, there was never any doubt in my mind that this work would succeed. The Section Editors proved a hardworking and dedicated group, and their choice of authors reflects their good judgment and persuasive abilities. I believe that you will appreciate the scope of knowledge and the erudition.

The editorship of this book provided me not only with an insight into the knowledge and thinking of some of the finest minds in ophthalmology but also with an insight into their lives. What an overwhelmingly busy group of people! Work was completed not through intimidation with deadlines but by virtue of their love of ophthalmology and their desire to share their knowledge and experience. The talent, commitment, persistence, and good humor of the authors are truly what made this book a reality.

It was our intent to present a work that was at once scholarly and pragmatic, that dealt effectively with the complexities and subtleties of modern ophthalmology, but that did not overwhelm the reader. We have worked toward a series of volumes that contained the relevant basic science information to sustain and complement the clinical facts. We wanted a well-illustrated set that went beyond the illustrations in any textbook or system previously published, in terms of quantity and quality and usefulnesss of the pictures.

In specific terms, in editing the book we tried to identify and eliminate errors in accuracy. We worked to provide as uniform a literary style as is possible in light of the numerous contributors. We attempted to make as consistent as possible the level of detail presented in the many sections and chapters. Related to this, we sought to maintain the length according to our agreed-upon plan. We tried, as far as possible, to eliminate repetition and at the same time to prevent gaps in information. We worked to direct the location of information into a logical and convenient arrangement. We attempted to separate the basic science chapters to the major extent into the separate **Basic Sciences** volume, but at the same time to integrate basic science information with clinical detail in other sections as needed. These tasks were made challenging by the size of the work, the number of authors, and the limited options for change as material was received close to publishing deadlines. We believe that these efforts have succeeded in providing ophthalmologists and visual scientists with a useful resource in their practices. We shall know in succeeding years the level of this success and hope to have the opportunity to improve all these aspects as the book is updated and published in future editions. Bacon wrote: "Reading maketh a full man, conference a ready man, and writing an exact man." He should have added: *Editing maketh a humble man.*

I am personally grateful to a number of individuals for making this book a reality. Nancy Robinson leads the list. Her intelligent, gracious, and unceasing effort as Managing Editor was essential to its successful completion. Mr. Lewis Reines, President of the W.B. Saunders Company, has a profound knowledge of publishing and books that makes him a worthy successor to John Dusseau. Richard Zorab, Senior Medical Editor, and Hazel N. Hacker, Developmental Editor, are thoroughly professional and supportive individuals with whom it was a pleasure to work. Many of the black-

and-white illustrations were drawn by Laurel Cook Lhowe and Marcia Williams; Kit Johnson provided many of the anterior segment photographs. Archival materials were retrieved with the aid of Richard Wolfe, Curator of Rare Books at the Francis A. Countway Library of Medicine, and Chris Nims and Kathleen Kennedy of the Howe Library at the Massachusetts Eye and Ear Infirmary.

The most exciting aspect of writing and editing a work of this type is that it puts one in touch with the present-day ophthalmologists and visual scientists as well as physicians training to be ophthalmologists in the future. We hope that this book will establish its own tradition of excellence and usefulness and that it will win it a place in the lives of ophthalmologists today and in the future.

"EXPLICIT," scribes wrote at the end of every book. EXPLICIT means *it has been unfolded.* Olmert notes in *The Smithsonian Book of Books,* "the unrolling or unfolding of knowledge is a powerful act because it shifts responsibility from writer to reader. . . . Great books endure because they help us interpret our lives. It's a personal quest, this grappling with the world and ourselves, and we need all the help we can get." We hope that this work will provide such help to the professional lives of ophthalmologists and visual scientists.

DANIEL M. ALBERT, M.D., M.S.
MADISON, WISCONSIN

PREFACE TO THE FIRST EDITION

Because of the pellucid beauty of the organ and tissues it studies, ophthalmology affords many pleasures and allurements. Although it might be more of a confessional than a verifiable statement, I have always believed that many individuals are also attracted to ophthalmology with the inchoate fantasy (later found to be erroneous) that it is an encapsulated and somewhat secessionist medical specialty one can totally master; this may indeed be an expression of the ophthalmic temperament's constitutive tropism toward control. Ophthalmology, furthermore, has long been a discipline that has generated exquisite teaching aids; most of the diseases and tissues we contend with are amenable to photographic documentation and elegant analysis by modern imaging and angiographic techniques. The quest for mastery in ophthalmology is marked by the periodic appearance of comprehensive textbooks, an example of which is the present enterprise.

If one person certainly could not do it today, is it possible for multiple authors to create a *Summa Ophthalmologica*? In my professional lifetime the most bruited effort was Duke-Elder's *System of Ophthalmology*, which encompassed 15 volumes, appearing ad seriatim from 1958 to 1976. As a resident-in-training, I remember anticipating the arrival of each new volume, and devouring it from cover to cover because of the spectacular tour d'horizon that was provided. Early in my career, I was privileged to become involved with the orbit section of Duane's five-volume *Clinical Ophthalmology* and subsequently with the anatomy, embryology, and teratology section of his three-volume *Biomedical Foundations of Ophthalmology*, both of which were intended to supersede Duke-Elder. Now, having acquired more experience and maturity, I am aware that it is impossible for an ophthalmic diorama to rival the timelessness of Thomas Aquinas' *Summa Theologica*, Immanuel Kant's *Kritiken*, or Bertrand Russell's *Principia Mathematica*, all of which self-reflexively proceed from deductions based on a priori axioms. Ophthalmology is a contingent, empirical, and non-oracular discipline, and its intellectual artifacts necessarily reflect the imperfections and messiness of human inductive knowledge. At their best, the present and predecessor efforts to produce comprehensive ophthalmic textbooks are temporary codifications, inventories, and snapshots of an ever-unfolding field, much as sequential photograph albums reveal the fructifying growth and evolution of families over generations.

Why, then, was the present project undertaken, and what are its distinctive features? Dan Albert and I began jointly planning this work in early 1989, shortly after I arrived in Boston from New York City to become Chief of Ophthalmology at the Massachusetts Eye and Ear Infirmary and Chairman of the Department of Ophthalmology at the Harvard Medical School. We felt the time was right for a new gesamtwerk for ophthalmology, fraught as it might be with the limitations alluded to previously. We believed that the Harvard environment would be especially conducive to producing an outstanding work of scholarship. Initially the **Principles and Practice of Ophthalmology** textbook carried the subtitle "The Harvard System"; this was reflected in the contract signed with the publisher as well as in the stationery that was used throughout the project in correspondence with the contributors. Whereas it is true that the vast majority of the 350 contributors are by design either present or past faculty or trainees of the Harvard Medical School, the Massachusetts Eye and Ear Infirmary, or the Schepens Eye Research Institute (now formally affiliated with the Harvard Department of Ophthalmology), it quickly became apparent that there was no single "Harvard" or systematic way of thinking about the various topics covered in these volumes. Even within the Harvard Department there are manifold approaches to basic science and clinical problems. Therefore, we were led to abandon the subtitle. Nonetheless, I personally am unabashedly proud that the high quality and erudition of the chapters derive from the intellectual formation that many contributors received from their association with the greater Harvard ophthalmic environment; well represented within this cadre are recent residents and fellows.

Of the six volumes, the longest (**Basic Sciences**) deals with the basic sciences of ophthalmology in ten sections. It is in this realm that one will expect the most rapid changes in subject matter in the immediate years ahead; on the other hand, this may be the most valuable of all the volumes, because there has not been a recent effort to synthesize the burgeoning of knowledge that has attended the revolutions in morphologic investigations, pharmacology, cell biology, immunology, and, lately, molecular genetics. Not every topic in the visual basic sciences could be covered: For example, an extensive and conventional repetition of the facts of embryology and anatomy has not been essayed, since there already exist serviceable references for these comparatively static subjects. The focus instead was on investigations that had been particularly rewarding and luminous over the past 10 years. My advice to readers is to approach each chapter in this volume as if it were an article in the *Scientific American* and to derive both knowledge and pleasure from these lapidary syntheses.

The five clinical volumes have been organized along the lines of standard anatomic and tissue-topographic demarcations. Additionally, there are systematic approaches to some established and newly emerging nodal points of knowledge: neuroophthalmology; the eye and systemic disease; pediatric ophthalmology; ocular oncology; ophthalmic pathology; trauma; diagnostic imaging; optical principles and applications; and psychological, social, and legal aspects of ophthalmology. Efforts were made to reduce unnecessary duplication from section to section in the coverage of various subjects; however, when it was felt that it would be profitable to have the same disease or topic covered from several perspectives, this was permitted. We are aware that, despite the length of our present undertaking, the end result is one of comprehensiveness but not exhaustiveness. It should be remembered that there already exist many published and revised multivolume treatises on subjects covered herein. What we have aimed for is to provide the generalist with a digestible up-to-date overview of ophthalmology and also to provide the superspecialist with readily accessible introductions to topics outside of his or her intensive areas of expertise.

Another distinctive feature of the present volumes is the prodigious number of illustrations, totaling well over 6000 if one includes tables, diagrams, and graphs. About half of these are in color, which enhances the aesthetic and teaching value of the entire project. The bibliographies are often daunting and will serve as pathfinders into the larger universe of their subjects. I would particularly like to thank Ms. Kit Johnson of the Infirmary for providing many of the color illustrations for diseases of the eyelids, conjunctiva, and anterior segment of the eye. For voluptuaries of ophthalmology, these and the fundus illustrations should provide a sumptuous feast.

It staggers the mind to contemplate the quotidian and oppressive amount of effort expended on this project—the incalculable atomistic acts of assemblage, the gently hectoring telephone calls, the background acquisition and scope of the basic science and clinical knowledge, the multiple textual revisions, the amassing of bibliographies and illustrations, and so on—and indeed the formidable cost of producing each of the individual chapters, much of which was borne by the authors themselves. Even as we are hopeful that these volumes will make a major positive impression on American and international ophthalmology, modesty in the face of our challenging task rather than arrogance has inspired the lofty goals that sustained the creation of the **Principles and Practice of Ophthalmology.** Still, I have no doubt that many of the chapters contained in these volumes are the most incandescent, scholarly, and useful summary presentations of their subjects that have been crafted up to now. In a many-authored textbook there will be some unevenness, the result of the idiosyncrasies of the contributors as well as the state of development of their subject matter. My own criterion for the success of this enterprise is a simple one: that 50% or more of the chapters will have achieved the status of being the best overviews and introductions for their subjects. Regarding topics that should have been covered but were somehow missed or that were surveyed inadequately, the chief editors, the section editors, the authors, and the publisher will look forward to hearing from readers and reviewers about any constructive criticisms on how to improve the textbook in its next edition. We are also exploring various mechanisms for issuing supplemental chapters to rectify some of these perceived and real deficiencies before the next edition.

Based on my familiarity with ophthalmic texts, I think the present work is the largest ophthalmic publication ever to appear *all at once as a complete set.* The W.B. Saunders Company is consequently to be congratulated for having maintained the highest standards of production in terms of copy editing, printing, paper quality, indexing, and reproduction of color and black-and-white illustrations. Mr. Richard Zorab, Senior Medical Editor, was a tireless and relatively humane flogger of myself and the other contributors to meet realistic deadlines; Mrs. Hazel N. Hacker was our highly expert Developmental Editor, and Mrs. Linda R. Garber kept the movement of manuscripts and galleys on schedule with minimal breakage. Ms. Nancy Robinson was a compassionate, patient, and effective intradepartmental Managing Editor. I particularly applaud the ability of the publisher to keep the price of the six volumes, with all their color illustrations, at a respectable level so that they are within the reach of trainees, basic scientists, and clinicians in an era of highly competitive National Institutes of Health funding and when ophthalmic reimbursements are being ratcheted down.

It is my compressed personal philosophy that we live to feel, think, and act and that the highest emanations of these faculties are enthusiasm, creativity, and love. This textbook is a manifestation of all six of these capacities, served up in superabundance. May the response of the ophthalmic community be commensurate with the spiritual and intellectual largesse lavished by the contributors on these volumes. Finally, although I somewhat iconoclastically do not fully subscribe to the notion of role models (because I believe that each person should construct his or her unique identity and excellence by cultivating one's intrinsic gifts while at the same time selectively interiorizing the finest qualities of many exemplars), I would like to thank my many professional friends and colleagues who have played salutary roles in the parturition of my own career, and who have taught me and/or supported me to this point in my professional life so that I could participate in this magnificent and bracing academic adventure: Dean James S. Adelstein, Dr. Henry Allen, Dr. Myles Behrens, Mr. Alexander Bernhard, Dr. Frederick Blodi, Dr. Sheldon Buckler, Dr. Alston Callahan, Dr. Charles J. Campbell, Dr. H. Dwight Cavanaugh, Mr. Melville Chapin, Dr. David Cogan, Dr. D. Jackson Coleman, Dr. Brian Curtin, Dr. Donald D'Amico, Dr. Arthur Gerard Devoe, Dr. Jack Dodick, Dr. Claes Dohlman, Dr. Anthony Donn, Ms. Cathleen Douglas-Stone, Dr. Thomas Duane, Dr. Howard Eggers, Dr. Robert Ellsworth, Dr. Andrew Ferry, Dr. Ramon L. Font, Dr. Max Forbes, Dr. Ephraim Friedman, Mr. Frank Garrity, Dr. Gabriel Godman, Dr. Evangelos Gragoudas, Dr. W. Richard Green, Dr. Winston Harrison, the late Dr. Paul Henkind, Dr. George M. Howard, Dr. Takeo Iwamoto, Dr. Ira Snow Jones, Mrs. Diane Kaneb, Dr. Donald West King, Dr. Daniel M. Knowles, Dr. Raphael Lattes, Dr. Simmons Lessell, Dr. Harvey Lincoff, Mr. Martin Lipton, Dr. Richard Lisman, Mr. Richard MacKinnon, Dr. Ian McLean, Dr. Julian Mansky, Dr. Norman Medow, Mr. August Meyer, Dr. George (Bud) Merriam, Sr., Dr. Carl Perzin, Dr. Katherine Stein Pokorny, Dr. Elio Raviola, the late Dr. Algernon B. Reese, Mr. William Renchard, Dr. Rene Rodriguez-Sains, Dr. Evan Sacks, Dr. Charles Schepens, Dr. James Schutz, the late Dr. Sigmund Schutz, Dr. John Shore, Dr. Jesse Sigelman, Mr. F. Curtis Smith, Dr. William Spencer, Dr. R. David Sudarsky, Dr. Myron

Tannenbaum, Dr. Elise Torczynski, Dean Daniel Tosteson, Dr. Arnold Turtz, Dr. Robert Uretz, the late Dr. Sigmund Wilens, Dr. Marianne Wolf, Dr. Myron Yanoff, and Dr. Lorenz E. Zimmerman.

I hope that this textbook will touch the lives of those who read it as much as these individuals have influenced my own.

Ad Astra Per Aspera!

FREDERICK A. JAKOBIEC, M.D., D.SC.(MED.)
BOSTON, MASSACHUSETTS

CONTENTS

VOLUME 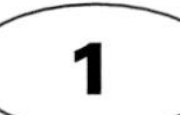

BASIC SCIENCES IN OPHTHALMOLOGY

VOLUME 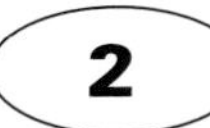

CLINICAL OPHTHALMOLOGY

SECTION VIII
Conjunctiva, Cornea, and Sclera, 609

Edited by DIMITRI T. AZAR and CLAES H. DOHLMAN

SECTION IX
Uveitis, 1149

Edited by WILLIAM J. POWER and FREDERICK A. JAKOBIEC

VOLUME 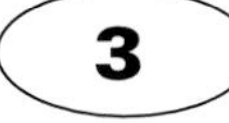

VOLUME

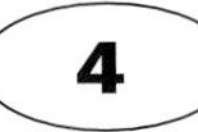

VOLUME

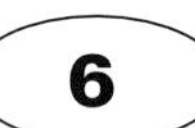

SECTION XVIII

Ocular Oncology, 5003

Edited by ANDREW P. SCHACHAT and DANIEL M. ALBERT

SECTION XIX

Trauma, 5177

Edited by WILLIAM F. MIELER

NOTICE

Ophthalmology is an ever-changing field. Standard safety precautions must be followed, but as new research and clinical experience broaden our knowledge, changes in treatment and drug therapy become necessary or appropriate. Readers are advised to check the product information currently provided by the manufacturer of each drug to be administered to verify the recommended dose, the method and duration of administration, and the contraindications. It is the responsibility of the treating physician, relying on experience and knowledge of the patient, to determine dosages and the best treatment for the patient. Neither the publisher nor the editor assumes any responsibility for any injury and/or damage to persons or property.

THE PUBLISHER

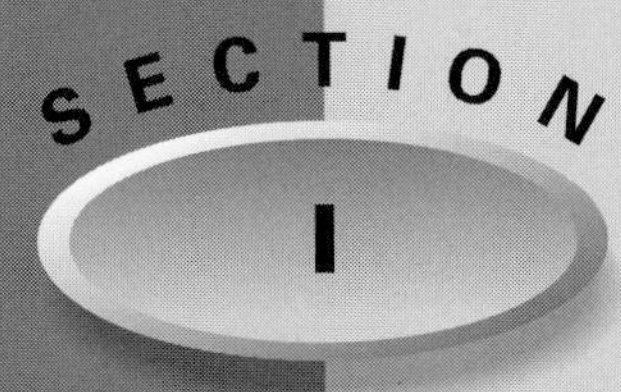

Genetics

Edited by

JANEY L. WIGGS

CHAPTER 1

Fundamentals of Genetics

Thaddeus P. Dryja

A Gene Is Defined by a Phenotype

Genes are the fundamental units used in the study of inherited traits or diseases. A gene is classically defined by the phenotype that is associated with it. For example, the gene causing choroideremia is the choroideremia gene, and the gene causing retinoblastoma is the retinoblastoma gene. However, in more recent years, many genes have been defined on the basis of the encoded protein product, irrespective of any phenotypes known to be associated with variations or mutations. For instance, a gene on chromosome 3 is named the "rhodopsin gene" because it encodes rhodopsin. Years after the isolation and characterization of the rhodopsin gene, it was discovered that mutations at this gene can cause retinitis pigmentosa or stationary night blindness. Rather than rename the locus as the retinitis pigmentosa gene or otherwise, this gene retains its name in most circles as the rhodopsin gene.

The term "gene" is actually somewhat ambiguous, because it can refer to the position on a chromosome (a locus) that governs a heritable trait or to a form of the DNA sequence at the locus (an allele) that is associated with a particular phenotype. Therefore, in common usage, one might state that a variation in iris color is due to a "gene," and it is also correct to state that a brown-eyed person has the "gene" for a brown iris. In the first case, one is stating that a genetic locus has alleles that specify iris color, and in the second case, one is referring to a particular allele at the iris color locus. To be more specific and unambiguous, one should state that a genetic *locus* controls iris color and that an individual with brown eyes carries a brown *allele* at that locus. The distinction is important, especially when one counsels a family with a hereditary disease such as retinoblastoma. The family may speak of the affected child as having the "retinoblastoma gene." They will be surprised to learn from the ophthalmologist that all family members have the "retinoblastoma gene," but that some relatives have normal versions of the gene that do not predispose to the cancer. Only those relatives with a mutant version have a high risk of being affected. Despite the ambiguities, the different uses for the word "gene" are so ingrained that any attempt to change them is futile.

Linear Polymers of DNA Are the Chemical Bases for Genes

The chemical material that contains genetic information is DNA. This is a linear polymer with two complementary strands. Each strand is made up of a linear array of purine bases, guanine (G) and adenine (A), and pyrimidine bases, cytosine (C) and thymine (T). Each base is linked covalently to a pentose; the combination is called a nucleoside. A single strand of DNA has a series of the four bases coupled through these carbohydrate moieties by phosphate bonds. The genetic information is contained in the specific sequence of the four bases in the 5′ to 3′ direction, where the 5′ and 3′ designations refer to the sites on the pentose moieties where phosphate bonds are linked. This strand is called the *sense* strand. The complementary strand, or *antisense* strand, runs in the opposite direction and invariably has nucleotides complementary to those in the sense strand as illustrated in Figure 1–1.

DNA-RNA-Protein. A gene is determined by the particular order of bases within a specified region (locus) in a molecule of DNA. Each gene codes for a protein. RNA is the chemical intermediate that conveys the base sequence in DNA to the protein-synthesizing machinery (ribosomes) in the cytoplasm of a cell. RNA is composed of the same purine and pyrimidine bases as DNA, except that the pyrimidine base thymine (T) present in DNA is instead uracil (U) in RNA. Another difference is that the pentose linked to each base is ribose rather than deoxyribose. The RNA molecules that transmit the DNA base sequence to the cytoplasm of a cell are called messenger RNA molecules, or mRNA. The synthesis of mRNA molecules from a DNA template is called transcription. The synthesis of strands of amino acids based on the sequence of bases in mRNA is called translation.

Organization of a Eukaryotic Gene. Eukaryotic genes, including human genes, are transcriptional units; that is, each gene is organized for the synthesis of a distinct mRNA sequence that codes for a distinct protein. Transcriptional units are organized in the following manner (Fig. 1–2). At the 5′ end is a region extending a few hundred bases called the promoter region. This region has sequences recognized by factors (typically proteins) that control the expression of the gene, as well as one or more binding sites for RNA polymerase. Besides the promoter region, other regions within a gene or at some distance from it can also have roles in determining the proper tissue-specific expression of a gene at the proper time during the life of the organism.[1]

Downstream of the promoter region is the transcription start site, which is a specific base at which the enzyme "RNA polymerase" initiates the synthesis of an RNA copy of the DNA sequence. The sequence of bases in the transcribed RNA molecule will be identical to the sequence in the sense strand of DNA, except that the base uracil (U) will be used instead of thymine (T), as noted earlier. Next comes the 5′ untranslated region, or the region of sequence that is in-

Thymine

Adenine

Guanine

Cytosine

A

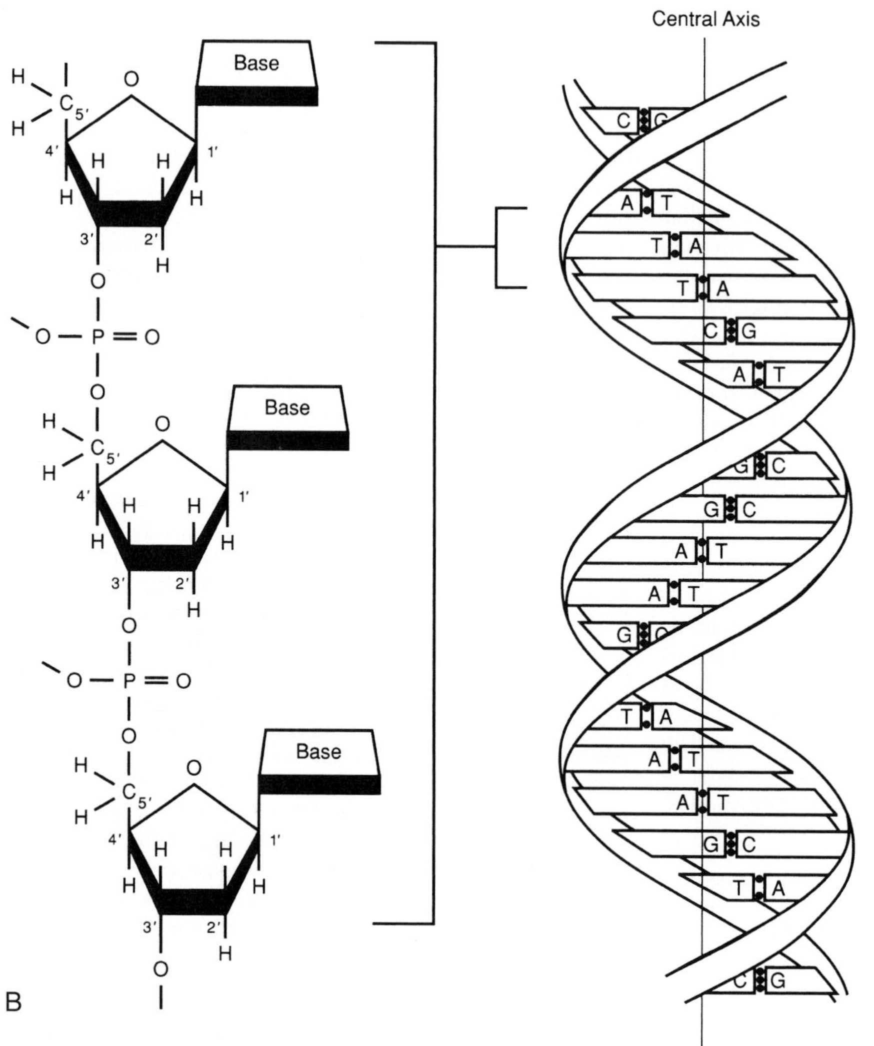

FIGURE 1–1. Chemical structure of DNA. *A,* Two hydrogen bonds *(dotted lines)* couple the bases thymine and adenine, and three hydrogen bonds couple guanine and cytosine. *B,* The double-helical structure of the linear DNA strands.

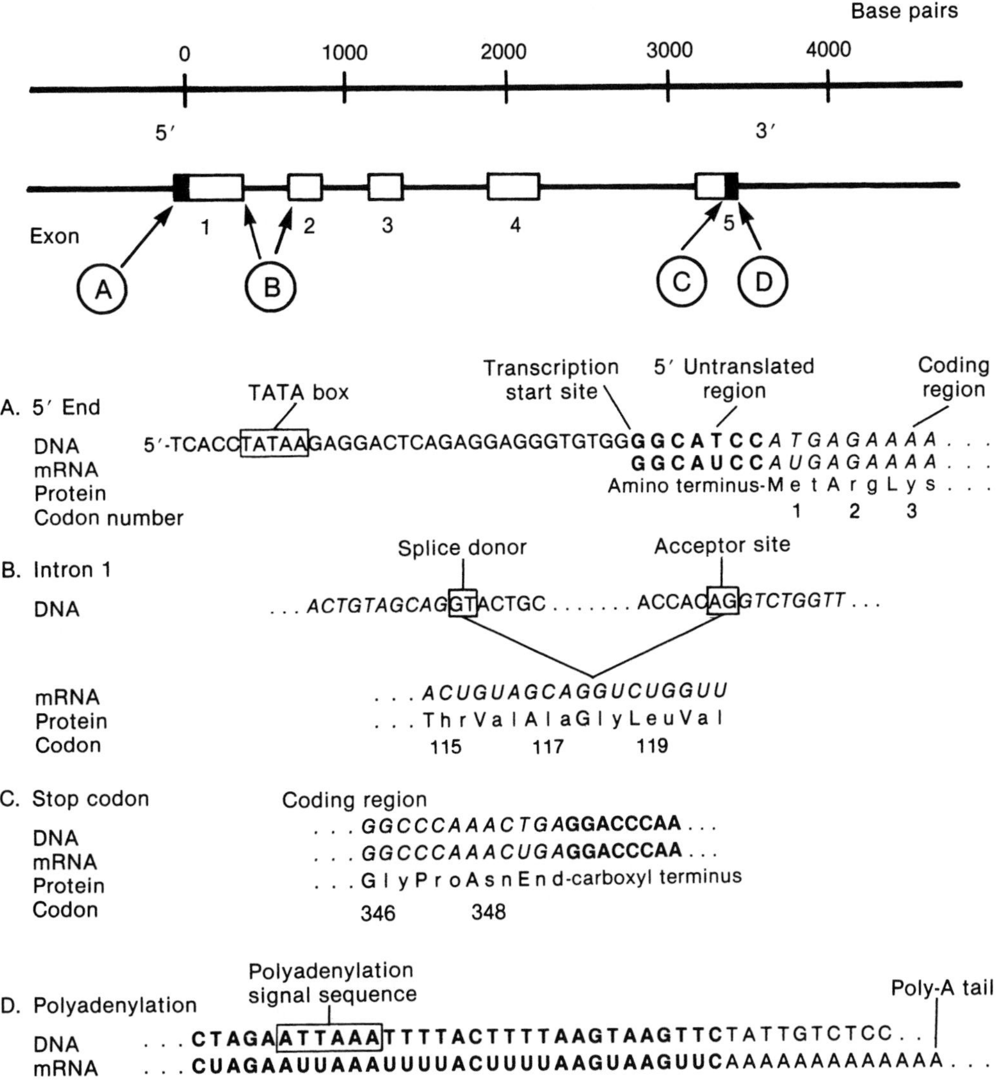

FIGURE 1–2. Functional organization of a transcriptional unit. The organization of the human blue cone opsin gene, which consists of approximately 4000 base pairs of DNA within human chromosome 7, is shown.[47] *Top,* Schematic representation of the position of each of the five exons. The letters A through D indicate the four regions illustrated in more detail below, where the DNA sequence (sense strand only) at each of the four positions is shown. *A,* The 5′ end of the gene. The TATA box is the sequence TATAA, which is an important recognition sequence for the binding of a factor that allows RNA polymerase to initiate transcription. The transcription start site is the point at which an RNA copy of the DNA sequence is begun. The RNA sequence differs from the DNA sequence only in that a U (uridine) is used instead of a T (thymine). The first segment of transcribed DNA is the 5′ untranslated region. Translation begins with the sequence AUG, which is called the initiation codon or the start codon. It specifies methionine, which will be at the amino terminus (N) of the resultant amino acid sequence. *B,* Intron 1. The first intron begins with the dinucleotide sequence GT and ends with the sequence AG. These dinucleotide sequences are almost invariably present at the ends of introns and are called the splice donor and splice acceptor sites, respectively. Notice that a codon is split by the intron. This is neither the rule nor the exception. *C,* Termination of translation. In the last exon (exon 5) a stop codon occurs—in this case the sequence TGA. Although transcription of RNA continues beyond this codon, the remaining RNA sequence is not translated into an amino acid sequence and therefore is called the 3′ untranslated region. *D,* Polyadenylation. The polyadenylation signal sequence, ATTAAA, is recognized by factors that cause the termination of transcription 20 bases downstream. At the end of the RNA sequence, a large string of As is added. The final RNA transcript, after the excision of the four introns and the addition of the poly-A sequence, is called a messenger RNA, or mRNA. It is transported to the cytoplasm for translation by the ribosomes.

cluded in the RNA transcript but is not used to code for a protein. The coding region begins with the initiation codon, which is always the triplet of bases "ATG" coding for methionine. The succeeding sequence of bases is called the coding region and is organized into codons or triplets of bases that specify the amino acids of the encoded protein. The coding region ends with a stop codon (either TGA, TAG, or TAA), which is followed by the 3′ untranslated region. Finally, a polyadenylation signal sequence registers the end of transcription by RNA polymerase.

A noteworthy feature of eukaryotic genes, but not prokaryotic genes, is that the coding region in genomic DNA is generally interrupted by one or more introns. After an RNA transcript is produced from a gene, these intron sequences are excised. This is one of the steps necessary to make mature messenger RNA or mRNA. The term cDNA is given to any DNA fragment with a sequence identical to that found in an mRNA molecule (i.e., a DNA sequence lacking intron sequences). cDNA molecules are not normally produced in living cells; instead, they are produced in research laboratories and are used as reagents helpful in studying genes.

Genetic Code. The DNA sequence that specifies the sequence of amino acids of a protein is in the form of a genetic "code." In the cytoplasm of cells, ribosomes translate the code (Fig. 1–3). Each set of three consecutive nucleotides, called a codon, in the coding region of an mRNA molecule specifies one amino acid.

Figure 1–4 shows the amino acid specified by each codon. The codon ATG, which specifies the amino acid methionine, is the only codon used by the ribosome to initiate translation. Hence, all proteins are first synthesized with the amino acid methionine at their amino terminus. (This amino acid may be subsequently removed as a post-translational modification of the protein.) Ribosomes recognize the correct ATG sequence present near the 5′ end of the mRNA for initiating translation; other ATG codons nearby are customarily ignored through mechanisms that remain unclear. Downstream from the initiating codon, every three bases specify one amino acid. There is no skipping or overlapping of codons. This process continues until one of the codons TAG, TGA, or TAA is encountered in the same frame as the initiating codon. These three codons are called stop or termination codons, because any one of them serves to terminate the translation of an mRNA molecule.

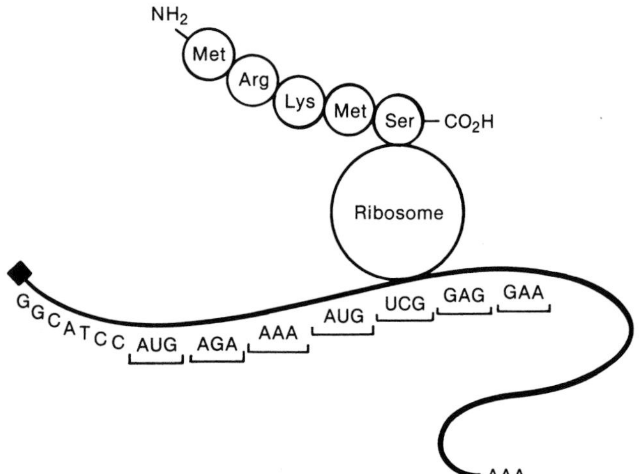

FIGURE 1–3. Translation of mRNA. A ribosome is depicted schematically in the process of synthesizing a molecule of blue cone opsin.

How Genes Are Organized in Human Cells

DNA molecules that carry genetic information are packaged into chromosomes. A *chromosome* is thought to be composed of a single long DNA molecule and numerous associated proteins and perhaps other substances. The complex of DNA and associated materials in chromosomes is called *chromatin*.

Human Chromosomes. Each nucleus of a human cell has 23 pairs of chromosomes (Fig. 1–5), corresponding to 46 molecules of DNA. The two chromosomes in each pair typically have an identical appearance and have the same complement of genetic loci in the same order. They are distinguished because they can carry different alleles at each locus. Each member of a pair of chromosomes is derived from a different parent. Of the 23 pairs of chromosomes, 22 are called *autosomes*; the remaining pair embodies the *sex chromosomes*. The 22 autosomes are numbered according to their size, with chromosome 1 being the largest chromosome, chromosome 2 the next in size, and so forth. The only exception to this rule involves chromosomes 21 and 22, because chromosome 21, not 22, is the smallest. The sex chromosomes are not named by numbers but instead are called the X and Y chromosomes.

Each chromosome has a centromere that divides it into two arms, the short arm and the long arm (Fig. 1–6). The short arm and long arm are called the *"p" arm* and the *"q" arm*, respectively. The *proximal* portion of a chromosome arm is the region close to the centromere; the *distal* portion is far from the centromere. A chromosome with a very small short arm is called an *acrocentric* chromosome. Acrocentric human chromosomes are numbers 13, 14, 15, 21, and 22. The short arms of acrocentric chromosomes contain multiple copies of the genes coding for ribosomal RNA rather than for proteins.

Until the early 1970s, chromosomes could only be distinguished on the basis of their overall size and the relative size of their short and long arms. Because of this, many human chromosomes could not be uniquely distinguished, and chromosomes of similar morphology were lumped into groups (e.g., the "A" group, "B" group, etc.). As an example, the "D" group included chromosomes 13, 14, and 15; all of these are acrocentric chromosomes of approximately the same size. A patient with a deletion of any of those three chromosomes was diagnosed as having a "D-deletion." A few cases of retinoblastoma with a deletion of a D group chromosome were reported in the 1960s, and this association was called "D-deletion retinoblastoma."[2, 3]

Improved chromosome banding techniques, using dyes such as quinacrine or Giemsa, became widely used by the early 1970s. A pattern of staining that is unique to each chromosome arm allowed the recognition of every human chromosome. There is now a standardized nomenclature for the set of darkly and lightly staining bands characteristic of each human chromosome arm. To continue the example of "D-deletion" retinoblastoma, after the new karyotyping techniques were developed, it was discovered that in all cases of "D-deletion retinoblastoma," the deleted chromo-

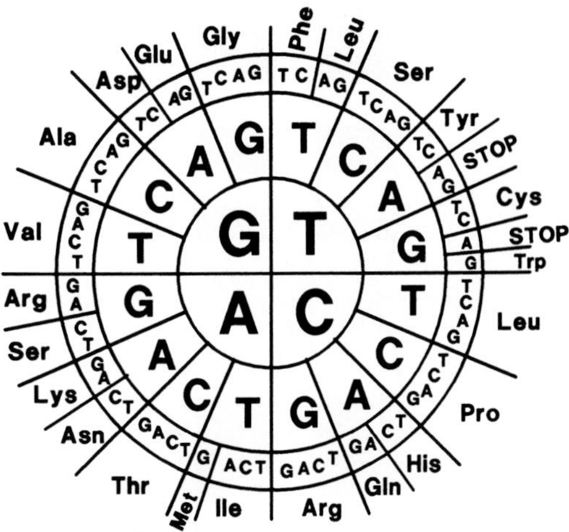

FIGURE 1–4. The genetic code. This wheel gives the amino acid specified by any three-base codon. The codon is read from the center to the periphery of the wheel. Amino acids are abbreviated using the standard three-letter code. At the *bottom* of the figure is the one-letter code, the three-letter code, and the full name of each amino acid. (Adapted from Ausubel FM, Brent R, Kingston RE, et al: Current Protocols in Molecular Biology. New York, John Wiley, 1991.)

One and Three Letter Codes

A	Ala	Alanine
R	Arg	Arginine
N	Asn	Asparagine
D	Asp	Aspartic acid
C	Cys	Cysteine
E	Glu	Glutamic acid
Q	Gln	Glutamine
G	Gly	Glycine
H	His	Histidine
I	Ile	Isoleucine
L	Leu	Leucine
K	Lys	Lysine
M	Met	Methionine
F	Phe	Phenylalanine
P	Pro	Proline
S	Ser	Serine
T	Thr	Threonine
W	Trp	Tryptophan
Y	Tyr	Tyrosine
V	Val	Valine

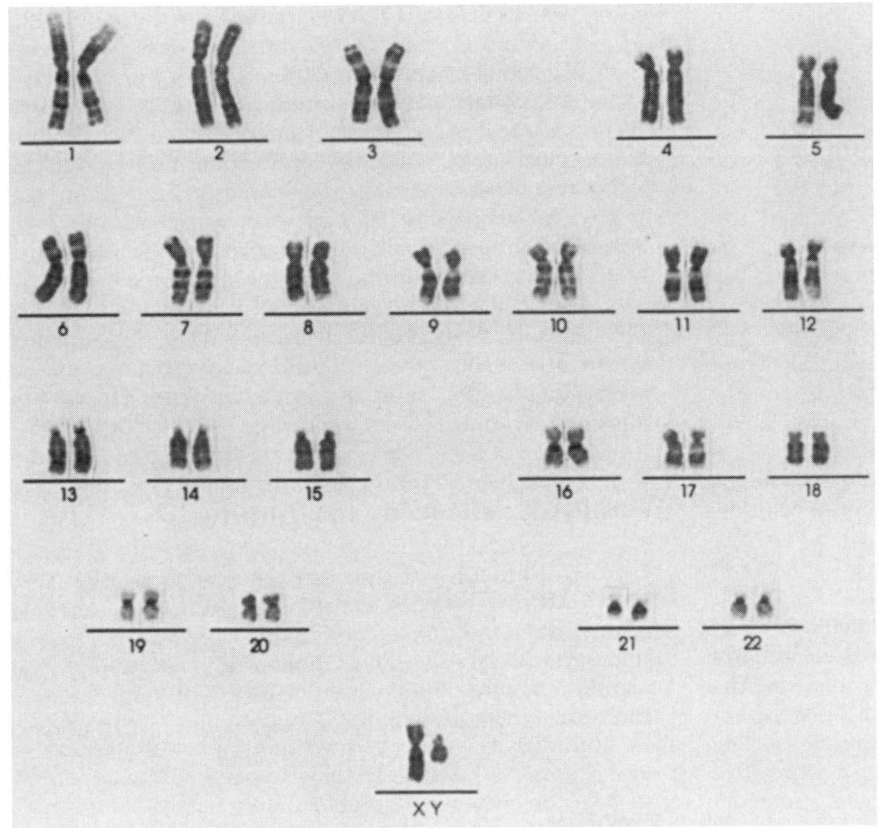

FIGURE 1–5. A normal human karyotype. Below the 22 pairs of autosomes are the sex chromosomes. Since both X and Y chromosomes are present, this karyotype is from a male. (Courtesy of Cynthia Morton, Ph.D.)

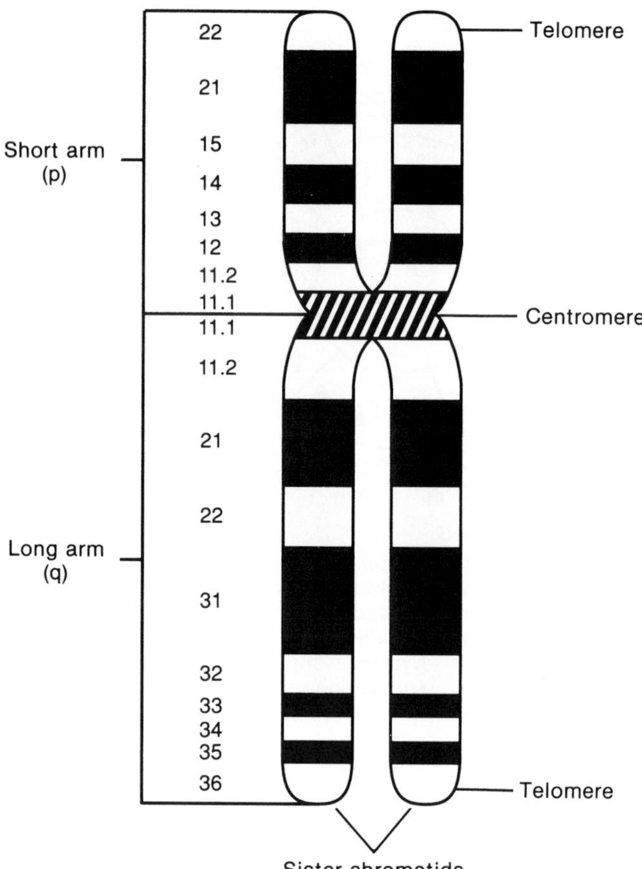

FIGURE 1–6. Anatomy of a chromosome, in this case human chromosome 7.

some was always chromosome 13, hence the name of the association was changed to "13-deletion retinoblastoma." Furthermore, in every case, the deletion included the band 14 on the long arm of the chromosome,[4] so that the term 13q14 deletion or 13q14− is more precise. Another important deletion associated with ophthalmologic and systemic abnormalities involves chromosome 11p13; deletions of this chromosomal segment cause a syndrome including aniridia and elevated predisposition to Wilms' tumor.[5]

Size of the Human Genome. A set consisting of one of each autosome as well as both sex chromosomes is called a *human genome.* It includes one copy of every human locus. The chromosomal molecules of DNA from one human genome, if tandemly arranged end to end, contain a sequence of approximately 3.2 billion base pairs. The amount of information contained within 3.2 billion base pairs can be instructively related to the quantity of information stored on modern desktop computers. At each position in DNA there is one of four possible bases (A, T, G, and C), which is equivalent to two bits of computer code. Since there are eight bits in a byte of computer memory, each byte could store the equivalent of four bases of DNA sequence. The DNA sequence of the human genome would occupy about 800 megabytes. The sequence could be stored on a 1-gigabyte hard drive (small by today's standards) with plenty of room to spare. Obtaining the complete sequence of the human genome within the first decade of the 21st century is one goal of the Human Genome Project.

In terms of the physical size of the human genome, the corresponding DNA would be 1 m long but only 2 nm in diameter. The total volume of a human genome, assuming the DNA is a cylinder, is about one hundred millionth of a microliter. Current estimates are that there are 60,000 to 100,000 genes embedded in this DNA sequence. On average, there is one gene about every 30,000 base pairs.

Haploidy, Diploidy, Triploidy. A set consisting of one of each autosome as well as an X *or* a Y chromosome is called a haploid set of chromosomes. The normal complement of two copies of each gene (or two copies of each chromosome) is called diploidy. In unusual circumstances, a cell or organism may have three copies of each chromosome; this is called triploidy. A triploid human is not viable; however, some patients have an extra chromosome or an extra segment of a chromosome. In such a situation, the abnormality is called trisomy for the chromosome involved. For example, patients with Down's syndrome have three copies of chromosome 21, also referred to as trisomy 21. Much the same phenotype can also result from trisomy of only the long arm of chromosome 21, or trisomy 21q.

If one copy of a pair of chromosomes is absent, the defect is called haploidy or deletion. Haploidy for an entire human chromosome is probably lethal, but individuals do exist who have a deletion of a segment of a chromosome.

Translocations. Occasionally a hybrid chromosome will be observed in the karyotype of an individual, with a mixture of material derived from two separate chromosomes. As a hypothetical example, a part of chromosome 1q might be fused to 3p. Depending on the number of normal chromosomes 1 and 3, an individual who carries a translocation (1q;3p) could be trisomic or monosomic for these chromosome arms. A translocation is "balanced" if there is a diploid amount of each chromosome band.

Sister Chromatids. Just before a cell divides, each chromosome arm is duplicated, so that chromosomes have two identical short arms and two identical long arms (see Fig. 1–6). At this point, there are four copies of each gene in a cell. Each chromosome has two short arms and two long arms, and each arm is called a *chromatid.* A pair of similar arms from the same chromosome is called a pair of *sister chromatids.* When one examines the "karyotype" of a cell, the chromosomes are observed just before the cell divides. Consequently, each chromosome has two sister chromatids corresponding to the short arm and two sister chromatids corresponding to the long arm. Sister chromatids always share the same alleles, whereas the two chromosome homologs in a human cell (one derived from each parent), can have different alleles at any locus.

Alleles Are Variations in the Nucleotide Sequence

An allele is a specific nucleotide sequence at a locus that is associated with an observable phenotype. The most common allele at a locus is called the *wild-type* allele, often abbreviated "+" or "wt." An allele that is different from the wild type is customarily given an abbreviated name that is somehow related to the phenotype or the nucleotide sequence. For example, an allele in the rhodopsin gene causing autosomal dominant retinitis pigmentosa could be labeled

Rho^{Pro23His} or rhodopsin, Pro23His, where Pro23His indicates that codon 23, which specifies proline in the wild-type allele, specifies histidine in the mutant allele.[6]

Although a genetic locus usually corresponds with a transcriptional unit, the boundaries of a locus in a DNA sequence are often not very precise. One reason for this is that DNA sequences many thousands of bases from the transcriptional unit can be important for the proper expression of a gene at the correct time during the development of a specific cell type.[1] It is conceivable that a mutation in such distant sequences can change the expression of a transcriptional unit and produce a phenotype associated with the locus. Hence, it is a simplification to state that alleles are the result of variations in the nucleotide sequence inside a transcriptional unit. In practice, however, this is usually the case.

If an allele has a frequency of 1 to 2% or higher and is not associated with a disease, it is called a *polymorphism*. Since humans have two alleles at each locus, the arbitrary criterion of a 1% allele frequency corresponds with a polymorphism for which about 2% of unrelated individuals are carriers. An example is the still unidentified locus on chromosome 19, where a polymorphism specifies the presence or absence of green iris color.[7] If an allele occurs with a frequency less than 1%, it is a *rare variant*. If an allele causes disease, it is customarily called a *mutation*. Most mutations are rare variants. However, at least one is at a frequency high enough to be considered a polymorphism: about 2% of whites carry the Phe508del mutation that causes cystic fibrosis.[8]

Genetic diseases are defined clinically before the underlying causative gene defects are known. Most clinically defined hereditary diseases turn out to be genetically heterogeneous. *Allelic heterogeneity* is the term used when different mutant alleles at the same locus can produce the same disease. For example, numerous mutations in the Rab escort protein gene have been found to produce choroideremia.[9] *Nonallelic heterogeneity* refers to the situation when mutations in different genes can produce the same clinically defined disease. An example of nonallelic heterogeneity is retinitis pigmentosa, which can be produced as a result of defects in any of dozens of different genes.[10] *Gene sharing* occurs if different mutations in the same gene can produce different phenotypes. For instance, defects in the Norrie disease gene can produce either Norrie disease, exudative vitreoretinopathy, or predisposition to retinopathy of prematurity.[11–13] Another example of two diseases sharing the same genes are retinitis pigmentosa and congenital stationary night blindness. Different defects in the rhodopsin gene can produce these two diseases[6, 14, 15]; so too can different defects in the gene encoding the β subunit of rod cGMP-phosphodiesterase.[16, 17]

Hereditary Transmission of Genetic Information

Somatic Cells Versus Germ Cells. Most of the cells in the human body are somatic cells. Somatic cells have a "diploid" set of chromosomes (i.e., two copies of each autosome, one derived from each parent) and two sex chromosomes (either XX or XY). Somatic cells are produced as a consequence of *mitosis* or cell division (Fig. 1–7). Before a cell divides into two daughter cells, the entire complement of chromosomes duplicates so that the cell has four copies of every autosomal gene. Each daughter cell receives a complete, diploid set of chromosomes with solitary short and long arms.

The second category of human cells involves those in the germ line; that is, cells whose descendants are "germ cells" (sperm and ova). Germ cells are haploid. The process that creates germ cells is called *meiosis*. Meiosis encompasses two cell divisions (see Fig. 1–7). In the first meiotic division, each daughter cell receives one member of each homologous pair. The daughter cells are therefore haploid. They, nevertheless, have two of each chromatid. The chromosomes separate during the second meiotic division to produce haploid germ cells with only one of each chromatid.

Recombination. In somatic cells, it is the general rule that each chromosome homolog has a set of alleles derived from one parent. After meiosis, a germ cell is haploid; that is, it has only one member of each pair of chromosomes. Hence, a germ cell could have the maternally derived chromosomes 1, 2, 4, 7, . . . , and the paternally derived chromosome 3, 5, 6, 8, and so forth.

This mixing of chromosomes is one source of the diversity that is provided by sexual reproduction. However, it is only half of the story. During the first meiotic division, chromatids from homologous chromosomes can recombine or *cross-over* (see Fig. 1–7). During this process, the chromatids exchange linear sets of alleles so that the daughter chromosomes have a mixture of maternal and paternal alleles. This is the second major source for new combinations of genes. The resultant germ cells receive a random mixture of these hybrid chromosomes.

Roughly 30 cross-overs occur during each meiosis. Cross-overs can take place anywhere along the length of a chromosome arm, although there appear to be regions that are especially susceptible to it (called "recombination hot spots"). Also, there is a relatively greater likelihood of a cross-over happening in the distal portion of a chromosome arm compared with the proximal portion. The rate of recombination occurring at any particular region of a chromosome can be different in males and females.

During oogenesis, the two X chromosomes carried by a female can recombine anywhere along their length just as with autosomes. In contrast, the X and Y chromosomes of a male usually do not recombine, and if they do, cross-overs occur only within the distal short arms.

Considering that during meiosis an average of 30 cross-overs occur among the 23 pairs of human chromosomes, most chromosomes in germ cells are recombinant. Furthermore, because there is also a random assortment of chromosomes during meiosis, there is the potential for a huge number of possible combinations of alleles. In effect, each gamete has a unique, haploid set of alleles. An individual conceived as the union between two such gametes is likewise unique.

Homozygotes and Heterozygotes

Since an individual has two copies of each autosome, he or she will have two copies of each autosomal locus. One copy is derived from the mother and one from the father. How similar are these two copies? Between any two chromosomes in a pair, the nucleotide sequence of the DNA is very similar:

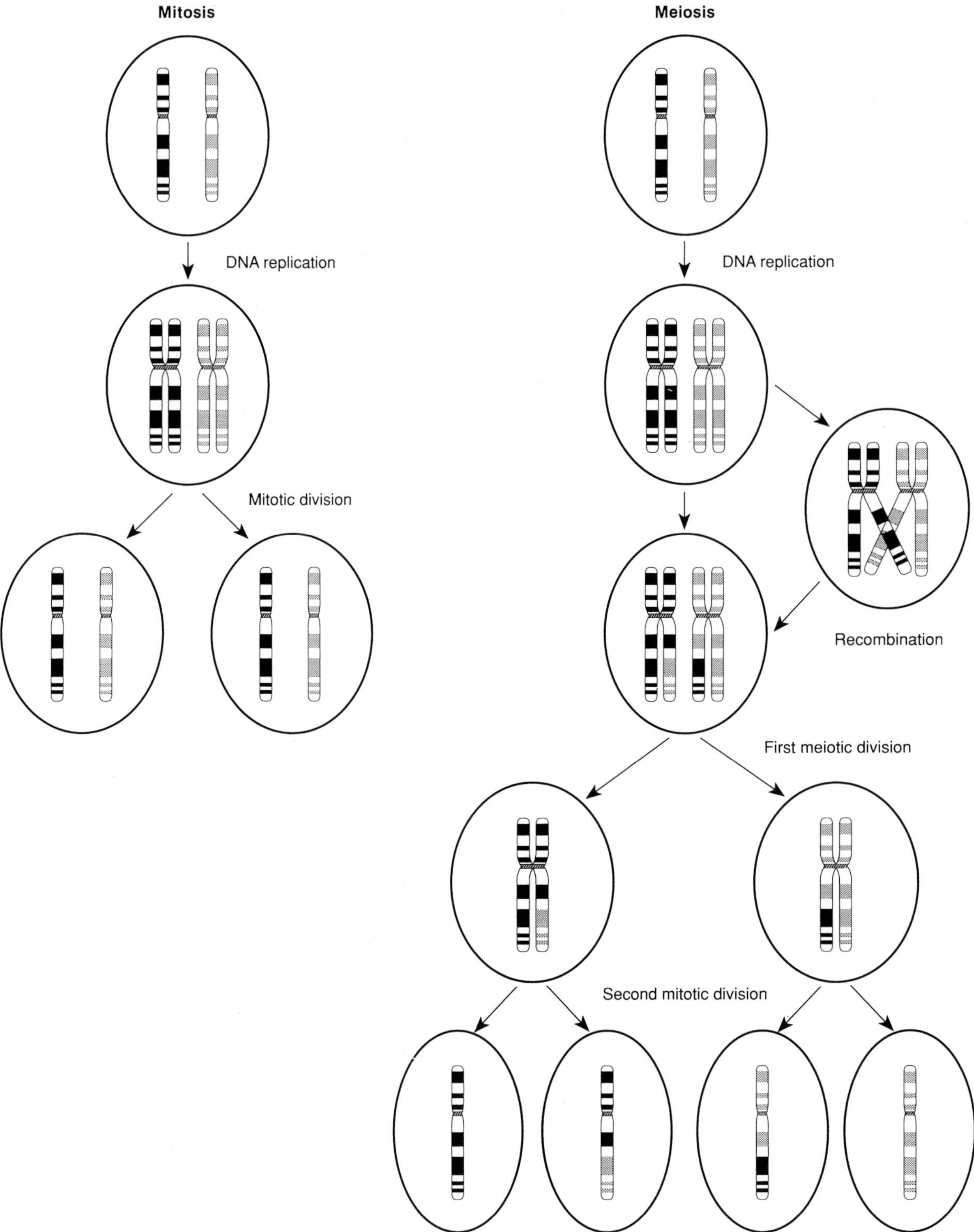

FIGURE 1–7. Steps involved in mitosis and meiosis. In both processes, the first step involves the replication of DNA so that each chromosome arm is duplicated, producing chromosomes with sister chromatids. In mitosis, the chromosomes divide so that each daughter cell receives a short and long chromatid from each chromosome in the pair. In meiosis, there is often recombination between chromatids from homologous chromosomes. After this, there is the first meiotic division, which segregates the chromosome pairs, followed by the second meiotic division which produces gametes with one set of chromatids from only one member of each pair of chromosomes.

more than 99 of 100 base pairs are identical. Most of the variations result in no observable phenotype and are therefore "silent" polymorphisms or rare variants. The less frequent variations in DNA sequence that correspond with a phenotype are the fundamental chemical basis for alleles.

The two copies of a given locus in an individual can by chance be identical, in which case the individual is *homozygous* for that particular allele. On the other hand, an individual can have two different alleles, one derived from each parent, and the individual is then *heterozygous*. An individual who is heterozygous for two different alleles, neither of which is wild-type, is called a *compound heterozygote*.

Uniparental disomy or *isodisomy* is the term given for the rare occasions when a locus is homozygous, but both identical alleles are derived from the same parent. As an illustration, some patients with cystic fibrosis have been found who are homozygous for a mutant allele that is present in only one parent.[18] A patient with rod monochromatism has been reported with isodisomy for chromosome 14q; this case possibly indicates that a recessive gene for the disease is on that chromosome.[19] Hydatidiform moles consist of cells that have uniparental disomy of the entire genome, where both copies of every gene are derived from the father.[20]

Patterns of Human Inheritance

The major types of inheritance of human disease are: dominant, recessive, X-linked, mitochondrial (also called maternal), digenic, and polygenic. Of these, the first four are the most commonly considered in ophthalmologic practice and will be discussed in most detail. For reference, Figure 1–8 provides schematic pedigrees illustrating each of these four inheritance patterns.

Dominant (Also Called Autosomal Dominant). If a mutation is present in one of the two gene copies at an autosomal locus, and if this heterozygous mutation produces a disease, the mutation is called dominant. For example, a patient with dominant retinitis pigmentosa will have a defect in one copy of one retinitis pigmentosa gene inherited from one parent who, in most cases, is also affected with retinitis pigmentosa. The other copy of that gene, the one inherited from the unaffected parent, is normal (wild type). The term "dominant" comes from the fact that the defective copy "dominates" over the wild-type gene copy to cause disease.

1. *Nature of a dominant gene defect.* Most dominant mutations cause disease through one of the following three general mechanisms.

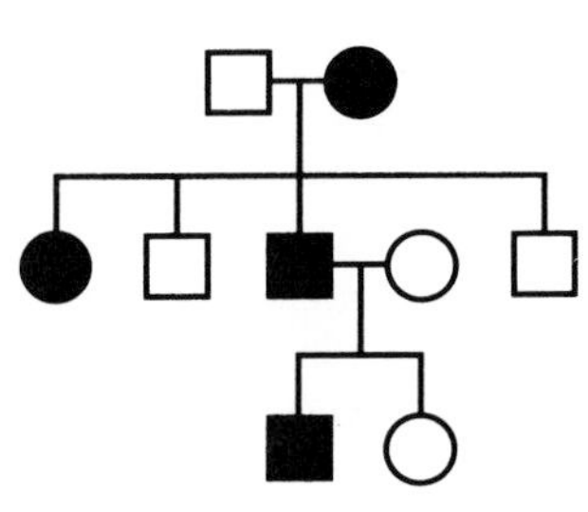

Autosomal Dominant

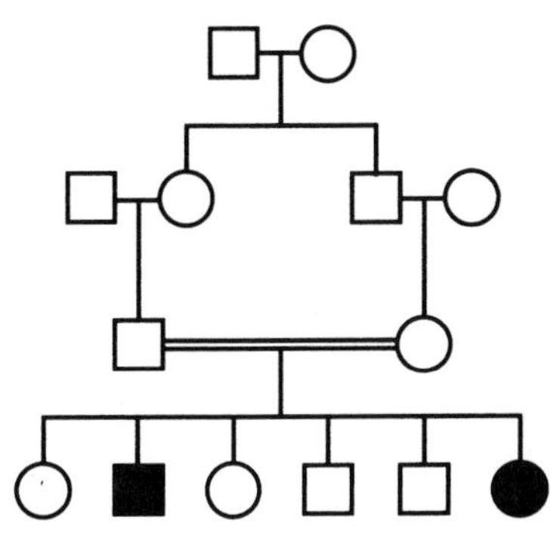

Autosomal Recessive

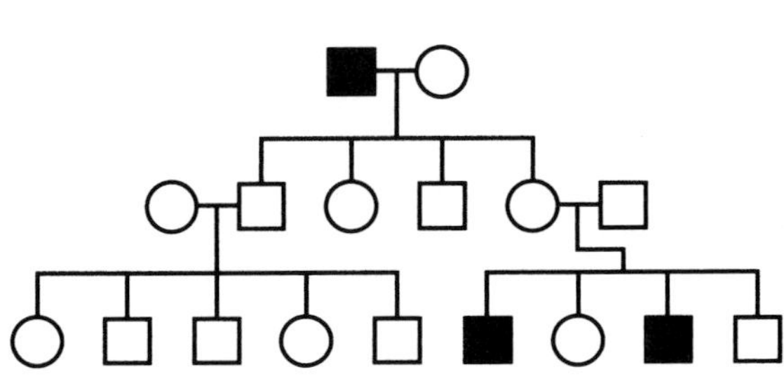

X-Linked

Mitochondrial

FIGURE 1–8. Factitious pedigrees illustrating various hereditary patterns. *Circles* represent females; squares represent males. *Filled-in circles* or *squares* represent individuals exhibiting a hypothetical hereditary trait.

a. *Novel function.* The mutant allele produces a protein that has a new function not present in the wild-type protein. The mutant protein might have a novel enzyme activity, or it might be toxic.

b. *Dominant-negative effect.* The mutant protein forms a complex with the wild-type protein encoded by the homologous wild-type allele and thus inactivates the wild-type protein. The phenotype is then a consequence of little or no functional protein remaining.

c. *Haplo-insufficiency.* The mutation produces no functional protein. The homologous wild-type allele produces functional protein, but because this is the only functional allele, the target tissues have only 50% of the normal level of the protein. This reduced level of functional protein results in disease.

2. *Note on the classical definition of a dominant allele.* It is customary in human genetics to view a dominant mutation as one that confers a disease or some other phenotype when present heterozygously. However, in the classic, mendelian lexicon, a dominant allele is one that produces its designated phenotype whether it is present homozygously or heterozygously. Proven examples of classically defined, dominant alleles in humans are uncommon. The Val30Met mutation in the transthyretin gene is a true dominant, because patients who are heterozygous for this allele have vitreous amyloidosis and polyneuropathy comparable in severity to those who are homozygous.[21] In contrast, most "dominant" human alleles are loosely categorized as such if they are known to produce phenotypes when present heterozygously, regardless of the phenotype produced in a homozygote or compound heterozygote. This definition is necessary because individuals who are homozygotes or compound heterozygotes for "dominant" alleles causing disease may be nonexistent. The disease alleles might be so rare that the likelihood that two affected heterozygous carriers mating, a precondition for the production of a homozygous offspring, is exceedingly low. Occasionally, the disease produced by a "dominant" mutation is so severe that affected heterozygotes do not reproduce at all; again, there would be little possibility for a homozygous individual to be conceived and the corresponding phenotype to be displayed. In some exceptional circumstances individuals who are homozygotes or compound heterozygotes for purportedly dominant ophthalmic disease alleles have been identified. They are sometimes found to have a phenotype that is markedly different from that found in heterozygotes. For example, a newborn with mutations of both copies of the aniridia gene had anophthalmia and severe developmental defects of the central nervous system that led to death soon after birth.[22] If a homozygote for a dominant allele has a more severe form of the same recognizable phenotype, the mutant allele is more appropriately called *semidominant.* Alleles in the PAX3 gene, causing Waardenburg's syndrome, are semidominant, exemplified by the report of a family in which a homozygote had very severe disease (very exaggerated dystopic canthorum and severely malformed upper limbs) compared with the heterozygote relatives with more typical disease.[23]

3. *Transmission of a dominant gene defect.* A patient with a dominant mutation at a disease locus can transmit the normal copy or the defective copy to a child. Each copy has an equal chance of being passed on, so that each child will have a 50/50 chance of getting the defective gene copy. Male and female children are equally likely to inherit the defective copy. A dominant disease can be inherited from a father or a mother. Unaffected individuals in a family do not carry the defective gene copy and therefore cannot pass a defective copy to their children.

4. *Features of a family with a dominant disease.* One can be fairly confident that a disease is dominant in a family if the following criteria are met:
   a. The disease is found in three consecutive generations, such as grandparents, parents, and children.
   b. Every affected member has an affected parent.
   c. There is at least one instance of transmission from an affected father to an affected son.

Many families with a dominant disease do not meet all three criteria. One will still be able to presume that a dominant mode of inheritance is likely if some of the criteria are met. For example, if there is transmission of the disease directly from a parent to a child, it is likely that the gene defect is a dominant one.

There are two common sources of error in cataloguing a dominant gene. First, in a family with two generations of affected individuals, there is the possibility that the allele under study is actually recessive, that the affected parent is homozygous for the allele, and that the unaffected parent carries the allele heterozygously. In this situation, offspring would invariably inherit the recessive, disease-inducing allele from the affected parent and would have a 50% chance of inheriting the recessive allele from the unaffected parent. This situation is called *pseudo-dominance* and is covered later. Pseudo-dominance is very unlikely if a family exhibits three consecutive generations of affected family members.

A second problem occurs when an X-linked allele is incorrectly designated as an autosomal dominant allele. Through a process called lyonization (discussed later), it is possible for females heterozygous for an X-linked recessive mutation to exhibit the corresponding phenotype. If such a female had two affected sons among four or five children in all, the pedigree would mimic that found for autosomal dominant retinitis pigmentosa. Suspicion of this type of mistake should be high whenever all affected children of an affected mother are male. This mistake is eliminated if one stipulates that a pedigree must show father-to-son transmission of a trait before autosomal dominant inheritance is diagnosed conclusively.

Recessive (Also Called Autosomal Recessive). A recessive disease arises if it is necessary for defects to be present in both gene copies at an autosomal locus. One wild-type allele together with one recessively defective allele does not cause disease. Hence a wild-type allele always dominates over a *recessive* one. The same recessive defect might affect both gene copies, in which case the patient is said to be a *homozygote.* Different recessive defects might affect the two gene copies, in which case the patient is a *compound heterozygote.*

1. *Nature of a recessive gene defect.* Most recessive mutations that have been functionally characterized result

in *null* alleles, which are defined as alleles that produce no functional protein. It is the lack of the protein's activity that causes disease. For example, patients with gyrate atrophy have recessive mutations in both copies of the locus normally encoding the enzyme ornithine aminotransferase. The disease is produced as a consequence of the lack of functional enzyme.

2. *Note on the classical definition of a recessive allele.* Classically defined recessive mutations are frequently encountered in human genetics. The heterozygote parents of an affected child (who is either a homozygote or a compound heterozygote) have a wild-type phenotype. In certain cases, however, recessive mutations are loosely defined. Consider alleles at the hemoglobin locus, where the sickle-cell allele is called recessive. However, an individual homozygous for a wild-type allele is not phenotypically equivalent to the heterozygote who carries one wild-type and one sickle allele. The latter individual, who has the "sickle trait," can become symptomatic if he or she visits an environment with low oxygen pressure such as the upper atmosphere.
3. *Transmission of a recessive gene defect.* In a family with recessive disease, both parents are unaffected carriers, each having one wild-type allele and one mutant allele. Each parent has a 50% chance of transmitting the defective allele to a child. Since a child must receive a defective allele from both parents to be affected, each child has a 25% chance of being affected (50% × 50% = 25%.)
4. *Features of a family with a recessive disease.* The following features make it likely that a family has a recessive disease.
   a. The parents are unaffected, and there is no previous family history of the disease. If the parents are blood relatives (e.g., cousins), the disease in the offspring is even more likely to be recessive.
   b. Male and female children are affected equally severely.

On average, one in four offspring of two carrier parents will be a homozygote and affected. Consanguineous mates tend to be carriers of the same rare alleles, so that children with recessive disease are often the product of such marriages. If a sibship with a presumed recessive disease has only affected males, the possibility of X-linked inheritance should be considered.

X-Linked (Also Called X-Linked Recessive). Mutations of the X chromosome produce distinctive inheritance patterns, because males have only one copy of the X chromosome whereas females have two. Almost all X-linked gene defects are of the X-linked recessive category. Carrier females are unaffected because they have one normal copy of the gene in question and one defective copy. Carrier males will be affected because their only copy is defective; that is, there is no normal copy to "compensate" for the recessive defect.

1. *Nature of an X-linked recessive defect.* Like recessive mutations involving autosomal loci, most recessive mutations of the X chromosome result in *null* alleles that produce no functional protein.
2. *Transmission of an X-linked recessive gene defect.* First consider the situation of a male affected with an X-linked disease. He has only one copy of any X-linked gene, thus he will transmit his defective X-linked gene to every daughter. All his daughters will be carriers. All his sons will be unaffected and will not be carriers, because fathers do not pass any X-linked genes to sons. Note that neither the daughters nor the sons of a male affected with an X-linked disease will be affected.

Next consider the situation of a carrier female who carries one defective allele at an X-chromosome locus. Each child of the carrier female has a 50% chance of inheriting the defective allele. If a son inherits the defective copy, he will be affected. If a daughter inherits the defective copy, she will be a carrier like her mother. If either a daughter or a son inherits the mother's normal gene copy, the child will be unaffected and will not be a carrier.

Ordinarily, no carrier females will be affected. However, for some X-linked diseases, female carriers can exhibit a phenotype that is usually less severe than that found in the affected male relatives. This could be due to the process of *lyonization.* In order for males (with one X chromosome) and females (with two X chromosomes) to have equal levels of expression of X-linked genes, female cells express genes from only one of the two X chromosomes that they have. The decision as to which X chromosome is expressed is made early in embryogenesis, and the line of cells descending from each decision-making progenitrix cell faithfully adheres to the choice of the active X chromosome of the progenitrix. Hence, females are mosaics with some of the cells in each tissue expressing the maternally derived set of X-linked alleles and the remainder expressing the paternally derived X-linked alleles. The proportion of cells that express the mutant versus the wild-type alleles in each tissue can vary. By chance a susceptible tissue might have a preponderance of cells expressing the mutant X chromosome, in which case the corresponding disease would become manifest. An example of this is offered by some female carriers of X-linked retinitis pigmentosa who develop symptoms, fundus signs, and electroretinographic abnormalities of the disease. Most females affected with X-linked retinitis pigmentosa because of lyonization have milder disease than that found in their male relatives.

Another explanation for a female affected with an X-linked disease involves the unusual situation in which the father is affected and the mother is a carrier. The father invariably will transmit his defective copy to every daughter. If the mother happens to transmit the defective copy to a daughter, the daughter will be a homozygote or compound heterozygote at the disease locus. This is the usual explanation for females who show protan or deutan color vision abnormalities due to defects in the genes encoding red and green cone opsins on the X chromosome. About 6% of X chromosomes in whites have defects in the red and green cone opsin genes, so about 6% × 6% = 0.36% of females, or about 1 in 280, would be homozygotes or compound heterozygotes. For most ophthalmic diseases, however, the proportion of female carriers is very low. For example, for X-linked retinitis pigmentosa, only approximately 1 in every 7000 women is a carrier. In view of this low proportion of carriers, it is very unlikely for an affected father to marry by chance a female carrier of X-linked retinitis pigmentosa. Hence, very few females with retinitis pigmentosa will be homozygotes or compound heterozygotes for mutations in an X-linked retinitis pigmentosa gene; most will have autosomal recessive or autosomal dominant retinitis pigmentosa instead.

3. *Features of a family with an X-linked recessive disease.* The following features of a family point to an X-linked recessive disease gene:
   a. The disease is found only in males. (In unusual circumstances, females may be affected; see the discussion earlier.)
   b. There is no instance of an affected male having an affected child.
   c. If the disease is present in more than one generation, the affected males are related through a carrier female. For example, an affected male might have an affected maternal uncle or an affected maternal grandfather, but he would not have affected relatives on his father's side.

Less Common Inheritance Patterns

1. *Maternal or mitochondrial inheritance.* The 23 pairs of human chromosomes described earlier are located in the nucleus of each cell. In addition, there is a small amount of DNA in the cytoplasm. This DNA is from the *mitochondrial chromosome*, a relatively tiny chromosome with only 16,569 base pairs of DNA. Thirteen mitochondrial proteins, 2 ribosomal RNAs, and 22 tRNAs are encoded by this chromosome. It is a clinically important chromosome because mutations are known to cause human disease (examples relevant to ophthalmology are Leber hereditary optic atrophy[24, 25] and Kearns-Sayre syndrome[26]). A noteworthy feature of these mutations is that they are maternally inherited, because almost all the mitochondria of a one-cell embryo are derived from the ovum. A father does not transmit mitochondria to his offspring. Mitochondrially inherited diseases are inherited invariably through the maternal lineage.

   One other peculiar feature of alleles in the mitochondrial genome is that an individual is neither homozygous nor heterozygous for them but rather is *heteroplasmic*. A typical cell has numerous mitochondria, each with about 2 to 10 copies of the mitochondrial genome. The proportion of mutant mitochondrial genomes in each mitochondrion, and the proportion of mutant mitochondria in a cell, can vary from one cell to another in an individual. Differences in the relative proportions of mutant mitochondria can partly explain the observed variable severity of mitochondrial diseases. In addition, the proportion of mutant mitochondria can change during the lifetime of a patient, which helps to explain the variable age of onset of mitochondrial diseases.

   Upon analysis of a pedigree with a mitochondrially inherited disease, one may note examples of mother-to-son and mother-to-daughter transmission, but one should never observe father-to-child transmission. In a particular family, the severity of disease can vary tremendously because of heteroplasmy and perhaps other factors, and one must be aware of possible asymptomatic carriers when scrutinizing a pedigree. In the case of Leber optic atrophy, a mitochondrially inherited disease, males tend to be affected more often than females for unknown reasons.[27]

2. *Pseudodominance.* This is the term given to an apparent dominant inheritance pattern due to recessive defects in a disease gene. Consider the situation in which an affected parent has recessive disease due to defects in both copies of a disease gene and the spouse happens to be a carrier with one normal gene copy and one copy that has a recessive defect. Children from this couple will always inherit a defective gene copy from the affected parent and will have a 50% chance of inheriting the defective gene copy from the unaffected carrier parent. On average, half of the children will inherit two defective gene copies and will be affected. The pedigree would mimic a dominant pedigree (Fig. 1–9) because of apparent direct transmission of the disease from the affected parent to affected children and because approximately 50% of the children will be affected. Pseudodominant transmission is uncommon, because few people are asymptomatic carriers for any particular recessive gene.
3. *Autosomal dominant with reduced penetrance.* In some pedigrees with an autosomal dominant disease, some individuals who carry the defective gene do not get disease. This would cause "skipped generations"; that is, cases where an unaffected offspring of an affected individual would have children with the disease. This phenomenon is typically locus-specific. For example, many families with dominant retinitis pigmentosa with reduced penetrance have a defective gene on chromosome 19q13[28]; those with dominant retinitis pigmentosa with full penetrance have mutations at other loci.
4. *X-linked dominant inheritance.* A few families with retinitis pigmentosa appear to have this distinctive inheritance pattern.[29] The inheritance pattern is similar to X-linked recessive inheritance, but all carrier females are affected rather than unaffected. All carrier males are affected as well. Other diseases with ophthalmic manifestations that are loosely considered to have X-linked dominant inheritance are Aicardi syndrome (frequent features are agenesis of the corpus callosum and patches of absent retinal pigment epithelium) and incontinentia pigmenti (irregularly pigmented atrophic

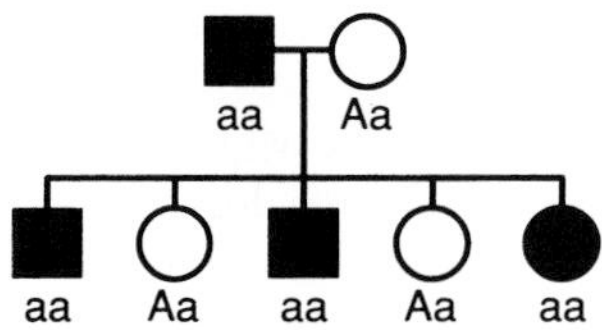

FIGURE 1–9. An example of pseudodominance. Beneath each schematic family member are the alleles of the disease locus under scrutiny. "A" is the dominant, wild-type allele; "a" is the recessive allele that causes the hypothetical disease. The parent-to-child transmission of the disease occurs because the unaffected parent is actually a carrier of the recessive allele.

scars on the trunk and the extremities, congenital avascularity in the peripheral retina with secondary retinal neovascularization). Both Aicardi syndrome and incontinentia pigmenti occur almost exclusively in females; it is likely that the X chromosome gene defects causing these diseases are embryonic lethals when present hemizygously in males.

5. *Digenic inheritance*. This is another rare form of inheritance, which till now has been found only in a few families with retinitis pigmentosa or ocular albinism.[30, 31] Digenic inheritance occurs when a patient has heterozygous defects in two different genes, and the combination of the two gene defects causes disease. Individuals who are heterozygous for a mutation only at one or the other locus are wild-type. Digenic inheritance is different from recessive inheritance, because the two mutations involve different gene loci. Affected individuals are called "double heterozygotes" rather than compound heterozygotes.
6. *Polygenic and multifactorial inheritance*. If the expression of a heritable trait or predisposition is influenced by the combination of alleles at three or more loci, it is polygenic. The contributing loci are considered "quantitative trait loci" to reflect the mathematical formulations used to calculate their relative impacts on the phenotype or the predisposition. If environmental factors contribute to a polygenic trait or disease, the term multifactorial is used. Examples of phenotypes in ophthalmology likely to be multifactorial are myopia, age-related macular degeneration, and adult-onset open-angle glaucoma.

Pedigree Analysis to Categorize Alleles

The classification of a genetic disease or trait can often be made by examining the relationships between the affected individuals in a pedigree. The following are general guidelines for using this method. It should be noted that in many circumstances, it is not possible to be certain of the mode of inheritance in a particular family because of the small size of the family or because of uncertainties in the diagnosis of key family members who might be too young, unavailable, or deceased.

Pedigree analysis is sometimes not necessary to determine the inheritance pattern in a family, because for some conditions there is only one known inheritance pattern. In those cases, the diagnosis will immediately provide the inheritance pattern. For example, all cases of choroideremia have an X-linked pattern of inheritance. For other diseases, such as hereditary cataract or hereditary retinal degeneration, many different inheritance patterns have been observed. In those cases, pedigree analysis can often be helpful. One constructs a family tree indicating which members in the family have the disease in question. It is important to make sure that the information on the pedigree is as complete and correct as possible. For example, if a distant relative is reported to have had "poor eyesight," one must know whether that report reflects the ophthalmic disease in question or simply the relative's need for eyeglasses. Examination of the pedigree rarely "proves" the type of inheritance beyond any doubt, but it can allow one to infer the most likely inheritance pattern.

Disease Is Present in Only One Family Member. "Isolate" or "simplex" cases of disease refer to families in which two parents with no previous family history of the disease in question have one affected child. In some cases, a simplex case might not have a hereditary disease at all. For example, about 80 to 90% of unilateral, simplex cases of retinoblastoma are not hereditary. Alternatively, simplex cases might represent autosomal recessive disease, with both parents being carriers and the affected child having inherited a defective gene copy from each parent. If the affected simplex case is a male, it is possible that he has X-linked disease, with the mother possibly being a carrier. For some diseases such as retinitis pigmentosa, a careful ophthalmologic evaluation including an electroretinogram of the mother might give clues as to her status in this regard. Another possibility is that the simplex case has a new gene defect not present in either parent. This is thought to be infrequent, because so few genes become mutant from one generation to the next.

Disease Present in Two or More Individuals in the Same Generation. An example of this situation would be a family with two or more siblings with a disease and no previous family history of the disease. In such families, the inheritance pattern is usually autosomal recessive. However, if the affected children are all males, the possibility of X-linked disease should be considered. Other unusual inheritance patterns, such as maternal, digenic, or multifactorial are possible.

Disease Present in Two Consecutive Generations. The disease is most likely to be autosomal dominant. If there is direct transmission from a father to a son, an autosomal dominant gene is inferred with even more certainty. Uncommon exceptions include pseudodominance or digenic inheritance. If there is direct transmission from a mother to a child, an autosomal dominant gene is still very likely, but maternal and X-linked inheritance should be considered as well.

Disease Present in Two Generations Separated by an Unaffected Generation. If the unaffected individual connecting the affected generations is a female and if all affected individuals are male, X-linked inheritance is likely. Alternatively, this could represent autosomal dominant inheritance with reduced penetrance.

Disease Present in Three or More Consecutive Generations. Dominant inheritance is most likely, although digenic and X-linked dominant inheritance are also possibilities.

Map of the Human Genome

Linkage. Because of the mixing of genes caused by meiotic cross-overs and the random assortment of chromosomes, alleles at two distinct loci are usually inherited together approximately 50% of the time. In the less common circumstance when alleles at two loci are inherited together more than 50% of the time, the two loci are *linked*. Linked loci are physically close to each other on the same chromosome.

The distance between two linked loci can be measured two ways: by the number of base pairs of DNA separating the loci (physical distance) or by the frequency of meiotic cross-overs occurring between the two loci (genetic distance or recombination distance). How are the two measures related? A haploid human genome contains about 3.2 billion base pairs of DNA. Since 30 cross-overs occur in a typical meiosis, there is an average of one cross-over per 100 million base pairs per meiosis. Between two loci physically separated by a distance of 1 million base pairs, there would be approximately one cross-over per 100 meioses, or a 1% cross-over rate. This distance is called 1 *centimorgan* (cM) and is one of the basic units in genetics for measuring the separation between two loci. The conversion of 1 cM/million base pairs is an overall average for the human genome, since the frequency of cross-overs is not equal throughout the length of each chromosome. The actual figure for a segment of a chromosome can be more than 10 times greater or less. Furthermore, it can be different in germ cells from males compared with females.

One of the major contemporary goals in the study of human genetics is the construction of a map of the physical position of every human gene and the correlation of that map with the recombination distances between linked loci. This "human genome project" is a formidable task, because the human genome is so large. The physical map that is part of this endeavor is started by physically assigning many human genes to their specific locations on chromosomes. Ultimately, the project will determine the DNA sequence of each chromosome.

DNA Polymorphisms. A major step in the human genome project is the construction of a linkage map of the human genome. This involves the determination of which human loci are linked and the recombination distances between them. This work is based on sites in the human genome where there is variation in the DNA sequence, called DNA *polymorphisms*. Most DNA polymorphisms are unrelated to clinically evident phenotypes.

Three major categories of DNA polymorphisms are used for linkage maps of the human genome: RFLPs (for restriction fragment length polymorphisms), VNTRs (for a variable number of tandem repeats), and microsatellites. RFLPs are the result of occasional variations that typically affect a single base pair in the DNA sequence. They are detectable with enzymes, called restriction endonucleases, that are purified from bacteria. A restriction endonuclease cleaves DNA at specific locations, usually specified by a particular stretch of four to six base pairs called the recognition sequence. If even a single base pair is altered at a recognition site, a restriction endonuclease will not cleave DNA at that site. For example, the restriction endonuclease *Eco*RI cleaves DNA at the sequence GAATTC (its recognition sequence) but would not cleave the sequence GAAGTC or GATTTC. Restriction endonucleases allow one to trace relatively easily the inheritance of a single-base polymorphism if a recognition sequence is created or destroyed by the variation.

VNTRs are sites in the human genome where there is a tandem repetition of a DNA sequence. The repeat unit is about 15 to 60 base pairs in length and typically has a core sequence that is common to all VNTRs.[32] The number of repeat units at a VNTR varies from a few to dozens, and this variation is the basis for the alleles specified by these polymorphisms. Microsatellites are like VNTRs in that they are tandemly repeated DNA sequences, but the repeated unit is much smaller, typically two to four base pairs. The most frequently used microsatellites are repeats of the dinucleotide sequence "CA"; these microsatellites are also known as "CA repeats." VNTRs and microsatellites are preferred for most linkage studies because they are generally easier to analyze than RFLPs. Also, RFLPs are biallelic (the recognition sequence is either present or absent at a locus) whereas VNTRs and microsatellites are multiallelic. A higher proportion of individuals are heterozygous for polymorphisms with numerous alleles, and therefore VNTRs and microsatellites provide more linkage data than RFLPs.

By following the inheritance of distinct DNA polymorphisms in human pedigrees, one can learn which are linked with each other and at what recombination distances. To date, linkage maps of each human chromosome are available with highly informative polymorphic markers distributed roughly every 1 to 3 cM or less.

With such a linkage map, it is possible to determine the location of a gene causing a human disease once one has a set of families with the disease available for study. DNA samples from family members are first obtained. Leukocyte DNA is typically used; DNA from 10 mL of venous blood is sufficient to assay hundreds of DNA polymorphisms distributed throughout the genome. The polymorphic site that most often correlates with the disease is the one that is closest to the disease gene (Fig. 1–10). By knowing the chromosomal location of that DNA polymorphism, one has the approximate chromosomal location for the disease gene. The strategies embodied in the term "positional cloning" allow one to proceed from the approximate chromosomal location of a disease gene, based on the data from the DNA polymorphisms, to the actual isolation of the gene. Positional cloning approaches are typically very labor-intensive, but they have been successful in identifying a number of genes causing ophthalmologic disease. Examples are the retinoblastoma gene (on chromosome 13), X-linked genes for choroideremia and one form of retinitis pigmentosa (RPGR), the aniridia gene (chromosome 11), and a gene for Usher syndrome type I (chromosome 11).

Mutations

Categories of Mutations. A new alteration in the DNA sequence of a gene is called a mutation. The word *mutant* can refer to the specific sequence abnormality (i.e., a mutant base pair), to the defective allele (mutant gene or mutant allele), to the gene product (mutant protein), or to the organism that is affected by the mutation (mutant mouse). There are various ways that mutations can be organized for didactic purposes. Mutations can be grouped according to whether they cause a dominant or a recessive phenotype, or no phenotype at all (*silent* mutations). Recessive mutations are often *loss-of-function*, or *null* mutations because they often interfere in some way with the production of an active protein product. On the other hand, the general rule is that dominant alleles represent *gain-of-function* mutations.

Types of Lesions in DNA. Another way to classify mutations is according to the type of lesion affecting the DNA sequence. A *point mutation* is the change of a single base for another. If a purine changes to another purine, or if a pyrimidine changes to another pyrimidine, the point mutation is called a *transition*. If a purine changes to a pyrimidine or vice versa, the mutation is a *transversion*. Although there are 12 possible transversions and four possible transitions (Fig. 1–11), transitions outnumber transversions at most human loci where naturally occurring mutations have been characterized. Among the transitions, the change from a C to a T is the most frequent and most commonly occurs if the C is part of the dinucleotide sequence CG.

A point mutation can change a codon so that it specifies a different amino acid. This is called a *missense* mutation. For example, a C-to-A transversion in codon 23 of the human rhodopsin gene, a cause of autosomal dominant retinitis pigmentosa, changes that codon from one that specifies proline (CCT) to one specifying histidine (CAT).

A *nonsense* mutation, also called a *premature stop codon*, is one that changes a codon that normally specifies an amino acid into a termination codon. For example, a C-to-T transition in codon 446 of the retinoblastoma gene, found to be the cause of hereditary retinoblastoma in one pedigree, changes the codon from CGA (arginine) to TGA (stop). During translation of the resultant mRNA, the encoded protein will have only the first 445 amino acid residues, whereas the normal protein product has 928 residues. The truncated, nonfunctional, mutant protein will not be able to prevent retinoblastoma.

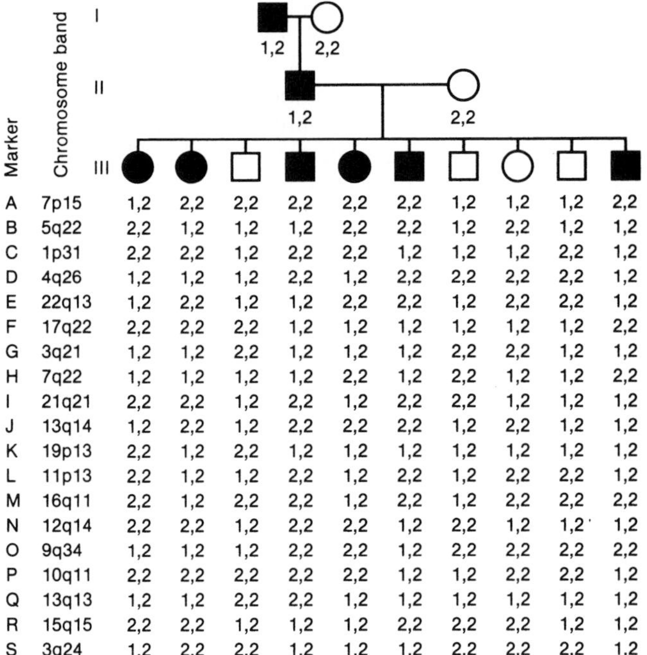

Marker	Chromosome band	III-1	III-2	III-3	III-4	III-5	III-6	III-7	III-8	III-9	III-10
A	7p15	1,2	2,2	2,2	2,2	2,2	2,2	1,2	1,2	1,2	2,2
B	5q22	2,2	1,2	1,2	1,2	2,2	2,2	1,2	2,2	1,2	1,2
C	1p31	2,2	2,2	1,2	2,2	2,2	1,2	1,2	1,2	2,2	1,2
D	4q26	1,2	1,2	1,2	2,2	1,2	2,2	2,2	2,2	2,2	1,2
E	22q13	1,2	2,2	1,2	1,2	2,2	2,2	1,2	2,2	2,2	1,2
F	17q22	2,2	2,2	2,2	1,2	1,2	1,2	1,2	1,2	1,2	2,2
G	3q21	1,2	1,2	2,2	1,2	1,2	1,2	2,2	2,2	1,2	1,2
H	7q22	1,2	1,2	1,2	1,2	2,2	1,2	2,2	1,2	1,2	2,2
I	21q21	2,2	2,2	1,2	2,2	1,2	2,2	2,2	1,2	1,2	1,2
J	13q14	1,2	2,2	1,2	2,2	2,2	2,2	1,2	2,2	1,2	1,2
K	19p13	2,2	1,2	2,2	1,2	1,2	1,2	1,2	1,2	1,2	1,2
L	11p13	2,2	1,2	1,2	2,2	1,2	2,2	1,2	2,2	2,2	1,2
M	16q11	2,2	1,2	2,2	2,2	1,2	2,2	1,2	2,2	2,2	2,2
N	12q14	2,2	2,2	1,2	2,2	2,2	1,2	2,2	1,2	1,2	1,2
O	9q34	1,2	1,2	1,2	2,2	2,2	1,2	2,2	2,2	2,2	2,2
P	10q11	2,2	2,2	2,2	2,2	2,2	1,2	1,2	2,2	2,2	1,2
Q	13q13	1,2	1,2	2,2	2,2	1,2	1,2	1,2	1,2	1,2	1,2
R	15q15	2,2	2,2	1,2	1,2	1,2	2,2	2,2	2,2	1,2	1,2
S	3q24	1,2	2,2	2,2	1,2	1,2	1,2	2,2	2,2	2,2	1,2

FIGURE 1–10. An example of a linkage study using RFLPs or other DNA markers. In this hypothetical example, a large pedigree with autosomal dominant retinitis pigmentosa is illustrated. Filled circles and squares indicated affected individuals. The numbers beneath each symbol are the alleles at marker loci that have been studied. This figure only shows the results of informative markers, i.e., for markers where the affected members of generations I and II are heterozygotes (1,2) and the unaffected spouses were homozygotes (2,2). (Note that any markers that are not heterozygous in the affected members of generations I and II would provide little useful information for this analysis.) Beneath the symbols for the members of the generation III are the alleles at the informative markers, as well as the chromosomal location of each marker.

At each of the marker loci, the "1" allele is defined as the allele that was transmitted from the affected male in generation I to the affected male in generation II. (This way of naming the "1" allele is done for pedagogic purposes for this figure.) If a marker locus is close to the disease gene, then the affected members of generation III should usually have marker "1" allele and the unaffected members should not. The markers G and S most closely fit this prediction. For both of these markers, nine out of the ten members of generation III fit the expected pattern for close linkage; the two members who do not probably are examples of meiotic recombination between the marker loci and the disease locus. Since both these markers come from the long arm of chromosome 3 (bands 3q21 and 3q24, respectively), these data indicate that the locus for the disease gene in this family is probably within or near this region. Data of this sort led to the search for mutations of the rhodopsin gene in patients with autosomal dominant retinitis pigmentosa, since the rhodopsin gene was known to lie in the region 3q21–q24.

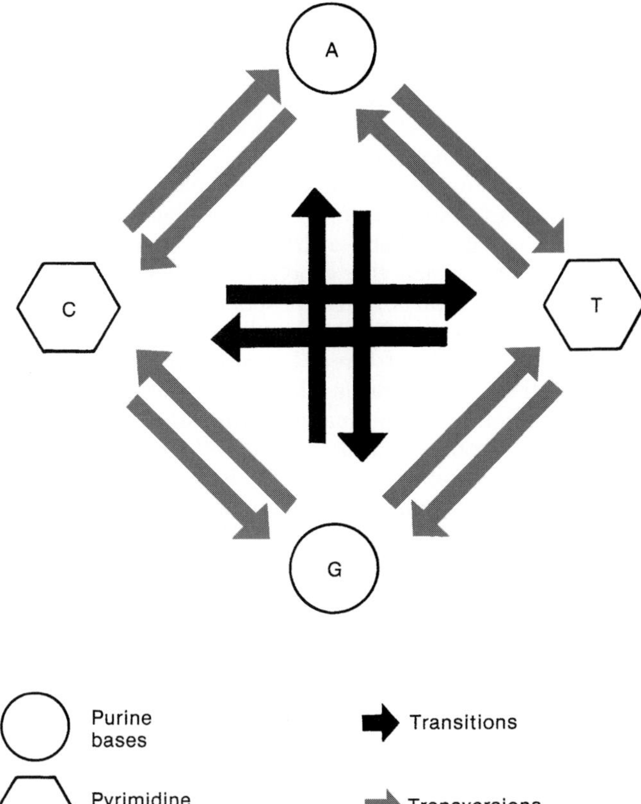

FIGURE 1–11. Transitions and transversions. The *black arrows* indicate base changes that would be termed transitions, because they involve an interchange of two bases of the same type (e.g., both purines). Transversions *(gray arrows)* involve the interchange of a purine and a pyrimidine.

A point mutation or other alteration affecting either of the ends of an intron will interfere with the proper splicing of the transcribed RNA. The 5′ end of an intron absolutely requires the dinucleotide sequence GT (called the splice donor sequence), and the 3′ end must have the dinucleotide sequence AG (the splice acceptor sequence). If a mutation changes either the splice acceptor or splice donor sequences, it is called a *splice site* mutation. The mRNA transcript will either improperly include sequence from the intron or will eliminate part or all of an exon. In either case, one expects a major alteration of the translated protein product.

Other areas of a transcriptional unit may be exquisitely sensitive to single base changes. For example, the promoter region upstream of a transcribed sequence has binding sites for factors necessary for the proper expression of a gene. A change in the sequence of these binding sites can bring about underexpression or overexpression of the protein product. Additional sequences that modulate the expression of a gene can be located in diverse regions of a transcriptional unit, such as within introns or within the 5′ or 3′ untranslated regions, or even many thousands of bases away from the cluster of exons and introns. Mutations in these regions can also affect the expression of a gene and cause an observable phenotype.

A *frameshift* mutation occurs when one or more bases are inserted into or deleted from the coding region of a gene. A frameshift mutation changes the reading frame of the encoded message. Since the genetic code uses consecutive, nonoverlapping triplets of DNA sequence, the number of bases that are inserted or deleted to cause a frameshift cannot be a multiple of three. Downstream of a frameshift mutation there is a drastic alteration of the amino acid sequence, often with a premature termination codon so that the encoded protein is truncated as well. If the number of base pairs removed or inserted in the coding region is a multiple of 3, the mutation is called an *in-frame* deletion or insertion. Only the amino acids encoded by the deleted or inserted codons will be affected.

Large deletions might remove a large portion of a transcriptional unit (an *internal* deletion), or the 5′ or 3′ end of a gene, or an entire transcriptional unit. Very large deletions might remove a number of closely linked genes. To be observable in a karyotype (i.e., to be detectable cytogenetically), a deletion must remove at least a few million base pairs of DNA. Since the density of genes in the human genome is approximately 1 per 30,000 to 50,000 base pairs, a cytogenetically detectable deletion usually affects dozens of genes. Like deletions, insertions can interfere with a gene if they interrupt a coding region or if they occur in a region that is important for proper RNA splicing or the proper expression of a gene.

This general categorization of mutations is not always applicable to naturally occurring defects in human DNA. Occasionally a single mutational event causes many single-base substitutions in a gene. Some deletions are not clean-cut, but instead a foreign segment of DNA is inserted where the normal sequence was deleted. More complex rearrangements have been documented, such as inversions where a segment of DNA is flipped backwards and relocated to a different region of the gene or to another gene. Such complex mutations represent a minority of the lesions that cause a disease.

Finally, because of our limited understanding of the molecular control of the regulation of transcription, splicing, and translation, the precise effect of a mutation sometimes cannot be deduced with certainty from inspection of the DNA sequence alone. The arrangement of bases in the coding region of a gene not only specifies the amino acid sequence of the protein product but also has some role in the recognition of splice sites and in maintaining the nuclear and cytoplasmic stability of the final mRNA product. Consequently, a point mutation labeled as a "missense" mutation, since it changes the amino acid specificity of a codon, might actually interfere with the splicing of an RNA transcript so that a very different protein product is produced. In some cases, considerable effort in a research laboratory is necessary to establish the exact biochemical consequences of a mutant allele of a known DNA sequence.

Origin of Mutations. Germline mutations either arise de novo in an individual or are inherited from a carrier parent. Actually, all mutations arise de novo in some individuals. Sometimes that individual is a distant ancestor who is called the *founder* or *progenitor* of the mutation.

Variability in the Rate of New Germline Mutations. For any given genetic disease, the proportion of patients who have a new germline mutation (as opposed to those who have inherited a mutation) is dependent on the mutation rate and the ability of those who carry the mutation to survive and reproduce. In practice, the quantification of both of these factors is difficult. Mutation rates at human loci extend over many orders of magnitude. New mutations at some loci, such as the Duchenne muscular dystrophy locus or the retinoblastoma locus, occur in more than 1 in 50,000 live births. For other diseases, such as tritanopia (due to a defect in the gene for blue cone opsin), the mutation rate is thought to be well below 1 in 10 million live births. The explanation for the wide range of mutation rates at different human loci is obscure. Possibilities include the size of the transcriptional unit (the Duchenne locus and the retinoblastoma locus are both large, encompassing 2 million and 180 thousand base pairs, respectively), limitations on the types of mutations that can cause a disease (almost all mutations of the rhodopsin gene causing dominant retinitis pigmentosa are missense mutations), or inherent variation in the mutability of loci based on their DNA sequences or their positions in the genome.

Mutation Spectrum of a Gene. An examination of mutations might provide clues to the mechanisms that are responsible for them. A *mutation spectrum* is a compilation of the frequency of each type of mutation at a specified locus; that is, the percentage of deletions, insertions, point mutations (broken down into transitions and transversions, or the specific nucleotide changes), frameshifts, and so forth. Tabulating the types of mutations causing a disease can give clues as to the functional domains of the encoded protein. Laboratory studies suggest that each class of mutagens causes certain types of mutations. For example, approximately half of the mutations resulting from gamma radiation are deletions and only about 20% are transitions. Ultraviolet light, on the other hand, induces deletions very infrequently but appears to facilitate transitions (about 50% of the resultant mutations). Thus, knowledge of the mutation spectrum can provide evidence implicating specific environmental mutagens as the cause of a disease. Indeed, ultraviolet light has been implicated by such evidence in the genesis of squamous cell carcinoma in sun-exposed skin.[33, 34] Unfortunately, the mutation spectrum of only a few genes is known with any accuracy. The available data do not implicate any specific environmental mutagen as the cause of most naturally occurring mutations in humans.

Parental Origin of New Mutations. An individual with a new germline mutation carries that mutation on the gene copy derived from either the mother or the father (except for males with a new mutation on the X chromosome, a chromosome necessarily derived from a son's mother). The parental origin of an autosomal allele with a new mutation can be determined in some situations. At many human loci, the general rule is that new germline mutations preferentially arise on a paternally derived allele. For example, approximately 80 to 90% of new germline mutations at the retinoblastoma locus[35–37] or the von Recklinghausen neurofibromatosis locus[38] affect the paternally derived allele. One attractive explanation for this bias relates to the fact that more than 300 cell divisions separate a one-cell male embryo from his resultant sperm (produced decades later) compared with approximately 20 cell divisions separating a one-cell female embryo from her resultant ova (produced while the female is still in utero).[39] The excess of mutant sperm may pertain to the fact that mutations chiefly arise during DNA replication.

Epigenetic Mutations. Defects that do not alter the sequence of DNA are called epigenetic. How such defects are transmitted through the germline, if at all, is open to speculation. One possible basis for epigenetic defects is that some bases of DNA are modified by the addition of methyl groups. The classic example of this involves the dinucleotide sequence CG. The cytosine in a CG dinucleotide sequence is customarily methylated in human DNA. However, in the vicinity of the promoter region at the 5′ end of a gene, cytosines are unmethylated in cells that express the gene.[40] If this region of a gene is aberrantly methylated, the gene will not be expressed. Despite no change in the DNA sequence, the allele will be inactive and thus equivalent to one with a null mutation. There is evidence that epigenetic defects in the retinoblastoma gene are one cause of retinoblastoma.[41–44]

Imprinting. Human cells have the capacity to distinguish the maternally derived allele from the paternally derived allele at some loci. This may be due to differences in the pattern of methylation of the two alleles or to differences in the configuration of DNA-binding factors that are present in chromatin. This *imprinting* of DNA has clinical importance because it explains peculiar patterns seen for some genetic diseases. For example, a deletion of q11-q13 of human chromosome 15 causes Prader-Willi syndrome if it affects the paternally derived chromosome 15, but Angelman syndrome if it affects the maternally derived chromosome homolog.[45] Also, the gene predisposing to glomus tumors must be inherited from a father to exert its tumor-predisposing influence.[46]

REFERENCES

1. Grosveld F, van Assendelft GB, Greaves DR, et al: Position-independent, high-level expression of the human beta-globin gene in transgenic mice. Cell 51:975, 1987.
2. Wilson MG, Towner JW, Fujimoto A: Retinoblastoma and D-chromosome deletions. Am J Hum Genet 25:57, 1973.
3. Lele KP, Penrose LS, Stallard HB: Chromosome deletion in a case of retinoblastoma. Ann Hum Genet 27:171, 1963.
4. Sparkes RS, Sparkes MC, Wilson MG, et al: Regional assignment of genes for human esterase D and retinoblastoma to chromosome band 13q14. Science 208:1042, 1980.
5. Francke U, Holmes LB, Atkins L, et al: Aniridia-Wilms' tumor association: Evidence for specific deletion of 11p13. Cytogenet Cell Genet 24:185, 1979.
6. Dryja TP, McGee TL, Reichel E, et al: A point mutation of the rhodopsin gene in one form of retinitis pigmentosa. Nature 343:364, 1990.
7. Eiberg H, Mohr J: Major genes of eye color and hair color linked to LU and SE. Clin Genet 31:186, 1987.
8. Kerem B, Rommens JM, Buchanan JA, et al: Identification of the cystic fibrosis gene: genetic analysis. Science 245:1073, 1989.
9. van den Hurk JAJM, Schwartz M, van Bokhoven H, et al: Molecular basis of choroideremia (CHM): Mutations involving the Rab escort protein-1 (REP-1) gene. Hum Mut 9:110, 1997.
10. Dryja TP, Li T: Molecular genetics of retinitis pigmentosa. Hum Mol Genet 4:1739, 1995.
11. Berger W, van de Pol D, Warburg M, et al: Mutations in the candidate gene for Norrie disease. Hum Mol Genet 1:461, 1992.
12. Chen ZY, Battinelli EM, Fielder A, et al: A mutation in the Norrie disease gene (NDP) associated with X-linked familial exudative vitreoretinopathy. Nature Genet 5:180, 1993.
13. Shastry BS, Pendergast SD, Hartzer MK, et al: Identification of missense mutations in the Norrie disease gene associated with advanced retinopathy of prematurity. Arch Ophthalmol 115:651, 1997.
14. Dryja TP, Berson EL, Rao VR, et al: Heterozygous missense mutation in the rhodopsin gene as a cause of congenital stationary night blindness. Nature Genet 4:280, 1993.
15. Sieving PA, Richards JE, Naarendorp F, et al: Dark-light: Model for nightblindness from the human rhodopsin Gly-90RAsp mutation. Proc Natl Acad Sci U S A 92:880, 1995.
16. McLaughlin ME, Sandberg MA, Berson EL, et al: Recessive mutations in the gene encoding the β-subunit of rod phosphodiesterase in patients with retinitis pigmentosa. Nature Genet 4:130, 1993.
17. Gal A, Orth U, Baehr W, et al: Heterozygous missense mutation in the rod cGMP phosphodiesterase β-subunit gene in autosomal dominant stationary night blindness. Nature Genet 7:64, 1994.
18. Voss R, Ben-Simon E, Avital A, et al: Isodisomy of chromosome 7 in a patient with cystic fibrosis: could uniparental disomy be common in humans? Am J Hum Genet 45:373, 1989.
19. Pentao L, Lewis RA, Ledbetter DH, et al: Maternal uniparental isodisomy of chromosome 14: Association with autosomal recessive rod monchromacy. Am J Hum Genet 50:690, 1992.
20. Jacobs PA, Wilson CM, Sprenkle JA, et al: Mechanism of origin of complete hydatidiform moles. Nature 286:714, 1980.
21. Sandgren O, Holmgren G, Lundgren E: Vitreous amyloidosis associated with homozygosity for the transthyretin methionine-30 gene. Arch Ophthalmol 108:1584, 1990.
22. Glaser T, Jepeal L, Edwards JG, et al: PAX6 gene dosage effect in a family with congenital cataracts, aniridia, anophthalmia, and central nervous system defects. Nature Genet 7:463, 1994.
23. Zlotogora J, Lerer I, Bar-David S, et al: Homozygosity for Waardenburg syndrome. Am J Hum Genet 56:1162, 1995.
24. Wallace DC, Singh G, Lott MT, et al: Mitochondrial DNA mutation associated with Leber's hereditary optic neuropathy. Science 242:1427, 1988.
25. Singh G, Lott MT, Wallace DC: A mitochondrial DNA mutation as a cause of Leber's hereditary optic neuropathy. N Engl J Med 320:1300, 1989.
26. Zeviani M, Moraes CT, DiMauro S, et al: Deletions of mitochondrial DNA in Kearns-Sayre syndrome. Neurology 38:1339, 1988.
27. Chalmers RM, Davis MB, Sweeney MG, et al: Evidence against an X-linked visual loss susceptibility locus in Leber hereditary optic neuropathy. Am J Hum Genet 59:103, 1996.
28. Al-Maghtheh M, Vithana E, Tarttelin E, et al: Evidence for a major retinitis pigmentosa locus on 19q13.4 (RP11), and association with a unique bimodal expressivity phenotype. Am J Hum Genet 59:864, 1996.
29. McGuire RE, Sullivan LS, Blanton SH, et al: X-linked dominant cone-rod degeneration: Linkage mapping of a new locus for retinitis pigmentosa (RP15) to Xp22.13-p22.11. Am J Hum Genet 57:87, 1995.
30. Kajiwara K, Berson EL, Dryja TP: Digenic retinitis pigmentosa due to mutations at the unlinked peripherin/RDS and ROM1 loci. Science 264:1604, 1994.
31. Morell R, Spritz RA, Ho L, et al: Apparent digenic inheritance of Waardenburg syndrome type 2 (WS2) and autosomal recessive ocular albinism (AROA). Hum Mol Genet 6:659, 1997.
32. Nakamura Y, Leppert M, O'Connell P, et al: Variable number of tandem repeat (VNTR) markers for human gene mapping. Science 235:1616, 1987.
33. Brash DE, Rudolph JA, Simon JA, et al: A role for sunlight in skin cancer: UV-induced p53 mutations in squamous cell carcinoma. Proc Natl Acad Sci U S A 88:10124, 1991.
34. Ziegler A, Jonason AS, Leffell DJ, et al: Sunburn and p53 in the onset of skin cancer. Nature 372:773, 1994.
35. Dryja TP, Morrow JF, Rapaport JM: Quantification of the paternal allele bias for new germline mutations in the retinoblastoma gene. Hum Genet 100:446, 1997.
36. Zhu X, Dunn JM, Phillips RA, et al: Preferential germline mutation of the paternal allele in retinoblastoma. Nature 340:312, 1989.
37. Kato MV, Ishizaki K, Shimizu T, et al: Parental origin of germ-line and somatic mutations in the retinoblastoma gene. Hum Genet 94:31, 1994.
38. Jadayel D, Fain P, Upadhyaya M, et al: Paternal origin of new mutations in von Recklinghausen neurofibromatosis. Nature 343:558, 1990.

39. Vogel F, Rathenberg R: Spontaneous mutation in man. Adv Hum Genet 5:223, 1975.
40. Antequera F, Boyes J, Bird A: High levels of de novo methylation and altered chromatin structure at CpG island in cell lines. Cell 62:503, 1990.
41. Greger V, Passarge E, Hopping W, et al: Epigenetic changes may contribute to the formation and spontaneous regression of retinoblastoma. Hum Genet 83:155, 1989.
42. Sakai T, Toguchida J, Ohtani N, et al: Allele-specific hypermethylation of the retinoblastoma tumor-suppressor gene. Am J Hum Genet 48:880, 1991.
43. Ohtani-Fujita N, Fujita T, Aoike A, et al: CpG methylation inactivates the promoter activity of the human retinoblastoma tumor-suppressor gene. Oncogene 8:1063, 1993.
44. Greger V, Debus N, Lohmann D, et al: Frequency and parental origin of hypermethylated RB1 alleles in retinoblastoma. Hum Genet 94:491, 1994.
45. Knoll JHM, Nicholls RD, Magenis RE, et al: Angelman and Prader-Willi syndromes share a common chromosome 15 deletion but differ in parental origin of the deletion. Am J Med Genet 32:285, 1989.
46. van der Mey AGL, Maaswinkel-Mooy PD, Cornelisse CJ, et al: Genomic imprinting in hereditary glomus tumours: Evidence for new genetic theory. Lancet i:1291, 1989.
47. Nathans J, Thomas D, Hogness DS: Molecular genetics of human color vision: The genes encoding blue, green, and red pigments. Science 232:193, 1986.

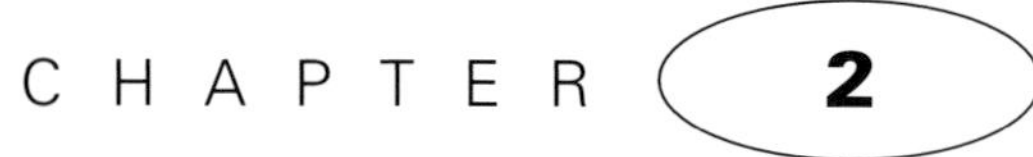

CHAPTER 2

Approaches to the Identification of Genes Responsible for Hereditary Ophthalmic Disease

Thaddeus P. Dryja

A major goal of the current generation of geneticists is to construct a table correlating genes with human phenotypes. The table will be large. One column will be composed of the approximately 5000 phenotypes that are currently known[1] (perhaps many more), and the second column will list approximately 60,000 to 70,000 transcriptional units now estimated to be in the human genome.[2] Gene-phenotype associations may be indicated by lines connecting entries in the "phenotype" column with loci in the "gene" column. At the moment, the table is only partially completed—a few hundred genes have been identified as causes for specific diseases or other phenotypes. Encyclopedic versions of the current state of this table exist, such as McKusick's *Mendelian Inheritance in Man.*[1] A list of identified genes causing some hereditary eye diseases is provided in Table 2–1.

There are two starting points for research aimed at identifying the connections between specific genes and phenotypes. One method begins with the phenotype column. Patients who have a particular phenotype are gathered and analyzed. Clues regarding the responsible genes are obtained from clinical findings and from biochemical and genetic analyses. Genes are evaluated until one is found with sequence abnormalities specific for the phenotype. Depending on the overall method, this approach may be referred to as "reverse genetics" or "positional cloning." It is the method responsible for most of the human gene-disease correlations discovered to date.

The second approach, less commonly used, is to start from the gene column. A gene is isolated, and its protein product is partially characterized. Work is then directed toward finding what human phenotype would result from mutations in it. This technique will be referred to as the "gene-oriented approach." With a gene-oriented mindset, the goal is to investigate the role of a particular gene in human disease.

Note that with either the phenotype- or gene-oriented approach, one does not actually scan the entire opposing column to discover a gene-phenotype association. This has been too time-consuming and therefore impractical to do. Rather, one narrows the search using various methods that are described in this chapter.

Phenotype-Oriented Approaches

1. *Detection of a biochemical abnormality.* If individuals with a particular phenotype are discovered to have a specific biochemical abnormality, that information can be used to narrow the scope of the gene scan to those genes expressing proteins in the defective biochemical pathway. Sometimes the biochemical abnormality pinpoints the responsible gene. For example, biochemical analyses showed that many albinos lacked tyrosinase activity, a key enzyme in the synthetic pathway for melanin. This knowledge made it logical to begin the search for genes causing albinism with the tyrosinase gene.[3] Similarly, the β-globin gene was the first to be analyzed as a cause for sickle cell anemia, because defects in this protein had already been discovered in patients.

   Gyrate atrophy of the choroid and retina provides

TABLE 2–1. **Identified Genes Causing Hereditary Ophthalmic Diseases***

Disease	Gene (Chromosomal Location)
Anterior Segment	
Lattice corneal dystrophy type I	Kerato-epithelin (5q31)[47]
Granular corneal dystrophy	Kerato-epithelin (5q31)[47]
Avellino corneal dystrophy	Kerato-epithelin (5q31)[47]
Reis-Bückler corneal dystrophy	Kerato-epithelin (5q31)[47]
Lattice dystrophy type II	Gelsolin (9q34)[48]
Meesman's corneal dystrophy	Keratin K3 (12q12–q13)[49]
Juvenile glaucoma	Trabecular meshwork protein (1q23–25)[50, 51]
Rieger's syndrome	RIEG (4q25)[52]
Aniridia	PAX6, homeobox gene (11p13)[16, 17]
Nonsyndromic cataract	γE-crystallin pseudogene (2q33–q35)[41]
	Galactokinase (17q24)[53]
	β-Crystallin (22q11.2–q12.1)[42]
Hyperferritinemia cataract	Ferritin L-subunit (19q13.3–qter)[54, 55]
Retina	
Tritanopia	Blue opsin (7q22–qter)[11, 12]
X-linked colorblindness	Red cone opsin (Xq22–q28)[8]
	Green cone opsin (Xq22–q28)[8]
Blue cone monochromacy	Red and green cone opsins (Xq22–q28)[9]
Retinitis pigmentosa, nonsyndromic	Rod opsin (3q21.3–q24)[36]
	Rod cGMP-phosphodiesterase, α subunit (5q31.2–q34)[56]
	Rod cGMP-phosphodiesterase, β subunit (4p16.3)[57–59]
	cGMP-gated channel protein, α subunit (4p14–q13)[60]
	Peripherin/RDS (6p12)[61, 62]
	ROM1 (11q13)[63]
	RPGR (Xp21.1)[64]
	RPE65 (1p31)[65]
	Cellular retinaldehyde binding protein (15q26)[66]
Leber's congenital amaurosis	Guanylate cyclase (17p13.1)[67]
	RPE65 (1p31)[68]
Usher syndrome type I	Myosin VIIa (11q13.5)[69]
Retinitis pigmentosa and ataxia	α-Tocopherol transport protein (8q13.1–q13.3)[70, 71]
Refsum disease	Phytanoyl-CoA α-hydroxylase (10pter–p11.2)[72, 73]
Batten disease	CLN3 (16p12.1)[74]
Kearns-Sayre syndrome	Mitochondrial proteins[75–77]
Abetalipoproteinemia	Microsomal triglyceride-transfer-protein (4q22–q24)[78]
X-linked retinoschisis	XLRS1 (Xp22.2)[79]
Congenital stationary nightblindness	Rod opsin (3q21.3–q24)[80, 81]
	Rod transducin, α subunit (3p21.3–p21.1)[82]
	Rod cGMP-phosphodiesterase, β subunit (4p16.3)[83]
Oguchi disease	Rod arrestin (2q37)[84]
	Rhodopsin kinase (13q34)[85]
Sorsby macular dystrophy	TIMP3 (22q12.1–q13.2)[86]
Stargardt disease	ABCR (1p21–p13)[87]
Norrie disease	Norrie disease gene (Xp11.4)[88–90]
X-linked vitreoretinopathy	Norrie disease gene (Xp11.4)[91]
Predisposition to retinopathy of prematurity	Norrie disease gene (Xp11.4)[92]
Gyrate atrophy	Ornithine amino transferase (10q26)[5]
Macular degeneration/dystrophy	Peripherin/RDS (6p12)[93–95]
Retinoblastoma	Cell cycle checkpoint protein (13q14)[21, 208]
von Hippel-Lindau disease	Tumor suppressor protein (3p25)[96]
Ocular albinism	Tyrosinase (11q14–q21)[97]
	OA1 (Xp22.3–p22.2)[98]
Neuroophthalmology	
Leber's optic atrophy	Mitochondria[99, 100]
Malformations	
Waardenburg syndrome type 1	Homeobox gene PAX3 (2q37)[101–103]
Waardenburg syndrome type 2	MITF (3p14.1–p12.3)[104, 105]
Optic nerve coloboma	Homeobox gene PAX2 (10q24–q25)[106]
Stickler syndrome	Type II procollagen (12q12–q13.2)[107]
Marfan syndrome	Fibrillin (15q21.1)[34]

*Ordered according to the region of the eye affected.

yet another example of this approach. The first clue to the genetic defect was that patients with the disease had elevated levels of ornithine in their blood and urine.[4] This led to a study of the enzymes involved in synthesizing and catabolizing ornithine. Within 5 years, a deficiency in ornithine-δ-aminotransferase (OAT) was discovered in various tissues from affected individuals. OAT is an enzyme responsible for consuming a major portion of the ornithine in human cells. Further evidence for OAT deficiency as a cause of gyrate atrophy came when the OAT gene was cloned and mutations in this gene were found in patients with gyrate atrophy.[5] Proof that these defects alone caused the disease came from the construction of transgenic mice with defects in the OAT gene: these mice had low OAT activity, high ornithine levels, and retinal degeneration.[6]

2. *Detection of a clinical abnormality.* In some cases, clinical findings give clues to the genes responsible for a hereditary trait. A frequently cited example is colorblindness. Individuals with anomalies or deficiencies in their red, green, or blue cone mechanisms might be expected to have abnormalities in genes encoding proteins specific to the red, green, or blue cone photoreceptors. This turns out to be the case. Defects in the genes encoding red or green cone opsins (both on the X chromosome) are found in males who have protan or deutan colorblindness.[7, 8] Blue cone monochromats are males who have defects in both the red and green cone opsin genes.[9] Tritanopia is due to defects in blue cone opsin.[10–12] No gene defect has yet been identified in rod monochromats, who have no functional cones, but it is likely that the responsible gene or genes encode protein(s) found in all three cone types but not in rods.
3. *Detection of a chromosome abnormality.* For most hereditary diseases in which the responsible gene is unknown, there are currently no known specific biochemical abnormalities and no clinical abnormalities that reliably point to one or a small set of genes as the likely cause. It is still possible to narrow down the list of genes possibly causing a given disease if one can determine approximately the chromosomal location for the disease gene. Only those genes in that region would remain as candidate genes for the disease. One way to determine a likely position for a disease gene is if affected individuals have similar chromosomal deletions or translocations detectable cytogenetically. One example relevant to ophthalmology is the aniridia–Wilms' tumor association. Patients with both aniridia and Wilms' tumor were often found to have a deletion of the short arm of chromosome 11p.[13, 14] It was later discovered that these deletions remove two genes that are near each other in the p13 band of chromosome 11; one gene is responsible for Wilms' tumor[15] and the other for aniridia.[16, 17] Similarly, deletions of chromosome 13 band q14 in patients with retinoblastoma[18, 19] and with Rieger's syndrome[20] pointed to that chromosome region as containing responsible genes for those two diseases.[21, 22]
4. *Linkage analysis.* The method most frequently used to find an approximate chromosomal location for a disease gene is called linkage analysis. For this method to work, one needs access at a minimum to one large family with numerous affected individuals, one large family with a few distantly related affected individuals, or many small families each with affected individuals all due to the same disease gene. DNA is obtained from blood samples from the affected and unaffected members.

The procedure next takes advantage of numerous sites in the human genome where there is variability in the DNA sequence, such as restriction fragment length polymorphisms, variable number of tandem repeats (VNTRs), and microsatellites (see Chapter 1, Fundamentals of Genetics). By assaying the DNA of two parents and their children, one can determine which alleles at each polymorphic site were transmitted to each child. Expanding this sort of analysis to all the members of a large, multigeneration family allows one to trace the inheritance of segments of each chromosome. For a linkage analysis, one compares the inheritance of each chromosomal segment with the inheritance of the disease in a large affected family (Fig. 2–1). If the family is large enough, there will be only one chromosomal region that perfectly "cosegregates" with the disease; that is, its inheritance matches the inheritance of the disease. For an autosomal dominant condition, perfect cosegregation occurs if all affected individuals in a given family have the same allele at a polymorphic site near the disease locus. For an autosomal recessive condition, unaffected family members may carry one or the other of the alleles that are linked to the disease gene, but only affected members will carry both. For an X-linked condition, all males will be hemizygous for the closely linked allele; female carriers will have that allele heterozygously.

The disease gene will be in the chromosomal region that perfectly cosegregates. The size of this region depends on the fortuitous discovery of meiotic recombinants in the families under study. If a nearby polymorphic site does not cosegregate in one branch of an affected family, then that polymorphic locus provides one boundary for the location of the disease gene. The goal is to find two boundary markers as close to each other as possible, with one on each side of the disease gene.

Initial reports of linkage of markers to human traits typically involve one or a few families with about 20 to 30 affected individuals and are able to narrow the disease interval to about 10 to 20 centimorgans (cM). A region this size corresponds to about 10 million base pairs of DNA, enough to include about 300 to 600 genes, or about 0.5 to 1% of all human genes. Such discoveries represent major advances, because they serve to rule out more than 99% of all human genes as the disease gene. Still, it is quite laborious to find and evaluate all the genes in an interval of 10 to 20 cM. Recruiting additional families for linkage analysis might permit the discovery of one or more recombinants that would further limit the disease interval. To have a 90% chance of limiting the disease interval to 2 cM or less (a region containing about 60 genes), one

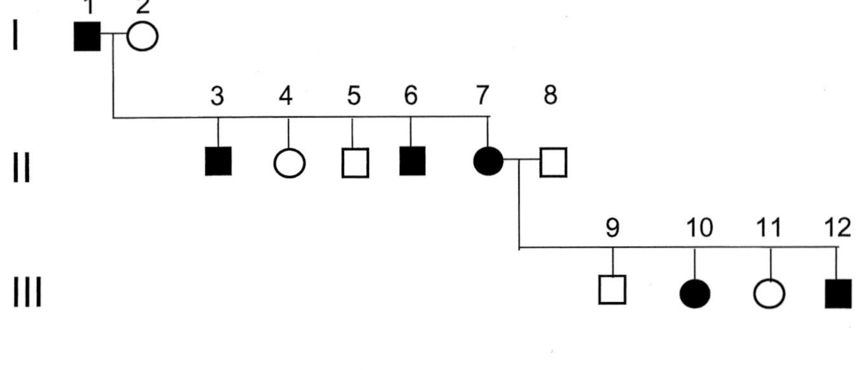

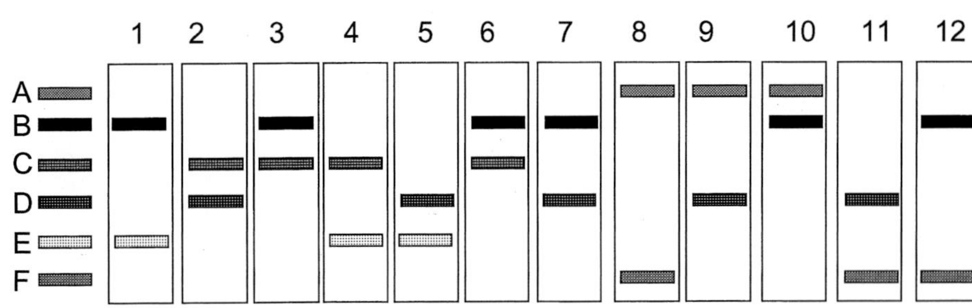

FIGURE 2–1. An example of linkage analysis in a three-generation family with a hereditary disease. Affected individuals are represented by *filled circles* (females) or *squares* (males). Stylized results from the analysis of a microsatellite marker locus are shown at the bottom. This marker has alleles labeled A through F. It turns out that the B allele is invariably transmitted with the disease. This result makes it likely that the marker locus is linked closely to the disease locus. (Courtesy of J. Wiggs.)

requires pedigrees that will in their totality provide 200 scorable meioses.[23]

Linkage analyses have mapped dozens of unidentified genes that cause a variety of hereditary eye diseases to specific regions of the human genome. A partial list is provided in Table 2–2.

It is still a formidable task to locate all the genes in an interval a few million base pairs in size. Repositories are available that have libraries of cloned human DNA fragments each about 80,000 to a few hundred thousand base pairs in length. These libraries are organized so that the overlapping fragments from any specified chromosomal interval can be requested. Once these are on hand, many transcriptional units (i.e., genes) can be located by searching for regions with a high content of the bases "C" and "G" and many CG dinucleotides; CG-rich regions are often present at the 5′ end of genes.[24, 25] Another method involves finding exons within the cloned DNA using a method called "exon-trapping."[26] Other valuable resources are libraries of partial sequences of the transcribed genes from specific tissues.[27] These sequences are in the process of being mapped to specific chromosomal intervals, so that it is now possible to obtain a list and partial sequence of many genes in a given interval through a search on databases available on the Internet.

5. *Search for mutations in candidate genes.* Regardless of the approach used, be it through the observation of a biochemical abnormality, clinical findings, abnormal karyotype, or linkage analysis, one eventually comes to a point where one gene or a handful of genes are likely candidates to be the disease gene for a given phenotype. The next step is to screen affected patients for mutations in those genes. Most methods for mutation screening of a gene require the knowledge of the normal sequence of the coding region of the gene, a map of where the introns interrupt the coding sequence, and the sequence of intron DNA flanking each exon. With this information, one can design assays using the polymerase chain reaction to amplify the coding sequence or to individually amplify the exons of the gene. The amplified DNA fragments are scanned for mutations using techniques such as denaturing gradient gel electrophoresis (DGGE) or single-strand conformation polymorphism (SSCP). Figure 2–2 illustrates how the SSCP technique detects mutations. These methods rapidly scan DNA fragments a few hundred base pairs in length for DNA sequence anomalies. Any variations in the DNA are subsequently evaluated through DNA sequence analysis, which is more laborious but provides the exact sequence of any fragment that is found to be variant through DGGE or SSCP analysis.

Gene-Oriented Approaches

The logic behind the gene-oriented approach begins with the assumptions that every gene mutates and that most genes have important functions. For any particular gene, there would be a high probability that some human has a mutation in that gene and a corresponding phenotype. To find correlations between genes and phenotypes, one picks a particular gene and then scans humans for mutations in it.

Gene-oriented approaches to discover the genetic causes of hereditary diseases have not been widely used, probably because they were not deemed attractive for several reasons. One argument against a gene-based approach is based on the smaller size of the phenotype column compared with the genotype column (5000 phenotypes versus approximately 60,000 to 70,000 genes). Assuming a one-to-one mapping, this discrepancy in size predicts that most genes have no companion in the phenotype column. It could be that the relatively low number of known human phenotypes (about

TABLE 2–2. **Linkage-Based Assignments of Unidentified Genes Causing Ophthalmic Diseases**

Disease	Chromosomal Location
Anterior Segment	
Megalocornea	Xq21–26[108]
Macular corneal dystrophy	16q[109]
Congenital hereditary endothelial dystrophy	20p13.1–12[110]
Dominant glaucoma	2cen–q13[51]; 3q21–24[111]
Recessive glaucoma	1p36[51]; 2p21[51]
Cataract	13cen–q12.1[112]; 17p13–12[113]; 17q11–12[114]; 17q24[115]
Nancy-Horan syndrome (microcornea and cataract)	Xp22.2–p22.3[116]
Dominant iridogoniodysgenesis	6p25[117, 118]
Dominant pigment dispersion syndrome	7q35–36[119]
Rieger's syndrome	13q14[22]
Blau's syndrome (uveitis, arthritis, skin rash)	16p21–q12[120]
Congenital microcoria	13q31–32[209]
Posterior Segment	
Nonsyndromic RP	Xp22.13–22.11 (X-linked dominant RP)[121]
	Xp11.3–11.2(RP2)[122, 123]
	Recessive 1q21–13[124]
	Dominant 1p13–q23[125]
	Recessive 6p21[126, 127]
	Dominant 7p13.3[128–130]
	Dominant 7q31–32 (RP10)[131–135]
	Dominant 8q11–q21[136, 137]
	Dominant 17p13.3[138–141]
	Dominant 17q22–24[142]
	Dominant 19q13.4[143–145]
	Recessive RP with preserved para-arteriolar retinal pigment epithelium 1q31–q32.1[146–148]
Syndromic RP	
Usher type I	10q[149]; 11p15[150–152]; 14q[153]; 21q21[154]
Usher type II	1q41[155–158]
Usher type III	3q21–25[158, 159]
Bardet-Biedl syndrome	3p12[160, 161]; 11q13[162–164]; 15q22–23[163–165]; 16q21[160, 163, 164, 166]
Atrophia areata	11p15[167]
Dominant juvenile macular degeneration	6q11–15[168]; 13q34[169]
Dominant cone dystrophy	17p13–12[170–172]
X-linked cone dystrophy	Xq27[173]
North Carolina macular dystrophy	6q14–16.2[174]
Progressive bifocal chorioretinal atrophy	6q14–16.2[175]
Cone-rod dystrophy	19q13.1–13.2[176, 177]
Rod monochromacy	2p11–q21
X-linked stationary nightblindness	Xp11.3[178]; Xp21.1[179, 180]
Dominant exudative vitreoretinopathy	11q14.3–21[181–183]
Recessive pseudoglioma and osteoporosis	11q12–13[184]
Best disease	11p12–q13.3[185–188]
Atypical vitelliform dystrophy	8q24.3[189]
Waardenburg syndrome	3p14.1–12[190]
Dominant cystoid macular edema	7p[191, 192]
Doyne dominant drusen (malattia leventinese)	2p16[193, 194]
Wagner syndrome	5q13–14[195]
Neuroophthalmology	
Congenital fibrosis of the extraocular muscles	12cen[196, 197]
Dominant congenital nystagmus	6p12[198]
Wolfram syndrome	4[199]
Kjer optic atrophy	3q28–29[200, 201]
Cerebellar ataxia with pigmentary macular dystrophy	3p21.1–12[202–205]
Congenital ataxia, myoclonic encephalopathy, and macular degeneration	Xpter–22.33[206]
Congenital ptosis	1p34.1–32[207]

Abbreviation: RP, retinitis pigmentosa.

one-tenth of the number of genes) occurs because many genes are essential for life, so that mutations in them are embryonic lethals. On the other hand, some sets of genes might have an overlapping or redundant function, so that defects in any one member of a set produce no phenotype or one that is too subtle to be recognized. If most human genes are essential to life or are redundant, studies of genes selected at random for evaluation in large sets of humans would frequently turn up nothing of value. However, the small size of the phenotype column could be primarily the result of our inability or failure to recognize many human phenotypes. There are probably a multitude of human per-

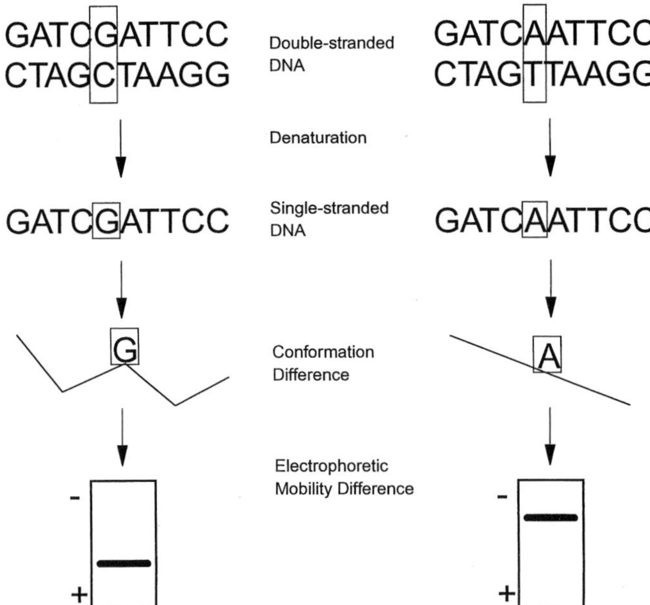

FIGURE 2–2. Basis for the single-strand conformation polymorphism (SSCP) technique to detect variations in DNA sequences. The polymerase chain reaction is used to amplify the gene sequence under investigation, producing double-stranded DNA fragments. These fragments are denatured, usually by heating to 90°C to 100°C for a few minutes, to produce single-stranded fragments. After rapid cooling on ice, these single-stranded fragments wrap themselves into specific conformations that are exquisitely dependent upon the DNA sequence. A single base change in a fragment 200 bases or more in length is usually sufficient to produce a change in the conformation of single-stranded DNA. The speed at which single-stranded DNA migrates through a gel will depend on its sequence-specific conformation. In practice, the SSCP technique has a sensitivity of about 90% in detecting novel single-base changes in DNA fragments of about 150 to 250 bases in length. (Courtesy of J. Wiggs.)

sonality traits that are genetic but are not yet individually listed in the phenotype column. Another reason for the small size of the phenotype column is our inability to distinguish similar phenotypes that are caused by different genes. There are numerous examples where a clinically defined disease is found to have underlying nonallelic heterogeneity in which defects in any of a number of genes can be the cause. As extreme examples, at least 30 genes are now known to be responsible for what is clinically defined as "congenital deafness,"[28, 29] and, as will be discussed below, perhaps 50 or more genes can cause hereditary forms of blindness such as congenital amaurosis and retinitis pigmentosa.[30–32] The actual number of genes responsible for just one of these phenotypes could be much higher, perhaps well over 100. Thus, the assumption of one-to-one genotype-phenotype mapping is false. Even for genes where mutations are embryonic lethals, there is a precedent for viable individuals with corresponding phenotypes. For example, mosaic individuals with defects in the ubiquitously expressed and essential G-protein Gsa have recognizable phenotypes such as McCune-Albright syndrome.[33] Some oncogenes provide special examples of phenotypes revealed only in mosaic individuals. In summary, it may be that a sizable proportion (and perhaps most human genes) corresponds with clinically evident phenotypes. There is a reasonable likelihood that, for any individual gene of interest, one could find some phenotype associated with alleles of it if one can evaluate a sufficiently large number of individuals including a wide range of phenotypes.

It may seem unsettling that, for any gene of interest, there would be a huge number of individuals and phenotypes to be scanned before one has a reasonable chance of finding a gene-phenotype correlation. However, just as for phenotype-based approaches, there are short-cuts that considerably reduce the amount of work involved.

1. *Tissue expression pattern*. The pattern of expression of a gene can provide an important insight: genes expressed only in the lens, for example, are most likely to be associated with hereditary forms of cataract.
2. *Biochemical pathway*. Knowledge of the physiologic role of the protein product of a gene can provide clues to the phenotype. For example, defects in a connective tissue protein are likely to be found in individuals with connective tissue diseases. For example, defects in fibrillin and various collagens cause Marfan's syndrome[34] and osteogenesis imperfecta,[35] respectively. Another example of the gene-oriented approach comes from a multi-year effort to understand the genes encoding the red, green, and blue opsins that enable color vision. This research first identified the responsible genes and then evaluated individuals with defective color vision to discover mutations.[7, 8]
3. *Chromosome maps*. Although the determination of chromosomal map positions is not an essential part of gene-based approaches, if a chosen gene happens to be from a region known to be implicated in a plausibly corresponding phenotype, researchers wisely screen individuals with that phenotype early on. For example, during a study of the rhodopsin gene,[36] an evaluation of patients with dominant retinitis pigmentosa was emphasized because of a report[37] that one family with dominant retinitis pigmentosa showed linkage between the disease gene and markers on chromosome 3q, the chromosome arm that contains the rhodopsin gene. Similarly, different families with hereditary cataract showed linkage to chromosomes 2q[38, 39] and 22q[40] in the vicinity of genes for γ-crystallin and β-crystallin, respectively. Responsible mutations in those genes were subsequently identified.[41, 42]
4. *Creation of animal models*. A more direct gene-oriented method is to study the phenotype of animals with transgenic or naturally arising mutations in the gene of interest; one then focuses the evaluation on humans with phenotypes similar to those in the homologously mutant animals. This is one currently active method for establishing phenotypes of genes encoding proteins specific to the central nervous system.[43, 44]

Evidence Required to Prove That a DNA Sequence Anomaly Is Pathogenic

For either a gene-based or phenotype-based approach, the allele-phenotype associations that are encountered will initially provide only tentative evidence of an etiologic relationship. Additional supporting evidence could come from the documentation of a statistically significant cosegregation of alleles with a phenotype in more than one family, the detection of new germ line or somatic mutations appearing together with the phenotype, the observation of a corresponding phenotype in lower animals with similar mutations in the homologous gene, or the demonstration of biochemical properties of the allelic variants of the protein product that reasonably explain the phenotype.

Gene Sharing

There are many cases where different alleles in a single gene cause different phenotypes or different inheritance patterns. Examples are provided by the genes encoding red opsin and green opsin. Defects in these can cause a deficiency in protan and deutan colorblindness,[8] blue cone monochromacy,[9] or a form of macular degeneration.[45] Another example is the rhodopsin gene, where some alleles cause dominant retinitis pigmentosa, others recessive retinitis pigmentosa, and still others dominant stationary night blindness. This phenomenon of gene sharing by phenotypes has been noted for other phenotypes not specific to the eye (e.g., the RET gene where different alleles can cause Hirschsprung's disease or multiple endocrine neoplasia type 2A or type 2B[46]). The implication is that evaluation of a gene cannot be considered complete just because one correlating phenotype is found.

REFERENCES

1. McKusick VA: Mendelian Inheritance in Man: Catalogs of Autosomal Dominant, Autosomal Recessive, and X-Linked Phenotypes, 11th ed. Baltimore and London, The Johns Hopkins University Press, 1994.
2. Fields C, Adams MD, White O, et al: How many genes in the human genome? Nature Genet 7:345, 1994.
3. Oetting WS, King RA: Molecular basis of type I (tyrosinase-related) oculocutaneous albinism: Mutations and polymorphisms of the human tyrosinase gene. Hum Mutat 2:1, 1993.
4. Simell O, Takki K: Raised plasma ornithine and gyrate atrophy of the choroid and retina. Lancet i:1031, 1973.
5. Mitchell G, Brody L, Looney J, et al: An initiator codon mutation in ornithine-δ-aminotransferase causing gyrate atrophy. J Clin Invest 81:630, 1988.
6. Wang T, Lawler AM, Steel G, et al: Mice lacking ornithine-delta-amino-transferase have paradoxical neonatal hypoornithinemia and retinal degeneration. Nature Genet 11:185, 1995.
7. Nathans J, Thomas D, Hogness DS: Molecular genetics of human color vision: The genes encoding blue, green, and red pigments. Science 232:193, 1986.
8. Nathans J, Piantanida TP, Eddy RL, et al: Molecular genetics of inherited variation in human color vision. Science 232:203, 1986.
9. Nathans J, Davenport CM, Maumenee IH, et al: Molecular genetics of human blue cone monochromacy. Science 245:831, 1989.
10. Li T, Zierath P, Went L, et al: Substitution of a highly conserved amino acid residue in the S-cone (blue) photopigment may be the cause of tritan defect in a Dutch pedigree. [Abstract] Invest Ophthalmol Vis Sci 32:783, 1991.
11. Weitz CJ, Miyake Y, Shinzato K, et al: Human tritanopia associated with two amino acid substitutions in the blue-sensitive opsin. Am J Hum Genet 50:498, 1992.
12. Weitz CJ, Went LN, Nathans J: Human tritanopia associated with a third amino acid substitution in the blue-sensitive visual pigment. Am J Hum Genet 51:444, 1992.
13. Riccardi VM, Sujansky E, Smith AC, et al: Chromosomal imbalance in the aniridia–Wilms' tumor association: 11p interstitial deletion. Pediatrics 61:604, 1978.
14. Francke U, Holmes LB, Atkins L, et al: Aniridia–Wilms' tumor association: Evidence for specific deletion of 11p13. Cytogenet Cell Genet 24:185, 1979.
15. Call KM, Glaser T, Ito CY, et al: Isolation and characterization of a zinc finger polypeptide gene at the human chromosome 11 Wilms' tumor locus. Cell 60:509, 1990.
16. Jordan T, Hanson I, Zaletayev D, et al: The human PAX6 gene is mutated in two patients with aniridia. Nature Genet 1:328, 1992.
17. Glaser T, Walton DS, Maas RL: Genomic structure, evolutionary conservation and aniridia mutations in the human PAX6 gene. Nature Genet 2:232, 1992.
18. Yunis JJ, Ramsay N: Retinoblastoma and subband deletion of chromosome 13. Am J Dis Child 132:161, 1978.
19. Sparkes RS, Sparkes MC, Wilson MG, et al: Regional assignment of genes for human esterase D and retinoblastoma to chromosome band 13q14. Science 208:1042, 1980.
20. Stathacopoulos RA, Bateman JB, Sparkes RS, et al: The Rieger syndrome and a chromosome 13 deletion. J Pediatr Ophthalmol Strabismus 24:198, 1987.
21. Friend SH, Bernards R, Rogelj S, et al: A human DNA segment with properties of the gene that predisposes to retinoblastoma and osteosarcoma. Nature 323:643, 1986.
22. Phillips JC, Del Bono EA, Haines JL, et al: A second locus for Rieger syndrome maps to chromosome 13q14. Am J Hum Genet 59:613, 1996.
23. Boehnke M: Limits of resolution of genetic linkage studies: Implications for the positional cloning of human disease genes. Am J Hum Genet 55:379, 1994.
24. Bird AP: CpG-rich islands and the function of DNA methylation. Nature 321:209, 1986.
25. Brown WR, Bird AP: Long-range restriction site mapping of mammalian genomic DNA. Nature 322:477, 1986.
26. Church DM, Stotler CJ, Rutter JL, et al: Isolation of genes from complex sources of mammalian genomic DNA using exon amplification. Nature Genet 6:98, 1994.
27. Adams MD, Dubnick M, Kerlavage AR, et al: Sequence identification of 2,375 human brain genes. Nature 55:632, 1992.
28. Petit C: Genes responsible for human hereditary deafness: Symphony of a thousand. Nature Genet 4:385, 1996.
29. Van Camp G, Willems PJ, Smith RJH: Nonsyndromic hearing impairment: Unparalleled heterogeneity. Am J Hum Genet 60:758, 1997.
30. Rosenfeld PJ, McKusick VA, Amberger JS, et al: Recent advances in the gene map of inherited eye disorders: Primary hereditary diseases of the retina, choroid, and vitreous. J Med Genet 31:903, 1994.
31. Dryja TP, Li T: Molecular genetics of retinitis pigmentosa. Hum Mol Genet 4:1739, 1995.
32. Daiger SP, Sullivan LA, Rodriguez JA: Correlation of phenotype with genotype in inherited retinal degeneration. Behav Brain Sci 18:452, 1995.
33. Shenker A, Weinstein LS, Sweet DE, et al: An activating Gsalpha mutation is present in fibrous dysplasia of bone in the McCune-Albright syndrome. J Clin Endocrinol Metab 79:750, 1994.
34. Dietz HC, Cutting GR, Pyeritz RE, et al: Marfan syndrome caused by a recurrent de novo missense mutation in the fibrillin gene. Nature 352:337, 1991.
35. Byers PH, Wallis GA, Willing MC: Osteogenesis imperfecta: Translation of mutation to phenotype. J Med Genet 28:433, 1991.
36. Dryja TP, McGee TL, Reichel E, et al: A point mutation of the rhodopsin gene in one form of retinitis pigmentosa. Nature 343:364, 1990.
37. McWilliam P, Farrar GJ, Kenna P, et al: Autosomal dominant retinitis pigmentosa (ADRP): Localization of an ADRP gene to the long arm of chromosome 3. Genomics 5:619, 1989.
38. Lubsen NH, Renwick JH, Tsui LC, et al: A locus for a human hereditary cataract is closely linked to the gamma-crystallin gene family. Proc Natl Acad Sci U S A 84:489, 1987.
39. Rogaev EI, Rogaeva EA, Korovaitseva GI, et al: Linkage of polymorphic congenital cataract to the gamma-crystallin gene locus on human chromosome 2q33-35. Hum Mol Genet 5:699, 1996.
40. Kramer P, Yount J, Mitchell T, et al: A second gene for cerulean cataracts maps to the β crystallin region on chromosome 22. Genomics 35:539, 1996.
41. Brakenhoff RH, Henskens HAM, van Rossum MWPC, et al: Activation of the gE-crystallin pseudogene in the human hereditary Coppock-like cataract. Hum Mol Genet 3:279, 1994.
42. Litt M, Carrero-Valenzuela R, LaMorticella DM, et al: Autosomal dominant cerulean cataract is associated with a chain termination mutation in the human β-crystallin gene CRYBB2. Hum Mol Genet 6:665, 1997.

43. Chen C, Tonegawa S: Molecular genetic analysis of synaptic plasticity, activity-dependent neural development, learning, and memory in the mammalian brain. Annu Rev Neurosci 20:157, 1997.
44. Lendent C, Vaugeois J-M, Schiffmann SN, et al: Aggressiveness, hypoalgesia and high blood pressure in mice lacking the adenosine A2a receptor. Nature 388:674, 1997.
45. Reichel E, Bruce AM, Sandberg MA, et al: An electroretinographic and molecular genetic study of X-linked cone degeneration. Am J Ophthalmol 108:540, 1989.
46. van Heyningen V. One gene—four syndromes. Nature 367:319, 1994.
47. Munier FL, Korvatska E, Djemaï A, et al: Kerato-epithelin mutations in four 5q31-linked corneal dystrophies. Nature Genet 15:247, 1997.
48. de la Chapelle A, Tolvanen R, Boysen G, et al: Gelsolin-derived familial amyloidosis caused by asparagine or tyrosine substitution for aspartic acid at residue 187. Nature Genet 2:157, 1992.
49. Irvine AD, Corden LD, Swensson O, et al: Mutations in cornea-specific keratin K3 or K12 genes cause Meesman's corneal dystrophy. Nature Genet 16:184, 1997.
50. Stone EM, Fingert JH, Alward WLM, et al: Identification of a gene that causes primary open angle glaucoma. Science 275:668, 1997.
51. Raymond V. Molecular genetics of the glaucomas: Mapping of the first five "GLC" loci. Am J Hum Genet 60:272, 1997.
52. Semina EV, Reiter R, Leysens NJ, et al: Cloning and characterization of a novel bicoid-related homeobox transcription factor gene, RIEG, involved in Rieger syndrome. Nature Genet 14:392, 1996.
53. Stambolian D, Ai Y, Sidjanin D, et al: Cloning of the galactokinase cDNA and identification of mutations in two families with cataracts. Nature Genet 10:307, 1995.
54. Girelli D, Corrocher R, Bisceglia L, et al: Molecular basis for the recently described hereditary hyperferritinemia cataract syndrome: A mutation in the iron-responsive element of ferritin L-subunit gene (the "Verona mutation"). Blood 86:4050, 1995.
55. Aguilar-Martinez P, Biron C, Masmejean C, et al: A novel mutation in the iron responsive element of ferritin L-subunit gene as a cause for hereditary hyperferritinemia-cataract syndrome. Blood 88:1895, 1996.
56. Huang SH, Pittler SJ, Huang X, et al: Autosomal recessive retinitis pigmentosa caused by mutations in the α subunit of rod cGMP phosphodiesterase. Nature Genet 11:468, 1995.
57. McLaughlin ME, Sandberg MA, Berson EL, et al: Recessive mutations in the gene encoding the β-subunit of rod phosphodiesterase in patients with retinitis pigmentosa. Nature Genet 4:130, 1993.
58. Danciger M, Blaney J, Gao YQ, et al: Mutations in the PDE6B gene in autosomal recessive retinitis pigmentosa. Genomics 30:1, 1995.
59. Valverde D, Solans T, Grinberg D, et al: A novel mutation in exon 17 of the β-subunit of rod phosphodiesterase in two RP sisters of a consanguineous family. Hum Genet 97:35, 1996.
60. Dryja TP, Finn JT, Peng Y-W, et al: Mutations in the gene encoding the α subunit of the rod cGMP-gated channel in autosomal recessive retinitis pigmentosa. Proc Natl Acad Sci U S A 92:10177, 1995.
61. Farrar GJ, Kenna P, Jordan SA, et al: A three-base-pair deletion in the peripherin-RDS gene in one form of retinitis pigmentosa. Nature 354:478, 1991.
62. Kajiwara K, Hahn LB, Mukai S, et al: Mutations in the human retinal degeneration slow gene in autosomal dominant retinitis pigmentosa. Nature 354:480, 1991.
63. Pittler SJ, Fliesler SJ, Fisher PL, et al: In vivo requirement of protein prenylation for maintenance of retinal cytoarchitecture and photoreceptor structure. J Cell Biol 130:431, 1995.
64. Meindl A, Dry K, Herrmann K, et al: A gene (RPGR) with homology to the RCC1 guanine nucleotide exchange factor is mutated in X-linked retinitis pigmentosa (RP3). Nature Genet 13:35, 1996.
65. Gu S, Thompson DA, Srikumari CRS, et al: Mutations in RPE65 cause autosomal recessive childhood-onset severe retinal dystrophy. Nature Genet 17:194, 1997.
66. Maw MA, Kennedy B, Knight A, et al: Mutation of the gene encoding cellular retinaldehyde-binding protein in autosomal recessive retinitis pigmentosa. Nature Genet 17:198, 1997.
67. Perrault I, Rozet JM, Calvas P, et al: Retinal-specific guanylate cyclase gene mutations in Leber's congenital amaurosis. Nature Genet 14:461, 1996.
68. Marlhens F, Bareil C, Griffoin J-M, et al: Mutations in RPE65 cause Leber's congenital amaurosis. Nature Genet 17:139, 1997.
69. Weil D, Blanchard S, Kaplan J, et al: Defective myosin VIIA gene responsible for Usher syndrome type Ib. Nature 374:60, 1995.
70. Gotoda T, Arita M, Arai H, et al: Adult-onset spinocerebellar dysfunction caused by a mutation in the gene for the α-tocopherol-transfer protein. N Engl J Med 333:1313, 1995.
71. Yokota T, Shiojiri T, Gotoda T, et al: Retinitis pigmentosa and ataxia caused by a mutation in the gene for the α-tocopherol transfer protein. N Engl J Med 335:1770, 1996.
72. Mihalik SJ, Morrell JC, Kim D, et al: Identification of PAHX, a Refsum disease gene. Nature Genet 17:185, 1997.
73. Jansen GA, Ofman R, Ferdinandusse S, et al: Refsum disease is caused by mutations in the phytanoyl-CoA hydroxylase gene. Nature Genet 17:190, 1997.
74. Lerner TJ, Boustany R-MN, Anderson JW, et al: Isolation of a novel gene underlying Batten disease, CLN3. Cell 82:949, 1995.
75. Zeviani M, Moraes CT, DiMauro S, et al: Deletions of mitochondrial DNA in Kearns-Sayre syndrome. Neurology 38:1339, 1988.
76. Lestienne P, Ponsot G: Kearns-Sayre syndrome with muscle mitochondrial DNA deletion. Lancet i:885, 1988.
77. Moraes CT, DiMauro S, Zeviani M, et al: Mitochondrial DNA deletions in progressive external ophthalmoplegia and Kearns-Sayre syndrome. N Engl J Med 320:1293, 1989.
78. Narcisi TME, Shoulders CC, Chester SA, et al: Mutations of the microsomal triglyceride-transfer-protein gene in abetalipoproteinemia. Am J Hum Genet 57:1298, 1995.
79. Sauer CG, Gehrig A, Warneke-Wittstock R, et al: Positional cloning of the gene associated with X-linked juvenile retinoschisis. Nature Genet 17:164, 1997.
80. Dryja TP, Berson EL, Rao VR, et al: Heterozygous missense mutation in the rhodopsin gene as a cause of congenital stationary night blindness. Nature Genet 4:280, 1993.
81. Sieving PA, Richards JE, Naarendorp F, et al: Dark-light: Model for nightblindness from the human rhodopsin Gly-90 R Asp mutation. Proc Natl Acad Sci U S A 92:880, 1995.
82. Dryja TP, Hahn LB, Reboul T, et al: Missense mutation in the gene encoding the α subunit of rod transducin in the Nougaret form of congenital stationary night blindness. Nature Genet 13:358, 1996.
83. Gal A, Orth U, Baehr W, et al: Heterozygous missense mutation in the rod cGMP phosphodiesterase β-subunit gene in autosomal dominant stationary night blindness. Nature Genet 1994; 7:64.
84. Fuchs S, Nakazawa M, Maw M, et al: A homozygous 1-base pair deletion in the arrestin gene is a frequent cause of Oguchi disease in Japanese. Nature Genet 10:360, 1995.
85. Millan JM, Fuchs S, Paricio N, et al: Gly114Asp mutation of rhodopsin in autosomal dominant retinitis pigmentosa. Mol Cell Probes 9:67, 1995.
86. Weber BHF, Vogt G, Pruett RC, et al: Mutations in the tissue inhibitor of metalloproteinases-3 (TIMP3) in patients with Sorsby's fundus dystrophy. Nature Genet 8:352, 1994.
87. Allikmets R, Singh N, Sun H, et al: A photoreceptor cell-specific ATP-binding transporter gene (ABCR) is mutated in recessive Stargardt macular dystrophy. Nature Genet 15:236, 1997.
88. Berger W, Meindl A, van de Pol TJR, et al: Isolation of a candidate gene for Norrie disease by positional cloning. Nature Genet 1:199, 1992.
89. Chen ZY, Hendriks RW, Jobling MA, et al: Isolation and characterization of a candidate gene for Norrie disease. Nature Genet 1:204, 1992.
90. Meindl A, Berger W, Meitinger T, et al: Norrie disease is caused by mutations in an extracellular protein resembling C-terminal globular domain of mucins. Nature Genet 2:139, 1992.
91. Chen ZY, Battinelli EM, Fielder A, et al: A mutation in the Norrie disease gene (NDP) associated with X-linked familial exudative vitreoretinopathy. Nature Genet 5:180, 1993.
92. Shastry BS, Pendergast SD, Hartzer MK, et al: Identification of missense mutations in the Norrie disease gene associated with advanced retinopathy of prematurity. Arch Ophthalmol 115:651, 1997.
93. Nichols BE, Drack AV, Vandenburgh K, et al: A 2 base pair deletion in the RDS gene associated with butterfly-shaped pigment dystrophy of the fovea. Hum Mol Genet 2:601, 1993.
94. Wells J, Wroblewski J, Keen J, et al: Mutations in the human retinal degeneration slow (RDS) gene can cause either retinitis pigmentosa or macular dystrophy. Nature Genet 3:213, 1993.
95. Kim RY, Dollfus H, Keen TJ, et al: Autosomal dominant pattern dystrophy of the retina associated with a 4-base pair insertion at codon 140 in the peripherin/RDS gene. Arch Ophthalmol 113:451, 1995.
96. Latif F, Tory K, Gnarra J, et al: Identification of the von Hippel-Lindau disease tumor suppressor gene. Science 260:1317, 1993.
97. Fukai K, Holmes SA, Lucchese NJ, et al: Autosomal recessive ocular

albinism associated with a functionally significant tyrosinase gene polymorphism. Nature Genet 9:92, 1995.
98. Bassi MT, Schiaffino MV, Renieri A, et al: Cloning of the gene for ocular albinism type 1 from the distal short arm of the X chromosome. Nature Genet 10:13, 1995.
99. Wallace DC, Singh G, Lott MT, et al: Mitochondrial DNA mutation associated with Leber's hereditary optic neuropathy. Science 242:1427, 1988.
100. Singh G, Lott MT, Wallace DC: A mitochondrial DNA mutation as a cause of Leber's hereditary optic neuropathy. N Engl J Med 320:1300, 1989.
101. Tassabehji M, Read AP, Newton VE, et al: Waardenburg's syndrome patients have mutations in the human homologue of the Pax-3 paired box gene. Nature 355:635, 1992.
102. Tassabehji M, Read AP, Newton VE, et al: Mutations in the PAX3 gene causing Waardenburg syndrome type 1 and type 2. Nature Genet 3:26, 1993.
103. Hoth CF, Milunsky A, Lipsky N, et al: Mutations in the paired domain of the human PAX3 gene cause Klein-Waardenburg syndrome (WS-III) as well as Waardenburg syndrome type I (WS-I). Am J Hum Genet 52:455, 1993.
104. Tachibana M, Perez-Jurado LA, Nakayama A, et al: Cloning of MITF, the human homolog of the mouse microphthalmia gene and assignment to chromosome 3p14.1-p12.3. Hum Mol Genet 3:553, 1994.
105. Tassabehji M, Newton VE, Read AP: Waardenburg syndrome type 2 caused by mutations in the human microphthalmia (MITF) gene. Nature Genet 8:251, 1994.
106. Sanyanusin P, Schimmenti LA, McNoe LA, et al: Mutation of the PAX2 gene in a family with optic nerve colobomas, renal anomalies and vesicoureteral reflux. Nature Genet 9:358, 1995.
107. Korkko J, Ritvaniemi P, Haataja L, et al: Mutation in type II procollagen (COL2AI) that substitutes aspartate for glycine alphaI-67 and that causes cataracts and retinal detachment: Evidence for molecular heterogeneity in the Wagner syndrome and the Stickler syndrome (arthro-ophthalmopathy). Am J Hum Genet 53:55, 1993.
108. Mackey DA, Buttery RG, Wise GM, et al: Description of X-linked megalocornea with identification of the gene locus. Arch Ophthalmol 109:829, 1991.
109. Vance JM, Jonasson F, Lennon F, et al: Linkage of a gene for macular corneal dystrophy to chromosome 16. Am J Hum Genet 58:757, 1996.
110. Toma NMG, Ebenezer ND, Inglehearn CF, et al: Linkage of congenital hereditary endothelial dystrophy to chromosome 20. Hum Mol Genet 4:2395, 1995.
111. Wirtz MK, Samples JR, Kramer PL, et al: Mapping a gene for adult-onset primary open-angle glaucoma to chromosome 3q. Am J Hum Genet 60:296, 1997.
112. Mackay D, Ionides A, Berry V, et al: A new locus for dominant "zonular pulverulent" cataract, on chromosome 13. Am J Hum Genet 60:1474, 1997.
113. Berry V, Ionides ACW, Moore AT, et al: A locus for autosomal dominant anterior polar cataract on chromosome 17p. Hum Mol Genet 5:415, 1996.
114. Padma T, Ayyagari R, Murty JS, et al: Autosomal dominant zonular cataract with sutural opacities localized to chromosome 17q11-12. Am J Hum Genet 57:840, 1995.
115. Armitage MM, Kivlin JD, Ferrell RE: A progressive early onset cataract gene maps to human chromosome 17q24. Nature Genet 9:37, 1995.
116. Lewis RA, Nussbaum RL, Stambolian D: Mapping X-linked ophthalmic diseases. IV. Provision assignment of the locus for X-linked congenital cataracts and microcornea (the Nancy-Horan syndrome) to Xp22.2-p22.3. Ophthalmology 97:110, 1990.
117. Mears AJ, Mirzayans F, Gould DB, et al: Autosomal dominant iridogoniodysgenesis anomaly maps to 6p25. Am J Hum Genet 59:1321, 1996.
118. Mirzayans F, Mears AJ, Guo S-W, et al: Identification of the human chromosomal region containing the iridogoniodysgenesis anomaly locus by genomic-mismatch scanning. Am J Hum Genet 61:111, 1997.
119. Andersen JS, Pralea AM, DelBono EA, et al: A gene responsible for the pigment dispersion syndrome maps to chromosome 7q35-q36. Arch Ophthalmol 115:384, 1997.
120. Tromp G, Kuivaniemi H, Raphael S, et al: Genetic linkage of familial granulomatous inflammatory arthritis, skin rash, and uveitis to chromosome 16. Am J Hum Genet 59:1097, 1996.
121. McGuire RE, Sullivan LS, Blanton SH, et al: X-linked dominant cone-rod degeneration: Linkage mapping of a new locus for retinitis pigmentosa (RP15) to Xp22.13-p22.11. Am J Hum Genet 57:87, 1995.
122. Teague PW, Aldred MA, Jay M, et al: Heterogeneity analysis in 40 X-linked retinitis pigmentosa families. Am J Hum Genet 55:105, 1994.
123. Thiselton DL, Hampson RM, Nayudu M, et al: Mapping the RP2 locus for X-linked retinitis pigmentosa on proximal Xp: A genetically defined 5-cM critical region and exclusion of candidate genes by physical mapping. Genome Res 6:1093, 1996.
124. Martínez-Mir A, Bayés M, Vilageliu L, et al: A new locus for autosomal recessive retinitis pigmentosa (RP19) maps to 1p13-1p21. Genomics 40:142, 1997.
125. Xu SY, Schwartz M, Rosenberg T, et al: A ninth locus (RP18) for autosomal dominant retinitis pigmentosa maps in the pericentromeric region of chromosome 1. Hum Mol Genet 5:1193, 1996.
126. Knowles JA, Shugart Y, Banerjee P, et al: Identification of a locus, distinct from RDS-peripherin, for autosomal recessive retinitis pigmentosa on chromosome 6p. Hum Mol Genet 3:1401, 1994.
127. Shugart YY, Banerjee P, Knowles JA, et al: Fine genetic mapping of a gene for autosomal recessive retinitis pigmentosa on chromosome 6p21. Am J Hum Genet 57:499, 1995.
128. Inglehearn CF, Carter SA, Keen TJ, et al: A new locus for autosomal dominant retinitis pigmentosa on 7p. Nature Genet 4:51, 1993.
129. Inglehearn CF, Keen TJ, Al-Maghtheh M, et al: Further refinement of the location for autosomal dominant retinitis pigmentosa on chromosome 7p (RP9). Am J Hum Genet 54:675, 1994.
130. Kojis TL, Heinzmann C, Flodman P, et al: Map refinement of locus RP13 to human chromosome 17p13.3 in a second family with autosomal dominant retinitis pigmentosa. Am J Hum Genet 58:347, 1996.
131. Jordan SA, Farrar GJ, Kenna P, et al: Localization of an autosomal dominant retinitis pigmentosa gene to chromosome 7q. Nature Genet 4:54, 1993.
132. McGuire RE, Gannon AM, Sullivan LS, et al: Evidence for a major gene (RP10) for autosomal dominant retinitis pigmentosa on chromosome 7q: Linkage mapping in a second, unrelated family. Hum Genet 95:71, 1995.
133. Millán JM, Martínez F, Vilela C, et al: An autosomal dominant retinitis pigmentosa family with close linkage to D7S480 on 7q. Hum Genet 96:216, 1995.
134. McGuire RE, Jordan SA, Braden VV, et al: Mapping the RP10 locus for autosomal dominant retinitis pigmentosa on 7q: Refined genetic positioning and localization within a well-defined YAC contig. Genome Res 6:255, 1996.
135. Mohamed Z, Bell C, Hammer HM, et al: Linkage of a medium sized Scottish autosomal dominant retinitis pigmentosa family to chromosome 7q. J Med Genet 33:714, 1996.
136. Blanton SH, Heckenlively JR, Cottingham AW, et al: Linkage mapping of autosomal dominant retinitis pigmentosa (RP1) to the pericentric region of human chromosome 8. Genomics 11:857, 1991.
137. Xu SY, Denton M, Sullivan L, et al: Genetic mapping of RP1 on 8q11-q21 in an Australian family with autosomal dominant retinitis pigmentosa reduces the critical region to 4 cM between D8S601 and D8S285. Hum Genet 98:741, 1996.
138. Greenberg J, Goliath R, Beighton P, et al: A new locus for autosomal dominant retinitis pigmentosa on the short arm of chromosome 17. Hum Mol Genet 3:915, 1994.
139. Goliath R, Shugart Y, Janssens P, et al: Fine localization of the locus for autosomal dominant retinitis pigmentosa on chromosome 17p. Am J Hum Genet 57:962, 1995.
140. Kojis TL, Heinzmann C, Heckenlively JR, et al: Map refinement of the autosomal dominant retinitis pigmentosa (adRP) locus RP13 to human chromosome 17p13.3 in a second adRP family: Evidence for a major gene. [Abstract] Am J Hum Genet 57:A216, 1995.
141. Tarttelin EE, Plant C, Wissenbach J, et al: A new family linked to the RP13 locus for autosomal dominant retinitis pigmentosa on distal 17p. J Med Genet 33:518, 1996.
142. Bardien S, Ebenezer N, Greenberg J, et al: An eighth locus for autosomal dominant retinitis pigmentosa is linked to chromosome 17q. Hum Mol Genet 4:1459, 1995.
143. Al-Maghtheh M, Inglehearn CF, Keen TJ, et al: Identification of a sixth locus for autosomal dominant retinitis pigmentosa on chromosome 19. Hum Mol Genet 3:351, 1994.
144. Xu SY, Nakazawa M, Tamai M, et al: Autosomal dominant retinitis pigmentosa locus on chromosome 19q in a Japanese family. J Med Genet 32:915, 1995.
145. Al-Maghtheh M, Vithana E, Tarttelin E, et al: Evidence for a major

retinitis pigmentosa locus on 19q13.4 (RP11), and association with a unique bimodal expressivity phenotype. Am J Hum Genet 59:864, 1996.
146. van den Born LI, van Soest S, van Schooneveld MJ, et al: Autosomal recessive retinitis pigmentosa with preserved para-arteriolar retinal pigment epithelium. Am J Ophthalmol 118:430, 1994.
147. van Soest S, van den Born LI, Gal A, et al: Assignment of a gene for autosomal recessive retinitis pigmentosa (RP12) to chromosome 1q31-q32.1 in an inbred and genetically heterogeneous disease population. Genomics 22:499, 1994.
148. Leutelt J, Oehlmann R, Younus F, et al: Autosomal recessive retinitis pigmentosa locus maps on chromosome 1q in a large consanguineous family from Pakistan. Clin Genet 47:122, 1995.
149. Wayne S, der Kaloustian VM, Schloss M, et al: Localization of the Usher syndrome type ID gene (Ush1D) to chromosome 10. Hum Mol Genet 5:1689, 1996.
150. Smith RJH, Lee EC, Kimberling WJ, et al: Localization of two genes for Usher syndrome type I to chromosome 11. Genomics 14:995, 1992.
151. Keats BJB, Nouri N, Pelias MZ, et al: Tightly linked flanking microsatellite markers for the Usher syndrome type I locus on the short arm of chromosome 11. Am J Hum Genet 54:681, 1994.
152. Marietta J, Walters KS, Burgess R, et al: Usher's syndrome type IC: Clinical studies and fine-mapping the disease locus. Ann Otol Rhinol Laryngol 106:123, 1997.
153. Kaplan J, Gerber S, Bonneau D, et al: A gene for Usher syndrome type I (USH1A) maps to chromosome 14q. Genomics 14:979, 1992.
154. Chaïb H, Kaplan J, Gerber S, et al: A newly identified locus for Usher syndrome type I, USH1E, maps to chromosome 21q21. Hum Mol Genet 6:27, 1997.
155. Kimberling WJ, Weston MD, Moller C, et al: Localization of Usher syndrome type II to chromosome 1q. Genomics 7:245, 1990.
156. Lewis RA, Otterud B, Stauffer D, et al: Mapping recessive ophthalmic diseases: Linkage of the locus for Usher syndrome type II to a DNA marker on chromosome 1q. Genomics 7:250, 1990.
157. Kimberling WJ, Weston MD, Moller C, et al: Gene mapping of Usher syndrome type IIa: Localization of the gene to a 2.1-cM segment on chromosome 1q41. Am J Hum Genet 56:216, 1995.
158. Pieke-Dahl S, van Aarem A, Dobin A, et al: Genetic heterogeneity of Usher syndrome type II in a Dutch population. J Med Genet 33:753, 1996.
159. Sankila EM, Pakarinen L, Kaariainen H, et al: Assignment of an Usher syndrome type III (USH3) gene to chromosome 3q. Hum Mol Genet 4:93–98, 1995.
160. Kwitek-Black AE, Carmi R, Duyk GM, et al: Bardet-Biedl syndrome: Mapping of a new locus to chromosome 3 and fine-mapping of the chromosome 16 linked locus. [Abstract] Am J Hum Genet 55:A191, 1994.
161. Sheffield VC, Carmi R, Kwitek-Black A, et al: Identification of a Bardet-Biedl syndrome locus on chromosome 3 and evaluation of an efficient approach to homozygosity mapping. Hum Mol Genet 3:1331, 1994.
162. Leppert M, Baird L, Anderson KL, et al: Bardet-Biedl syndrome is linked to DNA markers on chromosome 11q and is genetically heterogeneous. Nature Genet 7:108, 1994.
163. Beales PL, Warner AM, Hitman GA, et al: Bardet-Biedl syndrome: A molecular and phenotypic study of 18 families. J Med Genet 34:92, 1997.
164. Bruford EA, Riise R, Teague PW, et al: Linkage mapping in 29 Bardet-Biedl syndrome families confirms loci in chromosomal regions 11q13, 15q22.3-q23, and 16q21. Genomics 41:93, 1997.
165. Carmi R, Rokhlina T, Kwitek-Black AE, et al: Use of a DNA pooling strategy to identify a human obesity syndrome locus on chromosome 15. Hum Mol Genet 4:9, 1995.
166. Kwitek-Black AE, Carmi R, Duyk GM, et al: Linkage of Bardet-Biedl syndrome to chromosome 16q and evidence for non-allelic genetic heterogeneity. Nature Genet 5:392, 1993.
167. Fossdal R, Magnusson L, Weber JL, et al: Mapping the locus of atrophia areata, a helicoid peripapillary chorioretinal degeneration with autosomal dominant inheritance, to chromosome 11p15. Hum Mol Genet 4:479, 1995.
168. Stone EM, Nichols BE, Kimura AE, et al: Clinical features of a Stargardt-like dominant progressive macular dystrophy with genetic linkage to chromosome 6q. Arch Ophthalmol 112:765, 1994.
169. Zhang K, Bither PP, Park R, et al: A dominant Stargardt's macular dystrophy locus maps to chromosome 13q34. Arch Ophthalmol 112:759, 1994.
170. Balciuniene J, Johansson K, Sandgren O, et al: A gene for autosomal dominant progressive cone dystrophy (CORD5) maps to chromosome 17p12-p13. Genomics 30:281, 1995.
171. Small KW, Syrquin M, Mullen L, et al: Mapping of autosomal dominant cone degeneration to chromosome 17p. Am J Ophthalmol 121:13, 1996.
172. Kelsell RE, Evens K, Gregory CY, et al: Localisation of a gene for dominant cone-rod dystrophy (CORD6) to chromosome 17p. Hum Mol Genet 6:597, 1997.
173. Bergen AAB, Pinckers AJLG: Localization of a novel X-linked progressive cone dystrophy gene to Xq27: Evidence for genetic heterogeneity. Am J Hum Genet 60:1468, 1997.
174. Keen TJ, Inglehearn CF, Green ED, et al: YAC contig spanning the dominant retinitis pigmentosa locus (RP9) on chromosome 7p. Genomics 28:383, 1995.
175. Kelsell RE, Godley BF, Evans K, et al: Localization of the gene for progressive bifocal chorioretinal atrophy (PBCRA) to chromosome 6q. Hum Mol Genet 4:1653, 1995.
176. Evans K, Fryer A, Inglehearn C, et al: Genetic linkage of cone-rod retinal dystrophy to chromosome 19q and evidence for segregation distortion. Nature Genet 6:210, 1994.
177. Gregory CY, Evans K, Whittaker JL, et al: Refinement of the cone-rod retinal dystrophy locus on chromosome 19q. Am J Hum Genet 55:1061, 1994.
178. Musarella MA, Weleber RG, Murphey WH, et al: Assignment of the gene for complete X-linked congenital stationary night blindness (CSNB1) to Xp11.3. Genomics 5:727, 1989.
179. Bergen AAB, Ten Brink JB, Riemslag F, et al: Localization of a novel X-linked congenital stationary night blindness locus: Close linkage to the RP3 type retinitis pigmentosa gene region. Hum Mol Genet 4:931, 1995.
180. Bergen AAB, Ten Brink JB, Riemslag F, et al: Conclusive evidence for a distinct congenital stationary night blindness locus in Xp21.1. J Med Genet 33:869, 1996.
181. Li Y, Muller B, Fuhrmann C, et al: The autosomal dominant familial exudative vitreoretinopathy locus maps on 11q and is closely linked to D11S533. Am J Hum Genet 51:749, 1992.
182. Stone EM, Kimura AE, Folk JC, et al: Genetic linkage of autosomal dominant neovascular inflammatory vitreoretinopathy to chromosome 11q13. Hum Mol Genet 1:685, 1992.
183. Fuhrmann C, Duvigneau C, Müller B, et al: Autosomal dominant exudative vitreoretinopathy: Linkage analysis and its clinical application. German J Ophthalmol 4:43, 1995.
184. Gong Y, Vikkula M, Boon L, et al: Osteoporosis-pseudoglioma syndrome, a disorder affecting skeletal strength and vision, is assigned to chromosome region 11q12-13. Am J Hum Genet 59:146, 1996.
185. Stone EM, Nichols BE, Streb LM, et al: Genetic linkage of vitelliform macular degeneration (Best's disease) to chromosome 11q13. Nature Genet 1:246, 1992.
186. Weber BHF, Vogt G, Stöhr H, et al: High-resolution meiotic and physical mapping of the Best vitelliform macular dystrophy (VMD2) locus to pericentric chromosome 11. Am J Hum Genet 55:1182, 1994.
187. Stöhr H, Weber BHF: A recombination event excludes the ROM1 locus from the Best's vitelliform macular dystrophy region. Hum Genet 95:219, 1995.
188. Hou YC, Richards JE, Bingham EL, et al: Linkage study of Best's vitelliform macular dystrophy (VMD2) in a large North American family. Hum Hered 46:211, 1996.
189. Sohocki MM, Sullivan LS, Mintz-Hittner HA, et al: Exclusion of atypical vitelliform macular dystrophy from 8q24.3 and from other known macular degenerative loci. Am J Hum Genet 61:239, 1997.
190. Hughes AE, Newton VE, Liu XZ, et al: A gene for Waardenburg syndrome type 2 maps close to the human homologue of the microphthalmia gene at chromosome 3p12-p14.1. Nature Genet 7:509, 1994.
191. Kremer H, Pinckers A, van dem Helm B, et al: Localization of the gene for dominant cystic macular dystrophy on chromosome 7p. Hum Mol Genet 3:299, 1994.
192. Inglehearn C, Keen TJ, Al-Maghtheh M, et al: Loci for autosomal dominant retinitis pigmentosa and dominant cystoid macular dystrophy on chromosome 7p are not allelic. Am J Hum Genet 55:581, 1994.
193. Gregory CY, Evans K, Wijesuriya SD, et al: The gene responsible for autosomal dominant Doyne's honeycomb retinal dystrophy (DHRD) maps to chromosome 2p16. Hum Mol Genet 5:1055, 1996.
194. Héon E, Piguet B, Munier F, et al: Linkage of autosomal dominant radial drusen (malattia leventinese) to chromosome 2p16-21. Arch Ophthalmol 114:193, 1996.

195. Brown DM, Graemiger RA, Hergersberg M, et al: Genetic linkage of Wagner disease and erosive vitreoretinopathy to chromosome 5q13-14. Arch Ophthalmol 113:671, 1995.
196. Engle EC, Kunkel LM, Specht LA, et al: Mapping a gene for congenital fibrosis of the extraocular muscles to the centromeric region of chromosome 12. Nature Genet 7:69, 1994.
197. Engle EC, Marondel I, Houtman WA, et al: Congenital fibrosis of the extraocular muscles (autosomal dominant congenital external ophthalmoplegia): Genetic homogeneity, linkage refinement, and physical mapping on chromosome 12. Am J Hum Genet 57:1086, 1995.
198. Kerrison JB, Arnould VJ, Barmada MM, et al: A gene for autosomal dominant congenital nystagmus localizes to 6p12. Genomics 33:523, 1996.
199. Polymeropoulos MH, Swift RG, Swift M: Linkage of the gene for Wolfram syndrome to markers on the short arm of chromosome 4. Nature Genet 8:95, 1994.
200. Lunkes A, Hartung U, Magariño C, et al: Refinement of the OPA1 gene locus on chromosome 3q28-q29 to a region of 2–8 cM, in one Cuban pedigree with autosomal dominant optic atrophy type Kjer. Am J Hum Genet 57:968, 1995.
201. Votruba M, Moore AT, Bhattacharya SS: Genetic refinement of dominant optic atrophy (OPA1) locus to within a 2 cM interval of chromosome 3q. J Med Genet 34:117, 1997.
202. Benomar A, Krols L, Stevanin G, et al: The gene for autosomal dominant cerebellar ataxia with pigmentary macular dystrophy maps to chromosome 3p12-p21.1. Nature Genet 10:84, 1995.
203. Gouw LG, Kaplan CD, Haines JH, et al: Retinal degeneration characterizes a spinocerebellar ataxia mapping to chromosome 3p. Nature Genet 10:89, 1995.
204. Holmberg M, Johansson J, Forsgren L, et al: Localization of autosomal dominant cerebellar ataxia associated with retinal degeneration and anticipation to chromosome 3p12-p21.1. Hum Mol Genet 4:1441, 1995.
205. Jöbsis GJ, Weber JW, Barth PG, et al: Autosomal dominant cerebellar ataxia with retinal degeneration (ADCA II): Clinical and neuropathological findings in two pedigrees and genetic linkage to 3p12-p21.1. J Neurol Neurosurg Psychiatry 62:367, 1997.
206. Des Portes V, Bachner L, Brüls T, et al: X-linked neurodegenerative syndrome with congenital ataxia, late-onset progressive myoclonic encephalopathy and selective macular degeneration, linked to Xp22.33-pter. Am J Med Genet 64:69, 1996.
207. Engle EC, Castro AE, Macy ME, et al: A gene for isolated congenital ptosis maps to a 3-cM region within 1p32-p34.1. Am J Hum Genet 60:1150, 1997.
208. Kaelin WG: Recent insights into the functions of the retinoblastoma susceptibility gene product. Cancer Invest 15:243, 1997.
209. Rouillac C, Roche O, Marchant D, et al: Mapping of the congenital microcoria locus to 13q31-32. Am J Hum Genet 62:1117, 1998.

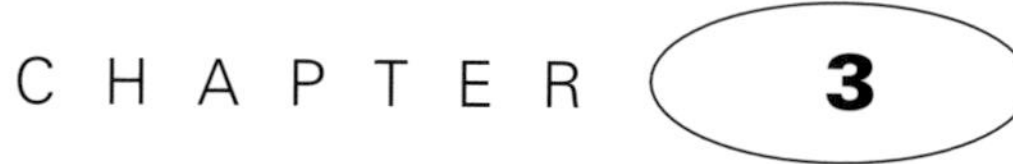

CHAPTER 3

Principles of Genetic Counseling

Bruce Korf, Pamela Hawley, and Gretchen Schneider

The rapid advance in knowledge about genetic diseases, the improvements in diagnostic testing, and the availability of some therapeutic options have greatly enhanced the usefulness of genetic counseling to families. The principles of genetic counseling can be readily appreciated from the definition recommended by an ad hoc committee of the American Society of Human Genetics.[1] The recommendation deals with issues of communication within a family when considering a genetic disorder, including understanding the medical implications of the disorder and the hereditary implications for the patient, parents, and, when indicated, other family members. Properly trained professionals must be prepared to help the individual and the family comprehend available options for dealing with recurrence risk and to appropriately guide and support them in choosing the best course of action.

Although the committee published this definition in 1974, these goals of genetic counseling still remain widely accepted and disseminated. What is changing rapidly are the diagnostic tools available to meet these goals. Because accurate genetic counseling is predicated on a correct diagnosis, knowledge of these new diagnostic tools and a consistent approach to clinical evaluation are essential to the process.

Who Provides Genetic Counseling?

The providers of genetic counseling have changed greatly in the past few decades. In the 1970s, when genetic counseling was growing in recognition, many counselors were MDs and PhDs who had no formal training. Physicians, nurses, and social workers have continued to provide genetic counseling, mostly by learning from experience. As genetic counseling became better defined, the need was recognized for persons trained specifically to deal with this process and its integration with medical science and psychology.

Master's level genetic counseling programs are designed to train medical professionals, called genetic counselors, who provide such a service. These 2-year programs have combined molecular and clinical genetics with counseling psychology in settings that emphasize clinical rotations to gain experience. More than 1000 genetic counselors have been trained at over 20 2-year programs. Genetic counselors often work with other health professionals, including board-certified geneticists, obstetricians, genetic fellows, nurses, social workers, and laboratory personnel. This team approach allows comprehensive genetic services in prenatal, pediatric, specialty clinic, and commercial settings.

Why Refer Patients for a Genetic Evaluation?

Accurate genetic counseling starts with a thorough genetic evaluation. It is important for both families and physicians to realize what is involved in the process and its value to the patient and immediate relatives. The genetic evaluation is important in two major ways:

1. It may help in understanding a patient's problems by providing a unifying diagnosis. When the diagnosis is a well-described entity, it can sometimes provide prognostic information. It may also change the clinical management of a patient.
2. A diagnosis may have genetic implications. Relatives may become similarly affected. In many instances, these relatives should be encouraged to receive genetic counseling. Future children in the family may be at risk. This risk is called the recurrence risk, and it sometimes can be mathematically quantified.

INDICATIONS FOR REFERRAL TO A GENETICS SPECIALIST

Although the need for a genetic evaluation or genetic counseling often is obvious, this is not always the case. A child born with multiple anomalies may have no clearly identifiable diagnosis until pedigree analysis reveals a pattern diagnostic of a genetic syndrome. This is particularly important whenever parents are planning additional children and are justifiably concerned about those children having similar problems. Even when a clinical diagnosis and the relevant genetic counseling may seem straightforward, unanticipated beneficial information might be gained from a visit to a genetics specialist.

Established Genetic Condition

For a child with an established diagnosis, the focus of a genetics visit might be to understand the hereditary implications of the diagnosis and the recurrence risks. For example, in a child with retinoblastoma and a positive family history, the diagnosis is clear. These families may be referred for genetic counseling to review recurrence risks in a setting separate from the ophthalmologist's office. An ophthalmologist may not feel well versed in the details of molecular testing and its use in testing other family members and in prenatal diagnosis. A genetics specialist can also discuss alternative reproductive options for those who may not want prenatal testing.

Genetic evaluation sometimes suggests a clinical diagnosis of a disorder that displays genetic heterogeneity. An example is oculocutaneous albinism. There are several types of albinism due to various mutations in any of several genes. A genetic evaluation might uncover relatives who clearly have albinism; this information might allow diagnosis with a mildly affected index patient. Confirmation of that diagnosis might require biochemical or molecular tests.

Eye Findings with Other Congenital Anomalies

A child is sometimes born with a number of malformations including ophthalmologic abnormalities. Some cases obviously fit a particular syndrome, but others do not. For example, a child might have microphthalmia, congenital heart disease, and delays in development, with no syndrome diagnosis immediately recognizable. Yet these multiple medical problems suggest a unifying explanation for these findings. This constellation of findings could be the syndrome of coloboma, heart defects, choanal atresia, retarded growth and development, genital hypoplasia in males, and ear anomolies—the CHARGE syndrome—or it could be caused by a chromosome anomaly such as 13q−. In these situations, the experience of a geneticist in recognizing malformation patterns and understanding the variability of genetic conditions can aid diagnosis. If an underlying cause is identified, relatives can then undergo genetic counseling.

Eye Findings with Other Minor Anomalies

Some patients referred to the ophthalmology clinic may have no obvious extraocular medical problems. During their visit, however, one may observe dysmorphic features or other seemingly unrelated minor medical signs or symptoms. For example, retinitis pigmentosa is a feature of a number of syndromes whose other signs and symptoms may be subtle. A child with retinitis pigmentosa, obesity, and polydactyly may have Bardet-Biedl syndrome, whereas one with prominent central incisors and slender hands and feet may have Cohen's syndrome. Similarly, a child referred for myopia who has micrognathia could have Stickler's syndrome. One with ectopia lentis due to Marfan's syndrome might be tall and lanky. Physical features that may not be classified as medical problems, when combined with eye findings, may lead to a syndrome diagnosis.

Specific Eye Diseases

A genetic evaluation may be important for patients with a purely ocular disease for a number of reasons. A family history might reveal similar eye disease or other findings that, when compared, may lead to a genetic diagnosis in the family. A comprehensive pedigree analysis sometimes reveals a genetic basis for such diseases. Many frequently encountered ophthalmologic diseases, such as cataracts or glaucoma, have a well-documented mendelian inheritance pattern. Identifying the inheritance pattern might lead to the identification of affected relatives who could be diagnosed and treated early in the course of disease. This is especially important in families with such conditions as dominantly inherited juvenile glaucoma.

Incidental Eye Findings

Eye findings with important genetic implications are sometimes observed incidentally during ophthalmologic evaluation. For example, a child may undergo ophthalmologic evaluation because of a failed eye test at school but be found to have Lisch nodules, which suggests neurofibromatosis type 1. Another child might have the stellate iris pattern of Williams' syndrome. Heterochromia irides indicates an examination for the possibility of Waardenburg's syndrome. Although such findings may not have any clinical implications, in some patients their strong association with genetic conditions indicates a genetic evaluation.

Despite the numerous situations in which it is important

to explore the possibility of a genetic etiology, an identifiable genetic condition is often not found. This does not exclude the possibility of a genetic etiology. Family members need to be aware of the possibility of recurrence risk even if no specific diagnosis is made.

What Is Involved in a Genetic Evaluation?

A genetic counselor begins a visit by ascertaining the client's understanding of the reason for the referral. The components of a genetics evaluation are described and, when appropriate, the client is cautioned that the evaluation does not always result in a definite diagnosis or establish a specific genetic etiology.

FAMILY HISTORY

A detailed pregnancy, medical, and developmental history is obtained, as is a three-generation family health history that includes the ethnic origins of the ancestors. The possibility of consanguinity should be explored. The family history is obtained not only to establish a hereditary pattern for the referring diagnosis but also to identify other conditions that could have hereditary implications. For example, if the parents of the patient are of Eastern European Jewish ancestry, their children are at increased risk for Tay-Sachs disease, a recessive neurodegenerative condition for which carrier testing is available. If the family history reveals developmental delay in a pattern suggestive of fragile X syndrome, carrier testing could be offered. Several modes of inquiry ascertain whether families could be at risk for certain conditions unrelated to the referring diagnosis (Table 3–1).

TABLE 3–1. **Family History Considerations Regardless of Reason for Referral**

Family History Positive for:	Consider:
Ancestry	
Eastern European Jewish	Tay-Sachs disease carrier testing Canavan's disease carrier testing Cystic fibrosis carrier testing
French Canadian	Tay-Sachs disease carrier testing
African American	Sickle cell anemia carrier testing
Mediterranean	β-Thalassemia carrier testing
Southeast Asian	α and β-thalassemia carrier testing
More than two miscarriages	Parental chromosome studies to rule out translocation
Birth defects in near relatives	Chromosome studies in parent
Developmental delay	Fragile X testing if family history indicates pattern. Because of the possibility of asymptomatic transmitting males and affected females, the inheritance is not the typical X-linked recessive pattern.
Maternal age over 35	Prenatal chromosome studies
Neonatal/childhood deaths in first-degree relative	Review of records, particularly autopsy
Known genetic disease	Possible carrier testing (i.e., cystic fibrosis, Duchenne's muscular dystrophy)

PHYSICAL EXAMINATION

A complete physical examination is performed with attention to subtle physical findings that can be important for establishing a syndrome diagnosis. Careful anthropometric measurements (e.g., inner canthal, outer canthal, and interpupillary distances; mid-finger/total hand length; and upper body:lower body ratios) may be obtained. Photographs also can be used to record nonmeasurable dysmorphic features.

Examination of other family members may be indicated to determine if a particular finding is hereditary. Sometimes this is incidental to the reason for referral. Findings such as fifth-finger clinodactyly, although a part of many syndromes, may also be isolated hereditary traits without other medical implications.

COMPUTER-ASSISTED DIAGNOSTICS

Many databases can be accessed as part of the genetics evaluation (Table 3–2). Pregnancy exposures may be assessed through REPROTOX, a computerized database of potential teratogens. Standard computer literature searches are performed. If findings are multiple and the patient's history and clinical findings do not suggest an obvious syndrome, the patient's information may be entered into genetic syndrome databases in an effort to diagnose a syndrome. If a specific syndrome is being considered or an isolated finding has been established, On-Line Mendelian Inheritance in Man (OMIM) is often useful. OMIM is a frequently updated catalog of more than 8400 human genetic conditions. It contains a historical summary of the condition, current information regarding available diagnostic and treatment options, and details of genetic etiology. It also provides references. HELIX is another database of up-to-date clinical and research diagnostic testing for specific conditions. When circumstances and time permit, computer searches are conducted prior to or during the initial visit.

ASSESSMENT

The initial assessment may include recommending testing or specialty consultations based on the history, examination, or

TABLE 3–2. **Computer-Assisted Diagnostics**

Program	Database
REPROTOX Reprotoxicology Center Columbia Hospital For Women Washington, DC	Teratogens
London Dysmorphology Oxford University Press	Syndrome identification
POSSUM Murdoch Institute for Research into Birth Defects Royal Children's Hospital Melbourne, Australia	Syndrome identification
OMIM http://www3.ncbi.nlm.nih.gov/omim/	Human genetic conditions
HELIX http://www.hslib.washington.edu/helix	Availability of clinical and research diagnostic testing
MEDLINE	Literature search

computer searches. Ophthalmologic examinations for relatives may be indicated to detect relevant eye findings. These examinations can be helpful in establishing familial patterns when autosomal dominant or X-linked conditions are being considered. For example, Best's disease is an autosomal dominant form of macular degeneration that causes a distinctive macular lesion in its early stage. Scarring at the site of the lesion can lead to decreased central vision. Macular lesions are not present in all affected patients, but all affected patients have abnormal electrooculogram findings. Ophthalmologic examinations of the parents of an affected child can help provide them with a recurrence risk assessment as well as identify which side of the family may have affected relatives. Another example is Lowe's syndrome, an X-linked condition with findings that include congenital cataracts, neurologic impairment, and renal tubular dysfunction. Female carriers typically show no neurologic or renal defects as detected by physical examination or laboratory testing. However, slit-lamp examination reveals specific lenticular changes in up to 94% of carriers.[2] Although molecular diagnostic capabilities are being developed for this condition, careful ophthalmologic examination is valuable to assess the carrier status and therefore the recurrence risk for this condition.

It may be necessary to obtain documentation of a previous chromosome analysis and to review the actual karyotype to confirm the adequacy of a chromosome study. Obtaining records to document a condition reported in a family member may be indicated. Review of the final assessment sometimes requires a follow-up visit.

At the completion of the genetic evaluation of a patient referred with a specific ocular finding, assessments can fall into one of three general areas:

1. Isolated ocular disease or anomaly
2. Nonocular findings with a pattern that fits no recognized genetic syndrome
3. Nonocular findings with a pattern that fits a recognizable syndrome or association

In the latter two situations, the ophthalmologist may not recognize other clinical implications. In any of these situations, a genetic component may be at work that influences the risk of disease in the patient's offspring, parents, and other family members.

Genetic counseling also involves explaining the assessment process and conclusions to the family, including what is known about the genetics of the patient's condition and any possible medical and developmental implications.

Medical and Developmental Implications

A genetic evaluation that results in a specific diagnosis may give rise to previously obscure medical or developmental implications to consider. It is important to discuss clinical variability in syndromes and to note that individuals do not usually develop all the findings associated with a given condition. Even if genetic testing has confirmed a diagnosis, it seldom provides information regarding the likelihood or severity of specific features of a genetic disease. However, for some syndromes, empirical data exist regarding the probability of the associated findings. A genetic specialist can explain the indications for medical monitoring or evaluations and can make appropriate referrals. The importance of age-appropriate developmental assessment and intervention programs in helping patients reach their maximum potential is also emphasized. An established diagnosis may have no additional medical or developmental implications, or no definitive diagnosis may be reached. In these cases, the focus is primarily on the genetic implications of the diagnosis.

Genetic Implications

PRECISION

The extent to which the genetic component of a disorder is understood can vary a great deal. This understanding affects the precision of recurrence risk assessment and the options available for modifying the recurrence risk. Some diseases have a definite inheritance pattern that permits recurrence risks to be calculated according to the laws of mendelian genetics. For example, in a patient with Marfan's syndrome, an autosomal dominant condition, there is high confidence in declaring a risk of 50% for offspring. Similarly, in a family with a child with an autosomal recessive disease such as Bardet-Biedl syndrome, the risk of recurrence in siblings is 1 in 4.

In contrast, in other diseases there is genetic heterogeneity, and various inheritance patterns are possible. This can complicate the prediction of recurrence risk. Instructive examples are nonsyndromic retinitis pigmentosa or congenital cataracts. The inheritance pattern can be autosomal recessive, autosomal dominant, or X-linked recessive. For an isolated male case of retinitis pigmentosa, empirical data suggest that his offspring have a 12% risk of recurrence.[3] In fact, the recurrence risk ranges from less than 1%, if it can be established that the patient has recessive retinitis pigmentosa, to 50% if he has dominant retinitis pigmentosa. In other scenarios, the recurrence risk differs from case to case. One example is when a syndrome whose genetic etiology is not well defined has been diagnosed in a child, but a recurrence risk of 2% has been reported. Another is when a child has a constellation of findings that has not previously been recognized. The actual recurrence in siblings could be negligible if the etiology is nongenetic, 25% if it is autosomal recessive, or nearly 50% if a parent carries the mutant gene but does not express it clinically (i.e., nonpenetrant).

Counselors must be cautious in providing recurrence risk in a well-established dominant syndrome if neither parent shows evidence of the disease. On first glance, we might assume that the affected child represents a new dominant mutation, in which case the parents are genetically normal and the recurrence risk for siblings is vanishingly small. However, two possibilities by which recurrence risk could be much higher need to be considered. One, nonpenetrance, is defined as the absence of phenotypic features in a person who has the mutant genotype. If one of the parents is a nonpenetrant carrier, the recurrence risk for subsequent children approaches 50%. Another possibility is gonadal mosaicism, in which the mutation has occurred during the growth and development in a parent, so that it is present in a proportion of that parent's germ cells. Although genetic testing or empirical data may be available to determine if a parent is a nonpenetrant carrier, testing is often not available to evaluate gonadal mosaicism, and empirical data on the frequency of gonadal mosaicism for specific conditions are rare.

PATIENT'S UNDERSTANDING OF RISKS AND OPTIONS

It is important to explain inheritance patterns and recurrence risks in ways that patients will understand. A patient's understanding of the recurrence risks can be aided by presenting the risk estimates in more than one way. Risk can be given as a fraction and as a percentage, and risks can be given for both affected and unaffected offspring. For example, one might explain that there is a 25%, or 1 in 4, chance that a disease would occur in the next child and a 75%, or 3 in 4, chance that it will not. The risk of recurrence can also be put into context by providing the general population risk for the particular condition, when available, as well as the general population risk for a newborn child to have a serious birth defect (3 to 4%).

A person's interpretation of a recurrence risk is affected by a number of factors, including personality (e.g., risk-taker versus risk-averse), family goals and beliefs, and perceived physical, emotional, and financial consequences of having a child with a particular condition. In addition, a patient's actual experience with the condition in question can significantly affect the perception of risk. The woman at risk for sons with Lowe's syndrome might feel differently about this condition if her uncle experienced the renal failure associated with this disorder and died before she was born than if her yet mildly affected son had been recently diagnosed.

It is not surprising, therefore, that a recurrence risk considered high by some will be viewed as low by others. Reviewing how these different factors affect interpretation of information and the choices that are made can help clients. The counselor also needs to be aware of his or her own perceptions of risk and burden. To the greatest extent possible, the information provided to a patient should emphasize the objective nature of risk figures and avoid the subjective nature of how people perceive risk and the consequences of a disease. There is no cut-off as to whether a given risk figure is high or low or whether a specific disease-given consequence is severe or minor. Clients also need to hear whether a specific disease is severe or mild. Patients should be told that decisions regarding having (more) children, seeking prenatal testing, or considering alternative ways to have families are their own decisions and are not based on perceived "orders" of their doctor or genetic counselor. Patients choose their future based on their own goals, beliefs, and values.

Risk Modification

PRENATAL DIAGNOSIS

One means of risk modification is prenatal diagnosis. For conditions in which a diagnosis can be confirmed with chromosome, biochemical, or molecular studies, three procedures can usually be offered:

1. Routine amniocentesis at 15 to 16 weeks' gestation
2. Early amniocentesis at 12 weeks' gestation
3. Chorionic villus sampling at 10 to 12 weeks' gestation

If diagnostic testing is not available for a condition that includes major congenital malformations, serial ultrasound examinations may be performed as a means of prenatal diagnosis. The examinations need to be performed by an ultrasonographer expert at detecting fetal malformations; even then, the rate of detection is not 100%.

If prenatal diagnosis is an option, a separate session should be arranged to discuss the information more thoroughly. The risks, benefits, and limitations of the procedures can be reviewed in detail. Couples need to be reminded that many conditions cannot be detected prenatally and that normal results from prenatal diagnostic evaluation do not guarantee a healthy child. All couples, regardless of their ages or family history, have a 3 to 4% risk of having a child with a birth defect. Also, many inherited conditions display considerable clinical variability. Couples need to be aware that prenatal diagnosis usually does not predict the severity of a condition.

In counseling for prenatal diagnosis, it is important to stress to parents that they are not committed in advance to any particular course of action in the event of an abnormal finding. Although termination of an affected pregnancy is available, this is clearly not an acceptable alternative for all couples. Some may wish to know in advance if the baby will be affected because this may affect delivery site and neonatal management. For others, early knowledge can help their families prepare and adjust for the baby. Many couples consider prenatal testing for the reassurance associated with the more likely event that the results are normal. Thus, prenatal diagnosis should not be summarily dismissed for those couples who indicate that they will not consider elective pregnancy termination.

A relatively recent option for some conditions is preimplantation diagnosis with in vitro fertilization (IVF). Conditions that can be diagnosed by polymerase chain reaction can be considered for this procedure. Following IVF, typically at the 8- to 16-cell blastomere stage, DNA from one or two separate cells is assayed using the polymerase chain reaction to amplify a minute amount of DNA. Only embryos lacking the mutation are then implanted into the mother's uterus. Although encouraging, experience to date is limited. Also, the procedure is expensive and may not be covered by insurance. Although some states require third-party payers to cover IVF, this is usually mandated for infertile couples, and those seeking preimplantation diagnosis are not infertile. Finally, because few facilities offer the procedure, logistics can preclude its availability.

ASSISTED REPRODUCTIVE TECHNOLOGIES AND ADOPTION

Some risk revision options do not involve prenatal testing. Assisted reproductive technologies offer a means for reducing risk, particularly for mendelian disorders or familial chromosome changes. IVF with donor egg when the mother has an autosomal dominant condition or is a carrier for an X-linked condition reduces the risk to the level of population incidence. Risk is similarly reduced with artificial insemination by donor if the father has an autosomal dominant condition. With recessive conditions, artificial insemination by donor usually reduces the risk to less than 1%. Adoption can be an alternative for couples who perceive the recurrence risk or consequences to be too high but whose personal goals include a (larger) family.

CARRIER TESTING

For some conditions, carrier testing is available to revise the recurrence risk. Often this means that prenatal diagnosis is available as well. However, assessment of carrier status sometimes helps a couple decide if they wish to pursue another pregnancy even if prenatal diagnosis is available. It could also have implications for other family members.

For example, if a child has microphthalmia and other congenital anomalies related to a translocation trisomy 13 and both parents have normal chromosomes, the risk of recurrence for their offspring and those born to other relatives is extremely low. In contrast, if one parent carries a balanced arrangement involving chromosome 13, the empirical recurrence risk data would be known for both parents and any sibling of the parent who carries the rearrangement. Fabry's disease is another example in which carrier testing is useful. This is an X-linked condition in which affected patients accumulate glycolipid as a result of an α-galactosidase deficiency. Onset is typically in childhood or adolescence and includes episodes of severe extremity pain, angiokeratomas, and characteristic corneal and lenticular opacities. Cardiac, renal, and cerebrovascular complications can occur later in life. Carrier assessment includes ophthalmologic examination. Corneal opacities detectable only by slit-lamp examination are present in about 80% of carriers.[4] Assaying α-galactosidase levels is another carrier testing option for this disorder. Both eye examination results and enzyme level can be normal in carriers, however, because of X-chromosome inactivation. Therefore, molecular testing may offer more definitive results to identify females in a family who are at risk of having affected sons.

MOLECULAR TESTING: DISTINCTIONS AND LIMITATIONS

Molecular testing often is used for prenatal testing and carrier detection. When newly developed technology is being considered, it is important that families be aware of whether the testing is provided on a clinical or research basis. Clinical testing implies well-established protocols with quality control measures and available data regarding sensitivity and specificity. The time required for testing is predictable, and a charge is often involved. Research testing is performed in an unpredictable time frame, and usually there is no charge.

Progress toward understanding the genetic basis of disease can be expected to affect diagnostic capabilities first. Treatment or management of a genetic disease generally lags behind considerably. Although "gene therapy" receives a great deal of media attention, clinical application is so far limited. Genetic counselors must explain this distinction between diagnostic and therapeutic interventions.

Even if a gene is mapped and DNA markers linked to the gene are available, linkage analysis in some families is not informative because of the limited size of the family. Studies should be performed on several family members before it is known whether linkage studies will be useful for carrier or prenatal assessment in that family. For those families in which study results are informative, the studies will provide a revised risk rather than a definitive answer, because with linkage studies, recombination is always possible. The degree of risk revision varies from family to family, depending on which markers are informative. Accuracy is highest for families with informative flanking markers. Another limitation of linkage studies is the possibility that an altered gene at a location unlinked to the markers could cause a similar clinical condition. If the gene mutation or product is not testable, this potential heterogeneity remains a concern.

Even when direct analysis of an actual gene mutation or gene product is possible, issues need to be discussed with families to help them understand how the information is useful to them. For example, if all possible mutations causing a condition cannot be identified, testing will not detect all cases. Although blood is an easily accessible source of genetic material and useful for linkage and mutation analysis, it may not be a good source for gene product testing. In this situation, additional tissue may be necessary, and the appropriateness of a more invasive test needs to be discussed with family members. The invasiveness of a test should be weighed against the additional information that will likely be obtained.

Documentation and Follow-Up

Clients who are counseled should receive a detailed written summary of the evaluation. Although writing clear and informative summaries can be extremely time-consuming, it is necessary for several reasons. It is unlikely that all the verbal information provided during the visit will be remembered, and what is remembered may be difficult for an individual to explain to others. A summary serves as an extension of the communication process that allows for review by the recipient.

Genetic counselors are available to clients on an ongoing basis to reexamine and clarify the issues covered during the visit(s) and in the written summary. They provide reassurance that the clients have received appropriate responses; this can be reinforced by providing families with information about support organizations. In addition, families need to be informed that genetics is a rapidly advancing area of medicine. Even if an evaluation has failed to identify a specific diagnosis, families who have received genetic counseling are encouraged to reestablish contact whenever planning a pregnancy to take advantage of any pertinent new developments.

Ethical Considerations in Genetic Counseling

The increased understanding of genetic disease and availability of testing bring many challenges to genetic counseling and raise a number of ethical issues. Although most genetic counseling situations do not give rise to these dilemmas, it is important for genetic counselors to be aware of these possibilities.

CONFIDENTIALITY

Issues of genetic privacy are much discussed in the genetics community and society as a whole. There is debate over who should have access to genetic information and how it can be used. Of particular concern is the potential for discrimination by insurance companies or employers. Insurance companies may use test results to deny coverage, claiming that a genetic disease is a preexisting condition. Alternatively, they may consider an affected individual to be an insurance risk if his or her condition could cause medical problems in the future. Employers may try to use genetic information to make hiring decisions, basing their assessment on risk for medical complications or disability.

These issues often lead families or individuals to be wary of genetic testing. Some decide to decline testing even if a positive test result could alter medical management. Others choose to pay for testing themselves to prevent the insurance company from having access to this information. Still others request that test results not be put in their medical record. Families may desire to have total control over the information.

Genetic professionals support the patients' right to privacy with regard to results of genetic testing. Those arranging testing should discuss the issues of confidentiality prior to the initiation of testing so there is consensus on how results are reported, who receives results, and where the information is documented.

CONTROVERSIAL USES OF GENETIC TESTING

Patients may want to use genetic testing for less traditional purposes in a number of situations. Because many patients have access to different types of genetic testing, particularly if they pay for it themselves, genetic counselors may be asked to arrange testing for reasons with which they do not necessarily agree. It is important for medical professionals to be aware of these scenarios, recognize their own opinions, and be able to refer patients to others if they do not feel that they can support such patients' wishes.

Sex Selection

A couple might wish to choose the sex of their child. Having a child of a particular gender has strong roots in some cultures. Other couples may simply wish to ensure that they have children of both sexes in their family. Although this is not illegal, it can make those providing the testing uncomfortable.

Presymptomatic Testing of Children

Because testing is available for a number of disorders with later onset, it is possible to test children or even fetuses for conditions that may not affect their lives for many years. Although parents may feel that this is in the best interest of their children, some fear it may cause stigmatization. Others argue that undergoing testing should be the decision of the individual, once he or she reaches adulthood, particularly if it would not affect medical management.

Testing for Selection of Affected Persons

Patients with certain conditions or physical limitations may desire to have similarly affected children. Patients with achondroplasia, for example, have wanted to have children with achondroplasia because this is what they have come to consider normal. This could lead them to choose prenatal diagnosis to "rule in" achondroplasia, possibly resulting in the termination of an unaffected pregnancy.

DISCOVERY OF UNANTICIPATED OR HARMFUL INFORMATION

Because genetic testing can involve studying a number of persons in a family, it can sometimes uncover information that family members did not anticipate or do not want to know. Prior to the initiation of testing, it is important to discuss not only the possible benefits of genetic testing but also the potential for unanticipated results.

Nonpaternity

Genetic testing can lead to the discovery of nonpaternity. Raising this as a possible outcome prior to testing may help to avoid an awkward situation when test results become available.

Disclosure of Disease Status

In large families studied by linkage analysis, a number of persons may learn a family member's disease status. Some such persons may have no relationship with the physician or genetic counselor that organized the testing. If possible, these persons should be referred to a qualified physician or local genetics center where they can learn about their disease status and discuss the implications of their test results. It is also best to determine which family members do not want to know their results before testing begins. Care must be taken to avoid divulging their status to other family members. Those not requesting information should have the option of obtaining it later, should they change their minds.

Nondisclosing Prenatal Diagnosis

A special situation surrounding genetic testing involves prenatal diagnosis for an autosomal dominant condition in which a parent is at risk but does not want to know his or her disease status. Prenatal diagnosis using linkage analysis is most accurate in families with affected individuals in more than one generation. In this scenario, if a fetus is found to be unaffected, the parent's status would not need to be conveyed (Fig. 3–1). However, the diagnosis of an affected fetus would indicate that the parent is also affected. This would necessarily prompt a couple to come to terms with the diagnosis in the parent.

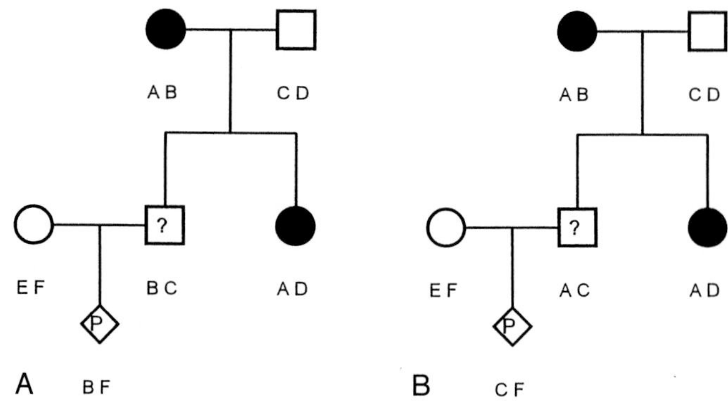

FIGURE 3–1. Linkage analysis with letters (A–E) represents specific RFLPs (see "Fundamentals of Genetics"). The fetus is unaffected in both scenarios. The father's disease state is determined but need not be disclosed. *A,* The fetus and father both have the nondisease allele of the affected grandmother. *B,* The fetus receives the allele of the unaffected grandfather, but the father has the disease allele from the affected grandmother.

Revision of Fetal Risk without Determining Parental Disease State

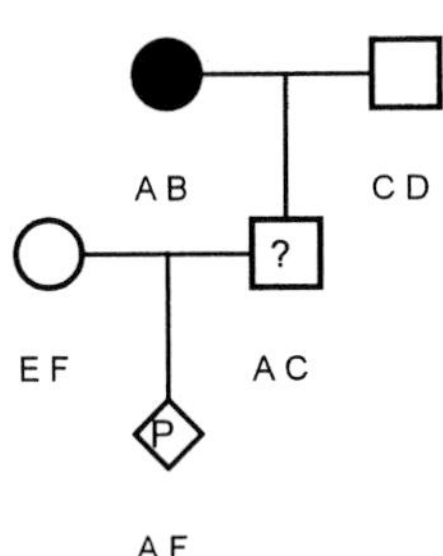

FIGURE 3–2. The risk of the fetus being affected is 50%. The father's risk remains unchanged. The fetus receives the grand-maternal allele, but testing cannot determine whether it is the disease allele.

Alternatively, testing to determine which grand-parental allele a fetus received without establishing linkage of the disease gene to a particular allele can be used when only one affected family member is available for testing and when parents want to guarantee that their status is not determined by testing. This could exclude (within the limits of recombination) a fetus being affected if it received an allele from the unaffected grandparent. If the fetus received the allele of the affected grandparent, this would not prove that the fetus is affected but would increase the risk from 25 to 50% (Fig. 3–2).

DUTY TO RECONTACT

In the era of rapid scientific discovery, particularly in molecular diagnostics, the question arises as to how to keep families informed of new information. Parents of a child with albinism seen years ago might now benefit from molecular testing. Therefore, what a family is told at a genetic counseling session could eventually become outdated. It is not generally possible for medical professionals to contact previous patients when new testing becomes available, however.

As discussed previously (see under Documentation and Follow-Up), genetic counselors must remain available to families. In addition, the importance of genetic counseling for affected children when they reach child-bearing age should be stressed. This allows for a review of the genetic implications as well as an update on the possibilities for diagnostic testing. Finally, periodic follow-up visits may be suggested to help families keep up-to-date on both clinical and molecular developments.

Conclusion

Genetic counseling involves the transfer of technical and conceptual information that is sometimes different from the information the family may have previously encountered. This information is often conveyed to persons who are feeling anxious, guilty, depressed, or overwhelmed. By recognizing and exploring the psychologic impact of genetic counseling issues, counselors can better integrate medical and genetic information so that families feel competent in making informed decisions. Such autonomy can reestablish their sense of control and aid in their psychologic adjustment.

REFERENCES

1. Fraser FC: Genetic counseling. Am J Hum Genet 26:636–659, 1974.
2. Charnas LR, Nussbaum RL: The oculocerebrorenal syndrome of Lowe (Lowe syndrome). *In* Scriver CR, Beaudet AL, Sly WS, et al (eds): The Metabolic and Molecular Bases of Inherited Disease, 7th ed, vol III. New York, McGraw-Hill, 1995.
3. Hereditary visual disorders. *In* Robinson A, Linden MG (eds): Clinical Genetics Handbook, 2nd ed. Boston, Blackwell Scientific, Boston, 1993.
4. Metabolic disorders. *In* Gorlin RJ, Cohen MM, Jr, Levin LS (eds): Syndromes of the Head and Neck, 3rd ed. New York, Oxford University, 1990.

SUGGESTIONS FOR FURTHER READING

Bernhardt BA: Empirical evidence that genetic counseling is directive: Where do we go from here? Am J Hum Genet 60:17–20, 1997.

Furu T, Kaarianinen H, Sankilla EM, et al: Attitudes towards prenatal diagnosis and selective abortion among patients with retinitis pigmentosa or choroideremia as well as among their relatives. Clin Genet 43:160–165, 1993.

Harper PS: Practical Genetic Counselling, 4th ed. Oxford, Butterworth-Heinemann, 1993.

Michie S, Bron F, Bobrow M, et al: Nondirectiveness in genetic counseling: An empirical study. Am J Hum Genet 60:40–47, 1997.

Reif M, Baitsch H: Psychological issues in genetic counselling. Hum Genet 70:193–199, 1985.

Sharpe NF: Psychological aspects of genetic counseling: A legal perspective. Am J Med Genet 50:234–238, 1994.

CHAPTER 4

Molecular Mechanisms of Inherited Disease

Janey L. Wiggs and Thaddeus P. Dryja

DNA mutations occurring in genes may result in the formation of a defective gene product. If the normal protein product of a mutated gene is necessary for a critical biologic function, then an alteration of the normal phenotype may occur. Many changes in phenotype are considered normal variations among humans, for example, brown hair instead of blond hair. However, some changes produce phenotypes that seriously affect health; these are the major focus of study in clinical genetics laboratories.

The type of mutation responsible for a disease usually determines the inheritance pattern. For example, mutations that create an abnormal protein that is detrimental to cells are typically dominant, because only one mutant gene is required to disrupt the normal functions of the cell. Mutations that result in proteins with reduced biologic activity (loss of function) may be inherited as dominant or recessive conditions depending on the number of copies of normal genes (and the amount of normal protein) required. Disorders caused by mutations in mitochondrial DNA have a characteristic inheritance pattern. Mutations in genes carried on the X chromosome also result in typical inheritance patterns. Examples of the types of mutations responsible for different inheritance patterns are described in the following sections.

Autosomal Dominant

Disorders inherited as autosomal dominant traits result from mutations that occur in only one copy of a gene (i.e., in heterozygous individuals). Usually the parental origin of the mutation doesn't matter. However, if the gene is subject to imprinting, then mutations in the maternal or paternal copy of the gene may give rise to different phenotypes.

HAPLOINSUFFICIENCY

Some cellular processes require a level of protein production that can only be furnished if both copies of a particular gene are active. Such proteins may be involved in a variety of biologic processes. If one copy of a gene is mutant and the protein level is reduced by half, a disorder may result.

ANIRIDIA—*PAX6*

Mutations in the *PAX6* gene cause disease through haploinsufficiency. Most of the mutations responsible for these disorders alter the paired-box sequence within the protein product, which is in the homeobox family of transcription factors (Fig. 4–1).[1] The paired box is an important region of the protein that participates in the regulation of expression of other genes.[2] *PAX6* plays a critical role in ocular development, presumably by regulating the expression of a set of genes that are essential for this process.[3] A reduction in the amount of active *PAX6* gene product changes the level at which these other genes operate.

There is extensive variation in the range of phenotypes exhibited by patients with *PAX6* mutations. Patients typically have various anterior segment abnormalities, such as aniridia,[4] Peters' anomaly,[5] or autosomal dominant keratitis.[6, 7] This spectrum of phenotypic abnormalities resulting from mutations in one gene is termed *variable expressivity* and is a common feature of disorders that result from haploinsufficiency. The variability of the mutant phenotype possibly results from the random activation of downstream genes that occurs when only half the required gene product is available. Another example of an eye disease caused by haploinsufficiency in a homeobox gene is Waardenburg's syndrome, which is due to defects in *PAX3*.[8]

LOSS OF FUNCTION

Autosomal dominant traits may result from mutations in one copy of a gene that increase the likelihood, but are not sufficient to cause the disease. For the disease to become manifest, a "second hit" that affects the remaining copy of the gene must occur. If the second hit is a common event, the inheritance of one mutant copy of the gene almost always results in the disease and the trait appears to be

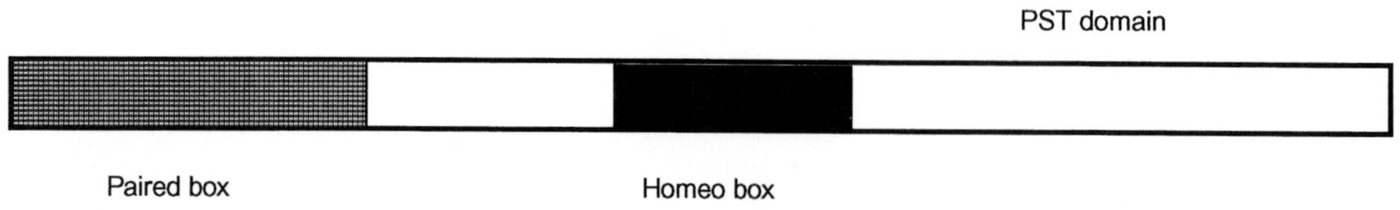

PST domain

Paired box

Homeo box

FIGURE 4–1. Schematic diagram of the *PAX6* gene.

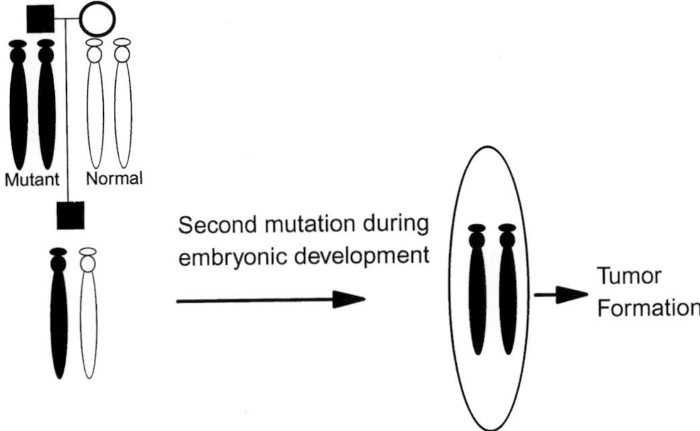

FIGURE 4–2. Inheritance of retinoblastoma. Individuals inheriting a mutation in the retinoblastoma gene are heterozygous for the mutation in all cells of their bodies. The "second hit" to the remaining normal copy of the gene occurs in a developing retinal cell and leads to tumor formation.

inherited in a dominant fashion. However, at the cellular level, the mutations appear recessive since cells must be homozygotes or compound heterozygotes to display the mutant phenotype.

RETINOBLASTOMA

Tumor suppressor genes such as the retinoblastoma gene provide good examples of loss-of-function dominant mutations. A gene responsible for retinoblastoma was identified in 1986 on chromosome 13q14.[9] The gene product is involved in regulating the cell cycle.[10] An absence of this protein in a sensitive embryonic retinal cell results in uncontrolled cell growth that eventually produces a tumor. Susceptibility to hereditary retinoblastoma is inherited as an autosomal dominant trait. Mutations in the retinoblastoma gene result in underproduction of the protein product or in production of an inactive protein product.[11] A retinal cell with only one mutant copy of the retinoblastoma gene will not become a tumor. However, inactivation of the remaining normal copy of the retinoblastoma gene is very likely in at least one retinal cell out of the millions present in each retina. Most individuals who inherit a mutant copy of the gene sustain a second hit to the remaining normal copy of the gene and develop the disease (Fig. 4–2).[12]

GAIN-OF-FUNCTION—DOMINANT NEGATIVE EFFECT

Autosomal dominant disorders can be caused by mutant proteins that have a detrimental effect on the native tissue. Under this scenario, mutations in one copy of a gene produce a mutant protein that may interfere with normal cellular processes or may accumulate as a toxic product, or both. This toxicity is a function not present in the wild-type protein; hence the mutation is termed a *gain-of-function* mutant. If the mutant protein interferes with the function of the wild-type protein expressed by the remaining normal copy of the gene, the mutation is described as *dominant negative.*[13]

CORNEAL DYSTROPHIES

The autosomal dominant corneal dystrophies are excellent examples of gain-of-function mutations that result in the formation of an aberrant protein. The four most common autosomal dominant corneal stromal dystrophies are: Groenouw's (granular) type 1,[14] lattice type 1,[15] Avellino's (combined granular-lattice),[16] and Reis-Bückler's.[17] Although all four corneal dystrophies affect the anterior stroma, the clinical and pathologic features differ. The granular dystrophies typically form discrete white localized deposits that progressively obscure vision. Histopathologically, these deposits stain bright red with Masson's trichrome bright red and have been termed *hyalin.* In lattice dystrophy, branching amyloid deposits gradually opacify the cornea. These deposits exhibit a characteristic birefringence and dichroism under polarized light after staining with Congo red. Avellino's dystrophy has features of both granular and lattice dystrophies. Reis-Bücklers primarily involves Bowman's layer and the superficial stroma.[18] All four dystrophies have been genetically mapped to a common interval on chromosome 5q31.[19–22] Mutations in a single gene, (beta)*ig-h3,* located in this region have been identified in a number of affected families.[23] The product of this gene, keratoepithelin, is probably an extracellular matrix protein that modulates cell adhesion. Four different missense mutations occurring at two arginine codons in the gene have been found (Fig. 4–3). Interestingly, different mutations at the same arginine codon cause lattice dystrophy type I or Avellino's dystrophy, the two dystrophies characterized by amyloid deposits. The mutations that cause Avellino's and lattice dystrophies abolish a putative phosphorylation site that is probably required for the normal structure of keratoepithelin. Destruction of this aspect of the protein structure leads to the formation of the amyloid deposits that cause opacification of the cornea. As a result, the mutant protein is destructive to the normal tissue. Mutations at the other arginine codon appear to result in either granular dystrophy or Reis-Bücklers dystrophy. The mutation analysis of this gene demonstrates that different mutations within a single gene can result in different phenotypes. Other examples of gain-of-function mutations causing ocular disease are transthyretin mutations causing vitreous amyloidosis,[24] and possibly *TIMP3* mutations causing Sorsby's dystrophy.[25]

RETINITIS PIGMENTOSA—RHODOPSIN

The rhodopsin locus is another example of a gene in which dominant gain-of-function mutations cause disease. Mutations in the gene for rhodopsin can cause retinitis pigmentosa.[26] To explore the pathogenic mechanisms relating to these mutations, transgenic mice were created that carried mutant copies of the gene.[27] Histopathologic studies of these mice showed an accumulation of vesicles containing rhodopsin at the junction between the inner and the outer segments of the photoreceptors. The vesicles probably interfere with the normal regeneration of the photoreceptors, causing photoreceptor degeneration.

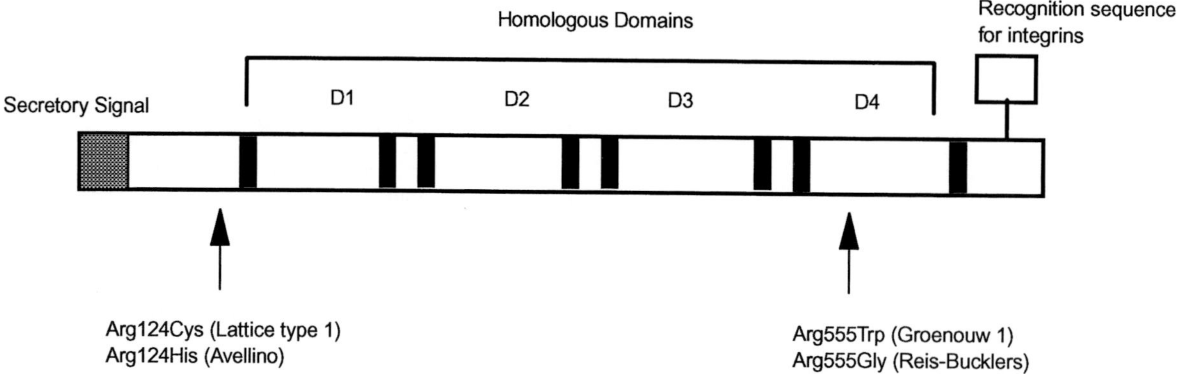

FIGURE 4–3. Schematic diagram of the keratoepithelin gene. D1 to D4, homologous domains. Arrows point to the location of the reported mutations.

OSTEOGENESIS IMPERFECTA

Osteogenesis imperfecta is an example of a dominant negative–type mutation. Osteogenesis imperfecta is a group of inherited disorders of type I collagen that predispose a patient to easy fracturing of bones, and skeletal deformity. Ocular findings include thinned sclera. The type I procollagen molecule is formed from two proalpha-1 chains and one proalpha-2 chain. To create a collagen molecule, the three chains form an α-helix beginning at the carboxyl terminus. Mutations that affect the amino acid sequence of an individual procollagen molecule disrupt the formation of the helix, and this results in the disease.[28]

ANTICIPATION—TRINUCLEOTIDE REPEATS

A new class of mutations responsible for autosomal dominant inheritance was discovered with the identification of the gene responsible for Huntington's disease.[29] Huntington's disease is a neurodegenerative disorder that results in motor, cognitive, and emotional disturbance. Huntington's disease demonstrates anticipation, which means that subsequent generations of affected individuals are more severely affected and are affected at an earlier age than their predecessors.[30] The gene defect responsible for this disease is an expanded and unstable trinucleotide repeat in the open-reading frame of the Huntington disease gene located on chromosome 4. The repeated DNA sequence causes the encoded protein to have a long span of the same amino acid residue repeated many times. A critical observation was made when the repeat lengths were correlated with the severity and the age of onset of the disease. Longer repeat lengths result in more severe disease at an earlier age of onset. The number of repeats within the gene expands with each subsequent generation and is likely to be the cause of the increased severity of the disease (Fig. 4–4).[31] Since the discovery of the Huntington gene a number of other disorders caused by unstable trinucleotide repeats have been recognized, such as myotonic dystrophy and fragile X syndrome. Although the mechanism of trinucleotide repeat disease is unknown, the autosomal dominant inheritance suggests that only one mutant copy of the gene is required and that the repeat in some way has a detrimental effect on the cell.

Autosomal Recessive

Autosomal recessive disorders result from mutations present on both the maternal and the paternal copies of a gene. Mutations responsible for recessive disease typically cause a loss of biologic activity, either because they create a defective protein product that has little or no biologic activity or because they interfere with the normal expression of the gene (regulatory mutations). Most individuals heterozygous for autosomal recessive disorders are clinically normal.

LOSS OF FUNCTION (ALBINISM)

Autosomal recessive diseases often result from defects in enzymatic proteins. Albinism is the result of a series of

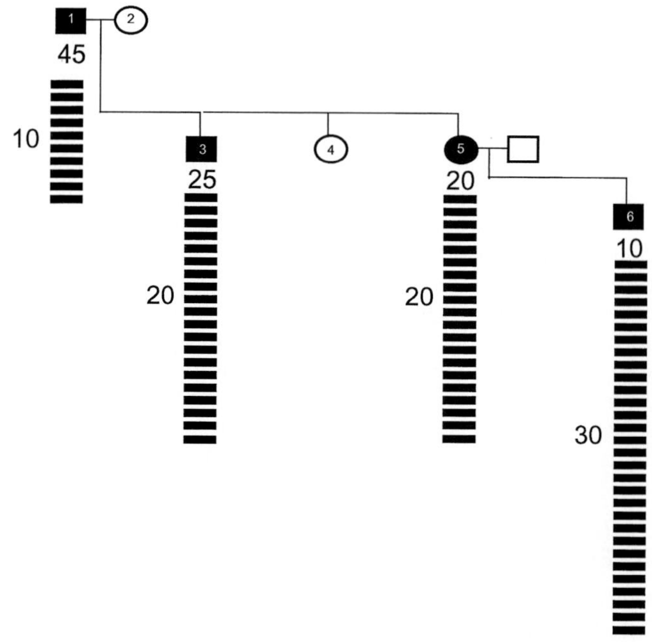

FIGURE 4–4. Pedigree illustrating anticipation associated with expansion of a trinucleotide repeat. Affected individuals are shown as solid circles or squares. The age of onset of the disease is shown beneath the pedigree symbol for each affected individual. The number of trinucleotide repeats within the disease gene (e.g., the gene responsible for Huntington's disease) are schematically represented beneath each affected individual. Successive generations have an earlier age of onset and a higher number of repeats (compare individual 1 with individual 6).

defects in the synthesis of melanin pigment.[32] Melanin is synthesized from the amino acid tyrosine, which is first converted to dihydroxyphenylalanine through the action of the copper-containing enzyme tyrosinase. An absence of tyrosinase results in one form of albinism. Mutations in the gene coding for tyrosinase are responsible for this disease cluster in the binding sites for copper, disrupting the metal ion–protein interaction necessary for enzyme function.[33] Both copies of the gene for tyrosinase must be mutated before a significant interruption of melanin production occurs. Heterozygous individuals do not have a clinically apparent phenotype, suggesting that one functional copy of the gene produces sufficient active enzyme that the melanin level is phenotypically normal.

X-Linked Recessive

X-linked recessive disorders, like autosomal recessive disorders, result from a mutant gene that causes a loss of a critical biologic activity. Because males have only one X chromosome, one mutant copy of a gene responsible for an X-linked trait results in the disease. Usually females are heterozygous carriers of recessive X-linked traits. In somatic cells of females, only one X chromosome is active; the second X chromosome is inactivated and becomes a Barr body. X inactivation has been associated with the geneticist Mary Lyon, and has been called Lyonization. Inactivation of either the maternal or the paternal X chromosome occurs early in embryonic life. In any one cell, the inactive X may be maternal or paternal, and once the X is inactivated, it remains inactive. Because females inherit two copies of the X chromosome, they can be homozygous for a disease allele at a given locus, heterozygous, or homozygous for the normal allele at the locus. Since only one X chromosome is active in any given somatic cell, about half the cells of a heterozygous female express the disease allele, and about half express the normal allele. Like autosomal recessive traits, the female heterozygote expresses about 50% of the normal level of the protein product. For recessive conditions, this is sufficient for a normal phenotype.

RETINOSCHISIS

Retinoschisis is a maculopathy that is caused by intraretinal splitting. The defect most likely involves retinal Müller's cells.[34] Retinoschisis is inherited as an X-linked recessive trait.[35] Female carriers with one normal and one abnormal copy of the gene do not demonstrate any clinical abnormalities. Fifty percent of the male offspring of female carriers are affected by the disease. Mutations in a gene located in the retinoschisis interval and expressed in the retina have been found in a protein that is implicated in cell-cell interaction and may be active in cell adhesion processes during retinal development. Mutational analysis of the retinoschisis gene (*XLRS1*) in affected individuals from nine unrelated families showed one nonsense, one frameshift, one splice acceptor, and six missense mutations.[36] Presumably these mutations all result in an inactive protein product.

X-Linked Dominant

X-linked dominant mutations are less common than X-linked recessive mutations. Clinically X-linked dominant inheritance is difficult to recognize because of the random inactivation of the X chromosome in females (Lyon's hypothesis).[37] The random inactivation of the X chromosome produces females who are X chromosome mosaics, with about 50% of the cells expressing genes from the paternally derived X and 50% of the cells expressing genes from the maternally derived X. If one of the X chromosomes has a mutant gene, these cells may display the phenotype; however, 50% of the female cells are normal, even for a "dominant" mutation. As a result, for recessive and dominant X-linked traits, the disease phenotype may not be evident in females carrying the mutation. X-linked dominant mutations could produce a protein that has a detrimental effect on normal biologic processes (gain-of-function or dominant negative effect). Mutations that result in haploinsufficiency of the X chromosome could also be X-linked dominant. X-linked dominant disorders include incontinentia pigmenti and X-linked hypophosphatemia rickets. A family with X-linked dominant retinitis pigmentosa has also been described.[38]

Digenic Inheritance

Digenic inheritance is a newly described pattern of inheritance in humans. A disease inherited as a digenic trait only develops when mutations are found in each of two independent genes simultaneously. Digenic inheritance is an example of the complex interactions that occur between multiple gene products in polygenic inheritance (see later).

RETINITIS PIGMENTOSA (PERIPHERIN AND *ROM1*)

One form of retinitis pigmentosa has been shown to be inherited as a digenic trait.[39] Although there was direct parent-to-child transmission of the disease, the affected families had unusual features for a dominantly inherited disease: the disease originated in the offspring of an ancestral mating between two unaffected individuals, and the affected individuals transmitted the disease to less than 50% of their offspring (about 25% rather than 50%). Mutation analysis of the peripherin gene and the *ROM1* gene showed that the affected individuals had specific mutations in both genes. Individuals who had a mutation in one copy of either gene were unaffected by the disease. Mutant copies of *ROM1* and peripherin can also cause autosomal dominant forms of retinitis pigmentosa.[40, 41] These results suggest that some mutant forms of peripherin and *ROM1* cause retinitis pigmentosa in a digenic pattern, whereas other mutations can independently cause autosomal dominant forms of the disease.

Mitochondrial Disease

Mutations in mitochondrial DNA can also result in human disease. The characteristic segregation and assortment of Mendelian disorders depends on the meiotic division of chromosomes found in the nucleus of cells. There are several hundred mitochondria in a cell, and each mitochondrion contains several copies of the mitochondrial genome. Mitochondria divide in the cellular cytoplasm by simple fission. Not all mitochondria present in a disease tissue carry DNA

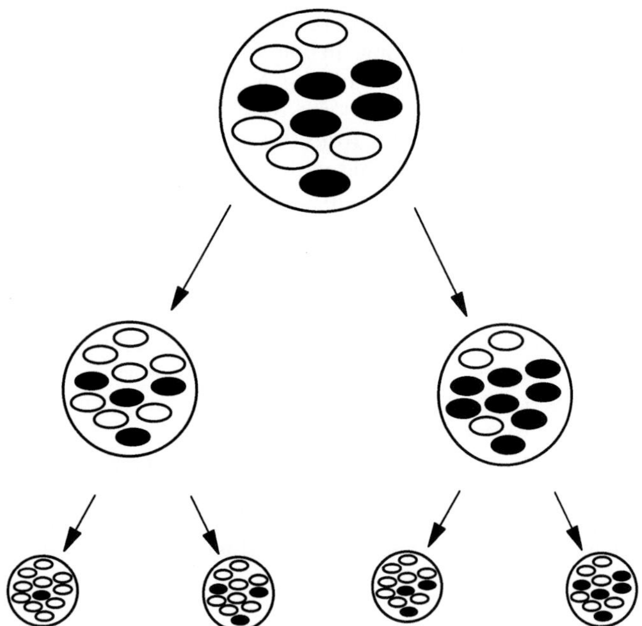

FIGURE 4–5. Heteroplasmy in mitochondria. Daughter cells resulting from the division of a cell containing mitochondria with mutant DNA may contain unequal numbers of mutant mitochondria. Subsequent divisions lead to a population of cells with varied numbers of normal and abnormal mitochondria.

mutations. During cell division, mitochondria and other cytoplasmic organelles are arbitrarily distributed to the daughter cells. Because each cell contains a population of mitochondrial DNA molecules, a single cell can contain DNA molecules that are normal as well as DNA molecules that are mutant (Fig. 4–5). This heterogeneity of DNA composition, called *heteroplasmy,* is an important cause of variable expression in mitochondrial diseases. As the diseased mitochondria are distributed to developing tissues, some tissues accumulate more abnormal mitochondria than others.

Disorders that result from mutations in mitochondrial DNA demonstrate a maternal inheritance pattern (see also Chapter 1—Fundamentals of Genetics). Maternal inheritance differs from Mendelian inheritance in that only affected females transmit the disease to their offspring. Unlike nuclear DNA that is equally contributed to the embryo by the mother and the father, mitochondria and mitochondrial DNA are derived solely from the maternal egg. A mutation occurring in mitochondrial DNA is present in cells containing mitochondria, including the female gametes. Sperm have few mitochondria, and they are not transmitted to the egg. A male carrying a mitochondrial DNA mutation will not transmit the disease to his offspring.

LEBER'S HEREDITARY OPTIC NEUROPATHY

Leber's hereditary optic neuropathy was one of the first diseases to be recognized as a mitochondrial DNA disorder.[42] For some time clinicians had observed maternal inheritance of this condition in affected families, but it wasn't until mutations in mitochondrial DNA of affected individuals were demonstrated that the cause of the inheritance pattern was understood. In familial cases of the disease, all affected individuals are related through the maternal lineage, consistent with the inheritance of human mitochondrial DNA.

Patients affected by Leber's hereditary optic neuropathy typically present with acute or subacute, painless, central vision loss leading to a permanent central scotoma and loss of sight. The manifestation of the disease can vary tremendously especially with respect to the onset of loss of vision and severity of the outcome.[43] The eyes can be affected simultaneously or sequentially. The vision may be lost rapidly over a period of weeks to months, or slowly over several years. Within a family the disease may also vary among affected family members. Several factors contribute to the variable phenotype of this condition. Certain mutations are associated with more severe disease. For example, the most severely affected patients with the 11,778-bp mutation may have no light perception,[44] whereas the most severely affected patients with the 3460-bp mutation may retain light perception.[45] Another important factor that affects the severity of the disease in affected persons is the heteroplasmic distribution of mutant and normal mitochondria. This partially explains why some patients develop a more severe optic neuropathy. Other genetic or environmental factors are likely to play a role as well.

Polygenic Inheritance

Human phenotypes inherited as polygenic or "complex" traits do not follow the typical patterns of Mendelian inheritance. Generally, complex traits are commonly found in the human population. Multiple genes are likely to contribute to the expression of the disease phenotype. Some genes may render an individual susceptible to a disease, and other genes or environmental conditions may influence the full expression of the phenotype. Secondary genes responsible for the modulation of the expression of a specific genetic mutation are called *modifier genes*; modifier genes may be inherited completely independently from the gene directly responsible for the disease trait. Not every individual who inherits a mutation partly responsible for a complex trait also inherits the set of modifier genes that is required for full expression of the disease. The digenic inheritance of retinitis pigmentosa seen by certain mutant alleles of peripherin and *ROM1* is an example of the simplest form of polygenic inheritance (see previous discussion). Certain conditions may require multiple genes or a combination of different genes and environmental conditions to be manifest. Examples of ocular disorders that are multifactorial are age-related macular degeneration, adult-onset primary open-angle glaucoma, and myopia.[46]

REFERENCES

1. Read AP: *Pax* genes—*Paired* feet in three camps. Nature Genet 9:333–334, 1995.
2. Ton CCT, Hirvonen H, Mira H, et al: Positional cloning and characterization of a paired box- and homeobox-containing gene from the aniridia region. Cell 67:1059–1074, 1991.
3. Richardson J, Cvekl A, Wistow G: *Pax-6* is essential for lens-specific expression of zeta-crystallin. Proc Natl Acad Sci USA 92:4676–4680, 1995.
4. Glaser T, Jepeal L, Edwards JG, et al: *PAX6* gene dosage effect in a family with congenital cataracts, aniridia, anophthalmia and central nervous system defects. Nature Genet 7:463–471, 1994.
5. Hanson IM, Fletcher JM, Jordon T, et al: Mutations at the *PAX6* locus are found in heterogeneous anterior segment malformations including Peters' anomaly. Nature Genet 6:168–173, 1994.

6. Mirzayans F, Pearce WG, MacDonald IM, et al: Mutation of the *PAX6* gene in patients with autosomal dominant keratitis. Am J Hum Genet 57:539–548, 1995.
7. Davis A, Cowell JK: Mutations in the *PAX6* gene in patients with hereditary aniridia. Hum Mol Genet 2:2093–2097, 1993.
8. Tassabehji M, Read AP, Newton VE, et al: Waardenburg's syndrome patients have mutations in the human homologue of the *Pax-3* paired box gene. Nature 355:635–636, 1992.
9. Friend SH, Dryja TP, Weinberg RA: Oncogenes and tumor-suppressing genes. N Engl J Med 318:618–622, 1988.
10. Weinberg RA: The retinoblastoma protein and cell cycle control. Cell 81:323–330, 1995.
11. Dryja TP, Cavenee W, White R, et al: Homozygosity of chromosome 13 in retinoblastoma. N Engl J Med 310:550–553, 1984.
12. Knudson AG Jr: Genetics of human cancer. Annu Rev Genet 20:231–251, 1986.
13. Herskowitz I: Functional inactivation of genes by dominant negative mutations. [Review] Nature 329:219–322, 1987.
14. Moller HU: Inter-familial variability and intra-familial similarities of granular corneal dystrophy Groenouw type I with respect to biomicroscopical appearance and symptomatology. Act Ophthalmol 67:669–677, 1989.
15. Klintworth GK: Lattice corneal dystrophy: An inherited variety of amyloidosis restricted to the cornea. Am J Pathol 50:371–399, 1967.
16. Folberg R, Alfonso E, Croxatto JO, et al: Clinically atypical granular corneal dystrophy with pathologic features of lattice-like amyloid deposits. Ophthalmology 95:46–51, 1988.
17. Rosenwasser GO, Sucheski BM, Rosa N, et al: Phenotypic variation in combined granular-lattice (Avellino) corneal dystrophy. Arch Ophthalmol 111:1546–1552, 1993.
18. Kuchle M, Green WR, Volcker HE, et al: Reevaluation of corneal dystrophies of Bowman's layer and the anterior stroma (Reis-Bücklers and Thiel-Behnke types): A light and electron microscopic study of eight corneas and a review of the literature. Cornea 14:333–354, 1995.
19. Eiberg H, Moller HU, Berendt I, et al: Assignment of granular corneal dystrophy Groenouw type I locus to within a 2 cM interval. Eur J Hum Genet 2:132–138, 1994.
20. Stone EM, Mathers WD, Rosenwasser GO, et al: Three autosomal dominant corneal dystrophies map to chromosome 5q. Nature Genet 6:47–51, 1994.
21. Gregory CY, Evans K, Bhattacharya SS: Genetic refinement of the chromosome 5q lattice corneal dystrophy to within a 2 cM interval. J Med Genet 32:224–226, 1995.
22. Small KW, Mullen L, Barletta J, et al: Mapping of Reis-Bücklers' corneal dystrophy to chromosome 5q. Am J Ophthalmol 121:384–390, 1996.
23. Munier FL, Korvatska E, Djemai A, et al: Kerato-epithelin mutations in four 5q31-linked corneal dystrophies. Nature Genet 15:247–251, 1997.
24. Sandgren O, Holmgren G, Lundgren E: Vitreous amyloidosis associated with homozygosity for the transthyretin methionine-30 gene. Arch Ophthalmol 108:1584–1586, 1990.
25. Felbor U, Suvanto EA, Forsius HR, et al: Autosomal recessive Sorsby fundus dystrophy revisited: Molecular evidence for dominant inheritance. Am J Hum Genet 60:57–62, 1997.
26. Dryja TP, McGee TL, Reichel E, et al: A point mutation of the rhodopsin gene in one form of retinitis pigmentosa. Nature 343:364–366, 1990.
27. Li T, Snyder WK, Olsson JE, et al: Transgenic mice carrying the dominant rhodopsin mutation P347S: Evidence for defective vectorial transport of rhodopsin to the outer segments. Proc Natl Acad Sci USA 93:14176–14181, 1996.
28. Stacey A, Bateman J, Choi T, et al: Perinatal lethal osteogenesis imperfecta in transgenic mice bearing an engineered mutant pro-alpha 1(I) collagen gene. Nature 332:131–136, 1988.
29. Richards RI, Sutherland GR: Dynamic mutations: A new class of mutations causing human disease. Cell 70:709–712, 1992.
30. Myers RH, Madden JJ, Teague JL, et al: Factors related to onset age of Huntington disease. Am J Hum Genet 34:481–488, 1982.
31. Ranen NG, Stine OC, Abbott MH, et al: Anticipation and instability of IT-15 $(CAG)_n$ repeats in parent-offspring pairs with Huntington disease. Am J Hum Genet 57:593–602, 1995.
32. Spritz RA: Molecular genetics of oculocutaneous albinism. Hum Mol Genet 3:1469–1475, 1994.
33. Spritz RA, Strunk K, Giebel LB, et al: Detection of mutations in the tyrosinase gene in a patient with type IA oculocutaneous albinism. N Engl J Med 322:1724–1728, 1990.
34. Yanoff M, Kertesz Rahn E, Zimmerman LE: Histopathology of juvenile retinoschisis. Arch Ophthalmol 79:49–53, 1968.
35. Pawar H, Bingham EL, Lunetta KL, et al: Refined genetic mapping of juvenile X-linked retinoschisis. Hum Hered 45:206–210, 1995.
36. Sauer CG, Gehrig A, Warneke-Wittstock R, et al: Positional cloning of the gene associated with X-linked juvenile retinoschisis. Nature Genet 17:164–170, 1997.
37. Krill AE: X-chromosome-linked disease affecting the eye: Status of the heterozygote female. Trans Am Ophthalmol Soc 67:535–608, 1969.
38. McGuire RE, Sullivan LS, Blanton SH, et al: X-linked dominate cone-rod degeneration: Linkage mapping of a new locus for retinitis pigmentosa (RP15) to Xp22.13-p22.11. Am J Hum Genet 57:87–94, 1995.
39. Kajiwara K, Berson EL, Dryja TP: Digenic retinitis pigmentosa due to mutations at the unlinked peripherin/*RDS* and *ROM1* loci. Science 264:1604–1608, 1994.
40. Kajiwara K, Hahn LB, Mukai S, et al: Mutations in the human retinal degeneration slow gene in autosomal dominant retinitis pigmentosa. Nature 354:480–483, 1991.
41. Bascom RA, Schappert K, NcInnes: Cloning of the human and murine *ROM1* genes: Genomic organization and sequence conservation. Hum Mol Genet 2:385–391, 1993.
42. Wallace DC, Singh G, Lott MT, et al: Mitochondrial DNA mutation associated with Leber's hereditary optic neuropathy. Science 242:1427–1430, 1988.
43. Brown MD, Voljavec AS, Lott MT, et al: Leber's hereditary optic neuropathy; a model for mitochondrial neurodegenerative diseases. FASEB J 6:2791–2799, 1992.
44. Johns DR, Smith KH, Savino PJ, et al: Leber's hereditary optic neuropathy. Clinical manifestations of the 15257 mutation. Arch Ophthalmol 110:981–986, 1993.
45. Johns DR, Smith KH, Miller NR: Leber's hereditary optic neuropathy. Clinical manifestations of the 3460 mutation. Arch Ophthalmol 110:1577–1581, 1992.
46. Wiggs JL: Complex disorders in ophthalmology. Sem Ophthalmol 10:323–330, 1995.

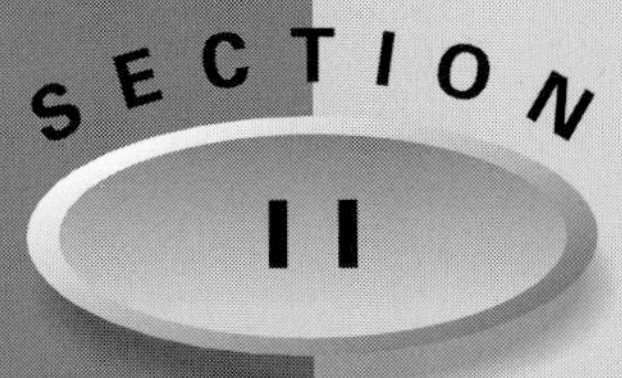

Immunology

Edited by

C. STEPHEN FOSTER AND J. WAYNE STREILEIN

CHAPTER 5

Immunology—An Overview

J. Wayne Streilein and C. Stephen Foster

All organisms live under the threat of attack from other living organisms. Among primitive single-celled eukaryotes, defense depends on physicochemical barriers at the cell surface and the capacity to engulf, phagocytize, and digest the attacking pathogen. As multicellular organisms evolved and individual cells assumed differentiated functions important to the well-being of the host, defense against invading pathogens became the responsibility of specialized cells and molecules. The multifaceted array of sophisticated cells and molecules of the mammalian immune system is the evolutionary descendant of these early forms of defense mechanisms.

The immune system found in mammals and higher vertebrates is divided into two functionally distinct components. One gives rise to innate immunity; the other provides adaptive immunity. Innate immunity is evolutionarily more ancient and provides the host organism with an immediate protective response. Adaptive immunity, by contrast, has arisen in early vertebrates and provides protection that takes time to develop, is remembered through time, and is exceedingly efficient. Whereas innate immunity has the capacity to recognize and respond to invading pathogens, the capacity to accurately distinguish between self-molecules and molecules of the pathogen (non-self) is much more highly developed in the adaptive immune system.

Innate Immunity

Innate, or natural, immunity consists of physicochemical barriers, erected at interfaces between the host and the environment, and a distinctive array of cells and molecules.[1–3] Intact body surfaces, such as skin with its stratum corneum and mucous membranes with tight junctions among adjacent epithelial lining cells, provide physical barriers to the entry of pathogens. In the case of the eye, mechanical phenomena such as the wiping action of eyelids or the bulk flow of tears across the ocular surface provide natural protection. The pH of body fluids, which include tears, and the chemical components of these fluids, including fatty acids, mucin, lysozyme, and complement components, make essential contributions to innate immunity. Finally, populations of bone marrow–derived cells, including neutrophils, macrophages, and natural killer cells, are mobilized in the natural defenses against invading pathogens.

Innate immunity is revealed when an invading bacterium, perhaps by releasing endotoxin, elicits a stereotypic inflammatory response in which microvascular dilatation, polymorphonuclear leukocytes, and serum complement proteins participate. Innate immunity is also revealed when a virus penetrates through the skin and evokes within the draining lymph node an accumulation of natural killer cells with the capacity to lyse virus-infected cells directly. In both of these examples, the cells and molecules responsible for innate immunity recognize and respond to the pathogen, but in neither case is the recognition specific for the particular organism. Moreover, if and when the attacker has been eliminated, the host is not protected against a second invasion from the same agent. Finally, the obligate inflammation associated with the innate immune response is poorly controlled, often excessive, and therefore damaging to surrounding host tissues.

Adaptive Immunity

Adaptive, or acquired, immunity depends on a highly developed, sophisticated set of lymphoid organs (thymus, spleen, lymph nodes, bone marrow, mucosa-associated lymphoid tissues), cells (T and B lymphocytes, antigen-presenting dendritic cells, and macrophages), and molecules (antibodies, cytokines, growth factors, and cell adhesion molecules).[1] The interactions between and among these elements allows the adaptive immune system to meet four important challenges:

1. To create a repertoire of recognition structures (antibodies by B cells, T cell receptors for antigen) that recognize all biologically important molecules in our universe
2. To eliminate or suppress lymphocytes whose recognition structures bind to self molecules and therefore threaten autoimmunity and autoimmune disease
3. To create a diversity of effector mechanisms designed to counter the diverse virulence strategies used by the many different potential pathogens
4. To fashion immune responses in individual organs and tissues such that protection is provided without interfering with the tissue's differentiated function

Cardinal Features of Adaptive Immunity

Certain features of the adaptive immune response set it apart from all other ways in which an organism can respond to its environment. First, adaptive immunity is acquired. Exposure of an adult individual to a foreign substance (antigen) for the first time leads to an immune response that is first detected (e.g., as antibody in the blood) within 5 to 7 days. During the "silent" interval after initial exposure, the adaptive immune system is "learning" about the presence of the antigen. Thus, adaptive immunity is **acquired.** Second, the immune response is absolutely specific for the eliciting antigen. The antibodies that form within 5 to 7 days react with eliciting antigen alone—not with any other molecule. Exposure of the same individual to a second (different) antigen elicits another antibody response that is absolutely specific for the second antigen and nonreactive with the first antigen. Thus, adaptive immunity is molecularly **specific.** Third, reexposure of an individual to an antigen for a second time elicits an antibody response that is accelerated in onset and exaggerated in amount—the so-called "anamnestic response." This means that what was **learned** by the immune system during its first exposure to an antigen is "remembered" through time, and the anamnestic response is the manifestation of that memory. Thus, adaptive immunity is "remembered." Fourth, adaptive immunity can be transferred from an individual who has it to another individual of the same species, thus conferring an identical immunity on the recipient. Both antibodies and specifically sensitized lymphocytes are capable of transferring adaptive immunity. Thus, adaptive immunity is **transferable.** Fifth, adaptive immunity can be specifically prevented by administering antigen under highly specialized, often experimental, conditions. Individuals treated with antigen in this manner may be rendered unable subsequently to acquire immunity to the same antigen if administered in a conventional fashion. Individuals rendered specifically unable to respond to a particular antigen are said to be immunologically **tolerant.** Thus, tolerance is a manifestation of adaptive immunity.

Benefits of Immunity

In mature mammals and higher vertebrates, both innate and adaptive immune systems exist. Virtually every immune response represents the summation of both innate and adaptive responses, and the two systems are inextricably entwined. Common sense dictates that these two complementary immune systems were designed evolutionarily to confer protection against exogenous and endogenous pathogens.[4] To describe briefly the interplay between innate and adaptive immunity, the following examples are given. Infection of the lung with *Streptococcus pneumoniae* is prevented from proceeding to consolidating pneumonia primarily by the innate immune response. Neutrophils and, to a lesser extent, macrophages form the primary defense system, aided by acute-phase reactants (e.g., C reactive protein) and members of the complement cascade of proteins. Adaptive immunity, in which *S. pneumoniae*–specific antibodies are produced, comes into play well after the primary infection has already been contained. However, reinfection with this organism rarely occurs, and antibodies play the key role in this protection. In influenza virus infections of the lung, natural killer cells act early to limit virus spread, but the infection appears to be terminated by virus-specific cytotoxic T cells that eliminate all virus-infected cells. In parasitic infections, where clearance and elimination of the organism may never be achieved, adaptive immunity plays the key role in containing the organism in situ.

While the importance of immunity in infectious disease is obvious, immunity is also believed to play a key role in the control of malignant neoplasms.[5, 6] Because tumors arise from host tissues, the antigenic differences between tumors (non-self) and self tissues are necessarily narrower. On the one hand, this makes it more difficult for the immune system to detect neoplastic cells, and, on the other hand, raises the possibility that immunity directed at antigens on tumor cells may spill over onto normal tissues because of shared antigenic moieties.

Hazards of Immunity

There are two important ways in which immunity proves to be a disservice to the host. First, most (if not all) immune responses that lead to elimination of a pathogen require the participation of nonspecific host defense mechanisms. Because they lack the high specificity of antibodies and T lymphocytes, neutrophils, macrophages, and natural killer cells are incapable of confining their destructive forces to pathogenic organisms. Similarly, activated proteases of the complement system are indiscriminate in their choice of substrates at the site of infection. Thus, host tissues adjacent to an infection are usually damaged, sometimes irreparably, by the intense inflammation taking place in their midst. This penchant for natural immunity to cause unwanted tissue damage is further enhanced by cells and molecules of the adaptive immune system.[1] The T cells that mediate delayed hypersensitivity secrete cytokines, which are powerful attractants and stimulants of macrophages. As a consequence, tissue injury and death is almost an invariant outcome of delayed hypersensitivity responses directed at infecting pathogens. Similarly, complement-fixing antibodies recruit and amplify the participation of neutrophils and macrophages at the site where they bind target pathogens, leading to exaggerated inflammation and necrosis. Thus, immunity can inadvertently produce injury to otherwise healthy host tissues, and immunopathogenic mechanisms are important causes of disease in many different organs and tissues.

Second, the adaptive immune response must meet the challenge of eliminating or suppressing T and B cells with recognition structures specific for self-antigens.[7] When this challenge is not met, autoimmunity can arise. In truth, not all autoimmunity is deleterious. Experimental and clinical evidence suggests that immunity against certain self-components may be a necessary part of the healing response to injury and infection. However, certain types of autoimmunity are destructive, and these can give rise to tissue-restricted inflammatory diseases. A hierarchy of self-antigens exists, dictated by the extent to which the antigens are accessible to lymphocytes of the systemic immune apparatus. For instance, circulating plasma proteins have an extremely low potential for evoking an autoimmune response. By contrast, proteins expressed on cells found only in the eye (e.g., photoreceptors) or testis (spermatozoa) have a high potential for eliciting an autoimmune response. In addition, tissue-restricted factors (e.g., blood:tissue barriers) influence whether a response that is autoimmune becomes immunopathogenic and therefore causes disease.

Special Case of the Eye: Immune Privilege

Most organs of the body can sustain substantial amounts of permanent damage from inflammatory reactions without losing significant amounts of function. For example, inflammation in skin, brain, heart, liver, kidney, and bone will be associated with the typical consequences of inflammation—damage to the normal cells of the organ and scarring from the compensatory reparative processes associated with injury. These organs are very forgiving in that they can each sustain substantial amounts of inflammation (provided that it is temporary) and still retain sufficient viability after the reparative processes to carry on the normal functions required for normal living activities. The same is not true for the eye.

Inflammation that in other tissues would be trivial is not tolerated by the eye. The vulnerability of the eye to even small amounts of inflammation derives from the need to preserve the anatomic integrity of the visual axis. Very slight alterations in components of the visual axis prevent light images from landing precisely on the retina, and blindness is the inevitable consequence. Thus, innocent bystander damage to ocular tissues during the course of inflammation is associated with a profound loss of function (i.e., blindness or substantial impairment of useful vision). Even slight temporary inflammation in the central part of the cornea can have substantial, long-term effects on functional visual acuity after resolution of the inflammation, simply because the reparative processes result in disorganization of the normally ordered arrangement of collagen fibrils within the corneal stroma, an organization that is critical to continued clarity in the cornea. Similarly, inflammation involving the retina (especially the macula), the vitreous, and the iris/ciliary body can also produce significant loss in visual function.

Thus, the eye is confronted with a dilemma. On the one hand, the eye needs to be protected from harmful agents such as microbes, and therefore the eye needs participation of the immune system in withstanding such invasions. On the other hand, immunity, whether innate or adaptive, is necessarily mediated in part by nonspecific host defense mechanisms that carry the threat of innocent bystander injury. To resolve this dilemma evolutionarily, the eye and the immune system have arranged a compromise in which certain forms of immunity are permitted, whereas others are suppressed. This compromise is expressed experimentally in the phenomenon of immune privilege.[8] It has been known for more than a century that foreign tissues implanted in the anterior chamber of the eye enjoyed prolonged survival compared with the fate of foreign tissues implanted at conventional body sites. In the 1950s, Medawar[9] correctly inferred that the ability of foreign grafts to survive in the eye was due to a failure of immunologic rejection. At the time, it was known that the eye lacked lymphatic vessels and contained a blood-ocular barrier. Medawar proposed that immune privilege resulted from sequestration of intraocular antigenic material from the systemic immune apparatus. The term *immunologic ignorance* has been used to identify this situation.

The past 25 years have witnessed a "renaissance" in our understanding of the phenomenon of immune privilege, and it is now clear that immunologic ignorance can only account for a small portion of this effect. Immune privilege is an actively acquired and maintained state in which ocular factors, acting on cells of the immune system, suppress the expression of immunity within the eye and alter the induction of systemic immunity to ocular antigens, leading to a stereotypic systemic immune response called *anterior chamber associated immune deviation (ACAID)*.[10] As a consequence, systemic immune responses to eye-derived antigens are deficient in T cells that mediate delayed hypersensitivity and in antibodies that activate complement components. At the same time, other immune effectors (e.g., cytotoxic T cells) and non–complement-fixing antibodies are enhanced. Thus, systemic immunity engendered by eye-derived antigens lacks the two effector modalities most closely linked to intense inflammation and innocent bystander injury—delayed hypersensitivity and complement-fixing antibodies.

It is important to emphasize that immune privilege in the eye is not simply the consequence of a completely failed immune response; rather, immune privilege results from stereotypic modifications in the immune response that afford immune protection for the eye that carries a minimal threat to nonspecific injury leading to blindness. The importance of this understanding lies in the implications that it holds for the diagnosis and treatment of ocular inflammatory and infectious disorders. The simple expedient of indiscriminate generalized suppression of inflammation, such as through the use of systemic or regional steroid therapy, is no longer the standard of care in modern societies. Rather, the logical pursuit of the underlying diagnosis, or at the very least, the pursuit of an understanding of the basic mechanisms of the patient's inflammation is what is required today, with subsequent selection of treatment based on the diagnosis and immunologic mechanisms responsible for the inflammation.

The sections and chapters that follow are designed to convince ophthalmologists of the value of this approach to the care of patients with inflammatory eye disease and are intended to provide an understanding of the basics of general immunology and of ocular immunology in particular.

REFERENCES

1. Janeway CA Jr, Travers P (eds): Immunobiology: The Immune System in Health and Disease, 3rd ed. New York, Current Biology, Ltd./Garland Publishing, Inc., 1997.
2. Fearon DT, Locksley RM: The instinctive role of innate immunity in the acquired immune response. Science 272:50, 1996.
3. Gallin JI, Goldstein IM, Snyderman R (eds): Inflammation—Basic Principles and Clinical Correlates, 2nd ed. New York, Raven Press, 1992.
4. Gibbons RJ: How microorganisms cause disease. *In* Gorbach SL, Bartlett JD, Blacklow NR (eds): Infectious Diseases. Philadelphia, WB Saunders, 1992.
5. Moller G: Tumor immunology. Immunol Rev 145:1, 1995.
6. Roth C, Rochlitz C, Kourilsky P: Immune response against tumors. Adv Immunol 57:281, 1994.
7. Burnet FM: The Clonal Selection Theory of Acquired Immunity. London, Cambridge University Press, 1959.
8. Streilein JW: Perspective: Unraveling immune privilege. Science 270:1158, 1995.
9. Medawar PB: Immunity to homologous grafted skin. III: The fate of skin homografts transplanted to the brain, to subcutaneous tissue, and to the anterior chamber of the eye. Br J Exp Pathol 29:58, 1948.
10. Streilein JW: Immune regulation and the eye: A dangerous compromise. FASEB J 1:199, 1987.

CHAPTER 6

A Cast of Thousands: The Cells of the Immune System

C. Stephen Foster

The cellular components of the immune system include lymphocytes, macrophages, Langerhans' cells, neutrophils, eosinophils, basophils, and mast cells. Many of these cell types can be further subdivided by subtypes and subsets. For example, lymphocytes include T lymphocytes, B lymphocytes, and non-T, non-B (null) lymphocytes. Each type can be further subcategorized, both by functional differences and by differences in cell surface glycoprotein specializations and uniqueness. The latter differentiating aspect of cell types and cell-type subsets has been made possible through the development of hybridoma-monoclonal antibody technology and through the pioneering work of Ortho Pharmaceuticals in collaboration with Dr. Stuart Schlossman and associates at Harvard Medical School. This phenomenon of cell surface glycoprotein specialization and uniqueness among cell types, and the technology for identifying those unique differences among cell types, are so important that a synopsis of the evolution and current understanding of this phenomenon follows.

Jeorges Kohler and Cesar Milstein, at Cambridge University, succeeded in immortalizing antibody-producing cells in 1975 by fusing them with myeloma tumor cells using a myeloma cell line with a selective deficiency of hypoxanthine phosphoribosyltransferase.[1] These researchers developed a technique for successfully recovering only the cells that had successfully fused to the myeloma cells (i.e., the hybridomas). Only the hybridoma cells survived in a tissue culture medium containing hypoxanthine, aminopterin, and thymidine, because the antibody-forming cell component of the hybridoma contributed enough hypoxanthine phosphoribosyltransferase to ensure survival of the hybrid. Selecting individual hybrids that produce the desired antibody against a particular immunogen (antigen or antigenic determinant or epitope) and then allowing that hybrid cell (hybridoma) to proliferate generated an immortal monoclonal cell population (i.e., a hybrid cell population derived from a single original cell) and thus produced a never-ending supply of highly specific antibody (monoclonal antibody) directed against the original immunogen of interest. For this innovative and important work, these researchers were awarded the Nobel Prize for Medicine in 1984.

Reinherz and Schlossman[2] exploited the monoclonal antibody technology in the late 1970s, first taking advantage of the fact that T lymphocytes possess well-known, unique cell surface determinants (e.g., a binding receptor for sheep erythrocytes), which made it possible to separate T lymphocytes into pure preparations from peripheral blood lymphocytes. Immunization of mice with such a purified preparation of T cells, with subsequent preparation of hybridomas from spleen cell populations harvested from those immunized mice, was followed by screening and selection of hybridomas that synthesize antibodies that would stick to the cell surface of T cells and by cloning of these hybridomas. This same strategy or similar strategies based on functional assays (e.g., beginning with cells that were efficient at helping an immune response to develop or beginning with cells that efficiently suppressed an immune response) resulted in the additional development of monoclonal antibody reagents that were specific for and identified the two major T lymphocyte subsets, helper-inducer T cells and suppressor-cytotoxic T cells.

Because the original work was performed in collaboration with Ortho Pharmaceuticals, the original designation of the cell surface determinants for T cells was OKT 3, the designation for helper-inducer T cells was OKT 4, and that for suppressor-cytotoxic T cells was OKT 8. As additional companies began to develop their reagents using the same technology, additional naming schemes developed, and the name game for cell surface determinants became extremely complicated. Investigator workshops have now generated a universal nomenclature system for cell surface glycoproteins, or "antigens," and this system is based on the so-called clusters of differentiation designation. Hence, the proper designation for the cell surface glycoprotein unique to T cells is now CD3, and the designation for the cell surface glycoprotein unique to helper/inducer T cells is CD4. Table 6–1 presents a partial list of current clusters of differentiation designations and the cell types that express these CD antigens.

Lymphocytes

Lymphocytes are mononuclear cells, round, 7 to 8 μm in diameter, found in lymphoid tissue (lymph node, spleen, thymus, gut-associated lymphoid tissue, mammary-associated lymphoid tissue, and conjunctiva-associated lymphoid tissue) and in blood. They ordinarily constitute approximately 30% of the total peripheral white blood cell count. The lymphocyte is the premier character in the immune drama; it is the primary recognition unit for foreign material, the principal specific effector cell type in immune reactions, and the cell exclusively responsible for immune memory.

T lymphocytes, or thymus-derived cells, compose 65 to 80% of the peripheral blood lymphocyte population, 30 to 50% of the splenocyte population, and 70 to 85% of the lymph node cell population. B lymphocytes compose 5 to 15% of peripheral blood lymphocytes, 20 to 30% of splenocytes, and 10 to 20% of lymph node cells.

TABLE 6–1. **Clusters of Differentiation (CD) Designations**

Clusters	Cell Specificity	Function
CD1	Thymocytes, Langerhans' cells	
CD2	T cells, NK subset	CD58 receptor/sheep erythrocyte receptor; adhesion molecule—binds to LFA-3
CD3	T cells	T-cell antigen-complex receptor
CD4	Helper-inducer T cells	MHC class II immune recognition; HIV receptor
CD5	T cells, B-cell subset	
CD6	T cell, subset	?
CD7	T cells, NK cells, platelets	?Fc receptor IgM
CD8	Cytotoxic suppressor T cells	MHC class I immune recognition
CD9	Pre-B cells	?
CD10	Pre-B cells, neutrophils	Neutrophil endopeptidase
CD11a	Leukocytes	Adhesion molecule (LFA-1) binds to ICAM-1
CD11b	Monocytes, granulocytes, NK cells	α-Chain of complement receptor CR3
CD11c	Monocytes, granulocytes, NK cells	Adhesion
CD13	Monocytes, granulocytes	Aminopeptidase N
CD14	Macrophages	Lipopolysaccharide receptor
CD15	Neutrophils, activated T cells	
CD16	Granulocytes, macrophages, NK cells	Fc receptor IgG (Fc-γ RIII); activation of NK cells
CD19	B cells	B-cell activation
CD20	B cells	B-cell activation
CD21	B cells	Complement receptor CR2—Epstein-Barr virus receptor
CD22	B cells	Adhesion; B-cell activation
CD23	Activated B cells, macrophages	Low-affinity Fc-ϵ receptor, induced by IL-4
CD25	Activated T cells, B cells	IL-2 receptor
CD28	T cells	Receptor for co-stimulator molecules B7.1 and B7.2
CD30	Activated B and T cells	?
CD31	Platelets, monocytes, and B cells	Role in leukocyte-endothelial adhesion
CD32	B lymphocytes, granulocytes, macrophages, eosinophils	Fc receptor IgG (Fc-γRIII) ADCC
CD35	B cells, erythrocytes, neutrophils, mononuclear cells	Complement receptor CR1
CD37	B cells	
CD38	Activated T and plasma cells	?
CD40	B cells	B-cell activation by T-cell contact
CD41	Megakaryocytes, platelets	Gp11b/111a platelet aggregation; Fn receptor
CD42	Megakaryocytes, platelets	Gp1b—platelet adhesion
CD43	Leukocytes	T-cell activation
CD44	Leukocytes	Pgp1 (Hermes) receptor; homing receptor for matrix components (e.g., hyaluronate)
CD45	All leukocytes	Leukocyte common antigen—signal transduction (tyrosine phosphatase)
CD45RA	Naive cells	
CD45RO	Activated/memory T cells	
CD45RB	B cells	
CD49 (VLA)	T cells, monocytes	Adhesion to collagen, laminin, Fn, VCAM
CD54 (ICAM-1)	Activated cells	Adhesion to LFA-1 and MAC-1
CD56	NK	NCAM—adhesion
CD58 (LFA-3)	B cells, antigen-presenting cells	Binds to CD2
CD62E E-selectin, ELAM-1	Endothelial cells	Adhesion
CD62L L-selectin, LAM-1	T cells	Adhesion
CD62P P-selectin, PADGEM	Platelets, endothelial cells	Adhesion
CD64	Monocytes, macrophages	Adhesion, FC-γ receptor; antibody-dependent, cell-mediated cytotoxicity
CD69	Activated lymphocytes	
CD71	Proliferating cells	Transferrin receptor
CD72	B cells	Ligand for CD5; B cell–T cell interactions
CD80 (B7-1)	B cells, dendritic cells, macrophages	Ligand for CD28; co-stimulator for T-cell activation
CD89 (Fc-α receptor)	Neutrophils, monocytes	IgA-dependent cytotoxicity
CD95 (Fas)	Multiple cell types	Role in programmed cell death
CD102 (ICAM-2)	Endothelial cells, monocytes	Ligand for LFA-1 integrin
CD103 (HML-1)	T cells	Role in T cell homing to mucosae
CD106 (VCAM-1)	Endothelial cells, macrophages	Receptor for VLA-4 integrin; adhesion

ELAM, endothelial leukocyte adhesion molecule; LAM, leukocyte adhesion molecule; MAC, macrophage; HIV, human immunodeficiency virus; ICAM, intercellular adhesion molecule; IL, interleukin; LPS, lipopolysaccharide; NCAM, neutrophil cellular adhesion molecule; NK, natural killer; MHC, major histocompatibility complex; LFA, $\alpha_2\beta_2$-integrins; VCAM, vascular cellular adhesion molecule; VLA, $\alpha_2\beta_1$-integrins.

T cells possess cell surface receptors for sheep erythrocytes and for the plant-derived mitogens concanavalin A and phytohemagglutinin. They do not possess surface immunoglobulin or surface membrane receptors for the Fc portion of antibody—two notable cell surface differences from B lymphocytes, which do possess these two entities. B cells also exhibit cell surface receptors for the third component of complement, for the Epstein-Barr virus, and for the plant mitogen known as pokeweed mitogen, as well as for the purified protein derivative of *Mycobacterium tuberculosis* and for lipopolysaccharide.

Null cells are lymphocytes that possess none of the aforementioned cell surface antigens characteristic of T cells or B cells. This cell population is heterogeneous, and some authorities include natural killer (NK) cells among the null cell population even though the origin of NK cells appears to be in monocyte/macrophage precursor lines rather than the lymphocyte lineage. Nonetheless, the morphologic characteristics and behaviors of NK cells, along with the ambiguity of their origin, allow one license to include them under the null cell rubric. NK cells are nonadherent (unlike macrophages, they do not stick to the surface of plastic tissue culture dishes) mononuclear cells present in peripheral blood, spleen, and lymph node. The most notable function of these cells is killing of transformed (malignant) cells and virus-infected cells. Because they do this without prior sensitization, they are an important component of the early natural response in the immune system. The cytotoxicity of NK cells is not major histocompatibility complex (MHC)-restricted, a dramatic contrast with cytotoxic T cells. (More about the MHC and the products of those gene loci later.) The large granules present in NK cells (the cells are sometimes called large granular lymphocytes) contain perforin and perhaps other cell membrane–lysing enzymes, and it is the enzymes in these granules that are responsible for the lethal-hit cytolysis for which NK cells are famous.

Killer cells are the other notable null cell subpopulation. These cells do have receptors for the Fc portion of immunoglobulin G (IgG) and thus can attach themselves to the Fc portion of IgG molecules. Through this receptor, they are a primary cell responsible for the cytolysis in the so-called antibody-dependent, cell-mediated cytotoxicity reaction. These cells probably participate in type II Gell and Coombs hypersensitivity reactions and are involved in immune removal of cellular antigens when the target cell is too large to be phagocytosed.

It is clear that both B cells and T cells can be further divided into specialized subsets. B cells, for example, are subdivided into the B cells that synthesize the five separate classes of immunoglobulin (IgG, IgA, IgM, IgD, and IgE). All B cells initially produce IgM specific for an antigenic determinant (epitope) to which it has responded, but some subsequently switch from synthesis of IgM to synthesis of other immunoglobulin classes. The details of the control of antibody synthesis and class switching are covered in Chapter 8 (B Lymphocyte Responses). Less known is the fact that functionally distinct subsets of B cells exist, in addition to the different B cells in terms of antibody class synthesis. The field of B-cell diversity analysis is embryonic, but it is clear that the exploitation of monoclonal antibody technology will distinguish, with increasingly fine specificity, differences in B-cell subpopulations. It is clear, for example, that a subpopulation of B lymphocytes possess the CD5 glycoprotein on the cell surface plasma membrane (a CD glycoprotein not ordinarily present on B lymphocytes but rather on the cell surface of T cells).[3] These cells appear to be associated with autoantibody production.[4]

It is also clear now that B cells are functionally important as antigen-presenting cells (APCs), a fact that startles most physicians who studied immunology before 1991. T-cell receptors (TCRs) cannot react with native antigen; rather they respond to processed antigenic determinants of that antigen. APCs phagocytose the antigen, process it, and display denatured, limited peptide sequences of the native antigen on the cell surface of the APC in association with cell surface class II MHC glycoproteins. B cells, as well as classic APCs, such as macrophages and Langerhans' cells, can perform this function. The antigen is endocytosed by the B cell and processed in the B-cell endosome (possibly through involvement of cathepsin D) to generate short, denatured peptide fragments, which are then transported to the B-cell surface bound to class II glycoprotein peptides, where the antigenic peptides are "presented" to CD4 helper T lymphocytes.

Finally, regarding B-cell heterogeneity, it is becoming apparent that some B lymphocytes also have suppressor or regulatory activity. The emerging data on B-cell functional and cell surface heterogeneity will be exciting to follow in the coming years.

Much more widely recognized, of course, is that subsets of T lymphocytes exist. Helper (CD4) T cells "help" in the induction of an immune response, in the generation of an antibody response, and in the generation of other, more specialized components of the immune response. Cytotoxic (CD8) T cells, as the name implies, are involved in cell killing or cytotoxic reactions. Delayed-type hypersensitivity (CD4) T cells are the classic participants in the chronic inflammatory responses characteristic of certain antigens such as the mycobacteria. Regulatory T cells (CD8) are responsible for modulating immune responses, preventing uncontrolled, host-damaging inflammatory responses. It is even likely that there are sub-subsets of these T cells. Excellent evidence exists, for example, that there are at least three subsets of regulatory T cells and at least two subsets of helper T cells.

Mosmann and Coffman[5] described two types of helper (CD4) T cells with differential cytokine production profiles. T_H1 cells secrete interleukin-2 (IL-2) and interferon-γ (IFN-γ) but do not secrete IL-4 or IL-5, whereas T_H2 cells secrete IL-4, IL-5, IL-10, and IL-13, but not IL-2 or IFN-γ. Furthermore, T_H1 cells can be cytolytic and can assist B cells with IgG, IgM, and IgA synthesis but not IgE synthesis. T_H2 cells are not cytolytic but can help B cells with IgE synthesis as well as with IgG, IgM, and IgA production.[6] It is becoming clear that CD4 T_H1 or CD4 T_H2 cells are selected in infection and in autoimmune diseases. Thus, T_H1 cells accumulate in the thyroid of patients with autoimmune thyroiditis,[7] whereas T_H2 cells accumulate in the conjunctiva of patients with vernal conjunctivitis.[8] The T cells that respond to *M. tuberculosis* protein are primarily T_H1 cells, whereas those that respond to *Toxocara canis* antigens are T_H2 cells. Romagnani has proposed that T_H1 cells are preferentially "selected" as participants in inflammatory reactions associated with delayed-type hypersensitivity reactions and low antibody production (as in contact dermatitis or tuberculosis), and T_H2 cells are preferentially selected in inflammatory reactions associated with persistent antibody production, including allergic responses in which IgE production is prominent.[9] Further, it is now clear that these two major CD4 T-lymphocyte subsets regulate each other through their cytokines. Thus, T_H2 CD4 lymphocyte cytokines (notably IL-10) inhibit T_H1 CD4 lymphocyte proliferation and cytokine secretion, and T_H1 CD4 lymphocyte cytokines (notably IFN-γ) inhibit T_H2 CD4 lymphocyte proliferation and cytokine production.

Macrophages

The macrophage ("large eater") is the preeminent professional APC. These cells are 12 to 15 μm in diameter, the largest of the lymphoid cells. They possess a high density of class II MHC glycoproteins on their cell surface, along with receptors for complement components, the Fc portion of Ig molecules, receptors for fibronectin, interferons-α, -β, and -γ, IL-1, tumor necrosis factor, and macrophage colony-stimulating factor. These cells are widely distributed throughout various tissues (when found in tissue, they are called histiocytes), and the microenvironment of the tissue profoundly influences the extent of expression of the various cell surface glycoproteins as well as the intracellular metabolic characteristics. It is clear that further compartmentalization of macrophage subtypes occurs in the spleen. Macrophages that express a high density of class II MHC glycoproteins are present in red pulp, and macrophages with significantly less surface class II MHC glycoprotein expression are in the marginal zone, where intimate contact with B cells exists. It is likely that just as in the murine system,[10] in humans one subclass of macrophage preferentially presents antigen to one particular subset of helper T cell responsible for induction of regulatory T-cell activation, whereas a different subset of macrophage preferentially presents antigen to a different helper T-cell subset responsible for cytotoxic or delayed-type hypersensitivity effector functions.

Macrophages also participate more generally in inflammatory reactions. They are members of the natural (early defense) immune system and are incredibly potent in their capacity to synthesize and secrete a variety of powerful biologic molecules, including proteases, collagenase, angiotensin-converting enzyme, lysozyme, IFN-α, IFN-β, IL-6, tumor necrosis factor-α, fibronectin, transforming growth factor-β, platelet-derived growth factor, macrophage colony-stimulating factor, granulocyte-stimulating factor, granulocyte-macrophage colony-stimulating factor, platelet-activating factor, arachidonic acid derivatives (prostaglandins and leukotrienes), and oxygen metabolites (oxygen free radicals, peroxide anion, and hydrogen peroxide). These cells are extremely important, even pivotal, participants in inflammatory reactions and are especially important in chronic inflammation. The epithelioid cell typical of so-called granulomatous inflammatory reactions evolves from the tissue histiocyte, and multinucleated giant cells form through fusion of many epithelioid cells.

Specialized macrophages exist in certain tissues and organs, including the Kupffer cell of the liver, dendritic histiocytes in lymphoid organs, interdigitating reticulum cells in lymphoid organs, and Langerhans' cells in skin, lymph nodes, conjunctiva, and cornea.

Langerhans' cells are particularly important to the ophthalmologist. They probably are the premier APC for the external eye. Derived from bone marrow macrophage precursors, like macrophages, their function is basically identical to that of the macrophage in antigen presentation. They are rich in cell surface class II MHC glycoproteins and have cell surface receptors for the third component of complement and for the Fc portion of IgG. Langerhans' cells are abundant in the mucosal epithelium of the mouth, esophagus, vagina, and conjunctiva. They are also abundant at the corneoscleral limbus, less so in the peripheral cornea; they are normally absent from the central third of the cornea.[11] If the center of the cornea is provoked through trauma or infection, the peripheral cornea Langerhans' cells quickly "stream" into the center of the cornea.[12] These CD1-positive dendritic cells possess a characteristic racket-shaped cytoplasmic granule on ultrastructural analysis, the Birbeck granule, whose function is unknown.

Polymorphonuclear Leukocytes

Polymorphonuclear leukocytes (PMNs) are part of the natural immune system. They are central to host defense through phagocytosis, but if they accumulate in excessive numbers, persist, and are activated in an uncontrolled manner, the result may be deleterious to host tissues. As the name suggests, they contain a multilobed nucleus and many granules. PMNs are subcategorized as neutrophils, basophils, or eosinophils, depending on the differential staining of their granules.

NEUTROPHILS

Neutrophils account for more than 90% of the circulating granulocytes. They possess surface receptors for the Fc portion of IgG (CD16) and for complement components, including C5a (important in chemotaxis) and CR1 (CD35) and CR3 (CD11b) (important in adhesion and phagocytosis). When appropriately stimulated by chemotactic agents (complement components, fibrinolytic and kinin system components, and products from other leukocytes, platelets, and certain bacteria), neutrophils move from blood to tissues through margination (adhesion to receptors or adhesion molecules on vascular endothelial cells) and diapedesis (movement through the capillary wall). Neutrophils release the contents of their primary (azurophilic) granules (lysosomes) and secondary (specific) granules (Table 6–2) into an endocytic vacuole, resulting in: (1) phagocytosis of a microorganism or tissue injury, (2) type II antibody-dependent, cell-mediated cytotoxicity, or (3) type III hypersensitivity reactions (immune complex–mediated disease). Secondary granules release collagenase, which mediates collagen degradation. Aside from the products secreted by the granules, neutrophils produce arachidonic acid metabolites (prostaglandins and leukotrienes) as well as oxygen free radical derivatives.

EOSINOPHILS

Eosinophils constitute 3 to 5% of the circulating PMNs. They possess surface receptors for the Fc portion of IgE

TABLE 6–2. **Neutrophil Granules and Their Contents**

Azurophil Granules	Specific Granules	Other Granules
Myeloperoxidase	Alkaline phosphatase	Acid phosphatase
Acid phosphatase	Histaminase	Heparinase
5′-Nucleotidase	Collagenase	β-Glucosaminidase
Lysozyme	Lysozyme	α-Mannosidase
Elastase	Vitamin B_{12}-binding proteins	Acid proteinase
Cathepsins B, D, G	Plasminogen activator	Elastase gelatinase
	Lactoferrin	
Proteinase 3		Glycosaminoglycans
β-Glycerophosphatase		
β-Glucuronidase		
N-acetyl-β-glucosaminidase	Cytochrome	
α-Mannosidase		
Arylsulfatase		
α-Fucosidase		
Esterase		
Histonase		
Cationic proteins		
Defensins		
Bactericidal permeability-increasing protein (BPI)		
Glycosaminoglycans		

(low affinity) and IgG (CD16) and for complement components, including C5a, CR1 (CD35), and CR3 (CD11b). Eosinophils play a special role in allergic conditions and parasitoses. They also participate in type III hypersensitivity reactions or immune complex–mediated disease following attraction to the inflammatory area by products from mast cells (eosinophil chemotactic factor of anaphylaxis), complement, and other cytokines from other inflammatory cells. Eosinophils release the contents of their granules to the outside of the cell after fusion of the intracellular granules with the plasma membrane (degranulation). Table 6–3 shows the known secretory products of eosinophils; the role these products of inflammation play, even in nonallergic diseases (such as Wegener's granulomatosis), is underappreciated.

BASOPHILS

Basophils account for less than 0.2% of the circulating granulocytes. They possess surface receptors for the Fc portion of IgE (high affinity) and IgG (CD16) and for complement components, including C5a, CR1 (CD35), and CR3 (CD11b). Their role, other than perhaps as tissue mast cells, is unclear.

TABLE 6–3. **Granular Contents of Eosinophils**

Lysosomal hydrolases	Cathepsin
Arylsulfatase	Histaminase
β-Glucuronidase	Peroxisomes
Acid phosphatase	Major basic proteins
β-Glycerophosphatase	Eosinophil cationic protein
Ribonuclease	Eosinophil peroxidases
Proteinases	Phospholipases
Collagenase	Lysophospholipases

Mast Cells

The mast cell is indistinguishable from the basophil in many respects, particularly its contents. There are at least two classes of mast cells based on their neutral protease composition, T-lymphocyte dependence, ultrastructural characteristics, and predominant arachidonic acid metabolites (Table 6–4). Mucosa-associated mast cells (MMC or MC-T) contain primarily tryptase as the major protease (hence, some authors designate these MC-T, or mast cells-tryptase) and prostaglandin D_2 as the primary product of arachidonic acid metabolism. MMCs are T-cell–dependent for growth and

TABLE 6–4. **Mast Cell Types and Characteristics**

Characteristic	Mucosal Mast Cell (MC-T, MMC)	Connective Tissue Mast Cell (MC-TC, CTMC)
Morphology		
Size	Small, pleomorphic	Large, uniform
Nucleus	Unilobed or bilobed	Unilobed
Granules	Few	Many
Location	Gut	Peritoneum, skin
Histochemistry		
Protease	Tryptase	Tryptase and chymase
Proteoglycans	Chondroitin sulfate	Heparin
Histamine	<1 pg/cell	≥15 pg/cell
IgE	Surface and cytoplasmic	Surface
Formalin sensitive	Yes	No
In Vitro Effect of:		
Compound 48/80	Proliferation	Degranulation
Polymyxin	Proliferation	Degranulation
Life Span	≤40 days	>40 days
Proliferation	Thymus-dependent	Thymus-independent
Secretagogues		
Antigen	Yes	Yes
Anti-IgE	Yes	Yes
Compound 48/80	No	Yes
Bee venom	No	Yes
Con A	Yes	Yes
Staining		
Alcian blue	Yes	Yes
Safranin	No	Yes
Berberine sulfate	No	Yes
Antiallergic Compounds		
Cromoglycate	No	Yes
Theophylline	No	Yes
Doxantrile	Yes	Yes
Enhancement of Secretion		
Phosphatidyl serine	No	Yes
Adenosine	Yes	Yes
Predominant Arachidonic Acid Metabolite	Prostaglandin D_2	Leukotrienes B_4, C_4, D_4
Ultrastructural Features of Granules	Lattice	Scroll

TABLE 6–5. **Mast Cell Contents**

Histamine
Serotonin
Rat mast-cell protease I and II
Heparin
Chondroitin sulfate
β-Hexosaminidase
β-Glucuronidase
β-D-Galactosidase
Arylsulfatase
Eosinophil chemotactic factor for anaphylaxis (ECF-A)
Slow reactive substance of anaphylaxis (SRS-A)
High molecular weight neutrophil chemotactic factor
Arachidonic acid derivatives
Platelet-activating factor

development (specifically IL-3–dependent), and they are located predominantly in mucosal stroma (e.g., gut). MMCs are small and short-lived (< 40 days). They contain chondroitin sulfate but not heparin, and their histamine content is modest (Table 6–5). MMCs degranulate in response to antigen-IgE triggering but not to exposure to compound 48/80, and they are not stabilized by disodium cromoglycate. They are formalin-sensitive, so formalin fixation of tissue eliminates or greatly reduces our ability to find these cells by staining technique. With special fixation techniques, MMC granules stain with alcian blue but not with safranin.

Connective tissue mast cells (CTMCs) contain both tryptase and chymase (so some authors designate them MC-TC), as well as leukotrienes B_4, C_4, and D_4, as the primary products of arachidonic acid metabolism. CTMCs are T-cell–independent. They are larger than MMCs and are located principally in skin and at mucosal interfaces with the environment. They contain heparin and large amounts of histamine, and they degranulate in response to compound 48/80 in addition to antigen-IgE interactions. CTMCs are stabilized by disodium cromoglycate. They stain with alkaline Giemsa, toluidine blue, alcian blue, safranin, and berberine sulfate.

The ultrastructural characteristics of MMCs and CTMCs are also different. Electron microscopy shows that the granules of MMCs contain lattice-like structures; the granules of CTMCs contain scroll-like structures. Mast cells play a special role in allergic reactions—they are the preeminent cell in the allergy drama. They also can participate in type II, III, and IV hypersensitivity reactions, however. Their role in these reactions, aside from notable vascular effects, is not well understood. Non–IgE-mediated mechanisms (e.g., C5a) can trigger mast cells to release histamine, platelet-activating factor, and other biologic molecules when antigen binds to two adjacent IgE molecules on the mast cell surface. Histamine and other vasoactive amines cause increased vascular permeability, allowing immune complexes to become trapped in the vessel wall.

Platelets

Blood platelets, cells well adapted for blood clotting, also are involved in the immune response to injury, a reflection of their evolutionary heritage as myeloid (inflammatory) cells. They possess surface receptors for the Fc portion of IgG (CD16) and IgE (low affinity), for class I histocompatibility glycoproteins (human leukocyte antigen-A, -B, or -C), and for factor VIII. They also carry molecules such as Gp11b/111a (CDw41), which bind fibrinogen, and Gp1b (CDw42), which binds von Willebrand's factor.

After endothelial injury, platelets adhere to and aggregate at the endothelial surface, releasing permeability-increasing molecules from their granules (Table 6–6). Endothelial injury may be caused by type III hypersensitivity. Platelet-activating factor released by mast cells after antigen-IgE antibody complex formation induces platelets to aggregate and release their vasoactive amines. These amines separate endothelial cell tight junctions and allow the immune complexes to enter the vessel wall. Once the immune complexes are deposited, they initiate an inflammatory reaction through activation of complement components and neutrophil lysosomal enzyme release.

Ontogeny of the Immune System

Cells of the hematologic system are derived from primordial stem cell precursors of the bone marrow. Embryonically, these cells originate in the blood islands of the yolk sac.[13] These cells populate embryonic liver and bone marrow.[14] All the blood elements are derived from these primordial stem cells: erythrocytes, platelets, PMNs, monocytes, and lymphocytes. These primordial stem cells are pluripotential, and the exact details of the influences that are responsible for a particular pluripotential primordial stem cell's evolving along one differentiation pathway (e.g., into a monocyte) as opposed to some other differentiation pathway (e.g., into a lymphocyte) are incompletely understood. It appears, however, that special characteristics of the microenvironment in the bone marrow, particularly with respect to the association with other resident cells in the bone marrow, contribute to or are responsible for the different pathways of maturation and differentiation. For example, specific cells in the bone marrow in the endosteal region promote the differentiation of hematopoietic stem cells into B lymphocytes.[15–21] In birds, primordial pluripotential stem cells that migrate to a gland near the cloaca of the chicken known as the bursa of Fab-

TABLE 6–6. **Platelet Granules and Their Contents**

α-Granules
Fibronectin
Fibrinogen
Plasminogen
Thrombospondin
von Willebrand factor
α_2-Plasmin inhibitor
Platelet-derived growth factor (PDGF)
Platelet factor 4 (PF4)
Transforming growth factor (TGF) α and β
Thrombospondin
β-Lysin
Permeability factor
Factors D and H
Decay-accelerating factor
Dense granules
Serotonin
Adenosine diphosphate (ADP)
Others
Arachidonic acid derivatives

TABLE 6–7. **Thymic Hormones**

Hormone	No. of Amino Acids
Thymosin	28
Thymopoietin	49
Thymic humoral factor	31
Facteur thymique serique	9

ricius (for reasons of probable stimuli in the bone marrow as yet not understood) are influenced by the epithelial cells in that gland to terminally differentiate into B lymphocytes.[22, 23] Interestingly, various candidates for the so-called bursal equivalent that is responsible for B-cell differentiation in humans were proposed for many years before the role of the bone marrow itself for this function became evident. Extra–bone marrow tissues that had been proposed as bursal equivalent candidates included the appendix, tonsils, liver, and Peyer's patch.

T-cell development results from pluripotential hematopoietic stem cell migration (stimulus unknown) from the bone marrow to the thymus. Thymic hormones (at least 20 have been preliminarily described) produced by the thymic epithelium initiate the complex series of events that result not only in differentiation of the hematopoietic stem cells into T lymphocytes but also in subdifferentiation of T lymphocytes into their various functional subsets; helper function, killer function, and suppressor function are acquired while the T cells are still in the thymus. Table 6–7 lists the four thymic hormones most rigorously studied to date. Note that all are involved in T-cell differentiation and in the development of helper T-cell function and that three of the four can be involved or are involved in the acquisition of suppressor T-cell activity. Clearly, the story is considerably more complex than the part we currently understand, and additional factors are undoubtedly responsible for the final differentiation of T lymphocytes into their functionally distinct subsets.

These various hormones are also undoubtedly responsible for the induction of cell surface glycoprotein expression on the surface of T cells. The cell surface expression of the various glycoproteins changes during T-cell maturation in the thymus. For example, the CD2 glycoprotein is the first that can be identified on the differentiating T cell, but this is eventually joined by CD5; these are both eventually replaced (CD2 completely and CD5 partially) by CD1 glycoprotein, which in turn is lost and replaced by the mature CD3 marker. CD4 and CD8 glycoproteins are acquired prior to emigration from the thymus of helper and cytotoxic-regulatory T cells, respectively.

Monocytes, NK cells, and killer cells evolve from pluripotential hematopoietic stem cells through influences that are incompletely understood. All three types of cells do arise from a common monocyte precursor and later subdifferentiate under unknown influences.

PRIMARY (CENTRAL) LYMPHOID ORGANS

The primary or central lymphoid organs are the bone marrow, thymus, and liver. The peripheral lymphoid organs include lymph nodes, spleen, gut-associated lymphoid tissue,

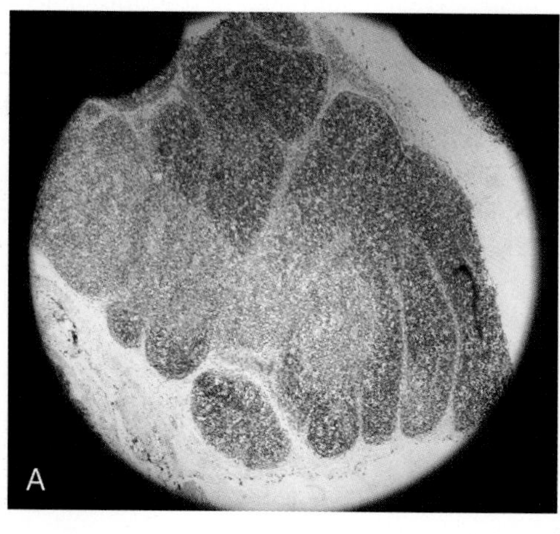

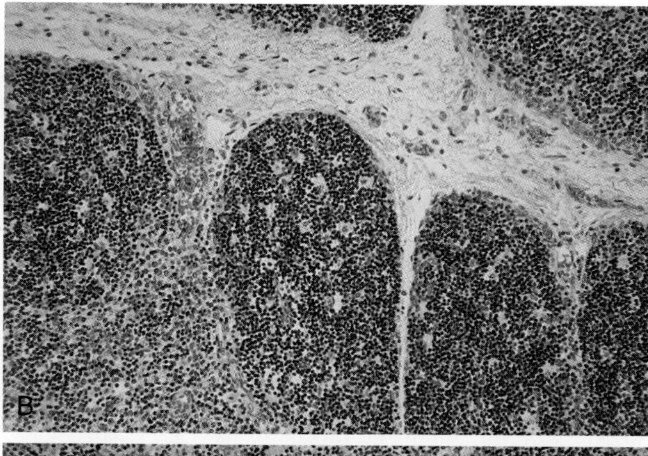

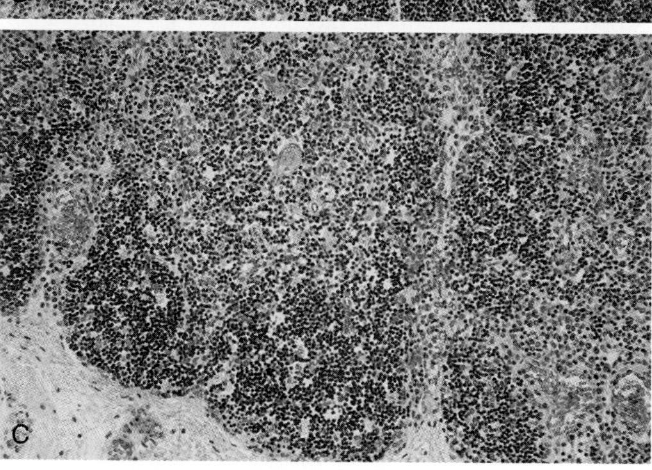

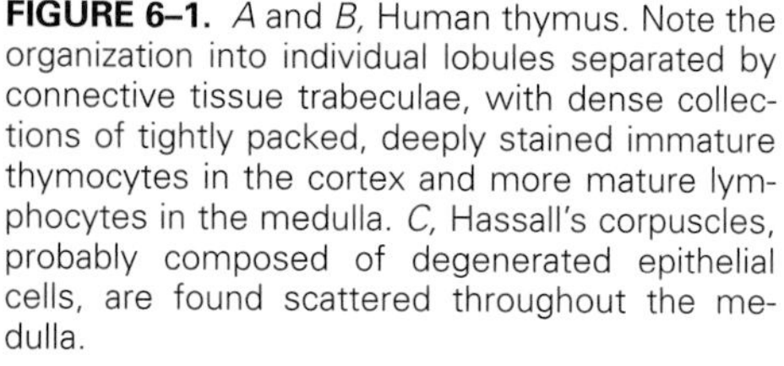

FIGURE 6–1. *A* and *B,* Human thymus. Note the organization into individual lobules separated by connective tissue trabeculae, with dense collections of tightly packed, deeply stained immature thymocytes in the cortex and more mature lymphocytes in the medulla. *C,* Hassall's corpuscles, probably composed of degenerated epithelial cells, are found scattered throughout the medulla.

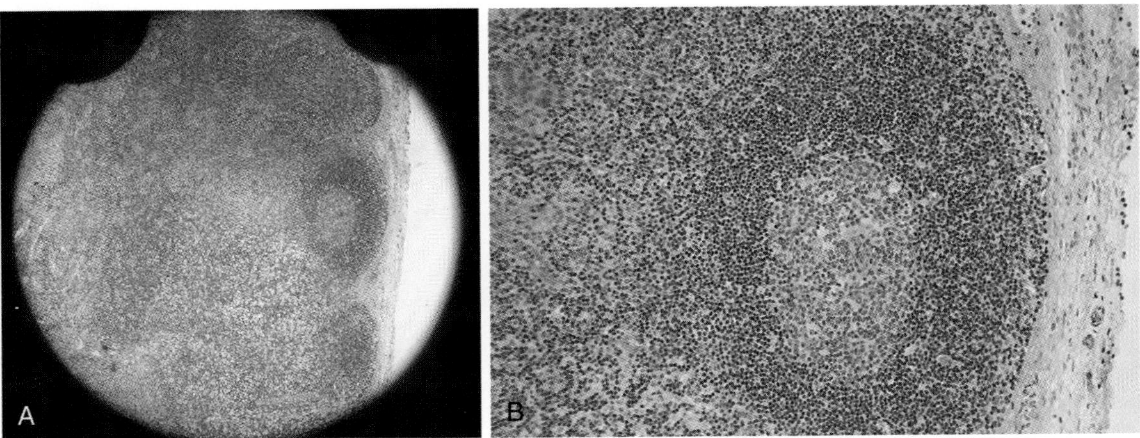

FIGURE 6–2. *A,* Human lymph node. Note the organization, in some respects similar to that of the thymus, into two predominant areas—the cortex and the medulla. The cortex is rich in B cells; the medulla contains cords of lymphoid tissue that contain both B and T cells; and an intermediate zone called the paracortex is rich in T cells. The paracortex, in addition to being rich in T cells, contains antigen-presenting cells. *B,* The medulla contains macrophages and plasma cells as well as B and T cells. The cortex contains the primary and secondary follicles, the distinction between the two being the germinal center (site of actively proliferating B cells) in the secondary follicles.

bronchus-associated lymphoid tissue, and conjunctiva-associated lymphoid tissue. The anatomic characteristics of the thymus, lymph node, and spleen are described briefly.

The thymus consists of a medulla, containing thymic epithelial tissue and lymphocytes, and a surrounding cortex densely packed with small, proliferating T lymphocytes (Fig. 6–1). The cells in the cortex emigrate from the thymus: The cell population turns over completely every 3 days. Only about 1% of the cells produced in the thymus, however, actually emigrate from it; 99% are destroyed locally, probably in a process designed to prevent autoreactive T lymphocytes from gaining access to the extrathymic regions of the organism. Thymic nurse cells, epithelial cells in the cortical region, may be responsible in part for some of the later events in T-lymphocyte differentiation (e.g., into helper and regulatory T cells).

Lymph nodes (Fig. 6–2) are also composed of medulla and cortex. The medulla, rich in the arterial and venous components of the lymph node, contains reticular cells that drain into the efferent lymphatic vessels. The cortex contains the primary lymphoid follicles, containing mature, resting B cells, secondary lymphoid follicles with their germinal centers (full of antigen-stimulated B cells and dendritic cells) and mantle, and lymphocytes. The paracortical region close to the medulla is rich in T cells, particularly $CD4^+$ T cells.

The arrangement of the spleen is similar to that of the thymus and lymph node, though lymph node–type follicles are not so clearly distinguished (Fig. 6–3). The lymphoid follicles and surrounding lymphocytes are called the white pulp of the spleen. The red pulp of the spleen is composed of the sinusoidal channels that typically contain a relatively large number of red blood cells. Popiernik has described the white pulp as being organized as a lumpy cylindrical sheath surrounding central arterioles. The arterioles curve back on the white pulp to develop it as the marginal sinus, which separates the white pulp from the red.[24] B cells predominate in the marginal zone, but $CD4^+$ T cells are present as well. T cells are clustered tightly around the central arteriole,

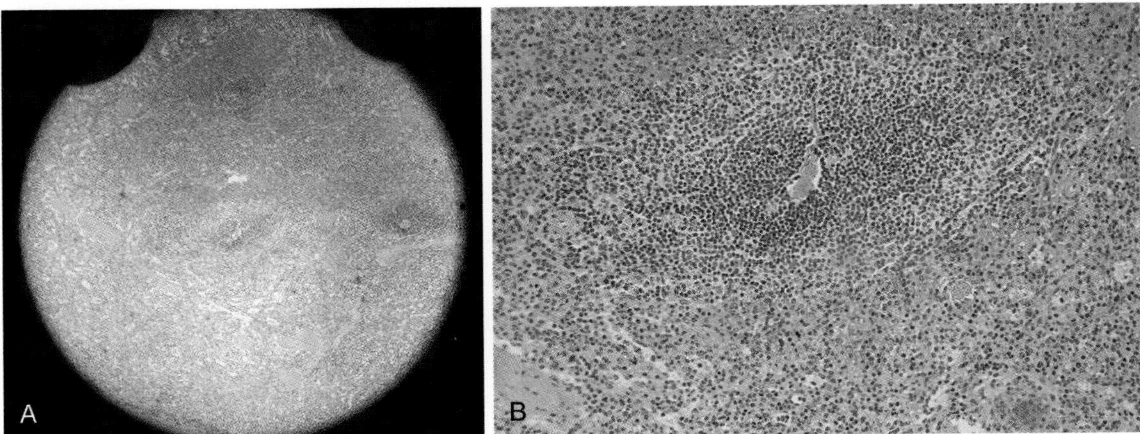

FIGURE 6–3. *A,* Human spleen. Note the red pulp, primarily involved in destruction of old red blood cells and red blood cells containing immune complexes, and white pulp, organized primarily around central arterioles and hence forming a "follicle" or a periarteriolar lymphoid sheath (PALS). *B,* T cells are particularly rich around the central arteriole of the PALS. B cells are particularly rich in the periphery of the PALS. The far periphery of the PALS, adjoining the red pulp, contains macrophages as well as B cells.

TABLE 6–8. **Lymphoid Organs**

Primary	Secondary
Thymus	Lymph nodes
Bone marrow	Spleen
	Mucosa-associated lymphoid tissue

where about 70% of the T cells are $CD4^+$. B cells also predominate in the lumpy eccentric follicle of white pulp. Table 6–8 outlines some of the characteristics of these three lymphoid organs and their organization. The spleen is the primary site of immune responses to intravenous and anterior chamber–introduced antigens.

LYMPHOID TRAFFIC

Lymphatic vessels and blood vessels connect these lymphatic organs to each other and to the other organs of the body. Lymphatic vessels drain every organ except the nonconjunctival parts of the eye, internal ear, bone marrow, spleen, cartilage, and some parts of the central nervous system. The interstitial fluid and cells entering this system are propelled (predominantly by skeletal muscle contraction) to regional lymph nodes. Efferent lymphatics draining these regional nodes converge to form large lymph vessels that culminate in the thoracic duct and in the right lymphatic duct. The thoracic duct empties into the left subclavian vein, carrying approximately three-quarters of the lymph, whereas the right lymphatic duct empties into the right subclavian vein.

The subject of lymphocyte traffic, like so many areas of immunology, has undergone intensive reexamination since the 1980s; since then, discoveries relating to homing receptors, addressins, and other adhesion molecules have revolutionized our understanding of how lymphoid cells migrate into and out of specific areas. For example, it is clear that one or more homing receptors is present on the surface of all lymphoid cells. These receptors can be regulated, induced, and suppressed. Furthermore, induction and suppression of other cell surface moieties that may regulate lymphoid cell exit from one location or another occurs. For example, cortical thymocytes rich in peanut agglutinin on their surface have a paucity of homing receptors, a fact that might ordinarily allow them to migrate out of the thymus to some other location. Butcher and Weissman have hypothesized that "terminal sialidation could release formerly peanut agglutinin–positive thymocytes from hypothetical peanut agglutinin–like lectins in the thymus, providing 'exit visas' for their release from the thymus."[25] In any event, one thing is clear: mature T cells emerging from the thymus cortex toward the medulla are rich in cell surface or plasma membrane–homing receptors, or adhesion molecules or "adhesomes," which are ligands for various addressins or adhesion molecules at other, remote loci. In the mouse, homing receptors on the surface of mature T cells have been identified for the lymph node (MEL-14 or L-selectin [LFA-1]) and for Peyer's patch (LPAM-1 $\alpha4\beta_7$ integrin, CD44). Equivalent homing receptors undoubtedly exist in humans, but work in this area is currently embryonic. A 90-kDa glycoprotein designated Hermes-3, however, has been identified as a specific heterotypic recognition unit on lymphocytes.[26] The Hermes glycoprotein has been shown to be identical to the CD44 molecule.[27] Antibodies to this glycoprotein prevent binding of lymphocytes to mucosal lymph node high endothelial venules.[28]

Table 6–9 summarizes many of the currently recognized adhesion molecules and their homing receptor ligands.

Immune Response

Professional APCs phagocytose foreign material (antigens), process it through protease endosomal-lysosomal degradation, "package" it with MHC molecules, and transport the peptide-MHC complex to the cell surface. B cells and dendritic cells (including Langerhans' cells) perform this function too, but differences in protease types and class II MHC molecules among these APCs may influence the type of T cell activated by an antigen. It is this unit of antigenic peptide determinant and self-MHC glycoproteins, along with the aid of adhesion molecules (ICAM-1 [CD54] and LFA-3 [CD58]) and co-stimulatory molecules (B7 [CD80]), that forms the recognition unit for the TCRs specific for the antigenic epitope of the foreign material. The TCR is composed of recognition units for the epitope and for the autologous MHC glycoprotein. Endogenous antigens, such as endogenously manufactured viral protein, typically result in cytoplasm, associate with class I MHC molecules, and are transported to the surface of the APC, where the class I MHC-peptide complex preferentially associates with the TCR of $CD8^+$ cells. Exogenous antigens that are phagocytized typically associate, as described earlier, in the endosomal, endoxytic, exocytic pathways with class II MHC molecules, and this type of complex preferentially associates with $CD4^+$ TCRs.

The $\alpha\beta$ heterodimer of the TCR is associated with CD3 and $\zeta\eta$ proteins and (for CD4 cells) the CD4 molecule, forming the TCR complex. Antigen presentation can then occur as the TCR complex interacts with the antigenic determinant/MHC complex on the macrophage, with simultaneous CD28-CD80 interaction. Macrophage secretion of IL-1 during this cognitive "presentation" phase of the acquired immune response to CD4 T cells completes the require-

TABLE 6–9. **Adhesion Molecules**

LFA-1α	(CD11a)
MAC-1	(CD11b)
GP150,95	(CD11c)
LFA-1β	(CD18)
Integrin α4	(CD49d)
TCR$\alpha\beta$	
TCRγ/δ	
LFA-2	(CD2)
CD 22	
NCAM	(CD56)
ICAM-1	(CD54)
LFA-3	(CD58)
LECAM-1	
CD5	
HCAM	(CD44)
HPCA-2	(CD34)
CD28	
88-1	
PECAM	(CD31)
GMP140	(CD62)
HNK-1	(CD57)

ments for successful antigen presentation to the helper T cell (see Fig. 6–1).

The CD3 and ζη proteins are the signal-transducing components of the TCR complex; transmembrane signaling via this pathway results in activation of several phosphotyrosine kinases, including those of the tyk/jak family and other signal transduction and activation of transcription molecules and phosphorylation of tyrosine residues in the cytoplasmic tails of the CD3 and ζη proteins, resulting in the creation of multiple sites that bind proteins (enzymes), like phosphatidylinositol phospholipase C-γ1 (PI-PLC-γ1) with SH2 binding domain. PI-PLC-γ1 in turn is phosphorylated (and thereby activated), and it catalyzes hydrolysis of plasma membrane phosphatidylinositol 4,5 bisphosphate into inositol 1,4,5 triphosphate (ID_3) and diacylglycerol. IP_3 then provokes the release of calcium from its endoplasmic reticulum storage sites. The increased intracellular calcium concentration that results from the release from storage in turn results in increased binding of calcium to calmodulin; this then activates the phosphatase, calcineurin. Calcineurin catalyzes the conversion of phosphorylated nuclear factor of activated T cells, cytoplasmic component (NFATc) to free NFATc. This protein (and probably others) then enters the cell nucleus, where gene transcription of cellular proto-oncogenes/transcription factor genes, cytokine receptor genes, and cytokine genes is then activated and regulated by it (or them). For example, NFATc translocates to the nucleus, where it combines with AP-1 proteins; this complex then binds to the NFATc binding site of the IL-2 promoter. This, coupled with NFκB binding by proteins *possibly* induced by the events stimulated by CD28-CD80 signal transduction, results in IL-2 gene transcription typical of T-cell activation (see Fig. 6–2). Thus, this activation phase of the acquired immune response is characterized by lymphocyte proliferation and cytokine production.

Expression of Immunity

The emigration of hematopoietic cells from the vascular system typically occurs at the region of postcapillary high endothelial venule cells. These cells are rich in the constitutive expression of so-called addressins, which are tissue- or organ-specific endothelial cell molecules involved in lymphocyte homing. These adhesion molecules are lymphocyte-binding molecules for the homing receptors on lymphocytes. Thus, the mucosal addressin[27] specifically binds to the Hermes 90-kDa glycoprotein. In the murine system, a 90-kDa glycoprotein (designated MECA-79) is a peripheral lymph-node addressin specifically expressed by high endothelial venules in peripheral lymph nodes.[29] MECA-367 and MECA-89 are additional addressin glycoproteins in the murine system that are specific for mucosal vascular high endothelial venules. In addition to the constitutive expression of addressins or adhesion molecules, expression of additional adhesion molecules is induced by a panoply of proinflammatory cytokines. It is this directed trafficking of inflammatory cells via adhesion molecules that gives the expression of an immune response its focus, its specifically directed, targeted expression.

Lymphocytes and monocytes and neutrophils preferentially migrate or "home" to sites of inflammation because of this upregulation of cytokines and the induction of adhesion molecules they promote. Thus, L-selectin (CD62L) on the neutrophil cell surface membrane does not adhere to normal vascular endothelium, but intercellular adhesion molecule (ICAM) and endothelial leukocyte adhesion molecule (ELAM) (CD62E) expression on the vascular endothelial cell surface induced by IFN-α, IFN-γ, IL-1, IL-17, or a combination thereof results in low-affinity binding of CD62L, with resultant slowing of neutrophil transit through the vessel, neutrophil "rolling" on the endothelial surface, and (with complement split product and IL-8–driven chemotaxis of increasing numbers of neutrophils) neutrophil margination in the vessels of inflamed tissue. Neutrophil LFA-1 (CD11a, CD18) activated expression (stimulated by IL-6 and IL-8) then results in stronger adhesion of the neutrophil to endothelial cell ICAM molecules, with resultant neutrophil spreading and diapedesis into the subendothelial spaces and into the surrounding tissue.

IMMUNOLOGIC MEMORY

The anamnestic capacity of the acquired immune response system is one of its most extraordinary properties. Indeed, it is this remarkable property that was the first to be recognized by the Chinese ancients and (later) by Jenner. We take it as axiomatic that our immunization in childhood with killed or attenuated smallpox and polio virus provoked not only a primary immune response but also the development of long-lived "memory" cells that immediately produce a rapid, vigorous secondary immune response whenever we might encounter smallpox or polio virus, thereby resulting in specific antibody and lymphocyte-mediated killing of the microbe and defending us from the harm the virus would otherwise have done. But just what do we know about the cells responsible for this phenomenon? What special characteristics enable memory cells to live for prolonged periods in the absence of continued or repeated antigen exposure?

Neils Jerne first hypothesized a clonal selection theory to explain at once the specificity and the diversity of the acquired immune response, and Macfarlene Burnet expanded on Jerne's original hypothesis, clearly predicting the necessary features that would prove the theory; many subsequent studies have done so. Clones are derived from the development of antigen-specific clones of lymphocytes arising from single precursors prior to and independent from exposure to antigen. Approximately 10^9 such clones have been estimated to exist in an individual, allowing him or her to respond to all currently known or future antigens. Antigen contact results in preferential activation of the preexisting clone with the cell surface receptors specific for it, with resultant proliferation of the clone and differentiation into effector and memory cells. The secondary or anamnestic immune response is greater and more rapid in onset than is the primary immune response because of the large number of lymphocytes derived from the original clone of cells stimulated by the primary contact with antigen, as well as the long-lived nature of many of the cells (memory cells). The memory cells can survive for very long periods, even decades. They express certain cell surface proteins not expressed by non-memory cells (CD45RO). In memory cells, the level of cell surface expression of peripheral lymph node homing receptors is low compared with the population of such re-

TABLE 6–10. **Cytokines and Target Cells**

Cytokine	Source	Target Cells
IL-1	Mϕ, T_H, FB, NK, B, Nϕ, EC	Pluripotent stem cells, or not T_CT_H, B, Mϕ, FB, Nϕ
IL-2	T_H1	T_CT_H, B, NK
IL-3	BM, T_H, MC	T_CT_H, B, MC, stem cells
IL-4	T_H2, MC	T_H1, B, Mϕ, MC, T_H2, NK, FC
IL-5	T_H2, MC, Eϕ	T_CT_H, B, Eϕ
IL-6	BM, Mϕ, MC, EC, B, T_H2, FB	Pluripotent stem cells, or not T_CT_H, B, FB, Nϕ
IL-7	FB, BM	Subcapsular and thymocytes, T_CT_H, F, FB
IL-8	BM, FB, EC, Mϕ, Nϕ, Eϕ	T_CT_H, Mϕ, Nϕ
IL-9	T_H2	Pluripotent stem cells, or not T_CT_H, MC
IL-10	T_H2, B, Mϕ	T_{CD2}, T_C, T_H1, MC
IL-11	BM	Pluripotent stem cells, or not T_CT_H, B
IL-12	Mϕ, Nϕ	NK, T_H–T_H1
IL-13	T_H2	T_H1, Mϕ, B
IL-14	T	B
IL-15	Mϕ, FB, BM	T, NK, B
IL-16	T, Eϕ	T
IL-17	T_H	FB, T
IL-18	Mϕ	T, NK
TNF-α	Mϕ	T_CT_H, B, Mϕ, FB
TNF-β	T_C, T_H1	EC, Nϕ
GM-CSF	TH, Mϕ, MC Null cells, FB	T_CT_H, Eϕ, Nϕ
G-CSF	BM, Mϕ, FB	T_CT_H, FB, Nϕ
M-CSF	BM, Mϕ, FB	
LIF	BM	Myeloid progenitor
SCF	BM	Myeloid progenitor Cortical thymocytes
IFN-γ	NK, T_H1	NK, T_C, T_H2, B, FB, MC
IFN-α	Mϕ	T_CT_H, B
IFN-β	FB	T_CT_H
TGF-β	Mϕ	T_CT_H, B, Mϕ, FB

B, B cell; BM, bone marrow; CSF, colony-stimulating factor; Eϕ, eosinophil; EC, endothelial cell; FB, fibroblast; GM, granulocyte, macrophage; IFN, interferon; IL, interleukin; LIF, leukocyte inhibitory factor; Mϕ, macrophage; MC, mast cell; Nϕ, neutrophil; NK, natural killer cell; SCF, stem cell factor; T_C, cytotoxic T cell; TGF, transforming growth factor; T_H, helper T cell; TNF, tumor necrosis factor.

ceptors on the surface of nonmemory cells; in contrast, the population of other adhesion molecules on the surface of memory cells is much greater than that of the surface of nonmemory cells. These adhesion molecules include CD11a, CD18 (LFA-1), CD44, and VLA molecules. Because of the constitutive expression of the cell surface adhesion molecules, memory T cells rapidly home to sites of inflammation, "looking" for antigen to which they might respond.

Summary

The evolutionary advantage of the immune system is obvious. The complexity of the system that has evolved to protect us, however, is extraordinary, and our understanding of the immune system is far from complete. The major cell types of the system are well known, but subtypes and sub-subtypes are still being identified. The primary products of one of the major cell types, the B lymphocytes, have been well characterized (antibody), but additional cellular products or cytokines from these cells, which in the 1980s were believed to secrete only immunoglobulins in their mature (plasma cell) state, are being discovered. Thus, the 18 interleukins and other cytokines listed in Table 6–10 will be an incomplete list of the known cytokines of the immune system by the time this edition is published. The seemingly never-ending story of immunologic discovery is at once as fascinating as any Shakespeare play and as frustrating as attempting to understand the universe and the meaning of life. Each year, a chapter brings new knowledge and new questions, and the wise physician will realize that schooling never ends in immunology as in so many other biologic sciences. Stay tuned.

REFERENCES

1. Kohler J, Milstein C: Continuous cultures of fused cells secreting antibody of predefined specificity. Nature 256:495, 1975.
2. Reinherz EL, Schlossman SF: The differentiation and function of human T lymphocytes. Cell 19:821, 1980.
3. Hardy RR, Hayakawa K, Parks DR, Herzenberg LA: Murine B cell differentiation lineages. J Exp Med 1959:1169, 1984.
4. Hardy RR, Hayakawa K, Schimizu M, et al: Rheumatoid factor secretion from human Leu-1 B cells. Science 236:81, 1987.
5. Mosmann TR, Coffman R: Two types of mouse helper T cell clones: Implications from immune regulation. Immunol Today 8:233, 1987.
6. Coffman R, O'Hara J, Bond MW, et al: B cell stimulatory factor-1 enhances the IgE response of lipopolysaccharide-activated B cell. J Immunol 136:4538, 1986.
7. Mariotti S, del Prete GF, Mastromauro C, et al: The autoimmune infiltrates of Basedow's disease: Analysis of clonal level and comparison with Hashimoto's thyroiditis. Exp Clin Endocrinol 97:139, 1991.
8. Maggi E, Biswas P, del Prete GF, et al: Accumulation of TH2-like helper T cells in the conjunctiva of patients with vernal conjunctivitis. J Immunol 146:1169, 1991.
9. Romagnani S: Human TH1 and TH2 subsets: Doubt no more. Immunol Today 12:256, 1991.
10. Murphy DB, Mamauchi K, Habu S, et al: T cells in a suppressor circuit and non-T:non-B cells bear different I-J determinants. Immunogenetics 13:205, 1981.
11. Gillette TE, Chandler JW, Greiner JV: Langerhans cells of the ocular surface. Ophthalmology 89:700, 1982.
12. Tagawa Y, Takeuchi T, Saga T, et al: Langerhans cells: Role in ocular surface immunopathology. *In* O'Connor GR, Chandler JW (eds): Advances in Immunology and Immunopathology of the Eye. New York, Masson, 1985, pp 203–207.
13. Le Douarin NM: Ontogeny of hematopoietic organ studies in avian embryo interspecific chimeras. Cold Spring Harbor Meeting on Differentiation of Normal and Neoplastic Hematopoietic Cells. Clarkson D, Marks PA, Till JE (eds): Cold Spring Harbor Laboratory, Cold Spring Harbor, NY, 1978, pp 5–32.
14. Metcalf D, Moore MAS: Hematopoietic cells. *In* Neuberger A, Tatum EL (eds): Frontiers of Biology, vol 24. Amsterdam, Elsevier North-Holland, 1971.
15. Hermans MJA, Hartsuiker H, Opstaelten D: An insight to study of B lymphocytopoiesis in rat bone marrow: Topographical arrangement of terminal yatsi nucleotidal transferase positive cells and pre-B cells. J Immunol 44:67, 1989.
16. Muller-Sieburg CL, Whitlock CA, Weissman YL: Isolation of two early B lymphocyte progenitors from mouse marrow: A committed pre-B cell and a clonogenic 5-1 hematopoietic stem cell. Cell 44:653, 1986.
17. Whitlock CA, Witte ON: Longterm culture of B lymphocytes and their precursors from murine bone marrow. Proc Natl Acad Sci U S A 79:3608, 1982.
18. Whitlock CA, Tidmarsh TS, Mueller C, et al: Bone marrow stromal cells with lymphoid activity express high levels of pre-B neoplasia-associated molecule. Cell 48:1009, 1987.
19. Hunt T, Robertson D, Weiss D, et al: A single bone marrow-derived stromal cell type supports the in vitro growth of early lymphoid and myeloid cells. Cell 48:997, 1987.
20. Dorshkind K, Johnson A, Collins A, et al: Generation of bone marrow stromal cultures that support lymphoid and myelocyte precursors. Immunol Methods 89:37, 1986.
21. Smith L, Weissman IL, Heimfeld S: Metapoietic stem cells give rise to

pre-B cells. *In* Paul W (ed): Fundamental Immunology, 2nd ed. New York, Raven Press, 1989, pp 41–67.
22. Szengerg A, Warner ML: Association of immunologic responsiveness in fowls with a hormonally arrested development of lymphoid material. Nature 194:146, 1962.
23. Cooper MD, Peterson RD, South MA, Good RA: The functions of the thymus system and the bursa system in the chicken. J Exp Med 123:75, 1966.
24. Popiernik M: Lymphoid organs. *In* Bach JF (ed): Immunology, 2nd ed. New York, John Wiley & Sons, 1982, pp 15–37.
25. Butcher EC, Weissman IL: Lymphoid tissues and organs. *In* Paul W (ed): Fundamental Immunology, 2nd ed. New York, Raven Press, 1989, pp 117–137.
26. Berg EL, Goldstein LA, Jutila MA, et al: Homing receptors and vascular addressins: Cell adhesion molecules that direct lymphocyte traffic. Immunol Rev 108:5, 1989.
27. Picker LJ, de los Toyos J, Tellen MJ, et al: Monoclonal antibodies against the CD 44 and Pgp-1 antigens in man recognize the Hermes class of lymphocyte homing receptors. J Immunol 142:2046, 1989.
28. Holzmann B, McIntyre BW, Weissman IC: Identification of a murine Peyer's patch–specific lymphocyte homing receptor as an integrin molecule with an a chain homologous to human VLA-4a. Cell 56:37, 1989.
29. Streeter PR, Rause ET, Butcher EC: Immunohistologic and functional characterization of a vascular addressin involved in lymphocyte homing into peripheral lymph nodes. J Cell Biol 107:1853, 1988.

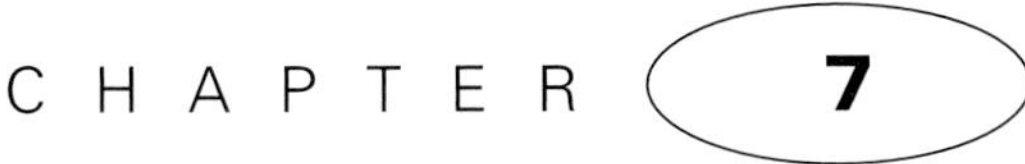

T-Lymphocyte Responses

J. Wayne Streilein

T lymphocytes stand at the center of the adaptive immune response.[1] In the presence of T cells, the entire array of immune effector responses and tolerance are possible, but in the absence of T cells, only primitive antibody responses and no cell-mediated immune responses can be made. T cells are leukocytes that originate from lymphocyte precursors in the bone marrow. The majority of T cells undergo differentiation in the thymus gland, and, upon reaching maturity, disseminate via the blood to populate secondary lymphoid organs and to circulate among virtually all tissues of the body. A second population of T cells undergoes differentiation extrathymically and has a somewhat different (and not yet completely defined) set of functional properties. T cells are exquisitely antigen-specific, a property conferred on them by unique surface receptors that recognize antigenic material in a highly distinctive manner. Once activated, T cells initiate or participate in the various forms of cell-mediated immunity, humoral immunity, and tolerance.

T-Lymphocyte Development

From the pluripotent hematopoietic stem cell, a lineage of cells emerges that becomes the oligopotent lymphocyte progenitor.[2] During fetal life, this lineage of cells is observed first in the liver, but as the fetus matures, the lymphocyte progenitors shift to the bone marrow. According to developmental signals not completely understood, lymphocyte progenitors in the bone marrow differentiate into (at least) three distinct lineages of committed precursor cells: pre-thymocytes, pre-B lymphocytes, and pre–natural killer lymphocytes. Pre-thymocytes, which give rise eventually to T lymphocytes, escape from the bone marrow (or fetal liver) and migrate via the blood primarily to the thymus, where cell adhesion molecules on microvascular endothelial cells direct them into the cortex. The differentiation process that thymocytes experience within the thymus accomplishes several critical goals in T-cell biology: (1) each cell acquires a unique surface receptor for antigen, (2) cells with receptors that recognize antigenic molecules in the context of *self* class I or class II molecules (encoded by genes within the major histocompatibility complex [MHC]) are positively selected,[3] (3) cells with receptors that recognize self-antigenic molecules in the context of self-MHC molecules are negatively selected (deleted or inactivated),[4] and (4) each mature cell acquires unique effector functions—the capacity to respond to antigen by secreting immunomodulatory cytokines or by delivering to a target cell a "lethal hit."[1]

Differentiation in the Thymic Cortex

Within the thymus cortex, pre-thymocytes receive differentiation signals from resident thymic epithelial cells and thus initiate the process of maturation.[2] A unique set of genes is activated, including: (1) genes that commit the cells to proliferation, (2) genes that encode the T-cell receptors for antigen, and (3) genes that code accessory molecules that developing and mature T cells use for antigen recognition and signal transduction. The genes that make it possible for T cells to create surface receptors for antigen are the structural genes that encode the four distinct polypeptide chains (α, β, γ, δ) from which the T-cell receptor (Tcr) for antigen is composed, as well as the genes that create genetic rearrangements that confer an extremely high degree of diversity on Tcr molecules. Each Tcr is a heterodimer of transmembrane polypeptides (αβ or γδ). The portion of the Tcr that is involved in antigen recognition resides at the ends of the peptide chains distal to the cell surface and is called the "combining site." The accessory genes encode, on the one hand, the CD3 molecular complex (γ, δ, ϵ, ζ), which enables a Tcr that has engaged antigen to signal the T cell across the plasma membrane, and, on the other hand, the CD4 and CD8 molecules that promote the affinity of the Tcr for antigenic peptides in association with class I and class II molecules, respectively, of the MHC. Thus, within the thymus cortex, individual pre-thymocytes proliferate, come to express a unique Tcr, and simultaneously express CD3, CD4, and CD8 on the cell surface. Each day, a very large number of thymocytes is generated and, therefore, an enormous diversity of Tcr is also generated. Conservative estimates place the number of novel Tcr produced each day in excess of 10^9!

Nature of Antigen Recognition by T Cells

Understanding the nature of the antigenic determinants detected by individual T-cell receptors for antigen is central to understanding the differentiation process that occurs among thymocytes in the thymus gland. Thymocytes acquire one of two types of T-cell receptors: αβ-Tcr are heterodimers composed of polypeptides encoded by the Tcr-α and Tcr-β chain genes; γδ-Tcr are heterodimers composed of polypeptides encoded by the Tcr-γ and Tcr-δ chain genes.[5] Because much is known about αβ-Tcr, whereas much remains to be learned about γδ Tcr, this discussion is limited to the former.

The αβ–T-cell receptor for antigen does not recognize a protein antigen in its native configuration. Rather, the Tcr recognizes peptides (ranging in size from 7 to 22 amino acids in length) derived from limited proteolysis of the antigen, and it recognizes these peptides when they are bound noncovalently to highly specialized regions of antigen-presenting molecules.[6] Two types of antigen-presenting molecules exist, and both are encoded within the MHC.[7] Class I molecules are transmembrane proteins expressed on antigen-presenting cells (APC). These molecules possess on their most distal domains a platform of two parallel α-helices separated by a groove. This groove accommodates peptides (generated by regulated proteolysis of antigenic proteins) ranging from seven to nine amino acids in length. Class II molecules are also transmembrane proteins expressed on APC, and the platforms on their distal domains contain similar grooves that accept peptides of 15 to 22 amino acids in length. The "combining site" of individual Tcrs possesses three contact points: a central point that interacts directly with an antigenic peptide in the groove, and two side points that interact directly with the platform (α-helices) of class I or class II molecules. Thus, the conditions that must be met for successful recognition of antigen by Tcr are: (1) a class I or class II molecule must be available on an APC, and (2) a peptide must occupy the groove of the presenting molecule's platform.

Other molecules promote the affinity of Tcr binding with antigenic peptides associated with class I and class II MHC molecules.[8] CD4 molecules that are expressed on certain T cells and thymocytes have the ability to bind class II molecules at a site distinct from the antigen presentation platform. As a consequence, CD4-bearing T cells whose Tcr has engaged a peptide-containing class II molecule are much more likely to be stimulated than T cells with similar receptors but that don't express CD4. Similarly, CD8-bearing T cells whose Tcr has engaged a peptide-containing class I molecule are much more likely to be stimulated than T cells without CD8.

Within the thymus cortex, epithelial cells express class I and class II molecules encoded by the individual's own MHC genes.[2, 3] When Tcr-bearing thymocytes are generated in the cortex, cells with Tcr that recognize peptide-containing self-class I or self-class II molecules are induced to undergo successive rounds of proliferation, leading to clonal expansion. By contrast, Tcr-bearing thymocytes that fail to recognize peptide-containing self-class I or self-class II molecules are not activated within the cortex. In the absence of this cognate signal, all such cells enter a default pathway, which ends inevitably in cell death (apoptosis). This process is called *positive selection*, because thymocytes with Tcr that have an affinity for self-MHC molecules (plus peptide) are being selected for further clonal expansion. Unselected cells simply die by apoptosis. At the completion of their sojourn in the thymus cortex, large numbers of positively selected Tcr^+, $CD3^+$, $CD4^+$, and $CD8^+$ thymocytes migrate into the thymus medulla.

Differentiation in the Thymic Medulla

In addition to epithelial cells, the thymic medulla contains a unique population of bone marrow–derived cells called *dendritic cells*.[4, 9] These nonphagocytic cells express large amounts of class I and class II molecules and actively endocytose proteins in their environment. Peptides derived from these proteins by proteolysis are loaded onto the grooves of MHC-encoded antigen presentation platforms. Within the thymic medulla, the vast majority of such endocytosed proteins are self proteins. As thymocytes enter the medulla from the cortex, a subpopulation expresses Tcr that recognize peptides of self proteins expressed on self-class I or self-class II molecules. By contrast, another subpopulation fails to recognize self-class I or self-class II molecules, because the Tcr is specific for a peptide not included among peptides from self proteins. The former population, comprising cells that recognize self exclusively, engage self-derived peptides plus MHC molecules on medullary dendritic cells. This engagement delivers a "death" signal to the T cell, and all such cells undergo apoptosis. This process is called *negative selection* because thymocytes with Tcr that have an affinity for self-peptides in self-MHC molecules are being eliminated. In part, this process plays a major role in eliminating autoreactive T cells that would be capable of causing autoimmunity if they should escape from the thymus. Many other thymocytes that enter the medulla express Tcr that are unable to engage self-class I or self-class II molecules on dendritic cells because the relevant peptide does not occupy the antigen-presenting groove. T cells of this type proceed to downregulate expression of either CD4 or CD8 and acquire the properties of mature T cells. The T cells that are ready at this point to leave the thymus are Tcr^+, $CD3^+$, and either $CD4^+$ or $CD8^+$ (but not both). Moreover, they are in G_0 of the cell cycle, that is, resting. The number of such cells exported from the thymus per day is very large; in humans, it is estimated that more than 10^8 new mature T cells are produced daily. These cells are fully immunocompetent and are prepared to recognize and respond to a large diversity of foreign antigens that are degraded into peptides and presented on self-class I or self-class II molecules on tissues outside the thymus. It is estimated that the number of different antigenic specificities that can be recognized by mature T cells (i.e., the T-cell repertoire for antigens) exceeds 10^9.

Properties and Functions of Mature T Lymphocytes

Mature, resting T cells with αβ-Tcr migrate from the thymus to any and all tissues of the body, but there are vascular specializations (postcapillary venules) in secondary lymphoid organs (lymph nodes, Peyer's patches, tonsils) that promote the selective entry of T cells into these tissues.[10] More than 99% of T cells in blood that traverse a lymph node are extracted into the parafollicular region of the cortex. This region of the nodal cortex is designed to encourage the interaction of T cells with APC. Because the encounter of any single, antigen-specific T cell with its antigen of interest on an APC is a rather rare event, most T cells that enter a secondary lymphoid organ fail to find their antigen of interest. In this case, the T cells disengage from resident APC and migrate into the effluent of the node, passing through lymph ducts back into the general blood circulation. An individual T cell may make journeys such as this numerous times during a single day, and countless journeys are accomplished during its lifetime (which may be measured in tens of years). Remarkably, this monotonous behavior changes dramatically if and when a mature T cell encounters its specific antigen via recognition of the relevant peptide in association with a class I or class II molecule on an APC in a secondary lymphoid organ. It is this critical encounter that initiates T-cell–dependent, antigen-specific immune responses.

T-Cell Activation by Antigen

There is a general rule regarding the minimal requirements for activation of lymphocytes, including T cells, which are normally in a resting state: two different surface signals received simultaneously are required to arouse the cell out of G_0.[8] One signal (referred to as *signal 1*) is delivered through CD3 and is triggered by successful engagement of the Tcr with its peptide in association with an MHC molecule. The other signal (referred to as *signal 2*) is delivered through numerous cell surface molecules *other than the Tcr*. Signals of this type are also referred to as co-stimulation, and co-stimulation is usually the result of receptor/ligand interactions in which the receptor is on the T cell and the ligand is expressed on the APC. For example, B7.1 and B7.2 are surface molecules expressed on APC; these molecules engage the receptor CD28 on T cells, thus delivering an activation signal to the recipient cells. Similarly, CD40 ligand on T cells and CD40 on APC function in a co-stimulatory manner. Another example of co-stimulation occurs when a cytokine produced by an APC, such as interleukin-1 (IL-1) or IL-12, is presented to T cells expressing the IL-1 or IL-12 receptor, respectively. When both conditions are met—signal 1 (Tcr binds to peptide plus MHC molecule) and signal 2 (e.g., B7.1 binds to CD28)—the T cell receives coordinated signals across the plasma membrane, and these signals initiate a cascade of intracytoplasmic events that lead to dramatic changes in the genetic and functional programs of the T cells.

Antigen-Activated T-Cell Responses

When a T cell encounters its antigen of interest along with a satisfactory signal 2, it escapes from G_0. Under these circumstances, the genetic program of the cell shifts in a direction that makes it possible for the cell to proliferate and to undergo further differentiation. *Proliferation* results in emergence of a "clone" of cells, all of the identical phenotype, including the Tcr. This process is called clonal expansion, results from the elaboration of growth factors (e.g., IL-2), is one hallmark of the process of immunization or sensitization, and accounts for why the number of T cells able to recognize a particular antigen increases dramatically after sensitization has taken place. The signal that triggers proliferation arises first from the APC, but sustained T-cell proliferation takes place because the responding T cell activates its own IL-2 and IL-2 receptor genes.[11, 12] IL-2 is a potent growth factor for T cells, and T cells expressing the IL-2R respond to IL-2 by undergoing repetitive rounds of replication. IL-2 is not the only growth factor for T cells; another important growth factor is IL-4, which is also made by T cells. Thus, once activated, T cells have the capacity to autocrine stimulate their own proliferation—so long as their Tcr remains engaged with the antigen (plus MHC) of interest.

In addition to proliferation, antigen-activated T cells proceed down pathways of further *differentiation*. The functional expressions of this differentiation include: (1) secretion of lymphokines that promote inflammation or modify the functional properties of other lymphoreticular cells in their immediate environment,[13] and (2) acquisition of the cytoplasmic machinery required for displaying cytotoxicity, that is, the ability to lyse target cells.[14] The list of lymphokines that an activated mature T cell can make is long: IL-2, IL-3, IL-4, GM-CSF, IL-5, IL-6, IL-10, interferon-γ (IFN-γ), tumor necrosis factor-α (TNF-α), transforming growth factor-β (TGF-β). The range of biologic activities attributable to these cytokines is extremely broad, and no single T cell produces all of these factors simultaneously. The pattern of cytokines produced by a T cell accounts in large measure for the functional phenotype of the cell (see later).

The ability of antigen-activated T cells to lyse antigen-bearing target cells is embodied in specializations of the cells' cytoplasm and cell surface. Cytotoxic T cells possess granules in their cytoplasm that contain a molecule, perforin, that can polymerize and insert into the plasma membrane of a target cell, creating large pores. The granules also contain a series of lytic enzymes (granzymes) that enter the target cell, perhaps through the perforin-created pores, and trigger programmed cell death. There is a second mechanism by which T cells can cause death of neighboring cells. Activated T cells express Fas or CD95, a cell surface glycoprotein. The co-receptor for Fas is called (appropriately) Fas ligand or CD95 ligand. It is a member of the TNF receptor superfamily and its cytoplasmic tail contains a "death domain." After sustained activation, T cells also express Fas ligand; when Fas interacts with Fas ligand, the cell bearing Fas undergoes programmed cell death. Thus, Fas ligand$^+$ T cells can trigger apoptotic death in adjacent cells that are Fas$^+$, including other T cells. In fact, the ability of antigen-activated T cells to elicit apoptosis among neighboring, similarly activated T cells may serve to downregulate the immune response to that particular antigen, that is, by eliminating responding T cells.

Imperfect Antigen-Activated T-Cell Responses

On occasion, T cells may encounter their antigen of interest (in association with an MHC molecule) under circumstances where an appropriate signal 2 does not exist.[15] This can be arranged in vitro, for example, by using paraformaldehyde-fixed APC. Not surprisingly, delivery of signal 1 alone fails to activate the T cells in question. However, if these same T cells are re-exposed subsequently to the same antigen/MHC signal 1 on viable APC capable of delivering a functional signal 2, activation of the T cells *still fails*. The inability of T cells first activated by signal 1 in the absence of signal 2 to respond subsequently to functional signal 1 and signal 2 is referred to as **anergy**. Although the phenomenon just described was discovered in vitro, there is evidence that anergy occurs in vivo and that this process is important in regulating the immune response and some forms of tolerance.

T-Lymphocyte Heterogeneity

The adaptive immune response is separable into a cell-mediated immune arm and an antibody or humoral immune arm.[1] T cells themselves initiate and mediate cell-mediated immunity, and they play a dominant role in promoting antibody-mediated responses. There is heterogeneity among T cells that function in cell-mediated immunity, and there is heterogeneity among T cells that promote humoral immunity.

Cell-mediated immunity arises when effector T cells are generated within secondary lymphoid organs in response to antigen-induced activation. Two types of effector cells are recognized: (1) T cells that elicit delayed hypersensitivity (DH), and (2) T cells that are cytotoxic for antigen-bearing target cells. T cells that elicit delayed hypersensitivity recognize their antigen of interest on cells in peripheral tissues and upon activation secrete pro-inflammatory cytokines such as IFN-γ and TNF-α. These cytokines act on microvascular endothelium, promoting edema formation and recruitment of monocytes, neutrophils, and other leukocytes to the site. In addition, monocytes and tissue macrophages exposed to these cytokines are activated to acquire phagocytic and cytotoxic functions. Since it takes hours for these inflammatory reactions to emerge, they are called "delayed." It is generally believed that the T cells that elicit delayed hypersensitivity reactions are CD4$^+$ and recognize antigen of interest in association with class II MHC molecules. However, ample evidence exists to implicate CD8$^+$ T cells in this process (especially in reactions within the central nervous system). Although the elicitation of delayed hypersensitivity reactions is antigen-specific, the inflammation that attends the response is itself nonspecific. This feature accounts for the high level of tissue injury and cell destruction that is found in DH responses. By contrast, effector responses elicited by cytotoxic T cells possess much less nonspecific inflammation. Cytotoxic T cells interact directly with antigen-bearing target cells and deliver a "lethal hit" that is clean and highly specific; there is virtually no innocent bystander injury in this response.

Humoral immunity arises when B cells produce antibodies in response to antigenic challenge.[1] Although antigen alone may be sufficient to activate B cells to produce IgM antibodies, this response is amplified in the presence of helper T cells. Moreover, the ability of B cells to produce more differentiated antibody isotypes, such as IgG or IgE, is dependent on helper signals from T cells. Within the past 10 years, immunologists have appreciated that helper T cells provide "help" in the form of lymphokines and that the pattern of lymphokines produced by a helper T cell plays a key role in determining the nature of the B cell antibody response. For example, one polar form of helper T cell—called Th1—responds to antigen stimulation by producing IL-2, IFN-γ, and TNF-α.[13] In turn, these cytokines influence B cell differentiation in the direction of producing complement-fixing IgG antibodies. By contrast, Th2 cells (the other polar form of helper T cell) respond to antigen stimulation by producing IL-4, IL-5, IL-6, and IL-10. In turn, these cytokines influence B-cell differentiation in the directions of producing non–complement-fixing IgG antibodies or IgA and IgE antibodies.

The discovery of two polar forms of helper T cells (as well as numerous intermediate forms) has already had a profound impact on our understanding of the immune response and its regulation. While the Th1/Th2 dichotomy was first described for CD4$^+$ T cells, recent evidence strongly suggests that a similar difference in cytokine profiles exists for subpopulations of CD8$^+$ T cells. Moreover, there is good experimental evidence to suggest that Th1-type cells mediate delayed hypersensitivity reactions and thus can function as effector cells, as well as helper cells. Th2-type cells do not mediate typical delayed hypersensitivity reactions, but these cells are not without immunopathogenic potential because they have been implicated in inflammatory reactions of the immediate and intermediate types. Much still remains to be learned about helper T cell subsets, but it is already clear that Th1-dependent immune responses are particularly deleterious in the eye.

T-Cell–Dependent Inflammation

Primarily by virtue of the lymphokines they produce, T cells can cause immunogenic inflammation if they encounter their antigen of interest in a peripheral tissue. This is equally true for CD4$^+$ and CD8$^+$ cells, although much more is known about the former. The requirement for signal 1 (peptide plus MHC class I or II molecules) must be fulfilled in order for effector T cells to be activated by antigen in the periphery. If the responding T cell is CD4$^+$, then an MHC class II–bearing professional APC (bone marrow–derived dendritic cell or macrophage) is usually responsible for providing signal 1. If the responding T cell is of the Th1 type, it produces IFN-γ along with other pro-inflammatory molecules. IFN-γ is a potent activator of microvascular endothelial cells and macrophages. Activated endothelial cells become "leaky," permitting edema fluid and plasma proteins to accumulate at the site. Activated endothelial cells also promote the immigration of bloodborne leukocytes, including monocytes, into the site, and it is the activated macrophages that provide much of the "toxicity" at the inflammatory site. These cells respond to IFN-γ by upregulating the genes responsible for nitric oxide (NO) synthesis. NO, together with newly generated reactive oxygen intermediates, creates much of the local necrosis associated with immunogenic inflammation. Because Th2 cells do not make IFN-γ in response to antigenic stimulation, one might expect that Th2 cells would not promote inflammatory injury, but this does not appear to be the case. Th2 cells have been directly implicated in immune inflammation, including that found in the eye. The offending lymphokine may be IL-10, although other cytokines may also participate.

T Cells in Disease: Infectious, Immunopathogenic, Autoimmune

T cells were presumably created via evolution to aid in the process by which invading pathogens are prevented from causing disease. It is generally believed that T cells were designed to detect intracellular pathogens, a belief based on the ability of T cells to detect peptides derived from degradation of intracellular or phagocytosed pathogens. This property is most obviously revealed in viral infections where $CD8^+$ T cells detect peptides on virus-infected cells derived from viral proteins in association with class I molecules. Once recognition has occurred, a "lethal hit" is delivered to the target cell, and lysis aborts the viral infection. T-cell immunity is also conferred when $CD4^+$ T cells detect peptides derived from bacteria (or other pathogens) phagocytosed by macrophages. Recognition in this case does not result in delivery of a "lethal hit"; instead, pro-inflammatory cytokines released by the activated T cells cause the macrophages to acquire phagocytic and cytotoxic functions that lead to the death of the offending pathogen.

To a limited extent with $CD8^+$ cells, but to a greater extent with $CD4^+$ cells, the inflammation associated with the immune attack on the invading pathogen can lead to injury of surrounding tissues.[16] If the extent of this injury is of sufficient magnitude, disease may result from the inflammation itself, quite apart from the "toxicity" of the pathogen. This is the basis of the concept of T-cell–dependent immunopathogenic disease. As previously mentioned, certain organs and tissues, especially the eye, are particularly vulnerable to immunopathogenic injury. In tissues of this type, the immune response may prove to be more problematic than the triggering infection.

In some pathologic circumstances, T cells mistakenly identify self molecules as "foreign," thus mediating an autoimmune response that can eventuate in disease. Although this idea is conceptually sound, it is often (usually) difficult to identify the offending self antigen. Because of this difficulty, it is frequently impossible to determine whether a particular inflammatory condition, initiated by T cells, is immunopathogenic in origin (and, therefore, triggered by an unidentified pathogen) or autoimmune in origin. This is a particular common problem in the eye.

REFERENCES

1. Janeway CA Jr, Travers P (eds): Immunobiology: The Immune System in Health and Disease, 3rd ed. New York, Current Biology, Ltd./Garland Publishing, Inc., 1997.
2. Von Boehmer H: The developmental biology of T lymphocytes. Annu Rev Immunol 6:309, 1993.
3. Moller G (ed): Positive T cell selection in the thymus. Immunol Rev 135:5, 1993.
4. Nossal GJV: Negative selection of lymphocytes. Cell 76:229, 1994.
5. Havran WL, Boismenu R: Activation and function of γδ T cells. Curr Opin Immunol 6:442, 1994.
6. Germain RN: MHC-dependent antigen processing and peptide presentation: Providing ligands for T lymphocyte activation. Cell 76:287, 1994.
7. Fremont DH, Rees WA, Kozono H: Biophysical studies of T cell receptors and their ligands. Curr Opin Immunol 8:93, 1996.
8. Janeway CA, Bottomly K: Signals and signs for lymphocyte responses. Cell 76:275, 1994.
9. Sprent J, Webb SR: Intrathymic and extrathymic clonal deletion of T cells. Curr Opin Immunol 7:196, 1995.
10. Picker LJ, Butcher EC: Physiological and molecular mechanisms of lymphocyte homing. Annu Rev Immunol 10:561, 1993.
11. Jain J, Loh C, Rao A: Transcription regulation of the IL-2 gene. Curr Opin Immunol 7:333, 1995.
12. Minami Y, Kono T, Miyazaki T, Taniguchi T: The IL-2 receptor complex: Its structure, function, and target genes. Annu Rev Immunol 11:245, 1993.
13. Mosmann TR, Coffman RL: T_H1 and T_H2 cells: Different patterns of lymphokine secretion lead to different functional properties. Annu Rev Immunol 7:145, 1989.
14. Griffiths GM: The cell biology of CTL killing. Curr Opin Immunol 7:343, 1995.
15. Mueller DL, Jenkins MK: Molecular mechanisms underlying functional T cell unresponsiveness. Curr Opin Immunol 7:325, 1995.
16. Maggi E, Romagnani S: Role of T cells and T cell-derived cytokines in the pathogenesis of allergic diseases. Ann N Y Acad Sci 725:2, 1994.

CHAPTER 8

B-Lymphocyte Responses

C. Stephen Foster

B-lymphocyte development from pluripotential bone-marrow stem cells influenced by endosteal region bone marrow interstitial cells is introduced in the Ontogeny of the Immune System section of Chapter 6, A Cast of Thousands: The Cells of the Immune System. This cell, thus committed, has been designated a *pre–B lymphocyte*. It contains cytoplasmic, but not membrane, immunoglobulin M (IgM) heavy chains that associate with "surrogate light chains" devoid of variable regions. These primitive immunoglobulin molecules in pre–B cells, composed of complete, mature heavy chains and surrogate light chains, are critical to the further development of the B cell into the immature B lymphocyte containing complete κ or λ light chains with suitable variable regions. IgM is then expressed on the immature B-cell surface. Interleukin-7 is important in the process of B-cell development, as is tyrosine kinase in bone marrow stromal cells and stem cells. When an antigen encounters cell-surface IgM that has binding specificities for the antigen (e.g., self-antigens), tolerance to the antigen is the typical result if such an encounter precedes emigration of the B cell from the bone marrow.

Once the immature B cell has acquired its "exit visa" (complete surface IgM), it leaves the bone marrow, residing primarily in the peripheral lymphoid organs (and blood), where it further matures to express both IgM and IgD on its cell surface. It is now a mature B cell, responsive to antigen with proliferation and antibody synthesis.

The hallmark of the vertebrate immune system is its ability to mount a highly specific response against virtually any foreign antigen, even those never before encountered. The ability to generate a diverse immune response depends on the assembly of discontinuous genes that encode the antigen-binding sites of immunoglobulin and T-cell receptors during lymphocyte development. Diversity is generated through the recombination of various germline gene segments, imprecise joining of segments with insertion of additional nucleotides at the junctions, and somatic mutations occurring within the recombining gene segments. Other factors, such as chromosomal position of the recombining gene segments and the number of homologous gene segments, may play a role in determining the specificities of the antigen-recognizing proteins produced by a maturing lymphocyte.

Antibody Diversity

The paradox of an individual possessing a limited number of genes but the capability to generate an almost infinite number of different antibodies remained an enigma to immunologists for a considerable time. The discovery of distinct variable (V) and constant (C) regions in the light and heavy chains of immunoglobulin molecules (Fig. 8–1) raised the possibility that immunoglobulin genes possess an unusual architecture. In 1965, Dreyer and Bennett proposed that the V and C regions of an immunoglobulin chain are encoded by two separate genes in embryonic (germline) cells *(germline gene diversity)*.[1] According to this model, one of several V genes becomes joined to the C gene during lymphocyte development. In 1976, Hozumi and Tonegawa discovered that variable and constant regions are encoded by separate, multiple genes far apart in germline DNA that become joined to form a complete immunoglobulin gene active in B lymphocytes.[2] Immunoglobulin genes are thus translocated during the differentiation of antibody-producing cells *(somatic recombination)* (Fig. 8–2).

STRUCTURE AND ORGANIZATION OF IMMUNOGLOBULIN GENES

The V regions of immunoglobulins contain three hypervariable segments that determine antibody specificity (Fig. 8–3).[3] Hypervariable segments of both the light (L) and heavy (H) chains form the *antigen-binding* site. Hypervariable re-

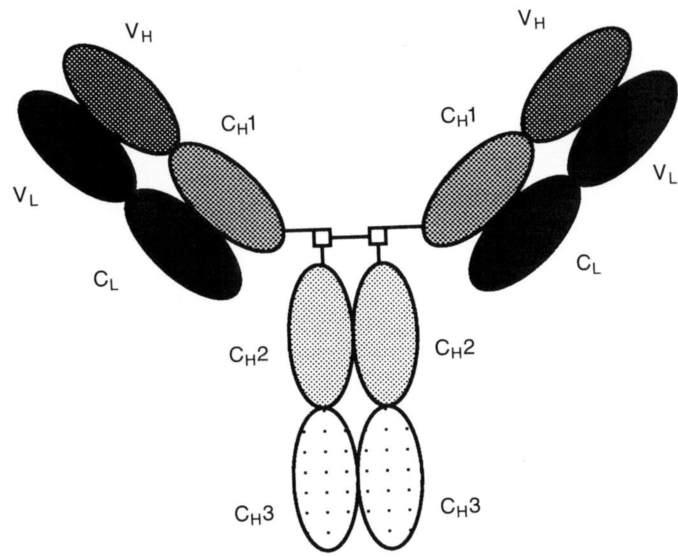

FIGURE 8–1. Structure of IgG showing the regions of similar sequence (domains).

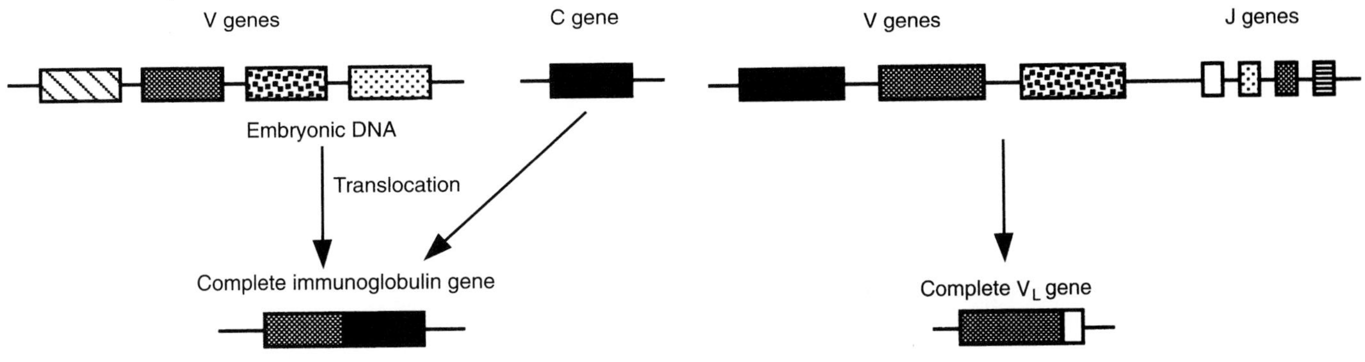

FIGURE 8–2. Translocation of a V-segment gene to a C gene in the differentiation of an antibody-producing B cell.

FIGURE 8–4. A V gene is translocated near a J gene in forming a light-chain V region gene.

gions are also called *complementarity-determining regions* (CDRs). The V regions of L and H chains have several hundred gene segments in germline DNA; the exact number of segments is still being debated but is estimated to range between 250 and 1000 segments.

Light-Chain Genes

A complete gene for the V region of a light chain is formed by the splicing of an incomplete V-segment gene with one of several J (joining)-segment genes, which encodes part of the last hypervariable segment (Fig. 8–4).[4–6] Additional diversity is generated by allowing V and J genes to become spliced in different joining frames *(junctional diversity)* (Fig. 8–5).[5] There are at least three frames for the joining of V and J. Two forms of light chains exist: kappa (κ) and lambda (λ). For κλ chains, assume that there are approximately 250 V-segment genes and four J-segment genes. Therefore, a total of 250 × 4 × 3 (for junctional diversity), or 3000, kinds of complete VK genes can be formed by combinations of V and J.

Heavy-Chain Genes

Heavy-chain V-region genes are formed by the somatic recombination of V, an additional segment called D (diversity), and J-segment genes (Fig. 8–6). The third CDR of the heavy chain is encoded mainly by a D segment. Approximately 15 D segments lie between hundreds of V_H and at least four J_H gene segments. A D segment joins a J_H segment; a V_H segment then becomes joined to the DJ_H to form the complete V_H gene. To further diversify the third CDR of the heavy chain, extra nucleotides are inserted between V and D and between D and J *(N-region addition)* by the action of *terminal deoxyribonucleotidyl transferase.*[7] Introns, which are noncoding intervening sequences, are removed from the primary RNA transcript.

The site-specific recombination of V, D, and J genes is mediated by enzymes *(immunoglobulin recombinase)* that recognize conserved nonamer and palindromic heptamer sequences flanking these gene segments.[8, 9] The nonamer and heptamer sequences are separated by either 12-base pair (bp) or 23-bp spacers (Fig. 8–7). Recombination can occur only between the 12- and 23-bp types but not between

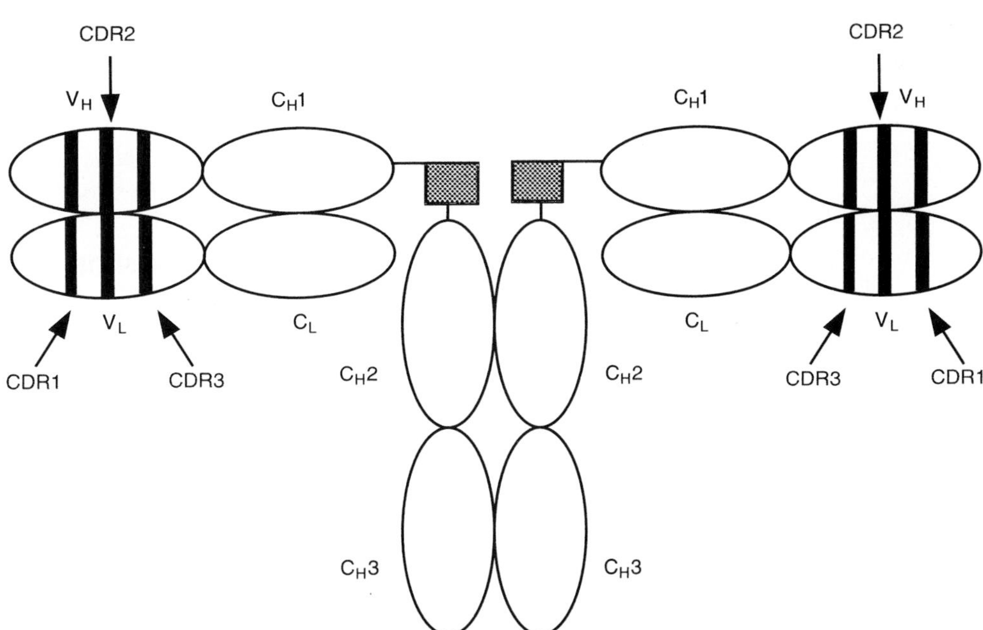

FIGURE 8–3. Hypervariable or complementarity-determining regions (CDRs) on the antigen-binding site of the variable regions of IgG.

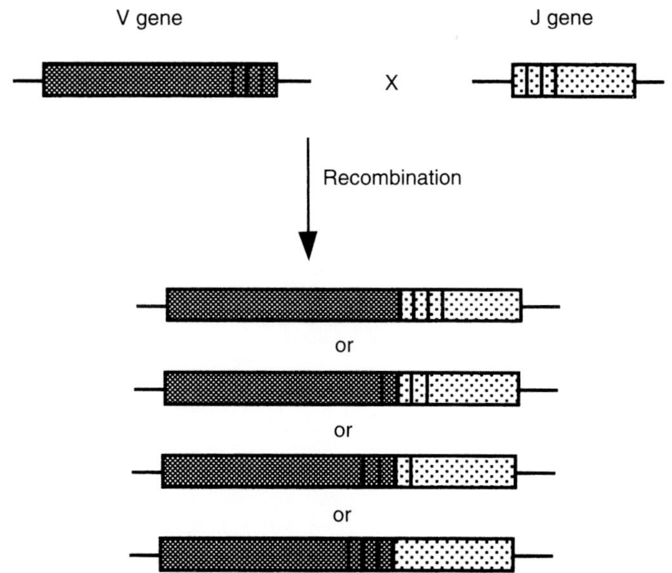

FIGURE 8–5. Imprecision in the site of splicing of a V gene to a J gene (junctional diversity).

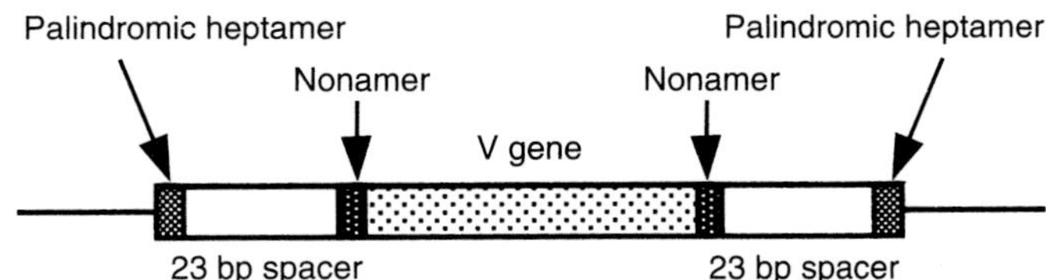

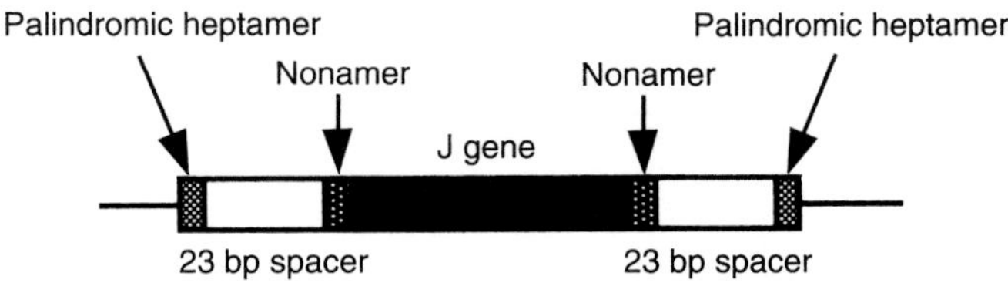

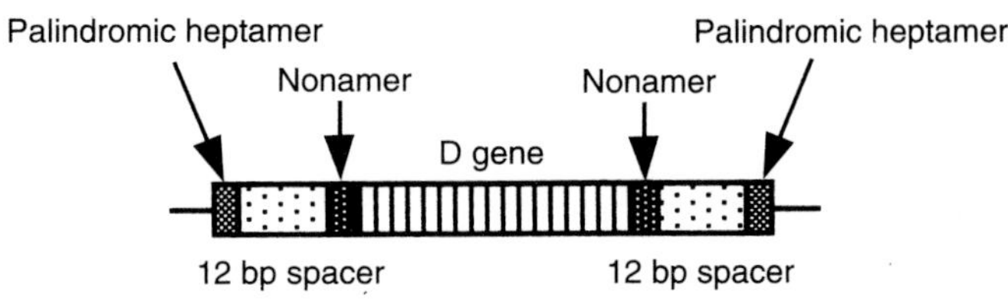

FIGURE 8–7. Recognition sites for the recombination of V-, D-, and J-segment genes. V and J genes are flanked by sites containing 23-bp spacers, whereas D-segment genes possess 12-bp spacers. Recombination can occur only between sites with different classes of spacers.

two 12-bp types or two 23-bp types (called the 12/23 rule of V-gene-segment recombination). For example, V_H segments and J_H segments are flanked by 23-bp types on both their 5′ and 3′ ends. Consequently, they cannot recombine with each other or among themselves. Instead, they recombine with D segments, which are flanked on both 5′ and 3′ ends by recognition sequences of the 12-bp type.

SOURCES OF IMMUNOGLOBULIN GENE DIVERSITY

For 250 V_H, 15 D_H, and 4 J_H gene segments that can be joined in three frames, at least 45,000 complete V_H genes can be formed. Therefore, more than 10^8 different specificities can be generated by combining different V, D, and J gene segments and by combining more than 3000 L and 45,000 H chains. If the effects of N-region addition are included, more than 10^{11} different combinations can be formed. This number is large enough to account for the immense range of antibodies that can be synthesized by an individual.

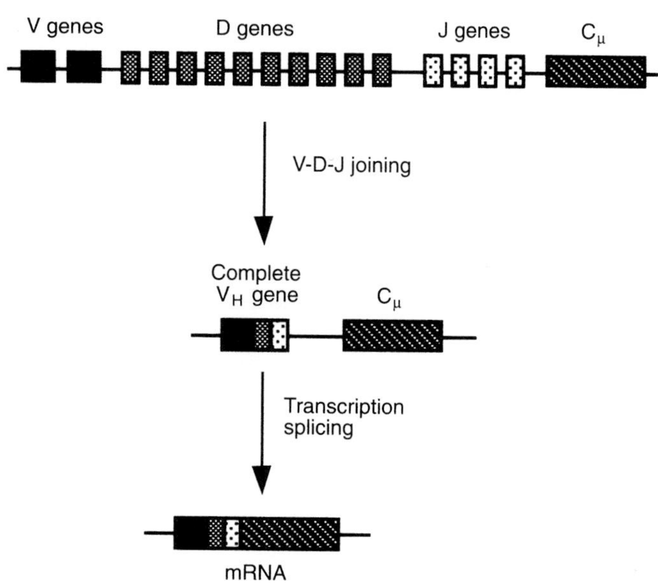

FIGURE 8–6. The variable region of the heavy chain is encoded by V-, D-, and J-segment genes.

Far fewer V genes than V_κ genes encode light chains. However, many more V amino-acid sequences are known.[10–12] It is therefore likely that mutations introduced somatically give rise to much of the diversity of λ light chains *(somatic hypermutation)*.[5] Likewise, somatic hypermutation further amplifies the diversity of heavy chains. To summarize, four sources of diversity are used to form the almost limitless array of antibodies that protect a host from foreign invasion: *germline gene diversity, somatic recombination, junctional diversity,* and *somatic hypermutation.*

REGULATION OF IMMUNOGLOBULIN GENE EXPRESSION

An incomplete V gene becomes paired to a J gene on only one of a pair of homologous chromosomes. Successful rearrangement of one heavy-chain V region prevents the process from occurring on the other heavy-chain allele. Only the properly recombined immunoglobulin gene is expressed. Therefore, all of the V regions of immunoglobulins produced by a single lymphocyte are the same. This is called *allelic exclusion.*[13, 14]

There are five classes of immunoglobulins. An antibody-producing cell first synthesizes IgM and then IgG, IgA, IgE, or IgD of the same specificity. Different classes of antibodies

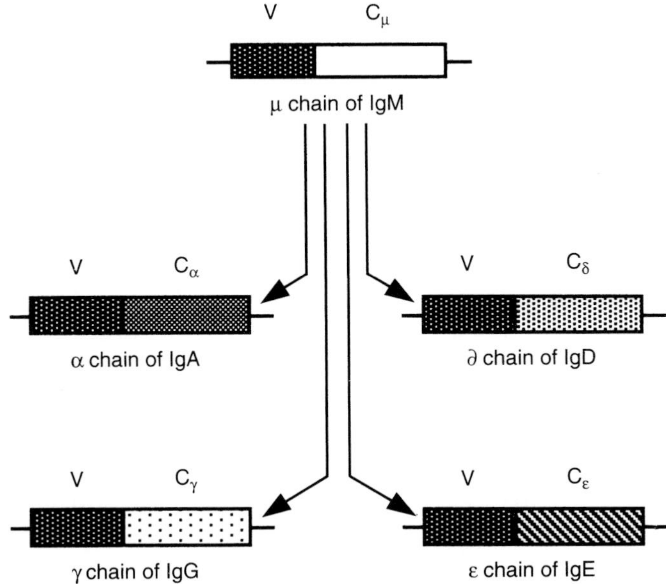

FIGURE 8–8. The V_H region is first associated with Cμ and then with another C region to form an H chain of a different class in the synthesis of different classes of immunoglobulins.

are formed by the translocation of a complete V_H (V_{HDH}) gene from the C_H gene of one class to that of another.[15] Only the constant region of the heavy chain changes; the variable region of the heavy chain remains the same (Fig. 8–8). The light chain remains the same in this switch. This step in the differentiation of an antibody-producing cell is called *class switching* and is mediated by another DNA rearrangement called *SS recombination* (Fig. 8–9).[16] This process is regulated by cytokines produced by helper T

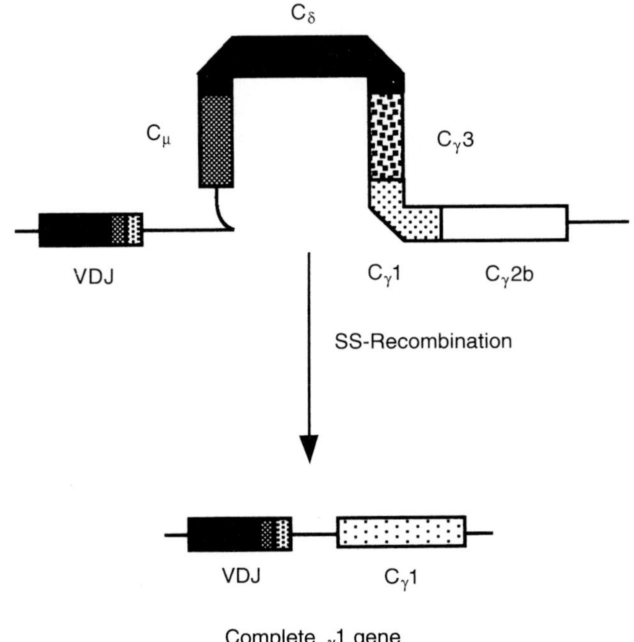

FIGURE 8–9. The V_HDJ_H gene moves from its position near Cμ to one near $C_γ1$ by SS recombination.

cells.[5] For example, switching to IgE class immunoglobulin production is provoked by the CD4 T_H2 cytokine, IL-4.

DETERMINATION OF B-CELL REPERTOIRE

V-segment genes can be grouped into families based on their DNA sequence homologies. In general, variable genes sharing greater than 80% nucleotide similarity are defined as a family.[17] There are 11 V_H gene families currently known in the mouse[17–20] and 6 in humans.[21–24] At least 29 families are known for the V of murine light-chain genes.[25, 26] In fetal pre–B cells, *chromosomal position* is a major determinant of V_H rearrangement frequency, resulting in a nonrandom repertoire that is biased toward use of V_H families closest to the J_H segments.[27–30] In contrast, random use of V_H families based on the *number of members in each family* occurs in mature B cells without bias toward J_H proximal families.[31–33] The preferential V_H gene rearrangement frequency seen in pre–B cells presumably becomes normalized when contact of the organism with a foreign antigen selects for the expression of the entire V_H gene repertoire. One can speculate that members of V_H families preferentially used in the pre–B cell encode antibody specificities that are needed in the early development of the immune system.[34]

Immunoglobulins are serum proteins that migrate with the globulin fractions by electrophoresis.[2] Although they are glycoproteins, the molecules' primary functions are determined by their polypeptide sequence.[3] At one end of the immunoglobulin, the amino terminus, is a region that binds a site (epitope) on an antigen with great specificity. At the other end, the carboxyl terminus, is a non–antigen-binding region responsible for various functions, including complement fixation and cellular stimulation via binding to cell-surface Ig receptors. The generalized structure of immunoglobulin is best understood initially by examining its most common class, IgG (see Fig. 8–1).

IgG is composed of four polypeptide chains: two identical heavy chains and two identical light chains. Heavy chains weigh about twice as much as light chains. The identical heavy chains are covalently linked by two disulfide bonds. One light chain is associated with each of the heavy chains by a disulfide bond and noncovalent forces. The two light chains are not linked. Asparagine residues on the heavy chains contain carbohydrate groups. The amino terminals of one light chain and its linked heavy chain compose the region for specific epitope binding. The carboxyl termini of the two heavy chains constitute the non–antigen-binding region.

Each polypeptide chain, whether light or heavy, is composed of regions that are called constant (C) or variable (V). A variable region on a light chain is called V_L, the constant region of a heavy chain is called C_H, and so forth. If the amino-acid sequence of multiple light or heavy chains is compared, the constant regions will vary little, whereas the variable regions differ greatly. The light chains are divided approximately equally into a constant (C_L) and variable (V_L) region at the carboxyl and amino terminals, respectively. The heavy chains also contain a similar length of variable region (V_H) at the amino terminals, but the constant region (C_H) is three times the length of the variable region (V_H). The variable regions are responsible for antigen binding, and it is this variability that accounts for the ability to bind to

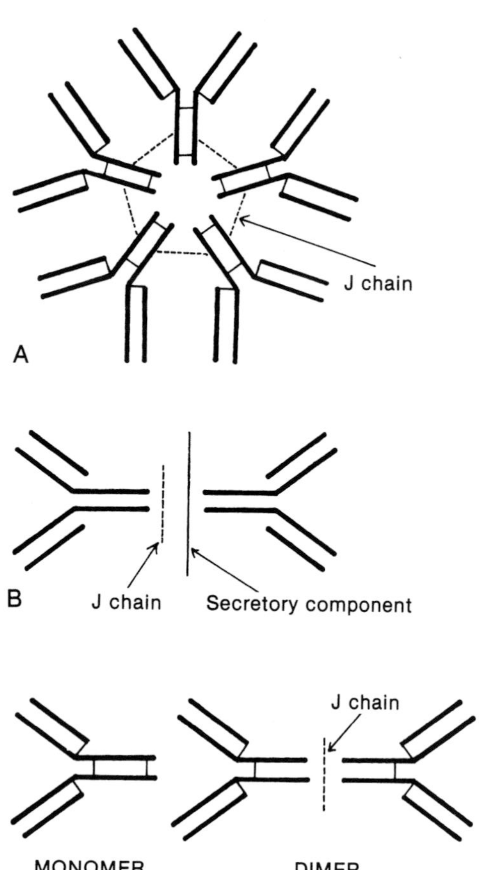

FIGURE 8–10. Schematic diagram of polymeric human immunoglobulins. *A,* IgM. *B,* Secretory IgA. *C,* Serum IgA.

millions of potential and real epitopes.[4] Because each antibody molecule has two antigen-binding sites with variable regions, cross-linking of two identical antigens may be performed by one antibody. The constant regions carry out effector functions that are common to all antibodies of a given class (e.g., IgG) without the requirement of unique binding sites.

The function of various regions of the immunoglobulin molecule was determined in part by the use of proteolytic enzymes that digest these molecules at specific locations. These enzymes have also been exploited for the development of laboratory reagents. The enzyme papain splits the molecule on the amino terminal side of the disulfide bonds that link the heavy chains, resulting in three fragments: two identical Fab fragments (each composed of the one entire heavy chain and a portion of the associated heavy chain) and one Fc fragment composed of the linked carboxyl terminal ends of the two heavy chains. In contrast, treatment with the enzyme pepsin results in one molecule composed of two linked Fab fragments known as F(ab′).[2] The Fc fragment is degraded by pepsin treatment.

Within some classes of immunoglobulins, whole molecules may combine with other molecules of the same class to form polymers with additional functional capabilities. J chains facilitate the association of two or more immunoglobulins (Fig. 8–10), most notably IgA and IgM. Secretory component is a polypeptide synthesized by nonmotile epithelium found near mucosal surfaces. This polypeptide may bind noncovalently to IgA molecules, allowing their transport across mucosal surfaces to be elaborated in secretions.

Five immunoglobulin classes are recognized in humans: IgG, IgM, IgA, IgE, and IgD (Table 8–1). Some classes are composed of subclasses as well. The class or subclass is determined by the structure of the heavy-chain constant region (C_H).[5] The heavy chains γ, μ, α, ϵ, and δ are found in IgG, IgM, IgA, IgE, and IgD, respectively. Four subclasses of IgG and two subclasses of both IgA and IgM exist (Table 8–2). The two light chains on any immunoglobulin are identical and, depending on the structure of their constant regions, may be designated kappa (κ) or lambda (λ). Kappa chains tend to predominate in human immunoglobulins regardless of the heavy chain–determined class. Whether an immunoglobulin is composed of two κ or two λ chains does not determine its functional capabilities. Heavy chain–determined class does dictate important capacities.[6]

IMMUNOGLOBULIN G (IgG)

The most abundant of the human classes in serum, IgG constitutes about three-quarters of the total serum immunoglobulins. Respectively, IgG_1 and IgG_2 make up about 60% and 20% of the total IgG. IgG_3 and IgG_4 are relatively

TABLE 8–1. **Diversity in TCR and Immunoglobulin Genes**

		Immunoglobulin		TCR			
		H	κ	α	β	γ	δ
Germline Segments	Variable (V)	250–1000	250	100	25	7	10
	Diversity (D)	15	0	0	2	0	2
	Joining (J)	4	4	50	12	3	2
Variable region combinations		62,500–250,000		2500		50	
	Use of different D and J segments	Yes	Yes	Yes	Yes	—	Yes
Junctional Diversity	Variability in 3′ Joining of V and J	Rarely	Rarely	Yes	No	Yes	Yes
	D joining in all three reading frames	Rarely	—	—	Often	—	Often
	N-region diversity	V-D, D-J	None	V-J	V-D, D-J	V-J	V-D, D1-D2
Junctional combinations		10^8		10^{15}		10^{18}	
Total repertoire		10^{11}		10^{17}		10^{19}	

The numbers of the V, D, and J gene segments in the murine genome are shown. Total repertoire produced by the various mechanisms for generating diversity was estimated.

TABLE 8–2. **Human Immunoglobulin Subclasses**

Immunoglobulin	Subclasses	Predominant Subclass	Unique Characteristics
IgG	1, 2, 3, and 4	1 (65%) and 2 (25%)	IgG2—crosses placenta poorly IgG3—aggregates spontaneously IgG4—blocks IgE binding; poor classic complement fixation
IgA	1 and 2	1	
IgM	1 and 2	1	

minor components. IgGs are the primary immunoglobulin providing immune protection in the extravascular compartments of the body. IgG is able to fix complement in the serum, an important function in inducing inflammation and controlling infection. IgG_3 and IgG_1 are most adept at complement fixation. IgG is the only immunoglobulin class to cross the placenta, an important aspect in fetal defense. Via their Fc portion, IgG molecules bind Fc receptors found on a host of inflammatory cells. Such binding activates cells such as macrophages and natural killer cells, enhancing cytotoxic activities important in the immune response.

IMMUNOGLOBULIN M (IgM)

Less abundant in the serum than IgG, IgM typically exists as a pentameric form, stabilized by J chains, theoretically allowing the binding of 10 epitopes. (In vivo, this is usually limited by steric considerations.) IgM appears early in the immune response to antigen and is especially efficient at initiating agglutination, complement fixation, and cytolysis. IgM probably preceded IgG in the evolution of the immune response and is the most important antibody class in defending the circulation.

IMMUNOGLOBULIN A (IgA)

IgA is found in secretions of mucosal surfaces as well as in the serum. In secretions, it exists as a dimer coupled by J chains and stabilized by secretory component. IgA protects mucosal surfaces from infections but may also be responsible for immunologic surveillance at the site of first contact with antigen. IgA in secretion is hardy, able to withstand the ravages of proteolytic degradation.

IMMUNOGLOBULIN D (IgD)

IgD is present in minute amounts in the serum and is the least stable of the immunoglobulins. Its function is not known, but it probably serves as a differentiation marker. IgD is found on the surface of B lymphocytes (along with IgM) and may have a role in class switching and tolerance.

IMMUNOGLOBULIN E (IgE)

IgE is notable for its ability to bind to mast cells; when cross-linked by antigen, it causes a variety of changes in the mast cell, including release of granule contents and membrane-derived mediators. Although recognized as a component of the allergic response, the role of IgE in protective immunity is speculative.

IMMUNOGLOBULIN INTRACLASS DIFFERENCES

Differences among the immunoglobulin classes are known as *isotypes*, because all of the normal individuals in a species possess all of the classes. *Allotype* refers to antigenic structures on immunoglobulins that may differ from one individual to another within a species. *Idiotype* refers to differences among individual antibodies and is determined by the variable domain. Just as the variable domain allows for antibodies to recognize many antigens (epitopes), these differences also allow individual antibodies to be recognized on the basis of their idiotype. In fact, antibodies directed against antibodies exist and are called anti-idiotypic antibodies. These anti-idiotypic antibodies are crucial to the regulation of the antibody response and constitute the basis for Jerne's idiotype network.

Complement

The complement system functions in the immune response by allowing animals to recognize foreign substances and defend themselves against infection.[23] The pathways of complement activation are complex (Fig. 8–11).[24] Activation begins with the formation of antigen-antibody complexes and the ensuing generation of peptides that lead to a cascade of proteolytic events. The particle that activates the system accumulates a protein complex on its surface that often leads to cellular destruction via disruption of membranes.

Two independent pathways of complement activation are known. The classic pathway is initiated by IgG- and IgM-containing immune complexes.[25] The alternative pathway is activated by aggravated IgA or complex polysaccharides from microbial cell walls.[26] One component, C3, is crucial to both pathways and in its proactive form can be found circulating in plasma in large concentrations. Deficiency or absence of C3 results in increased susceptibility to infection.[27] Cleavage of C3 may result in at least seven products (lettered a through g), each with biologic properties related to cellular activation and immune and nonimmune responses.[28] C3a, for instance, causes the release of histamine from mast cells, neutrophil enzyme release, smooth muscle contraction, suppressor T-cell induction, and secretion of macrophage IL-1, prostaglandin, and leukotriene.[29] C3e enhances vascular permeability. C3b binds to target cell surfaces and allows opsonization of biologic particles.

The alternative pathway probably is a first line of defense, because unlike the classic pathway, it may neutralize foreign material in the absence of antibody. The initiating enzyme of this pathway, factor D, circulates in an active form and may protect bystander cells from inadvertent destruction following activation of the pathway.

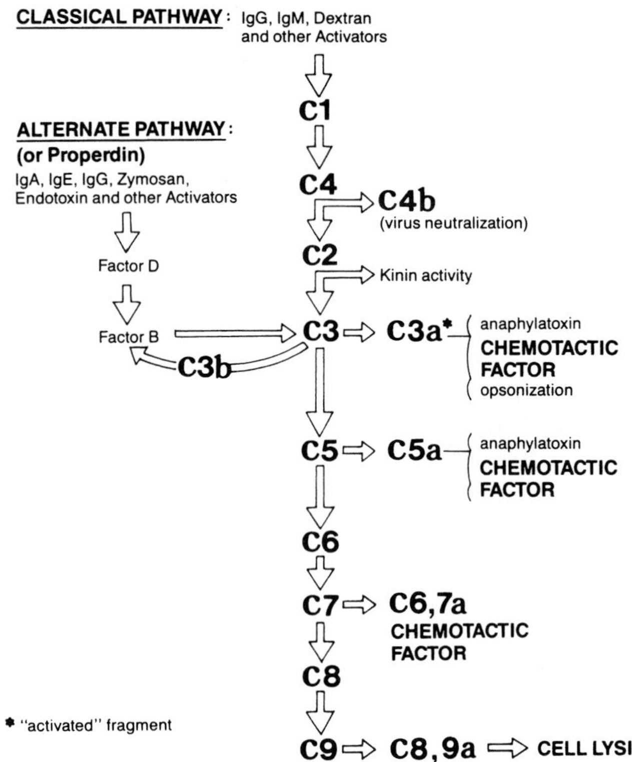

FIGURE 8–11. Simplified schematic of steps in classic and alternate complement cascades.

The final step of both pathways is membrane damage leading to cytolysis. Both pathways require the assembly of five precursor proteins to effect this damage: C5, C6, C7, C8, and C9. The mechanism of complement-mediated cell lysis is similar to that of cell-mediated cytotoxicity (as with natural killer cells). Membrane lesions result from insertion of tubular complexes into the membranes, leading to uptake of water with ion-exchange disruption and eventual osmotic lysis.

The complement system interfaces with a variety of immune responses, as outlined earlier, and with the intrinsic coagulation pathways.[30] Complement activity is usually measured by assessing the ability of serum to lyse sensitized sheep red blood cells.[31] Values are expressed as 50% hemolytic complement units per millimeter. The function of an individual component may be studied by supplying excess quantities of all the other components in a sheep red blood cell lysis assay.[32] Components are quantitated by radial diffusion or immunoassay. Complement may be demonstrated in tissue sections by immunofluorescence or enzymatic techniques.

Complement plays a role in a number of human diseases. Complement-mediated cell lysis is the final common pathologic event in type III hypersensitivity reactions. Deficiencies of complement exist in the following human disorders: systemic lupus erythematosus, glomerulonephritis, Raynaud's phenomenon, recurrent gonococcal and meningococcal infections, hereditary angioedema, rheumatoid disease, and others.[27]

B-Cell Response to Antigen

PRIMARY RESPONSE

Naive B cells respond to protein antigen in much the same way that T cells do, through the help of antigen-presenting cells and "helper" T cells. An antigen-presenting cell (usually a macrophage or dendritic cell) processes the antigen and presents it to an antigen-specific helper (CD4) T cell, generally in the T-cell–rich zones of the required lymph node. The T cell is thus activated, expresses the membrane protein gp39, secretes cytokines (e.g., IL-2 and IL-6), and binds to similarly activated antigen-specific B cells (activated by the binding cross-linking of antigen to surface IgM and IgD binding sites). The T-cell/B-cell proliferation and a cascade of intracellular protein phosphorylation events, together with T-cell cytokine signals, result in production of transcription factors that induce transcription of various B-cell genes, including those responsible for production of IgM light and heavy chains with paratopes specific to the antigen epitopes that initiated this primary B-cell response. The proliferating B cells form germinal centers in the lymph node follicles, and somatic hypermutation of the IgV genes in some of these cells results in the evolution of a collection of B cells in the germinal center with surface IgM of even higher antigen-binding affinity. This phenomenon is called affinity maturation of the primary antibody response. Those cells with the greatest antigen binding affinity survive as this primary B-cell response subsides, persisting as long-lived memory cells responsible for the classic distinguishing characteristics of the secondary humoral immune response.

SECONDARY RESPONSE

The development of the secondary humoral immune response is markedly accelerated compared with the primary response, and it is greatly amplified in terms of magnitude of antibody production (Fig. 8–12). The secondary response differs from the primary one in the isotype or isotypes of antibody produced, as well as in the avidity of the paratopes for the epitopes on the elicited antigen. IgG, IgA, and IgE isotypes may now be seen in the effector phase of this

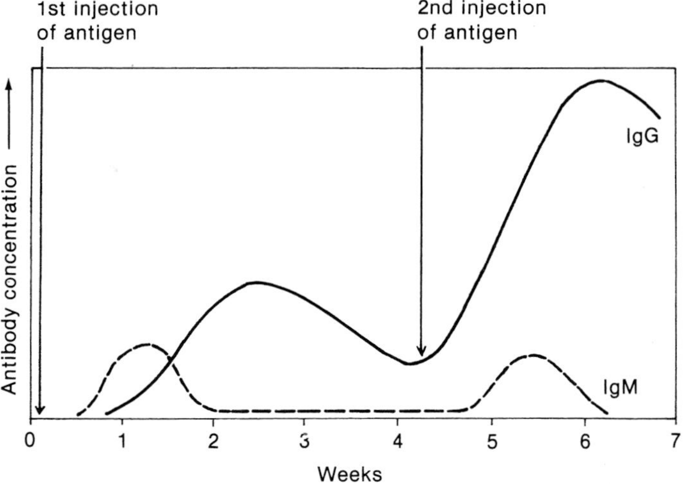

FIGURE 8–12. Relative synthesis of IgG and IgM following initial and subsequent antigen injection.

secondary humoral immune response, and the binding affinities of these antibodies are usually greater than that of the IgM elicited in the primary response.

The cellular and molecular events of the secondary B-cell response are considerably different from those of the primary response. Memory B cells themselves become the preeminent antigen-binding, processing, and presenting cells, presenting peptide fragments (antigenic determinants) to CD4 helper T cells in the typical major histocompatibility complex–restricted fashion, with "processed" peptide/human leukocyte antigen/DR motifs interacting with the appropriate elements of the T-cell receptor for antigen at the same time that B-cell CD40 and T-cell gp39 signaling occurs. Additionally, various T-cell cytokines induce the memory B cells to divide, proliferate, produce antibody, and switch the class of antibody being produced, depending on the sum total message being received by the B cell: the nature of the antigenic stimulus, the amount and the site of stimulation, and the site of the cells involved in the cognitive and activation phases of the secondary response. Memory cells of each immunoglobulin isotype involved in the secondary response will, of course, persist after devolution of the response.

References

1. Dreyer WJ, Bennett JC: The molecular basis of antibody formation: A paradox. Proc Natl Acad Sci U S A 54:864, 1965.
2. Hozumi N, Tonegawa S: Evidence for somatic rearrangement of immunoglobulin genes coding for variable and constant regions. Proc Natl Acad Sci U S A 73:3628, 1976.
3. Wu TT, Kabat EA: An analysis of the sequences of the variable regions of Bence Jones proteins and myeloma light chains and their implications for antibody complementarity. J Exp Med 132:211, 1970.
4. Leder P: The genetics of antibody diversity. Sci Am 246:102, 1982.
5. Tonegawa S: Somatic generation of antibody diversity. Nature 302:575, 1983.
6. Honjo T, Habu S: Origin of immune diversity: Genetic variation and selection. Annu Rev Biochem 54:803, 1985.
7. Alt FW, Baltimore D: Joining of immunoglobulin heavy chain gene segments: Implications from a chromosome with evidence of three D-JH fusions. Proc Natl Acad Sci U S A 79:4118, 1982.
8. Early P, Huang H, Davis M, et al: An immunoglobulin heavy chain variable region gene is generated from three segments of DNA: VH, D and JH. Cell 12:981, 1980.
9. Sakano H, Huppi K, Heinrich G, Tonegawa S: Sequences at the somatic recombination sites of immunoglobulin light-chain genes. Nature 280:288, 1979.
10. Weigert MG, Cesari IM, Yondovich SJ, Cohn M: Variability in the lambda light chain sequences of mouse antibody. Nature 228:1045, 1970.
11. Brack C, Hirama M, Lenhard-Schuller R, Tonegawa S: A complete immunoglobulin gene is created by somatic recombination. Cell 15:1, 1978.
12. Bernard O, Hozumi N, Tonegawa S: Sequences of mouse immunoglobulin light chain genes before and after somatic changes. Cell 15:1133, 1978.
13. Pernis BG, Chiappino G, Kelus AS, Gell PGH: Cellular localization of immunoglobulins with different allotypic specificities in rabbit lymphoid tissues. J Exp Med 122:853, 1965.
14. Cebra J, Colberg JE, Dray S: Rabbit lymphoid cells differentiated with respect to alpha-, gamma-, and mu-heavy polypeptide chains and to allotypic markers for Aa1 and Aa2. J Exp Med 123:547, 1966.
15. Kataoka T, Kawakami T, Takahasi N, Honjo T: Rearrangement of immunoglobulin g1-chain gene and mechanism for heavy-chain class switch. Proc Natl Acad Sci U S A 77:919, 1980.
16. Gritzmacher CA: Molecular aspects of heavy-chain class switching. Cri Rev Immunol 9:173, 1989.
17. Brodeur PH, Riblet R: The immunoglobulin heavy chain variable region (Igh-V) locus in the mouse I. One hundred Igh-V genes comprise seven families of homologous genes. Eur J Immunol 14:922, 1984.
18. Winter EA, Radbruch A, Krawinkel U: Members of novel VH gene families are found in VDJ regions of polyclonally activated B lymphocytes. EMBO J 4:2861, 1985.
19. Kofler R: A new murine Ig VH family. J Immunol 140:4031, 1988.
20. Reininger L, Kaushik A, Jaton JC: A member of a new VH gene family encodes anti-bromelinised mouse red blood cell autoantibodies. Eur J Immunol 18:1521, 1988.
21. Rechavi G, Bienz B, Ram D, et al: Organization and evolution of immunoglobulin VH gene subgroups. Proc Natl Acad Sci U S A 79:4405, 1982.
22. Rechavi G, Ram D, Glazer R, et al: Evolutionary aspects of immunoglobulin heavy chain variable region (VH) gene subgroups. Proc Natl Acad Sci U S A 80:855, 1983.
23. Matthyssens G, Rabbitts TH: Structure and multiplicity of genes for the human immunoglobulin heavy chain variable region. Proc Natl Acad Sci U S A 77:6561, 1980.
24. Berman JE, Mellis SJ, Pollock R, et al: Content and organization of the human Ig VH locus: Definition of three new VH families and linkage to the Ig CH locus. EMBO J 7:727, 1988.
25. Potter M, Newell JB, Rudikoff S, Haber E: Classification of mouse VK groups based on the partial amino acid sequence to the first invariant tryptophan: Impact of 14 new sequences from IgG myeloma proteins. Mol Immunol 12:1619, 1982.
26. D'Joostelaere LA, Huppi K, Mock B, et al: The immunoglobulin kappa light chain allelic groups among the Igk haplotypes and Igk crossover populations suggest a gene order. J Immunol 141:652, 1988.
27. Yancopoulos GD, Desiderio SV, Pasking M, et al: Preferential utilization of the most JH-proximal VH gene segments in pre-B cell lines. Nature 311:727, 1984.
28. Perlmutter RM, Kearney JF, Chang SP, Hood LE: Developmentally controlled expression of immunoglobulin VH genes. Science 227:1597, 1985.
29. Reth M, Jackson N, Alt FW: VHDJH formation and DJH replacement during pre-B differentiation: Non-random usage of gene segments. EMBO J 5:2131, 1986.
30. Lawler AM, Lin PS, Gearhart PJ: Adult B-cell repertoire is biased toward two heavy-chain variable region genes that rearrange frequently in fetal pre-B cells. Proc Natl Acad Sci U S A 84:2454, 1987.
31. Yancopoulos GD, Malynn B, Alt FW: Developmentally regulated and strain-specific expression of murine VH gene families. J Exp Med 168:417, 1988.
32. Dildrop R, Krawinkel U, Winter E, Rajewsky K: VH-gene expression in murine lipopolysaccharide blasts distributes over the nine known VH-gene groups and may be random. Eur J Immunol 15:1154, 1985.
33. Schulze DH, Kelsoe G: Genotypic analysis of B cell colonies by in situ hybridization. Stoichiometric expression of the three VH families in adult C57BL/6 and BALB/c mice. J Exp Med 166:163, 1987.
34. Krawinkel U, Cristoph T, Blankenstein T: Organization of the Ig VH locus in mice and humans. Immunol Today 10:339, 1989.

CHAPTER 9

Immune-Mediated Tissue Injury

C. Stephen Foster and J. Wayne Streilein

The immune response of an organism to an antigen may be either helpful or harmful. If the response is excessive or inappropriate, the host may incur tissue damage. The term "hypersensitivity reactions" has been applied to such excessive or inappropriate immune responses. Four major types of hypersensitivity reactions are described, and all can occur in the eye (Table 9–1). The necessary constituents for these reactions are already present in or can be readily recruited into ocular tissues. Immunoglobulins, complement components, inflammatory cells, and inflammatory mediators can, under certain circumstances, be found in ocular fluids (i.e., tears, aqueous humor, vitreous) and in the ocular tissues, adnexa, and orbit. Unfortunately, these tissues (especially the ocular tissues) can be rapidly damaged by inflammatory reactions that produce irreversible alterations in structure and function. Some authors have described a fifth type of hypersensitivity reaction, but this adds little to our real understanding of disease mechanisms and is unimportant to us as ophthalmologists in the study and care of patients with destructive ocular inflammatory diseases. For this reason, this discussion is confined to the classic four types of hypersensitivity reactions that were originally proposed by Gell, Coombs, and Lackmann.

Injury Mediated by Antibody

TYPE I HYPERSENSITIVITY

The antigens typically responsible for type I (immediate) hypersensitivity reactions are ubiquitous environmental allergens such as dust, pollens, danders, microbes, and drugs. Under ordinary cirsumstances, exposure of an individual to such materials is associated with no harmful inflammatory response. The occurrence of such a response is considered, therefore, out of place (Greek, *a topos*) or inappropriate, and it is for this reason that Cocoa and Cooke coined the word *atopy* in 1923 to describe individuals who develop such inappropriate inflammatory or immune responses to ubiquitous environmental agents.[1] The antibodies responsible for type I hypersensitivity reactions are homocytotropic antibodies, principally immunoglobulin E (IgE) but sometimes IgG4 as well. The mediators of the clinical manifestations of type I reactions include histamine, serotonin, leukotrienes (including slow-reacting substance of anaphylaxis [SRS-A]), kinins, and other vasoactive amines. Examples of type I hypersensitivity reactions include anaphylactic reactions to insect bites or to penicillin injections, allergic asthma, hay fever, and seasonal allergic conjunctivitis. It should be emphasized that in real life the four types of hypersensitivity reactions rarely are observed in pure form, in isolation from each other, and it is typical for hypersensitivity reactions to have more than one of the classic Gell and Coombs' responses as participants in the inflammatory problem. For example, eczema, atopic blepharokeratoconjunctivitis, and vernal keratoconjunctivitis have hypersensitivity reaction mechanisms of both type I and type IV. The atopic individuals who develop such abnormal reactions to environmental materials are genetically predisposed to such responses. The details of the events responsible for allergy

TABLE 9–1. **Gell, Coombs, and Lackmann Hypersensitivity Reactions**

Type	Participating Elements	Systemic Examples	Ocular Examples
Type I	Allergen, IgE, mast cells	Allergic rhinitis, allergic asthma, anaphylaxis	Seasonal allergic conjunctivitis, vernal keratoconjunctivitis, atopic keratoconjunctivitis, giant papillary conjunctivitis
Type II	Antigen, IgG, IgG3, or IgM, complement, neutrophils (enzymes), macrophages (enzymes)	Goodpasture's syndrome, myasthenia gravis	Ocular cicatricial pemphigoid, pemphigus vulgaris, dermatitis herpetiformis
Type III	Antigen, IgG, IgG3, or IgM, complement-immune complex, neutrophils (enzymes), macrophages (enzymes)	Stevens-Johnson syndrome, rheumatoid arthritis, systemic lupus erythematosus, polyarteritis nodosa, Behçet's disease, relapsing polychondritis	Ocular manifestations of diseases in Systemic Examples
Type IV	Antigen, T cells, neutrophils, macrophages	Transplant rejection, tuberculosis, sarcoidosis, Wegener's granulomatosis	Contact hypersensitivity (drug allergy), herpes disciform keratitis, phlyctenulosis, corneal transplant rejection, tuberculosis, sarcoidosis, Wegener's granulomatosis, uveitis, herpes simplex virus, stromal keratitis, river blindness

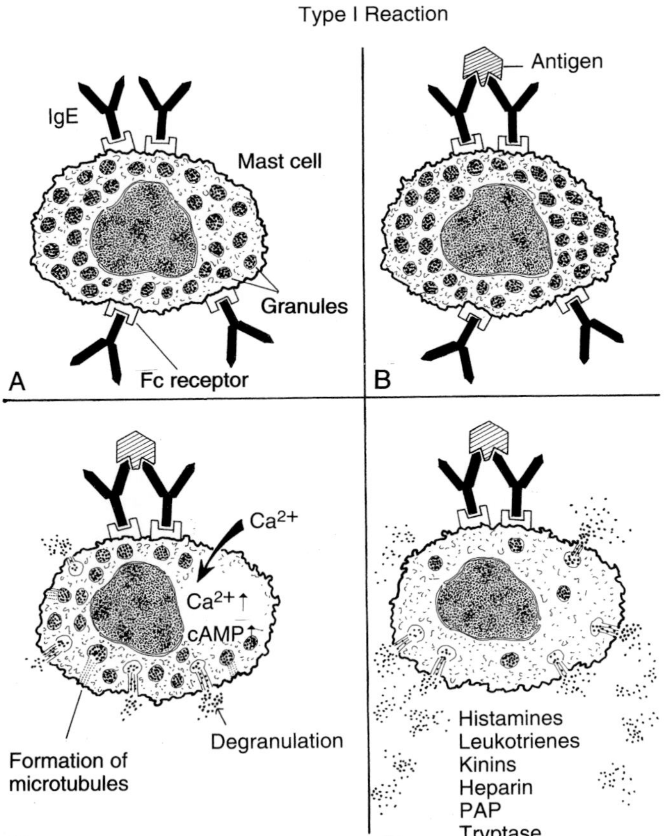

FIGURE 9–1. Type I hypersensitivity reaction mechanism. *A,* Mast cell Fc receptors have antigen-specific IgE affixed to them by virtue of the patient's being exposed to the antigen and mounting an inappropriate (atopic) immune response to that antigen, with resultant production of large amounts of antigen-specific IgE antibodies. The antibodies have found their way to the mucosal mast cell, have bound to the mast cells, but have not provoked allergic symptoms because the patient is no longer exposed to the antigen. *B,* Second (or subsequent) exposure to the sensitizing antigen or allergen results in a "bridging" binding reaction of antigen to two adjacent IgE antibodies affixed to the mast cell plasma membrane. *C,* The antigen-antibody bridging reaction shown in *B* results in profound changes in the mast cell membrane, with alterations in membrane-bound adenyl cyclase, calcium influx, tubulin aggregation into microtubules, and the beginning of the degranulation of the preformed mast cell mediators from their storage granules. *D,* The degranulation reaction proceeds, and newly synthesized mediators, particularly those generated by the catabolism of membrane-associated arachidonic acid, begin to work. The array of liberated and synthesized proinflammatory and inflammatory mediators is impressive.

(a term coined in 1906 by von Pirquet, in Vienna, meaning "changed reactivity") are clearer now than they were even a decade ago.[2]

Genetically predisposed allergic individuals have defects in the population of suppressor T lymphocytes responsible for modulating IgE responses to antigens. After the initial contact of an allergen with the mucosa of such an individual, abnormal amounts of allergen-specific IgE antibody are produced at the mucosal surface and at the regional lymph nodes. This IgE has high avidity, through its Fc portion, to Fc receptors on the surface of mast cells in the mucosa. The antigen-specific IgE antibodies, therefore, stick to the receptors on the surface of the tissue mast cells and remain there for unusually long periods. Excess locally produced IgE enters the circulation and binds to mast cells at other tissue locations as well as to circulating basophils. A subsequent encounter of the allergic individual with the antigen to which he or she has become sensitized results in antigen binding by the antigen-specific IgE molecules affixed to the surface of the tissue mast cells. The simultaneous binding of the antigen to adjacent IgE molecules on the mast cell surface results in a change in the mast cell membrane and particularly in membrane-bound adenyl cyclase (Fig. 9–1). The feature common to all known mechanisms that trigger mast cell degranulation (including degranulation stimulated by pharmacologic agents or anaphylatoxins like C3a and C5a and antigen-specific IgE-mediated degranulation) is calcium influx with subsequent aggregation of tubulin into microtubules, which then participate in the degranulation of vasoactive amines (see Fig. 9–1). In addition to the degranulation of the preformed mediators such as histamine, induction of synthesis of newly formed mediators from arachidonic acid also occurs with triggering of mast cell degranulation (Table 9–2). The preformed and newly synthesized mediators then produce the classic clinical signs of a type I hypersensitivity reaction: wheal (edema), flare (erythema), itch, and in many cases the subsequent, delayed appearance of the so-called late-phase reaction characterized by subacute signs of inflammation.

Control of IgE Synthesis

The Th2 subset of helper T cells bearing Fc_ϵ receptors produce, in addition to interleukin-4 (IL-4), IgE-binding factors after stimulation by interleukins produced by antigen-specific helper T cells activated by antigen-presenting cells and antigen. The two known types of IgE-binding factor that can be produced are IgE-potentiating factor and IgE-suppressor factor; both are encoded by the same codon, and the functional differences are created by posttranslational glycosylation. The glycosylation is either enhanced or suppressed by cytokines derived from other T cells. For example, glycosylation-inhibiting factor (identical to migration inhibitory factor) is produced by antigen-specific suppressor T cells. Glycosylation-enhancing factor is produced by an Fc receptor helper T cell (Fig. 9–2). The relative levels of these factors control the production of IgE-potentiating factor and IgE-suppressor factor by the central helper T cell and, thus, ultimately control the amount of IgE produced (see Fig. 9–2). They probably do so through regula-

TABLE 9–2. **Mast Cell Mediators**

Preformed in Granules	Newly Synthesized
Histamine	LTB_4
Heparin	LTC_4
Tryptase	LTD_4
Chymase	Prostaglandins
Kinins	Thromboxanes
Eosinophil chemotactic factor	Platelet-activating factor
Neutrophil chemotactic factor	
Serotonin	
Chondroitin sulfate	
Arylsulfatase	

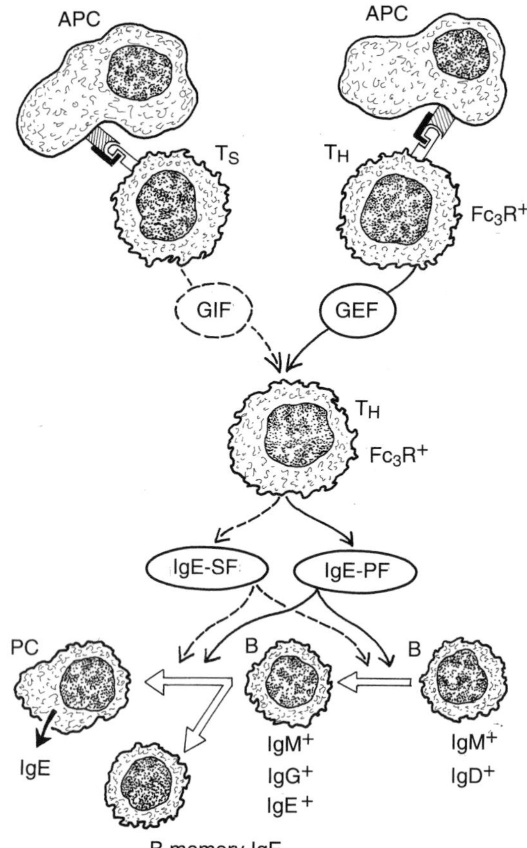

FIGURE 9–2. Diagrammatic display of IgE synthesis. Glycosylation-enhancing factor, glycosylation-inhibiting factor, IgE-promoting factor, IgE suppressor factor, and the helper and suppressor T lymphocytes specific for regulation of IgE synthesis are shown.

tion of IgE B lymphocyte proliferation and synthesis of IgE by these cells.

Mast Cell Subpopulations

It has become increasingly clear that at least two subpopulations of mast cells exist. Connective tissue mast cells (CTMCs) contain heparin as the major proteoglycan, produce large amounts of prostaglandin D_2 in response to stimulation, and are independent of T cell–derived interleukins for their maturation, development, and function. These cells stain brilliantly with toluidine blue in formalin-fixed tissue sections.

Mucosal mast cells (MMCs) do not stain well with toluidine blue. They are found primarily in the subepithelial mucosa in gut and lung; they contain chondroitin sulfate as the major proteoglycan; they manufacture leukotriene C4 as the predominant arachidonic acid metabolite after stimulation; and they are dependent on IL-3 (and IL-4) for their maturation and proliferation. Interestingly, MMCs placed in culture with fibroblasts rather than T cells transform to cells with the characteristics of CTMCs. Disodium cromoglycate inhibits histamine release from CTMCs but not from MMCs. Steroids suppress the proliferation of MMCs, probably through inhibition of IL-3 production.

Atopy Genetics and the Role of the Environment

Both genetic and environmental components are clearly involved in the allergic response. Offspring of marriages in which one parent is allergic have approximately 30% risk of being allergic, and if both parents are allergic the risk to each child is greater than 50%. At least three genetically linked mechanisms govern the development of atopy: (1) general hyperresponsiveness, (2) regulation of serum IgE levels, and (3) sensitivity to specific antigens. General hyperresponsiveness, defined as positive skin reactions to a broad range of environmental allergens, is associated HLA-B8/HLA-DW3 phenotypy, and this general hyperresponsiveness appears not to be IgE class specific. Total serum IgE levels are also controlled genetically, and family studies indicate that total IgE production is under genetic control. Finally, experimental studies using low molecular weight allergenic determinants disclose a strong association between IgE responsiveness to such allergens and HLA-DR/DW2 type, whereas for at least some larger molecular weight allergens, responsiveness is linked to HLA-DR/DW3. In mice at least, gene regulation of IgE production occurs at several levels, including: (1) regulation of antigen-specific, IgE-specific suppressor T cells, (2) manufacture of glycosylation-inhibiting factor or of glycosylation-enhancing factor by helper T cells, (3) at the level of IL-4 regulation of class switching to IgE synthesis, and (4) at the level of IgE-binding factors such as IgE-potentiating factor and IgE-suppressor factor.

The environment plays a major role in whether or not a genetically predisposed individual expresses major clinical manifestations of atopy. The "dose" of allergens to which the individual is exposed is a critical determinant of whether or not clinical expression of an allergic response develops. Less well recognized, however, is the fact that the general overall quality of the air in an individual's environment plays a major role in whether clinical expression of allergic responses to allergens to which the individual is sensitive does or does not develop. It has become unmistakably clear that as the general quality of the air in urban environments has deteriorated and as the air has become more polluted, the prevalence in the population of overt atopic clinical manifestations has increased dramatically. On a global level, the immediate environment in which an individual finds himself much of the time, the home, plays an important part in the expression of allergic disease. Allergically predisposed persons, at least one member of whose household smokes cigarettes, have enhanced sensitivity to allergens such as house dust, mites, and molds, among others. It is probably also true that the overall health and nutritional status of an individual influence the likelihood of that person developing a clinically obvious allergy.

Diagnosis of Type I Reactions

The definite diagnosis of type I hypersensitivity reactions requires the passive transfer of the reaction via a method known as the Prausnitz-Kustner reaction. Intradermal injection of the serum of a patient suspected of having a type I hypersensitivity-mediated problem into the skin of a volunteer is followed by injection of varying dilutions of the presumed offending antigen at the same intradermal sites as the patient's serum injection. A positive Prausnitz-Kustner reaction occurs when local flare and wheal formation follows the injection of the antigen. This method for proving type I reactions is not used clinically; therefore, diagnosis of type I mechanisms contributing to a patient's inflammatory disorder is always based on a collection of circumstantial evidence that strongly supports the hypothesis of a type I reaction. A typical history (e.g., of a family history of allergy or personal history of eczema, hay fever, asthma, or urticaria) elicitation of allergic symptoms following exposure to suspected allergens involves itching as a prominent symptom, elevated IgE levels in serum or other body fluids, and blood or tissue eosinophilia. In *Principles and Practice of Ophthalmology: Clinical Practice*, Section VIII, Chapter 11 (Ocular Bacteriology), these points in general are emphasized as well as the importance of the histopathologic characteristics of conjunctival biopsy tissue, in particular in the evaluation of patients with chronic cicatrizing conjunctivitis.

Therapy for Type I Reactions

Therapy for type I reactions must include scrupulous avoidance of the offending antigen. This is not easy, and it is a component of proper treatment that is often neglected by the patient and the physician alike. It is crucial, however, for a patient with an incurable disease such as atopy to recognize that throughout a lifetime he or she will slowly sustain cumulative permanent damage to structures affected by atopic responses (e.g., lung, eye) if he or she is subjected to repetitive triggering of the allergic response. Pharmacologic approaches to this disorder can never truly succeed for careless patients who neglect their responsibility to avoid allergens. A careful environmental history is, therefore, a critical ingredient in history taking, and convincing education of the patient and family alike is an essential and central ingredient in the care plan.

A careful environmental history and meticulous attention to environmental details can make the difference between relative stability and progressive inflammatory attacks that ultimately produce blindness. Elimination of pets, carpeting, feather pillows, quilts, and wool blankets and installation of air-conditioning and air-filtering systems are therapeutic strategies that should not be overlooked.[3]

One of the most important advances in the care of patients with type I disease during the past two decades has been the development of mast cell-stabilizing agents. Disodium cromoglycate, sodium nedocromil, and lodoxamide are three such agents. Topical administration is both safe and effective in the care of patients with allergic eye disease.[4, 5] This therapeutic approach is to be strongly recommended and is very much favored over the use of competitive H_1 antihistamines. Clearly, if the mast cells can be prevented from degranulating, the therapeutic effect of such degranulation-inhibiting agents would be expected to be vastly superior to that of antihistamines simply by virtue of preventing liberation of an entire panoply of mediators from the mast cell rather than competitive inhibition of one such mediator, histamine.

Histamine action-inhibition by H_1 antihistamines can be effective in patients with ocular allergy *provided that the drugs are administered systemically*. The efficacy of such agents when given topically is marginal at best, and long-term use can result in the development of sensitivity to ingredients in the preparations. The consistent use of systemic antihistamines, however, can contribute significantly to long-term stability, particularly of the newer noncompetitive antihistamines such as astemizole. Additionally, slow escalation of the amount of hydroxyzine used in the care of atopic patients can help to interrupt the itch-scratch-itch psychoneurotic component that often accompanies eczema and atopic blepharokeratoconjunctivitis.

Generalized suppression of inflammation, through use of topical corticosteroids, is commonly used for treatment of type I ocular hypersensitivity reactions, and this is appropriate for acute breakthrough attacks of inflammation. It is, however, completely inappropriate for long-term care. Corticosteroids have a direct effect on all inflammatory cells, including eosinophils, mast cells, and basophils. They are extremely effective, but the risks of chronic topical steroid use are considerable and unavoidable, thus chronic use is discouraged.

Although desensitization immunotherapy can be an important additional component to the therapeutic plan for a patient with type I hypersensitivity, it is difficult to perform properly. The first task, of course, is to document to which allergens the patient is sensitive. The second task is to construct a "serum" containing ideal proportions of the allergens that induce the production of IgG-blocking antibody and stimulate the generation of antigen-specific suppressor T cells. For reasons that are not clear, the initial concentration of allergens in such a preparation for use in a patient with ocular manifestations of atopy must often be considerably lower than the initial concentrations usually used when caring for a person with extraocular allergic problems. If the typical starting concentrations for nonocular allergies are employed frequently, a dramatic exacerbation of ocular inflammation immediately follows the first injection of the desensitizing preparation.

Plasmapheresis is an adjunctive therapeutic maneuver that can make a substantial difference in the care of patients with atopy, high levels of serum IgE, and documented *Staphlyococcus*-binding antibodies.[3] This therapeutic technique is expensive, is not curative, and must be performed at highly specialized centers, approximately three times each week, indefinitely. It is also clear, from our experience, that the aggressiveness of the plasmapheresis must be greater than that typically employed by many pheresis centers. Three to four plasma exchanges per pheresis session typically are required to achieve therapeutic effect for an atopic person.

Intravenous or intramuscular gamma globulin injections may also benefit selected atopic patients. It has been recognized that, through mechanisms that are not yet clear, gamma globulin therapy involves much more than simple passive "immunization" through adoptive transfer of antibody molecules. In fact, immunoglobulin therapy has a pronounced immunomodulatory effect, and it is because of this action that such therapy is now recognized and approved as effective therapy for idiopathic thrombocytopenic purpura.[6] The use of gamma globulin therapy is also being explored for other autoimmune diseases, including systemic lupus erythematosus and atopic disease.

Cyclosporine is being tested in patients with certain atopic diseases. Preliminary evidence suggests that topical cyclosporine can have some beneficial effect on patients with

TABLE 9–3. **Therapy of the Atopic Patient**

Environmental control
Mast cell stabilizers
Systemic antihistamines
Topical steroids (for acute intervention only)
Desensitization immunotherapy
Plasmapheresis
Intravenous gamma globulin
Cyclosporine (systemic and topical)
Psychiatric intervention for the patient and family

atopic keratoconjunctivitis and vernal keratoconjunctivitis.[7] Furthermore, in selected desperate cases of blinding atopic keratoconjunctivitis, we have demonstrated that systemic cyclosporine can be a pivotal component of the multimodality approach to the care of these complex problems.[3]

Finally, appropriate psychiatric care may be (and usually is) indicated in patients with severe atopy (and family members). It is not hyperbole to state that in most cases, patients with severe atopic disease and the family members with whom they live demonstrate substantial psychopathology and destructive patterns of interpersonal behavior. The degree to which these families exhibit self-destructive, passive-aggressive, and sabotaging behaviors is often astonishing. Productive engagement in psychiatric care is often difficult to achieve, but it can be extremely rewarding when accomplished successfully. Table 9–3 summarizes the components of a multifactorial approach to the care of atopic patients.

TYPE II HYPERSENSITIVITY REACTIONS

Type II reactions require the participation of complement-fixing antibodies (IgG1, IgG3, or IgM) and complement. The antibodies are directed against antigens on the surface of specific cells (i.e., endogenous antigens). The damage caused by type II hypersensitivity reactions, therefore, is localized to the particular target cell or tissue. The mediators of the tissue damage in type II reactions include complement as well as recruited macrophages and other leukocytes that liberate their enzymes. The mechanism of tissue damage involves antibody binding to the cell membrane with resultant cell membrane lysis or facilitation of phagocytosis, macrophage and neutrophil cell-mediated damage (Fig. 9–

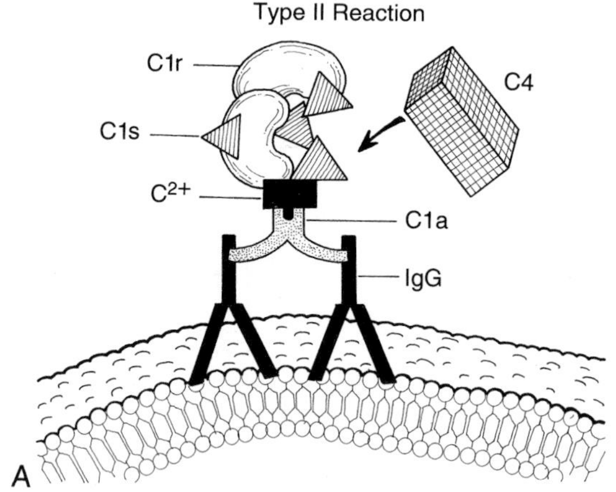

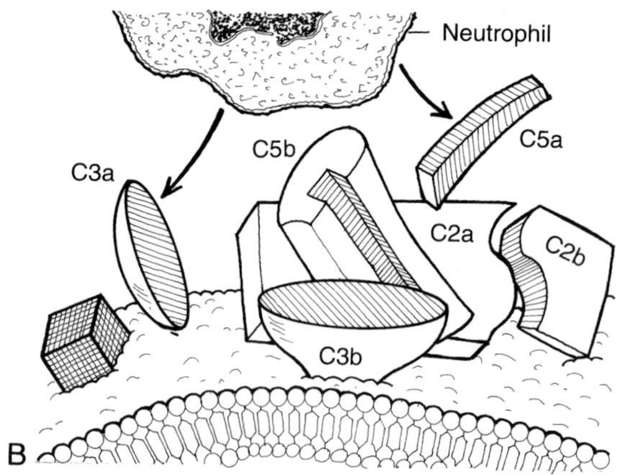

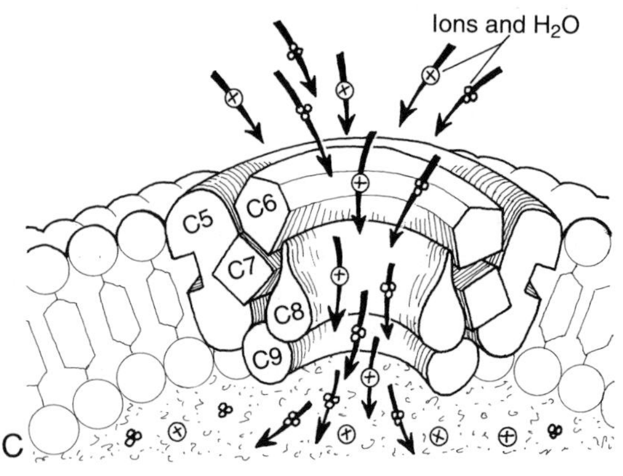

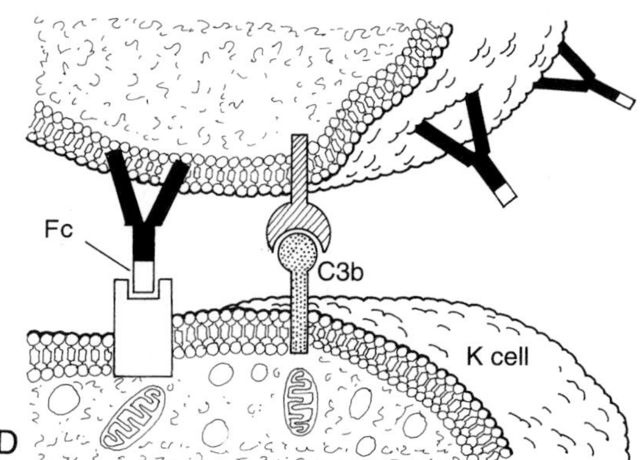

FIGURE 9–3. Type II hypersensitivity. *A,* A "sensitized" cell with two antibodies specific for antigenic determinants on the cell surface has attached to the target cell. C1q, C1r, and C1s complement components have begun the sequence that will result in the classical cascade of complement factor binding. *B,* The complement cascade has progressed to the point of C5 binding. Note that two anaphylatoxin and chemotactic split products, C3a and C5a, have been generated, and a neutrophil is being attracted to the site by virtue of the generation of these two chemotactic moieties. *C,* The complement cascade is complete, with the result that a pore has been opened in the target cell membrane, and osmotic lysis is the nearly instantaneous result. *D,* A variant of the type II hypersensitivity reaction is the antibody-dependent cellular cytotoxicity (ADCC) reaction. Target-specific antibody has attached to the target cell membrane, and the Fc receptor on a neutrophil, a macrophage, or a killer (K) cell is attaching to that membrane-affixed antibody. The result will be lysis of the target cell.

3A–C), and killer cell damage to target tissue through antibody-dependent cell-mediated cytotoxicity (ADCC) reaction (see Fig. 9–3D). It is important to remember (particularly in the case of type II hypersensitivity reactions that do not result in specific target cell lysis through the complement cascade with eventual osmotic lysis) that neutrophils are prominent effectors of target cell damage. Neutrophil adherence, oxygen metabolism, lysosomal enzyme release, and phagocytosis are tremendously "upregulated" by IgG-C3 complexes and by the activated split product of C5a. As mentioned in the description of type I hypersensitivity reactions, mast cells also participate in nonallergic inflammatory reactions, and type II hypersensitivity reactions provide an excellent example of this. The complement split products C3a and C5a both produce mast cell activation and degranulation. The result is the liberation of preformed vasoactive amines and upregulation of membrane synthesis of leukotriene B4, the most potent (and also other cytokines [e.g., TNF-α]) known chemoattractant for neutrophils, even more potent than IL-8/rantes, eosinophil chemotactic factor, and other arachidonic acid metabolites. Neutrophils and macrophages attracted to this site of complement-fixing IgG or IgM in a type II hypersensitivity reaction cannot phagocytose entire cells and target tissues, and thus liberate their proteolytic and collagenolytic enzymes and cytokines in "frustrated phagocytosis." It is through this liberation of tissue digestive enzymes that the target tissue is damaged. Direct target cell damage (as opposed to "innocent bystander" damage caused by liberation of neutrophil and macrophage enzymes) in type II hypersensitivity reactions may be mediated by killer (K) cells through the antibody-dependent cytotoxicity reaction. In fact, definitive diagnosis of type II reactions requires the demonstration of fixed antitissue antibodies at the disease site as well as a demonstration of killer cell activity in vitro against the tissue. No ocular disease has been definitively proved to represent a type II reaction, but several candidates, including ocular cicatricial pemphigoid, exist.

The classic human autoimmune type II hypersensitivity disease is Goodpasture's syndrome. Many believe ocular cicatricial pemphigoid is analogous (in mechanism at least) to Goodpasture's syndrome, in which complement-fixing antibody directed against a glycoprotein of the glomerular basement membrane fixes to the glomerular basement membrane. This action causes subsequent damage to the membrane by proteolytic and collagenolytic enzymes liberated by phagocytic cells, including macrophages and neutrophils.

Therapy for Type II Reactions

Therapy for type II reactions is extremely difficult, and immunosuppressive chemotherapy has, in general, been the mainstay of treatment. Experience with ocular cicatricial pemphigoid has been especially gratifying in this regard.[8–10] Progressive cicatricial pemphigoid affecting the conjunctiva was, eventually, almost universally blinding before the advent of systemic immunosuppressive chemotherapy for this condition. With such therapy now, however, 90% of cases of the disease are arrested and vision is preserved.[11]

TYPE III HYPERSENSITIVITY REACTIONS

Type III reactions, or immune complex diseases, require, like type II hypersensitivity reactions, participation of complement-fixing antibodies (IgG1, IgG3, or IgM). The antigens participating in such reactions may be soluble diffusible antigens, microbes, drugs, or autologous antigens. Microbes that cause such diseases are usually those that cause persistent infections in which not only the infected organ but also the kidneys are affected by the immune complex–stimulated inflammation. Autoimmune-immune complex diseases are the best known of these hypersensitivity reactions: the classic collagen vascular diseases and Stevens-Johnson syndrome. Kidney, skin, joints, arteries, and eyes are frequently affected in these disorders. Mediators of the tissue damage include antigen-antibody-complement complexes and the proteolytic and collagenolytic enzymes from phagocytes such as macrophages and neutrophils. As with type II reactions, the C3a and C5a split products of complement exert potent chemotactic activity for the phagocytes and also activate mast cells, which through degranulation of their vasoactive amines, TNF-α increase vascular permeability and enhance emigration of such phagocytic cells. It is again through frustrated phagocytosis that the neutrophils and macrophages liberate their tissue-damaging enzymes (Fig. 9–4).

Arthus' reaction, a special form of type III hypersensitivity, is mentioned for completeness. Antigen injected into the skin of an animal or individual previously sensitized with the same antigen, and with circulating antibodies against that antibody, results in an edematous, hemorrhagic, and eventually necrotic lesion of the skin. A passive Arthus reaction can also be created if intravenous injection of antibody into a normal host recipient is followed by intradermal injection of the antigen. An accumulation of neutrophils develops in the capillaries and venule walls after deposition of antigen, antibody, and complement in the vessel walls.

Immune complexes form in all of us as a normal consequence of our "immunologic housekeeping." Usually, however, these immune complexes are continually removed from

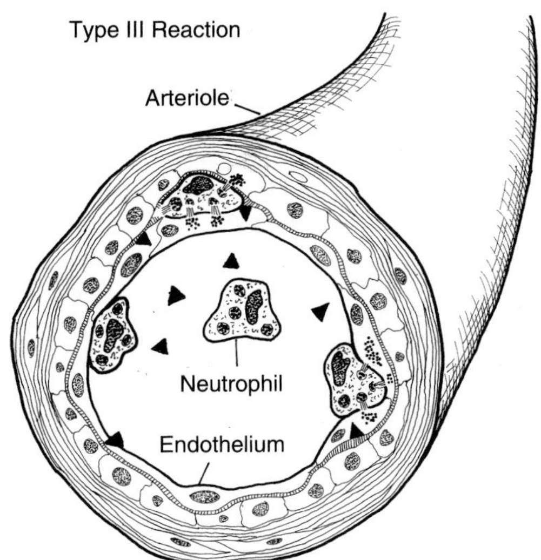

FIGURE 9–4. Type III hypersensitivity reaction. Circulating immune complexes (shown here as triangle-shaped moieties in the vascular lumen) percolate between vascular endothelial cells but become trapped at the vascular endothelial basement membrane. Neutrophils and other phagocytic cells are attracted to this site of immune complex deposition. These phagocytic cells liberate their proteolytic and collagenolytic enzymes and damage not only the vessel but also the surrounding tissue.

TABLE 9–4. **Types of Delayed Hypersensitivity Reactions**

Reaction Type	Example	Peak Reaction
Tuberculin contact	Tuberculin skin test	48–72 hr
Contact	Drug contact hypersensitivity	48–72 hr
Granulomatous	Leprosy	14 days
Jones-Mote	Cutaneous basophil hypersensitivity	24 hr

the circulation. In humans, the preeminent immune complex–scavenging system is the red blood cells, which have a receptor (CR1) for the C3b and C4b components of complement. This receptor binds immune complexes that contain complement, and the membrane-bound complexes are removed by fixed tissue macrophages and Kupffer cells as the red blood cells pass through the liver. Other components of the reticuloendothelial system, including the spleen and the lung, also remove circulating immune complexes. Small immune complexes may escape binding and removal, and not surprisingly, smaller immune complexes are principally responsible for immune complex–mediated hypersensitivity reactions. It is also true that IgA complexes (as opposed to IgG or IgM complexes) do not bind well to red blood cells. They are found in the lung, brain, and kidney rather than in the reticuloendothelial system.

The factors that govern whether or not immune complexes are deposited into tissue (and if so, where) are complex and rather incompletely understood. It is clear that the size of the immune complex plays a role in tissue deposition. It is also clear that increased vascular permeability at a site of immune system activity or inflammation is a major governor of whether or not immune complexes are deposited in that tissue. Additionally, it is clear that immune complex deposition is more likely to occur at sites of vascular trauma; this includes trauma associated with the normal hemodynamics of a particular site, such as the relatively high pressure inside capillaries and kidneys, the turbulence associated with bifurcations of vessels, and obviously at sites of artificial trauma as well. Excellent examples of the latter include the areas of trauma in the fingers, toes, and elbows of patients with rheumatoid arthritis, where subsequently vasculitic lesions and rheumatoid nodules form, and in the surgically traumatized eyes of patients with rheumatoid arthritis or Wegener's granulomatosis, where subsequently immune complexes are deposited and necrotizing scleritis develops.[12] It is likely that addressing or other attachment factors in a local tissue play a role in the "homing" of a particular immune complex. Antibody class and immune complex size are also important determinants of immune complex localization at a particular site, as is the type of the basement membrane itself.

Therapy for Type III Reactions

Therapy for type III reactions consists predominantly of large doses of corticosteroids, of immunosuppressive chemotherapeutic agents, or both. Cytotoxic immunosuppressive chemotherapy may or may not be necessary to save both the sight and the life of a patient with Behçet's disease, but it is categorically required to save the life of a patient with either polyarteritis nodosa[13] or Wegener's granulomatosis.[14] In the case of rheumatoid arthritis–associated vasculitis affecting the eye, it is likely that systemic immunosuppression will also be required if death from a lethal extraarticular, extraocular, vasculitic event is to be prevented.[15]

Injury Mediated by Cells

TYPE IV HYPERSENSITIVITY REACTIONS: IMMUNE-MEDIATED INJURY DUE TO EFFECTOR T CELLS

The original classification of immunopathogenic mechanisms arose in an era when considerably more was known about antibody molecules and serology than about T cells and cellular immunity. Out of this lack of knowledge, T cell–mediated mechanisms were relegated to the "type IV" category, and all manner of responses were unwittingly grouped together (Table 9–4).[16] We now know that T cells capable of causing immune-based injury exist in at least three functionally distinct phenotypes: cytotoxic T cells (typically CD8$^+$) and two populations of helper T cells (typically CD4$^+$) (Fig. 9–5). Since cytotoxic T lymphocytes (CTLs) were discovered well after the original Gell and Sell classification, they were, therefore, never anticipated in that classification system. As mentioned previously, CD4$^+$ T cells can adopt one of two polar positions with regard to their lymphokine secretions.[17] Th1 cells secrete IL-2, IFN-γ, and lymphotoxin, whereas Th2 cells were identified in the 1940s and 1950s as the initiators of delayed hypersensitivity reaction. The latter cells, in addition to providing helper factors that promote IgE production, also mediate tissue inflammation, albeit of a somewhat different type than Th1 cells.

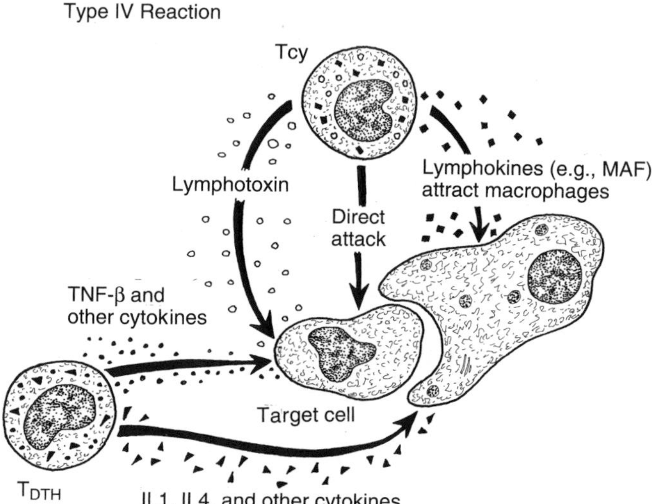

FIGURE 9–5. Type IV hypersensitivity reaction. DTH (CD4) T lymphocytes and cytotoxic (CD8 and CD4) T lymphocytes directly attack the target cell or the organism that is the target of the type IV hypersensitivity reaction. Surrogate effector cells are also recruited through the liberation of cytokines. The most notable surrogate or additional effector cell is the macrophage, or tissue histiocyte. If the reaction becomes chronic, certain cytokines or signals from mononuclear cells result in the typical transformation of some histiocytes into epithelioid cells, and the fusion of multiple epithelioid cells produces the classic multinucleated giant cell.

Immunopathogenic T Cells

CTLs exhibit exquisite antigen specificity in their recognition of target cells, and the extent of injury that CTLs effect is usually limited to target cells bearing the relevant instigating antigens. Therefore, if a CTL causes tissue injury, it is because host cells express an antigen encoded by an invading pathogen, an antigen for which the Tcr on the CTL is highly specific. Delivery of a cytolytic signal eliminates hapless host cells, and in so doing aborts the intracellular infection. Assuming that the infected host cell is one of many and can thus be spared (e.g., epidermal keratinocytes), there may be little or no physiologic consequence of this CTL-mediated loss of host cells. However, if the infected cell is strategic, limited in number, or cannot be replaced by regeneration (e.g., neurons, corneal endothelial cells), then the immunopathogenic consequences may be severe.

$CD4^+$ effector cells also exhibit exquisite specificity in recognition of target antigens. However, the extent of injury that these cells can effect is diffuse and is not limited to cells bearing the target antigen. $CD4^+$ effector cells secrete cytokines that possess no antigen specificity in their own right. Instead, these molecules indiscriminately recruit and activate macrophages, natural killer cells, eosinophils, and other mobile cells that form the nonspecific host defense network. It is this defense mechanism that leads to eradication and elimination of the offending pathogen. In other words, $CD4^+$ effector cells protect by identifying the pathogen antigenically, but they cause the elimination of the pathogen by enlisting the aid of other cells. The ability of $CD4^+$ effector cells to orchestrate this multicellular response rests with the capacity of these cells to secrete proinflammatory cytokines to arm inflammatory cells with the ability to "kill." Once armed, these "mindless assassins" mediate inflammation in a nonspecific manner that leads often, if not inevitably, to "innocent bystander" injury to surrounding tissues. For an organ that can scarcely tolerate inflammation of even the lowest amount, such as the eye, "innocent bystander" injury is a formidable threat to vision.

Autoimmune T Cells

The foregoing discussion addresses immunopathogenic injury due to T cells that develops among host tissues invaded by pathogenic organisms. However, there is another dimension to immunopathology. T cells can sometimes make a mistake and mount an immune attack on host tissues simply because those tissue cells express self molecules (i.e., autoantigens). Although an enormous amount of experimental and clinical literature is devoted to autoimmunity and autoimmune diseases, very little is known in a "factual" sense that enables us to understand this curious phenomenon. What seems clear is that T cells with receptors that recognize "self" antigens, as well as B cells bearing surface antibody receptors that recognize "self" antigens, exist under normal conditions.[16] Moreover, there are examples of T and B cells with "self"-recognizing receptors that become activated in putatively normal individuals. Thus, immunologists have learned to distinguish an autoimmune response (not necessarily pathologic) from an autoimmune disease. Whereas all autoimmune diseases arise in a setting where an autoimmune response has been initiated, we understand little about what causes the latter to evolve into the former. Whatever the pathogenesis, autoimmune disease results when effector T cells (or antibodies) recognize autoantigens in a fashion that triggers a destructive immune response.[18, 19]

The eye consists of unique cells bearing unique molecules. Moreover, the internal compartments of the eye exist behind a blood-tissue barrier. The very uniqueness of ocular molecules, and their presumed sequestration from the systemic immune system, has provoked immunologists to speculate that ocular autoimmunity arises when, via trauma or infection, eye-specific antigens are "revealed" to the immune system. Sympathetic ophthalmia is a disease that almost fits this scenario perfectly. Trauma to one eye, with attendant disruption of the blood-ocular barrier, and spillage of ocular tissues and molecules, leads to a systemic immune response that is specific to the eye. This response is directed not only at the traumatized eye but also at its putatively normal fellow eye. However, even in sympathetic ophthalmia, not every case of ocular trauma leads to this outcome; in fact, only in a few cases does this type of injury produce inflammation in the undamaged eye. Suspicion is high that polymorphic genetic factors may be responsible for determining who will, and who will not, develop sympathetic ophthalmia following ocular injury. However, environmental factors may also participate.

Range of Hypersensitivity Reactions Mediated by T Cells

Because a wealth of new information about T cell–mediated immunopathology has accrued within the past decade, our ideas about the range of hypersensitivity reactions that can be mediated by T cells have expanded. But, as yet, any attempt to classify these reactions must necessarily be incomplete. In the past, four types of delayed hypersensitivity reactions were described: (1) tuberculin, (2) contact hypersensitivity, (3) granulomatous, and (4) Jones-Mote. Delayed hypersensitivity reactions of these types were believed to be caused by IFN-γ–producing $CD4^+$ T cells and to participate in numerous ocular inflammatory disorders, ranging from allergic keratoconjunctivitis, through Wegener's granulomatosis, to drug contact hypersensitivity. Based on recent knowledge concerning other types of effector T cells, this list must be expanded to include cytotoxic T cells, and proinflammatory, but not IFN-γ–secreting, Th2 type cells, such as the cells that are believed to cause corneal clouding in river blindness.[20]

Herpes Simplex Keratitis As an Example of T Cell–Mandated Ocular Inflammatory Disease

Infections of the eye with herpes simplex virus are significant causes of morbidity and vision loss in developed countries. Although direct viral toxicity is damaging to the eye, the majority of intractable herpes infections appear to be immunopathogenic in origin. That is, the immune response to antigens expressed during a herpes infection leads to tissue injury and decompensation, even though the virus itself is responsible for little pathology directly. Herpes stromal keratitis (HSK) is representative of this type of disorder.[21]

Numerous experimental model systems have been developed in an effort to understand the pathogenesis of HSK.

Perhaps the most informative studies have been conducted in laboratory mice. Evidence from these model systems indicates that T cells are central to the corneal pathology observed in HSK.[21] At least four different pathogenic mechanisms have been discovered, each of which alone can generate stromal keratitis. Genetic factors of the host seem to play a crucial role in dictating which mechanism will predominate. First, HSV-specific cytotoxic T cells can cause HSK and do so in several strains of mice. Second, HSV-specific T cells of the Th1 type, which secrete IFN-γ and mediate delayed hypersensitivity, also cause HSK, but in genetically different strains of mice. Third, HSV-specific T cells of the TH2 type, that secrete IL-4 and IL-10, correlate with HSK in yet a different strain of mice. Fourth, T cells have been found in association with HSK that recognize an antigen uniquely expressed in the cornea. The evidence suggests that this corneal antigen is unmasked during a corneal infection with HSV, and an autoimmune response is evoked in which the cornea becomes the target of the attack.

Only time will tell whether similar immunopathogenic mechanisms will prove to be responsible for HSK in humans, but the likelihood is very great that this will be the case. Furthermore, it is instructive to emphasize that quite different pathologic T cells can be involved in ocular pathology, which implies that it will be necessary to devise different therapies in order to meet the challenge of preventing immunopathogenic injury from proceeding to blindness.

Summary

Faced with a patient who is experiencing extraocular or intraocular inflammation, the thoughtful ophthalmologist will try, to the best of his or her ability, to diagnose the specific cause of the inflammation, or at the very least to investigate the problem so that the mechanisms responsible for the inflammation are understood as completely as possible. Armed with this knowledge, the ophthalmologist is then prepared to formulate an appropriate therapeutic plan rather than to indiscriminately prescribe corticosteroids. It is clear as we move toward the 21st century that the past four decades of relative neglect of ocular immunology by mainstream ophthalmic practitioners is coming to an end. Most ophthalmologists are no longer satisfied to cultivate practices devoted exclusively to the "tissue carpentry" of cataract surgery or even to a broad-based ophthalmic practice that includes "medical ophthalmology" but is restricted to problems related exclusively to the eye (e.g., glaucoma) and divorced from the eye as an organ in which systemic disease is often manifested. More ophthalmologists than ever before are demanding the continuing education they need to satisfy intellectual curiosity and to prepare for modern care of the total patient when a patient presents with an ocular manifestation of a systemic disease. It is to these doctors that this chapter is directed. The eye can be affected by any of the immune hypersensitivity reactions, and understanding the mechanism of a particular patient's inflammatory problem lays the ground work for correct treatment. In the course of the average ophthalmologist's working life, the diagnostic pursuit of mechanistic understanding will also result in a substantial number of instances when the ophthalmologist has been responsible for diagnosing a disease that, if left undiagnosed, would have been fatal.

REFERENCES

1. Cocoa AF, Cooke RA: On the classification of the phenomena of hypersensitiveness. J Immunol 8:163, 1923.
2. von Pirquet C: Allergie. Munch Med Wochenschr 53:1457, 1906.
3. Foster CS, Calonge M: Atopic keratoconjunctivitis. Ophthalmology 97:992, 1990.
4. Foster CS, Duncan J: Randomized clinical trial of disodium cromoglycate therapy in vernal keratoconjunctivitis. Am J Ophthalmol 90:175, 1980.
5. Foster CS: Evaluation of topical cromolyn sodium in the treatment of vernal keratoconjunctivitis. Ophthalmology 95:194, 1988.
6. Bussel JB, Kimberly RP, Inamen RD, et al: Intravenous gamma globulin treatment of chronic idiopathic cytopenic purpura. Blood 62:480, 1983.
7. Bleik JH, Tabbara KS: Topical cyclosporine in vernal keratoconjunctivitis. Ophthalmology 98:1679, 1991.
8. Foster CS: Cicatricial pemphigoid. Thesis of the American Ophthalmological Society. Trans Am Ophthalmol Soc 84:527, 1986.
9. Foster CS, Wilson LA, Ekins MB: Immunosuppressive therapy for progressive ocular cicatricial pemphigoid. Ophthalmology 89:340, 1982.
10. Tauber J, Sainz de la Maza M, Foster CS: Systemic chemotherapy for ocular cicatricial pemphigoid. Cornea 10:185, 1991.
11. Neumann R, Tauber J, Foster CS: Remission and recurrence after withdrawal of therapy for ocular cicatricial pemphigoid. Ophthalmology 98:868, 1991.
12. Sainz de la Maza M, Foster CS: Necrotizing scleritis after ocular surgery: A clinical pathologic study. Ophthalmology 98:1720, 1991.
13. Leib ES, Restivo C, Paulus AT: Immunosuppressive and corticosteroid therapy of polyarteritis nodosa. Am J Med 67:941, 1979.
14. Wolf SM, Fauci AS, Horn RG, Dale DC: Wegener's granulomatosis. Ann Intern Med 81:513, 1974.
15. Foster CS, Forstot SL, Wilson LA: Mortality rate in rheumatoid arthritis patients developing necrotizing scleritis or peripheral ulcerative keratitis. Ophthalmology 91:1253, 1984.
16. Janeway CA Jr, Travers P (eds): Immunobiology: The immune system in health and disease. Third Edition. New York, Current Biology/Garland Publishing, 1997.
17. Mosmann TR, Coffman RL: TH_1 and TH_2 cells: Different patterns of lymphokine secretion lead to different functional properties. Ann Rev Immunol 7:145, 1989.
18. Steinman L: Escape from "horror autotoxicus": pathogenesis and treatment of autoimmune disease. Cell 80:7, 1995.
19. Tan EM: Autoantibodies in pathology and cell biology. Cell 67:841, 1991.
20. Pearlman E, Lass HJ, Bardenstein DS, et al: Interleukin 4 and T helper type 2 cells are required for development of experimental onchocercal keratitis (River Blindness). J Exp Med 182: 931, 1995.
21. Streilein JW, Dana MR, Ksander BR: Immunity causing blindness: Five different paths to herpes stromal keratitis. Immunol Today 18:443, 1997.

CHAPTER 10

Regulation of Immune Reponses

J. Wayne Streilein and C. Stephen Foster

Immunization with an antigen leads, under normal circumstances, to a robust immune response in which effector T cells and antibodies are produced with specificity for the initiating antigen. Viewed teleologically, the purpose of these effectors is to recognize and combine with antigen (e.g., on an invading pathogen) in such a manner that the antigen and pathogen are eliminated. Once the antigen has been eliminated, there is little need for the persistence of high levels of effector cells and antibodies, and what is regularly observed is that levels of these effectors in blood and peripheral tissues fall dramatically. Only the T cells and B cells that embody antigen-specific memory (anamnesis) are retained.

The ability of the immune system to respond to an antigenic challenge in a sufficient and yet measured manner such as this is a dramatic expression of the ability of the system to regulate itself. An understanding of the mechanisms of immune regulation is extremely important. Examples abound of unregulated immune responses that lead to tissue injury and disease, and therefore an understanding of the basis of immune regulation is an important goal.

Regulation by Antigen

Antigen itself is a critical factor in regulating an immune response.[1] When nonreplicating antigens have been studied, it has been found that the high concentration of antigen required for initial sensitization begins to fall through time. In part, this occurs because antibodies produced by immunization interact with the antigen and cause its elimination. As the antigen concentration falls, the efficiency with which specific T and B cells are stimulated to proliferate and differentiate also falls, and eventually, when antigen concentration slips below a critical threshold, further activation of specific lymphocytes stops. Thus, antigen proves to be a central player in determining the vigor and duration of the immune response. As a corollary, immune effectors (specific T cells and antibodies) also play a key role in terminating the immune response, in part by removing antigen from the system. The use of anti-Rh antibodies (RhoGAM) to prevent sensitization of Rh-negative women bearing Rh-positive fetuses is a clear, clinical example of the ability of antibodies to terminate (and in this particular case, even prevent) a specific (unwanted) immune response.

Regulation by Th1 and Th2 Cells

There are other, more subtle and more powerful, regulatory mechanisms that operate to control immune responses. More than 20 years ago, experimentalists discovered that certain antigen-specific T lymphocytes are capable of suppressing immune responses,[2] and the mechanism of suppression was found to be unrelated to the simple act of clearing antigen from the system. Although immunologists first suspected that a functionally distinct population of T lymphocytes (analogous to helper and killer cells) was responsible for immune suppression, it is now clear that there are a broad range of T cells that, depending on the circumstances, can function as suppressor cells. Moreover, the mechanisms by which these different T cells suppress are also diverse.

The concept has previously been introduced that helper T cells exist, cells that are responsible for enabling other T and B cells to differentiate into effector cells and antibody-producing cells, respectively. And it is now evident that the effectors of immunity include functionally diverse T cells (delayed hypersensitivity, cytotoxic) and antibodies (immunoglobulin [Ig]M, IgG1, IgG2, IgG3, IgG4, IgA, IgE). Any particular immunizing event does not necessarily lead to the production of the entire array of effector modalities, and one of the reasons for this is that helper T cells tend to polarize into one or the other of two distinct phenotypes.[3] Th1 cells provide a type of help that leads to the generation of T-cell effectors that mediate T-cell–dependent inflammatory responses (e.g., delayed hypersensitivity), and B cells that secrete complement-fixing antibodies. The ability of Th1 cells to promote these types of immune responses rests with their capacity to secrete a certain set of cytokines—interferon (INF)-γ, tumor necrosis factor (TNF)-β, large amounts of TNF-α and interleukin (IL)-2. It is these cytokines, acting on other T cells, B cells, and macrophages that shape proinflammatory responses. By contrast, Th2 cells provide a type of help that leads to the generation of B cells that secrete non–complement-fixing IgG antibodies, as well as IgA and IgE. Once again, the ability of Th2 cells to promote these types of antibody responses rests with their capacity to secrete a different set of cytokines—IL-4, IL-5, IL-6, and IL-10. These cytokines act on other antigen-specific B and T cells to promote the observed responses.

As it turns out, Th1 and Th2 cells can cross-regulate each other. Thus, Th1 cells with specificity for a particular antigen secrete IFN-γ, and in the presence of this cytokine, Th2 cells with specificity for the same antigen fail to become activated. Moreover, they are unable to provide the type of help for which they are uniquely suited. Similarly, if Th2 cells respond to a particular antigen by secreting their unique set of cytokines (especially IL-4 and IL-10), Th1 cells in the same microenvironment are prevented from responding to the same antigen. Thus, precocious activation of Th1 cells to an antigen, such as ragweed pollen, may prevent the activation of ragweed-specific Th2 cells and therefore prevent the production of ragweed-specific IgE antibodies. Alternatively, precocious activation of Th2 cells to an antigen (e.g., urushiol—the agent responsible for poison ivy dermatitis) may prevent the activation of urushiol-specific Th1 cells and thus eliminate the threat of dermatitis when the skin is exposed to the leaf of the poison ivy plant.

The discovery of Th1 and Th2 cell diversity has led to a profound re-thinking of immune regulation. It is still too early to know, on the one hand, whether the extent to which sensitization that leads to polarization in the direction of Th1- or Th2-type responses is responsible for human inflammatory diseases, and, on the other hand, whether the extent to which the ability to influence an immune response toward the Th1 or Th2 phenotypes will have therapeutic value in humans.

Regulation by Suppressor T Cells

Suppressor T cells are defined operationally as cells that suppress an antigen-specific immune response. Cells of this functional property were actually described before the discovery of Th1 and Th2 cells. It is now apparent that at least some of the phenomena attributed to suppressor T cells initially are actually explained by the cross-regulating abilities of Th1 and Th2 cells. However, it is also abundantly clear that there remain forms and examples of suppression of immune responses that depend on T cells that are neither Th1 nor Th2 cells.

Various experimental maneuvers have been described that lead to the generation of suppressor T cells. The list includes (but is not limited to): (1) injection of soluble heterologous protein antigen intravenously, (2) application of a hapten to skin previously exposed to ultraviolet B radiation, (3) ingestion of antigen by mouth, (4) injection of allogeneic hematopoietic cells into neonatal mice, (5) injection of antigen-pulsed antigen-presenting cells (APCs) that have been treated in vitro with transforming growth factor (TGF)-β (or aqueous humor, cerebrospinal fluid, or amniotic fluid), (6) engraftment of a solid tissue (e.g., heart, kidney) under cover of immunosuppressive agents.[4, 5] In each of these examples, T cells harvested from spleen or lymph nodes of experimentally manipulated animals induce antigen-specific unresponsiveness when injected into immunologically naive recipient animals. Cell transfers such as this have helped to define different types of suppressor cell activity. Since the immune response is functionally divided into its afferent phase (induction) and efferent phase (expression), it is no surprise that certain suppressor T cells suppress the afferent process by which antigen is first detected by specific lymphocytes, while other suppressor T cells inhibit the expression of immunity. Moreover, different suppressor T cells act on different target cells. Some suppressor cells inhibit the activation of $CD4^+$ helper or $CD8^+$ cytotoxic T cells, whereas other suppressor cells interfere with B-cell function. There are even suppressor cells that inhibit the activation and effector functions of macrophages and other APCs.

The mechanisms by which suppressor T cells function remain ill-defined. Certain suppressor T cells secrete immunosuppressive cytokines, such as TGF-β, whereas other suppressor cells inhibit only when they make direct cell surface contact with target cells. The notion that suppressor cells act by secreting suppressive factors (other than known cytokines) has been challenged and is a controversial topic in immunology. There is convincing evidence that suppressor T cells play a key role in regulating the normal immune response. The decay in the immune response that is typically observed after antigen has been successfully neutralized by specific immune effectors correlates with the emergence of antigen-specific suppressor T cells, and these cells have been found to be capable of secreting TGF-β.

Tolerance As an Expression of Immune Regulation

Immunologic tolerance is defined as the state in which immunization with a specific antigen fails to lead to a detectable immune response. In a sense, tolerance represents the ultimate expression of the effectiveness of immune regulation, because active mechanisms are responsible for producing the tolerant state. In another sense, tolerance is the obverse of immunity, and the fact that an antigen can induce either immunity or tolerance, depending on the conditions at the time of antigen exposure, indicates the vulnerability of the immune system to manipulation.

Originally described experimentally in the 1950s,[6, 7] but accurately predicted by Ehrlich and other immunologists at the end of the 19th century, immunologic tolerance has been the subject of considerable experimental study during the past 50 years. It has been learned that several distinct mechanisms contribute singly, or in unison, to creation of the state of tolerance. These mechanisms include clonal deletion, clonal anergy, suppression, and immune deviation.

MECHANISMS INVOLVED IN TOLERANCE

The term *clonal* refers to a group of lymphocytes that all have identical receptors for a particular antigen. During regular immunization, a clone of antigen specific lymphocytes responds by proliferating and undergoing differentiation. *Clonal deletion* refers to an aberration of this process in which a clone of antigen-specific lymphocytes responds to antigen exposure by undergoing apoptosis (programmed cell death).[8] Deletion of a clone of cells in this manner eliminates the ability of the immune system to respond to the antigen in question (i.e., the immune system is tolerant of that antigen). Subsequent exposures to the same antigen fail to produce the expected immune response (sensitized T cells and antibodies) because the relevant antigen-specific T and B cells are missing.

Clonal anergy resembles clonal deletion in that a particular clone of antigen-specific lymphocytes fails to respond to antigen exposure by proliferating and undergoing differentiation.[9] However, in clonal anergy, the lymphocytes within the clone are not triggered to undergo apoptosis by exposure to antigen. What has been learned experimentally is that lymphocytes exposed to their specific antigen under specialized experimental conditions enter an altered state in which their ability to respond is suspended, but the cells are protected from programmed cell death. Even though these cells survive this encounter with antigen, subsequent encounters still fail to cause their expected activation; that is, the immune system is tolerant of that antigen, and the tolerant cell is said to be anergic.

Antigen-specific *immune suppression*, as described earlier, is another mechanism that has been shown to cause immunologic tolerance. As in clonal deletion and anergy, immune suppression creates a situation in which subsequent encounters with the antigen in question fail to lead to signs of sensitization. However, in suppression, the failure to respond is actively maintained. Thus, suppressor cells actively inhibit antigen-specific lymphocytes from responding, even though the antigen-specific cells are present at the time antigen is introduced into the system.

Immune deviation is a special form of immune suppression.[10] Originally described in the 1960s, immune deviation refers to the situation where administration of a particular antigen in a particular manner fails to elicit the expected response. In the first such experiments, soluble heterologous protein antigens injected intravenously into naive experimental animals failed to induce delayed hypersensitivity responses. Moreover, subsequent immunization with the same antigens plus adjuvant injected subcutaneously also failed to induce delayed hypersensitivity. With respect to delayed hypersensitivity, one could say that the animals were tolerant. However, the sera of these animals contained unexpectedly large amounts of antibody to the same antigen, indicating that the so-called tolerance was not global. Thus, in immune deviation a preemptive exposure to antigen in a nonimmunizing mode prejudices the quality of subsequent immune responses to the same antigen. In other words, the immune response is deviated from the expected pattern, hence the term immune deviation.

FACTORS THAT PROMOTE TOLERANCE RATHER THAN IMMUNITY

Experimentalists have defined various factors that influence or promote the development of immunologic tolerance. The earliest description of tolerance occurred when antigenic material was injected into newborn (and therefore developmentally immature) mice. This indicates that exposure of the developing immune system to antigens before the system has reached maturity leads to antigen-specific unresponsiveness. In large part, maturation of the thymus gland during ontogeny correlates positively with development of resistance to tolerance induction. Much evidence reveals that the mechanism responsible for tolerance in this situation is clonal deletion of immature, antigen-specific thymocytes (see Chap. 5, Overview). In large measure, because cells within the thymus gland are normally expressing self-antigens, the thymocytes that are deleted represent those cells with T-cell receptors of high affinity for self-antigens. This mechanism undoubtedly contributes to the success with which the normal immune system is able to respond to all biologically relevant molecules, except those expressed on self-tissues—and therefore avoids autoimmunity.

However, tolerance can also be induced when the immune system is developmentally mature. The factors that are known to promote tolerance under these conditions include: (1) the physical form of the antigen, (2) the dose of antigen, and (3) the route of antigen administration. More specifically, soluble antigens are more readily able to induce tolerance than particulate or insoluble antigens. Very large doses of antigens, as well as extremely small quantities of antigens, are also likely to induce tolerance. This indicates that the immune system is disposed normally to respond to antigens within a relatively broad, but nonetheless defined, range of concentrations or amounts. Antigen administered in quantities above or below this range can induce tolerance. Injection of antigen intravenously also favors tolerance induction, whereas injection of antigen intracutaneously favors conventional sensitization. In a similar, but not identical, manner, oral ingestion of antigen produces a kind of immune deviation in which, on the one hand, delayed hypersensitivity to the antigen is impaired (i.e., tolerance), while, on the other hand, IgA antibody production to the antigen is exaggerated. (See the following discussion of ocular surface immunity.[11]) In addition, antigens injected with adjuvants induce conventional immune responses, whereas antigens administered in the absence of adjuvants may either promote tolerance or elicit no response whatever.

Additional factors influencing whether tolerance is induced concern the status of the immune system itself. For example, antigen X may readily induce tolerance when injected intravenously into a normal, immunologically naive individual. However, if the same antigen is injected into an individual previously immunized to antigen X, then tolerance will not occur. Thus, a prior state of sensitization mitigates against tolerance induction. Alternatively, if a mature immune system has been assaulted by immunosuppressive drugs, by debilitating systemic diseases, or by particular types of pathogens (the human immunodeficiency virus is a good example), it may display increased susceptibility to tolerance. Thus, when an antigen is introduced into an individual with a compromised immune response, tolerance may develop and be maintained, even if the immune system recovers.

Regional Immunity and the Eye

All tissues of the body requires immune protection from invading or endogenous pathogens. Because pathogens with different virulence strategies threaten different types of tissues, the immune system consists of a diversity of immune effectors. The diversity includes at least two different populations of effector T cells (that mediate delayed hypersensitivity and kill target cells) and seven different types of antibody molecules (IgM, IgG1, IgG2, IgG3, IgG4, IgA, and IgE). Thus, evolution has had to meet the challenge of designing an immune system that is capable of responding to a particular pathogen or antigen in a particular tissue with a response that is effective in eliminating the threat, while at the same time not damaging the tissue itself. Different tissues and organs display markedly different susceptibilities to immune-mediated tissue injury.[12, 13] The eye is an excellent example. Because integrity of the microanatomy of the visual axis is absolutely required for accurate vision, the eye can tolerate inflammation to only a very limited degree. Vigorous immunogenic inflammation, such as that found in a typical delayed hypersensitivity reaction in the skin, wreaks havoc with vision, and it has been argued that the threat of blindness has dictated an evolutionary adaptation in the eye that limits the expression of inflammation.

The conventional type of immunity that is generated when antigens or pathogens enter through the skin is almost never seen in the normal eye. Therefore, almost by definition, any immune responses that take place in or on the eye are regulated. On the ocular surface, immunity resembles that observed on other mucosal surfaces, such as the gastrointestinal tract, the upper respiratory tract, and the urinary tract. Within the eye, an unusual form of immunity is observed, and a description follows under ocular immune privilege.

OCULAR SURFACE IMMUNITY—CONJUNCTIVA, LACRIMAL GLAND, TEAR FILM, CORNEA, AND SCLERA

The normal human conjunctiva is an active participant in immune defense of the ocular surface against invasion by exogenous substances. The presence of blood vessels and lymphatic channels fosters transit of immune cells that can participate in the afferent and efferent arms of the immune response. The marginal and peripheral palpebral arteries and anterior ciliary arteries are the main blood suppliers of the conjunctiva. The superficial and deep lymphatic plexuses of the bulbar conjunctiva drain toward the palpebral commissures, where they join the lymphatics of the lids. Lymphatics of the palpebral conjunctiva on the lateral side drain into the preauricular and parotid lymph nodes. Lymphatics draining the palpebral conjunctiva on the medial side drain into the submandibular lymph nodes. Major immune cells found in normal human conjunctiva are dendritic cells, T and B lymphocytes, mast cells, and neutrophils. Dendritic cells, Langerhans and non-Langerhans, have been detected in different regions of the conjunctiva.[14] Dendritic cells act as APCs to T lymphocytes and may stimulate antigen-specific class II-region–mediated T-lymphocyte proliferation.[15] T lymphocytes, the predominant lymphocyte subpopulation in conjunctiva, are represented in the epithelium and in the substantial propria. T lymphocytes are the main effector cells in immune reactions such as delayed hypersensitivity or cytotoxic responses. B lymphocytes are absent except for rare scattered cells in the substantial propria of the fornices. Plasma cells are detected only in the conjunctival accessory lacrimal glands of Krause or minor lacrimal glands.[16] T and B lymphocytes and plasma cells are also present between the acini of the major lacrimal gland. Plasma cells from major and minor lacrimal glands synthesize Igs, mainly IgA.[17, 18] IgA is a dimer that is transported across the mucosal epithelium bound to a receptor complex. IgA dimers are released to the luminal surface of the ducts associated with a secretory component after cleavage of the receptor and are excreted with the tear film. Secretory IgA is a protectant of mucosal surfaces. Although secretory IgA does not seem to be bacteriostatic or bactericidal, it may blanket cell surface receptors that might otherwise be available for viral and bacterial fixation,[19] and it may modulate the normal flora of the ocular surface.[20] Foreign substances can be processed locally by the mucosal immune defense system. Somehow, after exposure to antigen, specific IgA helper T lymphocytes stimulate IgA B lymphocytes to differentiate into IgA-secreting plasma cells. Dispersed T and B lymphocytes and IgA-secreting plasma cells of the conjunctiva and lacrimal gland are referred to as the conjunctival and lacrimal gland–associated lymphoid tissue (CALT).[21] CALT is considered part of a widespread mucosa-associated lymphoid tissue (MALT) system, including the oral mucosa and salivary gland-associated lymphoid tissue, the gut-associated lymphoid tissue (GALT),[22] and the bronchus-associated lymphoid tissue (BALT).[23] CALT drains to the regional lymph nodes in an afferent arc; effector cells may return to the eye via an efferent arc.

The adaptive and the innate immune responses form part of an integrated system. Immunoglobulins and lymphokines produced by the lymphoid tissue of the conjunctiva help neutrophils and macrophages to destroy antigens. Macrophages in turn help the lymphocytes by transporting the antigens from the eye to the lymph nodes. Some immunoglobulins (e.g., IgE) bind to mast cells; others (IgG, IgM) bind complement. Mast cells and complement facilitate the arrival of neutrophils and macrophages.

Mast cells are located mainly perilimbally, although they can also be found in bulbar conjunctiva. Their degranulation in response to an allergen or an injury results in the release of vasoactive substances such as histamine, heparin, platelet-activating factor, and leukotrienes, which can cause blood vessel dilatation and increased vascular permeability.[24]

The tears contain several substances known to have antimicrobial properties. Lysozyme, immunoglobulins, and lactoferrin may be synthesized by the lacrimal gland. Lysozyme is an enzyme capable of lysing bacteria cell walls of certain gram-positive organisms.[25] Lysozyme may also facilitate secretory IgA bacteriolysis in the presence of complement.[26] The tear IgG has been shown to neutralize virus, lyse bacteria, and form immune complexes that bind complement and enhance bacterial opsonization and chemotaxis of phagocytes.[27] The tear components of the complement system enhance the effects of lysozyme and immunoglobulins.[28] Lactoferrin, an iron-binding protein, has both bacteriostatic and bactericidal properties.[29, 30] Lactoferrin may also regulate the production of granulocyte- and macrophage-derived colony-stimulating factor,[31] may inhibit the formation of the complement system component C3 convertase,[32] and may interact with specific antibody to produce an antibacterial effect more powerful than that of either lactoferrin or antibody alone.[33]

Autoimmune disorders that involve the conjunctiva include cicatricial pemphigoid, pemphigus vulgaris, erythema multiforme, and collagen vascular diseases. Autoimmune disorders that involve the lacrimal gland include Sjögren's syndrome. The mechanisms by which immunopathologic damage occurs in these diseases vary, depending on whether they are or are not organ-specific. When the antigen is localized in a particular organ, type II hypersensitivity reactions appear to be the main mechanisms (cicatricial pemphigoid and pemphigus vulgaris). In non–organ-specific diseases, type III and type IV hypersensitivity reactions are the more important (erythema multiforme, collagen vascular diseases).

The unique anatomic and physiologic characteristics of the human cornea explain on the one hand its predilection for involvement in various immune disorders and, on the other hand, its ability to express immune privilege. The peripheral cornea differs from the central cornea in several ways. The former is closer to the conjunctiva in which blood vessels and lymphatic channels provide a mechanism for the afferent arc of corneal immune reactions. Blood vessels derived from the anterior conjunctival and deep episcleral arteries extend 0.5 mm into the clear cornea.[34] Adjacent to these vessels, the subconjunctival lymphatics drain into regional lymph nodes. The presence of this vasculature allows diffusion of some molecules, such as immunoglobulins and complement components, into the cornea. IgG and IgA are found in similar concentrations in the peripheral and central cornea; however, more IgM is found in the periphery, probably because its high molecular weight restricts diffusion into the central area.[35] Both classic and alternative pathway components of complement and its inhibitors have been demonstrated in normal human corneas. However although most of the complement components have a peripheral-to-central cornea ratio of 1.2:1.0, C1 is denser in the periphery by a factor of 5. The high molecular weight of C1, the recognition unit of the classic pathway, may also restrict its diffusion into the central area.[36, 37] Normal human corneal epithelium contains small numbers of Langerhans cells, which are distributed almost exclusively at the limbus; very few cells are detected in the central cornea.[38] The peripheral cornea also contains a reservoir of inflammatory cells, including neutrophils, eosinophils, lymphocytes, plasma cells, and mast cells.[34] The presence of antibodies, complement components, Langerhans cells, and inflammatory cells makes the peripheral cornea more susceptible than the central cornea to involvement in a wide variety of autoimmune and hypersensitivity disorders, such as Mooren's ulcer and collagen vascular diseases. A discussion of corneal antigens and immune privilege follows.[39]

The sclera consists almost entirely of collagen and proteoglycans. It is traversed by the anterior and posterior ciliary vessels but retains a scanty vascular supply for its own use. Its nutrition is derived from the overlying episclera and underlying choroid[40]; similarly, both classic and alternative pathways components of complement are derived from these sources.[41] Normal human sclera has few if any lymphocytes, macrophages, Langerhans cells, or neutrophils.[42] In response to an inflammatory stimulus in the sclera, the cells pass readily from blood vessels of the episclera and choroid. Because of the collagenous nature of the sclera, many systemic autoimmune disorders, such as the collagen vascular diseases, may affect it.[42]

INTRAOCULAR IMMUNOLOGY: OCULAR IMMUNE PRIVILEGE

For more than 100 years, it has been known that foreign tissue grafts placed within the anterior chamber of an animal's eye can be accepted indefinitely.[43] The designation of this phenomenon as immune privilege had to await the seminal work of Medawar and colleagues, who discovered the principles of transplantation immunology in the 1940s and 1950s. These investigators studied immune privileged sites—the anterior chamber of the eye, the brain—as a method of exploring the possible ways to thwart immune rejection of solid tissue allografts.[44–47] It had been learned that transplantation antigens on grafts were carried to the immune system via regional lymphatic vessels and that immunization leading to graft rejection took place within draining lymph nodes. Because the eye and brain were regarded at the time as having no lymphatic drainage, and because both tissues resided behind a blood-tissue barrier, Medawar and associates postulated that immune privilege resulted from immunologic ignorance—although this was not a term that was used at the time. What these investigators meant was that foreign tissues placed in immune privileged sites were isolated by physical vascular barriers from the immune system and that they never alerted the immune system to their existence. During the past 25 years, immunologists who have studied immune privilege at various sites in the body have learned that this original postulate is basically untrue.[48–55] First, some privileged sites possess robust lymphatic drainage pathways—the testis is a good example. Second, antigens placed in privileged sites are known to escape and to be detected at distant sites, including lymphoid organs such as lymph nodes and the spleen. Third, antigens in privileged sites evoke antigen-specific, systemic immune responses, albeit of a unique nature. Thus, the modern view of immune privilege states that privilege is an actively acquired, dynamic state in which the immune system conspires with the privileged tissue or site in generating a response that is protective, rather than destructive. In a sense, immune privilege represents the most extreme form of the concept of regional immunity.

IMMUNE PRIVILEGED TISSUES AND SITES

Immune privilege has two different manifestations: privileged sites and privileged tissues (Table 10–1). Immune privileged sites are regions of the body where grafts of foreign tissue survive for extended, even indefinite, periods of time, compared with nonprivileged, or conventional sites. Immune privileged tissues, compared with nonprivileged tissues, are able to avoid, or at least resist, immune rejection when grafted into conventional body sites. The eye contains examples of both privileged tissues and sites, of which the best studied site is the anterior chamber, and the best studied tissue is the cornea.

Much has been learned about the phenomenon of immune privilege during the past 2 decades. The forces that confer immune privilege have been shown to act during both induction and expression of the immune response to antigens placed within, or expressed on, privileged sites and tissues. The forces that shape immune privileged sites and tissues include an ever-expanding list of microanatomic, biochemical, and immunoregulatory features. A short list of privilege-promoting features is displayed in Table 10–2. The eye expresses virtually every one of these features. Although passive features such as blood-ocular barrier, lack of lymphatics, and low expression of major histocompatibility complex (MHC) class I and II molecules are important, experimental attention has focused on immunomodulatory

TABLE 10–1. **Immune Privilege**

Sites	Tissues
Eye-cornea, anterior chamber	Cornea
Vitreous cavity, subretinal space	Lens
Brain	Cartilage
Pregnancy uterus	Placenta/fetus
Testis	Testis
Ovary	Ovary
Adrenal cortex	Liver
Hair follicles	
Tumors	Tumors

TABLE 10–2. **Features of Immune Privileged Sites**

Passive
Blood-tissue barriers
Deficient efferent lymphatics
Tissue fluid that drains into blood vasculature
Reduced expression of major histocompatibility complex class I and II molecules
Active
Constitutive expression of inhibitory cell surface molecules: Fas ligand, DAF, CD59, CD46
Immunosuppressive microenvironment: TGFb, α-MSH, VIP, CGRP, MIF, free cortisol

MIF, melanocyte-inhibiting factor; MSH, melanocyte-stimulating hormone; VIP, vasoinhibitory peptide; CGRP, calcitonin gene-related peptide.

molecules expressed on ocular tissues and present in ocular fluids.

REGULATION OF IMMUNE EXPRESSION IN THE EYE

As mentioned previously, activated T cells that express Fas on their surface are vulnerable to programmed cell death if they encounter other cells that express Fas ligand.[56] Constitutive expression of Fas ligand on cells that surround the anterior chamber has been shown to induce apoptosis among T cells and other leukocytes exposed to this ocular surface.[57] More important, Fas ligand expressed by cells of the cornea play a key role in rendering the cornea resistant to immune attack and rejection.[58, 59] Similarly, constitutive expression on corneal endothelial cells, as well as iris and ciliary body epithelium, of several membrane-bound inhibitors of complement activation are strategically located to prevent complement-dependent intraocular inflammation and injury.[60]

The realization that the intraocular microenvironment is immunosuppressive arises chiefly from studies of aqueous humor and secretions of cultured iris and ciliary body. Transforming growth factor-β_2, a normal constituent of aqueous humor,[61–63] is a powerful immunosuppressant, inhibiting various aspects of T cell and macrophage activation. However, it is by no means the only (or perhaps even the most) important inhibitor present. Although the list is still incomplete, other relevant factors in aqueous humor include α-melanocyte-stimulating hormone,[64] vasoactive intestinal peptide,[65] calcitonin gene–related peptide,[66] and macrophage migration inhibitory factor.[67] These factors account in part for the immunosuppressive properties of aqueous humor: inhibition of T-cell activation (proliferation) and differentiation (secretion of lymphokines such as INF-γ) after ligation of the T-cell receptor for antigen, suppression of macrophage activation (phagocytosis, generation of nitrous oxide),[68] and inhibition of natural killer (NK) cell lysis of target cells.[69] It is important to point out that aqueous humor does not inhibit all immune reactivity. For example, antibody neutralization of virus infection of target cells is not prevented in the presence of aqueous humor.[68] Moreover, cytotoxic T cells that are fully differentiated are fully able to lyse antigen-bearing target cells cultured in aqueous humor. The ability of the immune system to express itself within the eye is highly regulated by the factors just described, and suppression of immune expression that leads to inflammation and damage is one important dimension of ocular immune privilege.

REGULATION OF INDUCTION OF IMMUNITY TO EYE-DERIVED ANTIGENS

Another dimension to immune privilege is the ability of the eye to regulate the nature of the systemic immune response to antigens placed within it. It has been known for more than 20 years that injection of alloantigenic cells into the anterior chamber of rodent eyes evokes a distinctive type of immune deviation—now called anterior chamber–associated immune deviation (ACAID).[70–72] In ACAID, eye-derived antigens elicit an immune response that is selectively deficient in T cells that mediate delayed hypersensitivity and B cells that secrete complement-fixing antibodies. There is not, however, a global lack of response, because animals with ACAID display a high level of antigen-specific serum antibodies of the non–complement-fixing varieties[73, 74] and primed cytotoxic T cells.[75, 76] In ACAID, regulatory T cells are also generated which, in an antigen-specific manner, suppress both the induction and expression of delayed hypersensitivity to the antigen in question.[77–80] ACAID can be elicited by diverse types of antigens, ranging from soluble protein to histocompatibility to virus-encoded antigens. A deviant systemic response similar to ACAID can even be evoked by antigen injected into the anterior chamber of the eye of an individual previously immunized to the same antigen.[81]

Induction of ACAID by intraocular injection of antigen begins within the eye itself.[80–85] After injection of antigen into the eye, local APCs capture the antigen, migrate across the trabecular meshwork into the canal of Schlemm, and then traffic via the blood to the spleen. In the splenic white pulp, the antigen is presented in a unique manner to T and B lymphocytes, resulting in the spectrum of functionally distinct antigen-specific T cells and antibodies found in ACAID. The ocular microenvironment sets the stage for this sequence of events by virtue of the immunoregulatory properties of aqueous humor. This ocular fluid, or more precisely, TGF-β_2, confers upon conventional APCs the capacity to induce ACAID. Thus, the ocular microenvironment not only regulates the expression of immunity within the eye, but it also regulates the functions of eye-derived APCs and thus promotes a systemic immune response that is deficient in those immune effector modalities most capable of inducing immunogenic inflammation—delayed hypersensitivity T cells and complement-fixing antibodies.

RELATIONSHIP BETWEEN IMMUNE PRIVILEGE AND INTRAOCULAR INFLAMMATORY DISEASES

The rationale of immune privilege is that all tissues, including the eye, require immune protection. Immune privilege represents the consequence of interactions between the immune system and the eye in which local protection is provided by immune effectors that do not disrupt the eye's primary and vital function—vision. Because maintenance of a precise microanatomy is essential for vision, privilege allows for immune protection that is virtually devoid of immunogenic inflammation.

At the experimental level, ocular immune privilege has been implicated in: (1) the extraordinary success of corneal allografts,[86–89] (2) progressive growth of intraocular tumors,[90] (3) resistance to herpes stromal keratitis,[91] and (4) suppression of autoimmune uveoretinitis.[92–94] When immune privilege prevails within the eye, corneal allografts succeed; trauma to the eye heals without incident; and ocular infections are cleared without inflammation. However, in this case, ocular tumors may then grow relentlessly, and uveal tract infections may persist and recur.

The consequences of failed immune privilege have been explored experimentally and considered clinically. When privilege fails in the eye, blindness is a likely outcome. As examples, ocular trauma may result in sympathetic ophthalmia; ocular infections may produce sight-threatening inflammation; and corneal allografts may fail.

Corneal Transplantation Immunology

The cornea is an immune privileged tissue, and, in part, this attribute accounts for the extraordinary success of orthotopic corneal allografts in experimental animals and also in humans. It is pertinent that the corneal graft forms the anterior surface of a site that is also typically immune privileged (the anterior chamber). Despite the advances that have been made in corneal tissue preservation and surgical techniques, a significant proportion of grafts eventually fail.[95–98] The main cause of transplant failure is now immune-mediated graft rejection, which occurs in 16 to 30% of recipients in a large series after several years of follow-up. Certain recipients seem to be at increased risk of graft rejection.[99–101] Corneal vascularization, either preoperative from recipient herpetic, interstitial, or traumatic keratitis, or stimulated by silk or loose sutures, contact lenses, infections, persistent epithelial defects, and other disorders associated with inflammation, has been widely recognized as a clear risk factor for decreased graft survival. It is estimated that the failure rate is 25 to 50% in vascularized corneas and 5 to 10% in avascular ones. Other factors that increase the risk of allograft rejection include: (1) a history of previous graft loss,[102–104] (2) eccentric and large grafts, and (3) glaucoma. The reasons why corneal bed neovascularization is a dominant risk factor for cornea graft rejection remain to be elucidated. Evidence indicates that neovascularized corneas also contain neolymphatic vessels.[105] Moreover, the graft bed is heavily infiltrated with APCs, especially Langerhans cells. These factors are probably important for increasing the immunogenic potential of the allogeneic cornea graft.

TRANSPLANTATION ANTIGEN EXPRESSION ON CORNEAL TISSUE

In outbred species, such as humans, transplants of solid tissue grafts usually fail unless the recipient is immunosuppressed, and the reason for failure is the development of an immune response directed at so-called transplantation antigens displayed on cells of the graft. Immunologists have separated transplantation antigens into two categories: major and minor, primarily because major antigens induce more vigorous alloimmunity than do minor antigens.[106] The genes that encode the major transplantation antigens in humans are located within the MHC called human leukocyte antigen (HLA). Minor histocompatibility antigens are encoded at numerous loci spread throughout the genome. The HLA complex, which is a large genetic region, is situated on the short arm of the 6th human chromosome. HLA genes that encode class I and class II antigens are extremely polymorphic. Similarly, minor histocompatibility loci contain highly polymorphic genes. In the aggregate, polymorphisms at the major and minor histocompatibility loci account for the observation that solid tissue grafts exchanged between any two individuals selected at random within a species are acutely rejected.

The expression of HLA antigens on corneal cells is somewhat atypical.[107–111] Class I MHC antigens are expressed strongly on the epithelial cells of the cornea, comparable in intensity to the expression of epidermal cells of skin. Keratocytes express less class I than conventional fibroblasts, and corneal endothelial cells express small amounts of class I antigens under normal circumstances. Except at the periphery near the limbus, the cornea contains no adventitial cells (i.e., cells of bone marrow origin).[112, 113] In most solid tissues, class II HLA antigens are expressed primarily on these types of cells.[114] Therefore, under normal conditions, the burden of class II MHC antigens on corneal grafts is minimal. Corneal epithelial and endothelial cells resemble other cells of the body in responding to INF-γ by upregulation of class I antigen expression. Among INF-γ–treated epithelial cells, class II antigens are also expressed. However, corneal endothelial cells resist expression of class II antigens. Because class II antigens, especially those expressed on bone marrow–derived cells, are extremely important in providing solid tissue grafts with their ability to evoke transplantation immunity, the deficit of these antigens on corneal cells offers a significant barrier to sensitization.

A major accomplishment of modern immunology is the ability of contemporary clinical pathology laboratories to tissue type for HLA class I and class II antigens. With most solid tissue allografts, tissue typing that identifies HLA matching between a graft donor and recipient correlates with improved graft survival.[115] Thus, HLA-matched kidney grafts survive with fewer rejection episodes and with a reduced need for immunosuppressive therapy, compared to HLA-mismatched grafts. The evidence that HLA tissue typing similarly improves the fate of matched corneal allografts is conflicting.[116–123] There seems to be no controversy regarding the influence of tissue typing on grafts placed in eyes of patients with low risk. In this situation, virtually no studies suggest a positive typing effect. The rate of graft success is so high in low-risk situations with unmatched grafts that there is little opportunity for a matching effect to be seen. However, in high-risk situations, the literature contains reports that claim: (1) HLA matching, especially for class I antigens, has a powerful positive effect on graft outcome; (2) HLA matching has no effect on graft outcome; or (3) HLA matching may have a deleterious effect on graft outcome.

The reasons for confusion about the effects of HLA matching on corneal allograft success may relate to studies on orthotopic corneal allografts conducted in mice. It has been reported that minor transplantation antigens offer a significant barrier to graft success in rodents.[124–126] In fact, corneal allografts that display minor, but not major, transplantation antigens are rejected more vigorously and with a higher frequency than grafts that display MHC, but not minor, transplantation antigens. Two factors seem to be important in this outcome. First, the reduced expression of MHC antigens on corneal grafts renders these grafts less immunogenic than other solid tissue grafts. Second, corneal antigens are only detected by the recipient immune system when the recipient's own APCs infiltrate the graft and capture donor antigens. Graft cells are the source of donor antigens, and apparently in the cornea, minor transplantation antigens are quantitatively more numerous than MHC antigens. Therefore, the recipient mounts an immune response directed primarily at minor transplantation antigens. Because tissue typing is unable at present to match organs and donors for minor histocompatibility antigens, it is no surprise that current tissue typing has proved to be ineffectual at improving corneal allograft success.

CORNEAL ALLOGRAFT ACCEPTANCE—WHEN IMMUNE PRIVILEGE SUCCEEDS

The normal cornea is an immune-privileged tissue, and several features are known to contribute to the privileged status. First, as mentioned earlier, expression of MHC class I and class II molecules is reduced and impaired, especially on the corneal endothelium. The net antigenic load of corneal tissue is thus reduced compared with other tissues, which has a mitigating effect on both induction and expression of alloimmunity. Second, the cornea lacks blood and lymph vessels. The absence of these vascular structures isolates the cornea graft in a manner that prevents antigenic information from escaping from the tissue while at the same time prevents immune effectors from gaining access to the tissue. Third, the cornea is deficient in bone marrow–derived cells, especially Langerhans cells. Mobile cells of this type are one way in which antigenic information from a solid tissue graft alerts the immune system in regional lymph nodes to its presence. The absence of APCs from the cornea dramatically lengthens the time that it takes for the recipient immune system to become aware of the graft's existence. Fourth, cells of the cornea constitutively secrete molecules with immunosuppressive properties.[127–131] Cells of all three corneal layers secrete TGF-β, as well as yet-to-be-defined inhibitory molecules. In addition, corneal epithelial cells and keratocytes constitutively produce an excess of IL-1 receptor antagonist, compared with the endogenous production of IL-1γ.[129] These immunosuppressive molecules have powerful modulatory effects on APC, T cells, B cells, NK cells, and macrophages and can act during induction and expression of alloimmunity to prevent or inhibit graft rejection. Fifth, cells of the cornea constitutively express surface molecules that inhibit immune effectors. Corneal endothelial cells display on their surface DAF, CD59, and CD46—molecules that inhibit complement effector functions.[130] These inhibitors protect corneal endothelial cells from injury by complement molecules generated during an alloimmune response. Corneal cells have been found to express CD95L (Fas ligand), and expression of this molecule on mouse cornea grafts has been formally implicated in protecting the grafts from attack by Fas$^+$ T cells and other leukocytes.[58, 59, 131] Finally, the cornea graft forms the anterior surface of the anterior chamber; antigens released from the graft endothelium escape into aqueous humor. Experimental evidence indicates that allogeneic cornea grafts induce donor-specific ACAID in recipients,[124, 132] and the inability of these recipients to acquire donor-specific delayed hypersensitivity plays a key role in maintaining the integrity of accepted grafts.

When placed in low-risk (normal) eyes of mice, a high proportion of corneal allografts with the features listed earlier experience prolonged, even indefinite, survival in the complete absence of any immunosuppressive therapy. This dramatic expression of immune privilege is mirrored by the success of keratoplasties performed in low-risk situations in humans. However, in neither mice nor in humans are all such grafts successful. This observation indicates that immune privilege is by no means absolute and irrevocable.

PATHOGENESIS OF CORNEAL ALLOGRAFT REJECTION—WHEN IMMUNE PRIVILEGE FAILS

The high rate of failure of corneal allografts in high-risk situations in humans resembles the high rate of failure of orthotopic corneal allografts placed in high-risk mouse eyes.[133] Studies of the rejection process in experimental animals have begun to unravel the pathogenic mechanisms responsible. Sensitization develops in recipient animals with surprising rapidity when grafts are placed in high-risk eyes. Within 7 days of engraftment, immune donor-specific T cells can be detected in lymphoid tissues. Similar grafts placed in low-risk mouse eyes do not achieve T-cell sensitization until at least 3 weeks after engraftment. The reason for rapid sensitization when grafts are placed in high-risk eyes appears to be the speed with which recipient APCs (chiefly Langerhans cells) migrate into the graft from the periphery. Whereas migraton of Langerhans cells into allografts placed in low-risk eyes is detectable between 1 and 2 weeks after grafting, Langerhans cells can be detected in grafts in high-risk eyes within a few days of engraftment. It is very likely that the vulnerability to rejection of grafts placed in high-risk eyes is dictated by the efficiency with which recipient APCs enter the graft, capture antigens, and migrate to the regional lymph nodes where recipient T cells are initially activated. Support for this view is provided by the observation that Langerhans cell migration into the graft can be inhibited by topical application of IL-1 receptor antagonist.[134] Experiments indicate that grafts that have been treated with IL-1ra take longer to induce donor-specific sensitization, and the majority of such grafts avoid immune rejection.

When normal corneal grafts are placed in high-risk eyes, they are typically rejected. In this case, the inherent immune privileged status of the graft is clearly insufficient to overcome the fact that the graft site (a neovascularized eye) can no longer act as an immune privileged site. It is also possible to show that grafts that have lost their immune privileged status are vulnerable to rejection, even when placed in normal, low-risk eyes (which display immune privilege). A Langerhans cell can be induced to migrate into the central corneal epithelium by several different experimental maneuvers. When grafts containing Langerhans cells are placed in low-risk eyes, rapid recipient sensitization occurs, and the grafts are rejected. The tempo and vigor of rejection of these grafts strongly resemble the fate of normal grafts placed in high-risk eyes. These results indicate that both the privileged tissue (the cornea graft) and the privileged site (the low risk eye) make important contributions to the success of orthotopic corneal allografts.

Summary and Conclusion

The eye is defended against pathogens, just as is every other part of the body. Components of both the natural and the acquired immune systems respond to pathogens in the eye, but the responses are different from those following antigen encounter in most other places in the body, perhaps as a result of evolutionary pressures resulting in the survival of those species and species' members in which a blinding, exuberant inflammatory response was prevented by "regulation" of the response. In any event, we are left for the moment with an organ (the eye) in which special immunologic responsiveness allows us to enjoy a degree of "privilege" tolerance to transplanted tissue not experienced by other organs. It is clear now that this tolerance is an active process, not simply a passive one derived from the "invisibility" of the transplant from the recipient's immune system.

REFERENCES

1. Janeway CA Jr, Travers P: Immunobiology. Current Biology, 3rd ed. New York, Limited/Garland Publishing, 1997.
2. Qin S, Cobbold SP, Pope H, et al: Infectious transplantation tolerance. Science 259:974–977, 1993.
3. Mosmann TR, Coffman RL: Th1 and Th2 cells: Different patterns of lymphokine secretion lead to different functional properties. Ann Rev Immunol 7:145–173, 1989.
4. Asherson GL, Collizi V, Zembala M: An overview of T-suppressor cell circuits. Ann Rev Immunol 4:37, 1986.
5. Groux H, O'Garra A, Bigler M, et al: A CD4+ T-cell subset inhibits antigen-specific T-cell responses and prevents colitis. Nature 389:737–741, 1997.
6. Billingham RE, Brent L, Medawar PB: Actively acquired tolerance of foreign cells. Nature 172:603, 1953.
7. Burnet FM: The Clonal Selection Theory of Acquired Immunity. Cambridge, Cambridge University Press, 1959.
8. Kappler JW, Roehm N, Marrack P: T cell tolerance by clonal elimination in the thymus. Cell 49:273–280, 1987.
9. Jenkins MK, Pardoll DM, Mizguchi J, et al: RH: Molecular events in the induction of a non-responsive state in interleukin-2 producing helper lymphocyte clones. Proc Natl Acad Sci U S A 84:5409, 1987.
10. Asherson GL, Stone SH: Selective and specific inhibition of 24-hour skin reactions in the guinea-pig. I: Immune deviation: Description of the phenomenon and the effect of splenectomy. Immunology 9:205–211, 1965.
11. Khoury SJ, Hancock WW, Weiner HL: Oral tolerance to myelin basic protein and natural recovery from experimental autoimmune encephalomyelitis are associated with downregulation of inflammatory cytokines and differential upregulation of transforming growth factor β, interleukin 4, and prostaglandin E expression in the brain. J Exp Med 176:1355–1364, 1992.
12. Streilein JW: Regional immunology of the eye. *In* Pepose JW, Holland GN, Wilhemus KR (eds): Ocular Infection and Immunity. Philadelphia, Mosby–Year Book, 1996, pp 19–33.
13. Streilein JW: Regional Immunology. *In* Dulbecco R (ed): Encyclopedia of Human Biology, 2nd ed, vol 4. San Diego, Academic Press, 1997, pp 767–776.
14. Sacks E, Rutgers J, Jakobiec FA, et al: A comparison of conjunctival and nonocular dendritic cells utilizing new monoclonal antibodies. Ophthalmology 93:1089, 1986.
15. Murphy GF: Cell membrane glycoproteins and Langerhans cells. Hum Pathol 16:103, 1985.
16. Sacks E, Wieczorek R, Jakobiec FA, et al: Lymphocytic sub-populations in the normal human conjunctiva. Ophthalmology 93:1276, 1986.
17. Franklin RM, Remus LE: Conjunctival-associated lymphoid tissue: Evidence for a role in the secretory immune system. Invest Ophthalmol Vis Sci 25:181, 1984.
18. Wieczorek R, Jakobiec FA, Sacks E, et al: The immunoarchitecture of the normal human lacrimal gland. Ophthalmology 95:100, 1988.
19. Tomasi TB: The Immune System of Secretion. Englewood Cliffs, Prentice-Hall, 1976.
20. Gibbons RJ: Bacterial adherence to the mucosal surfaces and its inhibition by secretory antibodies. Adv Exp Med Biol 45:315, 1974.
21. Jackson DE, Lally ET, Nakamura MC, et al: Migration of IgA-bearing lymphocytes into salivary glands. Cell Immunol 63:203, 1981.
22. Parrott DM: The gut as a lymphoid organ. Clin Gastroenterol 5:211, 1976.
23. Bienenstock J, Johnston N, Perey DYE: Bronchial lymphoid tissue. I: Morphologic characteristics. Lab Invest 28:686, 1973.
24. Allansmith MR: The Eye and Immunology. St. Louis, CV Mosby, 1982.
25. Allansmith MR: Defense of the ocular surface. Int Ophthalmol Clin 12:93, 1979.
26. Fleming A: On a remarkable bacteriolytic element found in tissues and secretions. Proc R Soc Lond (Biol) 93:306, 1922.
27. Strober W, Hague HE, Lum LG, et al: IgA-Fc receptors on mouse lymphoid cells. J Immunol 121:2140, 1978.
28. Bluestone R: Lacrimal immunoglobulins and complement quantified by counter-immunoelectrophoresis. Br J Ophthalmol 59:279, 1975.
29. Masson PL, Heremans JF, Prignot JJ, et al: Immunohistochemical localization and bacteriostatic properties of an iron-binding protein from bronchial mucus. Thorax 21:358, 1966.
30. Arnold RR, Cole MF, McGhee JR: A Bactericidal effect for human lactoferrin. Science 197(297):263, 1977.
31. Badgy GC: Interaction of lactoferrin monocytes and lymphocyte subsets in the regulation in the regulation of steady-state granulopoiesis in vitro. J Clin Invest 68:56, 1981.
32. Kijlstra A, Jeurissen SHM: Modulation of classical C_3 convertase of complement by tear lactoferrin. Immunology 47:263, 1982.
33. Bullen JJ, Rogers HJ, Leigh L: Iron-binding proteins in milk and resistance of *Escherichia coli* infection in infants. BMJ 1:69, 1972.
34. Hogan MJ, Alvarado JA: The limbus. *In* Histology of the Human Eye: An Atlas and Textbook, 2nd ed. Philadelphia, WB Saunders, 1971.
35. Allansmith MR, McClellan BH: Immunoglobulins in the human cornea. Am J Ophthalmol 80:123, 1975.
36. Mondino BJ, Ratajczak HV, Goldberg DB, et al: Alternate and classical pathway components of complement in the normal cornea. Arch Ophthalmol 98:346, 1980.
37. Mondino BJ, Brady KJ: Distribution of hemolytic complement in the normal cornea. Arch Ophthalmol 99:1430, 1981.
38. Klaresjkog L, Forsum U, Tjernlund VM, et al: Expression of Ia antigen-like molecules on cells in the corneal epithelium. Invest Ophthalmol Vis Sci 18:310, 1979.
39. Mondino BJ: Inflammatory diseases of the peripheral cornea. Ophthalmology 95:463, 1988.
40. Watson PG, Hazleman BL: The Sclera and Systemic Disorders. Philadelphia, WB Saunders, 1976.
41. Brawman-Mintzer O, Mondino BJ, Mayer FJ: Distribution of complement in the sclera. Invest Ophthalmol Vis Sci 30:2240, 1989.
42. Fong LP, Sainz de la Maza M, Rice BA, et al: Immunopathology of scleritis. Ophthalmology 98:472, 1991.
43. van Dooremall JC: Die Entwicklung der in fremden Grund versetzten lebenden gewebe. Graefes Arch Clin Exp Ophthalmol 19:358–373, 1873.
44. Medawar P: Immunity to homologous grafted skin. III: The fate of skin homografts transplanted to the brain, to subcutaneous tissue and to the anterior chamber of the eye. Br J Exp Pathol 29:58–69, 1948.
45. Barker CF, Billingham RE: Immunologically privileged sites. Adv Immunol 25:1–54, 1977.
46. Streilein, JW: Immune privilege as the result of local tissue barriers and immunosuppressive microenvironments. Curr Opin Immunol 5:428–432, 1993.
47. Streilein JW: Perspective: Unraveling immune privilege. Science 270:1158–1159, 1995.
48. Streilein, JW: Immune regulation and the eye: A dangerous compromise. FASEB J 1:199–208, 1987.
49. Niederkorn JY: Immune privilege and immune regulation in the eye. Adv Immunol 48:191–226, 1990.
50. Tompsett E, Abi-Hanna D, Wakefield D: Immunological privilege in the eye: A review. Curr Eye Res 9:1141–1150, 1990.
51. Ksander BR, Streilein JW: Regulation of the immune response within privileged sites. *In* Granstein R (ed): Mechanisms Of Regulation Of Immunity Chemical Immunology. Basel, Switzerland, Karger, 1993, pp 117–145.

52. Streilein JW: Ocular regulation of systemic immunity. Reg Immunol 6:143–150, 1994.
53. Streilein JW: Ocular immune privilege and the Faustian dilemma. Invest Ophthalmol Vis Sci 37:1940–1950, 1996.
54. Streilein JW, Ksander BR, Taylor AW: Commentary: Immune privilege, deviation and regulation in the eye. J Immunol 158:3557–3560, 1997.
55. Streilein JW, Takeuchi M, Taylor AW: Immune privilege, T cell tolerance, and tissue-restricted autoimmunity. *In* Burlingham W (ed): Proceedings of Ray Owens Symposium on Tolerance. Hum Immunol 52:138–143, 1997.
56. Nagata S, Golstein P: The Fas death factor. Science 267:1449–1456, 1995.
57. Griffith TS, Brunner T, Fletcher SM, et al: Fas ligand-induced apoptosis as a mechanism of immune privilege. Science 270:1189, 1995.
58. Stuart PM, Griffith TS, Usui N, et al: CD95 ligand (FasL)-induced apoptosis is necessary for corneal allograft survival. J Clin Invest 99:396–402, 1997.
59. Yamagami S, Kawashima H, Tsuru T, et al: Role of Fas/Fas ligand interactions in the immunorejection of allogeneic mouse corneal transplantation. Transplantation 64(8):1107–1111, 1997.
60. Bora NS, Gobleman CL, Atkinson JP, et al: Differential expression of the complement regulatory proteins in the human eye. Invest Ophthal Vis Sci 34:3579–3584, 1993.
61. Granstein R, Stszewski R, Knisely T, et al: Aqueous humor contain transforming growth factor-β and a small (<3500 daltons) inhibitor of thymocyte proliferation. J Immunol 144:3021–3027, 1990.
62. Cousins SW, McCabe, MM, Danielpour D, et al: Identification of transforming growth factor-beta as an immunosuppressive factor in aqueous humor. Invest Ophthalmol Vis Sci 32:2201–2211, 1991.
63. Jampel HD, Roche N, Stark WJ, Roberts AB: Transforming growth factor-β in human aqueous humor. Curr Eye Res 9:963–969, 1990.
64. Taylor AW, Streilein JW, Cousins SW: Identification of alpha-melanocyte stimulating hormone as a potential immuno-suppressive factor in aqueous humor. Curr Eye Res 11:1199–1206, 1992.
65. Taylor AW, Streilein JW, Cousins SW: Vasoactive intestinal peptide (VIP) contributes to the immunosuppressive activity of normal aqueous humor. J Immunol 153:1080–1086, 1994.
66. Wahlestedt C, Beding N, Ekman R: Calcitonin gene-related peptide in the eye: Release by sensory nerve stimulation and effects associated with neurogenic inflammation. Regul Pept 16:107–115, 1986.
67. Apte RS, Niederkorn JY: MIF: A novel inhibitor of NK cell activity in the anterior chamber (AC) of the eye. J Allergy Clin Immunol 99:S467, 1997.
68. Kaiser CJ, Ksander BR, Streilein JW: Inhibition of lymphocyte proliferation by aqueous humor. Reg Immunol 2:42–49, 1989.
69. Apte RS, Niederkorn JY: Isolation and characterization of a unique natural killer cell inhibitory factor present in the anterior chamber of the eye. J Immunol 156:2667–2673, 1996.
70. Kaplan HJ, Streilein JW: Immune response to immunization via the anterior chamber of the eye. I: F_1 lymphocyte-induced immune deviation. J Immunol 118:809–814, 1977.
71. Kaplan HJ, Streilein JW: Immune response to immunization via the anterior chamber of the eye. II: An analysis of F_1 lymphocyte induced immune deviation. J Immunol 120:689–693, 1978.
72. Streilein JW, Niederkorn JY, Shadduck JA: Systemic immune unresponsiveness induced in adult mice by anterior chamber presentation of minor histocompatibility antigens. J Exp Med 152:1121–1125, 1980.
73. Niederkorn JY, Streilein JW: Analysis of antibody production induced by allogeneic tumor cells inoculated into the anterior chamber of the eye. Transplantation 33:573–577, 1982.
74. Wilbanks GA, Streilein JW: Distinctive humoral responses following anterior chamber and intravenous administration of soluble antigen: Evidence for active suppression of IgG2a-secreting B-cells. Immunology 71:566–572, 1990.
75. Niederkorn JY, Streilein JW: Alloantigens placed into the anterior chamber of the eye induce specific suppression of delayed type hypersensitivity but normal cytotoxic T lymphocyte responses. J Immunol 131:2670–2674, 1983.
76. Ksander BR, Streilein JW: Analysis of cytotoxic T cell responses to intracameral allogeneic tumors. I: Quantitative and qualitative analysis of cytotoxic precursor and effector cells. Invest Ophthalmol Vis Sci 30:323–329, 1989.
77. Waldrep JC, Kaplan HJ: Anterior chamber-associated immune deviation induced by TNP-splenocytes (TNP-ACAID). II: Suppressor T cell networks. Invest Ophthalmol Vis Sci 24:1339–1345, 1983.
78. Streilein JW, Niederkorn JY: Characterization of the suppressor cell(s) responsible for anterior chamber associated immune deviation (ACAID) induced in BALB/c mice by P815 cells. J Immunol 134:1381–1387, 1985.
79. Ferguson TA, Kaplan HJ: The immune response and the eye. II: The nature of T suppressor cell induction of anterior chamber-associated immune deviation (ACADI). J Immunol 139:352–357, 1987.
80. Wilbanks GA, Streilein JW: Characterization of suppressor cells in anterior chamber-associated immune deviation (ACAID) induced by soluble antigen: Evidence of two functionally and phenotypically distinct T-suppressor cell populations. Immunology 71:383–389, 1990.
81. Kosiewicz MM, Okamoto S, Miki S, et al: Imposing deviant immunity on the presensitized state. J Immunol 153:2962–2973, 1994.
82. Wilbanks GA, Streilein JW: Studies on the induction of anterior chamber associated immune deviation (ACAID). I: Evidence that an antigen-specific, ACAID-inducing, cell-associated signal exists in the peripheral blood. J Immunol 146:2610–2617, 1991.
83. Wilbanks GA, Mammolenti MM, Streilein JW: Studies on the induction of anterior chamber associated immune deviation (ACAID). II: Eye-derived cells participate in generating blood borne signals that induce ACAID. J Immunol 146:3018–3024, 1991.
84. Wilbanks GA, Mammolenti MM, Streilein JW: Studies on the induction of anterior chamber-associated immune deviation (ACAID). III: Induction of ACAID depends upon intraocular transforming growth factor-β. Eur J Immunol 22:165–173, 1992.
85. Hara Y, Okamoto S, Rouse B, et al: Evidence that peritoneal exudate cells cultured with eye-derived fluids are the proximate antigen presenting cells in immune deviation of the ocular type. J Immunol 151:5162–5171, 1993.
86. Maumanee AE: The influence of donor-recipient sensitization on corneal grafts. Am J Ophthalmol 34:142–152, 1951.
87. Sonoda Y, Streilein JW: Orthotopic corneal transplantation in mice: Evidence that the immunogenetic rules of rejection do not apply. Transplantation 54:694–703, 1992.
88. Streilein JW: Anterior chamber privilege in relation to keratoplasty. *In* Zierhut M (ed): Immunology Of Corneal Transplantation. Buren, Aeolus Press, 1994, pp 117–134.
89. Streilein JW: Immune privilege and the cornea. *In* Pleyer U, Hartmann C, Sterry W (eds): Proceedings of Symposium: Bullous Oculo-Muco-Cutaneous Disorders. Buren, Aeolus Press, 1997, pp 43–52.
90. Niederkorn J, Streilein JW, Shadduck, JA: Deviant immune responses to allogeneic tumors injected intracamerally and subcutaneously in mice. Invest Ophthalmol Vis Sci 20:355–363, 1980.
91. McLeish W, Rubsamen P, Atherton SS, et al: Immunobiology of Langerhans cells on the ocular surface. II: Role of central corneal Langerhans cells in stromal keratitis following experimental HSV-1 infection in mice. Reg Immunol 2:236–243, 1989.
92. Mizuno K, Clark AF, Streilein JW: Induction of anterior chamber associated immune deviation in rats receiving intracameral injections of retinal S antigen. Curr Eye Res 7:627–632, 1988.
93. Hara Y, Caspi RR, Wiggert B, et al: Suppression of experimental autoimmune uveitis in mice by induction of anterior chamber associated immune deviation with interphotoreceptor retinoid binding protein. J Immunol 148:1685–1692, 1992.
94. Gery I, Streilein JW: Autoimmunity in the eye and its regulation. Curr Opin Immunol 6:938–945, 1994.
95. Khodadoust AA: The allograft rejection reaction: The leading cause of late failure of clinical corneal grafts. *In* Porter R, Knight J (eds): Corneal Graft Failure. Ciba Foundation Symposium 15. Amsterdam, Associated Science Publishers, 1973.
96. Stark WJ: Transplantation immunology of penetrating keratoplasty. Trans Am Ophthalmol Soc 78:1079, 1980.
97. Epstein RJ, Seedor JA, Dreizen NG, et al: Penetrating keratoplasty for herpes simplex keratitis and keratoconus: Allograft rejection and survival. Ophthalmology 94:935, 1987.
98. Wilson SE, Kaufman HE: Graft failure after penetrating keratoplasty. Surv Ophthalmol 34:325, 1990.
99. Paque J, Poirier RH: Corneal allograft reaction and its relationship to suture site neovascularization. Ophthalmic Surg 8:71, 1977.
100. Vlker-Dieben HJM, D'Amaro J, Kok-van Alphen CC: Hierarchy of prognostic factors for corneal allograft survival. Aust N Z J Ophthalmol 15:11, 1987.
101. Boisjoly HM, Bernard P-M, Dube I, et al: Effect of factors unrelated

to tissue etching on corneal transplant endothelial rejection. Am J Ophthalmol 107:647, 1989.
102. Donshik PC, Cavanagh HD, Boruchoff SA, et al: Effect of bilateral and unilateral grafts on the incidence of rejections after keratoconus. Am J Ophthalmol 87:823, 1979.
103. Khodadoust AA, Karnema Y: Corneal grafts in the second eye. Cornea 3:17, 1984.
104. Meyer RF: Corneal allograft rejection in bilateral penetrating keratoplasty: Clinical and laboratory studies. Trans Am Ophthalmol Soc 84:664, 1986.
105. Dana M-R, Streilein JW: Loss and restoration of immune privilege in eyes with corneal neovascularization. Invest Ophthalmol Vis Sci 37:2485–2494, 1996.
106. Klein J: Natural History of the Major Histocompatibility Complex. New York, Wiley, 1986.
107. Fujikawa LS, Colvin RB, Bhan AK, et al: Expression of HLA-A/B/C and -DR locus antigens on epithelial, stromal and endothelial cells of the human cornea. Cornea 1:213, 1982.
108. Mayer DL, Daar AS, Casey TA, et al: Localization of HLA-A, B, C and HLA-DR antigens in the human cornea: Practical significance for grafting technique and HLA typing. Transplant Proc 15:126, 1983.
109. Whitsett CF, Stulting RD: The distribution of HLA antigens on human corneal tissue. Invest Ophthalmol Vis Sci 25:519, 1984.
110. Treseler PA, Foulks GN, Sanfilippo F: The expression of HLA antigens by cells in the human cornea. Am J Ophthalmol 98:763, 1984.
111. Abi-Hanna D, Wakefield D, Watkins S: HLA antigens in ocular tissues. I: In vivo expression in human eyes. Transplantation 45:610–613, 1988.
112. Streilein JW, Toews GB, Bergstresser PR: Corneal allografts fail to express Ia antigens. Nature 282:326–327, 1979.
113. William KA, Ash JK, Coster DJ: Histocompatibility antigen and passenger cell content of normal and diseased human cornea. Transplantation 39:265, 1985.
114. Austyn JM, Larsen CP: Migration patterns of dendritic leukocytes: Implications for transplantation. Transplantation 48:1–9, 1990.
115. Martin S, Dyer PA: The case for matching MHC genes in human organ transplantation. Nat Genet 5:210–213, 1993.
116. Batchelor JR, Casey TA, Gibbs DC, et al: HLA matching and corneal grafting. Lancet 1:551, 1976.
117. Kissmeyer-Nielsen F, Ehlers N: Corneal transplantation and matching for HLA-A and B. Scand J Urol Nephrol 42(Suppl):44, 1977.
118. Foulks GN, Sanfilippo FP, Locascio JA, et al: Histocompatibility testing for keratoplasty in high-risk patients. Ophthalmology 90:239, 1983.
119. Stark WJ, Taylor HR, Datiles M, et al: Transplantation antigens and keratoplasty. Aust J Ophthalmol 11:333, 1983.
120. Sanfilippo F, MacQueen JM, Vaughn WK, et al: Reduced graft rejection with good HLA-A and -B matching in high-risk corneal transplantation. N Engl J Med 315:29, 1986.
121. Boisjoly HM, Bernard P-M, et al: Association between corneal allograft reactions and HLA compatibility. Ophthalmology 97:1689, 1990.
122. Stark W, Stulting D, Maguire M, et al: The Collaborative Corneal Transplantation Studies (CCTS): Effectiveness of histocompatibility matching of donors and recipients in high risk corneal transplantation. Arch Ophthalmol 110:1392–1403, 1992.
123. Gore SM, Vail A, Bradley BA, et al: HLA-DR matching in corneal transplantation. Transplantation 60:1033–1039, 1995.
124. Sonoda Y, Streilein JW: Impaired cell mediated immunity in mice bearing healthy orthotopic corneal allografts. J Immunol 150:1727–1734, 1993.
125. Sonoda Y, Sano Y, Ksander B, et al: Characterization of cell mediated immune responses elicited by orthotopic corneal allografts in mice. Invest Ophthalmol Vis Sci 36:427–434, 1995.
126. Sano Y, Ksander BR, Streilein JW: Murine orthotopic corneal transplantation in "high-risk" eyes: Rejection is dictated primarily by weak rather than strong alloantigens. Invest Ophthalmol Vis Sci 38:1130–1138, 1991.
127. Wilson SE, Lloyd SA: Epidermal growth factor and its receptor, basic fibroblast growth factor, transforming growth factor beta-1, and interleukin 1 alpha messenger RNA production in human corneal endothelial cells. Invest Ophthalmol Vis Sci 32:2747–2756, 1991.
128. Kawashima H, Prasad SA, Gregerson DS: Corneal endothelial cells inhibit T cell proliferation by blocking IL-2 production. J Immunol 153:1982–1989, 1994.
129. Kennedy MC, Rosenbaum JT, Brown J: Novel production of interleukin-1 receptor antagonist peptides in normal human cornea. J Clin Invest 95:82–88, 1995.
130. Bora NS, Gobleman CL, Atkinson JP: Differential expression of the complement regulatory proteins in the human eye. Invest Ophthalmol Vis Sci 34:3579–3584, 1993.
131. Mohan RR, Liang Q, Kim W-J, et al: Apoptosis in the cornea: Further characterization of Fas/Fas ligand system. Exp Eye Res 65:575–589, 1997.
132. Yamada J, Streilein JW: Induction of anterior chamber-associated immune deviation by corneal allografts placed in the anterior chamber. Invest Ophthalmol Vis Sci 38(13):2833–2843, 1997.
133. Sano Y, Ksander BR, Streilein JW: Fate of orthotopic corneal allografts in eyes that cannot support ACAID induction. Invest Ophthalmol Vis Sci 36:2176–2185, 1995.
134. Dana M-R, Yamada J, Streilein JW: Topical IL-1 receptor antagonist promotes corneal transplant survival. Transplantation 63:1501–1507, 1997.

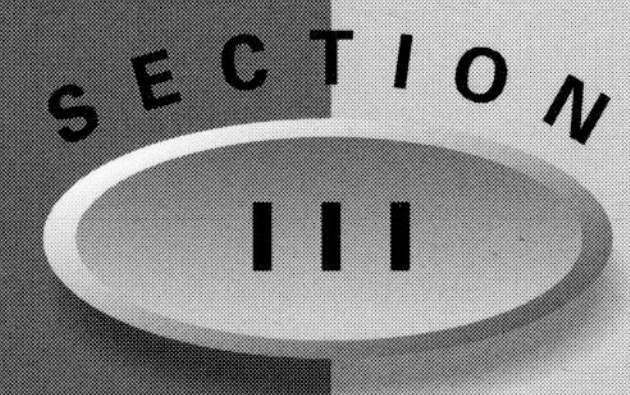

Microbiology

Edited by

DEBORAH PAVAN LANGSTON

CHAPTER 11

Ocular Bacteriology

R. Wayne Bowman and James P. McCulley

Bacterial infections comprise a complex and constantly changing group of ocular diseases. Various bacteriologic processes involve the eye and periocular structures, from something as simple as colonization of the skin and lashes alone without invasive disease to necrotizing bacterial keratitis. The site of infection may be the periocular skin or lid or an anaerobic environment such as the canalicular system or the capsular bag. The source of bacteria may be local (i.e., from the lids and lashes), or it may be from a remote site (as in metastatic endophthalmitis) or from the nasopharynx or sinuses. In recent years, significant advances in our understanding of the mechanisms of bacterial diseases have been made. Bacterial antibiotic resistance has been on the increase, and newer antibiotics that are more specific in their coverage have become available. We are constantly understanding more and more about the host-bacterial interaction, its effect on bacterial virulence and pathogenicity, and the resultant therapeutic implications. The method of identifying bacteria is gradually shifting away from traditional staining and culture techniques to newer automated or rapid-identification techniques. New patterns of infection, such as crystalline keratopathy, have become evident; new pathogens, such as *Acanthamoeba*, have been discovered. The ability to diagnose and treat infections correctly is critical. One might ask, "What should I know that will help me in the management of my patient with a bacterial infection?" In this chapter, we attempt to give the reader the basis for understanding this ever-changing field.

Anatomy, Physiology, and Life Cycle

Bacteria belong to the kingdom Protista, which encompasses fungi, protozoa, and algae as well. The more complex eukaryotic organisms are the fungi, protozoa, and algae; the simpler procaryotic organisms are the bacteria. The taxonomy of the bacteria is extensive, having undergone frequent revisions in the past but now requiring the approval of an official international body.[1] With newer techniques such as deoxyribonucleic acid (DNA) typing and sequencing, the heterogeneity of bacteria within their various groups becomes more apparent. The determination of DNA composition by identifying the G + C (the amino acids guanine, G, and cytosine, C) content of DNA has shown that the whole phylum of vertebrates ranges only from 36 to 44% G + C, whereas bacteria range from 25 to 75%. For example, in the genera *Staphylococcus* and *Micrococcus*, which are in the family Micrococcaceae, the former has 30 to 40% G + C, whereas the latter has 65 to 75% G + C.[2, 3] Such a variation in DNA sequencing among bacteria is now being used clinically to develop rapid diagnostic systems.

The most practical method of classifying bacteria still depends on their gram-staining properties and their cell morphology. Also important, however, are their fermentation products, their ability to metabolize various substrates, their sensitivity to different antibiotics, and their colonial morphology. Bacteria lack any nuclear or mitotic apparatus; their DNA is organized into a single, naked, circular chromosome. The structure of bacterial cells is termed prokaryotic; whereas those with a membrane-bounded nucleus are called eukaryotic. Owing to their small size, there is a limit to the number of molecules that can be present in the cell at any given time. Prokaryotic cells have come to regulate these syntheses by induction, regression, or end product inhibition to produce only what is required for metabolism or growth in a particular environment.[4] Cellular components that must be present all the time are not subject to underaction or suppression and their synthesis is called constitutive.[4]

Phospholipids and proteins make up the bacterial cell membrane, and in contrast to eukaryotic cells, bacterial cell walls (except for those of mycoplasmas) do not contain sterols. Because prokaryotic cells lack both mitochondria and an endoplasmic reticulum, electron transport systems are located in the cell wall itself.

The cell wall or cell envelope plays an important role in many bacterial cell functions. Besides containing the electron transport systems, the envelope also serves as an osmotic barrier and regulates the transport of solutes. Thus, the cell wall protects the cell against rupture from the high internal osmotic pressure. In hypertonic environments, bacteria may survive as spheroplasts, or L forms, without their rigid cell wall, but as a result they may lose their pathogenicity. A macromolecule unique to the cell wall of many bacteria is the peptidoglycan (PG). This component of the cell wall is responsible for shape definition and maintenance.[4]

The cell wall is the site of many antigenic determinants of the various bacteria. Moreover, when endotoxin is present, it is located in the cell wall. The cell envelope of gram-positive bacteria has only a thick (15- to 80-nm) PG layer surrounded by a polysaccharide capsule. PG is a cross-linked heteropolymer of amino acids and amino sugars that consists of approximately 50% of the cell wall by weight.[5] Teichoic acid (TA) is a negatively charged ribitol-phosphate polymer that attaches to PG by covalent bonds, accounting for 40% of the cell wall.[2] Another cell wall protein, protein A (SPA), comprises 5% of the cell wall mass.[2] The cell envelope of gram-negative bacteria is more complex than that of gram-positive bacteria. Although the PG layer is thinner (only 1 to 2 nm), there is a phospholipid outer membrane that forms a protective barrier, making gram-negative bacteria more resistant to hydrolytic enzymes and toxic substances. Membrane proteins that are present in the outer membrane serve to regulate transport through transmembrane prefixing, or porins, and are in part responsible for gram-negative bacterial antibiotic resistance. The number and diameter of the porin channels vary among different gram-negative species, which helps explain some of their intrinsic differences in antibiotic susceptibility.[6] Gram-negative bacteria possess a periplasma between the inner and outer walls of the cell membrane. The periplasma contains at least 50 different properties. Important among these may be β-lactamase and aminoglycoside phosphorylase that function to inactivate certain antibiotics.[4] Also found in the outer membrane of gram-negative bacteria is endotoxin, composed of lipopolysaccharide (LPS). It is endotoxin that confers virulence and species specificity. Variability of this surface polysaccharide allows serologic differentiation of bacterial isolates. The lipid A portion is mainly responsible for toxicity.[7] Mycoplasmas lack a rigid cell wall, and agents such as *Treponema, Borrelia,* and *Leptospira* have flexible thin walls.

The outer capsule that encloses many bacteria can be well organized, as in *pneumoniae*, or it can consist of a diffuse layer known as the slime layer, as in *Staphylococcus epidermidis*. This outer layer can prevent phagocytosis and aids in the adherence of bacteria to tissues and to artificial devices such as prostheses, catheters,[8] and intraocular lenses. Several species of bacteria have a capsule with a chemical structure that mimics host tissue, thus camouflaging the organism from the host's immune system.[9] The capsules of *Neisseria meningitidis* group B and the capsule of *Escherichia coli* are the two best known examples. Bacterial flagella allow bacteria to swim through liquid and move over solid surfaces (aprocytophaga exhibits gliding motility that may contribute to its potential to produce infections in immunocompromised patients).

Fimbriae also aid in bacterial adherence to tissues.[10] Shorter and more hairlike than the longer flagella that provide bacteria mobility, the fimbriae function as adhesins, mediating adhesion to specific surfaces. This is important in pathogenesis, especially for gonococcus and *E. coli*. In *N. gonorrhoeae*, at least two surface components have been identified aiding in attachment to genitourinary cells. These components are protein II and type-specific pili. Piliated strains attach much better than nonpiliated strains. New data show that in *E. coli* type 1 fimbriae potentiate the uptake of nutrients from and the delivery of toxins to eukaryotic cells.[11] Bacteria can shift rapidly between a form that possesses fimbriae and one that does not. Although the fimbriae help bacteria initially to establish colonization in a host, they also increase the bacteria's susceptibility to phagocytosis. Loss of the fimbriae after adherence may therefore aid in tissue invasion. Different types of fimbriae vary in specificity for the host glycoprotein receptor to which they attach. *S. pyogenes* also possess a nonfibrillar adhesin, protein F, which mediates attachment of the bacteria to fibronectin. Most adhesins are lectins and have a high affinity for binding to specific carbohydrates.

Biofilm is a nonspecific bacterial adhesin. Sometimes called glycocalyx, biofilm is an adhesive polymer containing a polysaccharide. This biofilm is potentially important in ophthalmology, because it prevents skin antisepsis. Even after a vigorous skin preparation, *S. epidermidis* cells can be seen embedded in keratin crypts surrounded by this biofilm. Biofilm may also play a role in staphylococcal adherence to plastic polymers such as intraocular and contact lenses. Streptococci appear to use biofilms to strengthen their adherence to mucosal surfaces.

The cytoplasm of bacteria contains ribosomes, or bodies of ribonucleic acid (RNA), and the chromosome that is a single closed loop. Smaller molecules of DNA known as plasmids are significant, because they may carry information for drug resistance or they may code for toxins that can affect human cellular functions.

Bacteria reproduce by an asexual process called binary fission. Cell division begins with an ingrowth of the cytoplasmic membrane, which eventually produces a complete cross-wall. Differences in cross-wall formation and cleavage account for the bacterial shape and arrangement. Incomplete cleavage results in bacterial chains. Streptococci form long chains by producing parallel cross-walls, whereas staphylococci form clumps by beginning each new septum perpendicular to the preceding one.[12]

Although much remains to be discovered about the growth of the individual bacterial organisms, we do know that bacterial growth depends on DNA synthesis controlled by RNA and that it depends on messenger RNA. Under unbalanced or adverse conditions such as are frequently present in the body, DNA synthesis can occur in the absence of RNA once the growth cycle has already begun. Typically, at least in the laboratory, the bacterial growth cycle has four phases: the lag phase, the logarithmic growth phase, the stationary growth phase, and a decline phase. Bacteria vary in their temperature requirements for growth and can be divided into three categories according to the temperature at which their growth or generation time is optimal. Psychrophiles grow best at a temperature of 0°C to 20.5°C; mesophiles thrive from 20°C to 40°C; and thermophiles multiply best at higher temperatures of 40°C to 90°C. Most bacteria are mesophiles; some important mesophiles can grow at temperatures below their normal range. Staphylococci grow slowly at 5°C and may contaminate donor corneas in preservative media or nonpreserved drops stored in the refrigerator. Because antibiotics may not inhibit the their growth at these low temperatures, it is recommended that corneal tissue and its storage media be allowed to come to room temperature before transplantation. Streptococci and *Proteus vulgaris* also possess the ability for psychrophilic growth.[13]

Iron is an essential nutrient for bacteria. In the human body, transferrin in the blood and lactoferrin in external secretions bind most of the iron.[14] Lactoferrin is able to bind iron even under the more acidic conditions that are present at sites of infection.[15] Organisms unable to obtain iron in vivo will not proliferate, but it is clear that pathogens can circumvent this problem. For example, the *Neisseria* species possess a major iron-regulated protein (MIRP) to help the pathogen in iron acquisition and subsequent pathogenicity.[16] Other organisms such as *Branhamella catarrhalis* possess iron-acquisition proteins that aid in virulence.[17] Iron availability may influence the nature of the disease and whether it stays in one place or disseminates; it may also determine whether the disease is extracellular or intracellular and the site of pathogenicity. Owing to its avascularity, the eye is iron deficient, and this may aid in its resistance to bacteria.[18] Bacteria undergo phenotypic changes in metabolism and outer membrane proteins that enable them to acquire iron. *N. meningitidis* becomes more virulent after growth in iron-restricted conditions at low pH.[19] Under conditions of iron-restricted growth, pathogenic bacteria appear to produce exotoxins.[20] These exotoxins include toxin A, elastase, alkaline phosphatase protease, and hemagglutinin from *Pseudomonas aeruginosa*, α-toxin from *Clostridium perfringens*, and β-toxin from *Serratia marcescens*.[21] Bacteria can break down almost any organic compound into usable components. For example, some *Pseudomonas* species can grow on camphor and naphthalene, and this may explain the propensity of *Pseudomonas* for growing in make-up.[22]

Classification of Common Ocular Bacteria

Identification of bacteria is a time-consuming and laborious task and not without controversy and debate. After a pure bacterial culture has been isolated and undergone a Gram stain, the bacterium is further identified as to genus and species by the results of various physiologic and biochemical tests. Commercially available kits are being used more and more, especially in nonreference laboratories for the rapid identification of bacteria; there are those who question the accuracy and cost of such methods. *Bergey's Manual* is the definite taxonomy source but cannot keep up with changes between its publication each decade. A list of all validated names is available on the internet at http://www.bdt.org.br/bdt/bacterianame/info. Recent developments have seen a shift from conventional phenotypic identification methods to modern molecular techniques.[23]

Conventional dehydration methods utilize morphology, cultured appearances, requirements for growth, metabolism and biochemical activities, and susceptibility to physical and chemical agents.

GRAM-POSITIVE COCCI

Staphylococci

Staphylococci belong to the family Micrococcaceae, which encompasses two genera: *Staphylococcus* and *Micrococcus*. The species in the genus *Staphylococcus* are divided into those that are coagulase-positive and those that are coagulase-negative.[24] Coagulase-positive staphylococci include *S. aureus, S. intermedius,* and *S. hyicus*.[25] At least 17 species of coagulase-negative staphylococci have been identified.[26] The best-known member of this family and the most common bacterium cultured from the eyelids and conjunctiva is *S. epidermidis*.[27] The absence of coagulase should not be equated with lack of virulence, because members of this group (e.g., *S. haemolyticus*) can have pathogenic potential.[28]

Both coagulase-positive and -negative staphylococci are responsible for various ocular diseases. That staphylococci are the organisms responsible for infection in some conditions such as dacryocystitis, keratitis, and endophthalmitis is obvious, but their role in blepharitis, marginal keratitis, and phlyctenulosis is more complex. McCulley and Dougherty have shown that blepharitis can be divided into several distinct clinical forms and that coagulase-negative staphylococci (CNS), as well as *S. aureus*, are important in the production of staphylococcal blepharitis and seborrheic blepharitis with a staphylococcal component.[29–31] Meibomian gland secretions from patients with meibomian gland involvement have an abnormality in the free fatty acid component that may be mediated by the normal ocular flora. Assays of the most common bacterial lid flora in normal subjects and patients with chronic blepharitis have shown that strains of coagulase-negative staphylococci isolated from patients with a meibomian gland abnormality more frequently produced both a fatty wax esterase and a cholesterol esterase.[32] These findings point out the important relationship among indigenous flora, environmental factors (e.g., temperature and pH), and bacterial virulence factors and exoenzyme production.

Streptococci

The genus belongs to the family Streptococcaceae. Species are classified according to the presence of certain surface antigenic and physiologic characteristics.[33] Important ophthalmic pathogens in this group include *S. pneumoniae* (formerly diplococcus), which is part of the respiratory flora, and β-hemolytic streptococci, group D (enterococci), which are part of the enteric flora. Streptococci can be classified based on the type of hemolysis produced on blood agar. *S. pneumoniae* is an α-hemolytic streptococcus (*Streptococcus viridans*) that can be separated from other viridans streptococci by its susceptibility to optochin and by its solubility in bile. Differentiation of the species and the sensitivity to various antibiotics have become crucial as α-streptococci have been found to be resistant to aminoglycoside and polymyxin B and they are becoming increasingly so to penicillin. A type of nutritionally deficient streptococci have recently been described: They require pyridoxine for growth and as a result will not grow on blood agar or in broth without the addition of pyridoxine. Nutritionally deficient streptococci are a known cause of endocarditis and can invade the eye as well, producing infectious crystalline keratitis.[34] Crystalline keratitis has also emerged as a new pattern of infection with other streptococci but also occurs with other bacteria such as *Pseudomonas* and coagulase-negative staphylococci.[35]

GRAM-NEGATIVE COCCI

Neisseriaceae

The family Neisseriaceae includes the genera *Neisseria, Branhamella, Moraxella, Kingella*, and *Acinetobacter*, all of which are potential ocular pathogens. The organisms are either diplococci or short bacilli. Their laboratory diagnosis is based on sugar fermentation reactions or serologic techniques.[36] All members of the Neisseriaceae are oxidase- and catalase-positive (except for *Acinetobacter*, which is oxidase-negative). *Neisseria* species and approximately 50% of *Acinetobacter* species ferment glucose. The differentiation of *Neisseria* from *Branhamella* can be difficult. *Branhamella* will typically grow on blood agar but not on Thayer-Martin medium, and it does not ferment glucose, dextrose, maltose, or lactose. Although the Centers for Disease Control and Prevention (CDC) recommend that all *Neisseria* isolates be tested for β-lactamase production,[37] testing is especially important for *Branhamella,* because up to 75% or more of *Branhamella* isolates produce β-lactamase.[38–40] *Acinetobacter* species are commensal organisms of the upper respiratory tract, skin, and genitourinary tract.[41] A negative oxidase test result will readily differentiate *Acinetobacter* from *Neisseria. Acinetobacter* species are frequently resistant to antibiotics, and treatment should consist of a combination of an enhanced-spectrum penicillin (e.g., carbenicillin) and an aminoglycoside.[42]

Moraxella species are either bacillary or coccobacilli, forming either pairs or short chains of pairs in smears. Presumptive identification in smears can usually be made owing to the large size and end-to-end configuration of *Moraxella* organisms, although they may appear to be gram-positive on thick smears. *Moraxella* species grow on MacConkey agar and do not ferment carbohydrates. All species are susceptible to penicillin. *Kingella* species were formerly classified as *Moraxella* and, like *Moraxella,* they can be the cause of angular blepharitis.[43] Both *Moraxella* and *Kingella* species can be confused with *N. gonorrhoeae,* and both are sensitive to penicillin, erythromycin, chloramphenicol, and gentamicin.[44]

GRAM-NEGATIVE BACILLI

Enterobacteriaceae

The family Enterobacteriaceae comprises at least 27 genera and 7 enteric groups, with more than 110 species.[45] Members of this family are either motile with peritrichous flagella or nonmotile, and they do not form spores. All members grow both aerobically and facultatively anaerobically. The Enterobacteriaceae ferment glucose, reduce nitrates to nitrites, and are oxidase-negative. They also lack cytochrome oxidase activity. Important genera include *Escherichia, Shigella, Salmonella, Klebsiella, Enterobacter, Serratia,* tribe Proteae (*Proteus, Morganella,* and *Providencia*), and *Yersinia.*

Escherichia coli association has rarely caused endogenous endophthalmitis following septicemia.[46] However, *E. coli* can acquire and transmit multiple antibiotic-resistant plasmids. *Serratia* was once considered to include a nonpathogen and was used to study air currents by being released from air balloons and blown through hospital ventilation systems.[47] Today, we know that *Serratia* causes a number of ocular infections, some of which are resistant to gentamicin.[48]

Members of the tribe Proteae, especially *Proteus mirabilis,* can produce ocular disease and are typically resistant to polymyxins and tetracycline.[49] On blood agar, *P. mirabilis* produces gray, swarming colonies that are oxidase- and indole-negative. *Yersinia pestis* causes bubonic plague, which had a devastating effect on Western civilization in the 14th century. Although now it is not commonly associated with ocular disease, *Yersinia* species have been cultured from patients with Parinaud's oculoglandular syndrome.[50]

Vibrionaceae

Members of the family Vibrionaceae are non–spore-forming gram-negative bacilli that are oxidase-positive. They move by means of a polar flagellum and are capable of aerobic or anaerobic growth. Although they are rarely found to be the cause of ocular disease, three genera, *Vibrio, Aeromonas,* and *Plesiomonas,* do sometimes cause endophthalmitis.[51, 52]

Pseudomonadaceae

The genus *Pseudomonas* comprises ubiquitous gram-negative bacilli. The presence of cytochrome oxidase distinguishes them from the Enterobacteriaceae. A polar flagella may be present. The growth requirements of *Pseudomonas* are simple: They can use a variety of compounds for nutrition, and some strains can even grow in distilled water. This may explain the incidence of *Pseudomonas* infections associated with homemade saline solution and soft contact lenses and inadequately sterilized intraocular lenses. *Pseudomonas* species are hemolytic on blood agar within 48 hours, which is unusual for gram-negative bacteria.[53] Capable of producing a rapidly progressive and destructive disease, members of *Pseudomonas* are especially virulent in patients with human immunodeficiency virus (HIV) infection.[54]

Pasteurellaceae

The bacteria of the family Pasteurellaceae are small non–spore-forming gram-negative bacilli. They are nonmotile and either aerobic or facultative anaerobic. Most are fastidious, requiring enriched media in the laboratory. The family has three genera: *Haemophilus, Actinobacillus,* and *Pasteurella. Haemophilus* species are the most common pathogens. They require hemin (X factor) and nicotinamide-adenine dinucleotide (NAD). The cell wall of *Haemophilus* is typical for a gram-negative bacterium showing endotoxic activity. Many *H. influenzae* possess a polysaccharide capsule and can be divided into serotypes based on the capsular reaction.

Many other species of the Pasteurellaceae can produce ocular disease, and they can be differentiated on the basis of their individual requirements for hemin and NAD. A variety of tests including indole production, urease activity, ornithine decarboxylase reactivity, and carbohydrate fermentation of glucose, sucrose, and lactose can also be used.[55] In clinical practice, species identification is not as important as the presence of β-lactamase production.[56] *Haemophilus ducreyi,* the cause of granuloma inguinale, is emerging as a major risk factor for acquisition of HIV-1 after heterosexual intercourse.[57] Erythromycin has proved to be extremely effective, whereas ceftriaxone and trimethoprim-sulfamethoxazole are effective alternatives.[58]

Actinobacillus species require carbon dioxide for growth. The only known pathogen of the genus is *A. actinomycetemcomitans,* which can cause endophthalmitis.[59] *Pasteurella* infections, which are usually transmitted through contact with animals that are carrying the bacilli, can cause conjunctivitis, corneal ulceration, and endophthalmitis.[60]

MISCELLANEOUS GRAM-NEGATIVE BACTERIA

Eikenella corrodens is a normal inhabitant of the human mouth and upper respiratory tract. It can cause infection following a human bite, and it can be the culprit in an opportunistic disease. *Eikenella* species are non–spore-forming, facultatively anaerobic, moderately sized, gram-negative bacilli. These bacteria grow slowly on common media with CO_2, and about half of the isolates form distinctive pits on the agar. Certain strains are mobile on moist surfaces and produce an endotoxin. *Eikenella corrodens* is susceptible to penicillin and ampicillin but resistant to aminoglycosides, first-generation cephalosporins, penicillinase-resistant penicillins, and clindamycin.[61] Another common member of the oral flora, *Capnocytophaga*, has been documented as the cause of a chronic corneal infection in a patient with HIV infection.[62, 63]

Although Debre first recognized cat-scratch disease in 1931, his findings were not reported until 1950.[64] And it was as recently as 1983 that the causative organism of cat-scratch disease, a delicate pleomorphic gram-negative bacillus, was identified.[65, 66] Ocular involvement typically takes the form of Parinaud's oculoglandular syndrome with a conjunctival granuloma at the inoculation site. Cat-scratch bacilli have been identified in conjunctival granulomas.[67] Treatment of cat-scratch disease is usually supportive with spontaneous resolution over 2 to 4 months. Oral cyprofloxicillin may speed resolution of the disease. When administered intravenously, trimethoprim-sulfamethoxazole may be effective in life-threatening cases.[68] The differential diagnosis of Parinaud's oculoglandular syndrome is quite long, including a number of bacterial and viral infections. Martin and associates have reviewed many of these possibilities.[69]

ANAEROBIC GRAM-NEGATIVE BACILLI

Anaerobic gram-negative bacilli are a group of non–spore-forming bacteria that comprises part of the normal anaerobic oral and intestinal flora. *Bacteroides fragilis* is the most commonly isolated organism. Unlike most anaerobes, *B. fragilis* is resistant to many antibiotics, including penicillin. Cuchural reviewed the antibiotic sensitivities of a number of strains of *B. fragilis*.[70] Resistance rates to imipenem and ticarcillin-clavulanic acid were 0.2 and 1.7%, respectively. No isolates were resistant to either metronidazole or chloramphenicol. The rate of resistance to clindamycin was 5% and to cefoxitin 11%.

GRAM-POSITIVE BACILLI

Gram-positive bacilli are comparatively large spore-forming bacilli that grow on nonselective media producing nonhemolytic rapidly growing colonies. They are ubiquitous and have been known to cause a severe endophthalmitis after trauma has occurred.[71] *Bacillus cereus* is the most common pathogen. Vancomycin, clindamycin, and the aminoglycosides are usually the drugs of choice.[72, 73]

The most important of the non–spore-forming gram-positive bacilli are the genera *Corynebacterium* and *Propionibacterium*. The organisms are small, nonmotile, and catalase-positive, and they ferment carbohydrates producing lactic acid (*Corynebacterium*) or propionic acid (*Propionibacterium*). *Propionibacterium* species are anaerobic and are a common isolate from the eyelid and the conjunctiva.[74] *P. acnes* is emerging as an important cause of indolent endophthalmitis.[75]

Anaerobic, gram-positive bacilli that are spore-forming belong to the genus *Clostridium*. They can cause several serious diseases, including botulism and tetanus. In addition, *C. difficile* causes pseudomembranous colitis.[76]

Listeria species are short, gram-positive, facultatively anaerobic (but not strictly) bacilli and they exhibit characteristic tumbling motility in suspension or in a hanging drop. *L. monocytogenes*, the most common species, is catalase–, methyl red–, and Voges-Proskauer–positive; it hydrolyzes esculin but does not produce hydrogen sulfide or reduce nitrite. *Listeria* species are known ocular pathogens. Zaidman and coworkers developed a rabbit model of *L. monocytogenes* infection and concluded that the best treatment is a combination of penicillin and gentamicin.[77]

Actinomyces and *Nocardia*

Actinomyces species are facultative anaerobic or strict anaerobic gram-positive bacilli that are usually arranged in hyphae but can fragment into short bacilli. *A. israelii*, the most common opportunistic species, grows on blood agar enriched with vitamin K. The organisms can cause a chronic canaliculitis. Penicillin remains the most effective treatment. Similar in appearance to *Actinomyces* and almost indistinguishable on Gram's stains is the genus *Nocardia*. *Nocardia* species are strict aerobic bacilli that are gram-positive, yet they may appear to be gram-negative with intracellular gram-positive beads. They have a cell wall similar to that of mycobacteria and are acid-fast with weak acids, which helps to distinguish them from *Actinomyces* species. Members of the *Nocardia* are catalase-positive and grow on nonselective media. Ocular infections usually consist of an indolent keratitis or an endophthalmitis.[78–81]

MYCOBACTERIA

Mycobacterium tuberculosis and *M. leprae* remain two of the most prevalent and serious causes of infections worldwide. They are acid-fast, although *M. leprae* is more sensitive to decolorization. The growth of these nonmotile slender rods is slow, with some species taking 2 to 6 weeks, although growth of fast-growing species can occur in 3 to 5 days. Runyon classified mycobacteria into four groups based on their rate of growth and chromogenicity. In ophthalmology, it is probably more practical to divide mycobacteria into two groups: *M. tuberculosis* and atypical mycobacteria. Atypical mycobacteria (especially *M. fortuitum* and *M. chelonei*) are usually resistant to standard antituberculous drugs. Topical amikacin has been effective in the treatment of corneal ulcers. Ciprofloxacin, erythromycin, cefoxitin, doxycycline, or the sulfonamides may be alternative choices.[82] The occurrence of *M. avium* infection is increasing, particularly in those infected with HIV, and it has been found to cause a metastatic endophthalmitis in at least one individual.[83]

MOLLICUTES

Mollicutes are a class of microorganisms bounded only by a membrane. The two most important genera are *Mycoplasma* and *Ureaplasma*. Mycoplasmas resemble chlamydiae, rickettsiae, and viruses in passing through 450-nm filters but, like bacteria, they are gram-negative, able to grow on artificial media, and capable of dividing by binary fission. Three pathogen strains have been identified: *M. pneumoniae*, *M.*

hominis, and *Ureaplasma urealyticum*. They can be differentiated by their ability to metabolize glucose (*M. pneumoniae*), arginine (*M. hominis*), or urea (*U. urealyticum*). Low birth weight infants frequently culture positive for *U. urealyticum*, a cause of nongonococcal urethritis.[84] Erythromycin and tetracycline are usually effective, although *M. hominis* is resistant to erythromycin.[85] Mollicute-like organisms (MLO) are found in chronic uveitis, especially gastrointestinal tract–associated disease.[86] Cell wall–deficient bacteria are also thought to play a role in cancer.[87] Some researchers have isolated cell wall–deficient bacteria from the blood and tumors of humans and animals with cancer. Furthermore, cancer can be induced by injecting these organisms into experimental animals.

Infection of the Host

Bacteria produce a variety of ocular diseases. Bacterial conjunctivitis and bacterial keratitis are commonly seen. Endophthalmitis presents a challenging clinical problem. Blepharitis in its various forms may constitute an imbalance in the normal relationship between bacteria and the skin of the eyelid. The exact roles of coagulase-negative staphylococci and their toxin production and of *Propionibacterium acnes* in meibomian gland dysfunction continue to be studied and defined. Infections of the periocular tissue include canaliculitis, dacryocystitis, and preseptal and orbital cellulitis. Bacteria also can have remote effects such as syphilitic interstitial keratitis and mycobacterial phlyctenulosis to possibly triggering HLA-B27 acute anterior uveitis.[88]

The virulence of a pathogenic organism depends on its potential to produce disease. One important factor is its ability to adhere to mucosal surfaces and to enter epithelial cells. Invasive properties are carried in various ways from plasmids to DNA segments in the bacterial chromosome.[89] These properties can be exchanged between bacteria, rendering noninvasive bacteria invasive. In addition to the virulence and invasiveness of an organism, the number of bacteria entering the host and their site of entry also determine the nature of an ocular infection. Finally, certain extracellular enzymes may be important in the establishment of infection and its spread throughout tissues. These enzymes include collagenase. Characteristics of bacteria important in ocular infections include virulence of the organism, the invasiveness of the organism, the number of organisms entering the host, and their site of entry. Certain extracellular enzymes may be important in the establishment of infection and in its spread through tissues. These include collagenase (*C. perfringens*), coagulase (staphylococci), hyaluronidases (staphylococci, streptococci, clostridia, pneumococci), streptokinase or fibrinolysis (hemolytic streptococci), hemolysins and leukocidins (streptococci, staphylococci, clostridia, gram-negative rods), and proteases (neisseriae, streptococci) that can hydrolyze immunoglobulins, such as secretory IgA.[90] In blepharitis, staphylococci and *P. acnes* produce lipases and esterases.

The host determines the effect of many virulence factors.[91] That is, certain characteristics of the host can influence the development of disease. For example, the host's age, use of drugs, and sexual habits can all determine the effect of virulence factors. The use of contact lenses or surgical trauma increase the risk of ophthalmic disease. Blepharitis, dry eye states, canaliculitis, chronic nasolacrimal duct obstruction, and previous ocular disease also increase the risk. Damaged epithelium in the cornea is particularly susceptible to bacterial adherence; bacteria adhere to the epithelial edge rather than the bare stroma.[92] Tissue injury results from the direct action of the bacteria, from microbial toxins, from indirect injury, from inflammation, or from immunopathologic processes. In response to an injury, polymorphonuclear cells, as well as macrophages and lymphocytes, enter the site. Tissue fluids provide plasma proteins, including immunoglobulins such as IgG, complement, and properdin. The primary mediators of inflammation include histamine, 5-hydroxytryptamine, and kinins.[93] Prostaglandins E and F seem to play a role in the termination of the response. The phagocytic cells play a key role in the interaction with the microorganism, ingesting and killing bacteria. Among the chemoattractant factors for phagocytosis are platelet-activating factor, leukotriene B4, C5a, and certain formyl peptides.[94]

ADHERENCE, COLONIZATION, AND INVASION

Cellular microbiology is a rapidly developing field that deals with the interaction of bacteria and their host cells. Epithelial cells with their tight cellular junctions act as a barrier to bacterial adherence, penetration, and the entry of soluble toxins. Epithelial cells may respond to bacterial adherence by secreting cytokines, causing a major cytoskeletal rearrangement and playing a major role in the mucosal immune response. However, the relationship between the host and the potential pathogen is complex and still incompletely understood regarding why some bacteria are invasive and others colonize the cell surface. Some produce exotoxins that destroy host cell functions, whereas others utilize the host cell to advance their pathogenic potential.[95] Pathogens cross-talk by sending molecular signals.[96]

Microbial adhesion to host tissue is a primary event in colonization and an important stage in microbial pathogenesis.[97] Adhesive ligands in bacteria range from rodlike structures (pili or fimbriae) to outer membrane proteins and polysaccharides. Individual bacteria may possess multiple adhesins that target distinct host cell molecules and deliver diverse signals resulting in extracellular location or internalization. Both the nature and the density of the target receptor on the host cell may be determining factors in the outcome of the bacteria-host interaction.[97]

The invasion of mucosal surfaces and ocular tissues by bacteria occurs in several steps. First, bacteria must establish themselves in close proximity to the ocular surfaces, such as the lids and lashes. This, by the way, is why the cleansing and isolation of these surfaces is so critical in ocular surgery. Second, the bacteria must avoid being swept away, which is one of several reasons why patients with severely dry eyes are at increased risk of infection. Next, bacteria must acquire essential nutrients for growth, especially iron, and be able to replicate at a rate sufficient to maintain or expand their population. Finally, the bacteria must resist local host defenses.[98] Before adherence can occur, association, that is, localization of bacteria on a surface must take place.[99] Motility of bacteria may enhance association.[100] Bacteria may associate with mucus or exudates, forming noncovalent bonds. Chemotaxis may help bacteria to penetrate the mucous barrier, thus enhancing contact with receptors on the epithelial surface.[101]

Bacterial attachment is essential in order for colonization to occur in environments with a surface exposed to a fluid flow.[102] Adhesion of bacteria to the epithelial surface depends upon adhesins, complex polymers on the bacterial surface. The attachment of *S. pneumoniae* to epithelial cells can result from a specific interaction between bacterial proteins and epithelial cell glycoconjugates.[103] The presence of fimbriae assist in bacterial adhesiveness.[104] These are frequently present on gram-negative organisms.[105–107] A variety of bacteria produce adhesins that tend to be outer membrane proteins. Outer membrane proteins, as well as fimbriae, aid in adhesion of *N. gonorrhoeae* to epithelial cells.[108, 109] Staphylococci and streptococci can adhere to epithelial cells and thus colonize skin and mucous membranes.[110] Their adherence to epithelial surfaces was once thought to relate to the presence of M protein.[111, 112] However, studies by Beachey and Ofek[113] subsequently demonstrated that cell wall lipoteichoic acid (LTA) was the critical element in binding of *S. pyogenes*. Furthermore, elimination of LTA-mediated binding by deacylation indicates that fatty acids on the LTA molecule are the essential components.[114] *S. aureus* produces a surface protein with specific affinity for fibronectin.[115] Numerous studies have shown that a variety of streptococci and staphylococci species can bind fibronectin, probably through affinity with their cell wall LTA.[116–119] The presence of fibronectin on the cell surface appears to enhance bacterial adhesion as well.[120] LTA can interfere with the killing of phagocytes by polymorphonuclear leukocytes.[121, 122] Some isolates of *S. epidermidis* can inhibit the bacterial activity of neutrophils, independent of adherence. This inhibition of neutrophils may represent another virulence factor.[123]

Adherence of *Pseudomonas aeruginosa* to the corneal epithelium may be the first step in the pathogenesis of infection.[124–126] *Pseudomonas* adheres to the basal epithelial cells through the interaction of a specific adhesion-receptor. In order for bacterial adherence to occur, several steps must take place. First, van der Waals forces produced by surface molecules overcome the normal repulsive forces of two similarly charged cells.[127] Then, once the cells become close enough, hydrophobic binding holds the bacteria to the surface, and strong bonds form between the exopolysaccharides of the bacteria and the substrate glycoprotein of the target cell. The significant differential adherence between basal and nonbasal corneal epithelial cells is probably the reason why superficial trauma or epithelial cell damage allows pseudomonal infections to develop.[128] This may play a significant role in contact lens–associated pseudomonal keratitis. Using a rabbit model, Koch and associates showed that a bacterial suspension of *P. aeruginosa* alone caused no inflammation but that corneal infection developed in 11 of 14 eyes wearing new or worn contaminated soft contact lenses.[129] Trancassini and associates demonstrated that strains of *P. aeruginosa* that produce alkaline protease and elastase adhere better.[130] Bacterial adherence may also depend on nonbacterial factors. Deighton and Balkau investigated the adherence of strains of *S. epidermidis* to glass and plastic material.[131] They found that the degree of adherence depended mainly on the growth media; adherence was enhanced by the addition of glucose or oleic acid and it was inhibited by serum. After attachment takes place, penetration of the epithelial cells must occur. In the case of *E. coli*, this is a process similar to phagocytosis.[132]

When they are present, bacterial cell wall capsules are important virulence factors.[133–135] While cell wall capsules are more commonly seen in gram-negative bacteria, encapsulated staphylococci may be seen in vivo.[136, 137] The primary virulence factor of *H. influenzae* surface antigen, the type b capsular polysaccharide, is polyribosylribitol phosphate (PRP).[138] Some bacteria, such as *Bacteroides* species, become encapsulated during an inflammatory process, further increasing their pathogenicity as a result.[139] The capsule thus formed inhibits phagocytosis by covering and thus making the recognition sites of opsonins (C3b and IgG) inaccessible to phagocytic cells.[140] M-protein inhibits opsonization[141]; it also impairs complement activation and binding of C3b to the bacterial cell wall.[142] Surface sialylation of the bacterial capsule also helps microorganisms to resist host defenses.[143] In a mouse model of *Campylobacter* infections, Pei and Blaser demonstrated that virulence was enhanced when S-protein was present on the bacterial cell surface as a capsule.[144]

Bacterial glycocalyx also may aid in colonization and infectivity by protecting the bacteria from antibiotics and from the host's immune system and phagocytic cells.[145] Glycocalyx production is important in the adhesion of certain *P. aeruginosa* strains to respiratory tissues.[146] For staphylococcal strains, protein A and clumping factor may be important mediators of adherence.[147, 148] Protein A interferes with opsonic activity of antibodies, because it binds to the Fc portion of IgG (except IgG3), and to a lesser extent, IgM and IgA2.[149, 150] Streptococci groups A, C, and G also carry an Fc binding protein on the cell wall.[151]

The ability of specific bacteria to adhere to the sites at which they produce clinical disease has been shown in various situations, including *S. pneumoniae* to human pharyngeal epithelial cells,[152] *S. pyogenes* to pharyngeal epithelial cells, and *E. coli* to bladder epithelium.[153] *S. aureus, P. aeruginosa, H. influenzae*, and *S. pneumoniae* adhere to mucus in the respiratory tract.[154] *S. aureus, S. pneumoniae*, and *P. aeruginosa*, three of the most common causes of corneal ulceration, exhibit markedly greater adherence to human corneal epithelial cells than do other bacterial species.[155] *S. aureus* produces a number of cell surface proteins that bind to host protein. These include fibronectin, fibrinogen, vitronectin, bone sialoprotein, thrombospondin, collagen, IgA, elastin, prothrombin, plasminogen, laminin, and mucin.[156] Protein A binds IgG in such a way that F_1-receptors on phagocytic cells cannot bind to the F_1 protein of the immunoglobulin. After establishing adhesion, some bacterial pathogens enter epithelial cells by endocytosis. Intracellular invasion provides a new source of nutrients and affords protection from some host defenses; however, the bacteria must survive inside an endocytic vacuole, and, while exposed to products such as lysozyme, they must multiply and spread to other cells.[157] Many pathogenic microbes may invade the host by inducing their own endocytosis. This phenomenon has been designated as parasite-directed endocytosis. Although still poorly understood for most pathogens, it is thought that in the case of most bacteria, this represents biologic mimicry, with the bacteria producing a molecule that resembles a natural host ligand for which there is a host cell receptor.[158] Organisms such as *Mycobacterium, Actinomyces, Corynebacterium, Lis-*

teria, and *Francisella* species contain large quantities of structural lipid that protects them from digestion by the lysosomes of phagocytes, probably because of their ability to scavenge oxygen radicals.[159]

The virulence of bacteria also depends on their ability to produce enzymes that are directed at host defenses. Coagulase produced by staphylococci forms a fibrin clot from fibrinogen, thus protecting the bacteria from phagocytosis. Streptococci can produce a streptokinase that dissolves fibrin clots and allows further spread of the bacteria. Streptokinase activation of plasminogen produces fibrinogen degradation products.[160, 161] Whitnack and coworkers showed that the binding of fibrinogen and fibrinogen degradation products to M-protein enhances its antiopsonic property.[162] *S. pneumoniae* pneumolysin inhibits polymorphonuclear leukocyte chemotaxis and the ability to kill opsonized pneumococcus.[163, 164] Neuraminidase may also be an important virulence factor of *S. pneumoniae*. Neuraminidase might alter glycoproteins on the ocular surface, thus enhancing bacterial attachment. Pneumococci can adhere to corneal epithelial cells in vitro.[165] Hyaluronidase digests hyaluronic acid, which is an important "tissue cement" and aids in the spread of some streptococci and staphylococci. Leukocidin, produced by some staphylococci and streptococci and some bacilli, disintegrates neutrophils and tissue macrophages. Catalase destroys the hydrogen peroxide present in lysosomes. *N. gonorrhoeae* produces an IgA protease that destroys immunoglobulin IgA1. Endotoxin activity is an important aspect of gram-negative virulence. *P. aeruginosa* produces an elastase, alkaline protease, exotoxin A, and LPS endotoxin. The *P. aeruginosa* exotoxin A has a cytopathic effect, and alkaline protease is active against collagen.[166–172] Burns and associates have shown that a metalloproteinase inhibitor (HSCH2) inhibits *P. aeruginosa* elastase and that, in a rabbit model, delayed the onset of corneal melting and perforation.[173]

Host Defenses

Several defense systems are important in the prevention of microbial infection. The first barrier consists of the skin and its indigenous flora that help to create a milieu inhospitable to most pathogens. Lactic acid and fatty acids in sweat and sebaceous glands serve to lower the pH to a point at which most pathogenic bacteria will not survive. The mechanical flushing action of the lids and tears, in addition to antibody, lactoferrin, β-lysin, and lysozyme present in tears, serve as the next major barrier to infection.[174] The conjunctiva and mucous membranes are important in preventing bacterial adherence and in allowing "natural antibodies" such as IgM, humoral immunity, and cell-mediated immunity access to the ocular surface.

NONSPECIFIC DEFENSES

The normal conjunctiva contains all immunologic components and high levels of inflammatory cells (about 300,000 per mm^2).[175] Although immunoglobulins and complement are the most important factors in the host's defense against bacteria, other factors include fibronectin, C-reactive protein, lysozyme, and transferrin. Immunoglobulins G and M (IgG and IgM) have the greatest bactericidal activity, whereas IgA is very effective in restricting bacterial adhesion on mucosal surfaces.[176, 177] These components contribute to specific as well as nonspecific defense mechanisms.[178] IgG is usually present, and IgM has been detected as well.[179] Secretory IgA, usually in conjunction with complement activated by the alternate pathway, can be bacteriolytic.[180, 181] Although the importance of IgA in preventing infections has been questioned, an increased incidence of staphylococcal infections has been observed in atopic disease with its associated defects in IgA and cell-mediated immunity.[182]

The complement system is also very important in defending against bacterial infections.[183] Complement assists phagocytic cells by depositing an opsonic protein (C3b) on the bacterial surface that then interacts with specific receptors on the phagocytic cell surface. It is clear that phagocytic killing by leukocytes is an important defense mechanism against bacterial infection, because patients with abnormalities of polymorphonuclear leukocyte function are susceptible to recurrent or persistent infections.[184–186] The PG component of the staphylococcal cell wall may be the key component required for their opsonization by neutrophils.[187] Other investigators have been unable to demonstrate any effect of PG in activating complement.[188] Pneumolysin can activate the classic complement pathway, whereas the alternate pathway may be activated by group A streptococci PG or the TA of *S. pneumoniae*.[189–191] In gram-negative infections, complement can be directly bactericidal through the assembly of a membrane attack complex (C5b-9) that can lyse susceptible gram-negative bacteria. Complement is also chemotactic, drawing leukocytes into the cornea. Typically, an antigen-antibody complex activates the complement reaction, but interaction of bacteria directly with C1q can also activate complement.[192, 193] Bacterial cell wall components such as LPS can activate the alternate complement pathway.[194] Deposition of LPS-antibody complexes may cause ring infiltrates in gram-negative corneal infections.[195] C-reactive protein (CRP) in vitro has shown several antibacterial activities, but its role in vivo is less certain.[196]

Neutrophils are the primary cells found at the site of bacterial corneal infections.[197] During phagocytosis they release prostaglandins, which increase vascular permeability and induce degranulation of mast cells and basophils. Mast cells in turn release histamine, eosinophil chemotactic factor, prostaglandins, and SRS-A.[198] Neutrophil lysosomal products include cationic proteins, acid proteases, and neutral proteases. The cationic proteins increase vascular permeability and are chemotactic for mononuclear phagocytes. The acid proteases degrade basement membrane, and neutral proteases degrade fibrin, elastin, and collagen. Neutrophils also contain collagenase.[199] New antimicrobial neutrophil peptides (defensins NP-1 and NP-5) have been isolated from rabbits. Cullor and associates have demonstrated that neutrophil defensins possess both bacteriostatic and bactericidal activity against various ocular pathogens.[200]

Fibronectin possesses opsonic activity and can bind both to gram-positive and gram-negative bacteria, although evidence that this aids in phagocytosis of bacteria is controversial.[201] Lanser reported that removal of fibronectin from serum decreased the phagocytosis of *S. aureus* by rat neutrophils and that the addition of fibronectin restored phagocytic activity.[202] However, Verbrugh found that neither fibronectin binding nor depletion significantly affected phagocytosis of *S. epidermidis* by human polymorphonuclear leukocytes.[203]

Fibronectin possesses specific binding sites for both streptococci and staphylococci. In streptococci, fibronectin can bind to LTA.[204] Protein A is the fibronectin receptor on staphylococci.[205] Proctor and Jacobs showed that fibronectin promoted attachment of bacteria to polymorphonuclear leukocytes but ingestion of bacteria did not occur unless classic opsonins such as IgG or complement were present.[206–208] Therefore, fibronectin's role as a substrate for bacterial attachment and colonization of tissue probably overshadows any effect on binding and phagocytosis of bacteria.

Lysozyme is an enzyme that can lyse certain bacteria by acting as a muramidase to cleave the glycosidic bond of the *N*-acetylmuramic acid residues in the bacterial cell wall.[209] Lysozyme is found in tears, with levels in normal adults ranging from 1.3 to 1.4 ± 0.6 mg/mL.[210, 211] The lysozyme content in tears decreases with age and decreases in several eye diseases, including keratoconjunctivitis sicca, chronic conjunctivitis, and nutritional deficiency with xerosis.[212–215] Lysozyme is primarily effective against saprophytic gram-positive bacteria such as micrococci. Some coagulase-positive staphylococcal strains can produce lysozyme,[216] which may help them overcome any inhibitory effect of the indigenous flora. Lysozyme may also interact with a recently described substance called lysostaphin. Certain staphylococcal strains produce lysostaphin. In contrast to lysozyme, lysostaphin inhibits many strains of staphylococci including *S. aureus*, but it does not inhibit micrococci.[217] Lysozyme appears to increase the antistaphylococcal activity of lysostaphin from 16- to 200-fold.[218] In gram-negative bacteria, lysozyme aids the action of complement on the cells cytoplasmic membrane.[219] The iron-binding protein lactoferrin can function to withhold iron that is necessary for microbial multiplication.[220]

RESISTANCE TO COMPLEMENT

Bacterial structure is closely linked to complement activation. The presence of various surface antigens appears to render bacterial cells resistant to complement activity.[221] Through its interaction with specific antibody, LPS can activate complement via both the classic and alternate pathways; LPS alone activates the alternate pathway.[222] Bacteria appear to alter their LPS to block complement.

HUMORAL IMMUNITY

Normal tears contain antibodies against bacteria. Local antibody synthesis takes place in the lacrimal gland, but some antibodies originate from lymphocyte sensitization in the mucosal immune system.[223] In *P. aeruginosa* infections, Berk and associates showed that mice develop IgM and IgG antibodies corresponding to their ability to recover from corneal infection.[224] Antibodies attach to the outer membrane proteins (porin protein F) and protect the cornea.[225] However, not all antibody responses are beneficial to the host. Griffiss and associates have reported that serum IgA directed against *N. meningitidis* blocks the lytic activity of IgG and IgM for this organism.[226]

Complement and opsins, discussed earlier, are necessary for the adherence of bacteria to polymorphonuclear leukocytes. Complement can destroy bacteria directly or by causing chemotaxis of neutrophils. Antibody-coated bacteria may be unable to adhere to corneal epithelium. Antibodies can also neutralize the exotoxins released by some bacteria. PG increases the responsiveness of mouse B lymphocytes to phytohemagglutinin and pokeweed mitogen, whereas cell wall preparation can either enhance or diminish human B- and T-cell responses to either purified protein derivative (PPD) or protein A.[227]

CELL-MEDIATED IMMUNITY

Cell-mediated immunity (CMI) contributes to the defense against microorganisms.[228] When a T lymphocyte becomes sensitized to a bacterial antigen, it releases a soluble factor (lymphokine) that can help to activate the macrophage and localize it at the site of an infection.[229] The sensitized lymphocyte can also release chemotactic factors for macrophages, neutrophils, basophils, and eosinophils.[230] PG, TA, and other cell wall components may be polyclonal activators of both B and T cells.[231, 232] Polyclonal activation of human lymphocytes may be useful to the host as a mechanism of resistance to infectious diseases; however, the process could also have adverse effects by triggering or perpetuating chronic inflammatory disease.[233–235] Studies in animals indicate that immunization with the capsular polysaccharide provides a T-cell–dependent immunity to abscess development when challenged with *Bacteroides fralis*. Also, it appears that the killing of *B. fragilis* is T-cell dependent.[236] Group A streptococcal cell membranes appear to enhance certain T-cell functions.[237]

Diagnostic Tests

The diversity of infectious processes that involve the eye makes it necessary for the ophthalmologist to be aware of a variety of basic microbiologic techniques. Jones and associates have written what still remains the most comprehensive approach to ocular laboratory diagnosis.[238] Both the ophthalmologist and laboratory must be aware that many pathogens in ocular disease for reasons iterated above are considered contaminants or normal flora. Frequently, the material obtained from cultures is small and must be inoculated onto media immediately. The specific technique to be used and the cultures taken will depend on the clinical diagnosis and setting; it is useful to have protocols written out beforehand in order to avoid needless errors. It is also helpful to maintain a culture tray that is readily available. Routine culture media can be stored in a refrigerator, but only fresh plates of media should be used. Media that appear dry or that have pulled back from the edges of the Petri dish should be replaced. Plates should be brought to room temperature before inoculating them with clinical material.

The method used to collect a specimen depends upon the site and etiology of the infection. Cultures of the cornea, conjunctiva, and lids can be done either with the Kimura platinum spatula or with swabs. For lid cultures, our procedure is to use a moistened calcium alginate swab. The use of a moistened swab to prevent drying of the material and to create a capillary attraction may enhance bacterial pickup. Furthermore, the moistened swab allows release of the material over several plates and avoids cutting into the media surface, which can make recognition and isolation of colonies more difficult. If the blepharitis is ulcerative, the platinum spatula may be used to remove the fibrin scale, and this material may be cultured as well. In cases of conjunctivitis, we will again use the swab moistened in sterile saline or nutrient broth, reserving the spatula to obtain specimens for cytology.

In cases of suspected microbial keratitis, a four-step approach to the culture is taken. First, a moistened swab is used to culture the ulcer base. Next the ulcer is scraped, usually with a platinum spatula, but in some cases a Bard-Parker No. 15 blade or a 21-gauge needle may be required to obtain sufficient material. The material obtained should then be immediately transferred to a moistened swab and streaked onto appropriate media. The spatula is used to obtain material for smears and slides, and finally a moistened swab is again applied to the ulcer in order to pick up any bacteria brought to the ulcer surface. It should be emphasized that this is the minimum number of samples that should be taken. Whenever there is a large, fulminating ulcer or sufficient material is available, separate scrapings of the ulcer should be done for each plate. In our laboratory, we have had more success using separate plates for each site cultured than we did by using the marking systems advocated by others.[239] Although it requires more plates and labeling, this technique facilitates the isolation and identification of individual pathogens, particularly in polymicrobial infections.[239]

In cases of endophthalmitis, both aqueous and vitreous should be cultured.[240, 241] Smears should also be performed. Although smears may not always agree with culture results, they may nevertheless be invaluable in confirming a bacterial process in cases of culture-negative endophthalmitis.

MEDIA

Media can be divided into two broad types: broad-spectrum and nonselective. All of the media used in ophthalmology are enriched, because selective media contain chemical substances or antibiotics to inhibit the growth of all but the desired organism. The basic media used for culture and identification of most ocular bacterial pathogens are listed in Table 11–1.

Blood Agar

Blood agar consists of a *Brucella* agar base with a peptic digest of animal tissue, dextrose, and yeast extract. Most aerobic bacteria (and fungi) will grow on it except for the more fastidious pathogens, especially *Neisseria, Haemophilus*, and *Moraxella*. When incubated under anaerobic conditions, most anaerobic organisms will grow on blood agar as well but it must be supplemented with hemin, vitamin K, and sometimes cysteine. It also has the advantage of revealing the hemolytic reaction of the organism. This is the best single general purpose culture medium for the diagnosis of ocular pathogens.

TABLE 11-1. **Bacterial Culture Media**

Routine
Blood agar
Chocolate agar
Enriched thioglycolate broth
Sabouraud dextrose agar (for fungi)
Optional (depends on availability and the clinical situation)
Brain-heart infusion broth

Chocolate Agar

Chocolate agar is prepared by using GC agar base and bovine hemoglobin. Growth factors, hemin (X factor), and nicotinamide adenine dinucleotide (V factor) are added to the agar.[242] These nutrients are essential for the growth of *Haemophilus, N. gonorrhoeae, N. meningitidis*, and *Moraxella*. When one suspects *N. gonorrhoeae*, Thayer-Martin medium should also be used. Thayer-Martin medium contains 3 mg of vancomycin, 7.5 mg of colistin, and 12.5 U of nystatin per milliliter of agar to inhibit other bacteria or yeasts that could inhibit the growth of gonococcus. However, Thayer-Martin medium is only a supplement to and not a replacement for chocolate agar, because potentially nongonococcal strains of *Neisseria* may be inhibited by the added antibiotics. Incubation of Thayer-Martin plates should be done in an atmosphere containing 3 to 10% CO_2.

Brain-Heart Infusion Broth

A highly nutritious and buffered liquid is a useful adjunct to solid media for several reasons. Material picked up by the swab but not released onto the solid agar thus has an opportunity to grow. Any antibiotics or other inhibitors of bacterial growth will be diluted and, therefore, have less effect. Inoculation of broth also allows the use of antimicrobial removal devices, such as those developed by Osato. However, they do not permit one to confirm that growth is occurring along the inoculum streak nor do they allow one to quantify the amount of growth.

Other useful selective media include eosin methylene blue (EMB) agar and MacConkey agar.[243, 244] These media are primarily useful for the isolation of gram-negative bacteria. Methylene blue agar inhibits gram-positive bacteria and has carbohydrates that can be fermented by *Escherichia coli* and other gram-negative bacteria. MacConkey agar contains the carbohydrate lactose, a fermentable carbohydride, as well as bile salts, which inhibit the growth of gram-positive bacteria.

Anaerobic cultures are routinely done in thioglycollate broth without indicator. The broth is supplemented with hemin and vitamin K.[245] At times, aerobes also grow in thioglycollate, usually near the surface; anaerobes, on the other hand, grow below the surface. A disadvantage is that an anaerobic pathogen can be overgrown by other anaerobic bacteria or by aerobic bacteria.[246] In cases in which anaerobic cultures are especially important, such as a possible *P. acnes* endophthalmitis or chronic canaliculitis, other anaerobic media should be used. Prereduced anaerobically sterilized media (PRAS), anaerobic blood agar, or chocolate agar can be used.[247] In cases in which one obtains a fluid sample, such as in endophthalmitis, the sample can be injected through the rubber stopper into a chopped meat glucose medium. Aerobic and anaerobic blood culture bottles can also be used.

Lowenstein-Jensen medium is used for the isolation of mycobacteria. It contains ribonucleic acid adequate for microbacterial growth, along with penicillin and nalidixic acid, which inhibit contaminating organisms. *Nocardia* species will also grow on this medium.[248]

Proper conditions during incubation are essential. Aerobic and anaerobic cultures should be kept at 35°C. Blood and chocolate agar should be incubated under higher carbon dioxide tension (3 to 10%). Routine cultures should be kept for 1 week, but anaerobic cultures should be incubated for 2 weeks. Fungal, actinomycete, and mycobacterial cultures should be held for 8 weeks. Mycobacteria grow best under a carbon dioxide tension of 5 to 10%.

STAINS

While they may not always agree with the final cultured organisms, smears are an important component of bacterial diagnosis. Although one could base initial therapy on Gram's stain findings, given the incongruity between smear and culture results, it would seem most prudent to use the smear results to add to therapy rather than delete from the standard initial treatment. Smears are also useful in identifying polymicrobial processes in which one type of bacteria may inhibit or delay the identification of other bacterial pathogens. Furthermore, smears may identify the presence of organisms that do not appear on culture for days or even weeks. Smears are invaluable whenever cultures prove to be negative, especially in patients who have previously received antibiotics. In the laboratory, stains are essential in order to identify cultured bacteria.

The proper preparation and examination of smears requires both experience and patience. Smears are prepared by spreading a thin film of the specimen over a defined area of the slide. Smears that are too thick can obscure many important details. Smears spread out over an entire slide increase the length of time required to completely examine the slide and increase the possibility of overlooking pathogens. The slide should be free of lint and fingerprints, air-dried, and gently heat-fixed. One must look at a large number of slides in order to be able to distinguish between the occasional bacteria of the "normal" flora and an actual pathogen. In repertory results, microbiologists should report only cell morphology and a Gram reaction, not whether they think they see "pathogens" or "normal flora."

One of the oldest and most commonly used stains is the Gram stain. As we have discussed earlier, this is a differential stain in that bacteria are either gram-positive (blue-purple) or gram-negative (orange-red). There are several theories to explain why bacteria respond differently to a Gram stain. One theory suggests that crystal violet and iodine form a chemical complex in the bacterial cytoplasm. Alcohol in the staining process may dissolve lipid, allowing the crystal violet–iodine complex to leak out of the cytoplasm. Gram-negative bacteria with their high lipid content in the cell wall would therefore lose more stain than would gram-positive bacteria. The cell walls of gram-positive bacteria are less permeable to small molecules than are those of gram-negative organisms. PG in the cell wall of gram-positive bacteria may trap the crystal violet–iodine complex. Because gram-negative bacteria have less PG, they would trap considerably less stain.[249] In any case, knowing whether an organism is gram-positive or gram-negative continues to have important diagnostic and therapeutic implications. Variable Gram's staining may occur with excessive decolorizing, with smears that are too thick, or with older cultures. Gram-positive organisms may appear gram-negative if there has been previous antibiotic treatment, leukocytic destruction, or excessive heating of the slide.[248] The safranin counterstain can replace crystal violet, thus the slide should not be counterstained for a prolonged time. Giemsa staining is not as important in bacterial infections, because it has no differential value, but its ability to delineate cellular types and detect inclusion bodies or multinucleated giant cells make it an important investigative tool in ocular diagnosis. Bacteria generally stain blue. The Brown-Hopps stain is a Gram stain modified for tissues. Aniline can be added to the Gram stain to improve identification of actinomycetes.

Acridine orange (AO) stains all DNA and RNA regardless of organism. AO has recently received renewed interest owing to its ability to stain *Acanthamoeba* species. The AO stain is very good for bacteria too and is more sensitive than a Gram stain, requiring fewer organisms to yield a positive result.[250] Bacteria can stain red, orange, or green depending on relative amounts of DNA versus RNA, whereas nonbacterial cells such as squamous cells and polymorphonuclear leukocytes stain green-yellow.[251] If bacteria are detected, then a Gram stain can be performed on the same slide without decolorization. The major disadvantage is that the AO stain requires a fluorescent microscope. Acid-fast staining is useful to detect *Mycobacterium* species. The brilliant green counterstain allows for improved contrast between acid-fast organisms and the background. If *Nocardia* is suspected, then an aqueous solution of 1% sulfuric acid rather than 3% hydrochloric acid in 95% ethanol must be used as the decolorizing agent. Fluorescein-conjugated lectins have been used to identify microorganisms, primarily fungi,[252] but do not offer any advantages over existing stains in bacteriologic diagnosis.

HIGH-TECHNOLOGY DIAGNOSTIC METHODS

Newer diagnostic methods may be used increasingly in bacteriologic diagnosis. Antigen detection tests have been developed utilizing a variety of techniques, including counterimmunoelectrophoresis (CIE), coagglutination (CoA), latex agglutination (LA), enzyme immunoassay (EIA), radioimmunoassay (RIA), solid-phase immunofluorescence and fluorescence polarization immunoassay (FPIA), and antigen detection tests. These tests have tremendous potential and to date have been useful in detecting cerebral spinal fluid pathogens, especially if there has been pretreatment with antibiotics.[253, 254] In ophthalmology, these tests are used most commonly for the detection of *Chlamydia*, viruses, fungi, and ocular protozoal disease.

DNA probes are particularly useful when looking for a particular organism such as a mycobacterium. These probes are also helpful for the detection of organisms that are present in small numbers or are fastidious and difficult to cultivate.[255] Radiolabeled DNA probes are more sensitive and more specific, but results take several days. Nonradioactive probes are generally less sensitive but faster. Various kits based upon the use of specific nucleic acid probes are now available commercially for identifying specific bacteria in a sample. They combine high specificity with speed.[256] These procedure do not distinguish between viable and nonviable bacteria, which may be an advantage, especially when prior antibiotic treatment has been used. The problem of sample size can be overcome by nucleic acid amplification. The most widely accepted method is the polymerase chain reaction (PCR). Despite the need for specific primers, the main problem with the use of PCR is its exquisite sensitivity, making contamination and the probability of the amplification of the wrong segment a real possibility. However, amplification of the 16S–23S rDNA region of bacterial chromosomes will eventually allow rapid identification of bacteria without any need for isolation and cultivation.[256] Monoclonal antibodies give rapid results but are very specific.[257] Gas-liquid chromatography (GLC) and high-pressure liquid chromatography (HPLC) have been useful in the clinical microbiology laboratory, especially in the identification of quinones and in carbohydrate analysis for taxonomic classification.[258] Also, analysis of cell wall phospholipid fatty acid has shown that each genus has a unique lipid fingerprint. Several automated bacteria identification systems are currently marketed. One approach developed by Biolog, Inc. (Hayward, CA), uses redox-based technology and the determination of what chemicals an organism can use as carbon and energy sources.[259] Once substrate profiles for organisms have been determined, then the process can be simplified by computerized microplate technology. Miller and Rhoden, at the Centers for Disease Control and Prevention, have reviewed this system.[260] They found the system to be versatile and easy to use with an error rate of 9.6% after 24 hours but concluded that the system is not yet ready to be used as the primary identification instrument for clinical laboratories.

ANTIBIOTIC SUSCEPTIBILITY AND SENSITIVITY

Susceptibility tests help to determine the most effective therapeutic agent available. These tests are somewhat artificial, because they do not consider the host's defenses and immune status, the number and accessibility of the organisms, and whether the bacteria are intra- or extracellular, all of which may influence antibiotic selection. In serious ocular infections, bactericidal rather than bacteriostatic antibiotics should be utilized whenever possible. In bacterial keratitis, sensitivity testing does not take into account the antibiotic levels obtainable through the use of fortified drops. Just as it is important for the clinical microbiology laboratory to report and identify all bacteria present in ocular cultures, it is vital to make sure that the clinical laboratory performing the sensitivity testing is aware of the specific agents available for ophthalmic use so that these antibiotics can be routinely tested. Antibiotics such as polymyxin B, bacitracin, and neomycin are no longer included in most clinical laboratories' sensitivity panel, but they remain important ocular therapeutic agents.

Susceptibility testing using either disc diffusion or dilutional tests should be performed on all potential pathogens. In order to accelerate the selection of appropriate antibiotics, direct susceptibility testing has been advocated.[261] A pure culture is required for the test to be reliable and several factors, including the density of the inoculum and the presence of other microorganisms, can make the results misleading. It is probably better to base initial therapy on the "cookbook" methods and then, once the microorganism has been identified, modify therapy, if necessary, based on previous antibiotic sensitivities of the organism. Disc diffusion tests are the most commonly used technique.[262] Antimicrobial-containing discs are placed on the agar surface inoculated with a pure culture of the organism. A zone of inhibition occurs around the disc. The extent of this inhibition determines whether the bacteria are sensitive to the particular antibiotic. The significant zone of inhibition is different for each antibiotic owing to differences in diffusion rates between antibiotics.[263, 264] Disc diffusion techniques do have some limitations. They depend upon rapidly growing organisms.[265, 266] The disc does not measure bactericidal activity, and combinations of agents cannot be assayed. The discs only reflect the usually obtainable serum concentrations and not the higher levels obtainable within the tear film or cornea or intraocularly. Therefore, organisms reported as resistant may be susceptible in the ophthalmic setting. The most common clinical setting in which this occurs is in the patient in the ICU or burn unit who is infected with multiple aminoglycoside-resistant *Pseudomonas* organisms and may respond to fortified aminoglycosides, especially when they are combined with carbenicillin or ticarcillin.[267, 268] A recently introduced BIOGRAM (Giles Scientific, New York, NY) translates disc diffusion zone sizes into minimal inhibitory concentrations (MICs), using regression line analysis. A printed report is produced that includes calculated MICs, Kirby-Bauer interpretations, and inhibitory quotients that are based on achievable serum, urine, bile, and cerebrospinal fluid concentrations.[269] Potential advantages include the ability to select from 34 antimicrobics, the ability to read results for many organisms in just 5 to 6 hours, and 90 to 95% correlation with reference laboratory results.[270, 271]

A third approach is an elution method. The antimicrobial elutes from paper discs into broth or agar, thus providing a desired concentration of the antimicrobial agent in the medium. This approach is used in some automated systems (Autobac and MS-2 or Avantage) for susceptibility testing of aerobic and facultatively anaerobic bacteria as well as in susceptibility testing of anaerobic bacteria and mycobacteria.[272] Paper diffusion methods are superior for the detection of methicillin-resistant strains, provided that either a medium with a high sodium chloride content is used or plates are incubated at 30°C for at least 24 hours.[273] The Kirby-Bauer test normally does not detect methicillin resistance nor do automated methods such as Autobac or MS-2.[274, 275]

Dilutional tests have several advantages over disc diffusion testing. Besides determining the MIC, the minimal lethal concentration (MLC), or minimal bactericidal concentration (MBC) can also be determined.[276, 277] Microdilution methods that place the antimicrobial agents in microtiter tray wells are more practical and lend themselves more to automation, because the trays can then be read photometrically. The small sample size may make detection of resistant subpopulations less likely, especially as incubation times are reduced. Clinically, this is important in detecting third-generation cephalosporin resistance because of depressed β-lactamase production in *Enterobacter, Serratia,* and *P. aeruginosa*.[278] In order to consider the organism susceptible, the peak obtainable concentration should be two to four times higher than the MIC. The MBC level assumes greater importance in clinical situations in which the cure of an infection depends entirely on the antibiotic and bactericidal activity.[279, 280] This is important for immune-deficient patients and for those with CNS infections, but it also may be an important consideration in endophthalmitis. Serum bactericidal activity can be measured by the Schlichter test.[281] Although not entirely standardized, this test considers other factors that influence antibiotic activity (especially serum protein binding) and has been used primarily in the treatment of endocarditis and osteomyelitis.[282] Interpretation of MIC data is confusing to many clinicians; one should encourage the laboratory to include interpretative data with the report. Other pharmacodynamic factors in bacterial infections of importance are the rate and extent of bactericidal action, postantibiotic effect, minimal antibiotic concentration, and postantibiotic leukocytic effect.[283]

Bacteria have shown great ability to develop resistance to antibodies usually by the transfer of DNA between bacteria of the same or different species. Much of the antibiotic resistance encoded by genes is carried on plasmids.[284]

The production of β-lactamase by *H. influenzae, N. gonorrhoeae*, and staphylococci correlates well with resistance to penicillin. Tests such as the nitrocefin test can provide results in a matter of minutes rather than overnight.[285] This is increasingly important as antibiotic resistance is seen more and more in clinical situations, for example, in coagulase-negative staphylococcal endophthalmitis.[286]

Pericellular resistance has now been found in *S. pneumoniae* not due to β-lactamase production but due to changes to the genes encoding the target enzymes.[287]

Antiseptics and Disinfection

Sterilization and disinfection are important concepts that are taken for granted every day. Sterilization implies destruction of all forms of life, including spores, and generally requires a physical agent such as pressurized steam or ethylene oxide. Disinfection refers to the destruction of pathogens and frequently involves the use of a chemical agent. Antimicrobial agents are used daily in ophthalmic practice to preserve medicines, sterilize instruments, and prepare the operative field for surgery. There are numerous factors to be considered in the selection of an appropriate antiseptic. The chemical must be bactericidal and nontoxic to the host. The length of exposure, pH, and temperature are also taken into account. Some methicillin-resistant strains of *S. aureus* (MRSA) containing plasmids encoding gentamicin resistance (MGRSA) also have increased MIC values toward biocides such as GACs, chlorhexidine, acridines, and propamidine isethionate.[288, 289] Gram-negative bacteria such as *Pseudomonas* are usually less sensitive to chemical antibactors than are gram-positive cocci. The main reason is due to the great complexity of the outer cell membrane.[290]

Skin asepsis is important in ophthalmic surgery, because, as noted earlier, most cases of endophthalmitis arise from the patient's own flora. Hendley and Ashe evaluated the effectiveness of various antimicrobial agents in eradicating coagulase-negative staphylococci from the surface and stratum corneum of the skin.[291] They evaluated five antiseptic solutions and four antimicrobial ointments. The skin surface was effectively sterilized by eight of the nine agents tested. A soap-and-water wash was ineffective, but solutions of povidone-iodine, chlorhexidine-ethanol, and 2% tincture of iodine eliminated surface bacteria. However, sterilization of the stratum corneum was much more difficult to accomplish. The rates of eradication of coagulase-negative staphylococci from the stratum corneum after surface treatment with chlorhexidine-ethanol and povidone-iodine were not different from the control sites. Only triple antibiotic ointment (neomycin, polymyxin B sulfate, and bacitracin) was effective initially and inhibited overnight repopulation from occurring.

Acknowledgment

Supported in part by an unrestricted grant from Research to Prevent Blindness, Inc., New York, New York.

REFERENCES

1. Krieg NR, Holt JG (eds): Bergey's Manual of Systematic Bacteriology, vol 1. Baltimore, Williams & Wilkins, p 13.
2. Meyer TE, Cusanovich MS, Kamen MD: Evidence against use of bacterial amino acid sequence data for construction of all-inclusive phylogenetic trees. Proc Natl Acad Sci U S A 83:217, 1986.
3. Muto A, Osawa S: The guanine and cytosine content of genomic DNA and bacterial evolution. Proc Natl Acad Sci U S A 84:166, 1987.
4. Holt SC, Leadbetter ER: Structure-function relationships in prokaryotic cells. *In* Balows A, Duerden BI (eds): Topley & Wilson's Microbiology and Microbial Infections. Vol 2: Systematic Bacteriology. Oxford, Oxford University Press, 1998, pp 11–44.
5. Wilkinson BJ, Kim Y, Peterson PK, et al: Activation of complement by cell surface components of *Staphylococcus aureus*. Infect Immun 20:388, 1978.
6. Hancock REW: Role of porins in outer membrane permeability. J Bacteriol 169:929, 1987.
7. Mims CA: The Pathogenesis of Infectious Disease, 3rd ed. New York, Academic Press/Grune & Stratton, 1987.
8. Christensen GD, Simpson WA, Bisno AL, Beachy E: Adherence of slime-producing strains of *Staphylococcus epidermidis* to smooth surfaces. Infect Immun 37:318, 1982.
9. Jann K, Jann B: Progress in allergy. Rev Infect Dis 9 (Suppl):S517, 1987.
10. Hoffman S, Sorkin BC, White PC, et al: Chemical characterization of a neural cell adhesion molecule purified from embryonic brain membranes. J Biol Chem 257:7720, 1982.
11. Eisenstein BI: Type 1 fimbriae of *Escherichia coli:* Genetic regulation, morphogenesis, and role in pathogenesis. Rev Infect Dis 10 (Suppl):S341, 1988.
12. Davis BD: Bacterial architecture. *In* Microbiology, 4th ed. Philadelphia, JB Lippincott, 1990, pp 38–39.
13. Alcamo IE: Fundamentals of Microbiology, 3rd ed. Menlo Park, CA, Benjamin Cummings, 1991, p 119.
14. Bexkorovainy A: Iron proteins. *In* Bullen JJ, Griffiths E (eds): Iron and Infection: Molecular, Physiological and Clinical Aspects. Chichester, England, John Wiley, 1987, pp 27–67.
15. Morgan EH: Transferrin, biochemistry, physiology and clinical significance. Mol Aspects Med 4:1, 1981.
16. Morse SA, Chen CY, LeFaou A, Mietzner TA: A potential role for the major iron-regulated protein expressed by pathogenic *Neisseria* species. Rev Infect Dis 10:(Suppl):S306, 1988.
17. Catlin BW: *Branhamella catarrhalis*: An organism gaining respect as a pathogen. Clin Microbiol Rev 3:293, 1990.
18. Tauber FW, Krause AC: The role of iron, copper, zinc, and manganese in the metabolism of the ocular tissues, with special reference to the lens. Am J Ophthalmol 26:260, 1943.
19. Brener D, DeVoe IW, Holbein BE: Increased virulence of *Neisseria meningitidis* after in vitro iron-limited growth at low pH. Infect Immun 33:59, 1981.
20. Griffiths E: The iron-uptake systems of pathogenic bacteria. *In* Bullen JJ, Griffiths E (eds): Iron and Infection: Molecular, Physiological and Clinical Aspects. Chichester, England, John Wiley, 1987, pp 69–137.
21. Brown V: Iron supply as a virulence factor. *In* Jackson GG, Thomas H (eds): The Pathogenesis of Bacterial Infections. Bayer-Symposium VIII. Berlin, Springer-Verlag, 1985, p 168.
22. World Health Organization: Methods of Assessment of Avoidable Blindness (WHO Offset Pub. No. 54). Geneva, 1980.
23. Townsor KJ, Cockayne A: Molecular Methods for Microbial Identification and Typing. London, Chapman and Hall, 1993.

24. Kloos WE, Scheifer KH: Simplified scheme for routine identification of human *Staphylococcus* species. J Clin Microbiol 1:82, 1980.
25. Hoover DG, Tatini SA, Maltais JB: Characterization of staphylococci. Appl Environ Microbiol 46:649, 1983.
26. Kloos WE: Natural populations of the genus *Staphylococcus*. Annu Rev Microbiol 34:592, 1980.
27. McCulley JP, Dougherty JM, Deneau DG: Classification of chronic blepharitis. Ophthalmology 89:1173, 1982.
28. Packer AJ, Koontz FP: Ocular staphylococcal infections. Am J Ophthalmol 97:645, 1984.
29. McCulley JP, Dougherty JM, Deneau DG: Classification of chronic blepharitis. Ophthalmology 89:1173, 1982.
30. Dougherty JM, McCulley JP: Comparative bacteriology of chronic blepharitis. Br J Ophthalmol 68:524, 1984.
31. McCulley JP, Dougherty JM: Bacterial aspects of chronic blepharitis. Trans Ophthalmol Soc U K 105:314, 1986.
32. Dougherty JM, McCulley JP: Bacterial lipases and chronic blepharitis. Invest Ophthalmol Vis Sci 27:486, 1986.
33. Bridge PD, Sneath PHA: Numerical taxonomy of *Streptococcus*. J Gen Microbiol 129:565, 1983.
34. Ormerod LD, Ruoff KL, Meisler DM, et al: Infectious crystalline keratopathy. Role of nutritionally variant streptococci and other bacterial factors. Ophthalmology 98(2):159, 1991.
35. Lubniewski AJ, Houchin KW, Holland EJ, et al: Posterior infectious crystalline keratopathy with *Staphylococcus epidermidis*. Ophthalmology 97:1454, 1990.
36. Ehret JM, Knapp JS: Gonorrhea. Clin Lab Med 9:445, 1989.
37. Centers for Disease Control: Antibiotic-resistant strains of *Neisseria gonorrhoeae*: Policy guidelines for detection, management, and control. MMWR 36(Suppl 5S):1S, 1987.
38. Hagar H, Verghese A, Alvarez S, Berk SL: *Branhamella catarrhalis* respiratory infections. Rev Infect Dis 9:1140, 1987.
39. Van Hare GF, Shurin PA, Marchant CD, et al: Acute otitis media caused by *Branhamella catarrhalis:* Microbiology and therapy. Rev Infect Dis 9:16, 1987.
40. Wright PW, Avery WG: *Branhamella catarrhalis* infections. Am Fam Physician 39:(2):125, 1989.
41. Retailliau HR, Hightower AW, Dixon RE, Allen JR: *Actinobacter calcoaceticus:* A nosocomial pathogen with an unusual seasonal pattern. J Infect Dis 139:371, 1979.
42. Murray PR, Drew WL, Kobayashi GS, Thompson JH (eds): Medical Microbiology. St. Louis, CV Mosby, 1990, p 98.
43. Van Bysterveld OP: A new *Moraxella* strain isolated from angular conjunctivitis. Appl Microbiol 20:405, 1970.
44. Brinser JH: Ocular bacteriology. *In* Tabbara KF, Hyndiuk RA (eds): Infections of the Eye. Boston, Little, Brown, 1986, p 139.
45. Brinser JH: Ocular bacteriology. *In* Tabbara KF, Hyndiuk RA (eds): Infections of the Eye. Boston, Little, Brown, 1986, p 133.
46. Shammas HF: Endogenous *E. coli* endophthalmitis. Surv Ophthalmol 21:429, 1977.
47. Alcamo IE: Fundamentals of Microbiology, 4th ed. Redwood City, CA, Benjamin Cummings, 1994, p 242.
48. Gammon JA, Schwab I, Joseph P: Gentamicin-resistant *Serratia marcescens* endophthalmitis. Arch Ophthalmol 98:1221, 1980.
49. Brinser JH: Ocular bacteriology. *In* Tabbara KF, Hyndiuk RA (eds): Infections of the Eye. Boston, Little, Brown, 1986, p 135.
50. Chin GN, Noble RC: Ocular involvement in *Yersinia enterocolitica* presenting as Parinaud's oculoglandular syndrome. Am J Ophthalmol 83:19, 1977.
51. Cohen KL, Holyk PR, McCarthy LR, Peiffer RL: *Aeromonas hydrophila* and *Plesiomonas shigelloides* endophthalmitis. Am J Ophthalmol 96:403, 1983.
52. Tacket CO, Barrett TJ, Sanders GE, Blake PA: Panophthalmitis caused by *Vibrio parahaemolyticus*. J Clin Microbiol 16:195, 1982.
53. Altenbern RA: Formation of hemolysin by strains of *Pseudomonas aeruginosa*. Can J Microbiol 12:231, 1966.
54. Nanda M, Pflugfelder SC, Holland S: Fulminant pseudomonal keratitis and scleritis in human immunodeficiency virus-infected patients. Arch Ophthalmol 109:503, 1991.
55. Barenkamp SJ: Outer-membrane protein subtypes of *Haemophilus influenzae* type b and spread of disease in day-care centers. J Infect Dis 144:210, 1981.
56. Doern GV, Jorgensen JH, Thornsberry C, et al: National collaborative study of the prevalence of antimicrobial resistance among clinical isolates of *Haemophilus influenzae*. Antimicrob Agents Chemother 32:180, 1988.
57. Ronald AR, Plummer FA: Chancroid and granuloma inguinale. Clin Lab Med 9:535, 1989.
58. Schmid G: The treatment of chancroid. JAMA 255:1757, 1986.
59. Lass JH, Varley MP, Frank KE, et al: *Actinobacillus actinomycetemcomitans* endophthalmitis with subacute endocarditis. Ann Ophthalmol 16:54, 1984.
60. Purcell JJ, Krachmer JH: Corneal ulcer caused by *Pasteurella multocida*. Am J Ophthalmol 93:540, 1977.
61. Klein B, Couch J, Thompson J: Ocular infections associated with *Eikenella corrodens*. Am J Ophthalmol 109:127, 1990.
62. Ticho BH, Urban RC Jr, Safran MJ, Saggan DD: Capnocytophaga keratitis associated with poor dentition and human immunodeficiency virus infection. Am J Ophthalmol 109:352, 1990.
63. de Smet MD, Chan CC, Nussenblatt RB, Palestine AG: *Capnocytophaga canimorsus* as the cause of a chronic corneal infection. Am J Ophthalmol 109:240, 1990.
64. Moriarty RA, Margileth AM: Cat-scratch disease. Infect Dis Clin North Am 1:575, 1987.
65. Wear DJ, Margileth AM, Hadfield TL, et al: Cat-scratch disease: A bacterial infection. Science 221:1403, 1983.
66. Kitchell CC, DeGirolami PC, Balogh K: Bacillary organisms in cat-scratch disease. N Engl J Med. 313:1090, 1985.
67. Wear DJ, Malaty RH, Zimmerman LE, et al: Cat-scratch disease bacilli in the conjunctiva of patients with Parinaud's oculoglandular syndrome. Ophthalmology 92:1282, 1985.
68. Black JR, Herrington DA, Hadfield TL, et al: Life-threatening cat-scratch disease in an immuno-compromised host. Arch Intern Med 146:394, 1986.
69. Martin X, Uffer S, Gailloud C: Ophthalmia nodosa and the oculoglandular syndrome of Parinaud. Br J Ophthalmol 70:536, 1986.
70. Cuchural GJ Jr, Tally JP, Jacobus NV, et al: Comparative activities of newer beta-lactam agents against members of the *Bacteroides fragilis* group. Antimicrob Agents Chemother 34:479, 1990.
71. Ho PC, O'Day DM, Head WS: Fulminating panophthalmitis due to exogenous infection with *Bacillus cereus*: Report of 4 cases. Br J Ophthalmol 66:205, 1982.
72. Boldt HC, Pulido JS, Blodi CF, et al: Rural endophthalmitis. Ophthalmology 96:1722, 1989.
73. Gigantelli JW, Torres Gomez J, Osato HS: In vitro susceptibilities of ocular *Bacillus cereus* isolates to clindamycin, gentamicin, and vancomycin alone or in combination. Antimicrob Agents Chemother 35:201, 1991.
74. Dougherty JM, McCulley JP: Comparative bacteriology of chronic blepharitis. Br J Ophthalmol 68:526, 1984.
75. Meisler DM, Mandelbaum S: *Propionibacterium*-associated endophthalmitis after extracapsular cataract extraction: Review of reported cases. Ophthalmology 96(1):54, 1989.
76. Barlett JG: Antibiotic-associated pseudomembranous colitis. Rev Infect Dis 1:530, 1979.
77. Zaidman GW, Coudron P, Piros J: *Listeria monocytogenes* keratitis. Am J Ophthalmol 109(3):334, 1990.
78. Ralph RA, Lemp MA, Liss G: *Nocardia asteroides* keratitis: A case report. Br J Ophthalmol 60:104, 1976.
79. Hirst LW, Merz WG, Green WR: *Nocardia asteroides* corneal ulcer. Am J Ophthalmol 94:123, 1982.
80. Lissner, GS, O'Grady R, Choromokos E: Endogenous intraocular *Nocardia asteroides* in Hodgkin's disease. Am J Ophthalmol 86:388, 1976.
81. Lass JH, Thoft RA, Bellows AR, Slansky HH: Exogenous *Nocardia asteroides* endophthalmitis associated with malignant glaucoma. Ann Ophthalmol 13:317, 1981.
82. Abrutyn E: New uses for old drugs. Infect Dis Clin North Am 3:653, 1989.
83. Cohen JI, Saragas SJ: Endophthalmitis due to *Mycobacterium avium* in a patient with AIDS. Ann Ophthalmol 22:47, 1990.
84. Sanchez PJ, Regan JA: Vertical transmission of *Ureaplasma urealyticum* from mothers to preterm infants. Pediatr Infect Dis J 9:398, 1990.
85. Murray PR, Drew WL: Medical Microbiology. St. Louis, CV Mosby, 1990, p 254.
86. Wirostko E, Johnson L, Wirostko B: Ulcerative colitis associated chronic uveitis, parasitization of intraocular leukocytes by mollicute-like organisms. J Submicrosc Cytol Pathol 22:231, 1990.
87. Macomber PB: Cancer and cell wall deficient bacteria. Med Hypotheses 32:1, 1990.
88. Saari KM: Acute anterior uveitis and HLA antigens. Acta Ophthalmol 165:18, 1984.

89. Urbaschek B, Urbaschek R: Introduction and summary: Perspectives on bacterial pathogenesis and host defense. Rev Infect Dis 9 (Suppl 5):S431, 1987.
90. Jawetz E, Melnick JL, Adelberg EA: Review of Medical Microbiology, 17th ed. Los Altos, CA, Lange, 1987, p 162.
91. Evans, AS: Bacterial infections of Humans. *In* Epidemiological Concepts. New York, Plenum Press, 1991, p 15.
92. Aly R, Shinefield HI, Strauss WG, Maich HI: Bacterial adherence to nasal mucosal cells. Infect Immun 17:546, 1977.
93. Mims CA: The Pathogenesis of Infectious Disease, 3rd ed. New York, Academic Press/Grune & Stratton, 1987, p 57.
94. Urbaschek, B, Urbaschek R: Introduction and summary: Perspectives on bacterial pathogenesis and host defense. Rev Infect Dis 9 (Suppl 5):S431, 1987.
95. Kolenbrander PE: Environmental sensing mechanisms and virulence factors of bacterial pathogens. *In* Balows A, Duerden BI (eds): Topley & Wilson's Microbiology and Microbial Infection. Vol 2: Systematic Bacteriology. Oxford, Oxford University Press, 1998, pp 307–326.
96. Galen JE: Molecular genetic basis of *Salmonella* entry into host cells. Mol Microbiol 20:263, 1996.
97. Virji M: Mechanisms of microbial adhesion; the paradigms of *Neisseriae*. *In* McCrae MA, Saunders JR, Smyth CJ, Stow ND (eds): Molecular Aspects of Host-Pathogen Interactions. Cambridge, Cambridge University Press, 1997, pp 95–110.
98. Roth JA: Virulence Mechanisms of Bacterial Pathogens. Washington, DC, American Society for Microbiology, 1988, p 3.
99. Marshall KC (ed): Microbial Adhesion and Aggregation. New York, Springer-Verlag, 1984, pp 397–399.
100. Costerton JW, Marrie TJ, Cheng KJ: Phenomena of bacterial adhesion. *In* Savage DC, Fletcher MM (eds): Bacterial Adhesion: Mechanisms and Physiological Significance. New York, Plenum, 1985, pp 3–43.
101. Freter R: Mechanisms of association of bacteria and mucosal surfaces, *In* Elliott K, O'Connor M, Whelan J (eds): Adhesion and Microorganism Pathogenicity. CIBA Foundation Symposium 80. London, Pitman Medical, 1981, pp 36–55.
102. Gibbons RJ: Bacterial adhesion to oral tissues: A model for infectious diseases. J Dent Res 68:750, 1989.
103. Andersson B, Svanborg-Eden C: Attachment of *Streptococcus pneumoniae* to human pharyngeal epithelial cells. Respiration 55 (Suppl 1):49, 1989.
104. Jann K, Hoschutzky H: Nature and organization of adhesins. Curr Top Microbiol Immunol 132:56, 1986.
105. Jones GW, Isaacson RE: Proteinaceous bacterial adhesins and their receptors. Crit Rev Microbiol 10:229, 1983.
106. Lark DL: Protein-Carbohydrate Integrations in Biologic Systems. New York, Academic Press, 1986.
107. Stephens DS: Gonococcal and meningococcal pathogenesis as defined by human cell, cell culture, and organ culture assays. Clin Microbiol Rev S2:S104, 1989.
108. Swanson J: Gonococcal adherence: Selected topics. Rev Infect Dis 5:S678, 1983.
109. Stephens DS: Gonococcal and meningococcal pathogenesis as defined by human cell, cell culture, and organ culture assays. Clin Microbiol Rev S2:S104, 1989.
110. Aly R, Shinefield HI, Strauss WG, Maich HI: Bacterial adherence to nasal mucosal cells. Infect Immun 17:546, 1977.
111. Ellen RP, Gibbons RJ: M protein-associated adherence of *Streptococcus pyogenes* to epithelial surface: Prerequisite for virulence. Infect Immun 5:826, 1972.
112. Ellen RP, Gibbons RJ: Parameters affecting the adherence and tissue tropisms of *Streptococcus pyogenes*. Infect Immun 9:85, 1973.
113. Beachey EH, Ofek I: Epithelial cell binding of group A streptococci by the lipoteichoic acid on fimbriae denuded of M protein. J Exp Med 143:759, 1976.
114. Carruthers MM, Kabat WJ: Mediation of staphylococcal adherence to mucosal cells by lipoteichoic acid. Infect Immun 40:444, 1983.
115. Espersen F, Clemmensen I: Isolation of a fibronectin-binding protein from *Staphylococcus aureus*. Infect Immun 37:526, 1982.
116. Courtney HS, Ofek I, Simpson WA, et al: Binding of *Streptococcus pyogenes* to soluble and insoluble fibronectin. Infect Immun 53:454, 1986.
117. Kuusela P: Fibronectin binds to *Staphylococcus aureus*. Nature 276:718, 1978.
118. Switalski LM, Ryden C, Rubin K, et al: Binding of fibronectin to *Staphylococcus* strains. Infect Immun 42:628, 1983.
119. Switalski LM, Ljungh A, Ryden C, et al: Binding of fibronectin to the surface of Group A, C, and G streptococci. Eur J Clin Microbiol 1:381, 1982.
120. Abraham SM, Beachey EH, Simpson WA: Adherence of *Streptococcus pyogenes, Escherichia coli*, and *Pseudomonas aeruginosa* to fibronectin-coated and uncoated epithelial cells. Infect Immun 412:1261, 1983.
121. Wicken JA, Know KW: Lipoteichoic acids: A new class of bacterial antigens. Science 187:1161, 1975.
122. Raynor RH, Scott DF, Best GK: Lipoteichoic acid inhibition of phagocytosis of *Staphylococcus aureus* by human polymorphonuclear leukocytes. Clin Immunol Immunopathol 19:181, 1981.
123. Noble MA, Grant SK, Hajen E: Characterization of a neutrophil-inhibitory factor from clinically significant *Staphylococcus epidermidis*. J Infect Dis 162:909, 1990.
124. Ramphal R, McNeice MT, Polack FA: Adherence of *Pseudomonas aeruginosa* to the mouse cornea: A step in the pathogenesis of corneal infections. Ann Ophthalmol 13:421, 1981.
125. Stern GA, Weitzenkorn D, Valenti J: Adherence of *Pseudomonas aeruginosa* to the mouse cornea: Epithelial vs stromal adherence. Arch Ophthalmol 100:1956, 1982.
126. Badenoch PR, Coster DJ: Antibiotics and corticosteroids: Functions and interaction in ocular disease. *In* Cavanagh HD (ed): The Cornea: Transactions of the World Congress on the Cornea III. New York, Raven Press, 1988, p 475.
127. Gristina AG, Oga M, Webb LX, Hobgood CD: Adherent bacterial colonization in the pathogenesis of osteomyelitis. Science 228:900, 1985.
128. Stern GA, Lubniewski A, Allen C: The interaction between *Pseudomonas aeruginosa* and the corneal epithelium: An electron microscopic study. Arch Ophthalmol 103:1221, 1985.
129. Koch JM, Refojo MF, Hanninen LA, et al: Experimental *Pseudomonas aeruginosa* keratitis from extended wear of soft contact lenses. Arch Ophthalmol 118:1453, 1990.
130. Trancassini M, Magni A, Ghezzi MC, et al: Role of alkaline protease and elastase in the adherence of *Pseudomonas aeruginosa* to WEHI cells. Microbiologica 12:257, 1989.
131. Deighton MA, Balkau B: Adherence measured by microtiter assay as a virulence marker for *Staphylococcus epidermidis* infections. J Clin Microbiol 28:2442, 1990.
132. Staley, TE, Jones EW, Corley LD: Attachment and penetration of *Escherichia coli* into the intestinal epithelium of the ileum of newborn pigs. Am J Pathol 56:371, 1969.
133. Melly MA, Duke LF, Liau DF, Hash JH: Biological properties of the encapsulated *Staphylococcus aureus*. Infect Immun 10:39, 1974.
134. Koenig MG, Melly MA, Rogers DE: Factors relating to the virulence of staphylococci: Observations on four mouse pathogenic strains. J Exp Med 116:589, 1962.
135. Yoshida K, Takeuchi Y: Comparison of compact and diffuse variants of strains of *Staphylococcus aureus*. Infect Immun 2:523, 1970.
136. Wiley BB: The incidence of encapsulated staphylococci and anticapsular antibodies in normal humans. Can J Microbiol 9:27, 1963.
137. Wiley BB, Maverakis NH: Capsule production and virulence among strains of *Staphylococcus aureus*. Ann N Y Acad Sci 236:221, 1974.
138. Munson RS Jr: *Haemophilus influenzae*: Surface antigens and aspects of virulence. Can J Vet Res 54 (Suppl):363, 1990.
139. Brook I: Pathogenicity of the *Bacteroides fragilis* group. Ann Clin Lab Sci 19:360, 1989.
140. Wilkinson BJ, Sisson SP, Kim Y, Peterson PK: Localization of the third component of complement on the cell wall of encapsulated *Staphylococcus aureus* M: Implications for the mechanisms of resistance to phagocytosis. Infect Immun 26:1159, 1979.
141. Peterson PK, Schmeling D, Cleary PP, et al: Inhibition of alternative complement pathway opsonization by group A streptococcal M-protein. J Infect Dis 139:575, 1981.
142. Gemmell CG, Peterson PK, Schmeling D, et al: Potentiation of opsonization and phagocytosis of *Streptococcus pyogenes* following growth in the presence of clindamycin. J Clin Invest 67:1249, 1981.
143. Wessels MR, Rubens CE, Benedi VJ, Kasper DL: Definition of a bacterial virulence factor: Sialylation of the group B streptococcal capsule. Proc Natl Acad Sci U S A 86(22): 8983, 1989.
144. Pei Z, Blaser MJ: Pathogenesis of *Campylobacter* fetus infections: Role of surface array proteins in virulence in a mouse model. J Clin Invest 85:1036, 1990.
145. Costerton JW, Lam J, Lam K, Chan R: The role of the microcolony mode of growth in the pathogenesis of *Pseudomonas aeruginosa* infections. Rev Infect Dis 5:S867, 1983.

146. Marcus H, Baker NR: Quantitation of adherence of mucoid and nonmucoid *Pseudomonas aeruginosa* to hamster tracheal epithelium. Infect Immun 47:723, 1985.
147. Austin RM, Daniels CA: The role of protein A in the attachment of staphylococci to infected cells. Lab Invest 39:128, 1978.
148. Barrett SP: Protein-mediated adhesion of *Staphylococcus aureus* to silicone implant polymer. J Med Microbiol 20:249, 1985.
149. Goding JW: Use of staphylococcal protein A as an immunological reagent. J Immunol Methods 20:241, 1978.
150. Richman DD: The use of staphylococcal protein A in diagnostic virology. Curr Top Microbiol Immunol 104:159, 1983.
151. Mjyhre EB, Kronvall G: Heterogeneity of nonimmune immunoglobulin Gc reactivity among gram-positive cocci: Description of three major types of receptors for human immunoglobulin G. Infect Immun 17:475, 1977.
152. Andersson B, Ericksson B, Falsen E, et al: Adhesion of *Streptococcus pneumoniae* to human pharyngeal epithelial cells in vitro: Differences in adhesive capacity among strains isolated from subjects with otitis media, septicemia, or meningitis or from healthy carriers. Infect Immun 32:311, 1981.
153. Ellen RP, Gibbons RJ: Parameters affecting the adherence of tissue tropisms of *Streptococcus pyogenes*. Infect Immun 9:85, 1974.
154. Ramphal R: The role of bacterial adhesion in cystic fibrosis including the staphylococcal aspect. Infection 18:61, 1990.
155. Reichert R, Stern G: Quantitative adherence of bacterial to human corneal epithelial cells. Arch Ophthalmol 102:1394, 1984.
156. Foster TJ, Hartford O and O'Donnell D: Host-pathogen protein-protein interactions in *Staphylococcus*. *In* McCrae MA, Saunders JR, Smyth CJ, Stow ND (eds): Molecular Aspects of Host-Pathogen Interactions. Cambridge, Cambridge University Press, 1997, pp 67–94.
157. Moulder JW: Comparative biology of intracellular parasitism. Microbiol Rev 49:298, 1985.
158. Gorby GL, Robinson EN Jr, Barley LR, et al: Microbial invasion: A covert activity? Can J Microbiol 34:507, 1988.
159. Chan J, Fujiwawara T, Brennan P, et al: Microbial glycolipids: Possible virulence factors that scavenge oxygen radicals. Proc Natl Acad Sci U S A 86:2453, 1989.
160. Whitnack E, Beachey E: Biochemical and biological properties of the binding of human fibrinogen to M protein in group A streptococci. J Bacteriol 164:350, 1985.
161. Whitnack E, Beachey EH: Inhibition of complement-mediated opsonization and phagocytosis of *Streptococcus pyogenes* by fragments of fibrinogen and fibrin bound to cell surface M protein. J Exp Med 162:1283, 1985.
162. Whitnack E, Beachey E: Biochemical and biological properties of the binding of human fibrinogen to M protein in group A streptococci. J Bacteriol 164:350, 1985.
163. Paton JC, Ferrante A: Inhibition of human polymorphonuclear leukocyte respiratory burst, bactericidal activity and migration by pneumolysin. Infect Immun 41:1212, 1983.
164. Johnson MK, Boese-Marrazzo D, Pierce WA Jr: Effects of pneumolysin on human polymorphonuclear leukocytes and platelets. Infect Immun 34:171, 1981.
165. Reichert R, Stern G: Quantitative adherence of bacteria to human corneal epithelial cells. Arch Ophthalmol 102:1394, 1984.
166. Howe TR, Iglewski BH: Alkaline protease deficient mutants of *Pseudomonas aeruginosa:* Isolation and characterization in vitro and in a mouse eye model. Infect Immun 43:1058, 1984.
167. Ohman DEA, Burns RP, Iglewski BH: Corneal infections of mice with toxin A and elastase mutants of *Pseudomonas aeruginosa*. J Infect Dis 142:547, 1980.
168. Liu PV: Extracellular toxins of *Pseudomonas aeruginosa*. J Infect Dis 130:94, 1974.
169. Berk RS, Brown D, Coutinho I, Meyers D: In vivo studies with two phospholipase C fractions from *Pseudomonas aeruginosa*. Infect Immun 55:1728, 1987.
170. Heck LW, Morihara K, Abrahamson D: Degradation of soluble laminin and depletion of tissue-associated basement membrane laminin by *Pseudomonas aeruginosa* elastase and alkaline protease. Infect Immun 54:149, 1986.
171. Johnson MK, Allen JH: The role of hemolysin in corneal infections with *Pseudomonas aeruginosa*. Invest Ophthalmol Vis Sci 17:480, 1978.
172. Nicas TI, Iglewski BH: The contribution of exoproducts to virulence of *Pseudomonas aeruginosa*. Can J Microbiol 31:387, 1985.
173. Burns FR, Paterson CA, Gray RD, Wells JT: Inhibition of *Pseudomonas aeruginosa* elastase and *Pseudomonas* keratitis using a thiol-based peptide. Antimicrob Agents Chemother 34(11):2065, 1990.
174. Lemp MA: Is the dry eye contact lens wearer at risk? Yes. Cornea 9 (Suppl 1): S48, 1990.
175. Baum JL: Current concepts in ophthalmology: Ocular infections. N Engl J Med 299:8, 1978.
176. Gibbons RJ: Bacterial adherence to mucosal surfaces and its inhibition by secretory antibodies. *In* Mestecky J, Lawton AR (eds): The Immunoglobulin A System. New York, Plenum Press, 1974, pp 315–321.
177. Williams RC, Gibbon RJ: Inhibition of bacterial adherence by secretory immunoglobulin A. Science 177:6897, 1972.
178. Chandler JW: Immunology of the ocular surface. Int Ophthalmol Clin 25:13, 1985.
179. Coyle PK, Sibony PA: Tear immunoglobulins measured by ELISA. Invest Ophthalmol Vis Sci 27:622, 1986.
180. Smolin G: Immunology of ocular infections. *In* Duane TD, Jaeger EA (eds): Biomedical Foundations of Ophthalmology, vol 2. Philadelphia, Harper & Row, 1985.
181. Burdon DW: The bactericidal action of immunoglobulin A. J Med Microbiol 6:131, 1973.
182. Luckasen JR, Sobad A, Goltz RW: T and B lymphocytes in atopic eczema. Arch Dermatol 110:375, 1974.
183. Gordon DL, Hostetter MK: Complement and host defense against microorganisms. Pathology 18:365, 1986.
184. Palestine AG, Meyern SM, Fauci AS, Gallin JI: Ocular findings in patients with neutrophil dysfunction. Am J Ophthalmol 95:598, 1983.
185. Rayner RH, Wary BB, et al: Neutrophil function studies in patients with elevated serum IgE levels and recurring *Staphylococcus aureus* infections. Clin Immunol Immunopathol 17:372, 1980.
186. Chastel C, Youinou P, Leglise MC, et al: Dissociated impairment of neutrophil dysfunctions and recurrent infections. Infection 10:125, 1982.
187. Peterson PK, Wilkinson BJ, Kim Y, et al: The key role of peptidoglycan in the opsonization of *Staphylococcus aureus*. J Clin Invest 61:597, 1978.
188. Wilkinson BJ, Kim Y, Peterson PK, et al: Activation of complement by cell surface components of *Staphylococcus aureus*. Infect Immun 20:388, 1978.
189. Paton JC, Rowan-Kelley B, Ferrante A: Activation of human complement by the pneumococcal toxin pneumolysin. Infect Immun 43: 1085, 1984.
190. Greenblatt J, Boackle RJ, Schwab JH: Activation of the alternative complement pathway by peptidoglycan from streptococcal cell wall. Infect Immun 19:296, 1978.
191. Winkelstein JA, Tomasz A: Activation of the alternative complement pathway by pneumococcal cell wall teichoic acid. J Immunol 120: 174, 1978.
192. Baker CJ, Edwards MS, Webb BJ, Kasper DL: Antibody-independent classical pathway mediated opsonophagocytosis of type 1a group B streptococcus. J Clin Invest 69:394, 1982.
193. Leist-Welsh P, Bjornson AB: Immunoglobulin-independent utilization of the classical complement pathway in opsonophagocytosis of *Escherichia coli* by human peripheral leukocytes. J Immunol 128:2643, 1982.
194. Fearson DT, Austen KF: The alternative pathway of complement: A system for host resistance to microbial infection. N Engl J Med 303:259, 1980.
195. Mondino BL, Rabin BS, Kessler E, et al: Corneal rings with gram-negative bacteria. Arch Ophthalmol 95:2222, 1977.
196. Gewurz HC, Mold J, Fiedel B: C-reactive protein and the acute phase response. Adv Intern Med 27:345, 1982.
197. Badenoch PR, Finlay-Jones JJ, Coster DJ: Enzymatic disaggregation of the infected rat cornea. Invest Ophthalmol Vis Sci 24:253, 1983.
198. Limberg MB, Margo CE, Lyman GH: Eosinophils in corneas removed by penetrating keratoplasty. Br J Ophthalmol 70:343, 1986.
199. Kao WWY, Ebert J, Kao CWC, et al: Development of monoclonal antibodies recognizing collagenase from rabbit PMN; the presence of this enzyme in ulcerating corneas. Curr Eye Res 5:801, 1986.
200. Cullor JS, Mannis MJ, Murphy CJ, et al: In vitro antimicrobial activity of defensins against ocular pathogens. Arch Ophthalmol 108:861, 1990
201. Van de Waters L, Destree AT, Hynes RO: Fibronectin binds to some bacteria but does not promote their uptake by phagocytic cells. Science 220:201, 1983.
202. Lanser MC, Saba TM: Fibronectin as a co-factor necessary for optimal granulocyte phagocytosis of *Staphylococcus aureus*. J Reticuloendothel Soc 30:414, 1981.

203. Verbrugh HA, Peterson PK, Smith DE, et al: Human fibronectin binding to staphylococcal surface protein and its relative inefficiency in promoting phagocytosis by human polymorphonuclear leukocytes, monocytes and alveolar macrophages. Infect Immun 33:811, 1981.
204. Courtney JS, Simpson WA, Beachey EH: Binding of streptococcal lipoteichoic acid to fatty acid-binding sites on human plasma fibronectin. J Bacteriol 153:763, 1983.
205. Ryden C, Rubin K, Speziale P, et al: Fibronectin receptors from *Staphylococcus aureus*. J Biol Chem 258:3396, 1983.
206. Proctor RA, Prendergast E, Mosher DF: Fibronectin mediates attachment of *Staphylococcus aureus* to human neutrophils. Blood 559: 681, 1982.
207. Proctor RA, Mosher DF, Olbrantz PJ: Fibronectin binding to *Staphylococcus aureus*. J Biol Chem 257:1478, 1982.
208. Jacobs PF, Kiel DP, Sanders ML, Steele RW: Phagocytosis of type III group B streptococci by neonatal monocytes: Enhancement by fibronectin and gamma globulin. J Infect Dis 152:695, 1985.
209. Chipman DM, Nathan S: Mechanism of lysozyme action. Science 165:454, 1969.
210. Velos P, Cherry PMH, Miller D: An improved method for measuring human tear lysozyme concentration. Arch Ophthalmol 103:31, 1985.
211. Sen DK, Sarin GS: Immunoassay of tear lysozyme in conjunctival diseases. Br J Ophthalmol 66:732, 1982.
212. Pietsch RL, Pearlman ME: Human tear lysozyme variable. Arch Ophthalmol 90:94, 1973.
213. Bonavida B, Sapse AT: Human tear lysozyme. Am J Ophthalmol 66:70, 1968.
214. Erickson OF: The absence of lysozyme in Sjögren's syndrome. Stanford Med Bull 13:292, 1955.
215. Mackie IA, Seal DV: Quantitative tear lysozyme assay in units of activity per microliter. Br J Ophthalmol 60:70, 1976.
216. Jay JM: Production of lysozyme by staphylococci and its correlation with three other extracellular substances. J Bacteriol 91:1804, 1966.
217. Schindler CA, Schudardt VT: Lysostaphin: A new bacteriolytic agent for the *Staphylococcus*. Proc Natl Acad Sci U S A 51:414, 1964.
218. Cisani G, Varaldo PE, Grazi G, Soro O: High-level potentiation of lysostaphin anti-staphylococcal activity by lysozyme. Antimicrob Agents Chemother 21:531, 1982.
219. Martinez RJ, Carroll SF: Sequential metabolic expression of the lethal process in human serum-tested *Escherichia* cells. Infect Immun 28:735, 1980.
220. Van Snick JL, Masson PL, Heremans JF: The involvement of lactoferrin in the hyposideraemia of acute inflammation. J Exp Med 140:1068, 1974.
221. Woolcock JB: Bacterial resistance to humoral defense mechanisms: An overview. *In* Roth JA (ed): Virulence Mechanisms of Bacterial Pathogens. Washington, DC, American Society for Microbiology, 1984, p 73.
222. Joiner KA, Brown EJ, Frank MM: Complement and bacteria: Chemistry and biology in host defense. Annu Rev Immunol 2:461, 1984.
223. Friedman MG: Antibodies in human tears during and after infection. Surv Ophthalmol 35:151, 1990.
224. Berk RS, Montgomery IN, Hazlett LD: Serum antibody and ocular responses to murine corneal infection caused by *Pseudomonas aeruginosa*. Infect Immun 56:3076, 1988.
225. Moon MM, Hazlett LD, Hancock RE, et al: Monoclonal antibodies provide protection against ocular *Pseudomonas aeruginosa* infection. Invest Ophthalmol Vis Sci 29:1277, 1988.
226. Griffiss JM, Bertram MA: Immunoepidemiology of meningococcal disease in military recruits. II: Blocking of serum bactericidal activity by circulating IgA early in the course of invasive disease. J Infect Dis 136:733, 1977.
227. Dziarski R: Modulation of mitogenic responsiveness by staphylococcal peptidoglycan. Infect Immun 30:431, 1980.
228. Orga PL, Wallace RB, Omana G: Implications of secretory immune system in viral infections. Adv Exp Med Biol 45:271, 1973.
229. David JR, David RR: Cellular hypersensitivity and immunity: Inhibition of macrophage migration and the lymphocyte mediators. Prog Allergy 16:300, 1972.
230. Baughn RE, Bonventre PF: Cell-mediated immune phenomena induced by lymphokines from splenic lymphocytes of mice with chronic staphylococcal infection. Infect Immunol 11:313, 1975.
231. Rasanen L, Arvilommi H: Cell walls, peptidoglycans, and teichoic acids of gram-positive bacteria as polyclonal inducers and immunomodulators of respiratory burst, bactericidal activity and migration by pneumolysin. Infect Immun 41:1212, 1983.
232. Levison AI, Dziarski A, Zweiman B, Dziarski R: Staphylococcal peptidoglycan. Infect Immun 39:290, 1983.
233. Clagget JA, Engle D: Polyclonal activation: A form of primitive immunity and its possible role in the pathogenesis of inflammatory disease. Dev Comp Immunol 2:235, 1978.
234. Moller E, Strom H, Al-Balaghi S: Role of polyclonal activation in specific immune responses. Scand J Immunol 12:177, 1980.
235. Rasanen L, Karhumaki E, Majuri R, Arvilommi H: Polyclonal activation of human lymphocytes by bacteria. Infect Immun 28:368, 1980.
236. Onderdonk AB, Cisneros RL, Finberg R, et al: Animal model system for studying virulence of and host response to *Bacteroides fragilis*. Rev Infect Dis 12 (Suppl 2):S169, 1990.
237. Toffaletti DL, Schwab JH: Modulation of lymphocyte functions by group A streptococcal membrane. Cell Immunol 42:3, 1979.
238. Jones DB, Liesegang TJ, Robinson NM: Laboratory diagnosis of ocular infections. *In* Washington JA II (ed): Cumitech 13, Cumulative Techniques and Procedures in Clinical Microbiology, Washington DC, American Society for Microbiology, 1981, p 10.
239. Dougherty J. Personal communication, 1991.
240. Forster RK, Zachary IG, Cottingham AJ Jr, Norton EWD: Further observations of the diagnosis, etiology and treatment of endophthalmitis. Trans Am Ophthalmol Soc 72:226, 1975.
241. Koul S, Philipson A, Arvidson S: Role of aqueous and vitreous cultures in diagnosing infectious endophthalmitis in rabbits. Acta Ophthalmol 68:466, 1990.
242. Thayer JD, Martin JE Jr: Improved medium selective for cultivation of *Neisseria gonorrhoeae* and *Neisseria meningitidis*. Public Health Rep 81:559, 1966.
243. MacConkey AT: Bile salt media and their advantages in some bacteriological examinations. J Hyg 8:322, 1908.
244. Bell H: Media, reagents and stains. *In* Wentworth BB (ed): Diagnostic Procedures for Bacterial Infections, 7th ed. Washington, DC, American Public Health Association, 1987, pp 773–835.
245. Finegold SM, Shepard WE, Spaulding EH: *In* Shepard WE (ed): Cumitech 5, Practical Anaerobic Bacteriology. Washington, DC, American Society for Microbiology, 1977.
246. Perry LD, Brinser JH, Kolodner H: Anaerobic corneal ulcers. Ophthalmology 89:636, 1982.
247. Brinser JH, Burd EM: Principles of diagnostic ocular microbiology. *In* Tabbara KF, Hynduik RA (eds): Infections of the Eye. Boston, Little Brown, 1977, p 77.
248. Grayson M: Diseases of the Cornea. St. Louis, CV Mosby, 1983, p 53.
249. Edward AI: Fundamentals of Microbiology, 3rd ed. Menlo Park, CA, Benjamin-Cummings, 1991, p 85.
250. Lauer BA, Reller LB, Mirrett S: Comparison of acridine orange and Gram stain for detection of microorganisms in cerebrospinal fluid and other clinical specimens. J Clin Microbiol 14:201, 1981.
251. Kronvall G, Myhre E: Differential staining of bacteria in clinical specimens using acridine orange buffered at low pH. Acta Pathol Microbiol Scand 85:249, 1977.
252. Robin JB, Arffa RC, Avni I, Rao NA: Rapid visualization of three common fungi using fluorescein-conjugated lectins. Invest Ophthalmol Vis Sci 27:500, 1986.
253. Baker CJ, Rench MA: Commercial latex agglutination for detection of group B streptococcal antigen in body fluid. J Pediatr 102:393, 1983.
254. Sobol WM, Gomez JT, Osato MS, Wilhelmus KR: Rapid streptococcal antigen detection in experimental keratitis. Am J Ophthalmol 107:60, 1989.
255. Paul PS: Applications of nucleic acid probes in veterinary infectious diseases. Vet Microbiol 24:409, 1990.
256. Duerden BI, Towner KJ, Mcgee JT: Isolation, description and identification of bacteria. *In* Balows A, Duerden BI (eds): Topley & Wilson's Microbiology and Microbial Infections. Vol 2: Systematic Bacteriology. Oxford, Oxford University Press, 1998, pp 65–84.
257. Romond C: New diagnostic methods for anaerobic bacteria. Scand J Infect Dis 62(Suppl):35, 1989.
258. Martin R, Schneider WA: Chromatography for the identification of microorganisms. *In* Wentworth BB (ed): Diagnostic Procedures for Bacterial Infections. Washington, DC, American Public Health Association, 1987, p 703.
259. Bochner B: "Breath prints" at the microbial level: An automated redox-based technology quickly identifies bacteria according to their metabolic capacities. ASM 55:536, 1989.
260. Miller JM, Rhoden DL: Preliminary evaluation of Biolog, a carbon source utilization method for bacterial identification. J Clin Microbiol 29:1143, 1991.

261. Barry AL, Joyce IJ, Aams AP, Benner EJ: Rapid determination of antimicrobial susceptibility for urgent clinical situations. Am J Clin Pathol 59:693, 1973.
262. Bauer AW, Kirby WMM, Sherris JC, Turck M: Antibiotic susceptibility testing by a standardized single disc method. Am J Clin Pathol 45:493, 1966.
263. Barry AL: Antimicrobial susceptibility testing. *In* Hoeprich PD, Jordan MC (eds): Infectious Diseases, 4th ed. Philadelphia, JB Lippincott, 1989, p 162.
264. Barry AL, Jones RN: A three-category system for interpretation of disk tests for *Pseudomonas*-active penicillins and β-lactamase hydrolysis/inhibition studies. J Antimicrob Chemother 9(Suppl A):35, 1982.
265. Barry AL, Carcia F, Trupp LD: An improved single disc method for testing the antibiotic susceptibility of rapidly growing pathogens. Am J Clin Pathol 53:149, 1970.
266. National Committee for Clinical Laboratory Standards: Approved Standard M2-A3. Performance Standards for Antimicrobial Disk Susceptibility Tests, 3rd ed. Villanova, PA, National Committee for Clinical Laboratory Standards, 1984.
267. Ormerod LD, Heseltine PN, Alfonso E, et al: Gentamicin-resistant pseudomonal infections. Cornea 8:195, 1989.
268. Gelender H, Rettich C: Gentamicin-resistant *Pseudomonas aeruginosa* corneal ulcers. Cornea 3:21, 1984.
269. Ellner PD, Neu HC: The inhibitory quotient: A method for interpreting minimum inhibitory concentration data. JAMA 246:1575, 1981.
270. D'Amato RF, Jochstein L, Vernaleo JR, Cleri JF: Evaluation of the BIOGRAM Antimicrobial Susceptibility Test System. 85th Annual Meeting of the American Society for Microbiology, Washington, DC, 1985, p 314.
271. Cohen RL: Instrument systems which utilize a conventional incubation period. *In* Jorgensen JH (ed): Automation in Clinical Microbiology. Boca Raton, FL, CRC Press, 1987, p 81.
272. Washington JA: In vitro testing of antimicrobial agents. Infect Dis Clin North Am 3:375, 1989.
273. Brumfitt W, Hamilton-Miller J: Methicillin-resistant *Staphylococcus aureus*. N Engl J Med 320:1188, 1989.
274. Brumfitt W, Hamilton-Miller J: Methicillin-resistant *Staphylococcus aureus*. N Engl J Med 320:1192, 1989.
275. Hansen SL, Freedy PK: Variation in abilities of automated, commercial, and reference methods to detect methicillin-resistant (heteroresistant) *Staphylococcus aureus*. J Clin Microbiol 20:494, 1984.
276. National Committee for Clinical Laboratory Standards: Standard Methods for Dilution Antimicrobial Susceptibility Tests for Bacteria Which Grow Aerobically. Approved Standard M7-A. Villanova, PA, National Committee for Clinical Laboratory Standards, 1985.
277. National Committee for Clinical Laboratory Standards: Methods for Determining Bactericidal Activity of Antimicrobial Agents. Approved Standard M-26P. Villanova, PA, National Committee for Clinical Laboratory Standards, 1986.
278. Sanders CC, Sanders WE Jr: Microbial resistance to newer generation β-lactam antibiotics: Clinical and laboratory implications. J Infect Dis 157:399, 1985.
279. Ernst JD, Sande MA: In vitro susceptibility testing and the outcome of treatment of infections. *In* Root RK, Sande MA (eds): New Dimensions in Antimicrobial Therapy. New York, Churchill Livingstone, 1984.
280. Neu HC: General concepts on the chemotherapy of infectious diseases. Med Clin North Am 76:1051, 1987.
281. Schlichter JG, MacLean H: A method of determining the effective therapeutic level in the treatment of subacute bacterial endocarditis with penicillin: A preliminary report. Am Heart J 34:209. 1947.
282. Jordon GW, Kawachi MM: Analysis of serum bactericidal activity in endocarditis, osteomyelitis and other bacterial infections. Medicine 60:49, 1981.
283. Levison ME, Bush LM: Pharmacodynamics of antimicrobial agents. Infect Dis Clin North Am 3:415, 1989.
284. Levin BR: Conditions for the evolution of multiple antibiotic resistance plasmids: A theoretical and experimental excursion. *In* Baumberg S, Young JPW, Willington EMH, Saunders JR (eds): Population Genetics of Bacteria Society for General Microbiol, Symposium 52. Cambridge, Cambridge University Press, 1995, pp 175–192.
285. O'Callaghan CH, Morris A, Kirby SM, Shingler AH: Novel method for detection of β-lactamase by using a chromogenic cephalosporin substrate. Antimicrob Agents Chemother 1:283, 1972.
286. Davis JL, Koidou-Tsiligianni A, Pflugfelder SC, et al: Coagulase-negative staphylococcal endophthalmitis, increased in antibiotic resistance. Ophthalmology 95:1404, 1988.
287. Spratt BG: Resistance to antibiotics mediated by target alterations. Science 264:388, 1994.
288. Lyon BR, Skurray RA: Antimicrobial resistance of *Staphylococcus aureus*: Genetic basis. Microbiol Res 51:89, 1987.
289. Cookson BD, Bolton MC, Platt JH: Chlorhexidine resistance in *Staphylococcus aureus* or just an elevated MIC? An in vitro and in vivo assessment. Antimicrob Agent Chem Ther 35:1997, 1993.
290. Russell AD: Microbial susceptibility and resistance to chemical and physical agents. *In* Balows A, Duerden BI (eds): Topley & Wilson's Microbiology and Microbial Infections. Vol 2: Systematic Bacteriology. Oxford, Oxford University Press, 1998, pp 149–184.
291. Hendley JO, Ashe KM: Topical antimicrobial treatment of aerobic bacteria in the human skin. Antimicrob Agents Chemother 35:627, 1991.

CHAPTER 12

Chlamydial Disease

Joseph M. Thomas, Alfred D. Heggie, and Jonathan H. Lass

Anatomy, Physiology, and Life Cycle of the Microorganism

TAXONOMY

The genus *Chlamydia* is composed of three species, *C. trachomatis, C. psittaci,* and *C. pneumoniae.* Humans are the natural hosts of *C. trachomatis* and *C. pneumoniae.* These species have no animal reservoirs, and transmission is from human to human. Birds and some mammals are the natural hosts of *C. psittaci.* Humans usually acquire infection by contact with infected birds. Although the three species have been considered to be related, the DNA homology among them is less than 10%.[1, 2] All three species produce intracytoplasmic inclusions that have different characteristics

(Table 12–1). Inclusions of *C. trachomatis* are single, contain fewer cells than inclusions of the other species, and therefore stain in a vacuolar pattern.[3, 4] Inclusions produced by *C. psittaci,* in contrast, are tightly packed with chlamydial cells and stain densely with Giemsa's stain. They are frequently multiple. The inclusions of *C. pneumoniae* are similar in density of staining to those of *C. psittaci* but are usually single.[5] Only the inclusions of *C. trachomatis* contain glycogen and stain brown with iodine.[4, 6] *C. trachomatis* can synthesize folate, whereas *C. psittaci* and *C. pneumoniae* use folate synthesized by the host cell. Consequently, only *C. trachomatis* is inhibited by folate antagonists such as sulfonamides.[7]

MICROBIAL CHARACTERISTICS

For many years *Chlamydia* organisms were considered viruses, because they can replicate only in living cells and are very small organisms with diameters of 200 to 1500 nm, depending on the stage of the developmental cycle. Technologic advances eventually revealed that, like bacteria but unlike viruses, *Chlamydia* have the following characteristics: (1) they contain both DNA and RNA,[8] (2) they replicate by binary fission, (3) they possess a cell wall, and (4) their replication is inhibited by several antimicrobial drugs. These characteristics clearly identify them as bacteria. Unlike other bacteria, however, they are unable to synthesize adenosine triphosphate or to otherwise produce metabolic energy.[9] Therefore, they have adapted to an intracellular existence, using the host cell for energy production. Although this dependence on the cell might appear to be restrictive, the high prevalence of chlamydial infections in humans and birds suggests that adaptation of *Chlamydia* to obligate intracellular parasitism offers some evolutionary advantage.

MORPHOLOGY AND LIFE CYCLE

The elementary body (EB) is the infectious particle of all chlamydial species. The EB of *C. trachomatis* and of *C. psittaci* is a spherical particle approximately 300 nm in diameter. The EB of *C. pneumoniae* is of similar size but is pear-shaped. All EBs are adapted for extracellular survival by being metabolically inactive and possessing a rigid, relatively impermeable cell wall (Fig. 12–1*A*). The structure of the EB cell wall is similar to that of gram-negative bacteria, except that it does not contain peptidoglycan.[10] Cross-linking of outer membrane proteins by disulfide bonds probably accounts for the rigidity and low permeability of the EB cell wall.[11–14] Examination of the inner structure of the EB reveals an electron-dense core of nucleic acids.[15] The chlamydial life cycle (Fig. 12–2) is initiated when EBs attach to cells of the susceptible host and enter the cell by a process of parasite-induced endocytosis.[16] Ingestion by the host cell results in formation of a phagosome containing the EB, but phagolysosomal fusion does not occur and the organism is protected from digestion by lysozymes.[17] The chlamydial phagosome, or inclusion body, is transported to a juxtanuclear position that corresponds to the peri-Golgi region. The inclusion body then intercepts cellular metabolites being transported from the Golgi apparatus to the cell membrane via the trans-Golgi exocytic pathway.[18, 19] Approximately 8 hours after entering the cell, the EB reorganizes into a reticulate body (RB), so-called because of the dispersed fibrillar pattern of its nucleic acids (see Fig. 12–1*B*).[20, 21] The RB is the replicative phase in the life cycle of *Chlamydia.* Transition of EB to RB is associated with loss of infectivity, an increase in diameter to 800 to 1000 nm, and an increase in ratio of DNA to RNA from 1:1 in the EB to 3:1 in the RB.[20] This change in DNA:RNA ratio corresponds to the increased rate of metabolic activity in the RB compared with the metabolically inert EB. Also during transition, the cell wall changes from rigid and impermeable in the EB to flexible and permeable in the RB. These changes are thought to result from reduction of cross-linked disulfide bonds in the outer membrane proteins by the intraphagosomal reducing conditions to which the EB is exposed after endocytosis.[13, 22, 23] The increased permeability of the RB cell wall permits uptake of adenosine triphosphate and nutrients from the host cell. RBs typically line the inner margin of the inclusion body membrane, probably to facilitate incorporation and use of intercepted cell metabolites. This contrasts with the metabolically inactive EBs that appear to be distributed randomly throughout the interior of the inclusion.[4, 24] RBs then replicate by binary fission until the original phagosome becomes distended by its content of several hundred to more than 1000 chlamydial cells. As RB replication proceeds, the reducing power of the microenvironment probably decreases, and free sulfhydryl groups are oxidized, forming disulfides. This restores the rigidity and impermeability of the cell wall and produces a decrease in the rate of metabolism coincident with reorganization of RB into EB.[13] At this point, approximately 48 hours after attachment of the infecting EB to the host cell, the cell and its one or more intracytoplasmic inclusions rupture, and the newly formed EBs are released into the extracellular milieu, from which they can infect other cells or a new host.[25]

TABLE 12–1. **Characteristics of Chlamydial Species**

Characteristic	*C. trachomatis*	*C. psittaci*	*C. pneumoniae*
Natural hosts	Humans	Birds, animals	Humans
Major human diseases	Trachoma, genital infections, neonatal conjunctivitis, infant pneumonia	Pneumonia	Pneumonia, bronchitis
Serovars (no.)	18	Unknown	1
Morphology of cytoplasmic inclusions	Single, vacuolar	Multiple, dense	Single, dense
Inclusions contain glycogen, stain with iodine?	Yes	No	No
Synthesize folate?	Yes	No	No
Inhibited by sulfonamides?	Yes	No	No

ANTIGENS

A microimmunofluorescence test using murine antisera and a radioimmunoassay using monoclonal antibodies have iden-

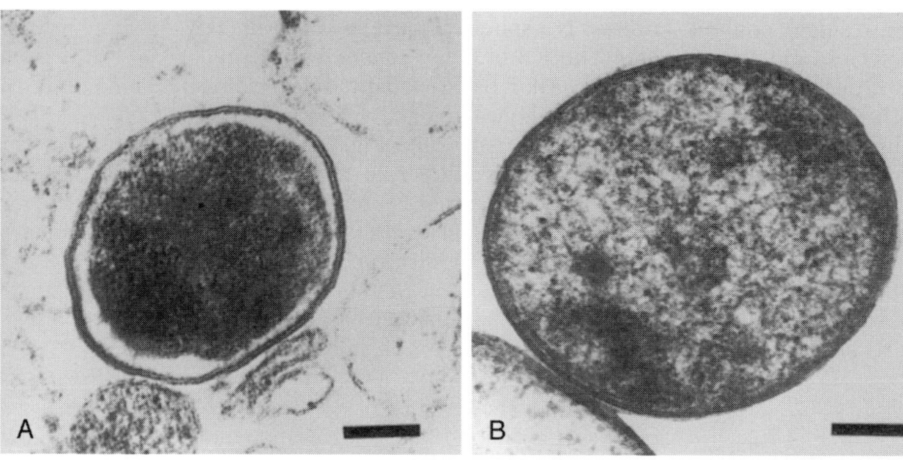

FIGURE 12–1. Electron micrographs of *Chlamydia trachomatis* showing *(A)* an EB with cell wall and electron-dense core of nucleic acids and *(B)* an RB with DNA and ribosomes distributed in a fibrillar pattern. RB is characteristically larger than EB (bars = 0.1 mm). (From Clark RB, Nachamkin I, Schatzki PF, et al: Localization of distinct surface antigens on *Chlamydia trachomatis* HAR-13 by immune electron microscopy with monoclonal antibodies. Infect Immun 38:1273, 1982.)

tified 15 serovars (i.e., serotypes) of *C. trachomatis*.[26, 27] Serovars A, B, Ba, and C are usually isolated from the eyes of persons living in areas of endemic trachoma and are seldom encountered in nontrachomatous areas.[28] Serovars D through K are seldom associated with trachoma but are the most prevalent sexually transmitted pathogens in industrialized societies.[29–31] They cause approximately 50% of cases of nongonococcal urethritis and are frequent causes of cervicitis, salpingitis, and epididymitis (Table 12–2). Ocular infection with these serovars results in inclusion conjunctivitis. Serovars L1, L2, and L3 are the agents of lymphogranuloma venereum.[28] Three additional serovars of *C. trachomatis* have more recently been identified.[32] Their proposed designations are Da, Ia, and L2a. Serologic subtypes of *C. psittaci* and *C. pneumoniae* have not been described.

Molecular evaluation of the major outer membrane protein (MOMP) gene (*omp*1) offers a more precise method of characterizing *C. trachomatis* than does immunotyping by microimmunofluorescence.[33] Allelic polymorphism at the *omp*1 locus is the basis for MOMP variation.[33] Determination of *omp*1 genotypes will be useful in epidemiologic studies to identify reservoirs and transmission patterns of *C. trachomatis* and to select candidate strains for vaccine development.[33]

Attachment of EB to cell
Endocytosis
Phagosome containing EB
Phagolysosoma fusion does not occur
Time 0
Reorganization and enlargement of EB into RB
8 hrs
Movement of phagosome toward nucleus and initial replication of RB by binary fission
18 hrs
Continued replication of RB lining phagosomal membrane
24 hrs
Reorganization of RB to EB
Mature cytoplasmic inclusion
40–72 hrs
Cell rupture with extrusion of EB
• = Elementary Body (EB)
o = Reticulate Body (RB)
N = Cell Nucleus
Life cycle of Chlamydia

FIGURE 12–2. Life cycle of *Chlamydia* organisms.

The genus-specific antigen shared by all chlamydiae is a glycoprotein that is similar in structure to the lipopolysaccharide found in the outer membranes of gram-negative bacteria.[34] It is present in the outer membranes of both EBs and RBs. Species-specific and type-specific antigens of *C. trachomatis* are located in another protein, designated as the MOMP.[35–37] MOMP, the principal protein surface component of this species, constitutes approximately 60% of its outer membrane and has a molecular mass of 38 to 42 kDa.[38–40] Genetic mapping has shown MOMP to consist of five conserved segments interspersed with four short variable domains.[35] The first and second variable domains contain serotype-specific epitopes. Epitopes of the fourth variable domain have species and subspecies specificity.[37] A number of other antigens associated with species and serotype specificity have also been identified in *C. trachomatis*;[41] however, the antigenic determinants in MOMP are immunodominant, because they are located on the surface of the organism and are probably more immunoaccessible than these other antigens.[42] Part of the reason that *C. trachomatis* evades the host's immunologic defenses is MOMP antigenic variation resulting from single-site mutation at the *omp*1 locus or recombination producing a novel mosaic antigen gene.[33] In addition to antigens incorporated into the chlamydial cell structure, soluble antigens that are released into the supernatant fluids of cell cultures infected by *C. trachomatis* have been described.[43, 44] These soluble antigens may be released into the microenvironment during infection in vivo and may provoke immunopathogenic responses in the host.[41]

TABLE 12–2. **Association of Serovars of *Chlamydia trachomatis* With Human Diseases**

Human Disease	Associated Serovars
Trachoma	A, B, Ba, C
Genital infections, conjunctivitis	D, Da, E, F, G, H, I, Ia, J, K
Lymphogranuloma venereum	L1, L2, L2a, L3

Systemic Infection of the Host

INFECTION AND INFLAMMATORY RESPONSE

The oculogenital serovars of *C. trachomatis* (A through K) can infect any squamocolumnar epithelial mucosa. Lymphogranuloma venereum serovars are more invasive and can infect lymph nodes and associated structures. *C. psittaci* can infect a wide variety of tissues and organs.[45] Chlamydial infections elicit an inflammatory response that consists initially of a mixture of lymphocytes and polymorphonuclear leukocytes (PMNs), the latter predominating.[46–50] Chemotaxis of PMNs probably results from activation of the complement cascade and generation of the chemotaxin C5a.[51] Sequential observations in animal models have shown that as infection with *C. trachomatis* progresses, the inflammatory response is characterized by a change from PMNs to a predominance of lymphocytes and by the formation of lymphoid follicles on infected mucosal surfaces.[52–55] Formation of lymphoid follicles is also a characteristic of human ocular and genital chlamydial infections.[56–58]

The inflammatory response probably serves as a defense mechanism to limit spread and hasten elimination of chlamydial infections. PMNs have been shown to ingest and kill chlamydial EBs.[59–61] PMNs probably serve as a first line of defense by phagocytosing EBs during initial exposure of the host and impede spread of infection by phagocytosing EBs released into the extracellular milieu during subsequent chlamydial growth cycles. The role of lymphocytes is incompletely understood, but intact lymphocyte function is apparently important, because duration of infection and infection-related mortality rates from the mouse pneumonitis strain of *C. trachomatis* were greater in athymic nude mice than in immunocompetent animals.[62–65] Genital infection by the same strain of *C. trachomatis* lasted longer in nude mice than in normal controls.[66] Similarly, guinea pigs treated with antithymocyte serum to suppress cell-mediated immune function were unable to eliminate genital infection by the guinea pig inclusion conjunctivitis strain of *C. psittaci*.[67]

ANTIBODY RESPONSE

C. trachomatis infections cause immunoglobulin M (IgM) and IgG antibodies to appear in the serum and IgG and IgA antibodies to appear in mucosal secretions.[68–70] These antibodies are directed against several chlamydial antigens, including MOMP, as well as 60-kDa and 75-kDa proteins.[71, 72] Monospecific antibodies against the 75-kDa protein neutralized *C. trachomatis* in cell culture.[73] Following a primary infection, IgM antibody against the chlamydial serovar involved persists for approximately a month. IgG antibody persists much longer.[68]

Our understanding of the role of antibody in natural infection is incomplete. In vitro, EBs that have been exposed to antibody fail to replicate in cell culture, although they attach to the cells and induce endocytosis.[74–76] In the mouse, high levels of serum antibody protect against the mouse pneumonitis strain of *C. trachomatis*.[65] In contrast, preexisting serum antibodies in humans do not appear to protect against infection. Most persons in groups at high risk for sexually transmitted infections have serum antibodies but are subject to repeated infections. Reinfection sometimes results from exposure to a previously unencountered chlamydial serovar or genotype; however, a study of recurrent infections with serovar E of *C. trachomatis* detected no relationship between preexisting serovar-specific antibody and reinfection.[71] Consistent with these findings is the observation that infants become infected with maternal serovars of *C. trachomatis* even if they acquired maternal IgG antibody transplacentally.[77]

Serum antibody appears to be important, however, in containment and resolution of chlamydial infections. In guinea pig inclusion conjunctivitis (GPIC), produced by a strain of *C. psittaci*, disease was more prolonged, severe, and invasive when the humoral antibody response was suppressed.[78, 79] In a study of women with cervical *C. trachomatis* infection who underwent elective abortion without prior antichlamydial treatment, ascending infection and salpingitis occurred less frequently in patients who had higher titers of serum antibodies.[72] Although infection occurs at birth in infants with congenital *C. trachomatis* infection, the incidence of pneumonia is highest during the second and third months of life, a period that coincides with the decline in titer of transplacentally acquired antibodies.[80]

CELL-MEDIATED IMMUNE RESPONSE

Cell-mediated immune responses (CMIs) to chlamydial infections, as detected by antigen-directed lymphocyte proliferation assays, have been demonstrated in both humans and animals.[60, 75–81] CMIs in animals have also been demonstrated by induction of footpad swelling in response to local antigen injection in the mouse pneumonitis model of chlamydial infection.[88] CMI appears to contribute to control and resolution of infection. For example, transfer of T cells from mice with normal immune function confers protection against the prolonged infection and high mortality otherwise observed in athymic mice infected with the mouse pneumonitis agent.[64] The same serovar of *C. trachomatis* also produces nonresolving genital infections in athymic mice but not in mice with an intact CMI.[66] Induction of cytotoxic T lymphocytes is another CMI mechanism that may be important in the resolution of chlamydial infections. In a study of mice previously infected with *C. psittaci*, spleen cells from the animals were found to be cytotoxic for cultures of L cells infected with the same organism.[89] Similarly, supernatant fluid from mutagen-treated suspensions of spleen cells from mice infected with *C. psittaci* was toxic for cultures of infected mouse fibroblasts.[90] In contrast, lymphoid cells from mice infected with *C. trachomatis* were not found to be cytotoxic for cultures of chlamydia-infected L929 cells.[91] It was speculated that absence of chlamydial antigens on the surfaces of infected L929 cells may have accounted for failure to induce cytotoxicity. Examination of *C. trachomatis*–specific cloned human T cells also demonstrated lack of toxicity against infected cells in culture.[92] Additional studies in mice infected with *C. trachomatis* have detected cytotoxicity mediated by the cytokine interferon-γ (IFN-γ).[93] Although cytotoxicity was directed principally against chlamydia-infected cells, nonspecific cytotoxicity against uninfected cells was also noted. Injury to uninfected cells was mediated by tumor necrosis factor-α (TNF-α).[94] Further studies are needed to delineate the role of CMI in chlamydial infections.

SPECTRUM OF *CHLAMYDIA TRACHOMATIS* INFECTIONS

Because *C. trachomatis* can infect columnar or transitional epithelium at any anatomic site, multiple-organ involvement is possible. The most frequently infected sites are those most accessible to contamination by infected mucosal secretions. Thus, the external genital tract, conjunctivae, and upper respiratory tract are most often involved. From these external sites, infection can spread within an organ system and result in infection of structures that are protected against primary contact with this pathogen (e.g., salpingitis, epididymitis, pneumonitis, perihepatitis).[26, 95–98] Infection can also spread from one infected external site to another (e.g., urethra, cervix, rectum, conjunctivae) by natural drainage of infected secretions or poor personal hygiene. Figure 12–3 summarizes frequently infected sites.

Susceptibility to Antimicrobial Drugs

Because chlamydial cell walls do not contain peptidoglycan, and because β-lactam antibiotics such as penicillin exert some of their antimicrobial action by inhibiting peptidoglycan synthesis, this class of antibiotics would be expected to have little effect on chlamydial replication. *Chlamydia* organisms have penicillin-binding proteins; in cell cultures infected by *C. psittaci*, penicillin inhibits replication of RBs and their reorganization into EBs.[99, 100] D-Cycloserine, another inhibitor of peptidoglycan synthesis, also interferes with chlamydial replication.[101, 102] This suggests that chlamydial cell walls contain peptides that are cross-linked to compounds other than peptidoglycan,[10] but despite their ability to inhibit chlamydial replication, β-lactam antibiotics are ineffective against chlamydial infections. This may be explained by two facts: Chlamydiae are intracellular parasites and penicillin penetrates poorly into intracellular spaces, and the effect of penicillin on *Chlamydia* is only inhibitory, not chlamydicidal.[103] In cell culture, the inhibitory effect of penicillin on replication of *C. trachomatis* can be reversed by replacing the penicillin medium with an antibiotic-free one.[104]

Erythromycin and the tetracyclines block chlamydial protein synthesis by inhibition of the 50S and 30S ribosomal subunits, respectively.[105] They achieve much greater intracellular concentrations than β-lactam antibiotics, and although their action is bacteriostatic, they are effective therapeutic agents in the treatment of chlamydial infections.[103]

More recently, a multicenter study showed that azithromycin is an effective single-dose treatment of adult urethral and endocervical infections caused by *C. trachomatis*. The drug belongs to a group of antibiotics known as azolides. It differs structurally from the macrolide erythromycin, by the insertion of a methyl-substituted nitrogen at position 9a in the lactose ring, creating a 15-member ring structure.[99a]

The study involved 299 female and 158 male patients with uncomplicated genital infections and test-proven *C. trachomatis* infection. They were randomly assigned to receive either a single dose of 1 g of azithromycin orally or 100 mg of doxycycline orally twice a day for 7 days. Of the patients evaluated at 21 to 35 days after treatment, cultures were positive in none of the 112 treated with azithromycin and in 1 of the 102 patients treated with doxycycline.[106]

A randomized, single-blind study of two Gambian villages assessed the effectiveness and safety of a single oral dose of 20 mg/kg of azithromycin compared with conventional treatment (6 weeks of topical tetracycline plus oral erythromycin for severe cases) in ocular *C. trachomatis* infection. By 6 months' follow-up, trachoma had resolved in 76 (78%) of 97 subjects who received azithromycin compared with 70 (72%) of 97 who were treated conventionally. Of note, pregnant and lactating women were excluded from the study because no adequate or well-controlled studies have involved the use of azithromycin on this population. In addition, although more than 92% of the patients treated were 11 years of age or younger, azithromycin is not yet approved for treatment of persons younger than 16 years of age.[107]

Host-Microbe Interaction in the Eye

NATURAL HISTORY OF TRACHOMA

Blinding trachoma, the end-stage of a chronic process caused by repeated infections with *C. trachomatis*, occurs in impoverished and uneducated populations living under conditions of poor personal and community hygiene.[108–110] The disease is particularly prevalent in the Middle East and parts of southeast Asia. In hyperendemic areas, infection is acquired during infancy, and most children are infected by age 2 years.[111] Primary infection induces purulent follicular conjunctivitis (except during the neonatal period). The follicles consist of lymphoid germinal centers.[112] Because lymphoid tissue is absent from the conjunctivae of neonates, lymphoid follicles do not form. Infection at this age produces acute purulent conjunctivitis, but the tissue reaction is one of papillary hypertrophy.[113] The primary infection resolves spontaneously and induces transient protective immunity. In endemic areas, however, reinfection is inevitable. The same serovar of *C. trachomatis* is often transmitted reciprocally among members of a household.[114] With repeated infections, healing is associated with central degeneration and necrosis

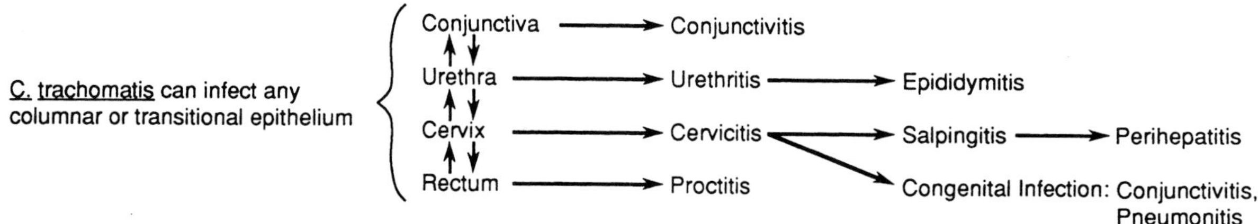

FIGURE 12–3. Spectrum and routes of spread of *Chlamydia trachomatis* infections. Because *C. trachomatis* can infect any columnar or transitional epithelium, infection may involve several organ systems.

of lymphoid follicles, thinning of the overlying conjunctival epithelium, and proliferation of fibroblasts, resulting in fibroses and scarring.[115] Uninterrupted progression of this process eventually converts the normally smooth and lubricating conjunctival epithelium into one that is xerotic and cicatrized. Extensive fibrosis produces entropion and trichiasis. End-stage blindness is the result of corneal drying, ulceration, and scarring.

PATHOGENESIS OF TRACHOMA

Studies in Humans

The observation that repeated chlamydial infections are characteristic of the course of blinding trachoma has led to the concept that the disease constitutes an immunopathologic response of the host to *C. trachomatis* infections.[28, 114, 116] The initial infection presumably induces immune sensitization of the host but only transient or incomplete protective immunity. Reinfections or relapses result in intensified inflammatory reactions, fibrosis, scarring, and pannus formation. Clinical observations support this hypothesis. In vaccine studies using inactivated EB as antigen, recipients immunized with an antigen dose that proved to be inadequate to induce immunity against infection developed more severe disease with subsequent infections than did unvaccinated controls.[117] Reinfection also frequently results in exacerbation of trachoma.[114–116] Consistent with this observation is a report that trachoma did not progress further in persons who moved from an endemic to a nonendemic area where they were no longer exposed to the pathogen.[118] Immunopathogenesis is further evidenced by the finding that in trachoma-endemic areas, proliferative responses of peripheral blood lymphocytes to stimulation by chlamydial antigens, a marker of CMI, are more common in patients with trachoma than in controls without disease.[119]

The apparent genetic susceptibility to trachoma further supports this concept. In a study in Gambia, the frequencies of the human leukocyte antigen (HLA) complex class I antigen, HLA-A28, and the A′6806 allele were significantly greater in patients with trachoma than in age-, sex-, and location-matched controls.[120] Immunopathology may be associated with HLA-A′6802–restricted T-lymphocyte responses. In chlamydia-associated involuntary tubal infertility, another disease of suspected immunopathogenic origin, antibodies to the 60-kDa *C. trachomatis* heat shock protein, a putative immunopathogenic antigen, are more common in affected individuals than in controls.[70, 121–124] Heat shock or stress proteins are produced by all prokaryotic and eukaryotic cells in response to damaging stimuli such as elevated environmental temperature.[125] They are major antigens of many pathogens and appear to be important to the immune response, including immune surveillance and autoimmunity.[125, 126] In mice, the immune response to the 60-kDa heat shock protein of *C. trachomatis* is genetically controlled.[127] This observation adds support to the concept that the outcome of chlamydial infections in humans may also have a genetic component.

Studies in Animals

Animal experiments support the hypothesis that trachoma is an immunopathologic process induced by repeated ocular infections with *C. trachomatis*. In studies with *Macaca cyclopis* monkeys that received conjunctival inoculations of yolk sac preparations of *C. trachomatis*, Wang, Grayston, and Alexander reported that progressive conjunctival and limbal scarring and pannus formation occurred only in animals that had received more than one chlamydial inoculation or that had previously been immunized with an experimental trachoma vaccine.[128–130] These investigators were the first to suggest that hypersensitivity to the trachoma agent, which then was classified as a virus, is an important factor in the pathogenesis of this disease. Monnickendam and Darougar also produced progressive ocular disease in guinea pigs by repeated conjunctival inoculation with the GPIC strain of *C. psittaci*.[131]

In 1981, Taylor and coworkers developed a primate model in which trachoma could be induced by repeated weekly conjunctival inoculations of live *C. trachomatis* serovar E, a frequent cause of genital infections in humans.[53] Both rhesus and cynomolgus monkeys were used. The latter species developed more severe disease with a progressive course that mimics human disease. Initial infection produced follicular conjunctivitis. Infiltration with T and B lymphocytes occurred. B lymphocytes were localized to conjunctival follicles, whereas T lymphocytes showed a perifollicular distribution.[132, 133] Ten to 100 times more chlamydia-specific lymphocytes accumulated in the conjunctivae than in the peripheral circulation during the peak inflammatory response.[134] Fine linear conjunctival scarring occurred 3 to 6 weeks after the initial infection, and fine "basketweave" conjunctival scarring developed between 7 and 21 weeks. Conjunctival scarring continued to progress throughout the 54-week course of the experiment. Dilatation of limbal blood vessels and early pannus formation occurred at approximately 6 weeks, but these abnormalities resolved during the next 4 to 5 weeks. At 16 weeks, the animals developed midstromal corneal haze and opacification of corneal nerves at the point of entry into the cornea. All monkeys were seronegative prior to infection and became seropositive for *C. trachomatis* during the study. Similar results were reported when the experiment was repeated using *C. trachomatis* serovar A instead of serovar E.[135] In trachoma-endemic areas, serovar A is a frequent cause of ocular infections. This suggests that repeated ocular infection induces trachoma, regardless of what serovar is involved. In studies of both serovars, the inflammatory reaction decreased in severity with repeated inoculations, and *Chlamydia* could not be reisolated from the eyes after six to eight weekly inoculations, despite continuation of the inoculations. This is consistent with the fact that *C. trachomatis* can seldom be isolated from the eyes of humans with advanced trachoma. As in humans, chronic eye changes continued to progress in the monkeys. This progression of disease in the absence of detectable *Chlamydia* organisms suggests that the immune response is partially protective, but continued antigenic stimulation elicits a pathologic immune response. Repeated inoculation with live organisms was essential to development of chronic disease. The response to substitution of formalin-inactivated EBs for inoculation following initial infection with live organisms was only minimal.[136]

Conjunctivitis caused by ocular pathogens other than *C. trachomatis* is prevalent in trachoma-endemic areas and has been suspected of increasing the severity and hastening the progression of trachoma.[137, 138] Nonchlamydial bacterial conjunctivitis has even been suggested to be an essential component of the disease process.[139] To examine the role of ocular superinfection in the pathogenesis of trachoma, researchers inoculated the conjunctivae of monkeys that had experimentally induced trachoma with *Haemophilus influenzae, Haemophilus aegyptius,* or *Streptococcus pneumoniae.* The severity of trachoma did not increase, indicating that in this model, chronic chlamydial infection alone is sufficient to produce trachoma.[140]

Because formalin inactivation of chlamydial EBs does not alter their surface antigens, failure of inactivated EBs to produce trachoma in the monkey model implies that surface antigens are not the stimuli essential to induction of trachoma.[140, 141] To identify the stimulating antigens, Taylor and coworkers initially infected cynomolgus monkeys with *C. trachomatis* and subsequently challenged them with MOMP, lipopolysaccharide, or a soluble triton extract prepared from EBs of *C. trachomatis* serovar B.[142, 143] MOMP and lipopolysaccharide failed to produce inflammation, but the soluble triton extract rapidly elicited an inflammatory response in the eyes of previously infected monkeys. Inoculation of the extract into the eyes of control animals (i.e., animals not previously infected with *C. trachomatis*) had no effect. This suggests that internal antigens rather than surface antigens are the stimuli involved in the pathogenesis of trachoma. Ocular delayed hypersensitivity was similarly demonstrated in guinea pigs previously infected with the GPIC strain of *C. psittaci* and then challenged by conjunctival instillation of triton extracts of GPIC or *C. trachomatis* EB.[144, 145] Extracts of both GPIC agent and *C. trachomatis* elicited inflammatory responses in the eyes of previously sensitized guinea pigs but not in unsensitized controls. A triton extract of GPIC EBs also produced an inflammatory response in the eyes of monkeys previously infected with *C. trachomatis,* suggesting that the sensitizing antigen is genus-specific rather than species-specific.[142] Lymphocytes in the inflammatory response were antigen-specific for *Chlamydia.*[133] In guinea pigs, infection of the conjunctivae, vagina, or intestine, but not intramuscular injection of live GPIC EBs, resulted in ocular sensitization and a delayed hypersensitivity reaction on subsequent conjunctival challenge with triton-extracted antigen. [145] This suggests that ocular hypersensitivity can be induced by prior infection of mucosal surfaces, not only of the eye but of other anatomic sites.

These observations in monkeys suggest that soluble products derived from chlamydial EBs may be important to the pathogenesis of trachoma. These products are genus-specific, because they can be extracted from EBs of both *C. trachomatis* and the GPIC strain of *C. psittaci.* Additional studies have identified 57- and 45-kDa proteins in the triton extract. In guinea pigs, only the 57-kDa protein elicits an ocular delayed hypersensitivity reaction.[146, 147] Other investigators have reported the release of soluble antigens into the microenvironment in studies of *C. trachomatis* in cell cultures.[43, 44] These antigens may also elicit responses that contribute to the immunopathogenesis of trachoma.[41]

Cytokines elaborated by the host in response to chlamydial infections may also be important to the progression of trachoma (Table 12–3). In animal studies, chlamydial infections induce host production of both IFN-γ and TNF-α.[93, 94] TNF-α stimulates collagenase, prostaglandin E_2, and hyaluronic acid production by human fibroblasts.[148, 149] IFN-γ also stimulates hyaluronic acid production, both alone and synergistically with TNF-α.[149] These observations suggest mechanisms by which chlamydial infections, particularly if they are recurrent or persistent, may result in destruction, fibrosis, and distortion of infected tissues.

TABLE 12–3. **Summary of Evidence for Immunopathogenesis of Trachoma**

Development of trachoma requires repeated ocular infections.
Reinfections cause intensified inflammatory reactions.
Subsequent ocular infections cause more severe inflammation in immunized humans and animals than in unimmunized controls.
A 57-kDa protein prepared from triton extracts of *C. trachomatis* and GPIC agent produces ocular inflammation in monkeys sensitized by prior chlamydial infection.
Chlamydial infections induce cytokine production that stimulates fibroblasts to produce collagenase, prostaglandin E_2, and hyaluronic acid.

Peeling and Brunham have written a useful review of chlamydiae as pathogens.[150]

INCLUSION CONJUNCTIVITIS

Neonatal Inclusion Conjunctivitis

C. trachomatis is the most frequent cause of neonatal conjunctivitis.[151–153] When a pregnant woman has cervical infection with *C. trachomatis* at the time of labor and delivery, the infant born per vaginam has an 18 to 50% chance of becoming infected, as determined by culture of various anatomic sites.[154] When measured by seroconversion, the rate of infection may be as high as 70%.[77] The conjunctivae of the infant delivered via an infected birth canal appear to be the usual site of initial infection; subsequently, infection spreads to the nasopharynx.[155] If untreated, the infection may involve the lower respiratory tract and cause pneumonia.[154, 156] The rectum and vagina may also become colonized.[157, 158] Almost all infants with conjunctival infection develop conjunctivitis within the first 3 weeks of life, which, even if it is not treated, is usually self-limited.[155] In industrialized nations, infants seldom become reinfected, and progression to trachoma does not occur. In cases of persistent or untreated infection, however, corneal micropannus and palpebral conjunctival scarring occur occasionally.[159–161]

Inclusion Conjunctivitis in Adults

In studies of adults in western Europe and in the United States that used culture techniques for detection of *C. trachomatis*, this organism was identified as the pathogen in as many as 9% of cases of acute conjunctivitis and 19% of cases of chronic conjunctivitis.[162–168] In one study that focused on patients 20 to 25 years of age, the isolation rate was 23%.[164] Adults with chlamydial conjunctivitis frequently have a concurrent genital infection. Presumably, poor personal hygiene results in contamination of the conjunctivae by infected genital secretions. Because repeated ocular infections are rare, corneal scarring, although reported, appears to be unusual.

Laboratory Diagnosis

CHLAMYDIA TRACHOMATIS

Cytologic Examination

C. trachomatis was discovered in 1907 by cytologic examination of conjunctival cells from patients with trachoma.[169] Until 1957, when *C. trachomatis* was successfully cultured in the yolk sacs of embryonated eggs, the only laboratory diagnostic test available to detect this agent was cytologic examination of stained smears of cells from tissues suspected to be infected.[170] The technique is still useful in the diagnosis of ocular chlamydial infections, especially when laboratory facilities are limited. In patients with trachoma or acute chlamydial conjunctivitis, the juxtanuclear cytoplasmic inclusions of *C. trachomatis* can often be detected in Giemsa-stained smears of conjunctival cells.[171] The test has the advantage of requiring a minimum of supplies and equipment; however, in chlamydial conjunctivitis, it is only 20 to 60% as sensitive as culture or other newer detection techniques discussed later in this chapter.[172–174] The Giemsa stain technique for detection of chlamydial inclusions in smears of conjunctival cells from cases of adult chlamydial conjunctivitis is particularly insensitive, although results are positive in as many as 95% of cases of neonatal chlamydial conjunctivitis.[168, 175] In a study of genital infections, the Giemsa method detected only 15% of infections of the male urethra and 41% of cervical infections.[175] Papanicolaou-stained cervical smears are also insensitive and nonspecific for detection of cervical infections.[176, 177]

Detection by Cell Culture

Because *C. trachomatis* is an obligate intracellular parasite, it replicates only in living cells. Although the organism was first successfully cultivated in the cells lining the yolk sacs of embryonated eggs, this method is labor-intensive and less sensitive than the cell culture technique that was developed several years later.[170, 178] The cell types most frequently used for cultivation and detection of *C. trachomatis* are McCoy cells, a mouse heteroploid line, and HeLa 229 cells, a line derived from a human epithelioid cervical carcinoma.[179, 180] A nutrient-rich cell culture medium is employed, and the cultures are treated with metabolic inhibitors such as cycloheximide or cytochalasin B to prevent the cells from competing with the parasite for nutrients.[181, 182] Despite this favorable microenvironment, *C. trachomatis*—except for serovars L1, L2, and L3—does not readily infect cell cultures. Infection requires enhancement by centrifugation of inoculated cultures at 2500 to 3000 × g for 60 minutes.[183, 184] Two explanations for such enhancement by centrifugation are that centrifugal force overcomes repellent electrostatic forces by precipitating chlamydial EBs onto cell surfaces, or that centrifugal force somehow alters cell membranes to make them more receptive to attachment by the organism.[185] In the case of HeLa 229 cells, pretreatment of cultures with the positively charged polycation, diethylaminoethyl (DEAE)-dextran, further enhances susceptibility of the cells to infection.[180, 186] DEAE-dextran pretreatment enhances the susceptibility of uncentrifuged McCoy cells but not of centrifuged ones.[187, 188] After inoculation, cultures are usually incubated for 72 hours at 35°C and then stained and examined for chlamydial cytoplasmic inclusion bodies. Giemsa's or iodine stains can be used to stain the inclusions; however, the sensitivity of the method is increased by staining with fluorescein-conjugated monoclonal antibody prepared against *C. trachomatis*.[189, 190] Chlamydial inclusions fluoresce with a bright apple-green color. Figure 12–4*A* shows an example of inclusions in an infected McCoy cell culture stained with fluorescein-conjugated monoclonal antibody.

The methods used for collection, transport, and storage of specimens containing *C. trachomatis* are critical to the success of detection by cell culture. If the organism dies during these procedures, attempts at culture are useless, because detection depends on infection and replication of viable organisms in the cell culture. Because *Chlamydia* organisms are present in infected epithelial cells and not in the exudate produced by infection, the specimen should contain as many epithelial cells as possible. To collect conjunctival specimens, one should cleanse the eye of exudate and swab the conjunctival surface with pressure sufficient to exfoliate cells. Swabs with metal or plastic shafts rather than

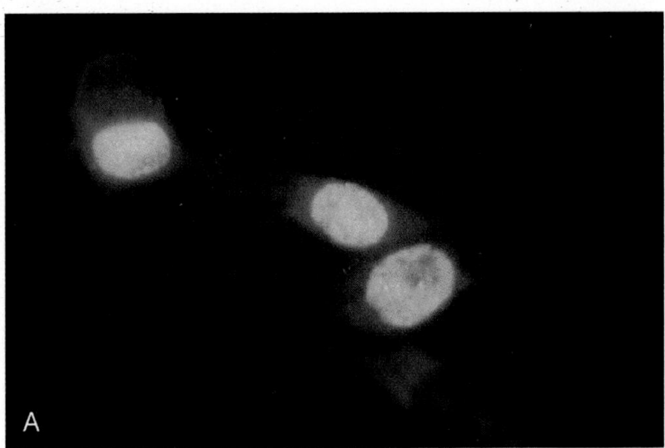

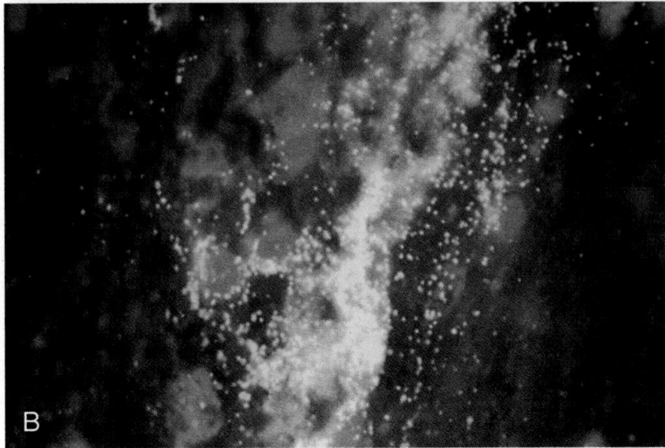

FIGURE 12–4. Diagnosis of *Chlamydia trachomatis* infections by immunofluorescence test with monoclonal antibodies. *A*, Fluorescein-conjugated antibody was reacted with McCoy cell culture 48 hours after infection with *C. trachomatis*. Fluorescing structures are intracytoplasmic chlamydial inclusions (×400). *B*, A direct cervical specimen from a patient with culture-confirmed chlamydial infection. Fluorescing material consists of single or clumped chlamydial EBs or RBs from infected and disrupted cervical mucosal cells (×630). (From Tam MR, Stamm WE, Handsfield HH, et al: Culture-independent diagnosis of *Chlamydia trachomatis* using monoclonal antibodies. N Engl J Med 310:1146, 1984.)

wood shafts are preferred, because toxic products from wood may be leached into the collection medium and have toxic effects on the cell culture into which it is inoculated. Sucrose phosphate buffer is frequently used as a collection medium.[175] Antibiotics to which *C. trachomatis* organisms are resistant are usually incorporated into the collection medium to inactivate contaminating bacteria that otherwise would grow in and destroy inoculated cell cultures. Viral collection media should not be used because they commonly contain antibiotics to which *Chlamydia* organisms are susceptible. After collection, specimens may be stored at 40°C if they are to be cultured within 24 to 48 hours. Specimens that cannot be cultured within that time frame should be stored at −70°C to retard inactivation.[191] Isolation rates are highest when specimens are cultured promptly after collection.

Cell cultures are considered the gold standard for detection of *C. trachomatis.* The sensitivity and specificity of all other tests for detection of the organism are compared with the results of isolation in cell culture. The principal disadvantages of cell culture are that (1) it may give false-negative results if the organism is inactivated by improper collection, transport, or storage; (2) it requires special laboratory facilities and experienced personnel, neither of which is generally available; (3) it takes several days to perform the test and obtain results; and (4) it is expensive.

Antigen Detection

Direct Staining of Specimens by Fluorescein-Conjugated Monoclonal Antibody (DFA). In this test, smears of cells obtained by swabbing infected mucous membranes are stained with fluorescein-conjugated monoclonal antibodies prepared against *C. trachomatis.* When examined under a fluorescent microscope, intact inclusion bodies or scattered EBs from ruptured cells fluoresce a bright apple-green. The technique was first used to detect urethral and cervical infections, but it is equally useful for detection of conjunctival infections.[192–197] Figure 12–4*B* shows a positive cervical smear. The test can also be used for rectal specimens, but the typically high concentrations of other bacteria in such specimens sometimes produce false-positive results from cross-reactive staining.[198] Compared with cell culture, the sensitivity of DFA testing in various reports has ranged from 70 to 100%, and specificity appears to be greater than 95%.[199] A study of neonatal conjunctivitis reported sensitivity of 100% and specificity of 94%.[152]

DFA testing has the following advantages: (1) Unlike cell culture, DFA detects both viable and nonviable *Chlamydia* organisms. Therefore, the rigorous transport and storage conditions that are essential for prevention of inactivation are unnecessary. (2) The test is more rapid than culture. Results are available in hours rather than days. (3) The cost of a DFA test is approximately a fourth that of culture. (4) The adequacy of the specimen can be assessed during the procedure by noting the presence or absence of columnar or cuboidal epithelial cells. Absence or paucity of these cells indicates an inadequate specimen. The technique also has certain disadvantages: (1) It requires a fluorescent microscope and an experienced microscopist. Evaluation of fluorescence is subjective, and smears can be misread by inexperienced workers. Reading requires intense concentration, and errors can result from examiner fatigue. (2) Cross-reactive staining sometimes occurs in specimens that contain large numbers of other bacteria. This is most common with rectal specimens and is seldom a problem in conjunctival specimens.

Enzyme Immunoassay. In enzyme immunoassay (EIA), *C. trachomatis* antigen is detected by a colorimetric signal generated by antigen-antibody reactions. Microscopy is not involved. The procedure is as follows: (1) The specimen is collected by swabbing, as was described for the DFA test, and the swab is immersed in collection medium. (2) Rabbit antichlamydial monoclonal antibody is permitted to bind to any chlamydial antigen in the specimen. (3) Antirabbit antibody conjugated to an enzyme is allowed to bind to the rabbit antibody that is bound to the chlamydial antigen. (4) A chemical substrate is added, which reacts with the enzyme conjugated to the antirabbit antibody. This reaction generates a color signal, the end-point of the test, that is read in a photometer. Washes are performed at critical points during the procedure to wash away unbound antibodies, so that if the specimen does not contain *C. trachomatis,* no color signal will be generated and the test result will read as negative.

Like DFA, EIA is quicker and less expensive than culture, and the viability of *C. trachomatis* organisms in the specimen is irrelevant to the validity of the test. The test has an objective end-point (photometric measurement of color intensity), in contrast with the subjective interpretation required by microscopic examination in DFA. However, the adequacy of the specimen (presence of epithelial cells) cannot be assessed by EIA. The sensitivity and specificity of EIA and DFA are approximately equivalent.[200–202] EIA has been reported to compare favorably with culture for the detection of ocular *Chlamydia* infections.[203, 204] Like DFA, EIA is less sensitive and specific than isolation of the organism in cell culture by an experienced laboratory.[205] Because the EIA procedure includes three 1-hour incubation periods, it takes approximately 5 hours for completion.[200] DFA, in contrast, can be performed in 30 to 60 minutes. Therefore, EIA is impractical for processing single or small numbers of specimens. When large numbers of specimens are processed, however, EIA requires less technologist time per specimen than DFA does because the objective (photometric) end-point of EIA makes the test much less labor-intensive than the microscopic examination required by DFA.

Nucleic Acid Probes

Nucleic acid probes for detection of bacteria utilize the principle that, under appropriate conditions, nucleic acids of a bacterial species hybridize with nucleic acids from that species but not with nucleic acids from other sources.[206] Very small amounts of nucleic acids can be detected by this technique. Therefore, diagnostic tests that apply this principle should be very sensitive and very specific. The application of this technology to the detection of *C. trachomatis* is new, and few studies have been performed. An assay in which a cryptic plasmid present in all serovars of *C. trachomatis* was used as a DNA probe was compared with culture and DFA for detection of ocular *C. trachomatis* infection in a trachoma-endemic area of Nepal.[207–209] Compared with chlamydial isolation by culture, the DNA probe had 87% sensitivity and 91% specificity. In another assay, the target of the chlamydial DNA probe is the ribosomal RNA of *C. trachomatis*.[210] For detection of the organism in cervical specimens, two studies found this assay to be 60% and 80% sensitive and 95% and 98% specific, respectively.[211, 212] Additional studies are required to determine the clinical utility of this technique.

Serologic Diagnosis

Chlamydial antibodies can be detected by complement fixation (CF), microimmunofluorescence (MIF) testing, and enzyme-linked immunosorbent assay (ELISA).[199] The CF test is relatively insensitive and detects antibodies to lymphogranuloma venereum (caused by serovars L1, L2, and L3) but not other serovars of *C. trachomatis*. MIF, in contrast, is a sensitive and specific test that detects both IgG- and IgM-class antibodies in serum, tears, and genital secretions.[213] Acute- and convalescent-phase serum antibody titers can be compared to demonstrate diagnostic rises in primary infections. However, many patients in groups at high risk of infection have experienced primary infections in the past and already have appreciable titers of IgG antibodies.[213] Reinfection with the same serovar of *C. trachomatis* does not induce an IgM-class response, and the anamnestic IgG-class antibody response may not be strong enough to be diagnostic. Another potential difficulty is that it is often impractical to obtain appropriately timed acute- and convalescent-phase serum samples. Therefore, although the MIF test is useful in epidemiologic studies, it has limited diagnostic application in *C. trachomatis* infections. Two exceptions are that detection of IgM-class antibodies has been shown to be a useful method for diagnosis of chlamydial pneumonia in infants, and the presence of IgG or IgA chlamydial antibodies in tears appears to correlate with disease activity in ocular infections with *C. trachomatis*.[213–216]

ELISA is sensitive in detecting *C. trachomatis* antibodies.[217–220] However, although correlation of ELISA results with MIF is good for IgG-class antibodies, discrepancies between results of the two tests are reported with IgM-class antibodies.[221, 222] This suggests that the ELISA IgM test lacks specificity. An improved solid-phase immunoassay for IgM-class antibodies has been reported to be 100% sensitive and specific for infants but only 85% sensitive and 76% specific for adults.[223] ELISA usually detects genus-specific rather than species-specific antibodies, and cross-reactivity among species-specific antibodies may occur,[199] which can prevent the technique from differentiating between antibody to *C. trachomatis* and to *C. pneumoniae*.

Amplified DNA Techniques

Nucleic acid amplification techniques such as polymerase chain reaction (PCR) and ligase chain reaction (LCR) involve exponential amplification of well-defined DNA targets, resulting in better sensitivity of detection than with other nonculture methods.[224] The precision of nucleic acid hybridization and the rapid amplification of a single gene target facilitated the design of diagnostic tests with specificities in excess of 99% and lower detection limits of 1 to 10 elementary bodies.[150] Another advantage of these tests is that the increased sensitivity allows for noninvasive methods, such as urine collection, which may likely improve compliance for diagnostic testing.[224]

In one study, a total of 530 male urine specimens were obtained from 322 symptomatic men with urethral symptoms and 208 asymptomatic men attending two sexually transmitted disease clinics. The prevalence of *C. trachomatis* by urethral culture was 9.8% and, compared with culture, the sensitivity of PCR was 95% and specificity was 99.8%.[224] Another study evaluated 472 asymptomatic men and evaluated PCR performance on urethral swab specimens as well as first void urine (FVU). Patients were considered infected if they were culture-positive or positive by PCR with both plasmid and major outer membrane protein-based primers. This extended gold standard revealed a prevalence of infection of 7.6%. The results showed sensitivities of 72% and 91%, respectively, with specificity higher than 99.7%. Cervical swab specimens were taken from 242 asymptomatic women. The prevalence of infection was 7.9%. PCR had 90% sensitivity and 99.3% specificity.[224]

A multicenter study compared detection of *C. trachomatis* plasmid DNA by LCR with detection by culture in 542 men attending sexually transmitted disease clinics (Study A). The second part of this study (Study B) compared LCR of FVU with urethral swab cultures from 1043 men. Discordant results were resolved with DFA staining of sediments from the FVU or urethral culture specimen with a second LCR directed against a fragment of the major outer membrane protein gene. The LCR plasmid assay had a sensitivity of 98.0% in Study A and 93.5% in Study B. Specificity was 99.8 to 100%. The sensitivity of culturing urethral swabs from all study centers was 68.2%.[226]

Another multicenter study evaluated cervical swab LCR to detect *C. trachomatis* in 2132 women from sexually transmitted disease clinics. The cell culture sensitivities varied from 53% to 92% among study sites, and the LCR sensitivity showed less variability with a range of 87 to 89%. The specificity of each test was greater than 99.9%.[227] A study of 447 women based the presence of infection on an expanded gold standard whereby a patient was determined to be infected by culture or by a confirmed nonculture test. The prevalence of infection was 6%. The sensitivity of urine LCR was 96% compared with 37% for urine EIA. Cervical swab culture was the least sensitive approach to diagnosis, with 56% and 78% sensitivity for cervical swab EIA.[228]

The excellent performance of molecular amplification techniques in detecting *C. trachomatis* suggests that they may become the test of choice for diagnosing and screening FVU in both men and women, urethral infection in men, and cervical swab specimens in women.

CHLAMYDIA PSITTACI AND *CHLAMYDIA PNEUMONIAE*

C. psittaci can be isolated from respiratory tract secretions, blood, and tissue biopsy specimens (spleen, liver) from patients with ornithosis (psittacosis). The organism can be isolated by inoculation of the yolk sac of embryonated eggs or of cell cultures of L cells or McCoy cells. *C. psittaci* inclusion bodies are detected by Giemsa staining of infected cell culture monolayers or impression smears of infected yolk sac membranes. The genus-specific CF test can be used for serologic diagnosis.

For isolation of *C. pneumoniae,* throat swabs or specimens of respiratory tract secretions are obtained and placed in the same transport medium that is used for *C. trachomatis. C. pneumoniae* was originally isolated in HeLa 229 cells, but HL, HEp-2, and H292 cell cultures have been reported to be more sensitive.[229–234] Inclusions in infected cells can be specifically identified by staining with fluorescein-conjugated monoclonal antibodies. Antibody responses specific for *C. pneumoniae* can be measured by a microimmunofluorescence test.[235] Methods for serologic diagnosis are being refined.[236]

Summary

Chlamydiae are specialized bacteria that have no capacity for producing metabolic energy and, therefore, are obligate intracellular parasites. Unlike other bacteria, their cell walls do not contain a peptidoglycan. Hence, β-lactam antibiotics are ineffective against chlamydial infections. *C. trachomatis* and *C. pneumoniae* are pathogens of humans and have no animal reservoirs. *C. trachomatis* is the most prevalent sexually transmitted pathogen in Western societies and an important cause of acute and chronic conjunctivitis, including trachoma. Protective immunity is transient; repeated infections often cause fibrosis and scarring of affected tissues, probably as the result of an immunopathologic process. *C. pneumoniae* is a recently described human pathogen that infects the upper and lower respiratory tract. *C. psittaci* is principally a pathogen of birds that causes pneumonia and systemic infection when transmitted to humans. Several recent reviews of the biology and pathogenesis of chlamydial infections have appeared in the literature.[237–240] If untreated, chlamydial infections tend to be persistent. Tetracyclines and erythromycin arrest chlamydial protein synthesis and are effective therapeutic agents. Development of vaccines for prevention of chlamydial disease requires a more complete understanding of the immunology and pathogenesis of chlamydial infections.

REFERENCES

1. Kingsbury DT, Weiss E: Lack of deoxyribonucleic acid homology between species of the genus *Chlamydia.* J Bacteriol 96:1421, 1968.
2. Campbell LA, Kuo C-C, Grayston JT: Characterization of the new *Chlamydia* agent, TWAR, as a unique organism by restriction endonuclease analysis and DNA-DNA hybridization. J Clin Microbiol 25:1911, 1987.
3. Gordon FB, Quan AL: Occurrence of glycogen in inclusions of the psittacosis–lymphogranuloma venereum–trachoma agents. J Infect Dis 115:186, 1965.
4. Matsumoto A: Structural characteristics of chlamydial bodies. *In* Barron AL (ed): Microbiology of Chlamydia. Boca Raton, FL, CRC Press, 1988, pp 21–45.
5. Kuo C-C, Chen H-H, Wang S-P, et al: Identification of a new group of *Chlamydia psittaci* strains called TWAR. J Clin Microbiol 24:1034, 1986.
6. Rice CE: Carbohydrate matrix of the epithelial cell inclusion in trachoma. Proc Soc Exp Biol Med 33:317, 1935.
7. Lin HS, Moulder JW: Patterns of response to sulfadiazine, D-cycloserine, and D-alanine in members of the psittacosis group. J Infect Dis 116:372, 1966.
8. Tamura A, Higashi N: Purification and chemical composition of meningopneumonitis virus. Virology 20:596, 1963.
9. Weiss E, Wilson NN: Role of exogenous adenosine triphosphate in catabolic and synthetic activities of *Chlamydia psittaci.* J Bacteriol 97:719, 1969.
10. Garret AJ, Harrison MJ, Manire GP: A search for the bacterial mucopeptide component, muramic acid, in *Chlamydiae.* J Gen Microbiol 80:315, 1974.
11. Hatch TP, Vance DW, Al-Hossainy E: Identification of a major protein in *Chlamydia* species. J Bacteriol 146:426, 1981.
12. Newhall WJ, Jones RB: Disulfide-linked oligomers of the major outer membrane protein of chlamydiae. J Bacteriol 154:998, 1983.
13. Bavoil P, Olin A, Schachter J: Role of disulfide bonding in outer membrane structure and permeability in *Chlamydia trachomatis.* Infect Immun 44:479, 1984.
14. Wilbert J, Newhall V: Biosynthesis and disulfide cross-linking of outer membrane components during the growth cycle of *Chlamydia trachomatis.* Infect Immun 55:162, 1987.
15. Matsumoto A: Electron microscopic observations of surface projections and related intracellular structures of *Chlamydia* organisms. J Electron Microsc 30:315, 1981.
16. Byrne GI, Moulder JW: Parasite-specified phagocytosis of *C. psittaci* and *C. trachomatis* by L and HeLa cells. Infect Immun 19:598, 1978.
17. Friis RR: Interaction of L cells and *Chlamydia psittaci:* Entry of the parasite and host response to its development. J Bacteriol 110:706, 1972.
18. Hackstadt T, Scidmore MA, Rocky DD: Lipid metabolism in *Chlamydia trachomatis*–infected cells: Directed trafficking of Golgi-derived sphingolipids to the chlamydial inclusion. Proc Natl Acad Sci U S A 92:4877, 1995.
19. Hackstadt T, Rockey DD, Heinzen RA, Scidmore MA: *Chlamydia trachomatis* interrupts an exocytic pathway to acquire endogenously synthesized sphingomyelin in transit from the Golgi apparatus to the plasma membrane. EMBO J 15:964, 1996.
20. Tamura A, Matsumoto A, Higashi N: Purification and chemical composition of reticulate bodies of the meningopneumonitis organisms. J Bacteriol 93:2003, 1967.
21. Tamura A, Matsumoto A, Manire GP, et al: Electron microscopic observations on the structure of the envelopes of mature elementary bodies and developmental reticulate forms of *Chlamydia psittaci.* J Bacteriol 105:355, 1971.
22. Hatch TP, Allan I, Pearce JH: Structural and polypeptide differences between envelopes of infective and reproductive life cycle forms of *Chlamydia* species. J Bacteriol 157:13, 1984.
23. Hatch TP, Miceli M, Sublett JE: Synthesis of disulfide-bonded outer membrane proteins during the developmental cycle of *Chlamydia psittaci* and *Chlamydia trachomatis.* J Bacteriol 165:379, 1986.
24. Todd WJ, Caldwell HD: The interaction of *Chlamydia trachomatis* with host cells: Ultrastructural studies of the mechanism of release of a biovar II strain from HeLa 229 cells. J Infect Dis 151:1037, 1985.
25. Ward ME: The chlamydial developmental cycle. *In* Barron AL (ed): Microbiology of Chlamydia. Boca Raton, FL, CRC Press, 1988, pp 71–95.
26. Wang S-P, Kuo C-C, Grayston JT: A simplified method for immunological typing of trachoma–inclusion conjunctivitis–lymphogranuloma venereum organisms. Infect Immun 7:356, 1973.
27. Newhall WJ, Terho P, Wilde CE, et al: Serovar determination of *Chlamydia trachomatis* isolates by using type-specific monoclonal antibodies. J Clin Microbiol 23:333, 1986.
28. Grayson JT, Wang S-P: New knowledge of chlamydiae and the diseases they cause. J Infect Dis 132:87, 1975.
29. Thompson JE, Washington AE: Epidemiology of sexually transmitted *Chlamydia trachomatis* infections. Epidemiol Rev 5:96, 1983.
30. Kuo C-C, Wang S-P, Holmes KK, et al: Immunotypes of *Chlamydia trachomatis* isolates in Seattle, Washington. Infect Immun 41:865, 1983.
31. Barnes RC, Wang S-P, Kuo C-C, et al: Immunotyping of *Chlamydia trachomatis* with monoclonal antibodies in a solid-phase enzyme immunoassay. J Clin Microbiol 22:609, 1985.
32. Wang S-P, Grayston JT: Three new serovars of *Chlamydia trachomatis:* Da, Ia, and L2a. J Infect Dis 163:403, 1991.
33. Dean D, Schachter J, Dawson CR, Stephens RS: Comparison of the major outer membrane protein variant sequence regions of B/Ba isolates: A molecular epidemiologic approach to *Chlamydia trachomatis* infections. J Infect Dis 166:383, 1992.
34. Nurminen M, Leinonen M, Saikku P, et al: The genus-specific antigen of *Chlamydia:* Resemblance to the lipopolysaccharide of enteric bacteria. Science 220:1279, 1983.
35. Stephens RS, Sanchez-Pescador R, Wagar EA, et al: Diversity of *Chlamydia trachomatis* major outer protein genes. J Bacteriol 169:3879, 1987.

36. Stephens RS, Wagar EA, Schoolnik GK: High-resolution mapping of serovar-specific and common antigenic determinants of the major outer membrane protein of *Chlamydia trachomatis.* J Exp Med 167:817, 1988.
37. Baehr W, Zhang YX, Joseph T, et al: Mapping antigenic domains expressed by *Chlamydia trachomatis* major outer membrane protein genes. Proc Natl Acad Sci U S A 85:4000, 1988.
38. Caldwell HD, Kromhout J, Schachter J: Purification and partial characterization of the major outer membrane protein of *Chlamydia trachomatis.* Infect Immun 31:1161, 1981.
39. Caldwell HD, Schachter J: Antigenic analysis of the major outer membrane protein of Chlamydia species. Infect Immun 35:1024, 1982.
40. Batteiger BE, Newhall WJ, Terho P, et al: Antigenic analysis of the major outer membrane protein of *Chlamydia trachomatis* with murine monoclonal antibodies. Infect Immun 53:530, 1986.
41. MacDonald AB: Antigens of *Chlamydia trachomatis.* Rev Infect Dis 7:731, 1985.
42. Zhang YX, Stewart S, Joseph T, et al: Protective monoclonal antibodies recognize epitopes located on the major outer membrane protein of *Chlamydia trachomatis.* J Immunol 138:575, 1987.
43. Richmond SJ, Stirling P: Localization of chlamydial group antigen in McCoy cell monolayers infected with *Chlamydia trachomatis* or *Chlamydia psittaci.* Infect Immun 34:561, 1981.
44. Stuart ES, MacDonald AB: Genus glycolipid exoantigen from *Chlamydia trachomatis:* Component preparation, isolation and analyses. *In* Oriel D, Ridgway G, Schachter J, et al (eds): Chlamydial Infections. Proceedings of the 6th International Conference on Human Chlamydial Infections. Cambridge, Cambridge University, 1986, pp 122–125.
45. Krieg NR, Holt JG (eds): Bergey's Manual of Systematic Bacteriology. Baltimore, Williams & Wilkins, 1984, p 737.
46. Stenson S, Newman R, Fedukowicz H: Conjunctivitis in the newborn: Observations on incidence, cause, and prophylaxis. Ann Ophthalmol 13:329, 1981.
47. Quinn TC, Goodell SE, Mkrtichian PAC, et al: *Chlamydia trachomatis* proctitis. N Engl J Med 305:195, 1981.
48. Mardh P-A, Svensson L: Chlamydial salpingitis. Scand J Infect Dis 32(Suppl):64, 1982.
49. Kraus SJ: Semiquantitation of urethral polymorphonuclear leukocytes as objective evidence of nongonoccocal urethritis. Sex Transm Dis 9:52, 1982.
50. Wilhelmus KR, Robinson NM, Tredici LL, et al: Conjunctival cytology of adult chlamydial conjunctivitis. Arch Ophthalmol 104:691, 1986.
51. Megran DW, Stiver HG, Bowie WR: Complement activation and stimulation of chemotaxis by *Chlamydia trachomatis.* Infect Immun 49:670, 1985.
52. Kuo C-C, Chen W-J: A mouse model of *Chlamydia trachomatis* pneumonitis. J Infect Dis 141:198, 1980.
53. Taylor HR, Prendergast RA, Dawson CR, et al: An animal model for cicatrizing trachoma. Invest Ophthalmol Vis Sci 21:422, 1981.
54. Patton DL, Kuo C-C, Wang S-P, et al: Chlamydial salpingitis in subcutaneous fimbrial transplants in monkeys. *In* Oriel D, Ridgway G, Schachter J, et al (eds): Chlamydial Infections. Proceedings of the 6th International Symposium on Human Chlamydial Infections. Cambridge, Cambridge University, 1986, pp 367–370.
55. Quinn TC, Kappus EW, James SP: The immunopathogenesis of lymphogranuloma venereum rectal infection in primates. *In* Oriel D, Ridgway G, Schachter J, et al (eds): Chlamydial Infections. Proceedings of the 6th International Symposium on Human Chlamydial Infections. Cambridge, Cambridge University, 1986, pp 404–407.
56. Dunlop EMC, Hare MJ, Darougar S, et al: Chlamydial infection of the urethra in men presenting because of nonspecific urethritis. *In* Nichols RL (ed): Trachoma and Related Disorders. Amsterdam, Excerpta Medica, 1971, pp 494–500.
57. Schachter J, Dawson CR: Human Chlamydial Infections. Littleton, MA, PSG, 1978, pp 63–109.
58. Dunlop EMC, Garner A, Darougar S, et al: Colposcopy, biopsy and cytology results in women with chlamydial cervicitis. Genitourin Med 65:22, 1989.
59. Zvillich M, Sarov I: Interaction between human polymorphonuclear leukocytes and *Chlamydia trachomatis* elementary bodies: Electron microscopy and chemiluminescent response. J Gen Microbiol 131:2627, 1985.
60. Yong EC, Chi EY, Chen W-J, et al: Degradation of *Chlamydia trachomatis* in human polymorphonuclear leukocytes: An ultrastructural study of peroxidase positive phagolysosomes. Infect Immun 53:427, 1986.
61. Register KB, Davis CH, Wyrick PB, et al: Non-oxidative antimicrobial effects of human polymorphonuclear leukocyte granule proteins on *Chlamydia* species *in vitro.* Infect Immun 55:2420, 1987.
62. Williams DM, Schachter J, Drutz DJ et al: Pneumonia due to *Chlamydia trachomatis* in the immunocompromised (nude) mouse. J Infect Dis 143:238, 1981.
63. Williams DM, Schachter J, Grubbs B, et al: The role of antibody in host defense against the agent of mouse pneumonitis. J Infect Dis 145:200, 1982.
64. Williams DM, Schachter J, Coalson JE, et al: Cellular immunity to the mouse pneumonitis agent. J Infect Dis 149:630, 1984.
65. Williams DM, Schachter J, Weiner MH et al: Antibody in host defense against mouse pneumonitis agent (murine *Chlamydia trachomatis*). Infect Immun 45:674, 1984.
66. Rank RG, Soderberg LSF, Barron AL: Chronic chlamydial genital infection in congenitally athymic nude mice. Infect Immun 48:847, 1985.
67. Rank RG, Barron AL: Effect of antithymocyte serum on the course of chlamydial genital infection in female guinea pigs. Infect Immun 41:876, 1983.
68. Wang S-P, Grayston JT: Microimmunofluorescence antibody responses in *Chlamydia trachomatis* infection: A review. *In* Mardh P-A, Holmes KK, Oriel JD, et al (eds): Chlamydial Infections. Proceedings of the 5th International Conference on Human Chlamydial Infections. Amsterdam, Elsevier Biomedical, 1982, pp 301–316.
69. Williams DW: Stimulator of the immune response. *In* Barron AL (ed): Microbiology of Chlamydia. Boca Raton, FL, CRC Press, 1988, pp 209–216.
70. Wager EA, Schachter J, Bavoil P, Stephens, RS: Differential human serologic response to two 60,000 molecular weight *Chlamydia trachomatis* antigens. J Infect Dis 162: 922, 1990.
71. Jones RB, Batteiger BE: Human immune responses to *Chlamydia trachomatis* infections. *In* Oriel D, Ridgway G, Schachter J, et al (eds): Chlamydial Infections. Proceedings of the 6th International Symposium on Human Chlamydial Infections. Cambridge, Cambridge University, 1986, pp 423–432.
72. Brunham RC, Maclean I, MacDowell J, et al: *Chlamydia trachomatis* antigen specific serum antibodies among women who did and did not develop acute salpingitis following therapeutic abortion. *In* Oriel D, Ridgway G, Schachter J, et al (eds): Chlamydial Infections. Proceedings of the 6th International Symposium on Human Chlamydial Infections. Cambridge, Cambridge University, 1986, pp 221–224.
73. Maclean IW, Peeling RW, Brunham RC: Characterization of *Chlamydia trachomatis* antigens with monoclonal and polyclonal antibodies. Can J Microbiol 34:141, 1988.
74. Howard LV: Neutralization of *Chlamydia trachomatis* in cell culture. Infect Immun 11:698, 1975.
75. Caldwell HD, Perry LJ: Neutralization of *Chlamydia trachomatis* infectivity with antibodies to the major outer membrane protein. Infect Immun 38:745, 1982.
76. Peeling R, Maclean IW, Brunham RC: In vitro neutralization of *Chlamydia trachomatis* with monoclonal antibody to an epitope on the major outer membrane protein. Infect Immun 46:484, 1984.
77. Schachter J, Grossman M, Holt J, et al: Prospective study of chlamydia infection in neonates. Lancet 2:377, 1979.
78. Rank RG, White HJ, Barron AL: Humoral immunity in the resolution of genital infection in female guinea pigs infected with the agent of guinea pig inclusion conjunctivitis. Infect Immun 26:573, 1979.
79. White HJ, Rank RG, Soloff BL, et al: Experimental chlamydial salpingitis in immunosuppressed guinea pigs infected in the genital tract with the agent of guinea pig inclusion conjunctivitis. Infect Immun 26:728, 1979.
80. Kunimoto E, Brunham RC: Human immune response and *Chlamydia trachomatis* infection. Rev Infect Dis 7:665, 1985.
81. Hanna L, Schmidt L, Sharp M, et al: Human cell-mediated immune response to chlamydial antigens. Infect Immun 23:412, 1979.
82. Brunham RC, Martin DH, Kuo C-C, et al: Cellular immune response during uncomplicated genital infection with *Chlamydia trachomatis* in humans. Infect Immun 34:98, 1981.
83. Hanna L, Kerlan R, Senyk G, et al: Immune response to chlamydial antigens in humans. Med Microbiol Immunol 171:1, 1982.
84. Qvigstad E, Skaug K, Thorsby E: Proliferative human T-cell response to *Chlamydia trachomatis* in vitro. Acta Pathol Microbiol Immunol Scand 91:203, 1983.
85. Heggie AD, Wyrich PB, Chase PA, et al: Cell mediated immune

response to *Chlamydia trachomatis* in mothers and infants. Proc Soc Exp Biol Med 181:586, 1986.

86. Senyk G, Sharp M, Stites DP, et al: Cell-mediated immune responses to chlamydial antigens in guinea pigs injected with inactivated chlamydiae. Med Microbiol Immunol 168:91, 1980.
87. Senyk G, Kerlan R, Stites DP, et al: Cell-mediated and humoral immune responses to chlamydial antigens in guinea pigs infected ocularly with the agent of guinea pig inclusion conjunctivitis. Infect Immun 32:304, 1981.
88. Barron AL, Rank RG, Moses EB: Immune response in mice infected in the genital tract with mouse pneumonitis agent (*Chlamydia trachomatis* serovar). Infect Immun 44:82, 1984.
89. Lammert JK: Cytotoxic cells induced after *Chlamydia psittaci* infection in mice. Infect Immun 35:1011, 1982.
90. Byrne GI, Krueger DA: In vitro expression of factor-mediated cytotoxic activity generated during the immune response to *Chlamydia* in the mouse. J Immunol 134:4189, 1985.
91. Pavia CS, Schachter J: Failure to detect cell-mediated cytotoxicity against *Chlamydia trachomatis*–infected cells. Infect Immun 39:1271, 1983.
92. Qvigstad E, Hirschberg H: Lack of cell-mediated cytotoxicity towards *Chlamydia trachomatis* infected target cells in humans. Acta Pathol Microbiol Immunol Scand [Copenh] 92:153, 1984.
93. Byrne GI, Grubbs B, Marshall TJ, et al: Gamma-interferon–mediated cytotoxicity related to murine *Chlamydia trachomatis* infection. Infect Immun 56:2023, 1988.
94. Williams DM, Bonewald LF, Roodman GD, et al: Tumor necrosis factor alpha is a cytotoxin induced by murine *Chlamydia trachomatis* infection. Infect Immun 57:1351, 1989.
95. Berger RE, Alexander ER, Monda GD, et al: *Chlamydia trachomatis* as a cause of acute "idiopathic" epididymitis. N Engl J Med 298:301, 1978.
96. Thompson SE, Dretler RH: Epidemiology and treatment of chlamydial infections in pregnant women and infants. Rev Infect Dis 4:747, 1982.
97. Wolner-Hanssen P, Westrom L, Mardh P-A: Perihepatitis and chlamydial salpingitis. Lancet 1:901, 1986.
98. Wang S-P, Eschenbach DA, Holmes KK, et al: *Chlamydia trachomatis* infection in Fitz-Hugh-Curtis syndrome. Am J Obstet Gynecol 139:1034, 1980.
99. Barbour AG, Amato K-I, Hackstadt T, et al: *Chlamydia trachomatis* has penicillin-binding proteins but not detectable muramic acid. J Bacteriol 151:420, 1982.
100. Matsumoto A, Manire GP: Electron microscopic observations on the effects of penicillin on the morphology of *Chlamydia psittaci.* J Bacteriol 101:278, 1970.
101. Moulder JW, Novasel DL, Officer JE: Inhibition of the growth of agents of the psittacosis group by D-cycloserine and its specific reversal by D-alanine. J Bacteriol 85:707, 1963.
102. Lin H-S, Moulder JW: Patterns of response to sulfadiazine, D-cycloserine, and D-alanine in membranes of the psittacosis group. J Infect Dis 116:372, 1966.
103. Gerding DN, Peterson LR, Hughes CE, et al: Extravascular antimicrobial distribution in man. *In* Lorian V (ed): Antibiotics in Laboratory Medicine. Baltimore, Williams & Wilkins, 1986, pp 938–994.
104. Johnson FWA, Hobson D: The effect of penicillin on genital strains of *C. trachomatis* in tissue culture. J Antimicrob Chemother 3:49, 1977.
105. Edwards DI: Antimicrobial Drug Action. Baltimore, University Park, 1980, pp 200–216.
106. Martin DH, Mroszkowski TF, Dalu ZA, et al: A controlled trial of a single dose of azithromycin for the treatment of chlamydial urethritis and cervitis. N Engl J Med 327:921, 1992.
107. Bailey RL, Arullendran P, Whittle HC, Mabey DCW: Randomised controlled trial of single-dose azithromycin in treatment of trachoma. Lancet 342:453, 1993.
108. Assaad FA, Sundaresan T, Maxwell-Lyons F: The household pattern of trachoma in Taiwan. Bull WHO 44:605, 1971.
109. Jones BR: Prevention of blindness from trachoma. Trans Ophthalmol Soc UK 95:16, 1975.
110. Dawson CR, Jones BR, Tarizzo ML: Guide to Trachoma Control. Geneva, World Health Organization, 1981, pp 12–24.
111. Dawson CR, Daghfous M, Messodi M, et al: Severe endemic trachoma in Tunisia. Br J Ophthalmol 60:245, 1976.
112. Schachter J, Dawson CR: Human Chlamydial Infections. Littleton, MA, PSG, 1978, p 65.
113. Thygeson PL: The etiology of inclusion blenorrhea. Am J Ophthalmol 17:1019, 1934.
114. Grayston JT, Wang S-P, Yeh L-J, et al: Importance of reinfection in the pathogenesis of trachoma. Rev Infect Dis 7:717, 1985.
115. Kuo C-C: Host response. *In* Barron AL (ed) Microbiology of Chlamydia. Boca Raton, FL, CRC Press, 1988, pp 193–208.
116. Grayston JT, Yeh L-H, Wang S-P, et al: Pathogenesis of ocular *Chlamydia trachomatis* infections in humans. *In* Hobson D, Holmes KK (eds): Nongonoccocal Urethritis and Related Infections. Washington, DC, American Society for Microbiology, 1977, pp 113–125.
117. Grayston JT, Wang S-P, Lin HM, et al: Trachoma vaccine studies in volunteer students of the National Defense Medical Center. II: Response to challenge eye inoculation of egg grown trachoma virus. Chin Med J 8:312, 1961.
118. Detels R, Alexander ER, Dhir SP: Trachoma in Punjabi Indians in British Columbia: A prevalence study with comparisons to India. Am J Epidemiol 84:81, 1966.
119. Mabey DCW, Holland MJ, Bailey RL, et al: *In vitro* studies of cell mediated immunity to chlamydial antigens in trachoma. *In* Bowie WR, Caldwell HD, Jones RP, et al (eds): Chlamydial Infections. Cambridge, Cambridge University, 1990, pp 283–286.
120. Conway DJ, Holland MJ, Campbell AE, et al: HLA class I and II polymorphisms and trachomatous scarring in a *Chlamydia trachomatis*–endemic population. J Infect Dis 174:643, 1996.
121. Brunham RC, Peeling R, Maclean I, et al: *Chlamydia trachomatis*–associated ectopic pregnancy: Serologic and histologic correlates. J Infect Dis 165:1076, 1992.
122. Toye B, Laferriere C, Claman P, et al: Association between antibody to the chlamydial heat-shock protein and tubal infertility. J Infect Dis 168:1236, 1993.
123. Arno JN, Yuan Y, Cleary RE, Morrison RP: Serologic responses of infertile women to the 60-kd chlamydial heat shock protein (hsp60). Fertil Steril 64:730, 1995.
124. Kimani J, Maclean IW, Bwayo JJ, et al: Risk factors for *Chlamydia trachomatis* pelvic inflammatory disease among sex workers in Nairobi, Kenya. J Infect Dis 173:1437, 1996.
125. Young RA, Elliot TJ: Stress proteins, infection, and immune surveillance. Cell 59:5, 1989.
126. Kaufmann SHE: Heat shock proteins and the immune response. Immunol Today 11:129, 1990.
127. Zhong G, Brunham RC: Antibody responses to the chlamydial heat shock proteins hsp 60 and hsp 70 are H-2 linked. Infect Immun 60:3143, 1992.
128. Wang S-P, Grayston JT: Trachoma in the Taiwan monkey, *Macaca cyclopis.* Ann N Y Acad Sci 98:177, 1962.
129. Wang S-P, Grayston JT: Pannus with experimental trachoma and inclusion conjunctivitis agent infection of Taiwan monkeys. Am J Ophthalmol 63:1133, 1967.
130. Wang S-P, Grayston JT, Alexander ER: Trachoma vaccine studies in monkeys. Am J Ophthalmol 63:1615, 1967.
131. Monnickendam MA, Darougar S: An animal model for hyperendemic trachoma: A study of immunity and hypersensitivity to *Chlamydia. In* Silverstein AM, O'Connor GR (eds): Immunology and Immunopathology of the Eye. New York, Masson, 1979, pp 375–380.
132. Whittum-Hudson JA, Taylor HR, Farazdaghi M, et al: Immunohistochemical study of the local inflammatory response to chlamydial ocular infection. Invest Ophthalmol Vis Sci 27:64, 1986.
133. Whittum-Hudson JA, Taylor HR: Antichlamydial specificity of conjunctival lymphocytes during experimental ocular infection. Infect Immun 57:2977, 1989.
134. Whittum-Hudson JA, Zhang P, Pal S, et al: Chlamydia-specific lymphocytes in conjunctiva in a model of trachoma. *In* Bowie WR, Caldwell HD, Jones RP, et al (eds): Chlamydial Infections. Proceedings of the 7th International Symposium on Human Chlamydial Infections. Cambridge, Cambridge University, 1990, pp 287–290.
135. Taylor HR, Johnson SL, Prendergast RA, et al: An animal model of trachoma. II: The importance of repeated infection. Invest Ophthalmol Vis Sci 23:507, 1982.
136. Taylor HR, Prendergast RA, Dawson CR, et al: Animal model of trachoma. III: The necessity of repeated exposure to live chlamydia. *In* Mardh PA, Holmes KK, Oriel JD, et al (eds): Chlamydial Infections. Proceedings of the 5th International Symposium on Human Chlamydial Infections. Amsterdam, Elsevier Biomedical, 1982, pp 387–390.
137. Dawson CW: Lids, conjunctiva, and lacrimal apparatus. Arch Ophthalmol 93:854, 1975.

138. Jones BR, Darougar S, Mohsenine H, et al: Communicable ophthalmia: The blinding scourge of the Middle East. Yesterday, today and tomorrow. Br J Ophthalmol 60:492, 1976.
139. Vastine DW, Dawson CR, Daghfous T, et al: Severe endemic trachoma in Tunisia. 1. Effect of topical chemotherapy on conjunctivitis and ocular bacteria. Br J Ophthalmol 58:833, 1974.
140. Taylor HR, Kolarczyk RA, Johnson SL, et al: Effect of bacterial secondary infection in an animal model of trachoma. Infect Immun 44:614, 1984.
141. Wang S-P, Grayston JT: Immunologic relationship between genital TRIC, lymphogranuloma venereum, and related organisms in a new microtiter indirect immunofluorescence test. Am J Ophthalmol 70:367, 1970.
142. Taylor HR, Johnson SL, Schachter J, et al: Pathogenesis of trachoma: The stimulus for inflammation. J Immunol 138:3023, 1987.
143. Taylor HR, Schachter J, Caldwell HD: The stimulus for conjunctival inflammation in trachoma. *In* Oriel D, Ridgway G, Schachter J, et al (eds): Chlamydial Infections. Proceedings of the 6th International Symposium on Human Chlamydial Infections. Cambridge, Cambridge University, 1986, pp 167–170.
144. Watkins NG, Caldwell HD: Delayed hypersensitivity as a pathogenic mechanism in chlamydial disease. *In* Oriel D, Ridgway G, Schachter J, et al (eds): Chlamydial Infections. Proceedings of the 6th International Symposium on Human Chlamydial Infections. Cambridge, Cambridge University, 1986, pp 408–411.
145. Watkins NG, Hadlow WJ, Moos AB, et al: Ocular delayed hypersensitivity: A pathogenetic mechanism of chlamydial conjunctivitis in guinea pigs. Proc Natl Acad Sci U S A 83:7480, 1986.
146. Morrison RP, Lyng K, Caldwell HD: Chlamydial disease pathogenesis. Ocular hypersensitivity elicited by a genus-specific 57-kD protein. J Exp Med 169:663, 1989.
147. Morrison RP, Belland RJ, Lyng K, et al: Chlamydial disease pathogenesis. The 57-kD chlamydial hypersensitivity antigen is a stress response protein. J Exp Med 170:1271, 1989.
148. Dayer J-M, Beutler B, Cerami A: Cachectin/tumor necrosis factor stimulates collagenase and prostaglandin E_2 production by human synovial cells and dermal fibroblasts. J Exp Med 162:2163, 1985.
149. Elias JA, Krol RC, Freundlich B, et al: Regulation of human lung fibroblast glycosaminoglycan production by recombinant interferons, tumor necrosis factor, and lymphotoxin. J Clin Invest 81:325, 1988.
150. Peeling RW, Brunham RC: Chlamydiae as pathogens: New species and new issues. Emerg Infect Dis 2:307, 1996.
151. Heggie AD, Jaffe AC, Stuart LA, et al: Topical sulfacetamide vs oral erythromycin for neonatal chlamydial conjunctivitis. Am J Dis Child 139:564, 1985.
152. Rapoza PA, Quinn TC, Kiessling LA, et al: Epidemiology of neonatal conjunctivitis. Ophthalmology 93:456, 1986.
153. Fisher MC: Conjunctivitis in children. Pediatr Clin North Am 34:1447, 1987.
154. Alexander ER, Harrison HR: Role of *Chlamydia trachomatis* in perinatal infection. Rev Infect Dis 5:713, 1983.
155. Heggie AD, Lumicao GG, Stuart LA, et al: *Chlamydia trachomatis* infection in mothers and infants. Am J Dis Child 135:507, 1981.
156. Beem MO, Saxon EM: Respiratory-tract colonization and a distinctive pneumonia syndrome in infants infected with *Chlamydia trachomatis.* N Engl J Med 296:306, 1977.
157. Schachter J, Dawson CR: Is trachoma an ocular component of a more generalized chlamydial infection? Lancet 1:702, 1979.
158. Schachter J, Grossman M, Sweet RL, et al: Prospective study of perinatal transmission of *Chlamydia trachomatis.* JAMA 225:3374, 1986.
159. Forster RK, Dawson CR, Schachter J: Late follow-up of patients with neonatal conjunctivitis. Am J Ophthalmol 69:467, 1970.
160. Goscienski PJ, Sexton RR: Follow-up studies in neonatal inclusion conjunctivitis. Am J Dis Child 124:180, 1972.
161. Mordhorst CH: Clinical epidemiology of oculogenital chlamydia infection. *In* Hobson D, Holmes KK (eds): Nongonococcal Urethritis and Related Infections. Washington, DC, American Society for Microbiology, 1977, pp 126–134.
162. Ronnerstam R, Personn K: Chlamydial conjunctivitis in a Swedish population. *In* Mardh PA, Holmes KK, Oriel JD, et al (eds): Chlamydia Infections. Proceedings of the 5th International Symposium on Human Chlamydial Infections. Amsterdam, Elsevier Biomedical, 1982, pp 87–90.
163. Wishart PK, James C, Wishart MS, et al: Prevalence of acute conjunctivitis caused by chlamydia, adenovirus, and herpes simplex virus in an ophthalmic casualty department. Br J Ophthalmol 68:653, 1984.
164. Bialasiewicz AA, Jahn GJ: Epidemiology of chlamydial eye diseases in a mixed rural/urban population of West Germany. Ophthalmology 93:757, 1986.
165. Potts MJ, Paul ID, Roome APCH, et al: Rapid diagnosis of *Chlamydia trachomatis* infection in patients attending an ophthalmic casualty department. Br J Ophthalmol 70:677, 1986.
166. Fitch CP, Rapoza PA, Owens S, et al: Epidemiology and diagnosis of acute conjunctivitis at an inner-city hospital. Ophthalmology 96:1215, 1989.
167. Heggie AD: Incidence and etiology of conjunctivitis in Navy recruits. Milit Med 155:1, 1990.
168. Rapoza PA, Quinn TC, Terry AC, et al: A systematic approach to the diagnosis and treatment of chronic conjunctivitis. Am J Ophthalmol 109:138, 1990.
169. Halberstaedter L, von Prowazek S: Uber Zelleinschlusse parasitarer Natur beim Trachom. Arb Kaiserlichen Gesundheitsamte 26:44, 1907.
170. T'ang FF, Chang HL, Huang YT, et al: Studies on the etiology of trachoma with special reference to isolation of the virus in chicken embryo. Chin Med J 75:429, 1957.
171. World Health Organization: Guide to the Laboratory Diagnosis of Trachoma. Geneva, World Health Organization, 1975.
172. Schachter J, Dawson CR: Comparative efficacy of various diagnostic methods for chlamydial infection. *In* Hobson D, Homes KK (eds): Nongonococcal Urethritis and Related Infections. Washington, DC, American Society for Microbiology, 1977, pp 337–341.
173. Darougar S, Woodland RM, Jones BR, et al: Comparative sensitivity of fluorescent antibody staining of the conjunctival scrapings and irradiated McCoy cell culture for the diagnosis of hyperendemic trachoma. Br J Ophthalmol 64:276, 1980.
174. Sandstrom KI, Bell TA, Chandler JW, et al: Microbial causes of neonatal conjunctivitis. J Pediatr 105:706, 1984.
175. Smith TF, Wentworth BB: Chlamydial infections. *In* Wentworth BB, Judson FN (eds): Laboratory Manual for the Diagnosis of Sexually Transmitted Diseases. Washington, DC, American Public Health Association, 1984, pp 81–104.
176. Dorman SA, Danos LM, Wilson DJ, et al: Detection of chlamydial cervicitis by Papanicolaou stained smears and culture. Am J Clin Pathol 79:421, 1983.
177. Quinn TC, Gupta PK, Burkman RT, et al: Detection of *Chlamydia trachomatis* cervical infection: A comparison of Papanicolaou and immunofluorescent staining with cell culture. Am J Obstet Gynecol 157:394, 1987.
178. Gordon FB, Harper IA, Quan AL, et al: Detection of Chlamydia (Bedsonia) in certain infections of man. I. Laboratory procedures: Comparison of yolk sac and cell culture for detection and isolation. J Infect Dis 120:451, 1969.
179. Gordon FB, Quan AL: Isolation of the trachoma agent in cell culture. Proc Soc Exp Biol Med 118:354, 1965.
180. Kuo C-C, Wang S-P, Wentworth BB, et al: Primary isolation of TRIC organisms in HeLa 229 cells treated with DEAE-dextran. J Infect Dis 125:665, 1972.
181. Ripa KT, Mardh P-A: Cultivation of *Chlamydia trachomatis* in cycloheximide-treated McCoy cells. J Clin Microbiol 6:328, 1977.
182. Sompolinsky D, Richmond S: Growth of *Chlamydia trachomatis* in McCoy cells treated with cytochalasin B. Appl Microbiol 28:912, 1974.
183. Darougar S, Cubitt S, Jones BR: Effect of high-speed centrifugation on the sensitivity of irradiated McCoy cell culture for the isolation of *Chlamydia.* Br J Vener Dis 50:308, 1974.
184. Reeve P, Owen J, Oriel JD: Laboratory procedures for the isolation of *Chlamydia trachomatis* from the human genital tract. J Clin Pathol 28:910, 1975.
185. Allan I, Pearce JH: Modulation by centrifugation of cell susceptibility to chlamydial infection. J Gen Microbiol 111:87, 1979.
186. Kuo C-C, Grayston JT: Interaction of *Chlamydia trachomatis* organisms and HeLa 229 cells. Infect Immun 13:1103, 1976.
187. Rota TR, Nichols RL: Infection of cell culture by trachoma agent. Enhancement by DEAE-dextran. J Infect Dis 124:419, 1971.
188. Smith TF, Brown SD, Weed LA: Diagnosis of *Chlamydia trachomatis* infections by cell cultures and serology. Lab Med 13:92, 1982.
189. Stevens RS, Kuo C-C, Tam MR: Sensitivity of immunofluorescence with monoclonal antibodies for detection of *Chlamydia trachomatis* inclusions in cell culture. J Clin Microbiol 16:4, 1982.
190. Stamm WE, Tam M, Koester M, et al: Detection of *Chlamydia*

trachomatis inclusions in McCoy cell cultures with fluorescein-conjugated monoclonal antibodies. J Clin Microbiol 17:666, 1983.
191. Mahony JB, Chernesky MA: Effect of swab type and storage temperature on the isolation of *Chlamydia trachomatis* from clinical specimens. J Clin Microbiol 22:865, 1985.
192. Tam RT, Stamm WE, Handsfield HH, et al: Culture-independent diagnosis of *Chlamydia trachomatis* using monoclonal antibodies. N Engl J Med 310:1146, 1984.
193. Stamm WE, Harrison HR, Alexander ER, et al: Diagnosis of *Chlamydia trachomatis* infections by direct immunofluorescence staining of genital secretions—A multicenter trial. Ann Intern Med 101:638, 1984.
194. Bell TA, Kuo C-C, Stamm WE, et al: Direct fluorescent monoclonal antibody stain for rapid detection of infant *Chlamydia trachomatis* infections. Pediatrics 74:224, 1984.
195. Taylor HR, Rapoza PA, Kiessling A, et al: Rapid detection of *Chlamydia trachomatis* with monoclonal antibodies. Lancet 2:38, 1984.
196. Mabey DCW, Booth-Mason S: The detection of *Chlamydia trachomatis* by direct immunofluorescence in conjunctival smears from patients with trachoma and patients with ophthalmia neonatorum using a conjugated monoclonal antibody. J Hyg 96:83, 1986.
197. Rapoza PA, Quinn TC, Kiessling LA, et al: Assessment of neonatal conjunctivitis with a direct fluorescent monoclonal antibody stain for *Chlamydia*. JAMA 255:3369, 1986.
198. Rompalo AM, Suchland RJ, Price CB, et al: Rapid diagnosis of *Chlamydia trachomatis* rectal infection by direct fluorescence staining. J Infect Dis 155:1075, 1987.
199. Barnes RC: Laboratory diagnosis of human chlamydial infections. Clin Microbiol Rev 2:119, 1989.
200. Baselski VS, McNeeley SG, Ryan G, et al: A comparison of nonculture-dependent methods for detection of *Chlamydia trachomatis* infections in pregnant women. Obstet Gynecol 70:47, 1987.
201. Lefebvre J, Laperriere H, Rousseau H, et al: Comparison of three techniques for detection of *Chlamydia trachomatis* in endocervical specimens from asymptomatic women. J Clin Microbiol 26:726, 1988.
202. Kellogg JA: Clinical and laboratory considerations of culture vs antigen assays for detection of *Chlamydia trachomatis* from genital specimens. Arch Pathol Lab Med 113:453, 1989.
203. Hammerschlag MR, Roblin PM, Cummings C, et al: Comparison of enzyme immunoassay and culture for diagnosis of chlamydial conjunctivitis and respiratory infections in infants. J Clin Microbiol 25:2306, 1987.
204. Mabey DCW, Robertson JN, Ward ME: Detection of *Chlamydia trachomatis* by enzyme immunoassay in patients with trachoma. Lancet 2:1491, 1987.
205. Hipp SS, Yangsook H, Murphy D: Assessment of enzyme immunoassay and immunofluorescence test for detection of *Chlamydia trachomatis*. J Clin Microbiol 25:1938, 1987.
206. Enns RK: DNA probes: An overview and comparison with current methods. Lab Med 5:295, 1988.
207. Horn JE, Hammer ML, Faldow S, et al: Detection of *Chlamydia trachomatis* in tissue culture and cervical scrapings by in situ DNA hybridization. J Infect Dis 153:1155, 1986.
208. Horn JE, Quinn T, Hammer M, et al: Use of nucleic acid probes for the detection of sexually transmitted infectious agents. Diagn Microbiol Infect Dis 4(Suppl):101, 1986.
209. Dean D, Palmer L, Pant CR, et al: Use of a *Chlamydia trachomatis* probe for detection of ocular Chlamydiae. J Clin Microbiol 27:1062, 1989.
210. Kohne DE: Application of DNA probe tests to the diagnosis of infectious disease. Am Clin Prod Rev Nov 20–29, 1986.
211. Peterson EM, Oda R, Alexander R, et al: Molecular techniques for the detection of *Chlamydia trachomatis*. J Clin Microbiol 27:2359, 1989.
212. Woods GL, Young A, Scott JC, et al: Evaluation of a nonisotopic probe for detection of *Chlamydia trachomatis* in endocervical specimens. J Clin Microbiol 28:370, 1990.
213. Wang S-P, Grayston JT: Micro-immunofluorescence antibody responses in *Chlamydia trachomatis* infection: A review. *In* Mardh P-A, Holmes KK, Oriel JD, et al (eds): Chlamydial Infections. Proceedings of the 5th International Symposium on Human Chlamydial Infections. Amsterdam, Elsevier Biomedical, 1982, pp 301–316.
214. Schachter J, Grossman M, Azimi PH: Serology of *Chlamydia trachomatis* in infants. J Infect Dis 146:530, 1982.
215. Darougar S, Treharne JD, Minassian D, et al: Rapid serologic test for diagnosis of chlamydial ocular infections. Br J Ophthalmol 62:503, 1978.
216. Treharne JD, Dwyer RS, Darougar S, et al: Antichlamydial antibody in tears and sera. Br J Ophthalmol 62:509, 1978.
217. Lewis VJ, Thacker WL, Mitchell SH: Enzyme-linked immunosorbent assay for chlamydial antibodies. J Clin Microbiol 6:507, 1977.
218. Evans RT, Taylor-Robinson D: Development and evaluation of an enzyme-linked immunosorbent assay (ELISA), using chlamydial group antigen to detect antibodies to *Chlamydia trachomatis*. J Clin Pathol 35:1122, 1982.
219. Saikku P, Paavonen J, Vaananen P, et al: Solid-phase enzyme immunoassay for chlamydial antibodies. J Clin Microbiol 17:22, 1983.
220. Jones RB, Bruins SC, Newhall WJ: Comparison of reticulate and elementary body antigens in detection of antibodies against *Chlamydia trachomatis* by an enzyme-linked immunosorbent assay. J Clin Microbiol 17:466, 1983.
221. Finn MP, Ohlin A, Schachter J: Enzyme-linked immunosorbent assay for immunoglobulin G and M antibodies to *Chlamydia trachomatis* in human sera. J Clin Microbiol 17:848, 1983.
222. Mahony JB, Schachter J, Chernesky MA: Detection of antichlamydial immunoglobulin G and M antibodies by enzyme-linked immunosorbent assay. J Clin Microbiol 18:270, 1983.
223. Mahony JB, Chernesky MA, Bromberg K, et al: Accuracy of immunoglobulin M immunoassay for diagnosis of chlamydial infection in infants and adults. J Clin Microbiol 24:731, 1986.
224. Toye B, Peeling RW, Jessamine P, et al: Diagnosis of *Chlamydia trachomatis* infections in asymptomatic men and women by PCR assay. J Clin Microbiol 34:1396–1400, 1996.
225. Jaschek G, Gaydos CA, Welsh LE, Quinn TC: Direct detection of *Chlamydia trachomatis* in urine specimens from symptomatic and asymptomatic men by using a rapid polymerase chain reaction assay. J Clin Microbiol 31:1209, 1993.
226. Chernesky MA, Lee H, Schachter J, et al: Diagnosis of *Chlamydia trachomatis* urethral infection in symptomatic and asymptomatic men by testing first void urine in a ligase chain reaction assay. J Infect Dis 170: 1308, 1994.
227. Schachter J, Stamm WE, Quinn TC, et al: Ligase chain reaction to detect *Chlamydial trachomatis* infection of the cervix. J Clin Microbiol 32:2540, 1994.
228. Chernesky MA, Jang D, Lee H, et al: Diagnosis of *Chlamydia trachomatis* infections in men and women by testing first-void urine by ligase chain reaction. J Clin Microbiol 32:2682, 1994.
229. Grayston JT, Kuo C-C, Wang S-P, et al: A new *Chlamydia psitacci* strain, TWAR, isolated in acute respiratory tract infections. N Engl J Med 315:161, 1986.
230. Cles LD, Stamm WE: Use of HL cells for improved isolation and passage of *Chlamydia pneumoniae*. J Clin Microbiol 28:938, 1990.
231. Kuo C-C, Grayston JT: A sensitive cell line, HL cells, for isolation and propagation of *Chlamydia pneumoniae*. J Infect Dis 162:755, 1990.
232. Theunissen JJH, van Heijst BYM, Wagenvoort JHT, et al: Factors influencing the infectivity of *Chlamydia pneumoniae* elementary bodies on HL cells. J Clin Microbiol 30:1388, 1992.
233. Wong KH, Skelton SK, Chan YK: Efficient culture of *Chlamydia pneumoniae* with cell lines derived from the human respiratory tract. J Clin Microbiol 30:1625, 1992.
234. Grayston JT: Infections caused by *Chlamydia pneumoniae* strain TWAR. Clin Infect Dis 15:757, 1992.
235. Wang S-P, Grayston JT: Microimmunofluorescence serological studies with the TWAR organism. *In* Oriel JD, Ridgway G, Schachter J, et al (eds): Chlamydial Infections. Proceedings of the 6th International Symposium on Human Chlamydial Infections. Cambridge, Cambridge University, 1986, pp 329–332.
236. Campbell LA, Kuo C-C, Wang S-P, et al: Serological response to *Chlamydia pneumoniae* infection. J Clin Microbiol 28:1261, 1990.
237. Batteiger BE, Jones RB: Chlamydial infections. Infect Dis Clin North Am 1:55, 1987.
238. Schachter J: The intracellular life of *Chlamydia*. Curr Top Microbiol Immunol 138:109, 1988.
239. Schachter J: Pathogenesis of chlamydial infections. Pathol Immunopathol Res 8:206, 1989.
240. Wyrick PB, Richmond SJ: Biology of *Chlamydia*. J Am Vet Med Assoc 195:1507, 1989.

CHAPTER 13

The Spirochetes

Mark D. Oberlander and Stefan D. Trocme

The spirochetes belong to the eubacterial phylum and are unicellular, mobile, coil-shaped bacteria with a morphology different from that of other bacterial organisms. Many spirochetes are not cultivable and range from anaerobes to aerobes and from free-living organisms to obligate parasites. Spirochetes (Greek *spira,* "coil," + *chaete,* "hair") are long, slender, flexible organisms appearing as helical coils or as undulating waves of varying amplitude. Many can be observed only by dark-field microscopy or by staining with silver salts. Examination of spirochetes by dark-field illumination reveals a motility characteristic of the organism, including apparent rotation around its axis, flexion, and boring corkscrew motion. All spirochetes contain a central protoplasmic cylinder consisting of cytoplasmic and nuclear regions surrounded by a cytoplasmic membrane[1] and closely adherent cell wall (Fig. 13–1). Filamentous structures called axial fibrils, periplasmic flagella, or endoflagella are located between the protoplasmic cylinder and outer envelope. These structures are similar to flagella of other bacteria, both chemically and morphologically. They probably play a role in motility, because nonmotile mutant spirochetes contain flagella that are straight, rather than coiled, as in motile spirochetes. The outer envelope of spirochetes is similar to that of gram-negative bacteria: Large spirochetes stain gram-negative but do not contain endotoxin.

Three genera of spirochetes cause human disease: *Treponema,* which includes the pathogens that cause syphilis *(T. pallidum),* yaws *(T. pertenue),* and pinta *(T. carateum); Borrelia,* which includes the agents of epidemic relapsing fever *(B. recurrentis)* and Lyme disease *(B. burgdorferi);* and *Leptospira,* a variety of small spirochetes that cause mild to severe systemic human illness. The following review is limited to *T. pallidum* and *B. burgdorferi,* the two spirochetes that produce human disease that has significant ocular manifestations.

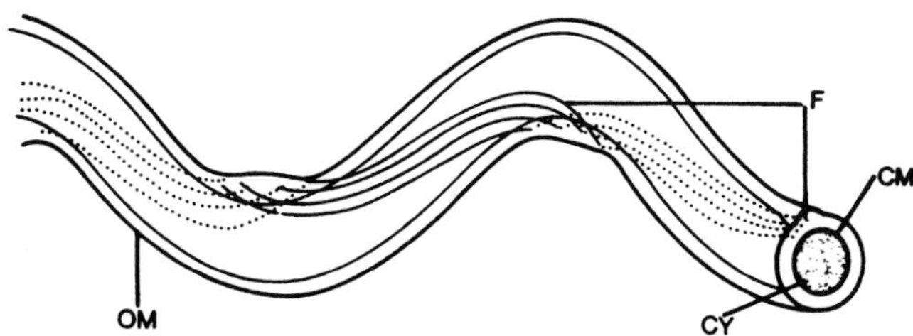

FIGURE 13–1. Diagram of a generalized basic structure of spirochetes. CM, cytoplasmic membrane–peptidoglycan complex; CY, cytoplasm; F, axial fibrils; OM, outer membrane.

Treponema Pallidum

HISTORY AND EPIDEMIOLOGY OF SYPHILIS

The first descriptions of syphilis date back to the pandemic in Europe and Asia at the end of the 15th century. Unexplained virulence of *T. pallidum,* seldom seen today, frequently caused death during the secondary stage. The disease was particularly malignant for approximately 60 years, starting in the 1490s; after this time it became less severe, though the late consequences were still serious. The primary and secondary stages of the disease were recognized early during the pandemic, as was the sexual mode of transmission. Interestingly, gonorrhea and syphilis were long viewed as one disease, an erroneous concept explained in part by John Hunter's self-inoculation with a patient's gonorrheal pus in 1767, after which he developed syphilis; the patient probably suffered concurrently from gonorrhea and syphilis. It was only in the mid-1800s that the two were recognized to be separate entities, although the cause remained elusive until the beginning of the 20th century. Schaudinn and Hoffman discovered *T. pallidum* in serum from secondary syphilitic lesions in 1905.[2] In 1910, Wassermann developed a diagnostic complement fixation test for syphilis, and in the same year an arsenic derivative, arsphenamine (Salvarsan), was introduced as an effective treatment for syphilis.

The exact prevalence of syphilis cannot be established with certainty, but it is well known that the number of reported cases has varied over the years. Incidence peaked in the early 1940s, then declined until 1955. The number of recorded cases increased again until it reached a steady level in the early 1960s.[3] Since 1977, reported cases have increased annually. The increased incidence of syphilis has closely paralleled the acquired immunodeficiency syndrome (AIDS) epidemic. Recent studies of patients presenting with ocular syphilis revealed that 44 to 70% were found to be human immunodeficiency virus (HIV)–positive on serologic testing.[4] These patients have more extensive ocular disease at presentation, a higher incidence of bilaterality, a more fulminant course, and an increased incidence of central nervous system involvement compared with HIV-negative patients.[4] Syphilis epidemiology also bears out two important points: first, the disproportionately large number of cases in homosexual and bisexual males, and second, the predominance of syphilis in urban areas.

ANATOMY AND METABOLISM

T. pallidum measures 5 to 20 mm in length and less than 0.2 mm in thickness; it is morphologically indistinguishable from other pathologic treponemes. The organism is best recognized in dark-field illumination, because this permits observation of the characteristic motility. The pathogenic treponemes are pointed at each end; nonpathogens have blunt, rounded ends.

Experimental animals such as rabbits are readily infected with *T. pallidum.* Testicular infections of rabbits can yield considerable numbers of viable spirochetes for physiologic studies. It is generally agreed that virulent *T. pallidum* organisms able to cause disease have not yet been cultured in artificial media; cultivable strains have all been nonvirulent. All cultured strains have been anaerobic and slow-growing; division times range from 4 to 18 hours. Successful attempts to cultivate *T. pallidum* in tissue-cultured rabbit epithelial cells have been reported.[5] Subsequent studies on tissue-culture infection have demonstrated that virulent *T. pallidum,* but not nonvirulent treponemes, adhere to cells in culture and rapidly become intracellular.[6] A terminal end-structure of the spirochete anchors the organism to the cell membrane, after which the spirochete can be observed to wave and flex.[7] The treponemes are frail microorganisms that quickly die outside the host. They are rapidly destroyed by soap and water or by drying. The organism is unusually susceptible to heat and is killed in a matter of hours at 41°C. Although infection occasionally has been transmitted through blood products, the risk of such transmission is small, because the spirochete dies in 3 or 4 days at refrigerator temperature and rapidly in lyophilized plasma.

CLINICAL MANIFESTATIONS OF SYPHILIS

Primary Stage

After penetrating the skin or mucous membrane, *T. pallidum* rapidly invades tissue.[8] The primary lesion, often called the hunterian chancre, appears 10 to 30 days later. The chancre is indolent and typically has a hard base; *T. pallidum* can frequently be demonstrated in the "serum" expressed from the chancre. Evidence from both rabbit and human infections indicates that systemic dissemination occurs soon after entry; treponemes appear in draining lymph nodes in a short time and are spread to other tissues within hours. At the entry site, treponemes multiply, causing hemorrhage, vascular damage, and necrosis within a few days and producing a characteristic chancre with accumulation of mucoid material. The chancre typically heals within weeks, but the disseminated infection continues.

Secondary Stage

During this phase, which occurs approximately 4 to 8 weeks after the appearance of the primary chancre, the generalized nature of the disease becomes evident. Cutaneous lesions; bone, joint, and ocular lesions; enlargement of the lymph nodes; and other phenomena occur. *T. pallidum* is present in large numbers in the blood and in lesions on mucous membranes and skin. An immune response often leads to healing of the lesions but not necessarily elimination of the spirochetes. The effectiveness of the immune response is indicated by the observation that only about one-fourth of patients develop secondary syphilis, and of these only about half progress to the tertiary stage.

Tertiary Stage

Cutaneous ulcerations and visceral gummatous lesions may develop during this phase; clinical symptoms depend on localization of lesions. *T. pallidum* is present in tertiary lesions, but only in small numbers. Neurosyphilis may develop during the third or even the second stage, but it is mostly a manifestation of late tertiary syphilis and formerly was called quaternary or parasyphilitic disease; the most common clinical forms are tabes dorsalis and general paresis. Treponemes may be found in the central nervous system and cerebrospinal fluid of patients suffering from neurosyphilis.

Latent Syphilis

Diagnosis of latent syphilis requires a positive specific treponemal antibody test result for syphilis, with normal cerebrospinal fluid and absence of clinical manifestations or history of manifestations of syphilis. The early phase of latent syphilis that encompasses the first 2 years after infection may be marked by intermittent occurrence of primary lesions. The late latent syphilis, which follows 2 years after infection, is frequently associated with some degree of immunity to reinfection, although seeding of *T. pallidum* into the patients' blood may still occur, and fetal infection is a risk in pregnant women. The spirochete and the immune system of the host appear to reach a steady state in which the organism survives although the infection remains latent. It is unclear whether patients with latent syphilis ever experience spontaneous cure of their disease; however, 50 to 70% of untreated patients never develop clinically evident syphilis.

Congenital Syphilis

During the fifth month of gestation, the placenta reaches a developmental stage that permits transmission of the spirochetes to the fetus. Syphilis may cause developmental arrest of the fetus, with intrauterine death, or it may continue to develop to term. Often, however, the child is born with generalized syphilis and with lesions characteristic of the secondary stage. In early maternal syphilis, the risk of the fetal infection may be as high as 80 to 95%; the risk of transmission decreases in later stages of maternal syphilis. Clinically, the most common problem is a healthy baby who has a mother with positive serology; fulminant cases of congenital syphilis in newborns certainly occur, and the prognosis for the afflicted child is poor. The characteristic stigmata of congenital syphilis include Hutchinson's teeth; an abnormal facies with frontal bossing, saddle nose, and poorly developed maxilla; nerve deafness; and ocular disease, such as chorioretinitis, optic atrophy, and interstitial keratitis.

Ocular Syphilis

The manifestations of ocular syphilis were discussed in a recent report[9] and are discussed extensively elsewhere (see Chap. 80, Keratoprosthesis, and Chap. 249, Anatomy of the Eyelids and Lacrimal Drainage System). Syphilis was once considered one of the most common causes of intraocular inflammation, although the epidemiology of syphilis changed with the advent of antibiotic therapy. Reported cases have surged since the 1970s. Ocular syphilis lacks pathognomonic signs and can mimic almost any ocular inflammatory condition. Reported ocular diseases associated with syphilis include iritis, chorioretinitis, interstitial keratitis, retinal vasculitis, papillitis, iris papules, episcleritis, scleritis, and exudative retinal detachment.

IMMUNITY AND LABORATORY DIAGNOSIS OF SYPHILIS

Syphilitic infection produces an immune response and prevents reinfection. Once the first chancre has appeared, reinfection does not produce a second initial lesion. Histologically, the lesion shows a mononuclear and histiocytic infiltrate with obliterative periarteritis of small vessels. By electron microscopy, *T. pallidum* organisms can be seen in interstitial and perivascular spaces. Although the host infected with *T. pallidum* does develop immunity, it is not completely protective: Elimination of the spirochete does not always occur. The importance of a competent immune system to the infected host is underscored by recent reports of syphilis in HIV-infected persons, which appears to have an accelerated course, frequently involving the central nervous system and responding less favorably to standard therapy.[10] Infection with *T. pallidum* produces a delayed type of hypersensitivity; a typical delayed hypersensitivity skin reaction can be elicited in the late stages of the disease. A humoral immune response is also induced by *T. pallidum* infection, with both antilipoidal (reaginic) and specific antitreponemal antibodies. The protective role of humoral immunity is ill understood. In the presence of complement, spirochetes are killed by specific antibodies, although passive immunization of rabbits with immune serum does not confer immunity to infection. The virulence factors that give *T. pallidum* the ability to produce syphilitic disease are incompletely understood, because of difficulty of culturing the organism. Two virulence factors have been proposed: first, the mucopolysaccharide surface component, which may protect against specific antibodies, and second, the mucopolysaccharidase, which may be used to adhere to host cells.

Dark-field examination of fresh exudate from open lesions can be used for diagnosis of the primary or secondary stage of syphilis; dark-field examinations must be interpreted with care, and a skilled observer can often differentiate *T. pallidum* from other spiral organisms on the basis of its characteristic morphology and motility. Immunofluorescence staining techniques can also be employed to identify the organism in fluid from active lesions.

Several serologic tests developed[11] for the diagnosis of syphilis can be categorized as either nonspecific (reagin) antibody tests or specific treponemal antibody tests (Table 13–1). The nontreponemal (reaginic) antibodies in syphilis are directed against a lipoidal antigen resulting from the interaction between *T. pallidum* and host tissues. The most commonly used nonspecific antibody tests are the rapid plasma reagin (RPR) tests and the Venereal Disease Research Laboratories (VDRL) slide flocculation test; reagin titer reflects disease activity. Unfortunately, other diseases–including malaria, lupus erythematosus, and leprosy–may produce a false-positive reaction. Reaginic antibody is usually present in detectable amounts 1 to 3 weeks after the primary lesion erupts, and it reaches peak levels during the secondary stage of infection. The antibody may remain at high levels or fall below detectable levels in serum. VDRL results are positive in only 75% of cases of late (tertiary) syphilis; thus, a negative VDRL result does not exclude late syphilis.

TABLE 13–1. **Common Serologic Tests for Syphilis**

Nonspecific antibody tests
Flocculation: Venereal Disease Research Laboratories (VDRL)
Agglutination: rapid plasma reagin (RPR)
Specific treponemal antibody tests
Immunofluorescence: fluorescent treponemal antibody absorption (FTA-ABS)
Immobilization: *Treponema pallidum* immobilization (TPI)
Hemagglutination: *T. pallidum* hemagglutination assay (TPHA)

Specific treponemal antibody tests, such as the *T. pallidum* immobilization (TPI) test, are more specific than the VDRL test but are not generally available. A more widely performed assay is the fluorescent treponemal antibody absorption (FTA-ABS) test, which uses an extract of the Reiter treponeme to adsorb cross-reacting antibodies. This test yields positive results in only about 80% of patients with primary syphilis but in almost all patients with secondary or tertiary syphilis. A hemagglutination test (*T. pallidum* hemagglutination assay [TPHA]) for treponema antigen is also available and is similar to the FTA-ABS in sensitivity and specificity. After treatment, antitreponemal antibodies decline more slowly than reaginic antibodies and may cause positive reactions for years after treatment.

TREATMENT OF SYPHILIS

Although several antibiotics—tetracyclines, erythromycin, cephalosporins—may be effective, penicillin G is still the drug of choice for all stages of syphilis. *T. pallidum* is killed by fairly small amounts of penicillin G, but a long period of exposure to penicillin is required for treatment because of the slow multiplication rate of the organism. Penicillin acts on growing bacterial cells by interfering with the synthesis of peptidoglycans of the cell wall. For any given treatment regimen, the recurrence rate increases as the infection evolves from incubating syphilis to secondary and late syphilis. Although it has not been proved, it may well be that a longer course of treatment may be required as the disease progresses to later phases. No well-controlled studies exist on optimal dose and duration of therapy with penicillin G, although certain treatment guidelines for syphilis have been advanced by the Centers for Disease Control and Prevention (CDC).

Lyme Disease

HISTORY AND EPIDEMIOLOGY OF LYME DISEASE

In 1977, a cluster of children in Lyme, Connecticut, appeared to have contracted juvenile rheumatoid arthritis. It soon became apparent that their ailment was a spirochetal infection that involved multiple systems, including the skin, nervous system, heart, and joints.[12] This disease was later called Lyme disease. The skin manifestation, erythema migrans, linked Lyme disease with certain syndromes previously described in Europe. Lipschutz in Austria[13] and Afzelius in Sweden[14] described a slowly expanding skin lesion, erythema chronicum migrans, produced by tick bites. Tick-borne meningopolyneuritis[15] (Bannwarth's syndrome) could also be preceded by erythema migrans. These syndromes were united in 1982 when Burgdorfer and Barbour isolated a spirochete previously unknown, later named *Borrelia burgdorferi*, from *Ixodes dammini* ticks.[16] The clinical manifestations of this spirochetal infection appear to be subject to regional variations, although the basic features are shared. Lyme disease and syphilis have striking similarities: Both mimic other diseases and occur in stages.

Lyme disease is the most common vectorborne infection in the United States. According to the CDC, Lyme disease accounted for 81% of all reported cases of arthropod-transmitted diseases in the United States between 1986 and 1991.[17] Since the 1980s, the number of reported cases has increased 10-fold, with 13,043 cases reported in 1994 compared with only 523 cases in 1982.[17] Most recently, in 1996, a total of 16,461 cases of Lyme disease were reported to the CDC by 45 states and the District of Columbia. The disease remains concentrated in Eastern and North Central states—Connecticut, Rhode Island, New York, New Jersey, Delaware, Pennsylvania, Maryland, and Wisconsin accounted for 91% of all cases. Nantucket Island, off the coast of Massachusetts, recorded the highest per-capita caseload, with over 1200 persons afflicted per 100,000 population.[17] Many European countries have also reported a large number of cases. The infection usually occurs when the nymphal ticks feed between May and July (Fig. 13–2). Adult ticks occasionally transmit the disease when they feed in the autumn; the ticks that propagate *B. burgdorferi* are part of the *Ixodes ricinus* complex, including *I. dammini*, *I. pacificus*, *I. ricinus*, and *I. persulcatus*. The preferred host for both the nymphal and larval stages of *I. dammini*, which dominates in the midwestern and northeastern United States, is the white-footed mouse. The white-tailed deer, although not involved in the life cycle of the spirochete, is the preferred host of the adult form of *I. dammini* and appears to be critical to the survival of the ticks.

One can only speculate about the reasons for the spread and focal epidemics of Lyme disease in the northeastern United States in recent years. It is possible that the habitat for deer improved in some areas of the northeast as abandoned farmland reverted to woodland, resulting in migration of deer that brought the tick with them. Other rural areas where both deer and deer ticks reside may also have become more heavily populated, resulting in exposure of susceptible urban dwellers to the spirochete.

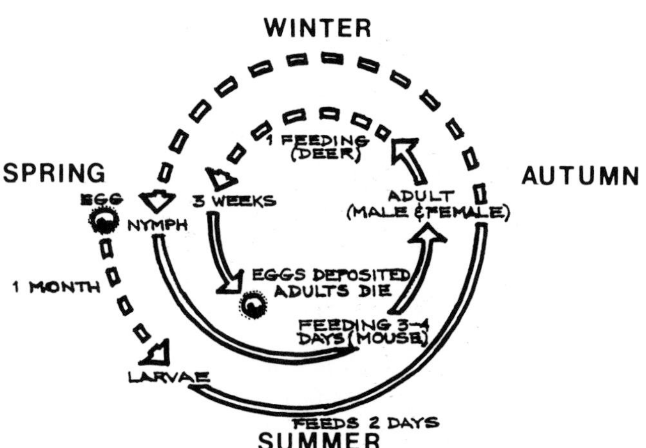

FIGURE 13–2. Life cycle of *Ixodes dammini* tick.

ANATOMY AND CULTIVATION

B. burgdorferi is the longest (20 to 30 mm) and narrowest (0.2 to 0.3 mm) of the *Borrelia* species and, like all spirochetes, is made up of a protoplasmic cylinder, a cell membrane, a flagellum, and an outer membrane. *Borrelia* organisms differ from other spirochetes, because they are longer and more loosely coiled than others. *B. burgdorferi* is fastidious but cultivable in a complex liquid medium called Barbour-Stoenner-Kelly medium,[18] although the organism loses its pathogenicity in culture after 10 to 15 passages. The spirochete is easy to obtain as a primary isolate from ticks but difficult to isolate from patients. The *Borrelia* species grow slowly and elongate for 12 to 24 hours before dividing into two cells.

Differences in morphology and surface proteins have been noted among American and European isolates of *B. burgdorferi*. European strains have been more diverse than American ones; some of this diversity may explain variations in clinical disease in different geographic regions. Currently, there is no accepted system for subclassifying different subtypes of *B. burgdorferi*.

CLINICAL MANIFESTATIONS OF LYME DISEASE

Lyme disease usually evolves in stages and has different clinical characteristics at each. A classification plan, analogous to that used in syphilis, has been advanced by Asbrink and Hovmark[19]: stage 1 with localized erythema migrans; stage 2 with disseminated infection; and stage 3 with chronic infection. An infected person may not exhibit all stages, and the disease may not cause symptoms until the later stages.

Stage 1

Erythema migrans develops in 60 to 80% of patients after *B. burgdorferi* has been inoculated into the skin by the tick. Sometimes the skin manifestations are accompanied by fever and regional lymphadenopathy. The spirochete can sometimes be cultivated from the skin lesions at this stage. The erythema migrans lesion fades within 3 to 4 weeks but can recur.

Stage 2

The spirochete rapidly spreads in the patient's blood to multiple sites. The disseminated infection is often associated with symptoms affecting the skin, nervous system, and musculoskeletal apparatus (Table 13–2). The characteristic annular skin lesion of this stage, which occurs in 50% of patients, is generally smaller and migrates less than that of erythema migrans. The patient may complain of headache, stiff neck, and migrating pain in joints, bursae, muscle, and bone. The symptoms are typically intermittent and changing. After weeks to months, the infection starts to localize, and about 15 to 20% exhibit neurologic involvement; meningitis with

TABLE 13–2. **Lyme Disease by Stage**

Organ	Stage 1	Stage 2	Stage 3
Skin	Erythema migrans	Secondary annular lesions, malar rash, diffuse erythema or urticaria, evanescent lesions, lymphocytoma	Acrodermatitis chronica atrophicans, localized scleroderma-like lesions
Musculoskeletal system		Migratory pain in joints, tendons, bursae, muscle, bone; brief arthritis attacks; myositis, osteomyelitis; panniculitis	Prolonged arthritis attacks, chronic arthritis, peripheral enthesopathy, periostitis or joint subluxations below lesions of acrodermatitis
Neurologic system		Meningitis, cranial neuritis, Bell's palsy, motor or sensory radiculoneuritis, subtle encephalitis, mononeuritis multiplex, myelitis, chorea, cerebellar ataxia	Chronic encephalomyelitis, spastic paraparesis, ataxic gait, subtle mental disorders, chronic axonal polyradiculopathy, dementia
Lymphatic system	Regional lymphadenopathy	Regional or generalized lymphadenopathy, splenomegaly	
Heart		Atrioventricular nodal block, myopericarditis, pancarditis	
Eyes		Conjunctivitis, iritis, choroiditis, retinal hemorrhage or detachment, panophthalmitis	Keratitis
Liver		Mild or recurrent hepatitis	
Respiratory system		Nonexudative sore throat, nonproductive cough, adult respiratory distress syndrome	
Kidney		Microscopic hematuria or proteinuria	
Constitutional symptoms	Minor	Severe malaise and fatigue	Fatigue

superimposed cranial or peripheral neuropathy is common. The spirochete has been cultured from spinal fluid from patients with meningitis. Unilateral or bilateral facial palsy is the most common cranial neuropathy, and it may be the only neurologic sign. The neurologic abnormalities of stage 2 last weeks to months but can recur and become chronic. Some 4 to 8% of patients suffer cardiac complications, such as atrioventricular block or acute myocarditis. Many of the ocular manifestations of Lyme disease occur during stage 2.

Stage 3

Arthritic episodes become longer in duration in the second and third year of the illness and may become chronic. One or a few large joints are affected, usually the knees. Late in the disease, progressive encephalomyelitis may develop, characterized by spastic paraparesis, bladder dysfunction, ataxia, seventh or eighth cranial nerve deficit, and dementia.[20] Another late manifestation of Lyme disease is acrodermatitis chronica atrophicans. This skin lesion, which has been observed principally in Europe, begins with a bluish red discoloration and swollen skin, which lasts for years and gradually leads to skin atrophy.

CONGENITAL LYME DISEASE

Transplacental transmission of *B. burgdorferi* has been reported in infants of mothers who have Lyme disease during early pregnancy; potentially lethal congenital malformations sometimes result. Although *B. burgdorferi* can cause serious fetal infections and malformations, they appear to be rare.

OCULAR LYME DISEASE

The ocular complications of Lyme disease, which were recently reviewed,[21, 22] include such diverse manifestations as papilledema associated with pseudotumor cerebri, ischemic optic neuropathy, oculomotor or abducens nerve paresis, bilateral keratitis, panophthalmitis, diffuse choroiditis, and exudative retinal detachment. In stage 1, mild follicular conjunctivitis and photophobia have been reported in up to 11% of patients.[23]

It is in late stage 2 (disseminated infection) or stage 3 (persistent infection) that most of the severe ocular manifestations of Lyme disease occur. One series reported that 10.6% of patients had seventh-nerve paresis or Bell's palsy; nearly one-fourth of these patients had bilateral Bell's palsy.[23] In general, patients presenting with cranial neuropathy (Bell's palsy in particular), idiopathic chronic uveitis, pars planitis, unexplained bilateral keratitis, optic nerve inflammation, or papilledema should be questioned about a history of a tick bite, skin rash, arthritis, or meningitis, and serologic testing for Lyme disease should be initiated if the answer to any of these questions is yes.

LABORATORY DIAGNOSIS OF LYME DISEASE

Cultivation and visualization of tissue-bound *B. burgdorferi* organisms are not practical diagnostic modalities, because the recovery rate is low owing to the paucity of organisms in tissue. Diagnosis of Lyme disease typically depends on serologic methods (Table 13–3). The most commonly used serologic tests are the immunofluorescence assay and the

TABLE 13–3. **Serologic Tests for Lyme Disease**

Indirect immunofluorescent assay (IFA)
Enzyme-linked immunosorbent assay (ELISA)
ELISA (IgG)
ELISA (IgM)
with ELISA *Treponema reiteri* adsorption

enzyme-linked immunosorbent assay (ELISA). Currently, the ELISA is preferred because it is more sensitive and specific for all stages of Lyme disease.[24] Even the ELISA, however, lacks sensitivity during the first weeks of infection, and it has been modified to include a *Treponema reiteri* adsorption step that decreases background activity in normal control serum, which enhances the sensitivity of the test.[25] Another pitfall of serologic testing is that the results obtained on the same patient can vary from laboratory to laboratory because of a lack of standardization.

In untreated patients, the immunoglobulin M (IgM) antibody peaks first, 3 to 6 weeks after infection, and gradually decreases thereafter. The IgG antibody response follows that of IgM and becomes the predominant late antibody. Patients exhibiting the manifestations of stage-2 and -3 disease typically have strongly positive serology for IgG. Determining the isotype of the antibody response is seldom advantageous and can be reserved for unusual or difficult cases; a polyvalent conjugate can be used for routine testing.[26]

False-negative results may occur during the first several weeks of infection because most patients have not yet developed a sufficient antibody response to Lyme disease to give a positive serologic result. However, by 5 weeks after disease onset, 90% of patients yield positive results with either the ELISA or the immunofluorescence assay.[27] Other important causes of false-negative results include patients who have been partially or inadequately treated with oral antibiotics early in the course of Lyme disease. These patients may develop chronic symptoms yet never yield positive serologic results. Finally, immunosuppressed patients may never develop an adequate antibody response to Lyme disease and thus continue to yield false-negative results.

False-positive results due to cross-reactivity have been reported between Lyme disease and syphilis, Rocky Mountain spotted fever, leptospirosis, relapsing fever, some autoimmune diseases, and neurologic disorders. The cross-reaction between Lyme disease and syphilis has been reported in 22 to 54% of patients.[28]

A positive or equivocal ELISA assay result should be followed up with a corresponding Western blot assay. The Western blot is a qualitative assay based on the individual visualization of a patient's unique antibody against the various *Borrelia* antigens. This type of assay is more sensitive and specific than the ELISA test; it provides detection before the peak of the response. Cross-reactions have been reported to be due to rheumatoid factor, other flagellar diseases, and mononucleosis.[29] Other tests in current use include the Lyme Urine Antigen Test and the polymerase chain reaction, which is used to amplify minute amounts of DNA in clinical specimens.[30]

TREATMENT OF LYME DISEASE

B. burgdorferi's antibiotic sensitivity has been assessed in vitro and in experimental animals. There is general agreement that the spirochete is highly sensitive to tetracycline but only moderately sensitive to penicillin. For early Lyme disease (stage 1 or 2), tetracycline or doxycycline is generally effective. Amoxicillin is the best choice for children and an alternative to tetracycline for adults. Topical corticosteroids may be given for anterior segment inflammation (keratitis, episcleritis). Patients with severe disease (i.e., meningitis, carditis, or severe neuroophthalmic disease) must be treated with parenteral therapy, either intravenous penicillin G or ceftriaxone, for 14 days.[31] The role of systemic corticosteroids in the treatment of Lyme disease remains controversial; however, it is generally accepted that systemic corticosteroids should not be used without the concomitant use of antibiotics. Researchers are currently at work on a vaccine against Lyme disease. In the meantime, CDC officials advise the public to wear light-colored clothes, tuck long pants into socks, and use insecticides to keep ticks at bay. Another preventative measure is to avoid low, dense foliage when walking in tick-prone areas.[32]

Summary

Two genera of spirochetes have pathogens that can cause human ocular disease: *Treponema,* with the pathogen *T. pallidum,* which can cause the protean ocular manifestations of syphilis; and *Borrelia,* with the pathogen *B. burgdorferi,* which can produce the many ophthalmic findings of Lyme disease. Both *T. pallidum* and *B. burgdorferi* can give rise to ocular and systemic disease, which may lack pathognomonic signs and symptoms and may mimic most any ocular or general inflammatory condition. The diagnosis is often uncovered only after serologic testing. Both *T. pallidum* and *B. burgdorferi* are sensitive to appropriate antibiotics, although despite treatment the organisms may survive in the host in a latent state.

REFERENCES

1. Canale-Parola E: Physiology and evolution of spirochetes. Bacteriol Rev 41:181, 1977.
2. Schaudinn F, Hoffman E: Vorlanfiger Bericht uber das Vorkommen von Spirochaeten in syphilitischen Krankheitsproducten und bei papillomen. Arb Gsundhtsamte 22:527, 1904–1905.
3. Syphilis trends in the United States. MMWR 30:441, 1981.
4. Williams JK, Kirsch LS, Russack V, Freeman WR: Rhegmatogenous retinal detachments in HIV-positive patients with ocular syphilis. Ophthalmic Surg Laser 27(8):699–705, 1996.
5. Fieldsteel AH, Cox DL, Moeckli RA: Cultivation of virulent *Treponema pallidum* in tissue culture. Infect Immun 32:908, 1981.
6. Fitzgerald TJ: Interaction of *Treponema pallidum* (Nichols strain) with cultured mammalian cells: Effects of oxygen, reducing agents, serum supplements, and different cell types. Infect Immun 15:444, 1977.
7. Hayes HS, et al: Parasitism by virulent *Treponema pallidum* of host cell surfaces. Infect Immun 17:174, 1977.
8. Treponemal Infections. WHO Technical Report Series No. 674. Geneva, World Health Organization, 1982.
9. Tamesis RR, Foster CF: Ocular syphilis. Ophthalmology 97:1281, 1990.
10. Passo MS, Rosenbaum JT: Ocular syphilis in patients with human immunodeficiency virus infection. Am J Ophthalmol 106:1, 1988.
11. Balows A, Feely JL, Jaffe HW: Laboratory diagnosis of treponematoses (with emphasis on syphilis). *In* Johnson RC (ed): The Biology of Parasitic Spirochetes. New York, Academic Press, 1976.
12. Steere AC, Malawista SR, Hardin JA, et al: Erythema chronicum migrans and Lyme arthritis: The enlarging clinical spectrum. Ann Intern Med 86:685, 1977.
13. Lipschutz B: Weiterer Betrag zur Kenntnis des "Erythema chronicum migrans." Arch Dermatol Syphilol 143:365, 1923.
14. Afzelius A: Erythema chronicum migrans. Acta Dermatol Venereol (Stockh) 2:120, 1921.
15. Bannwarth A: Zur Klinik und Pathogenese der "Chronischen lymphocytaren meningitis." Arch Psychiatr Nervenkr 117:161, 1944.
16. Burgdorfer W, Barbour AG, Hayes SF, et al: Lyme disease: A tick-borne spirochetosis. Science 216:1317, 1982.
17. Lyme disease in the United States. MMWR 46(23), 1997.
18. Barbour AG: Isolation and cultivation of Lyme disease spirochetes. Yale J Biol Med 57:521, 1984.

19. Asbrink E, Hovmark A: Early and late cutaneous manifestations of *Ixodes*-borne borreliosis (erythema migrans borreliosis, Lyme borreliosis). Ann N Y Acad Sci 539:4, 1988.
20. Ackermann R, Rhese-Kupper B, Gottmer E, Schmidt R: Chronic neurologic manifestations of erythema migrans borreliosis. Ann N Y Acad Sci 539:16, 1988.
21. Winward KE, Smith JL, Culbertson WW, Paris-Hamelin A: Ocular Lyme borreliosis. Am J Ophthalmol 108:651, 1989.
22. Kornmehl EW, Lesser RL, Janos P, et al: Bilateral keratitis in Lyme disease. Ophthalmology 96:1194, 1989.
23. Bergloff J, Gasser R, Feigl B: Ophthalmic manifestations in Lyme borreliosis. A review. J Neuroophthalmol 14(1):15–20, 1994.
24. Craft JE, Grodzicki RL, Steere AC: Antibody response in Lyme disease: Evaluation of diagnostic tests. J Infect Dis 149:789, 1984.
25. Mertz LE, Wobig GH, Duffy J, Katzmann JA: Improved sensitivity in a Lyme disease enzyme-linked immunosorbent assay using a *Treponema reiteri* adsorbent [Abstract]. Arthritis Rheum 30(Suppl):17, 1987.
26. Mertz LE, Wobig G, Duffy J, Katzmann JA: A comparison of test procedures for the detection of antibody to *Borrelia burgdorferi*. Ann N Y Acad Sci 539:474, 1988.
27. Lesser RL, Kornmehl EW, Pachmer AR, et al: Neuroophthalmologic manifestations of Lyme disease. Ophthalmology 97:699–706, 1990.
28. Winward KE, Lawton Smith J: Ocular disease in Caribbean patients with serologic evidence of Lyme borreliosis. J Clin Neuroophthalmol 9:65–70, 1989.
29. Berg D, Abson KG, Prose NS: The laboratory diagnosis of Lyme disease. Arch Dermatol 127:866–870, 1991.
30. Hilton E, Smith C, Sood S: Ocular Lyme borreliosis diagnosed by polymerase chain reaction on vitreous fluid. Ann Intern Med 125(5):424–425, 1996.
31. Zaidman GW: The ocular manifestations of Lyme disease. Int Ophthalmol Clin 33(1):9–22, 1993.
32. Lyme disease in the United States. MMWR 46(23), 1997.

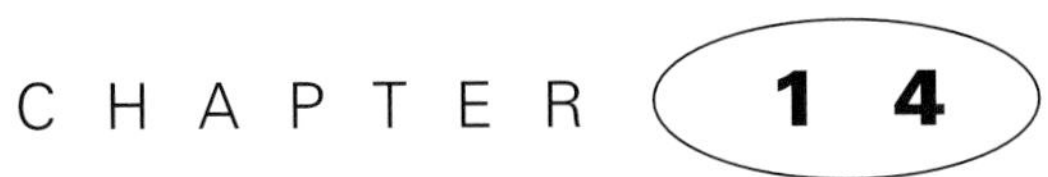

Parasitic and Rickettsial Ocular Infections

Juan-Carlos Abad

Introduction to Parasitology

TERMINOLOGY

Parasitology is the study of different species from the animal kingdom that live together or in close association (on or in the body of another). Symbiosis is the term used to describe this association, each organism called a symbiont. There are various types of symbiosis: Commensalism occurs when one member of the associating pair, usually the smaller, receives all the benefit and the other member is neither benefited or harmed; mutualism exists when both organisms benefit from the association; and parasitism exists when a symbiont lives at the expense of and injures the host.[1] A parasite living on the surface of its host is an ectoparasite; an internal parasite is an endoparasite. Infestation is associated with ectoparasitism and infection with endoparasitism. Parasites are either obligate (they exist only as a parasites) or facultative (they may also exist in a free-living state). Parasites can be permanent (complete life cycle within the host) or temporary.

Hosts can be classified as definitive (the parasite reproduces within the host), intermediate (partial parasite development within the host), or paratenic (no further development of the parasite, yet it remains infectious). A *vector* is the intermediate host that carries and transmits the infectious stage of a parasite to the definitive host. A reservoir host is the source of human infection. An animal-to-human parasite transmission is called zoonosis.

PARASITE CLASSIFICATION

Morphology, life cycle, genetics, reproduction, and aspects of parasite growth and development are used to classify and categorize parasitic species. Serology, biochemistry, electron microscopy, isoenzyme electrophoresis, DNA, RNA, and protein analysis techniques may be required to differentiate members of a species that are otherwise indistinguishable. Various studies and various authors classify parasites by different schema.

The single-celled Protozoa, long considered to be one phylum, have recently been divided into a number of groups assigned phylum rank.[2] These phyla are: Sarcomastigophora, Labyrinthomorphorpha, Apicomplexa, Microspora, Acetospora, Myxozoa, and Ciliophora. Examples of human parasitic protozoans are *Acanthamoeba, Trypanosoma, Leishmania, Giardia, Toxoplasma,* and *Plasmodium.*

The phylum Platyhelminthes are worms characterized by bilateral symmetry with rudimentary development of sensory and motor nerve elements. Platyhelminthes are divided into four classes: Turbellaria, Monogenea, Cestoidea, and Trematoda. Adult cestodes, commonly called tapeworms, have a head (scolex) and a segmented body (strobila) and live within the digestive tract of their host. Examples of Cestoidea are *Taenia, Echinococcus,* and *Spirometra.* Adult trematodes in the subclass Digenea are commonly called flukes, and their

The author wishes to acknowledge Denise de Freitas, M.D., and Edmund C. Dunkel, Ph.D., for their extensive work in this chapter in the first edition of this book.

TABLE 14–1. **Ocular Parasitic Diseases in Humans**

Parasite	Ocular Lesions	Geographic Distribution	Laboratory Tests	Therapy
Protozoa				
Acanthamoeba	Indolent, painful corneal ulcer and infiltrates, iridocyclitis	Worldwide	Calcoflour white stain, culture on *Escherichia coli*	Polyhexamethylene biguanide or chlorhexidine; propamidine or hexamidine; itraconazole
American trypanosomiasis (*Tripanosoma cruzi*)	Bipalpebral edema, unilateral conjunctivitis, Romaña's sign	Central and South America	Blood smears	Nifurtimox
Giardia lamblia	Retinal vasculitis	Worldwide	Cysts and trophozoites in stool	Metronidazole
Leishmania tropica, braziliensis (oriental sore, espundia)	Lid ulcer	Middle East, Asia Minor, Central and South America	Scrapings of skin lesions	Antimony sodium gluconate, allopurinol, or ketoconazole
Malaria (*Plasmodium* species)	Retinal hemorrhages, papilledema, retinal edema	Equatorial region	Blood smear	Chloroquine, primaquine
Microsporidiosis (*Encephalitozoon* species in immunosuppressed patients)	Superficial epithelial keratopathy	Worldwide	Corneal scrapings	Débridement, topical fumagillin, itraconazole
(*Nosema* species in immunocompetent patients)	Stromal keratitis	Worldwide	Corneal scrapings and biopsy	Trimethoprim-sulfamethoxazole
Pneumocystis carinii	Choroidal granulomas	Worldwide	Bronchial washings, sputum cultures, tissue biopsy	Pentamidine isothionate, trimethroprim-sulfamethoxazole
Toxoplasma gondii	Retinochoroiditis, papillitis, retinal vasculitis, uveitis, secondary glaucoma	Worldwide	Serum ELISA, aqueous or vitreous PCR	Pyrimethamine, trisulfapyrimidine or sulfadiazine, clindamycin; steroids, laser, cryotherapy
Intestinal Nematodes				
Ascaris lumbricoides	Rare intraocular worm, vitamin A deficiency	Worldwide	Eggs in stool, complement fixation larva in ocular granuloma or histopathology	Mebendazole, piperazine
Extraintestinal Nematodes				
Baylisascaris procyonis	Diffuse unilateral subacute retinitis	Southeastern United States and Caribbean	Direct observation	Laser photocoagulation; thiabendazole or ivermectin
Dracunculus medinensis	Eyelid and orbital mass	Africa and India	Examination of the worm	Surgical excision
Filariasis				
1. *Dirofilaria* species	Periorbital or intraocular worm	Worldwide	ELISA	Surgical excision
2. Lymphatic filariasis (*Wuchereria bancrofti, Brugia malayi, Brugia timori*)	Elephantiasis, anterior chamber or subretinal microfilaria (rare)	Tropical areas, Far East	Peripheral blood	Diethylcarbamazine
3. *Loa loa*	Subcutaneous nodule, subconjunctival worm, periorbital swelling and pain	Central Africa	Blood smear, tissue biopsy	Diethylcarbamazine
4. *Onchocerca volvulus*	Skin and eye nodules, keratitis, uveitis, chorioretinitis, optic atrophy	Africa, Central and South America	Skin snip, nodule biopsy	Ivermectin
Thelazia callineda or *californiensis*	Conjunctivitis, extraocular muscle paresis, orbital granuloma	Central America	Biopsy lesion for worm	Surgical excision
Toxocara canis, cati	Posterior and peripheral retinal granuloma, panuveitis	Worldwide	ELISA on serum, aqueous or vitreous; CT	Thiabendazole, mebendazole
Trichinella spiralis	Lid and periorbital edema, extraocular muscle paresis and pain	Worldwide	Serology, skin biopsy	Thiabendazole and steroids

TABLE 14–1. **Ocular Parasitic Diseases in Humans** *Continued*

Parasite	Ocular Lesions	Geographic Distribution	Laboratory Tests	Therapy
Trematodes (Flukes)				
Paragonimus westermani	Periocular cyst	Far East, India, Africa, Central and South America	Eggs in feces or sputum, serum ELISA	Praziquantel
Schistosoma haematobium and *japonicum* (bilharzia, schistosomiasis)	Dacryoadenitis, conjunctival and orbital granulomas	Africa, Middle East, Far East	Eggs in urine, lesion biopsy, CT	Praziquantel, niridazole
Tapeworms				
Coenuriasis (*Multiceps multiceps, Taenia brauneri*)	Lids and intraocular cyst	Sheep-raising areas (Africa)	Casoni's intradermal test	Surgical excision
Echinococcus granulosus	Orbital cyst (common), intraocular cyst (rare)	Sheep-raising areas (New Zealand, Argentina, California)	Skin test, indirect hemagglutination or immunofluorescent serology, radiography, CT	Praziquantel
Sparganum proliferum	Orbit or anterior chamber cyst	Far East	Direct observation	Surgical excision
Cysticercus cellulosae	Intraocular granuloma	Worldwide	Skin test, radiograph for calcified cysts	Praziquantel, niridazole
Arthropods				
Demodex folliculorum	Chronic blepharitis	Worldwide	Direct observation	Lid hygiene
Myasis				
1. Ophthalmomyasis externa (*Dematobia hominis, Chrysomia bezziana*)	Lid furuncule and cellulitis, orbital invasion	Central and South America, Old World	Direct observation	Mechanical removal
2. Ophthalmomyasis interna (*Hypoderma lineatum*)	Subretinal tracks, intravitreal invasion	Tropical areas	Direct observation, parasite recovery	Laser photocoagulation, removal of the parasite
Ophthalmia nodosa (Caterpillar hairs)	Conjunctival nodule	Worldwide	Histopathology	Surgical excision
Phthirus pubis	Chronic blepharitis	Worldwide	Direct observation	Lid hygiene, antibiotic or eserine ointment

CT, computed tomography; ELISA, enzyme-linked immunosorbent assay; PCR, polymerase chain reaction.

development occurs in at least two hosts. Examples of Trematoda are *Schistosoma* and *Paragonimus*.

The phylum Nematoda comprises a large number of organisms commonly known as roundworms. Nematodes are divided into two classes, Phasmidia and Aphasmidia, based on the presence or absence of cuticle-lined organs (phasmids). Examples of nematodes are *Trichinella, Ascaris, Toxocara, Dracunculus, Loa,* and *Onchocerca.*[3]

The phylum Arthropoda includes organisms from the classes Arachnida, Insecta, and Crustacea; all have a hard cuticle exoskeleton. Examples of Arthropoda are *Sarcoptes, Demodex, Phthirus, Oestrus, Dermatobia,* and *Hypoderma.*

Table 14–1 is a summary of parasites that cause major ocular diseases.

HOST-PARASITE INTERACTIONS

Interactions between the host and the parasite are crucial for maintenance and continued transmission of parasitic infections. Morphologic, physiologic, and life-cycle modifications have evolved in both host and parasite that have ensured continued disease transmission. Of central importance are adaptations of the parasites that avoid eliciting the host immune response. These parasitic adaptations include the following: (1) different life-cycle stages (eggs, larvae, adult organisms, cysts) evoke different host immune responses, (2) parasite surface composition changes in which alteration of surface antigens render specific host antibodies ineffective,[4] and (3) parasite location within the host (i.e., intracellular versus extracellular) escaping from the immune surveillance mechanisms.

In addition to these parasite adaptations, in certain circumstances the host immune response to parasitic infection can be altered. They include the following: (1) host nutritional status wherein malnourished patients usually have an altered immune response, (2) special host susceptibility: A relative resistance to *Plasmodium vivax* occurs in African Americans, and it has been attributed to the Duffy-negative phenotype present in this population,[5] and (3) altered immune responses such as the case of endogenous or exogenous immunosuppression.

Protozoa

ACANTHAMOEBA

Several genera of free-living amebae cause disease in humans. *Acanthamoeba* infections are the most important; they has been associated with keratitis in healthy persons. In immunosuppressed patients, *Acanthamoeba* infections may result in granulomatous amebic encephalitis (GAE) and disseminated infections. *Vahlkampfia* and *Hartmannella* have also been implicated as a cause of infectious keratitis.[6] *Naegleria* causes primary amebic encephalitis in healthy persons without an ocular component.

DISTRIBUTION

Acanthamoeba species are widespread in nature. They are found in all kinds of water, including fresh, sea, tap, bottled, and brackish,[7] as well as in dust, sewage, sludge, swimming pools, hot tubs, air conditioning ducts, dialysis units, human and animal feces, human oral cavities, and contact lenses and associated paraphernalia. The organisms are found more frequently in thermally enriched water, heated swimming pools, and during the warmer months of the year.[7] *Acanthamoeba* cysts were found to be still infective after being stored in water at 4°C for 24 years.[8]

Acanthamoeba keratitis affects healthy persons and has been associated with corneal trauma, exposure to contaminated water and dust,[9] and contact lens wear. The use of homemade saline solutions, improper contact lens care, and eye exposure to contaminated water while wearing lenses are responsible for the association of *Acanthamoeba* with contact lens use.[10] Males and females are affected equally. Since the first documented case of *Acanthamoeba* keratitis was reported in 1973,[11, 12] the number of cases has increased steadily.[3, 13] A recent series using a confocal microscope as a diagnostic aid suggests that *Acanthamoeba* keratitis may be more common than previously thought.[14]

GAE remains infrequent.[15] Several cases of disseminated *Acanthamoeba* infection in patients with acquired immunodeficiency syndrome (AIDS) with mainly cutaneous manifestations have been reported.[16]

MORPHOLOGY, BIOLOGY, AND LIFE CYCLE

Acanthamoeba exists in two stages: trophozoite and cyst. Trophozoites are the proliferative, active forms; size depends on species (20 to 40 μm).[7] They have irregular shape and pseudopodia with characteristic spine-like processes, Acanthopodina (Fig. 14–1). The cytoplasm contains a single nucleus with a large, dense, central nucleolus surrounded by a clear zone called the zona pellucida. Cytoplasmic organelles

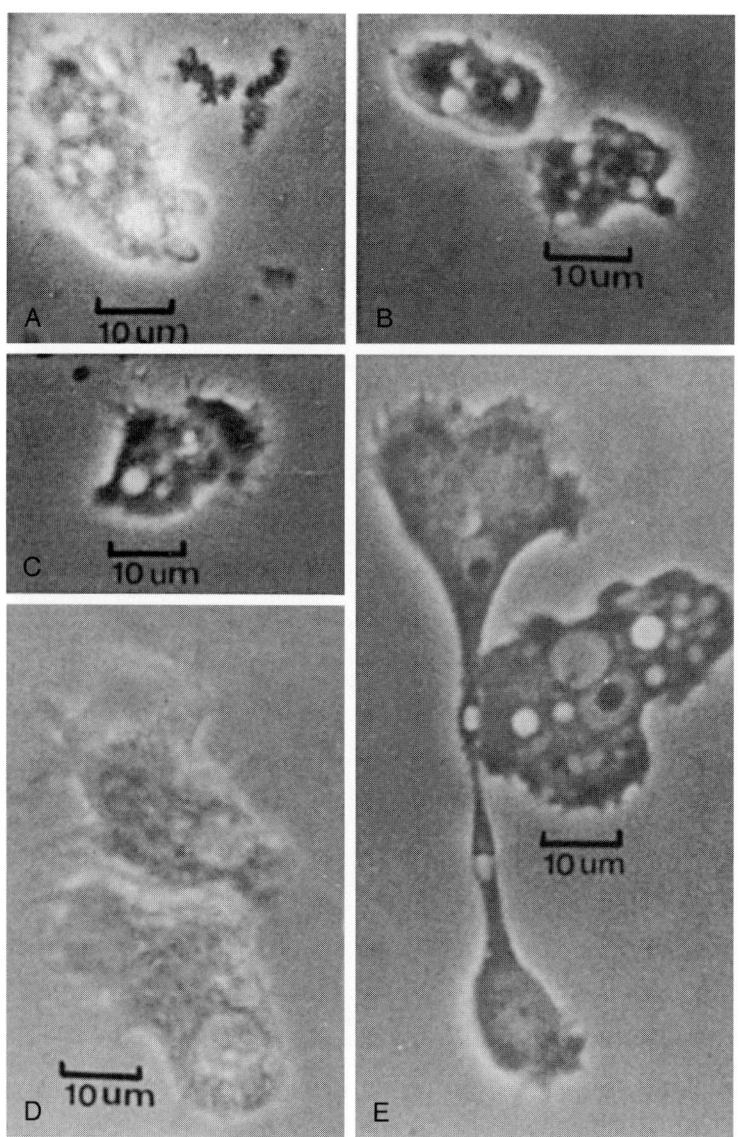

FIGURE 14–1. *Acanthamoeba* trophozoites; unstained culture, fresh wet preparation, phase contrast (×400). *Acanthamoeba* species *(A)*, *A. polyphaga (B)*, *A. culbertsonii (C)*, *A. astronyxis (D)*, *A. castellani (E)*.

are evident, as is a characteristic large contractile vacuole. Trophozoites move by gliding in straight lines and feed on *Escherichia coli* and other enteric gram-negative bacilli. The trophozoite, when exposed to unfavorable conditions (desiccation, lack of food, contact with toxic substances or solutions), undergoes immediate encystment. *Acanthamoeba* proliferate by binary fission.

Acanthamoeba cysts are the resistant, dormant stage of this parasite. Cysts are characterized by a double-walled envelope. The outer wall, the exocyst, is wrinkled, and the inner wall, the endocyst, is smooth. There is a space between the two walls except at the ostiole, where the exocyst is joined to the endocyst. Cyst morphology and size are species-specific (12.5 to 19.2 μm), and encystment states can be differentiated by shape (e.g., spherical, polygonal).[7] The cytoplasm of the cyst contains a single nucleus located centrally, several lipid droplets, mitochondria, and other cytoplasmic organelles but lacks a functioning contractile vacuole. Excystment occurs when favorable environmental conditions return.

INFECTION OF THE HOST

The mechanism for development of *Acanthamoeba* keratitis may be related to epithelial trauma, strain virulence, the number of organisms present, and favorable ameba-cornea contact conditions.[17] The proliferation and binding of *Acanthamoeba* to contact lenses is enhanced by co-contamination of the contact lens care system with gram-negative bacteria.[18] *Acanthamoeba* infection causes destruction of the corneal epithelium and stroma, with subsequent infiltration of inflammatory cells, descemetocele formation, and corneal perforation.[19] The cellular reaction around necrotic organisms may be more intense.[20] *Acanthamoeba castellani* has been shown to produce a plasminogen activator[21] and nonspecific collagenases,[22] which might be related to its pathogenicity. In cases of GAE, the route of central nervous system (CNS) invasion appears to be hematogenous, probably from a primary infection focus in the skin or respiratory tract.[15] Infection with *Acanthamoeba* produces a granulomatous reaction with multinucleated giant cells and a necrotizing angiitis with trophozoites and cysts present within the CNS lesions.

DIAGNOSIS

In cases of *Acanthamoeba* keratitis, smears and culture isolation are the initial diagnostic steps. Recovery of *Acanthamoeba* depends on sampling techniques and organism depth in the cornea. Generally, deep corneal scrapes are necessary to detect *Acanthamoeba.* The confocal microscope has been used for in vivo diagnosis of *Acanthamoeba* keratitis.[23, 24] If these diagnostic measures are unrewarding and clinical suspicion is high, corneal biopsy is recommended.[25]

In cases of CNS infection, cerebrospinal fluid can be centrifuged at low speed and the sediment transferred to a slide to be examined fresh, stained, or transferred to appropriate culture media. Amebic cysts and trophozoites can be identified on histologic sections of brain tissue stained with hematoxylin and eosin (H&E), periodic acid–Schiff, or fluorescent antibody.

Corneal Smears

In Giemsa-stained or Gram-stained samples, *Acanthamoeba* may resemble leukocytes, macrophages, and other mononuclear cells (Fig. 14–2). Gomori-methenamine silver (stains the cyst wall black) as well as periodic acid–Schiff (stains the cyst wall red) may help in identifying the organisms. Calcofluor white, a chemofluorescent dye, has proved useful in detecting *Acanthamoeba* cysts.[26] Smear preparations can be fixed in methyl alcohol and processed using an aqueous solution of 0.1% calcofluor white with Evans blue counterstain. The slides are examined by fluorescent microscopy. The cyst wall appears bright apple-green; trophozoites and other cells appear red-brown. Fluorescent antibody staining of corneal scrapes can also provide a rapid diagnosis of *Acanthamoeba* keratitis with the added advantage of species differentiation.[27] Slides can be fixed in 10% buffered formaldehyde, incubated with diluted rabbit anti-*Acanthamoeba* serum, followed by second-labeled anti-rabbit serum. Cysts and trophozoites fluoresce brightly. More recently, isoenzyme profiles[28] and restriction fragment length polymorphisms of mitochondrial DNA[29] have been used in differentiating *Acanthamoeba.*

Acanthamoeba Culture

Acanthamoeba grows at 25°C to 35°C. For corneal culture recovery, non-nutrient agar overlaid with *E. coli* is a common culture medium. The scraped specimen is placed on the agar surface without streaking or cutting the agar. The plates are sealed with adhesive tape to prevent dehydration and observed for a minimum of 2 weeks. If culture plates are not available, transport solutions can be used. Page's saline solution (a low-osmolarity solution) allows trophozoites to survive transportation at ambient temperature for up to 48 hours.[30] Small aliquots of the solution can be inoculated directly onto the agar.

Corneal Biopsy

If corneal smears and cultures from the corneal scrapings are negative, corneal biopsy is the next viable diagnostic approach. A 3- to 4-mm dermatologic punch is used to make a half-thickness corneal trephination straddling the lesion

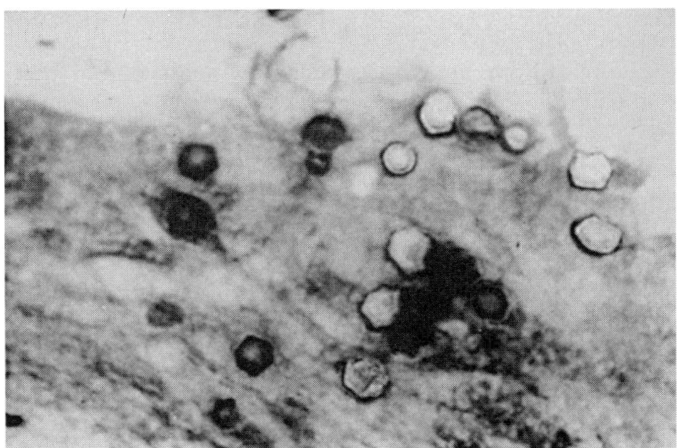

FIGURE 14–2. Corneal scraping from a patient with *Acanthamoeba* keratitis shows double-walled polygonal cysts. Giemsa stain ×400.

and normal cornea. The tissue is resected in a lamellar fashion with a crescent blade. The specimen is split in half. One part is fixated in glutaraldehyde for light and electron microscopy studies. The other half is hand-carried to the microbiology laboratory for bacteria, fungi, and *Acanthamoeba* culture. The same diagnostic stains and culture media used in the scrapings are used in addition to fluorescent antibody stains. Electron microscopy could be used as well.[31]

PREVENTION

Acanthamoeba keratitis, because of its association with contact lenses, may be prevented by meticulous lens care and sterilization precautions. Ophthalmologists should explain to their patients the appropriate care of contact lenses and review the instructions periodically. Tap water and unpreserved saline solutions must be avoided. Thermal disinfection solutions are effective against *Acanthamoeba.*[32] For lenses requiring chemical disinfection, solutions containing chlorhexidine killed *Acanthamoeba* in 30 minutes, benzalkonium chloride systems required at least 1 hour, and hydrogen peroxide systems required up to 2 hours.[33] Solutions containing sorbate, polyaminopropylbiguanide, or polyquaternium-1 may not be effective in killing *Acanthamoeba* organisms.[33] Contact lenses should not be worn during activities that may increase exposure to potentially contaminated water. Prevention of GAE is difficult owing to the opportunistic nature of the infection.

TREATMENT

Cationic antiseptics such as polyhexamethylene biguanide (Baquacil)[34–36] and chlorhexidine[37] are effective against *Acanthamoeba* cysts and trophozoites by disrupting the parasite's plasmalemma. Aromatic diamidines, such as propamidine isethionate (Brolene)[36] and hexamidine (Desomedine),[38] inhibit the parasite's DNA synthesis and can be used in combination with the cationic antiseptics to potentiate their effect. The antibiotic aminoglycosides (neomycin, paromomycin) and the antifungal imidazoles (miconazole, clotrimazole[39]) have some efficacy in tolerable doses as topical agents. Oral itraconazole has been used by some authors.[40] Early animal work suggested that corticosteroids block the conversion of trophozoites to cysts, hence enhancing the effect of the amebicidal medications.[41] Further work has failed to confirm this.[42] Steroids suppress the host's immune response and decrease inflammatory signs, making the patient more comfortable,[43] but they may be associated with a poor outcome.[44] A subconjunctival vaccine composed of *Acanthamoeba* antigens was successfully evaluated in a pig model.[45]

American Trypanosomiasis

American trypanosomiasis (Chagas' disease) is caused by the protozoan *Trypanosoma cruzi.* Sleeping sickness, or African trypanosomiasis, is caused by *T. brucei rhodesiense* (East Africa) and *T. brucei gambiense* (West Africa). There is no direct ocular involvement in African trypanosomiasis.

DISTRIBUTION

South and Central America are endemic areas of Chagas' disease.

MORPHOLOGY, BIOLOGY, AND LIFE CYCLE

In Chagas' disease, triatomid insects are infected with the parasite during a blood meal from a contaminated human. They are also called *besadores* ("kissing bugs") because of their tropism to bite in the head region. During the next blood meal, the insect defecates near the bite wound; the host experiences a mild itching sensation and rubs the feces contaminated with trypomastigotes into the insect bite. If the insect bites near the eye or mouth, the parasites can penetrate directly into the host via mucosal membranes. Trypomastigotes enter a wide variety of cells (cardiac, striated muscle fibers, and cells of the reticuloendothelial system), where they transform into amastigotes (1.5 to 5 μm in length; aflagellated). Intracellularly, the amastigotic forms replicate by binary fission and destroy the cell. Amastigotic forms released in the peripheral blood rapidly transform into trypomastigotes and infect other cells or are ingested by triatomid insects. American trypanosomiasis can be transmitted congenitally and in blood transfusion.

INFECTION OF THE HOST

In Chagas' disease, acute-phase reactions depend on the route of entry of the parasite. When the trypanosomes enter via the conjunctiva, Romaña's sign (unilateral bipalpebral edema with conjunctivitis and lymphadenopathy) may be observed.[46] If trypanosomes enter through the skin, a hypersensitivity reaction, called chagoma (furuncle-like lesion with swelling of the regional lymph nodes), may be present. There is a mild febrile illness that usually goes unnoticed. In the chronic phase, cardiomyopathy and motility alterations of the digestive tract (megaesophagus and megacolon) are common complications.

DIAGNOSIS

During the acute stage in Chagas' disease, direct examination of peripheral blood smears can confirm the diagnosis of trypanosomiasis. Fresh anticoagulated blood may demonstrate motile trypomastigotes, or the parasite may be identified on Giemsa-stained blood smears. During chronic disease, the parasite is rarely found in the peripheral blood. Xenodiagnosis (the feeding of uninfected triatomids on an infected patient and subsequent demonstration of parasites in the insect), hemoculture, or animal inoculation are limited by the time lag until they become positive.[47] Serologic examinations are affected by cross-reactivity with antileishmaniasis antibodies.[48] Clinical findings of cardiac arrhythmias, right bundle branch block, and heart failure in conjunction with megaesophagus and megacolon in a patient from an endemic area suggest trypanosomiasis.

PREVENTION

For Chagas' disease, elimination of triatomid insects in endemic areas is useful. Chemoprophylaxis is controversial. The use of insect repellents and appropriate clothing decreases the chances of acquiring the infection.

TREATMENT

Nifurtimox and benznidazole can be used in the treatment of acute trypanosomiasis.[49] They have no proven effect on the chronic manifestations of the disease.

Giardiasis

Giardiasis is an infection of the upper digestive tract caused by the protozoa *Giardia lamblia.*

DISTRIBUTION

Giardiasis occurs worldwide, with a higher prevalence associated with poor sanitary practices. Persons of all ages can be affected, although infection is more frequent in children. Humans are the primary reservoir for the parasite.

MORPHOLOGY, BIOLOGY, AND LIFE CYCLE

Giardiasis is caused by *Giardia lamblia,* a flagellated binucleate protozoan with trophozoite (9 to 21 × 6 to 12 μm) and cyst (8 to 12 × 7 to 10 μm) stages. The trophozoites have a flat pear shape and are bilaterally symmetric. The cyst is the infectious form, because trophozoites are destroyed rapidly in the external environment or by gastric acid. Infection occurs by transmission of *Giardia* cysts in drinking water and food or by direct fecal-oral contamination.

INFECTION OF THE HOST

In humans, *G. lamblia* inhabits the duodenum, where it can be asymptomatic or cause acute, subacute, or chronic diarrhea. Extraintestinal manifestations, such as pulmonary infiltrates and lymphadenopathy, have been reported. Clinical and therapeutic observations have related eye disease, including retinal arteritis and iridocyclitis, to giardiasis.[50]

DIAGNOSIS

Diagnosis can be made by identification of cysts or trophozoites in feces, duodenojejunal aspirates, or biopsy specimens. The parasite is more easily detected during the acute infection stage. Trophozoites are usually found in unformed stools and cysts in formed stools.[51] Immunoelectrophoresis and the enzyme-linked immunosorbent assay (ELISA) allow rapid detection of *G. lamblia* antigens in stool specimens.[52]

PREVENTION

Prevention of giardiasis is ensured by boiling water (cysts are quickly destroyed by heating to 122°F) because standard chlorination practices may not be sufficient to inactivate the cysts. Untreated or unpeeled fruits and vegetables should be avoided in endemic areas.

TREATMENT

Nitro-imidazoles such as metronidazole and tinidazole can be used in the treatment of giardiasis.[49] Alternatives such as quinacrine (Atabrine) are associated with a higher incidence of side effects and are no longer available in the United States. Furazolidone is especially useful in children. The disease may recur after treatment.

Leishmaniasis

Leishmaniasis is a cutaneous, mucocutaneous, or visceral infection caused by protozoa of the genus *Leishmania* (family Trypanosomatidae).

DISTRIBUTION

Four major clinical syndromes are caused by several species of leishmania: cutaneous leishmaniasis of the Old (*L. tropica*) and New (*L. mexicana* and *L. braziliensis*) Worlds; mucocutaneous leishmaniasis or espundia (*L. braziliensis braziliensis*); diffuse cutaneous leishmaniasis in patients with decreased immunity; and visceral leishmaniasis, or kala-azar (*L. donovani*).

MORPHOLOGY, BIOLOGY, AND LIFE CYCLE

Leishmania organisms are found in two stages: promastigote (flagellated) and amastigote (nonflagellated). The life cycle alternates between the vector sandfly *Phlebotomus* (Old World) or *Lutzomyia* (New World) and a mammal host. The female fly acquires the parasite during a blood meal from an infected host. The promastigotic form (infectious stage for humans) proliferates extracellularly in the intestine of the sandfly and is introduced into the mammalian host by the fly bite. Promastigotes in the host enter macrophages and transform into obligate intracellular amastigotes (2 to 5.5 × 1 to 2 μm). Disease spread occurs through infection of new macrophages, following lysis of parasite-infected cells.

INFECTION OF THE HOST

The human cutaneous infection, in the early form of the disease, is a single nodule at the site of the bite. The nodule can progress centrifugally, ulcerate, and scar. Mucocutaneous leishmaniasis is characterized by lesions involving the lower extremities, followed by lesions of mucous membranes and cartilage of the oral cavity, nasal septum, and larynx. Ocular infection may result in eyelid edema, ulceration, and scarring. Conjunctival granuloma and interstitial keratitis have been reported.[46, 53] Kala-azar is manifested by recurrent fever, pancytopenia, and massive splenomegaly.

DIAGNOSIS

Definitive diagnosis of leishmaniasis is by direct identification of the parasite. Stained smears (Wright's or Giemsa stain) or biopsy (H & E or Wilder's reticulin stain) may demonstrate amastigotic or intracellular forms. Needle aspiration culture from the lesion edge or inoculation of a tissue biopsy specimen in appropriate culture media may demonstrate the promastigotic form. Serologic tests provide only indirect evidence of *Leishmania* infection. The leishmanin skin test (Montenegro test) is a delayed hypersensitivity reaction to dead promastigotes injected intradermally. Test results are variable. Negative hypersensitivity results occur in cases of diffuse cutaneous leishmaniasis, and strongly positive results occur in leishmaniasis recidivans. In visceral leishmaniasis, the leishmanin skin test result is negative during active disease and positive in most patients several months to 1 year after recovery.

PREVENTION

Insect repellents, appropriate clothing, and fly netting may provide protection.

TREATMENT

The drugs of choice for all forms of the disease are pentavalent antimonials: sodium stibogluconate or meglumine antimoniate (Glucantime). Alternatives for cutaneous leishmaniasis include allopurinol[54, 55] or ketoconazole.[56] Amphotericin B and pentamidine can be used in severe cases.[49]

Malaria

Malaria is an infection caused by the protozoan *Plasmodium.* Four species have been identified as human pathogens: *P. falciparum, P. vivax, P. ovale,* and *P. malariae. P. vivax,* the species most commonly infecting humans, causes benign tertian malaria. *P. falciparum* is the most dangerous species, causing malignant tertian malaria.

DISTRIBUTION

Malaria is endemic in hot and humid (tropical or subtropical) regions of Africa, Asia, and Central and South America, affecting an estimated 200 million people and causing over 1 million deaths every year, especially among children.[57]

MORPHOLOGY, BIOLOGY, AND LIFE CYCLE

The parasites are transmitted through the bite of the infected female anopheline mosquito, the definitive host for all *Plasmodium* species. The mosquito becomes infected when it ingests the macrogametocytic and microgametocytic forms of the parasite in the peripheral blood of an infected human, the intermediate host. After fusion of the gametocytes (sexual cycle), a zygote develops into an ookinete, forms an oocyst, and then differentiates into sporozoites. The sporozoites (2 to 3 μm), the infectious form of the parasite, remain in the mosquito's salivary glands and are inoculated into humans along with the salivary secretions during blood feeding. The sporozoites, once in the human circulatory system, rapidly enter the hepatic parenchymal cells, differentiate into merozoites (1.5 μm), replicate, rupture the cells, and are released back into the circulatory system. Alternatively, in infections by *P. vivax* and *P. ovale,* hepatic merozoites can differentiate into hypnozoites, a dormant form that can cause disease relapse many years later. Merozoites released into the circulatory system cannot enter new parenchymal cells but enter red blood cells instead, initiating the erythrocytic cycle. In red blood cells, merozoites transform into trophozoites, which enlarge and then give rise to multiple merozoites (schizogony) that rupture the red blood cells and are released into the circulatory system to enter new red blood cells. Trophozoites can also differentiate into macrogametocytes (female presexual stage, 10 μm) or microgametocytes (male presexual stage). The macrogametocytes and microgametocytes are ingested by the anopheles mosquito during the blood feeding and reinitiate the sexual life cycle.

INFECTION OF THE HOST

Sudden attacks of headaches, spiking fever, perspiration, and shaking chills, interspersed with asymptomatic normal periods, are clinical symptoms of acute-phase malaria. Subacute, chronic, and recurrent forms of the disease also can occur. Ocular manifestations of malaria include blotchy preretinal and retinal hemorrhages believed to be caused by cytoaggregation of the parasitized erythrocytes.[58, 59] In children with cerebral malaria, papilledema or retinal edema beyond the arcades are markers of a poor prognosis.[60]

DIAGNOSIS

Malaria is diagnosed by detection of the trophozoite or gametocyte in blood smears. Several smears should be collected at hourly intervals and stained with Giemsa or Gram's stain. Two smears should be prepared at each time interval, one thick, for parasite detection, and another thin, for morphologic analysis. Diagnostic serologic techniques are not routinely available.[61]

PREVENTION

Prevention of malaria is achieved by personal protection from mosquito exposure and by the use of insecticides. Chemoprophylaxis can also be used in endemic areas. Blood banks should follow the American Association of Blood Banks regulations in screening donors for preexisting malarial infection.[61] A malaria vaccine against the merozoite has shown variable results.[62, 63]

TREATMENT

Chloroquine is the drug of choice for the erythrocytic phase of the infection. In cases of chloroquine-resistant *P. falciparum,* quinine or the antiarrhythmic quinidine could be used. Alternatives include mefloquine and pyrimethamine/sulfadoxine (Fansidar). Primaquine is used to eradicate the hypnozoites in cases of infections by *P. vivax* or *P. ovale.* Caution should be taken in patients with glucose-6-phosphate deficiency. A number of antibiotics, including the tetracyclines, rifampin, clindamycin, trimethoprim, sulfonamides, and doxycycline, have some effect.[49]

Microsporidiosis

"Microsporidia" is the nontaxonomic term given to a group of eukaryotic, obligate intracellular protozoan parasites. They infect a wide variety of life forms, ranging from protozoa to humans. Five genera of Microsporidia are infective to humans: *Encephalitozoon*, *Nosema*, *Enterocytozoon*, *Septata*, and *Pleistophora*. Only the first two affect the ocular tissues.

MORPHOLOGY, BIOLOGY, AND LIFE CYCLE

Microsporidia are endemic in the tropics,[64] but it seems that not all healthy people are susceptible to this disease. Recognition of this disease has increased because of the AIDS pandemic. Horizontal transmission is believed to take place in animals and possibly in humans. Infection with Microsporidia is believed to occur after ingestion or inhalation of spores from fecal or urine contamination. The spores that infect humans usually measure 1 to 2 μm by 2 to 4 μm.[65] Organisms usually infect the epithelial cells in the intestinal or respiratory tracts, and from there they could disseminate to other organ systems.[66] The most common presentation of Microsporidia in humans is chronic diarrhea in AIDS patients.[66] Two forms of keratitis are recognized. The first type is caused by *Nosema,* which affects immunocompetent people and produces stromal keratitis.[67, 68] Only four cases have been reported. The second type is caused by *Encephalitozoon,* and it affects the corneal epithelium in the form of punctate epithelial keratitis in AIDS and immunosuppressed patients. Fifteen cases have been reported.[69–71]

DIAGNOSIS

In corneal scrapes, the acid-fast and Gomori-methenamine silver stains demonstrate the organism well.[68] Electron microscopy might be required for the diagnosis. Histopathologic features of keratoplasty specimens in patients with corneal nosematosis demonstrate invasion of the stroma by multiple organisms, areas of necrosis, and multinucleated giant cells. In cases of AIDS, the parasites seem to be confined to the corneal epithelium with absent inflammation.[72]

TREATMENT

In cases of *Encephalitozoon* keratitis, local débridement[72] could be combined with topical fumagillin.[73] Oral itraconazole or albendazole[74] has been used as an adjuvant.

Pneumocystosis

Pneumocystosis is an infection caused by *Pneumocystis carinii,* a eukaryotic microorganism of unclear taxonomic classification.

DISTRIBUTION

P. carinii is an extracellular parasite that causes pneumonia in patients with impaired immunity resulting from AIDS, other immunodeficiency syndromes, protein malnutrition, or drug therapy.[75] Few cases of extrapulmonary *Pneumocystis* infection (lymph nodes, spleen, liver, and eye) have been described.[76, 77] The prevalence of the disease is poorly known, but presumably *P. carinii* infection occurs worldwide, with primary exposure occurring early in life (most children have positive antibody titers to the parasite by the age of 3).[78] Pneumocystosis is the most common infection in AIDS patients, with more than 60% of AIDS cases presenting *P. carinii* pneumonia as the initial opportunistic infection.[79]

MORPHOLOGY, BIOLOGY, AND LIFE CYCLE

Pneumocystis has properties similar to those of fungi[80] and reacts with fungal stains (methenamine silver); however, it has structural characteristics resembling those of protozoans and is sensitive to antiprotozoal agents (pentamidine isethionate). *P. carinii* can assume three morphologic forms: trophozoite, precyst, and cyst. The latter is spherical (4 to 6 μm in diameter), with a thick wall containing one to four nuclei and six to eight pear-shaped bodies (1 to 2 μm long) called sporozoites (believed to give rise to trophozoites). The mode of transmission, life cycle, and reproduction of the parasite are poorly understood. In animals, *P. carinii* pneumonia can be transmitted via airborne particles.[81] This may also be true for human transmission, although in patients with AIDS the disease appears to be the result of reactivation of subclinical infection.

INFECTION OF THE HOST

The infection in the immunocompetent host is generally asymptomatic[78] with occasional clinical manifestations demonstrated in sporadic outbreaks.[82] In the immunosuppressed patient, pneumonia is the most frequent clinical manifestation. Eye disease in the form of large patches of choroiditis has been described in AIDS patients.[76]

DIAGNOSIS

Diagnosis is made by demonstration of *P. carinii* via bronchoalveolar lavages, in smears from needle aspirations, or in tissue from biopsy specimens. Occasionally, organisms can be found in sputum and tracheal and pharyngeal aspirations. The stain of choice is Gomori-methenamine silver, although several different stains have been used.[83] Monoclonal antibodies and the polymerase chain reaction (PCR) test can help in detecting low levels of *P. carinii* infection.[84, 85] Serologic tests are useful in epidemiologic studies but not in the diagnosis and management of the disease.[86]

PREVENTION

Pneumocystosis can be prevented by administration of high protein-caloric nutrition to premature and marasmic infants. Prophylactic chemotherapy for *P. carinii* pneumonia is indicated in high-risk patients (e.g., AIDS), either in the form of aerosolized pentamidine or oral sulfonamides with or without trimethoprim.[87] Dapsone seems to be associated with a higher incidence of side effects.[88]

TREATMENT

Trimethoprim-sulfamethoxazole and pentamidine are the drugs of choice for treatment of pneumocystosis.

Toxoplasmosis

Toxoplasmosis is an infection caused by the protozoan *Toxoplasma gondii.* Cats are the only known definitive host of the parasite, but intermediate hosts, including humans, are at risk of infection.

DISTRIBUTION

Both animals and humans demonstrate serologic evidence of *Toxoplasma* infection worldwide. Prevalence varies markedly in different populations and is related directly to exposure to the parasite, food preparation habits, and climate. Toxoplasmosis can be congenital or acquired. In the United States, 30 to 60% of adults have positive serology results for *Toxoplasma.*[89] In developing countries, acquired toxoplasmosis occurs at a younger age with a higher prevalence in the adult population.[89] In congenital toxoplasmosis, 45% of untreated women that develop primary toxoplasmosis during gestation give birth to infected infants; 8% of these infants are severely affected.[90] Estimates of fetal infection in the United States range from 4200 to 16,800 cases per year.[91] *Toxoplasma* encephalitis has been reported in immunocompromised patients and occurs predominantly in patients with AIDS.[92, 93] *T. gondii is* one of the most frequent causes of retinochoroiditis and posterior uveitis,[94] occurring mainly in the second and third decades of life.[95] In contrast with intracranial disease, toxoplasmic retinochoroiditis appears to be uncommon in patients with AIDS.[96]

MORPHOLOGY, BIOLOGY, AND LIFE CYCLE

T. gondii exists in three forms: Trophozoites (tachyzoites) are the propagative form of the parasite. Tissue cysts (bradyzoites) occur in the chronic stage of the disease. Oocysts are shed in the cat's feces after sexual reproduction of the parasite (Fig. 14–3).

Intestinal Phase

When cats are infected by ingestion of bradyzoite cysts from an infected intermediate host, such as rodents and birds, bradyzoites rapidly transform into tachyzoites, penetrate the cat's intestinal mucosa, and undergo an enteroepithelial cycle of sexual proliferation, resulting in the development of oocysts. Oocysts detach from the intestinal epithelium and are shed in the feces. Each oocyst (11 to 14 × 9 to 11 μm) contains four sporozoites. In the external environment, the oocyst undergoes sporulation within 1 to 3 days and then becomes infectious. Cats can shed 3 to 100 million oocysts after primary infection.

Tissue Phase

Intermediate hosts (as well as cats) can be infected by: (1) ingesting bradyzoites or tachyzoites from uncooked meat, unpasteurized milk, or contaminated water from an intermediate host, (2) ingesting or inhaling oocysts shed in the cat's feces, and (3) congenital transmission of tachyzoites (see Fig. 14–3). After exposure, the host immune defenses are initiated, and the proliferative stage of the infection is curtailed. Organisms encyst and remain viable in the cell tissues, where they can reactivate at a later date.

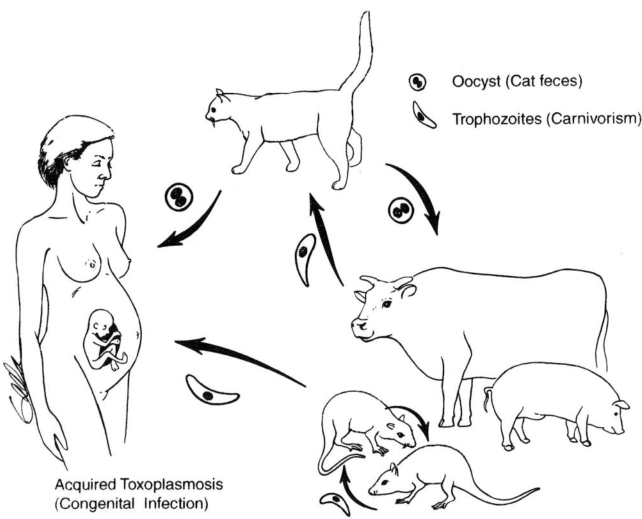

FIGURE 14–3. Toxoplasmosis. Life cycle of *Toxoplasma gondii.* The human as an intermediate host could get infected by ingesting oocysts shed in the cat's feces, by eating meat contaminated with tissue cysts, or by transplacental (congenital) infection.

INFECTION OF THE HOST

Toxic products from *Toxoplasma* and hypersensitivity reactions are responsible for the tissue damage. Inflammatory reactions are not usually observed around the bradyzoite cysts, owing possibly to incorporation of host elements into the cyst walls, masking the parasite antigens.[97] The infection recurs when a cyst ruptures, releasing parasites that proliferate and invade neighboring cells. Bradyzoite cysts can be located in many tissues and are most numerous in the brain, skeletal muscle, myocardium, and retina.[89]

Infection in Immunocompetent Patients

The acute infection in healthy persons leads to a mononucleosis-like clinical picture with fever, malaise, headache, arthralgia, hepatosplenomegaly, and lymphadenopathy. It is transient and usually of no consequence, except in cases of placental transmission or delayed retinochoroiditis.

Infection in Immunocompromised Patients

Toxoplasmosis in the immunocompromised host is most probably reactivation of a previous latent infection,[93] although in certain circumstances (leukemia and organ transplantation), infection can be acquired from blood transfusions and contaminated donor tissue. The cell-mediated immune response is an important mechanism for resistance to *T. gondii* infection. Chronic immunosuppression can reactivate latent infection.

Retinochoroiditis

The most common form of retinal involvement is necrotizing retinochoroiditis, although cases of neuroretinitis[98] and progressive panophthalmitis[99] have been reported. Elderly patients seem to be prone to a particularly severe form of *Toxoplasma* retinochoroiditis.[100] Ocular disease in healthy persons is mainly the result of reactivation of encysted organisms after congenital infection,[95] although several cases of acquired retinochoroiditis have been reported from endemic areas.[101–103] Ruptured retinal cells sensitize lymphocytes and initiate the production of autoantibodies that may contribute to the retinitis.[104]

Congenital Infection

Congenital transmission of toxoplasmosis occurs when a *Toxoplasma* infection is acquired during pregnancy or 6 months before. The neonate of a woman with previous antibodies to *Toxoplasma* will not have congenital toxoplasmosis.[95] The disease is usually more severe in the fetus than in the mother. Transplacental transmission of *Toxoplasma* increases when the infection is acquired in the second and third trimesters of pregnancy. Severe fetal disease, however, is more prevalent when the infection is acquired in the first trimester of pregnancy.[90]

DIAGNOSIS

Laboratory diagnosis of *T. gondii* infection includes serologic analysis and its histologic identification.

Serologic Tests

The high prevalence and persistence of *Toxoplasma* antibodies in the general population makes interpretation of serologic test results difficult. Diagnosis of acquired infection requires demonstration of seroconversion and a rise in antibody titer in samples taken 4 to 6 weeks apart. The presence of *Toxoplasma*-specific gamma immunoglobulin M (IgM) antibodies indicates a recently acquired infection. Because IgM antibodies do not cross the placenta, an increase in the IgM antibody titers in the neonatal period is an indicator of congenital toxoplasmosis. Recurrent *Toxoplasma* chorioretinitis may not increase IgG levels, and IgM antibody is not detected. When ocular lesions suggest toxoplasmosis, serum antibodies are considered to be significant at any level of detection, although a positive serologic test result is not conclusive proof of toxoplasmosis. A negative serologic test result in an undiluted sample should exclude the diagnosis of toxoplasmosis, although exceptions have occurred, especially in patients with AIDS.[105] No association between serologic *Toxoplasma* antibody titers and eye disease severity has been reported.[102] The Sabin-Feldman dye or methylene blue test[105] is of historical interest, but the most commonly used test nowadays is the ELISA, which can identify and quantify IgM and IgG antibodies individually. *Toxoplasma* antibodies can be detected in ocular fluids, and the ELISA can demonstrate local ocular production of antibodies, thus aiding in the diagnosis of difficult ocular toxoplasmosis cases.[106, 107] Other serologic tests, such as complement fixation, hemagglutination, latex agglutination, and immunofluorescent antibody, have been largely replaced by the ELISA test. The PCR may be useful in detecting *Toxoplasma* parasite DNA when cysts cannot be visualized.[108, 109] In cases of retinochoroiditis, the diagnostic yield of PCR is higher in the vitreous than in the aqueous.[110]

Histologic Identification

The parasite is identified by routine microscopic examination of H & E-stained or Giemsa-stained tissue sections. Identification of tachyzoites indicates an active infection; detection of cysts indicates a chronic stage of the disease (except for identification of cysts in placental or fetal tissues). Fluorescent antibodies[111] and peroxidase-antiperoxidase techniques[112] are reliable methods for *Toxoplasma* detection.

PREVENTION

Oocyst Contamination

Toxoplasma oocysts can be destroyed by exposure to heat in excess of 60°C; chemical disinfectants are usually ineffective. Hand washing is indicated after contact with soil contaminated by cat feces and when changing cat litter boxes. Dried cat litter should be disposed of without shaking to avoid dispersing oocysts into the air. The litter should be changed daily (freshly deposited oocysts are not infectious for 1 to 3 days).

Bradyzoite Contamination

Bradyzoite cysts in tissues may remain viable in meat for several days at room and refrigerator temperatures. All bradyzoites are destroyed by cooking meat to 70°C. Hands should be washed after handling raw meat. Soap, alcohol, and chemical disinfectants inactivate bradyzoites on the skin.

Congenital Toxoplasmosis

Pregnant women should be cautioned about exposure to *Toxoplasma.* Seronegative pregnant women in high-incidence areas may be tested repeatedly; if seroconversion is detected, prompt therapy should be initiated with nonmutagenic drugs. To facilitate early diagnosis and treatment, pregnant women in high-incidence areas should be familiarized with the clinical symptoms of acquired toxoplasmosis.

Cats

Cats should be kept indoors as much as possible to minimize contact with birds and mice. When cats are fed meat, it should be dried, canned, or cooked. Contact with stray cats should be avoided.

TREATMENT

Although *Toxoplasma* eye disease is self-limiting, some cases may require treatment. The combination of sulfadiazine and pyrimethamine[113] (given concomitantly with folinic acid) is usually the first line of treatment in cases of toxoplasmic retinochoroiditis. Clindamycin,[114] spiramycin, and trimethoprim-sulfamethoxazole are alternative drugs. Steroids can be added to the antimicrobial therapy if the ocular lesions threaten the macula or the optic nerve. Cryotherapy and laser photocoagulation may be indicated in special cases.

Intestinal Nematodes

ASCARIASIS

Ascariasis is a nematode infection caused by *Ascaris lumbricoides.*

Distribution

Ascariasis occurs worldwide, more frequently where hygiene and sanitary conditions are inadequate.

Morphology, Biology, and Life Cycle

Ascaris infection occurs when fertilized eggs (45 to 70 × 35 to 50 μm) are ingested from contaminated soil or vegetables. Ingested eggs hatch in the host intestine after the outer coating is dissolved by gastric acid. The larvae penetrate the intestinal mucosa and are disseminated via the lymphatic and circulatory systems. The larvae become trapped in the lung's circulation, penetrate the alveolar wall, migrate to the trachea and esophagus, and are swallowed. In the small intestine, the larvae mature and mate. Adult *A. lumbricoides* are large parasites (female, 20 to 40 cm × 3 to 6 mm; male, 15 to 30 cm × 2 to 4 mm). The female passes an average of 200,000 eggs a day.

Infection of the Host

The adult parasite inhabits the small intestine, where it can cause symptoms that range from vague abdominal pain to complete intestinal obstruction. Single worms can migrate to the biliary tree, pancreatic duct, or appendix, causing obstruction. In cases of massive ascaris infection, vitamin A absorption may be decreased, which in turn causes xerophthalmia.[115] Systemic manifestations can occur during the larval migration stage, including fever, pneumonitis, and even invasion of the intraocular or periocular tissues.

Diagnosis

The diagnosis of ascariasis is made by identification of eggs in feces or, more rarely, larvae in sputum. Occasionally, adult worms are expelled from the mouth or rectum. Abdominal radiographs may demonstrate parasites as worm outlines; chest radiographs may show fleeting infiltrates (Löffler's pneumonia) owing to migrating larvae. The ELISA test can also be used.[116]

Prevention

Adequate hygienic and sanitary conditions contribute to prevention of ascariasis. Water should be boiled and uncooked vegetables avoided in endemic areas.

Treatment

Mebendazole and albendazole inhibit glucose uptake by the parasite.[117, 118] Mebendazole is slowly and only slightly absorbed from the gastrointestinal tract.[119] Mebendazole is teratogenic in rats and should not be given to pregnant women.[119] In cases of massive parasite load, these drugs should be used with caution because they might promote parasite migration (i.e., biliary duct or appendix obstruction). Pyrantel pamoate is effective against *Ascaris*. It produces spastic paralysis and could lead to intestinal obstruction in cases of massive infection. In these cases, piperazine citrate, which produces flaccid paralysis of the parasite, should be used. Most of the anthelmintics kill the adult parasite, not the larvae, so a second course of treatment is often given 2 weeks after the first to allow time for the larvae to complete the pulmonary cycle and mature into adult parasites.[116]

Extraintestinal Nematodes

DRACUNCULIASIS

The guinea worm, *Dracunculus medinensis*, lives in the subcutaneous tissues of humans, usually in the lower extremities. Occasionally, it affects other parts of the body, including the eyelids and orbit.[120] The gravid female measures 1 m and is 2 mm in diameter. When the feet come in contact with water, multiple first-stage larvae are liberated that subsequently are ingested by copepods of the genera *Cyclops*, among others. Humans are infected by contaminated water, and the cycle repeats again. Few cases of ocular dracunculiasis have been reported, mostly from rural communities of India and Africa. Diagnosis and therapy involve surgical excision of the worm. Supportive treatment with thiabendazole, metronidazole, and mebendazole has been attempted.[121]

DIFFUSE UNILATERAL SUBACUTE NEURORETINITIS

Diffuse unilateral subacute neuroretinitis[122, 123] is a syndrome caused by the subretinal migration of the larval or adult form of a parasite of the class Nematoda. Most reported cases have been from the southeastern United Stated and the Caribbean, although increased awareness of this entity will lead to more cases being diagnosed in other parts of the world. Several nematodes have been implicated, including *Toxocara* species and *Ancylostoma caninum*. Recent reports have implicated the raccoon and skunk roundworm *Baylisascaris procyonis*.[124–126] The migration of the parasite causes unilateral damage to the retina, pigment epithelium, and optic nerve along with vitreal inflammation. There is usually severe loss of visual acuity. If the parasite is seen, photocoagulation is an effective means of treatment.[126, 127] If no parasite is seen and clinical suspicion is high, thiabendazole[128] or ivermectin[129] can be used.

FILARIASIS

Human filarial parasites infect an estimated 200 million people and cause a range of disease manifestations. Adult filarial worms are threadlike, live in the subcutaneous tissues and lymphatics, and reproduce sexually to produce microfilariae, the first larval stage. Microfilariae are ingested by hematophagous arthropods, in which they develop into infective larvae that molt in the vertebrate host and mature into male or female worms.

Dirofilariasis

Dirofilaria immitis is the heartworm of dogs; *D. repens* is found in cats and dogs in Asia, Europe, and South America; and *D. tenuis* infects raccoons in North America. They are accidentally transmitted to humans by the same vectors that infect the animal hosts, *Aedes* and *Culex* mosquitos. The parasite is unable to produce microfilariae in the human host. Subcutaneous nodules and cardiopulmonary "coin" lesions have been reported. Ophthalmic dirofilarial infections are more common in the eyelids and periorbital tissues,[130] conjunctiva,[131] orbit,[132] vitreous,[133] and anterior chamber, in that order. The most common clinical presentation is a well-encapsulated nonviable parasite, although an occasional viable parasite has been detected. Diagnosis is serologic using a highly specific ELISA test.[134] Surgical removal is the mainstay of therapy.

Lymphatic Filariasis

Wuchereria bancrofti, *Brugia malayi*, and *Brugia timori* are filarial nematodes with a propensity for lymphatic invasion.

W. bancrofti is distributed throughout Africa, Asia, the Caribbean, Latin America, and Western and South Pacific Islands. *B. malayi* and *B. timori* are found in the Far East. Infection of the mosquito vector occurs when the insect takes a blood meal of an infected host. Infection in humans seems to occur only after repeated inoculations with infective larvae. Larvae migrate to the lymphatics, where they produce elephantiasis. Ocular filariasis is rare. Adult *B. malayi* worms have been found in the conjunctiva and probably result from direct inoculation to the eye rather than migration. Elephantiasis of the eyelid has been reported. One case of a subretinal worm,[135] and a second of an immature *W. bancrofti* in the iris,[136] represent rare intraocular cases. The finding of living adult worms in lymphatic vessels is suggestive. A single dose of 100 mg of diethylcarbamazine (DEC) provokes the emergence of microfilariae into the peripheral circulation—blood should be drawn 1 hour after the administration of DEC. Treatment consists of a 21-day regimen of DEC, although infection may recur. Topical 1% atropine solution has been described as an agent capable of killing microfilariae in the anterior chamber.[136]

LOIASIS

Loiasis is a nematode infection caused by the filaria *Loa loa.*

Distribution

Endemic areas of loiasis are the rain forests of West and Central Africa.

Morphology, Biology, and Life Cycle

The vectors, female flies of the genus *Chrysops* (family Tabanidae), are infected by ingesting human blood contaminated with the parasitic microfilariae. The larvae become infectious in the arthropod and penetrate the host skin during the next blood meal. Larvae develop into adult roundworms (male, 4 to 7 cm in length; female, 2 to 3 cm) in the subcutaneous tissues of the host. After mating, gravid females release microfilariae, which enter the circulatory system and, after transmission to another fly, initiate a new life cycle. The microfilariae exhibit diurnal activity, appearing in the peripheral blood only from dawn to dusk.

Infection of the Host

The disease is often asymptomatic, although transient pruritic or painful subcutaneous swellings (known as Calabar swellings) are a classic manifestation of the disease. Adult worms can sometimes be observed beneath the skin or conjunctiva[137] (Fig. 14–4).

Diagnosis

Definitive diagnosis is made by identification of either microfilariae in the blood or adult worms in subcutaneous tissues or conjunctiva. Blood should be drawn during daylight because of the diurnal periodicity of microfilaremia. Serologic testing for specific IgG immunoglobulin may be useful in the diagnosis of *L. loa* in amicrofilaremic cases.[138]

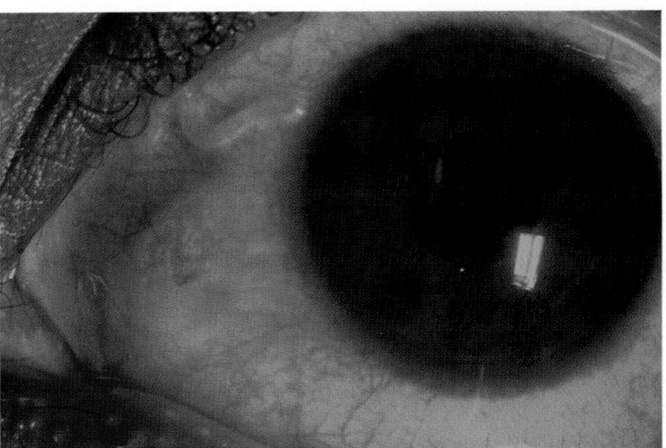

FIGURE 14–4. *Loa loa.* Note the adult worm in the subconjunctival space. (Courtesy of Roberto Pineda II, M.D., and Susannah Rowe, M.D.) (Photo by Kit Johnson.)

Prevention

Loiasis is prevented by protection against fly bites (appropriate clothing, insect repellents).

Treatment

Diethylcarbamazine citrate is the drug of choice in the treatment of loiasis. Adult worms should be surgically removed from the subconjunctiva.[139]

ONCHOCERCIASIS

Onchocerciasis, or river blindness, is a chronic filarial disease caused by the nematode *Onchocerca volvulus.* It is one of the major causes of infectious blindness worldwide.

Distribution

Onchocerciasis is an endemic disease with over 18 million infected persons worldwide, of whom around 2 million have some form of visual impairment and approximately 400,000 suffer from blindness.[140] Endemic areas include Equatorial Africa and several foci in Central America, South America, and the Arabian peninsula. All age groups are affected. The intensity of infection increases with host age and reaches a plateau during the second decade of life. In hyperendemic areas in West Africa, approximately one-third of people over the age of 15 years have microfilariae in the anterior chamber of the eye, and half of those over the age of 40 become blind from the disease.[141] Men are more commonly affected than women because of occupational exposure.[140]

Morphology, Biology, and Life Cycle

Black flies, members of the family Simuliidae (order Diptera), are the only known vectors for *O. volvulus.* The flies are found mostly near fast-flowing rivers in tropical and subtropical regions. Female black flies are blood feeders, and it is during the blood meal that the fly can transmit or receive the infection from humans. When a black fly (1 to 5 mm long; black, gray, or tan) bites an infected person, microfilariae in the circulatory system are ingested along with the blood meal (Fig. 14–5). In the insect vector, microfilariae (300 to 360 × 5 to 9 μm, unsheathed) develop into infectious larvae and are retransferred to human skin during the next blood meal. They enter humans via the fly bite wound and develop into adult nematodes within 2 to 3 months (see Fig. 14–5). Adult worms (females, 25 to 50 cm × 0.25 to 0.50 mm; males, 1.9 to 4.2 × 0.13 to 0.15 mm) are white or cream-colored, threadlike roundworms, living in the subcutaneous tissues, deep fasciae, or joints, commonly in clusters; they may be encapsulated (onchocercoma) by a host immune response. The worms reproduce sexually, and new microfilariae appear within a year after primary infection (see Fig. 14–5). The adult female can produce millions of microfilariae during her lifetime (15 years). *O. volvulus* can be transmitted congenitally from severely infected mothers, but this is rare. Parasitic nodules are usually concentrated in the area of the original black fly bites. African black flies more frequently bite on the hips and legs; Central and South American black flies usually bite the head area.

Infection of the Host

Living *Onchocerca* microfilariae cause little adverse reaction in humans and appear to be undetected by the host immune system. Damage caused by onchocerciasis is due to dead or dying microfilariae. The pathogenicity varies with the species of *Onchocerca*.[142, 143] If a large number of microfilariae die at the same time (e.g., after DEC treatment in heavily infected persons), an inflammatory/immune response called the Mazzotti reaction may result.[144] The reaction causes a localized or generalized skin pruritic rash, fever, lymph node inflammation, headache, nausea, joint and muscle pain, tachycardia, respiratory distress, and hypotension. Deaths caused by the Mazzotti reaction have been reported. The anterior segment manifestations of ocular onchocerciasis, such as sclerosing keratitis and iritis, as well as the presence of optic neuritis and atrophy, are sometimes reversible after ivermectin therapy.[145] The chorioretinitis caused by *Onchocerca* keeps progressing despite therapy and might be related to a cross-reactivity between a microfilarial antigen and the retinal pigment epithelium.[146, 147]

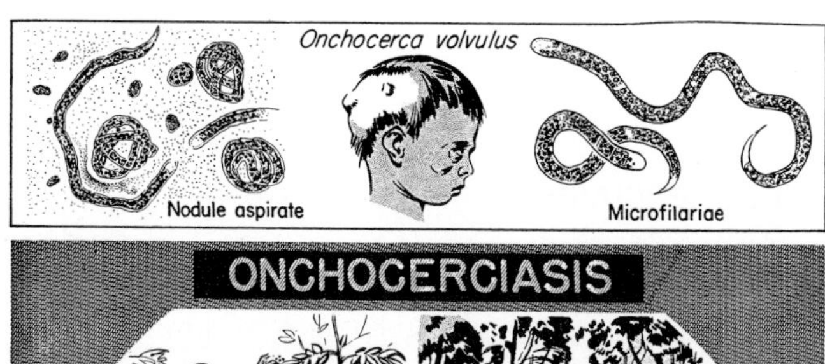

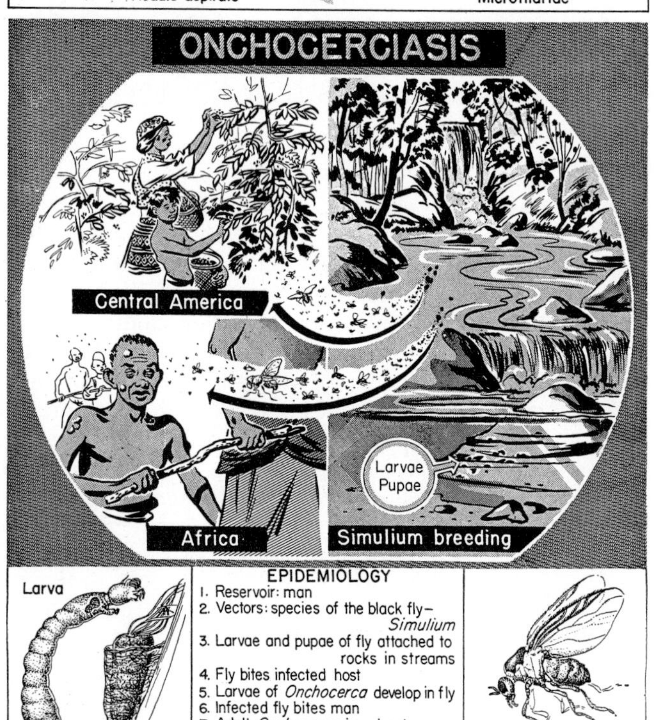

FIGURE 14–5. Epidemiology of onchocerciasis. (From Hunter EW III, Schwartzwelder JC, Clyde J: A Manual of Tropical Medicine. Philadelphia, WB Saunders, 1960.)

Diagnosis

Clinical Diagnosis

Detection of typical subcutaneous nodules suggests the diagnosis of onchocerciasis, which must be confirmed by histologic examination.[148] Detection of intraocular *O. volvulus* microfilariae is diagnostic for onchocerciasis.[141] Serologic tests for onchocerciasis are sensitive but nonspecific; blood analysis usually reveals moderate eosinophilia.

Skin Biopsy

Skin biopsy is used not only for diagnosis but also to assess the intensity of infection (number of microfilariae per milligram of skin).[116] Usually, 1 mg of healthy skin is sliced to a depth of 0.5 mm from several sites (shoulders, buttocks). The skin snips are placed immediately into 0.5 mL of saline solution, where they are held for 3 hours to allow the microfilariae sufficient time to migrate from the tissue. Detection of a single microfilaria is a definitive diagnosis; a moderately infected patient has 20 to 100 microfilariae per milligram of skin.

Prevention

Areas of black fly infestation should be avoided because no prophylactic drug is effective against the infectious larvae. Personal protection, such as appropriate clothing and insect repellents, should be used. Both black fly larvae and adults can be eliminated by spraying DDT along rivers in fly breeding sites. The Onchocerciasis Control Program established by the World Health Organization has been effective in reducing transmission of onchocerciasis in a 700,000-km^2 area involving seven countries in Central and West Africa.[140]

Treatment

Ivermectin is the drug of choice.[145, 149] It causes a spastic paralysis of microfilariae, thus reducing the side effects of treatment related to migration of the parasites. It does not affect adult worms.[141] The drugs formerly used in the treatment of onchocerciasis, suramin and DEC, can cause severe reactions related directly to the patient load of microfilariae and are not currently recommended. Nodulectomy may be useful to decrease the adult worm load.

Thelaziasis

Nematode members of the family Spiruroidea, genus *Thelazia,* are parasites of birds and mammals and are usually located in the conjunctiva and lacrimal gland ducts. Adult worms are cream-colored and measure 0.75 × 17 mm. Some species (*T. callipaeda,* Asia, China, and Korea; *T. californiensis,* North America) have been reported in humans. Flies of the genera *Musca* and *Fannia* are the intermediate hosts for this parasite. Definitive hosts include dogs, cats, horses, sheep, bear, and deer. In humans, the worms invade the conjunctiva, causing pain and watery conjunctivitis.[150] They can be seen as creamy white, threadworm masses coiled in the conjunctival sac or migrating over the cornea. Eyelids and extraocular muscles can also be compromised. Intraocular penetration does not occur. Therapy for ocular thelaziasis is surgical removal of the parasite.

Toxocariasis

Dogs and cats are the definite hosts for *Toxocara canis* and *Toxocara cati,* which are members of the nematode family Ascarididae. Toxocariasis in humans (an intermediate host) is caused predominantly by *T. canis,* and it is manifested clinically as either visceral larva migrans (VLM) or ocular larva migrans (OLM).

DISTRIBUTION

T. canis has a worldwide distribution in dogs and is uniformly prevalent in North America.[151] Pregnant and lactating dogs are the most important factors in *Toxocara* infection. In puppies, intestinal infection rates can reach 100%; in adult dogs, the rate falls to less than 20%.[152] *T. cati* infection also appears to occur worldwide in cats, with a prevalence in North America varying between 24% and 67%.[151] *Toxocara* infection in humans is sporadic but widespread. Demographic factors, such as socioeconomic status, hygiene practices, and association with dogs, influence infection rates.[153] Environmental factors, such as moist soil and grass that favor the persistence of *Toxocara* eggs for long periods, are also important in transmission of the parasite. Seroprevalence rates of toxocariasis in children (1 to 11 years) in different geographic regions of the United States range between 4.6% and 7.3% and are higher in warmer climates.[153] The frequency of seropositive titers declines markedly with increasing age; peak infection occurs at 1 to 5 years. Children with geophagic behavior and who are exposed to dogs are most likely to develop OLM.[154]

MORPHOLOGY, BIOLOGY, AND LIFE CYCLE

Dogs and other canines (definitive hosts) are infected by several routes: ingestion of infectious eggs, ingestion of late-stage larvae or immature adult worms (during maternal grooming of the litter), ingestion of larvae in tissues of paratenic hosts (e.g., mice), and transplacental or transmammary transmission (Fig. 14–6). Transplacental migration occurs because dormant larvae in somatic tissues of female dogs are reactivated to migratory forms during pregnancy, probably associated with hormonal changes.[155] Transmammary transmission of larvae occurs soon after parturition and peaks during the second week of lactation. Infection in cats is similar to that in dogs, although there is no evidence of transplacental infection. The life cycle in puppies is similar to the life cycle of *A. lumbricoides* in humans, which initiates with ingestion of *Toxocara* eggs (75 to 85 μm, spherical with a thick shell) that hatch in the stomach or small intestine of the definitive host and release infectious larvae (20 × 400 μm). The larvae burrow into the intestinal mucosa, enter the lymphatic and circulatory systems, and migrate to the lung capillary bed within 3 to 5 days. In the lungs, the larvae enter the bronchioles, trachea, and pharynx and are swallowed to develop into adult worms (*T. canis,* 4 to 18 cm; *T. cati,* 3 to 12 cm) in the intestine. Adult worms produce eggs (200,000/day)[156] that are shed in the feces 4 to 5 weeks after infection. Eggs are noninfective when shed and require appropriate soil conditions for development of the infectious larvae.

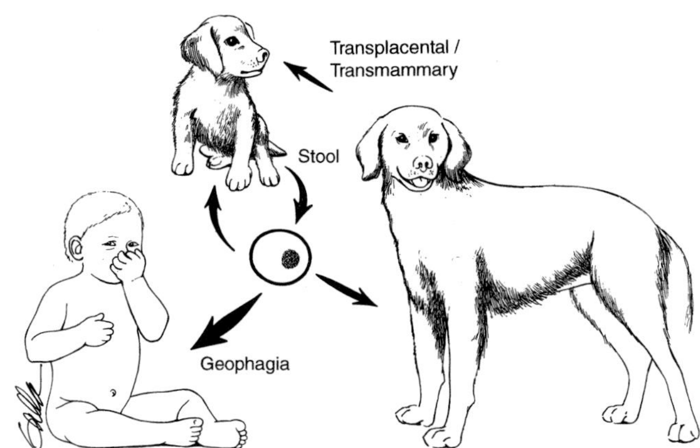

FIGURE 14–6. Toxocariasis. Life cycle of *Toxocara canis.* The toddler gets infected by ingesting soil contaminated with puppy's feces (geophagia).

Transmission to humans may occur by ingestion of eggs from the soil, contaminated hands, and fomites, or less frequently by ingestion of the larval stage from undercooked meat (see Fig. 14–6). If the host is large enough (adult dogs and humans), larvae pass through the pulmonary capillaries and are distributed to somatic tissues instead of being trapped in the alveoli. Humans are paratenic hosts, with larvae migrating aimlessly in the tissues for varying time periods. The larvae reach the eye via the choroidal blood vessels, where they migrate into the subretinal space or vitreous cavity.[157]

INFECTION OF THE HOST

The tissue damage observed in toxocariasis results from larva migration (mechanical) and immune reaction. Clinical manifestation of the disease depends on the organ and the number of invading larvae. Several larvae in the liver may cause no disease, whereas a single larva in the eye can cause blindness.

DIAGNOSIS

Serology

The serologic test of choice for toxocariasis is the ELISA. Specificity of the ELISA is enhanced by preabsorption of test sera with *Ascaris* antigens. Titers may be equal[158] but are usually lower[159] in patients with ocular infections compared with patients with systemic disease. ELISA titers of 1:32 are indicative of VLM (78% sensitivity, 92% specificity),[160] and titers of 1:8 are indicative of OLM (90% sensitivity, 91% specificity).[161] ELISAs can also be used on intraocular fluids.[162, 163] High titers can be detected in the aqueous humor and the vitreous when concomitant serum titers are low or absent, suggesting localized antibody production.[164, 165] Aqueous humor (especially when cells are observed at the clinical examination) and vitreous cytology can demonstrate eosinophils, suggesting a parasitic infection.[166]

Immunodiagnostic tests (e.g., bentonite flocculation, fluorescent antibody, and skin tests) for toxocariasis may lack sensitivity and specificity, mainly because the antigens are prepared from adult *Toxocara,* which may result in a false-positive reaction in patients infected concomitantly with *Ascaris* or other helminths.[167]

Blood Analysis

Patients with VLM may have leukocytosis, hypereosinophilia, and hypergammaglobulinemia (IgG, IgM, or IgE); blood findings are usually normal in patients with OLM.

Ocular Imaging Studies

Detection of intraocular calcifications by computed tomography may provide a differential diagnosis with retinoblastoma, although small retinoblastomas can remain uncalcified, and cases of toxocariasis with calcium deposits have been reported.[168] Echographic findings such as a solid, highly reflective peripheral mass; a vitreous band or membranes extending between the posterior pole and the mass; and a traction retinal detachment or fold from the posterior pole to the mass suggest ocular toxocariasis.[169]

Histopathology

In tissue sections, circumscribed granulomatous reactions with neutrophil and eosinophil infiltrates are seen, occasionally with the larvae located in the center of the reaction (Fig. 14–7). Fibrinoid necrosis may occur in the central area of recent lesions, whereas older lesions may reveal fibrous encapsulation. Giant cells, epithelioid cells, macrophages, and lymphocytes are usually present around degenerating larvae.[170]

Stool Examination

Human stool examinations are of no use because the parasite does not mature in the human intestine.

PREVENTION

Children should be supervised with respect to geophagia and placing foreign objects in their mouths. Stray dogs and cats should not be permitted in yards and playgrounds. Newborn litters and lactating dogs and cats should be dewormed at regular intervals. Because deworming medication does not eradicate all somatic larvae, pregnant dogs require repetitive prophylaxis and deworming with each new litter.

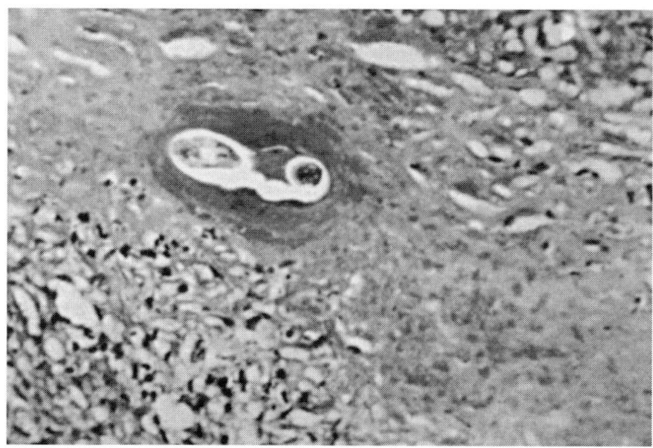

FIGURE 14–7. Intraocular toxocariasis. Fibrotic mass with many eosinophils. *Toxocara canis* larvae within the fibrotic proliferation. Masson's trichrome stain ×250. (Courtesy of Miguel Burnier, Jr., M.D.)

TREATMENT

Thiabendazole is controversial because the death of the parasite entices an intense inflammatory response.[171] Steroids are frequently used to decrease it. Photocoagulation, cryopexy, and vitrectomy have been employed.

Trichinosis

Trichinosis is a nematode infection caused by the roundworm *Trichinella spiralis.* Humans are infected by eating raw or improperly cooked meat, especially pork.

DISTRIBUTION

Trichinosis is endemic in the Western hemisphere and Western Europe. It occurs worldwide wherever pork is consumed. Several cases have been attributed to the consumption of wild carnivores, such as bear and wild boar. Between 1982 and 1986, the annual average number of cases in the United States was 57.[172]

MORPHOLOGY, BIOLOGY, AND LIFE CYCLE

There are no intermediate hosts, and both the adult and larval stages develop in the same animal. After ingestion of contaminated meat, encysted *Trichinella* larvae (0.4 × 0.26 mm) are freed by gastric digestion of the cyst wall. The larvae develop into adult worms (females, 2 to 3.6 mm × 75 to 90 μm, are approximately twice the length of males) in the small intestinal mucosa. Following copulation, the male dies, and within a week the viviparous female releases larvae (100 to 160 μm × 6 to 7 μm), which enter the mucosal vascular channels and are distributed throughout the body. Larviposition continues for about 4 to 6 weeks. Only larvae that encyst in skeletal muscles mature and become infectious. The muscles of the diaphragm, tongue, and eye are mostly affected. Calcification of cysts begins in 6 to 18 months. The cycle is repeated when the host is eaten by another carnivore.

INFECTION OF THE HOST

Disease severity is directly related to the numbers of larvae ingested, varying from completely asymptomatic to neurologic, pulmonary, and cardiovascular complications. In the intestine, the adult worms cause inflammation and mucus production. Muscle invasion by the larvae can cause myalgia and weakness and can involve the diaphragm, tongue, masseter, intercostal, extraocular, and laryngeal muscles. Encysted larvae, localized in extraocular muscles cause periorbital inflammation with conjunctivitis, hemorrhage, edema, pain, and photophobia.[3] Eosinophilia is frequent.

DIAGNOSIS

Definitive diagnosis is made by direct observation of encysted, coiled larvae in tissue biopsy specimens. Serologic test results are positive after the third week of infection.

PREVENTION

Trichinosis is prevented by proper cooking of pork. Pigs should be isolated and fed only cooked meat and grains.

TREATMENT

Mebendazole and thiabendazole are available for the treatment of trichinosis. Thiabendazole therapy has been associated more frequently with side effects, such as dizziness, mental changes, rash, nausea, and Stevens-Johnson syndrome in children.[173] The administration of corticosteroids is indicated for the treatment of the allergic reaction to dead parasites.

Trematodes (Flukes)

PARAGONIMIASIS

Paragonimiasis is a disease caused by trematodes of the genus *Paragonimus.* Most human cases are due to infection with *P. westermani.*

Distribution

Paragonimiasis is prevalent in Japan, Korea, China, India, Africa, and Central and South America.

Morphology, Biology, and Life Cycle

Adult worms (6 to 8 mm × 4 to 8 mm) live in the lung of the definitive host, where they shed eggs. Eggs (80 to 120 μm × 50 to 65 μm) reach the host's mouth through the bronchi, are swallowed, and are shed subsequently in the feces. In water, eggs hatch into miracidium forms of the parasite, invade snails (first intermediate host), differentiate into sporocysts, and mature into cercariae. Cercariae leave the snail and penetrate crustaceans—crabs or crayfish (second intermediate hosts). Cercariae become encysted in tissues and develop into metacercariae. When infected crabs or crayfish are eaten by the definitive host, the metacercariae excyst in the small intestine, pass through the intestinal wall into the abdominal cavity, and migrate to the pleural cavity through the diaphragm. In the lungs, metacercariae develop into adult worms and mate, and gravid females lay their eggs.

Infection of the Host

During acute disease, symptoms range from none to moderate to severe fever, chills, and gastrointestinal (diarrhea, abdominal pain) and pulmonary (chest pain, cough, dyspnea) clinical symptoms. Chronic stages of pulmonary paragonimiasis include symptoms of chronic bronchitis with hemoptysis. Extrapulmonary paragonimiasis occurs when worms lodge in other tissues (brain, gastrointestinal, and subcutaneous tissues, including periocular areas [ocular paragonimiasis]). CNS paragonimiasis is characterized by symptoms of meningoencephalitis, cerebral hemorrhage, visual disturbances, and optic nerve atrophy.

Diagnosis

Diagnosis is made by isolation of *Paragonimus* eggs in feces or sputum. ELISA and complement fixation serologic tests are sensitive and specific for paragonimiasis diagnosis.

Prevention

Paragonimiasis can be prevented by avoiding raw or undercooked crustaceans.

Treatment

The drug of choice for the treatment of paragonimiasis is praziquantel.[121] Corticosteroids are indicated mainly in cases of cerebral involvement, because the death of the parasites may initiate an inflammatory reaction.

SCHISTOSOMIASIS

Schistosomiasis is an infection caused by three species of *Schistosoma: S. mansoni, S. japonicum,* and *S. haematobium.*

Distribution

S. mansoni is prevalent in Africa, the Middle East, and South and Central America; *S. japonicum* in the Far East; and *S. haematobium* in the Middle East and Africa.

Morphology, Biology, and Life Cycle

The intermediate host of *Schistosoma is* the snail *(Biomphalaria* species). Humans are the only definite host and only significant disease reservoir. *Schistosoma* eggs in fresh water release miracidium larvae that enter the snail and differentiate into cercariae (final larval stage). Cercariae pass from the snail to the water and penetrate the human skin. After penetration, the cercariae migrate to the lungs and then to the liver as worms, where they mature and mate. Females of *S. mansoni* and *S. japonicum* lay their eggs in the smallest venules of the intestinal wall, and the eggs are shed with the feces. Females of *S. haematobium* lay their eggs in the smallest vessels of the vesical plexuses, and the eggs are shed in the urine. The eggs reach fresh water, and the cycle is repeated again.

Infection of the Host

The prepatent period in humans (from cercaria penetration until appearance of eggs in the feces or urine) is about 50 days.[174] Local dermatitis after contact with infested water is common ("swimmer's itch"). In cases of *S. mansoni* or *S. japonicum* infection, the acute phase may include abdominal pain, chills, fever, cough, diarrhea, and eosinophilia; during chronic phases, hepatosplenomegaly, ascites, and esophageal varices, with recurrent episodes of hematemesis, can occur. In cases of *S. haematobium* infection, dysuria, hematuria, and suprapubic pain, as well as obstructive uropathy, may occur. Infection of the eye includes granulomatous choroiditis,[175, 176] dacryoadenitis,[177] and conjunctivitis,[178] and lid masses[179] in endemic areas.

Diagnosis

Definitive diagnosis is made by detecting the eggs in feces or urine. Biopsy of the rectal or urinary bladder mucosa is rarely indicated.

Prevention

Prevention can be accomplished by improving sanitation and reducing egg contamination in fresh water. Snail control with molluscicides may be useful in endemic areas.

Treatment

Praziquantel, oxamniquine, metrifonate, and niridazole are available for the specific treatment of schistosomiasis.[49]

Tapeworms

COENURIASIS

The definite host of *Multiceps multiceps* and *Taenia brauneri* is the dog, where the adult tapeworm lives in the intestinal tract. Eggs shed in the feces are ingested by sheep, where the larval form *Coenurus cerebralis* mostly affects the CNS of sheep, producing the syndrome of "blind staggers." Coenurosis rarely affects humans, attacking the CNS and occasionally the eye[180] and subcutaneous tissues, particularly in Africa. The diagnosis is made by finding an expanding cyst in a person from an endemic area. The Casoni intradermal test can be used.[121] Surgical excision is the only therapeutic option.

ECHINOCOCCOSIS

Echinococcosis is an infection caused by tapeworms of the genus *Echinococcus*. Three species (*E. granulosus, E. multilocularis,* and *E. vogeli*) cause disease in humans, with *E. granulosus* (cystic hydatid disease) being most widespread.

Distribution

Echinococcosis is prevalent in South America, the former Soviet Union, Asia, Africa, Australia, and New Zealand. In the United States, it is found in the sheep-raising regions of Utah, Arizona, New Mexico, and California.[181]

Morphology, Biology, and Life Cycle

Definitive hosts (dogs and cats) are infected by eating the viscera of intermediate hosts (sheep and pigs). Humans (an intermediate host) are contaminated by ingesting the parasite eggs shed in dog feces, either directly in a hand-to-mouth transmission or indirectly from water and vegetables contaminated with *Echinococcus* eggs. After ingestion, the eggs hatch, release embryos, penetrate the host intestinal wall, pass to the lymphatic and circulatory systems, and are disseminated to the liver and other organs. In the tissues, the embryos develop and produce spherical, slow-growing cysts. Scoleces during the larval stage are formed in the cyst by asexual division. When scoleces are ingested by a definitive host, adult worms (2 to 10 mm) develop, mate, and initiate a new cycle.

Infection of the Host

In humans, clinical manifestations of echinococcosis are secondary to slow-growing cysts or from hypersensitivity reactions to cyst fluid. Liver and lungs are the most frequently affected tissues, although the peritoneum, CNS, kidney, bone, spleen, heart, orbit, muscles, and subcutaneous tissues may also be infection sites.

Diagnosis

Serologic tests (ELISA, indirect hemagglutination, and latex agglutination) can be diagnostic, although cross-reactions with cysticercosis have been noted. Radiographic imaging techniques such as computed tomography and magnetic resonance can be used to demonstrate the thick-walled, spherical, fluid-filled cysts.

Prevention

Personal hygiene and limiting contact with infected dogs are preventive measures.

Treatment

Surgical removal of the entire hydatid cyst is the recommended treatment in human disease. Mebendazole and albendazole can be used with varied success in the clinical treatment of disease that is irresectable (owing to cyst localization or extension).[121]

SPARGANOSIS

Sparganosis is the infection with the larvae of the tapeworm *Spirometra,* which reaches maturity in dogs and cats. The eggs hatch in water, they are ingested by copepods of the genus *Cyclops,* where they develop into procercoid larvae. Humans, birds, and snakes can be infected, but the parasite only matures in cats and dogs. Humans are infected by drinking water contaminated with *Cyclops,* or by eating raw flesh of contaminated frogs, snakes, or birds. The practice of poulticing open wounds with flesh of frogs or snakes, common in the Far East, is another way of acquiring the infection. In ocular sparganosis, the cyst is found in the conjunctiva, the orbit, or the anterior chamber.[182] Treatment is by surgical excision, although oral praziquantel and mebendazole have been attempted.[183]

TAENIASIS AND CYSTICERCOSIS

Tapeworms of the genus *Taenia* can cause two different human diseases: taeniasis and cysticercosis. Taeniasis is an intestinal infection caused by the adult *T. solium* and *T. saginata.* Cysticercosis is a tissue infection caused by the larval form of *T. solium (Cysticercus cellulosae).*

Distribution

Taeniasis and cysticercosis occur where sanitary conditions are poor and where raw or undercooked contaminated pork and beef are routinely consumed. Endemic foci of the disease are South and Central America and Africa.

Morphology, Biology, and Life Cycle

Taeniasis is acquired by ingestion of raw or poorly cooked meat contaminated with the larval form of the parasite (cysticerci). *Taenia* larvae attach to the host intestinal mucosa and develop into adult worms (3 to 9 m) in the intestinal lumen. Terminal gravid segments of the worm, called proglottids *(T. saginata,* 20 × 5 to 7 mm; *T. solium,* 12 × 5 mm), are shed in feces and contain 50,000 to 100,000 viable eggs. Eggs (30 to 40 μm) in proglottids are infectious immediately after shedding. Ingestion of eggs by intermediate hosts (pigs, cattle, or humans) results in hatching of the eggs into larvae (5 × 10 mm, with a scolex) and penetration through the intestinal wall. The larvae are transmitted through the lymphatic and circulatory systems, where they invade various organs and develop into cysticerci (infectious form). Humans develop cysticercosis via ingestion of *T. solium* eggs, either from exogenous sources or from their own stools. Only larvae of *T. solium* penetrate the human intestine; *T. saginata* does not cause human cysticercosis because the larvae cannot penetrate the intestinal wall.

Infection of the Host

Patients with taeniasis are usually asymptomatic. Patients with cysticercosis may also be asymptomatic, although clinical manifestations of neurocysticercosis (epilepsy, intracranial hypertension, and mental disturbances), ophthalmocysticercosis (loss of vision, periorbital pain, scotoma, and photopsia),[184] and subcutaneous and muscular cysticercosis (subcutaneous nodules) may be noted. In the eye, the cysticercus cyst may be localized in the orbit,[185] the subconjunctival space, or intraocularly in the anterior or posterior chamber. Larvae can be identified in the subretinal space, where they cause hemorrhage and edema.[186]

Diagnosis

Taeniasis is diagnosed by isolation and identification of the proglottids in feces. If *T. solium* proglottids are identified, additional evaluation for potential cysticercosis is warranted. Clinical findings, such as brain calcifications, cystic lesions in the CNS, and demonstration of larvae with scoleces within the eye, are diagnostic of cysticercosis. Ocular ultrasonography may be an alternative to computed tomography and magnetic resonance imaging in the evaluation of patients of suspected intraocular or orbital cysticercosis.[187] Indirect hemagglutination and ELISA may be helpful, although false-positive results can occur.[188]

Prevention

Appropriate sanitation and personal hygiene are important in the control of fecal contamination of water and food. Raw or improperly cooked pork should be avoided, especially in endemic areas.

Treatment

Anthelminthic drugs used in the treatment of taeniasis and cysticercosis include praziquantel (drug of choice), niclosamide, and paromomycin. Mebendazole and albendazole are effective against *Taenia* but not against *Cysticercus.* In cases of ocular cysticercosis, surgical removal of cysts is usually necessary.[189, 190]

Arthropods

DEMODICOSIS

Demodex folliculorum and *D. brevis* are two species of follicle mites causing demodicosis in humans. *D. folliculorum* lives on hair follicles in the facial region, and *D. brevis* inhabits sebaceous glands. The disease is extremely common, with infestation rates reaching 97% in endemic areas.[191] Demodicosis is usually a benign infestation, although follicle mites have been associated with blepharitis.[191]

MYIASIS

Ophthalmomyiasis refers to the involvement of the ocular tissues by larvae from flies of the order Diptera.

Distribution

Myiasis is a worldwide disease, occurring more frequently in warm climates. The prevalence of the different species of flies varies according to the locale. *Dermatobia hominis* is endemic in transequatorial coffee-growing areas of South America. *Chrysomyia bezziana* is primarily a cattle parasite in the Old World. *Calliphora vomitoria* organisms are present in decaying animal or vegetable matter worldwide. Ophthalmomyiasis is the infestation that occurs in the ocular or periocular tissues.

Morphology, Biology, and Life Cycle

Larvae from several fly species can cause ophthalmomyiasis. These larvae are usually obligatory parasites, requiring host tissue for completion of their larval stages. Eggs or larvae may be transported to the eye by the adult fly, by a secondary vector such as a tick or mosquito, or by the patient's hands. *D. hominis*, *C. vomitoria,* and *Chrysomyia bezziana* infection occurs via oviposition on periocular tissue. *Hypoderma lineatum* larvae, a cattle parasite, penetrate the skin and migrate aimlessly, causing painful abscesses.

Infection of the Host

Ocular disease may be external or internal. In external ophthalmomyiasis, lid edema,[192] furuncular lesions,[193] orbital involvement,[194] and even loss of the eye[195, 196] can occur (Fig. 14–8). Internal ophthalmomyiasis is caused predominantly by larvae of *H. lineatum.* Subretinal tracks (trails of depigmentation in the retinal pigment epithelium) are the result of maggot migration in the subretinal spaces and are pathognomonic of internal ophthalmomyiasis.[197] The larvae could migrate into the vitreal cavity. Visual compromise varies from nonexistent[198] to severe visual loss.[199]

Diagnosis and Treatment

Myiasis is diagnosed on the basis of recovery or visualization of the larvae. In cases of ophthalmomyiasis externa, covering of the skin lesion with bland medicinal oil or petroleum jelly forces the larvae to the skin surface, facilitating removal with a forceps. In cases of ophthalmomyiasis interna, laser photocoagulation of the subretinal larvae[200] or extraction by vitrectomy of the intravitreal larvae has been attempted.

OPHTHALMIA NODOSA

Ophthalmia nodosa is a condition caused by an immune reaction to caterpillar hairs or other insect matter. Caterpillar hairs are acquired by direct contact or via airborne transmission. The hairs induce a granulomatous inflammatory response with pain and foreign body sensation. The most commonly affected tissue is the conjunctiva, where nodules have been occasionally reported.[201, 202] The caterpillar hairs may penetrate into the deeper ocular tissues, causing keratitis, iridocyclitis, and even endophthalmitis.[203] Ophthalmia nodosa is treated by surgically removing the caterpillar hair and by topical steroids.

PHTHIRIASIS

Phthiriasis is a lice infestation caused by the arthropod *Phthirus pubis.*

Distribution

Lice infestation is cosmopolitan; transmission occurs by direct physical contact with infected persons. The 15- to 40-year-old age group is more commonly affected. In children, infestation with *P. pubis* results from contamination from an adult.[204]

Morphology, Biology, and Life Cycle

Phthiriasis is considered a venereal disease. The source of lice is generally the hair in the pubic area of an affected person. The lashes become infected by either direct contact or by contact with contaminated bedding and clothes. Other species of lice, such as *P. humanus capitis* (head louse) and *P. humanus humanus* (body louse), do not affect the eyelashes. The reason the lashes are affected by *P. pubis* seems to be related to the parasite's arm span. There is itching and erythema of the lid margin. Chronic follicular conjunctivitis is common. The oval and transparent parasite's eggs or nits are glued to the eyelashes. The adult louse is frequently overlooked because of its transparency.

Diagnosis

The diagnosis of lice infestation is based on the demonstration of nits and adult lice in the lashes. Wood-light illumination can be used to demonstrate the fluorescence of the nits.[205]

Treatment

Physostigmine (Eserine) ointment can be used to suffocate the parasite.[206, 207] Lindane should be used in the pubic area.

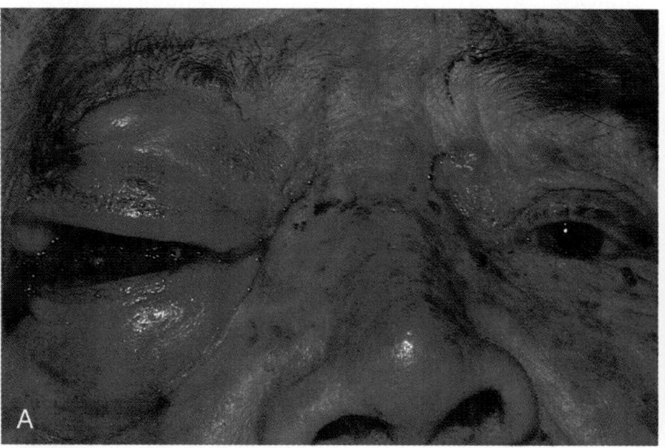

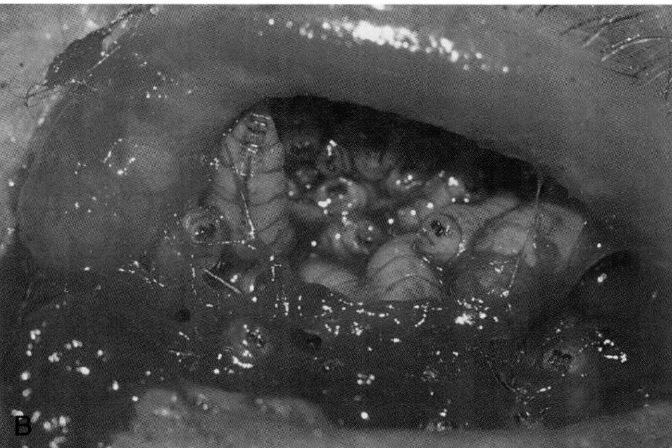

FIGURE 14–8. Ophthalmomyasis externa. A 94-year-old woman from Cundinamarca (Colombia) with altered mental status found with massive orbital infestation by *Dermatobia hominis*. Note the marked lid edema and distorted anterior segment *(A)*. The larvae had destroyed all the intraocular contents *(B)*. (Courtesy of Pedro I. Navarro, M.D.)

Rickettsial Diseases

Rickettsial infection is an acute disease caused by the bacteria-like microorganisms of the family Rickettsiaceae. Three genera are involved: *Rickettsia, Rochalimaea,* and *Coxiella,* with human infections caused primarily by *Rickettsia prowazekii, Rickettsia typhi, Rickettsia rickettsii, Rickettsia tsutsugamushi, Coxiella burnetii,* and *Rochalimaea quintana. Rickettsia* can infect a wide number of hosts, from invertebrates to vertebrates. Rickettsial diseases in humans can be divided clinically into the typhus group (epidemic typhus, murine typhus), the spotted fever group (Rocky Mountain spotted fever, boutonneuse fever, rickettsialpox), and other rickettsial diseases (scrub typhus or chigger-borne typhus, Q fever, trench fever).

DISTRIBUTION

Rickettsial infections occur worldwide. Improved treatment and prevention methods have decreased the incidence of rickettsioses, but they have not been completely eliminated.

MORPHOLOGY, BIOLOGY, AND LIFE CYCLE

Rickettsia are pleomorphic, gram-negative organisms (0.2 to 0.5 μm × 0.8 to 2 μm) that resemble bacteria in their structural and chemical characteristics but are distinct organisms, because several species have an obligate intracellular nature. They multiply by binary fission in the cytoplasm of infected cells or, as with the spotted fever group organisms, replication can also occur in the cell nucleus. *R. prowazekii* replicates until the cell lyses, whereas *R. rickettsii* does not cause cell lysis and leaves the host cell early in the course of infection to infect other cells.[208] Disease transmission is via arthropods.

Lice *(Pediculus humanus)* are the vectors of the epidemic typhus caused by *R. prowazekii.* The organisms invade the louse's intestinal epithelial cells and multiply, causing cell lysis. The louse does not survive more than 10 days after the primary infection, and during this period it sheds rickettsiae in its feces. Contaminated louse feces are deposited on the skin during insect blood meals, and the rickettsia gains entrance into the body via wounded or scratched skin. Humans are an important reservoir host for epidemic typhus.

Ticks (several *Dermacentor* species) are the vectors of the Rocky Mountain spotted fever caused by *R. rickettsii.* The vector is contaminated by feeding on infected animals (e.g., rodents), with rickettsiae remaining in the arthropod salivary glands. Humans are only accidentally infected. *R. rickettsii* are not pathogenic for the ticks; infection is maintained among ticks by transovarial transmission.

Several species of *Leptotrombidium* (mites) are the vectors of the scrub, or chigger-borne, typhus, caused by *R. tsutsugamushi.* Adult mites and larvae (chiggers) are infected by feeding on contaminated vertebrates (e.g., mice). Rickettsiae are located in the arthropod salivary glands and are inoculated into the host during the blood meal. *R. tsutsugamushi is* not harmful to the mites; infection is maintained among mites by transovarial passage. The mites function as both reservoirs and vectors of the disease. Because *R. tsutsugamushi* has strain variations, some patients may experience a second attack of scrub typhus.

Lice *(P. humanus)* are the vectors of the trench fever caused by *R. quintana.* The body louse acquires and passes the infection by feeding on a rickettsemic human. Organisms grow extracellularly in the louse intestinal lumen; humans are contaminated through louse feces deposited on the skin. Humans are reservoirs for trench fever. Transovarial transmission of *R. quintana* among lice has not been observed.

Fleas *(Xenopsylla cheopis)* are the vectors of the murine typhus caused by *R. typhi.* Humans are accidentally infected. Organisms proliferate in the flea intestinal cells, and the disease is transmitted by contaminated flea feces deposited on the skin. Fleas do not transmit *R. typhi* to offspring transovarially.[209]

Mites *(Allodermanyssus sanguineus)* are the vectors of the rickettsialpox caused by *R. akari.* Humans are only accidentally infected. The mite also transmits the infection transovarially.

Q fever is caused by *C. burnetii.* Ticks transmit the infection to domestic animals that shed the rickettsia in milk, urine, feces, and placental products. *C. burnetii is* highly resistant to extremes of temperature and desiccation. Humans and other animals are infected by inhalation or mucosal contact with dust containing the rickettsiae. In ticks, infection with one species may prevent subsequent infection with other rickettsial species.[210]

INFECTION OF THE HOST

In humans, rickettsiae multiply in endothelial cells of small blood vessels, causing endothelial proliferation and perivascular infiltration, subsequent extravasation of fluid with edema, and hypotension. If untreated, the disease can progress to gangrene and disseminated intravascular coagulation. Formation of a typhus nodule or glial nodule (a perivascular aggregation of mononuclear cells such as lymphocytes and macrophages) in the CNS is characteristic of the disease.[211] Skin and several other organ tissues (kidney, heart, lung) can be involved, causing skin rash, encephalitis, and renal and liver failure, and may lead ultimately to death of the host. Rickettsial infection may induce resistance to reinfection or, in contrast, persistent lymphoid tissue disease as in Q fever and recrudescent epidemic typhus. Table 14–2 summarizes the epidemiology and clinical findings of some human rickettsial diseases.

CLINICAL FINDINGS

The clinical spectrum of rickettsial disease varies widely according to the organism involved and the host response. Fever, rash, and history of arthropod exposure suggest the disease, although these signs are not always present.[212] Other signs, including prostration, nausea, vomiting, abdominal and back pain, myalgia, arthralgia, cough, photophobia, and conjunctivitis, may be present. A primary cutaneous lesion (eschar) may be observed at the site of the insect bite or attachment. In epidemic typhus, a recrudescent mild form of the disease, called Brill-Zinsser disease, can occur. Classic Q fever presents as atypical pneumonia or with influenza-like symptoms. Ocular findings in all rickettsial diseases may include sore, red eyes with conjunctival papillae, chemosis, and petechiae; iritis, retinitis (edema, hemorrhage, exudate);

TABLE 14–2. **Epidemiology and Clinical Characteristics of Rickettsial Diseases**

Organism	Transmission	Mammalian Reservoir	Geographic Distribution	Disease	Incubation (Days)	Clinical Signs*
Rickettsia prowazekii	Louse feces	Humans	North and South America, Africa, Asia	Epidemic typhus	5–23	Generalized maculopapular rash; central nervous system involvement, myocarditis, renal insufficiency; no eschar; may be recrudescent
Rickettsia typhi	Flea feces	Rodents	Worldwide	Murine typhus	4–15	Generalized maculopapular rash; no eschar
Rickettsia rickettsii	Tick bite, dogs	Rodents	Western hemisphere	Rocky Mountain spotted fever	2–14	Maculopapular (petechial) rash on extremities and later on trunk, eschar
Rickettsia tsutsugamushi	Mite bite	Rodents	Asia	Scrub typhus	8–12	Maculopapular rash on trunk spreading to palms and soles; eschar
Coxiella burnetii	Inhalation, goats	Cattle, sheep	Worldwide	Q fever	8–39	Interstitial pneumonia; no eschar; rare rash; chronic form: hepatitis and endocarditis
Rickettsia akari	Mite bite	Mice	USA, former USSR, Korea	Rickettsialpox	10–24	Mild condition; vesicular lesions on initial papular rash; eschar
Rochalimaea quintana	Louse feces	Humans	Europe and Africa	Trench fever	8–30	Splenomegaly; macular rash

*All patients usually present with high fever and headache that may be accompanied by prostration, myalgia, arthralgia, and conjunctivitis.

venous engorgement; arteriole occlusion; and optic nerve edema.[213–216]

DIAGNOSIS

Demonstration of rising antibody titers to rickettsial antigens using paired acute and convalescent sera is the most widely used method of clinical diagnosis of rickettsial infection. A fourfold or higher rise in titer suggests acute disease. Serologic methods include indirect immunofluorescent antibody, complement fixation, indirect hemagglutination, and ELISA. The Weil-Felix reaction is an agglutination test using *Proteus mirabilis* strains OX19, OX2, or OXk with antigens similar to those of *Rickettsia*. The Weil-Felix reaction is not completely reliable, and rickettsialpox and Q fever are not associated with Weil-Felix antibody rises.

Rickettsiae stain poorly with Gram's stain but can be visualized using Giemsa or Macchiavellos stain. Culture using enriched blood-agar media can be used for recovery of *R. quintana*. All other rickettsiae require living cells (embryonated eggs or other tissue culture systems) for culture.

PREVENTION

Personal protection against vector contact (protective clothing) and use of insect repellents in endemic areas are preventive measures. Lice infestation can be avoided by frequent changes of clothing or by application of insecticides. Forceps and hand protection while removing ticks are recommended because both tissues and fluids from crushed ticks are contaminated. Vector and reservoir control may be indicated in endemic areas. Milkborne transmission, observed in Q fever, can be prevented by pasteurization. Chemoprophylaxis is not recommended.[212] Effective vaccines for the major rickettsial infections (e.g., Rocky Mountain spotted fever) have been developed but are not used frequently[210] because rickettsial diseases, if promptly recognized and treated, are no longer lethal.[211]

TREATMENT

Tetracyclines are preferred drugs in the treatment of rickettsiosis. Chloramphenicol is also effective.[216]

REFERENCES

1. Noble ER, Noble GA. Parasitology. The Biology of Animal Parasites. Philadelphia, Lea & Febiger, 1982.
2. Markell EK, Voge M, John DT: Medical Parasitology, 7th ed. Philadelphia, WB Saunders, 1992.
3. Kean BH, Sun T, Ellsworth RM: Color Atlas/Text of Ophthalmic Parasitology. New York, Igaku-Shoin, 1991.
4. Borst P, Cross GAM: Molecular basis for trypanosome antigenic variation. Cell 29:291, 1982.
5. Wyler DJ: Malaria—Resurgence, resistance, and research (second of two parts). N Engl J Med 308:934, 1983.
6. Aitken D, Hay J, Kinnear FB: Amebic keratitis in a wearer of disposable contact lenses due to a mixed *Vahlkampfia* and *Hartmannella* infection. Ophthalmology 103:485, 1996.
7. Martinez AJ: Free-Living Amebas: Natural History, Prevention, Diagnosis, Pathology, and Treatment of Disease. Boca Raton, CRC Press, 1985.
8. Mazur T, Hadas E, Iwanicka I: The duration of cyst stage and the viability and virulence of *Acanthamoeba* isolates. Trop Med Parasitol 46:106, 1996.
9. Chynn EW, Lopez MA, Pavan-Langston D, Talamo JH: *Acanthamoeba* keratitis: Contact lens and noncontact lens characteristics. Ophthalmology 102:1369, 1995.
10. Talamo JH, Larkin DS: Bilateral *Acanthamoeba* keratitis and gas-permeable contact lenses. [Letter] Am J Ophthalmol 116:651, 1993.
11. Jones DB, Visvesvara GS, Robinson NM: *Acanthamoeba polyphaga* keratitis and *Acanthamoeba* uveitis associated with fatal meningoencephalitis. Trans Ophthal Soc U K 95:221, 1975.
12. Naginton J, Watson PG, Playfair TJ: Amoebic infection of the eye. Lancet 2:1537, 1974.
13. Stehr-Green JK, Bailey TM, Visvesvara G: The epidemiology of *Acanthamoeba* keratitis in the United States. Am J Ophthalmol 107:331, 1989.
14. Mathers WD, Sutphin JE, Folberg R: Outbreak of keratitis presumed to be caused by *Acanthamoeba*. Am J Ophthalmol 121:129, 1996.
15. Ma P, Visvesvara GS, Martinez AJ: *Naegleria* and *Acanthamoeba* infection: Review. Rev Infect Dis 12:490, 1990.
16. Murakawa GJ, McCalmont T, Altman J: Diseminated acanthamoebi-

asis in patients with AIDS: A report of five cases and a review of the literature. Arch Dermatol 131:1291, 1995.
17. Moore MB, McCulley JP, Newton C: *Acanthamoeba* keratitis: A growing problem in soft and hard contact lens wearers. Ophthalmology 94:1654, 1987.
18. Gorlin AI, Gabriel MM, Wilson LA, Ahearn DG: Effect of adhered bacteria on the binding of *Acanthamoeba* to hydrogel lenses. Arch Ophthalmol 114:576, 1996.
19. Garner A: Pathogenesis of acanthamoebic keratitis: Hypothesis based on a histological analysis of 30 cases. Br J Ophthalmol 77:366, 1993.
20. Blackman HJ, Rao NA, Lemp MA: *Acanthamoeba* keratitis successfully treated with penetrating keratoplasty: Suggested immunogenic mechanisms of action. Cornea 3:125, 1984.
21. Mitra MM, Alizadeh H, Gerard RD, Niederkorn JY: Characterization of a plasminogen activator produced by *Acanthamoeba castellani.* Mol Biochem Parasitol 73:157, 1995.
22. Mitro K, Bhagavathiammai A, Zhou OM: Partial characterization of the proteolytic secretions of *Acanthamoeba polyphaga*. Exp Parasitol 78:377, 1994.
23. Cavanagh HD, Petroll WM, Alizadeh H: Clinical and diagnostic use of in vivo confocal microscopy in patients with corneal disease. Ophthalmology 110:1433, 1993.
24. Cavanagh HD, McCulley JP: In vivo confocal microscopy and *Acanthamoeba* keratitis. [Editorial] Am J Ophthalmol 121:207, 1996.
25. Tay-Kearney ML, McGhee CN, Crawford GJ, Trown K: *Acanthamoeba* keratitis: A masquerade of presentation in six cases. Aust N Z J Ophthalmol 21:237, 1993.
26. Wilhelmus KR, Osato MS, Font RL: Rapid diagnosis of *Acanthamoeba* keratitis using calcofluor white. Arch Ophthalmol 104:1309, 1986.
27. Epstein RJ, Wilson LA, Visvesvara GS: Rapid diagnosis of *Acanthamoeba* keratitis from corneal scrapings using indirect fluorescent antibody staining. Arch Ophthalmol 104:1318, 1986.
28. Matias R, Schottelius J, Raddatz CF, Michel R: Species identification and characterization of an *Acanthamoeba* strain from human cornea. Parasitol Res 77:469, 1991.
29. Kilvington S, Beeching JR, White DG: Differentiation of *Acanthamoeba* strains from infected corneas and the environment by using restriction endonuclease digestion of whole-cell DNA. J Clin Microbiol 29:310, 1991.
30. Gradus MS, Koenig SB, Hyndiuk RA: Filter-culture technique using amoeba saline transport medium for the noninvasive diagnosis of *Acanthamoeba* keratitis. Am J Clin Pathol 92:682, 1989.
31. Mathers WD, Stevens GJ, Rodriguez M: Immunopathology and electron microscopy of *Acanthamoeba* keratitis. Am J Ophthalmol 103:626, 1987.
32. Ludwig IH, Meisler DM, Rutherford I: Susceptibility of *Acanthamoeba* to soft contact lens disinfection systems. Invest Ophthalmol Vis Sci 27:626, 1987.
33. Silvany KE, Dougherty JM, McCulley JP: The effect of currently available contact lens disinfection systems on *Acanthamoeba castellani* and *Acanthamoeba polyphaga.* Ophthalmology 97:286, 1990.
34. Dawson MW, Brown TJ, Till DG: The effect of Baquacil on pathogenic free-living amoebae (PFLA). 1. In axenic conditions. N Z J Mar Freshwater Res 17:305, 1983.
35. Larkin DFP, Kilvington S, Dart JKG: Treatment of *Acanthamoeba* keratitis with polyhexamethylene biguanide. Ophthalmology 99:1985, 1992.
36. Varga JH, Wolf TC, Jensen HG: Combined treatment of *Acanthamoeba* keratitis with propamidine, neomycin, and polyhexamethylene biguanide. Am J Ophthalmol 115:466, 1993.
37. Hay J, Kirkness CM, Seal DV, Wright P: Drug resistance and *Acanthamoeba* keratitis: The quest for alternative antiprotozoal chemotherapy. Eye 8:555, 1994.
38. Brasseur G, Favennec L, Perrine D: Successful treatment of *Acanthamoeba* keratitis by hexamidine. Cornea 13:459, 1994.
39. Driebe WT, Stern GA, Epstein RJ: *Acanthamoeba* keratitis: Potential role for topical clotrimazole in combination chemotherappy. Arch Ophthalmol 106:1196, 1988.
40. Ishibashi Y, Matsumoto Y, Dabata T: Oral itraconazole and topical miconazole with debridement for *Acanthamoeba* keratitis. Am J Ophthalmol 109:121, 1990.
41. Osato MS, Robinson NM, Wilhelmus KR, Jones DB: Morphogenesis of *Acanthamoeba castellani.* Titration of the steroid effects. [Abstract] Invest Ophthalmol Vis Sci 27(Suppl 5):37, 1986.
42. John T, Lin J, Sahm D, Rockey JH: Effects of corticosteroids in experimental *Acanthamoeba* keratitis. [Abstract] Rev Infect Dis 13(Suppl):440, 1991.
43. Horsburgh B, Hirst LW, Carey T: Steroid sensitive *Acanthamoeba* keratitis. Aust N Z J Ophthalmol 19:349, 1991.
44. Ravinovitch T, Weissman SS, Ostter HB: *Acanthamoeba* keratitis: Clinical signs and analysis of outcome. [Abstract] Rev Infect Dis 13(Suppl):427, 1991.
45. Alizadeh H, He Y, McCulley JP: Successful immunization against *Acanthamoeba* keratitis in a pig model. Cornea 14:180, 1995.
46. Lam S: Keratitis caused by leishmaniasis or trypanosomiasis. Ophthalmol Clin North Am 7:635, 1995.
47. Schmidt GD, Roberts LS: Foundations of Parasitology, 3rd ed. St. Louis, Times Mirror/Mosby College Publishing, 1985.
48. Malchiodi EL, Chiaramonth MG, Taranto N: Cross-reactivity studies and differential serodiagnosis of human infections caused by *Tripanosoma cruzi* and *Leishmania* spp: Use of immunoblotting and ELISA with a purified antigen (Ag163B6). Clin Exp Immunol 97:417, 1994.
49. Pavan-Langston D, Dunkel EC: Handbook of Ocular Drug Therapy and Ocular Side Effects of Systemic Drugs. Boston, Little, Brown, 1991.
50. Knox DL, King JJ: Retinal arteritis, iridocyclitis, and giardiasis. Ophthalmology 89:1303, 1982.
51. Turner JA: Giardiasis and infections with *Dientamoeba fragilis*. Pediatr Clin North Am 32:865, 1985.
52. Pickering IK, Engelkirk PG: *Giardia lamblia.* Pediatr Clin North Am 35:565, 1988.
53. Roizenblatt J: Interstitial keratitis caused by American (mucocutaneous) leishmaniasis. Am J Ophthalmol 87:175, 1979.
54. Martinez S, Marr JJ: Allopurinol in the treatment of American cutaneous leishmaniasis. N Engl J Med 326:741, 1992.
55. Saenz RE: Treatment of American cutaneous leishmaniasis with orally administered allopurinol riboside. J Infect Dis 160:153, 1989.
56. Saenz RE, Paz H, Berman JD: Efficacy of ketoconazole against *Leishmania braziliensis panamensis* cutaneous leishmaniasis. Am J Med 89:147, 1990.
57. Powell RD: Malaria and babesiosis. *In* Goldsmith R, Heyneman D (eds): Tropical Medicine and Parasitology. Norwalk, CT, Appleton & Lange, 1989, p 303.
58. Hidayat AA, Nalbandian RM, Sammons DW: The diagnostic histopathologic features of ocular malaria. Ophthalmology 100:1183, 1993.
59. Biswas J, Fogla R, Srinivasan P, et al: Ocular malaria: A clinical and histopathologic study. Ophthalmology 103:1471, 1996.
60. Lewallen S, Taylor TE, Molyneux ME: Ocular fundus findings in Malawian children with malaria. Ophthalmology 100:857, 1993.
61. Randall G, Seidel JS: Malaria. Pediatr Clin North Am 32:893, 1985.
62. Valero MV, Amador LR, Galindo C: Vaccination with SPf66, a chemically synthesized vaccine, against *Plasmodium falciparum* malaria in Colombia. Lancet 341:705, 1993.
63. Nosten F, Luxemburger C, Kyle DE: Randomized double-blind placebo-controlled trial of SPf66 malaria vaccine in children in northwestern Thailand. Shoklo SPf66 Malaria Vaccine Trial Group. Lancet 348:701, 1996.
64. WHO Parasitic Diseases Surveillance: Antibody to *Encephalitozoon cuniliculi* in man. WHO Weekly Epidem Rec 58:30, 1983.
65. Davis RM, Font RL, Keisler MS, Shadduck JA: Corneal microsporidiosis: A case report including ultrastructural observations. Ophthalmology 97:953, 1990.
66. Weiss LM: ...And now microsporidiosis. Ann Intern Med 123:954, 1995.
67. Ashton N, Wirasinha PA: Encephalitozoonosis (nosematosis) of the cornea. Br J Ophthalmol 57:669, 1973.
68. Pinnolis M, Egbert PR, Font RL: Nosematosis of the cornea: Case report, including electron microscopy studies. Arch Ophthalmol 99:1044, 1981.
69. Friedberg DN, Stenson SM, Orenstein JM, et al: Microsporidial keratoconjunctivitis in acquired immunodeficiency syndrome. Arch Ophthalmol 108:504, 1990.
70. Lowder CY, Meiler DM, McMahon JT, et al: Microsporidia infection of the cornea in an HIV-positive man. Am J Ophthalmol 109:242, 1990.
71. Metcalfe TW, Doran RM, Rowlands PL: Microsporidial keratoconjunctivitis in a patient with AIDS. Br J Ophthalmol 76:177, 1992.
72. Yee RW, Tio FO, Martinez JA: Resolution of microsporidial epithelial keratopathy in a patient with AIDS. Ophthalmology 98:196, 1991.
73. Diesenhouses MC, Wilson LA, Corrent GF: Treatment of microspori-

dial keratoconjunctivitis with topical fumagillin. Am J Ophthalmol 115:293, 1993.
74. Molina J, Oksenhendler E, Beauvaia B, et al: Disseminated microsporidiosis due to *Septata intestinalis* in patients with AIDS: Clinical features and response to albendazole therapy. J Infect Dis 171:245, 1994.
75. Walzer PD: *Pneumocystis carinii:* New clinical spectrum? N Engl J Med 324:263, 1991.
76. Rao NA, Zimmerman PL, Boyer D: A clinical, histopathologic, and electron microscopy study of *Pneumocystis carinii* choroiditis. Am J Ophthalmol 107:218, 1989.
77. Raviglione MC: Extrapulmonary pneumocystosis: The first 50 cases. Rev Infect Dis 12:1127, 1990.
78. Pifer LL, Hugher Wt, Stagno S: *Pneumocystis carinii* infection: Evidence for high prevalence in normal and immunosuppressed children. Pediatrics 61:35, 1978.
79. Telzak EE, Cote RJ, Gold JWM: Extrapulmonary *Pneumocystis carinii* infections. Rev Infect Dis 12:380, 1990.
80. Edman JC, Kovacs JA, Masur H: Ribosomal RNA sequence shows *Pneumocystis carinii* to be a member of the Fungi. Nature 334:519, 1988.
81. Hughes WT: Natural mode of acquisition for the novo infection with *Pneumocystis carinii.* J Infect Dis 145:842, 1982.
82. Jacobs JL, Libby DM, Winters RA: A cluster of *Pneumocystis carinii* pneumonia in adults without predisposing illness. N Engl J Med 324:246, 1991.
83. Sun T: Opportunistic parasitic infections in patients with acquired immunodeficiency syndrome. Pathol Annu 23:1, 1988.
84. Wakefield AE, Pixley FJ, Banerji S: Detection of *Pneumocystis carinii* with DNA amplification. Lancet 2:451, 1990.
85. Miyawaki H, Fujita J, Hojo S: Detection of *Pneumocystis carinii* in serum by polymerase chain reaction. Resp Med 90:153, 1996.
86. Pifer LL: *Pneumocystis carinii*: A diagnostic dilemma. Pediatr Infect Dis J 2:177, 1983.
87. Hughes WT, Killmar J: Monodrug efficacies of sulfonamides in prophylaxis for *Pneumocystis carinii* pneumonia. Antimicrob Agent Chem 40:962, 1996.
88. Salmon-Ceron D, Fontbonne A, Saba J: Lower survival of AIDS patients receiving dapsone compared with aerosolized pentamidine for secondary prophylaxis of *Pneumocystis carinii* pneumonia. Study Group. J Infect Dis 172:656, 1995.
89. Frenkel JK: Transmission of toxoplasmosis and the role of immunity in limiting transmission and illness. J Am Vet Med Assoc 196:233, 1990.
90. Daffos F, Forestier F, Capella-Pavlovsky M: Prenatal management of 746 pregnancies at risk for congenital toxoplasmosis. N Engl J Med 318:271, 1988.
91. Roberts T, Frenkel JK: Estimating income losses and other preventable costs caused by congenital toxoplasmosis in people in the United States. J Am Vet Med Assoc 196:249, 1990.
92. Hooper DC, Pruitt A, Rubin RH: Central nervous system infection in the chronically immunosuppressed. Medicine 61:166, 1982.
93. Wong B, Gold JWM, Brown AE: Central-nervous-system toxoplasmosis in homosexual men and parenteral drug abusers. Ann Intern Med 100:36, 1984.
94. Henderly DE, Genstler AJ, Smith RE: Changing patterns of uveitis. Am J Ophthalmol 103:131, 1987.
95. Perkins ES: Ocular toxoplasmosis. Br J Ophthalmol 57:1, 1973.
96. Holland GN, Engstrom REJ, Glasgow BJ: Ocular toxoplasmosis in patients with the acquired immunodeficiency syndrome. Am J Ophthalmol 106:653, 1988.
97. Dutton GN, McMenamin PG, Flay J: The ultrastructural pathology of congenital murine toxoplasmic retinochoroiditis. Part II: The morphology of the inflammatory changes. Exp Eye Res 43:545, 1986.
98. Fish RH, Hoskins JC, Kline LB: Toxoplasma neuroretinitis. Ophthalmology 100:1177, 1993.
99. Moorthy RS, Smith RE, Rao NA: Progressive ocular toxoplasmosis in patients with acquired immunodeficiency syndrome. Am J Ophthalmol 115:742, 1993.
100. Johnson MW, Greven CM, Jaffe GJ, et al: Atypical, severe toxoplasmic retinochoroiditis in elderly patients. Ophthalmology 104:48, 1997.
101. Silveira C, Belfort R Jr, Burnier M Jr: Acquired toxoplasmic infection as the cause of toxoplasmic retinochoroiditis in families. Am J Ophthalmol 106:362, 1988.
102. Akstein RB, Wilson LA, Teutsch SM: Acquired toxoplasmosis. Ophthalmology 89:1299, 1982.
103. Ronday MJ, Luyendijk L, Baarsma GS, et al: Presumed acquired ocular toxoplasmosis. Arch Ophthalmol 113:1524, 1995.
104. Abrahams W, Gregerson DS: Longitudinal study of serum antibody responses to retinal antigens in acute ocular toxoplasmosis. Am J Ophthalmol 93:224, 1982.
105. Rothova A, van Knapen F, Baarsma GS: Serology in ocular toxoplasmosis. Br J Ophthalmol 70:615, 1986.
106. Desmonts G: Definitive serological diagnosis of ocular toxoplasmosis. Arch Ophthalmol 76:839, 1966.
107. Rollins DF, Tabbara KF, O'Connor GR: Detection of toxoplasmal antigen and antibody in ocular fluids in experimental ocular toxoplasmosis. Arch Ophthalmol 101:455, 1983.
108. Brezin AP, Egwuagu CE, Burnier M Jr: Identification of *Toxoplasma gondii* in paraffin-embedded sections by the polymerase chain reaction. Am J Ophthalmol 110:599, 1990.
109. Norose K, Tokushima T, Yano A: Quantitative polymerase chain reaction in diagnosing ocular toxoplasmosis. Am J Ophthalmol 121:441, 1996.
110. Garweg J, Boehnke M, Koerner F: Restricted applicability of the polymerase chain reaction for the diagnosis of ocular toxoplasmosis. Ger J Ophthalmol 5:104, 1996.
111. Rao NA, Font RL: Toxoplasmic retinochoroiditis. Arch Ophthalmol 95:273, 1977.
112. Dutton GN, Hay J, Flair DM: Clinicopathological features of a congenital murine model of ocular toxoplasmosis. Graefes Arch Clin Exp Ophthalmol 224:256, 1986.
113. Colebunders R, Mathis R: Ocular toxoplasmosis treated with pyrimetamine. Am J Ophthalmol 93:371, 1982.
114. Araujo FG, Remington JS: Effect of clindamycin on acute and chronic toxoplasmosis in mice. Antimicrob Agents Chemother 5:647, 1974.
115. Curtale F, Pokhrel RP, Tilden RL, Higashi G: Intestinal helminths and xerophthalmia in Nepal: A case-control study. J Trop Pediatr 41:334, 1995.
116. Markell EK: Intestinal nematode infections. Pediatr Clin North Am 32:971, 1985.
117. Keystone JS, Murdoch JK: Mebendazole. Ann Intern Med 91:582, 1979.
118. Lacey E: Mode of action of benzimidazole. Parasitol Today 6:112, 1990.
119. Burd EM: Antiparasitic agents. *In* Tabbara KF, Hyndiuk RA (eds): Infections of the Eye, 2nd ed. Boston, Little, Brown, 1996, p 281.
120. Burnier MJ, Hidayat AA, Neafie RC: Dracunculiasis of the orbit and eyelid. Light and electron microscopic observations of two cases. Ophthalmology 98:919, 1991.
121. Tabbara KF: Other parasitic infections. *In* Tabbara KF, Hyndiuk RA (eds): Infections of the Eye, 2nd ed. Boston, Little, Brown, 1996, p 697.
122. Gass JDM, Scelfo R: Diffuse unilateral subacute neuroretinitis. J R Soc Med 71:95, 1978.
123. Gass JDM, Gilbert WRJ, Guerry RK, Scelfo R: Diffuse unilateral subacute neuroretinitis. Ophthalmology 85:521, 1978.
124. Kazacos KR, Vestre WA, Kazacos EA, Raymond LA: Diffuse unilateral subacute neuroretinitis syndrome: Probable cause. Arch Ophthalmol 102:967, 1997.
125. Kazacos KR, Raymond LA, Kazacos EA, Vestre WA: The racoon ascarid: A probable cause of human ocular larva migrans. Ophthalmology 92:1735, 1985.
126. Goldberg MA, Kazacos KR, Boyce WM, et al: Diffuse unilateral subacute neuroretinitis: Morphometric, serologic, and epidemiologic support for *Baylisascaris* as a causative agent. Ophthalmology 100:1695, 1993.
127. Raymond LA, Gutierrez Y, Strong LE, et al: Living retinal nematode (filarial-like) destroyed with photocoagulation. Ophthalmology 85:944, 1978.
128. Gass JDM, Callanan DG, Bowman CB: Oral therapy in diffuse unilateral subacute neuroretinitis. Arch Ophthalmol 110:675, 1992.
129. Callanan D, Davis JL, Cohen SM, et al: The use of ivermectin in diffuse unilateral subacute neuroretinitis. Ophthalmology 100(Suppl):114, 1993.
130. Font RL, Neafie RC, Perry HD: Subcutaneous dirofilariasis of the eyelid and ocular adnexa: Report of six cases. Arch Ophthalmol 98:1079, 1980.
131. Orsani JG, Coggiola G, Minazzi P: Filaria conjunctivae. Ophthalmologica 4:243, 1985.
132. Brumback GF, Marrison HM, Weatherly NF: Orbital infection with *Dirofilaria.* South Med J 61:188, 1968.

133. Moorhouse DE: *Dirofilaria immitis:* A case of human intraocular infection. Infection 6:192, 1978.
134. Sun S, Sugane K: Immunodiagnosis of human dirofilariasis by enzyme-linked immunosorbent assay using recombinant DNA-derived fusion protein. J Helminthol 66:220, 1992.
135. Gupta A, Agarwal A, Dogra MR: Retinal involvement in *Wuchereria bancrofti* filariasis. Acta Ophthalmol 70:832, 1992.
136. Tham MH, Hall IB: Impacted microfilaria in the lens capsule. Br J Ophthalmol 55:484, 1971.
137. Lee BYP, McMillan R: Loa loa: Ocular filariasis in an African student in Missouri. Ann Ophthalmol 16:456, 1984.
138. Akue JP, Hommel M, Devaney E: Markers of Loa loa infection in permanent residents of a loiasis endemic area of Gabon. Trans R Soc Trop Med Hyg 90:115, 1996.
139. Gendelman D, Blumberg R, Sadun A: Ocular *Loa loa* with cryoprobe extraction of subconjunctival worm. Ophthalmology 91:300, 1984.
140. WHO Expert Committee on Onchocerciasis: Third Report. Geneva, World Health Organization, 1987.
141. Taylor HR: Onchocerciasis. Int Ophthalmol 14:189, 1990.
142. Earttmann K, Unnasch T, Greene B: A DNA sequence specific for forest form *Onchocerca volvulus.* Nature 327:415, 1987.
143. Zimmerman P, Dadzie K, DeSole G: *Onchocerca volvulus* DNA probe classification correlates with epidemiologic patterns of blindness. J Infect Dis 165:964, 1992.
144. Gleich GJ, Ottesen EA, Leiferman KM: Eosinophils and human disease. Int Arch Allergy Appl Immunol 88:59, 1989.
145. Mabey D, Whitworth JA, Eckstein M: The effects of multiple doses of ivermectin on onchocerciasis: A six-year follow up. Ophthalmology 103:1001, 1996.
146. Chan CC, Nussenblatt RB, Kim MK: Immunopathology of ocular onchocerciasis. 2. Anti-retinal autoantibodies in serum and ocular fluids. Ophthalmology 94:439, 1987.
147. McKechnie NM, Braun G, Connor V: Immunologic cross-reactivity in the pathogenesis of ocular onchocerciasis. Invest Ophthalmol Vis Sci 34:2888, 1993.
148. Albiez EJ, Buttner DW, Duke BOL: Diagnosis and extirpation of nodules in human onchocerciasis. Trop Med Parasitol 39(Suppl 4):331, 1988.
149. Aziz MA, Diallo S, Diop IM: Efficacy and tolerance of ivermectin in human onchocerciasis. Lancet 2:171, 1982.
150. Kirshner BI, Dunn JP, Ostler HB: Conjunctivitis caused by *Thelazia californiensis.* Am J Ophthalmol 110:573, 1990.
151. Glickman LT, Schantz PM: Epidemiology and pathogenesis of zoonotic toxocariasis. Epidemiol Rev 3:230, 1981.
152. Glickman LT, Schantz PM, Cypess RH: Canine and human toxocariasis: Review of transmission, pathogenesis, and clinical disease. J Am Vet Med Assoc 175:1265, 1979.
153. Herrmann N, Glickman LT, Schantz PM: Seroprevalence of zoonotic toxocariasis in the United States: 1971–1973. Am J Epidemiol 122:890, 1985.
154. Schantz PM, Weis PE, Pollard ZF: Risk factors for toxocaral ocular larva migrans: A case-control study. Am J Public Health 70:1269, 1980.
155. Scothorn MW, Koutz FR, Groves HF: Prenatal *Toxocara canis* infection in pups. J Am Vet Med Assoc 146:45, 1965.
156. Schantz PM, Glickman LT: Toxocaral visceral larva migrans. N Engl J Med 298:436, 1978.
157. Kielar RA: *Toxocara canis* endophthalmitis with low ELISA titer. Ann Ophthalmol 15:447, 1983.
158. Schantz PM, Meyer D, Glickman LT: Clinical, serologic, and epidemiologic characteristics of ocular toxocariasis. Am J Trop Med Hyg 28:24, 1979.
159. Pollard ZF: Long-term follow-up in patients with ocular toxocariasis as measured by ELISA titers. Ann Ophthalmol 19:167, 1987.
160. Glickman LT, Schantz P, Dombrsoke R: Evaluation of serodiagnostic tests for visceral larva migrans. Am J Trop Med Hyg 27:492, 1978.
161. Pollard ZF, Jarret WH, Hagler WS: ELISA for diagnosis of ocular toxocariasis. Ophthalmology 86:743, 1979.
162. Feldberg NT, Shields JA, Federman JL: Antibody to *Toxocara canis* in the aqueous humor. Arch Ophthalmol 99:1563, 1981.
163. Benitez del Castillo JM, Herreros G, et al: Bilateral ocular toxocariasis demonstrated by aqueous humor enzyme-linked immunosorbent assay. Am J Ophthalmol 119:514, 1995.
164. Biglan AW, Glickman LT, Lobes LAJ: Serum and vitreous *Toxocara* antibody in nematode endophthalmitis. Am J Ophthalmol 88:898, 1979.
165. Felberg NT, Shields JA, Federman JL: Antibody to *Toxocara canis* in the aqueous humor. Arch Ophthalmol 99:1563, 1981.
166. Shields JA, Lerner HA, Felberb NT: Aqueous cytology and enzymes in nematode endophthalmitis. Am J Ophthalmol 84:319, 1977.
167. Shields JA: Ocular toxocariasis: A review. Surv Ophthalmol 28:361, 1984.
168. Howard GM, Ellsworth RM: Differential diagnosis of retinoblastoma: A statistical survey of 500 children. 1: Relative frequency of the lesions which simulate retinoblastoma. Am J Ophthalmol 60:610, 1965.
169. Wan WL, Cano MR, Pince KJ: Echographic characteristics of ocular toxocariasis. Ophthalmology 98:28, 1991.
170. Dent JH, Nichols RL, Beaver PC: Visceral larva migrans: With a case report. Am J Pathol 32:777, 1956.
171. Sturchler D, Schubarth P, Gualzata M, et al: Thiabendazole vs albendazole in treatment of toxocariasis: A clinical trial. Ann Trop Med Parasitol 83:473, 1989.
172. Bailey TM, Schantz PM: Trends in the incidence and transmission patterns of trichinosis in humans in the United States: Comparisons of the periods 1975–1981 and 1982–1986. Rev Infect Dis 12:5, 1990.
173. Frierson JG: Trichinosis. *In* Goldsmith R, Heyneman D (eds): Tropical Medicine and Parasitology. Norwalk, CT, Appleton & Lange, 1989, p 423.
174. Cline BL: Schistosomiasis mansoni. *In* Goldsmith R, Heyneman D (eds): Tropical Medicine and Parasitology. Norwalk, CT, Appleton & Lange, 1989, p 434.
175. Orefice F, Simal CR, Pittella JEH: Schistosomotic choroiditis. I: Fundoscopic changes and differential diagnosis. Br J Ophthalmol 69:294, 1985.
176. Pittella JEH, Orefice F: Schistosomotic choroiditis. II: Report of first case. Br J Ophthalmol 69:300, 1985.
177. Jakobiec FA, Gess L, Zimmerman LE: Granulomatous dacryoadenitis caused by *Schistosoma haematobium.* Arch Ophthalmol 95:278, 1977.
178. Welsh NH: Bilharzial conjunctivitis. Am J Ophthalmol 66:933, 1968.
179. Kabo AM, Warter A: [A propos of 1 case of ophthalmologic manifestations of bilharziasis]. Bull Soc Pathol Exot 86:174, 1993.
180. Williams PH, Tempelton AC: Infection of the eye by tapeworm *Coenurus.* Br J Ophthalmol 55:766, 1971.
181. Bryan RT, Schantz PM: Echinococcosis (hydatid disease). J Am Vet Med Assoc 195:1214, 1989.
182. Sen DK, et al: Cestoda larva (*Sparganum*) in the anterior chamber of the eye. Trop Geogr Med 41:270, 1989.
183. Torres JR, et al: Treatment of proliferative sparganosis with mebendazole and praziquantel. Trans R Soc Trop Med Hyg 75:864, 1981.
184. Topilow HW, Yimoyines DJ, Freeman HM: Bilateral multifocal intraocular cysticercosis. Ophthalmology 88:1166, 1981.
185. Stewart CR, Salmon JF, Murray AD, Sperry C: Cysticercosis as a cause of severe medial rectus muscle myositis. Am J Ophthalmol 116:510, 1993.
186. Kruger-Leite E, Jalkh AE, Quiroz H: Intraocular cysticercosis. Am J Ophthalmol 99:252, 1985.
187. Atul K, Kumar TH, Mallika G, Sandip M: Socio-demographic trends in ocular cysticercosis. Acta Ophthalmol Scand 73:438, 1995.
188. Brown WJ, Voge M: Cysticercosis: A modern day plague. Pediatr Clin North Am 32:953, 1985.
189. Arciniegas A, Gutierrez F: Our experience in the removal of intravitreal and subretinal cysticerci. Ann Ophthalmol 20:75, 1988.
190. Santos R, Chavarria M, Aguirre AE: Failure of medical treatment in two cases of intraocular cysticercosis. Am J Ophthalmol 97:249, 1984.
191. English FP, Nutting WB: Demodicosis of ophthalmic concern. Am J Ophthalmol 91:362, 1981.
192. Wilhelmus KR: Myasis palpebrarum. [Letter] Am J Ophthalmol 101:496, 1986.
193. Savino DF, Margo CE, McCoy ED, Friedl FE: Dermal myasis of the eyelid. Ophthalmology 93:1225, 1986.
194. Kersten RC, Shoukrey NM, Tabbara KF: Orbital myasis. Ophthalmology 93:1228, 1986.
195. Wood TR, Slight JR: Bilateral orbital myasis: Report of a case. Arch Ophthalmol 84:692, 1970.
196. Navarro P, Vera Cristo L: Miasis multilarvaria orbitaria interna. Rev Soc Col Oftalmol 23:28, 1990.
197. Gass JDM, Lewis RA: Subretinal tracks in ophthalmolmyasis. Arch Ophthalmol 94:1500, 1976.
198. Slusher MM, Holland WD, Weaver RG, Tyler ME: Ophthalmomyasis interna posterior. Subretinal tracks and intraocular larvae. Arch Ophthalmol 97:885, 1979.

199. Edwards KM, Meredith TA, Hagler WS, Healy GR: Ophthalmomyasis interna causing visual loss. Am J Ophthalmol 97:605, 1984.
200. Fitzgerald C, Rubin M: Intraocular parasite destroyed by photocoagulation. Arch Ophthalmol 91:162, 1974.
201. Watson PG, Sevel D: Ophthalmia nodosa. Br J Ophthalmol 50:209, 1966.
202. Lertchavanakul A, Pearce WG, Nigam S: Ophthalmia nodosa. Can J Ophthalmol 10:86, 1975.
203. Haluska FG: Experimental gypsy moth (*Lymantria dispar*) ophthalmia nodosa. Arch Ophthalmol 101:799, 1983.
204. Gurevitch AW: Scabies and lice. Pediatr Clin North Am 32:987, 1985.
205. Couch JM, Green WR, Hirst LW, De La Cruz ZC: Diagnosing and treating *Phthirus pubis* palpebrum. Surv Ophthalmol 26:219, 1982.
206. Cogan DG, Grant WM: Treatment of pediculosis ciliaris with anticholinesterase agents. Arch Ophthalmol 41:627, 1949.
207. Mathew M, D'Souza P, Mehta DKA: A new treatment for phthiriasis palpebrum. Ann Ophthalmol 14:439, 1982.
208. Wisseman CL Jr: Selected observations on rickettsiae and their host cells. Acta Virol 30:81, 1986.
209. Brezina R, Murray ES, Tarizzo ML: Rickettsiae and rickettsial diseases. Bull WHO 49:433, 1973.
210. Weiss E: The biology of rickettsial diseases. Annu Rev Microbiol 36:345, 1982.
211. Walker DH: Diagnosis of rickettsial diseases. Pathol Annu 23(Pt 2):69, 1988.
212. WHO Working Group on Rickettsial Disease: Rickettsioses: A continuing disease problem. Bull WHO 60:157, 1982.
213. Presley GD: Fundus changes in Rocky Mountain spotted fever. Am J Ophthalmol 67:263, 1969.
214. Raab EL, Leopold IH, Hodes HL: Retinopathy in Rocky Mountain spotted fever. Am J Ophthalmol 68:42, 1969.
215. Smith TW, Burton TC: The retinal manifestations of Rocky Mountain spotted fever. Am J Ophthalmol 84:259, 1977.
216. Duffey RJ, Hammer ME: The ocular manifestations of Rocky Mountain spotted fever. Ann Ophthalmol 19:301, 1987.

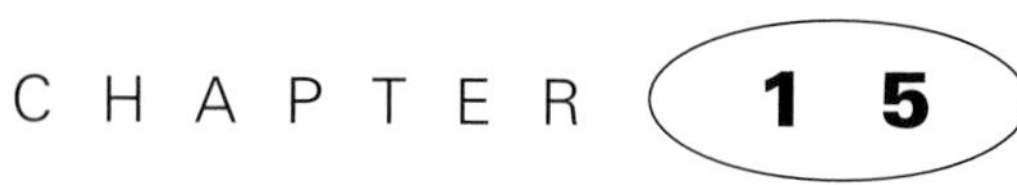

Fungal Infections of the Eye

Wiley A. Schell, Gary N. Foulks, and John R. Perfect

The first case of fungal infection of the cornea was reported in 1879, involving a farmer who was struck in the eye by oat chaff with resultant keratomycosis caused by *Aspergillus glaucus*.[1] Physicians and microbiologists subsequently have realized the unique relationship between fungi and human ocular disease. The frequent association of fungal ocular infection with occupational trauma and exposure to vegetable material is well documented.[2, 3] Increasing recognition of fungal ocular infection in the 1950s and 1960s concurrent with the increased use of topical antibiotics and corticosteroids on the eye led to more than 148 case reports by 1962 and firmly established the association of fungal infection with impaired host defenses or physical trauma.[4] Subsequent work has confirmed the importance of impaired host defenses or broken anatomic barriers and has examined fungal growth characteristics as they relate to expression of clinical disease, providing insight into improved therapy against these infrequent but extremely tenacious invaders.

Many fungal species have been identified in human ocular disease.[5, 6] Chorioretinal or orbital disease is most often a result of systemic mycoses contracted through respiratory tract exposure *(Histoplasma, Cryptococcus, Blastomyces, Coccidioides)* or dissemination from the gastrointestinal tract or an intravascular catheter (*Candida*).[7–15] In contrast, the fungal species associated with lacrimal, corneal, or traumatic intraocular infections are found in soil and vegetable matter and can be cultured from 2.5 to 52% of normal eyes, depending on climate and occupation. Fungi are probably not part of the normal flora of the lids or conjunctiva of normal eyes but are only transient colonizers. When specimens are taken from the conjunctiva or lids, the same fungus is rarely isolated sequentially in an individual, and most cultures grow only one or two fungal colonies, suggesting a very low burden of organisms.[16, 17] Almost half of the reported cases of ocular surface infection are attributed to environmentally common species of the genera *Aspergillus, Penicillium,* and *Fusarium,* and to *Candida albicans,* a commensal of humans. This finding correlates with epidemiologic studies in which these fungi have been transiently isolated from normal eyes.

Typically, environmental fungi cause keratitis after penetrating into the cornea through trauma. Also, topical therapy with antibiotics and corticosteroids generally increases fungal colonization of the eyelids and conjunctiva and is thus a major predisposing factor for oculomycosis through superinfection.[18, 19] Isolation of fungal species in eyes with known underlying abnormalities such as dacryocystitis has increased. An association of seborrheic blepharitis with *Malassezia furfur* colonization or infection has been suggested. Finally, an increase in colonization of eye structures may result from exogenous factors, such as the use of mascara contaminated by fungi such as *Candida parapsilosis.*

Mycologic Characteristics of Fungi

Fungi are eukaryotic organisms characterized in part by a cell wall surrounding a cell membrane that encloses an

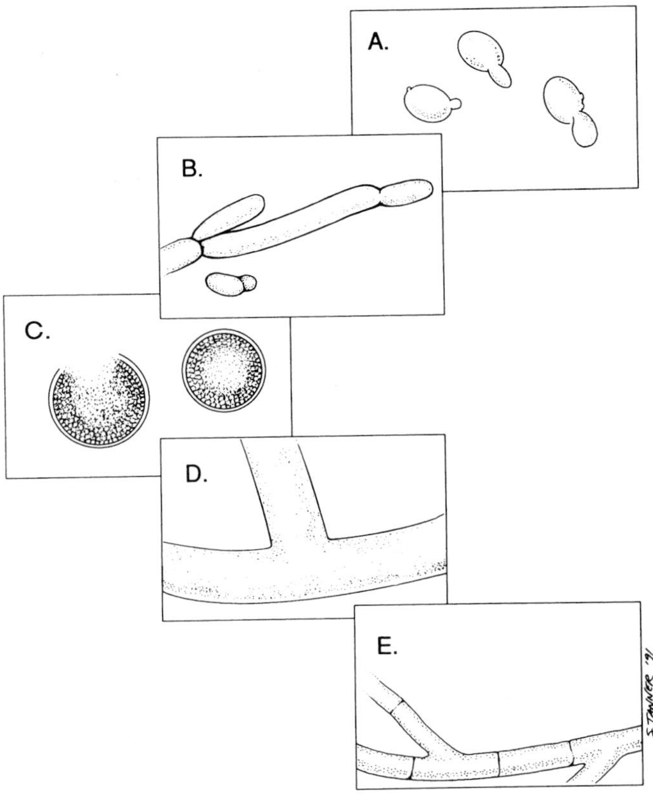

FIGURE 15–1. Basic fungal morphology as seen in infected tissue. *A,* Budding yeast cells. *B,* Pseudohyphae and budding yeast cell. *C,* Spherules with endospores *(Coccidioides immitis). D,* Nonseptate hypha. *E,* Septate hypha.

array of membranous endoplasmic reticulum studded with ribosomes, a nucleus enclosed by a nuclear membrane, and mitochondria resembling those of animals and plants. They may grow as aggregations of single cells (yeasts) or as multicellular, filamentous organisms (molds). The cell wall in many molds and yeasts contains chitin, composed of *N*-acetyl-glucosamine residues linked by γ-1,4-glycosidic bonds similar to the glucose residues in cellulose.[20] Yeasts also contain an insoluble glucan and a soluble mannan in the cell wall. These cell wall structures have become unique targets for antifungal therapies. For example, antifungal drugs, such as echinocandin B analogs or pneumocandins, 1–3 β-glucan synthesis inhibitors, and nikkomycin Z (chitin synthase inhibitor), are prototype agents in the exploration of new antifungal compounds that selectively inhibit fungal cell wall synthesis. These agents are being used in clinical trials. The fungal cell membrane contains ergosterol as well as other lipids and glycoproteins. The primary mode of action of both polyenes and azoles is on ergosterol biosynthesis.

Morphologically, yeasts are unicellular, elliptical to spherical cells, about 3 to 5 μm in diameter, that usually reproduce by a budding process. In some yeast species, cells may remain attached after budding, with subsequent elongation of the buds. These filamentous forms are known as pseudohyphae. The molds are composed of branching, tubular filaments called hyphae. They are mostly 3 to 15 μm in diameter, grow by apical synthesis, and intertwine to form a mycelium that constitutes an entire colony. In most species, the hyphae are partitioned by cross-walls, called septa, which occur regularly in conjunction with nuclear division. Septa have one or more small pores that allow cytoplasmic continuity between cells (Fig. 15–1). Although most fungi live either as yeasts or as molds, many species can grow in either form (dimorphism), depending on the environment, or they may combine budding, pseudohyphal, and hyphal forms simultaneously (pleomorphism). The form of growth is influenced by temperatures within the fungal environment and the availability of nutrients and oxygen, along with genetic factors; hence, morphology of the fungus may vary in clinical infections (Table 15–1).

Fungus grows by simple mitosis of somatic nuclei, with budding or apical extension of the cell wall. The reproductive cycle of fungi can be complex and may be sexual, asexual, or both, depending on the species (Fig. 15–2). The sexual form is called the teleomorph, the asexual form the anamorph. The entire fungus, consisting of all its known forms, is called the holomorph. In sexual reproduction, propagules arise through a process of plasmogamy, followed by

TABLE 15–1. **In Vivo Morphology of Fungi**

Typical Features	Likely Fungi
Hyphae	
Hyaline (colorless) Diameter varying (6–20 μm) Thin-walled Folded, twisted, or ribbon-like Septations absent or sparse	*Rhizopus* *Absidia* *Mucor* *Rhizomucor* *Pythium*
Hyaline Mainly uniform diameter (3–5 μm) Septations evenly spaced	*Aspergillus* *Fusarium* *Scedosporium** *Paecilomyces*† Bipolaris* *Alternaria** *Lasiodiplodia**
Dematiaceous (brown) Septations evenly spaced Yeast-like forms and pseudohyphae may be present	*Exophiala* *Wangiella* *Phialophora*
Yeast Cells (Hyaline)	
3–5 μm diameter Elliptical shape Pseudohyphae present Hyphae may be present	*Candida*
2.5–4 μm diameter Elliptical to subglobose shape No pseudohyphae or hyphae present	*Candida* *Torulopsis* *Histoplasma* *Sporothrix*
3–10 μm diameter Spherical shape Buds rarely are seen attached Capsule evident via India ink	*Cryptococcus*
8–20 μm (or larger) diameter Broad base of attachment between parent cell and bud Thick-walled parent cell	*Blastomyces*
Spherules	
20–60 μm diameter Internal endospores 2–5 μm diameter	*Coccidioides*

*Mature in vitro colonies are dematiaceous, but hyphae in vivo are usually hyaline.
†*P. lilacinus* can produce globose conidia as well as rare yeast-like cells in vivo and may be mistaken for *Candida*.

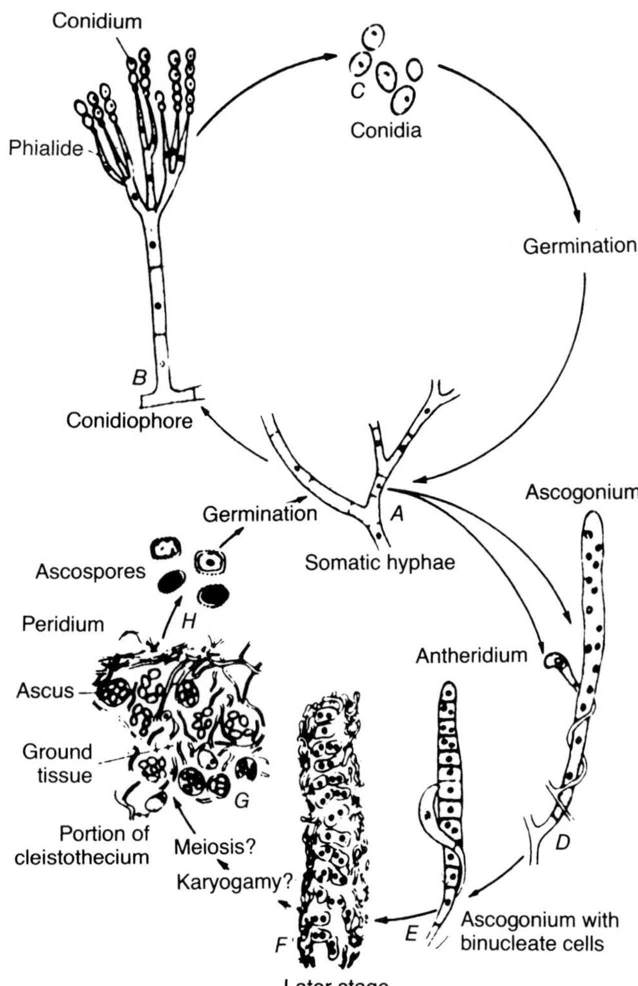

FIGURE 15–2. Life cycle of *Talaromyces vermiculatus* (anamorph, *Penicillium vermiculatum*), representative of sexual reproduction in some ascomycetes, and asexual reproduction in some of the Fungi Imperfecti. *A*, Vegetative hyphal growth. *B* and *C*, Asexual reproduction. *D–H*, Sexual reproduction. (From Alexopoulos CJ, Mims CW: Introductory Mycology, 3rd ed. New York, John Wiley, 1979.)

karyogamy of compatible nuclei and subsequent meiosis (the point at which meiosis occurs varies among species). In contrast, asexual reproduction is characterized by propagules that form directly from existing nuclei through mitosis. Spores are dispersed chiefly by air currents, water, and animals. Most fungi have an aerobic metabolism. Some fungi, notably yeasts, are capable of fermentative respiration as well. Fungi lack chlorophyll and must obtain nutrition by secreting enzymes and absorbing the digested substrate.

Previously classified as plants, fungi are now placed in the kingdom Fungi. Medically important fungi occur mainly within the phyla Basidiomycota, Ascomycota, and Zygomycota, and in the group known as the Fungi Imperfecti. The first three phyla are delineated by characteristics of sexual reproductive structures and thus reflect phylogeny as it is currently interpreted. Imperfect fungi are so named because they are not characterized by a sexual form and thus must be more artificially classified by features of their asexual reproductive structures. Molecular phylogeny continues to be used to define relationships among fungal groups. For instance, sequencing of ribosomal DNA genes now suggests that *Pneumocystis carinii* is most closely related to the fungi.

Interestingly, the life cycle of certain medically important fungi includes a teleomorph as well as one or more anamorphs. These forms of a given fungus may not always occur together, however; furthermore, a given teleomorph may be connected to one or more anamorphs, and vice versa. This is why mycologists have applied a parallel system of names to accommodate teleomorphs and anamorphs separately. As one result, pathogens such as *Pseudallescheria boydii* (anamorph *Scedosporium apiospermum*), *Cryptococcus neoformans* (teleomorph *Filobasidiella neoformans*), or *Histoplasma capsulatum* (teleomorph *Ajellomyces capsulatus*) sometimes appear in the literature under the teleomorph name as well as the anamorph name. Virtually all mycotic infections of humans, including oculomycosis, are caused by fungi that are recovered in their anamorphic form. Most of these species have ascomycetous connections, but others have zygomycetous or basidiomycetous affiliations or characteristics (Table 15–2).

Host-Fungi Interactions in the Eye

Ocular defenses to fungal infection are numerous, and oculomycosis is only common when anatomic structures are breached. Normal flora of the eyelids, the conjunctival sac with normal lacrimation, and the mechanical movements of the eyelids create an unfavorable environment for the growth of most opportunistic fungi, such as *Aspergillus* and *Candida* species. Alteration of the normal flora with systemic or topical antibacterial agents or corticosteroids, however, can decrease this barrier and allow colonization and growth of fungi. Because many fungi do not grow at elevated temperatures, normal body temperature is high enough to prevent many environmental fungi from becoming pathogenic. The lower temperature of the cornea relative to the rest of the body and eye may partially explain why keratomycosis is the most common ocular fungal infection. The intact corneal epithelium is generally resistant to fungal penetration and infection; this affords great protection. Breach of the epithelial barrier is often a prerequisite for keratomycosis, which

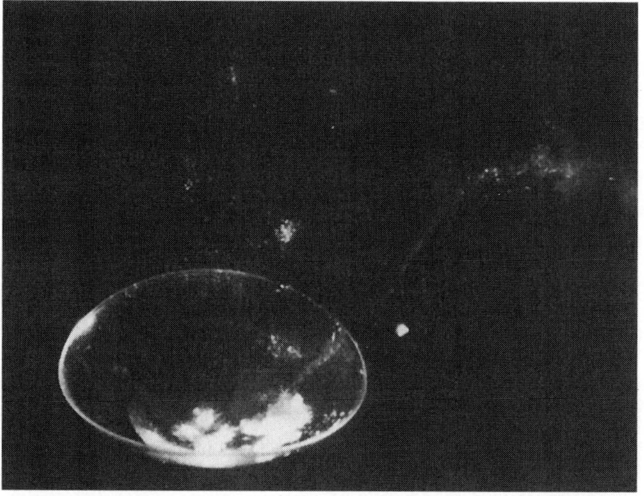

FIGURE 15–3. *Fusarium solani* growing from soft contact lens.

TABLE 15–2. **Fungi Reported to Cause Ocular Infection***

Anamorph	Teleomorph/Affinity	Anamorph	Teleomorph/Affinity
Absidia	Zygomycota	*Penicillium*	Ascomycota
Mucor		*Periconia*	*(Continued)*
Rhizopus†		*Phaeococcomyces*[90]	
Pythium[83, 84]‡	Oomycota	*Phialophora*	
		Phoma	
Acremonium	Ascomycota	*Pseudallescheria*†	
Alternaria		*Scedosporium*†	
Aspergillus†		*Scopulariopsis*	
Aureobasidium		*Sporothrix*†	
Bipolaris (as *Drechslera*)†		*Torulopsis*	
Blastomyces		*Trichoderma*[90]	
Botrytis		*Trichothecium*[91]	
Candida†		*Tubercularia*[92]	
Cladorrhinum		*Volutella*	
Cladosporium		*Wangiella*[93]	
Coccidioides†			
Colletotrichum		*Cryptococcus*†	
Curvularia		*Rhizoctonia*	Basidiomycota
Cylindrocarpon		*Rhodotorula*	
Exophiala		*Trichosporon*	
Fusarium†		*Acrophialophora*	
Fusidium		*Beauveria*[94, 95]	Unknown
Geotrichum		*Cephaliophora*[96–98]	
Gibberella		*Dichotomophthora*[99]	
Gliocladium[85]		*Dichotomophthoropsis*[100]	
Graphium		*Epicoccum*	
Histoplasma[86]		*Phaeotrichonis*[101]	
Lasiodiplodia (as *Botryodiplodia*)†		*Pneumocystis*[102]	
Malbranchea[87]		*Rhinosporidium*[103, 104]†	
Myrothecium[88]		*Scytalidium*[105]	
Oedemium[85]		*Sphaeropsis*[106]	
Paecilomyces†		*Tetraploa*	
Papulospora[89]		*Tritirachium*	

Data from Nachamkin I: Eye specimens. *In* Dalton HP, Nottebard HC Jr (eds): Interpretive Microbiology. New York, Churchill Livingstone, 1986, p 805; and Schell WA: Oculomycosis caused by dematiaceous fungi. Pan American Health Organization 479:106, 1986. References are cited for those not included in these two publications.

*More than one species is reported for most of these genera.

†More than a dozen cases reported in the literature.

‡*Pythium insidiosum* is a member of the phylum Oomycota but is characterized by in vivo morphologic features identical to those of the Zygomycota (Zygomycetes).

explains its association with trauma through occupational, recreational, or surgical exposures. First, direct inoculation by trauma may occur when the fungus is carried on a projectile. Second, colonizing fungi may invade the wound after trauma; such invasion is particularly enhanced by the use of antibacterials, corticosteroids, or both. Third, surgical procedures such as keratoplasty, corneal transplantation, or radial keratotomy are occasionally associated with introducing fungi into the eye via transplant or contaminated irrigating solutions.[21–23] Several well-described outbreaks of ocular fungal infections with *C. parapsilosis* and *Paecilomyces lilacinus* have been associated with lens implants and contaminated irrigation solutions.[24–27] Finally, soft contact lenses can act as a nidus for fungal invasion into the cornea if they are not properly cleaned and disinfected (Fig. 15–3).[28] Corneal infection allows extension to the sclera or intraocular space because there are few subsequent tissue barriers. The role of local antibodies and complement in protection against fungal infections of the eye is uncertain. The polysaccharide nature of the fungal cell wall can activate complement, and secretory immunoglobulin A (IgA) can protect against mucosal infection with *Candida* species, but the importance of such local immunity protection in the eye is not well understood. On the other hand, clinical experience demonstrates that topical and systemic corticosteroids enhance the risk of ocular fungal infections and clearly suggests that local immunity factors are important in protecting the eye from fungal invasion.

The second avenue for fungal invasion is through the blood stream (endogenous rather than exogenous). This oculomycosis generally occurs when there is some systemic host immune depression. The most common example is white blood cell defects, particularly chemotherapy-induced neutropenia. During neutropenia, invasion of the eye is particularly difficult to diagnose because general hallmarks of infection, such as an inflammatory response in the chorioretina or vitreous body, are not always visible.[29] *Candida* and *Aspergillus* species, however, can reach the retina in the presence of a normal granulocyte count if the systemic inoculum is high, as occurs in certain human infections and in experimental animal models. For example, fungal ocular infections have occurred during hyperalimentation, post partum, during prolonged antibiotic therapy, in the neonatal period, and with intravenous drug use.[30–34]

The cell-mediated immune system is a well-characterized protective system against fungal infection and obviously is important in preventing and fighting established ocular fungal infections. Debilitating diseases or generalized impairments of the immune system are predilecting factors for fungal infection, both systemically and ophthalmically. Rhinoorbital zygomycosis in the diabetic or cancer patient represents invasion of blood vessels within the orbit secondary to an underlying immune depression. *C. neoformans* invasion of the orbit or chorioretinal area has become more common in severely immunocompromised hosts with cell-mediated defects, such as patients with acquired immunodeficiency syndrome (AIDS) and those on high-dose corticosteroids.

Although ocular involvement with *C. neoformans* has increased during the AIDS epidemic, infection with this fungus was frequently reported in prior years. One study found ocular signs and symptoms in 45% of all patients with meningitis.[9] Manifestations range from ocular palsies to involvement of the choroid-retina.[9, 35] In one-fourth of cases, eye involvement is diagnosed before meningitis.[36] Simultaneous infections with *C. neoformans* and other pathogens such as human immunodeficiency virus and cytomegalovirus can occur in severely immunosuppressed patients.[37] Although most cases of ocular cryptococcosis arise from blood stream dissemination, the eye has been the direct portal of entry in such cases as donor transmission through a corneal transplant[21] and cryptococcal keratitis after a keratoplasty procedure.[23] Thus, some cases of disseminated cryptococcosis might originate in the eye rather than the lung.

Ocular cryptococcosis can lead to visual loss. In fact, most cases of cryptococcal endophthalmitis lead to severe visual loss; successful management is rare.[38] The AIDS epidemic has given rise to reports of catastrophic loss of vision in patients with cryptococcosis without evidence of endophthalmitis.[39, 40] The funduscopic examination yields either normal results or evidence of papilledema. The clinical manifestations suggest two pathogenic processes. First, some patients experience rapid visual loss within 12 hours to a few days. This clinical syndrome suggests optic neuritis in which the optic nerve and its vessels are infiltrated by large numbers of yeast cells. No successful therapeutic strategies are known for this form of visual loss. Other patients can present with slow visual loss that generally begins later during antifungal therapy and gradually progresses over weeks to months. Symptoms may be related to increased intracranial pressure in these patients, and treatment with central nervous system shunts or optic nerve fenestrations may halt the progression of visual loss.[40]

In contrast with infections, in which ocular defenses clearly fail to prevent fungal inoculum from replicating, is a syndrome called presumed ocular histoplasmosis, which is characterized by chorioretinal scars, hemorrhage, and neovascularization. Although it has been suggested that these host reactions are due to the presence of the yeast cells or antigens of *H. capsulatum*, viable organisms have not been documented for this syndrome, and there is no evidence that growth of *H. capsulatum* is involved. Therefore, the thrust of treatment has been corticosteroids or laser therapy to stop the lesion's advancement;[41] antifungal therapy has not been helpful.

When oculomycosis occurs, the fungus tends to invade directly into tissue planes. This is particularly apparent in keratomycosis, as demonstrated in Figure 15–4, a case of *C. parapsilosis* infection in a keratoplasty patient on long-term topical steroid therapy. The host response to the organism can be acute suppurative inflammation, chronic inflammation, or granulomatous inflammatory reaction, depending on the fungal species and tissue location (Fig. 15–5). The organism can actively damage host tissue by stimulating the host to elaborate inflammatory mediators such as oxidative products. The fungus may also secrete products that injure the eye. For example, a potential virulence factor for *C. albicans* is its production of extracellular acid proteases and phospholipases, which may further aid in tissue destruction.[42] *Aspergillus* species can produce elastase, which likely facilitates hyphal invasion into blood vessels and may further contribute to damage of eye tissue.[43] Because certain fungi produce mycotoxins under specific conditions, such products might someday be detected and shown to contribute to destruction of ocular tissue.

Fungi possess poorly understood factors that allow a certain tropism for eye structures during blood stream invasion. For instance, during fungemia with *C. albicans* in the rabbit model of candidiasis, yeast cells consistently localize in the eye and kidney when other tissues are spared. In humans, the propensity for ocular invasion during candidemia is high.[32] This may be related to the unique vascular arrange-

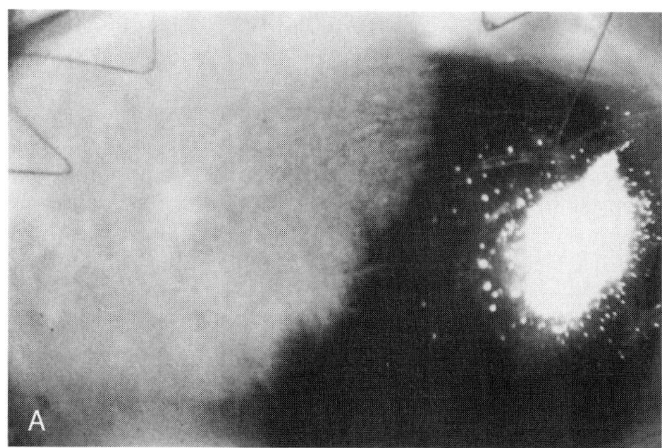

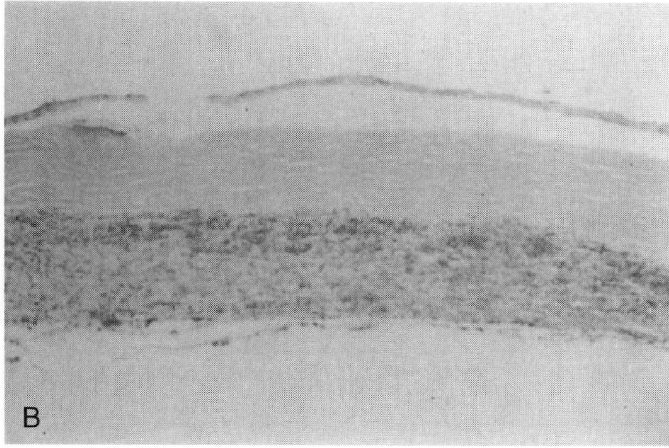

FIGURE 15–4. *A,* Clinical picture of stromal keratitis in corneal graft *(Candida parapsilosis). B,* Histologic section demonstrating deep lamellar infiltration of yeast *(C. parapsilosis)* with acute and chronic inflammatory cellular infiltrate. Methenamine silver stain, ×33.

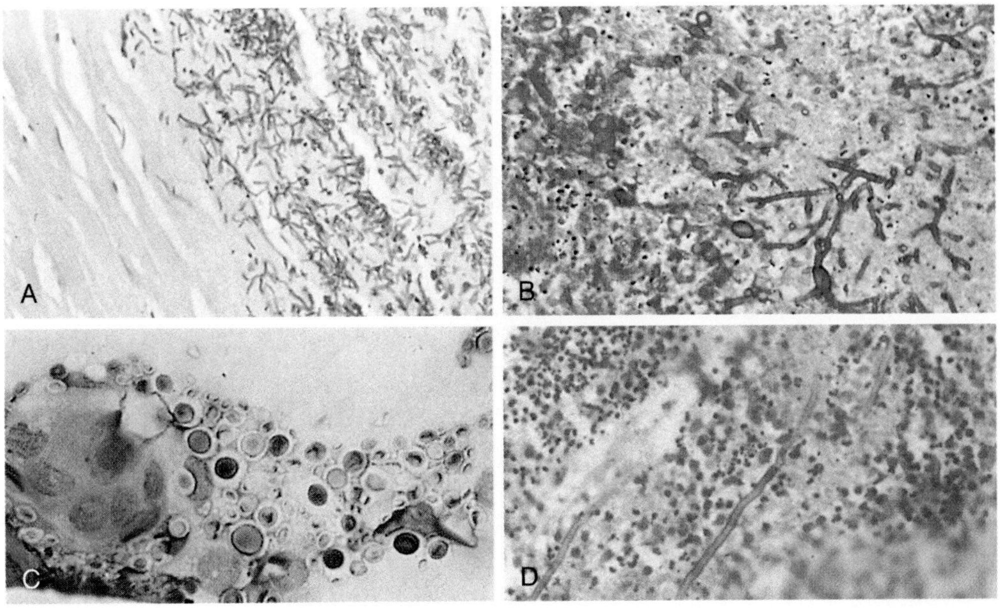

FIGURE 15–5. Histopathology of mycotic ocular infections. *A,* Stromal keratitis due to *Candida parapsilosis* with acute and chronic inflammatory infiltrate. Methenamine silver stain, ×132. *B,* Keratitis with infiltration by *Cryptococcus neoformans* showing granulomatous reaction. Papanicolaou stain, ×600. (*A* and *B,* Reprinted from Perry HD, Donnenfeld ED: Cryptococcal keratitis after keratoplasty. Am J Ophthalmol 110:320, 1990. With permission from Elsevier Science.) *C,* Endophthalmitis due to a zygomycetous fungus. H&E, ×132. *D,* Chorioretinitis due to *Aspergillus* species. PAS, ×132.

ments of the eye, but specific fungal factors for this localization also are likely. In rabbits, it is difficult to produce eye infections with *Candida* species other than *C. albicans* by the hematogenous route.[44] These findings suggest that early pseudohyphal formation plays a role in establishing an endogenous ocular infection. This propensity for *C. albicans* ocular infections has been corroborated in human infections, of which the vast majority are associated with this *Candida* species. However, other *Candida* species occasionally cause endogenous eye infection, particularly when the inoculum is as large as can occur with *C. parapsilosis* infection during hyperalimentation. Spores from *Aspergillus* species, which are found on fomites such as drug paraphernalia, can reach ocular structures and establish infection when inoculated intravenously.[45, 46]

Diagnostic Testing

The diagnosis of fungal etiology in ocular infection can be difficult. Certain clinical characteristics may be helpful to ophthalmologists, including duration and features of the ocular lesions. These are reviewed elsewhere in this book. However, it must be emphasized that there remains no substitute for the proper collection of specimens for histologic and cultural identification (Fig. 15–6). Superficial infections can be identified by scraping surface lesions, with organisms identified by culture and often corroborated by microscopy of stained smears prepared from the scrapings. Definitive diagnosis of deep keratitis or intraocular infection requires culture of an aspirate, because direct smears do not reliably correlate with culture-proved infection.[47] Biopsy of deep corneal lesions may be required to demonstrate the organism by special histologic stains.

Various techniques can be used to examine direct smears. Calcofluor white/KOH can be an extremely sensitive technique. It is rapid and easy to perform but is not a permanent preparation. Giemsa stain, periodic acid–Schiff, and methenamine silver stain are sensitive and permanent preparations. Gram's stain detects yeasts such as *Candida* and *Torulopsis* species but is not reliable for other fungi such as molds and should not be relied on for detecting mycotic infection. Gram-stained slides can be decolorized and restained with one of the preferred stains. Stains may reveal yeast or hyphae of the infecting organism, but specific identification of the species of fungus requires culture. When culture is not possible, fluorescein-conjugated lectins or fluorescent antibody conjugates may allow differentiation among species such as *Candida, Aspergillus,* and *Fusarium,* but these stains are not commercially available.[48] Certain molds, particularly *Paecilomyces lilacinus,* sometimes form spores within the infected tissue, and this can be a useful differential characteristic.[49] These spore forms can be mistaken for *Candida* species.

Because ocular infections are often caused by common saprobes in the environment and access to tissue or other diagnostic specimens is limited, special techniques for specimen evaluation must be used to diagnose fungal infections of the eye. The clinician and laboratory personnel must communicate effectively to agree on protocols for using media that do not inhibit fungal growth, inoculation techniques that help differentiate infective organisms from contaminants, and prolonged incubation times and optimal temperature to allow for the slow growth of some fungal species.

Media for culture should not include cycloheximide, which inhibits fungal growth, but inclusion of gentamicin or chloramphenicol may be needed to suppress bacterial overgrowth. A streak inoculation technique on media with specimens obtained in the examining room or operative suite should allow laboratory personnel to determine whether growth is on or off the inoculation streaks and thus differentiate possible pathogens from airborne contaminants. Specimens should be collected from external ocular surface infections or lacrimal infections with a moist applicator and inoculated by streaking directly onto culture media.[50] Scrapings from corneal ulcers in cases of keratomycosis or aspirates from the anterior chamber and the vitreous cavity in cases of endophthalmitis should be directly inoculated onto both Sabouraud's (or similar) agar media and brain-

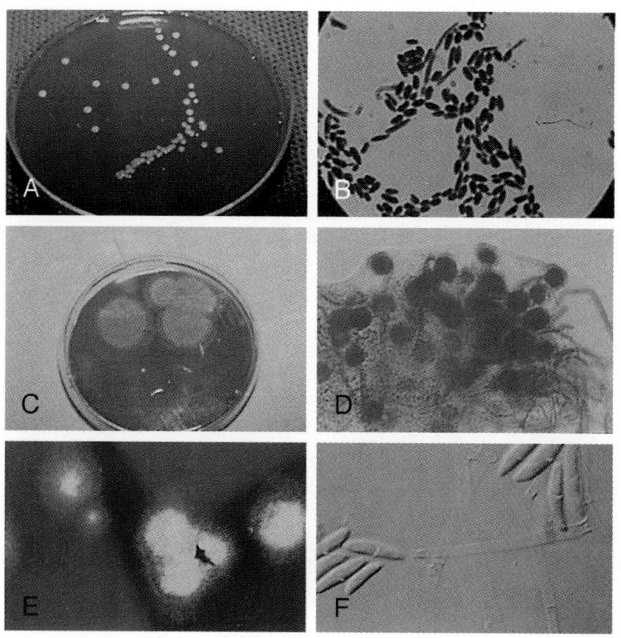

FIGURE 15–6. Colony and microscopic appearance of pathogenic fungi. *A,* Creamy, round colony growth of *Candida albicans. B,* Gram's stain of yeast cells, *Candida* species. *C,* Filamentous colony of *Aspergillus fumigatus,* with characteristic blue-green color due to sporulation. *D,* Cotton blue stain of hyphae and sporulating structures of *A. fumigatus. E,* Filamentous white colonies of *Fusarium solani. F,* Microscopic view of spores of *F. solani.*

heart infusion broth medium as well as blood agar plates.[47, 50] Incubation should be at 24°C to 30°C (30°C is preferred) and should be prolonged. Although species of some genera, such as *Candida, Fusarium, Paecilomyces, Curvularia,* and *Alternaria,* normally are visible within 3 days, as many as 25% of fungal isolates may require up to 2 weeks of incubation.[50] When *Histoplasma* or *Blastomyces* is suspected, cultures must be incubated for at least 4 weeks.

In deep infections of the cornea, superficial scraping may not yield enough organisms to identify or culture. Corneal biopsy with histopathologic examination may be required. In such situations, the use of periodic acid–Schiff, methenamine silver, or calcofluor white stains is helpful in demonstrating the organism; detection with fluorescein-conjugated lectins or fluorescent antibody conjugates also is possible.[51]

Therapeutic Concepts

Therapy of fungal infections can be difficult and prolonged. The difficulty in treatment is due to a combination of the growth characteristics of fungi, the limited availability of effective antifungal agents, and the poor tissue penetration of these agents. Until 1950, safe and reliable treatment for deep fungal infections did not exist, and treatment of superficial infections depended on empirical topical preparations. Nystatin was first introduced in the mid-1950s, and amphotericin B came to dominate treatment of deep mycoses in the 1960s. In the 1970s, 5-fluorocytosine was introduced as treatment for candidiasis and cryptococcosis, but drug resistance became a problem. Since the mid-1980s, several *N*-substituted imidazole or triazole compounds have been introduced and modified with significant improvement in activity and pharmacokinetics.

The most useful antifungal agents are of two groups: those affecting cell walls or membranes and those interrupting nucleic acid or protein synthesis. Table 15–3 summarizes some characteristics of the available and experimental antifungal agents. The polyene macrolide antibiotics interact with the sterols in the fungal cell membranes to impair their barrier function and thus produce leaking of cellular substances with subsequent metabolic disturbance and resulting cell death. The toxicity of amphotericin B, however, is related to similar interactions with sterols in host cells. Resistance of fungi to amphotericin B is rare and probably occurs by alterations in the sterol composition of the cell membrane.[52] The azole antifungals share an imidazole or

TABLE 15–3. **Antifungal Agents**

Class	Agent	Mechanism of Action
Polyene	Amphotericin B Nystatin Natamycin	Interacts with sterol (ergosterol) in cell membrane, resulting in leakage of vital constituents
Pradimincins/ benanomycins	BMS 181184	Binds to cell-membrane mannoproteins
Pyrimidine	5-Fluorocytosine	Inhibits RNA synthesis by intracellular conversion to 5-fluorouracil
Imidazole/triazoles	Miconazole Econazole Clotrimazole Ketoconazole Itraconazole Fluconazole Voriconazole SCH56592	Inhibits demethylation of lanosterol, preventing formation of ergosterol and damaging cell membrane
Grisan	Griseofulvin	Binds to tubulin, preventing microtubule assembly
Glutaramide	Cycloheximide	Inhibits protein synthesis at ribosomal level
Allylamine/ thiocarbanates	Terbinafine/ tolnaftate	Inhibits squalene epoxidase for sterol metabolism of cell membrane
Morpholines	Amorolfine	Inhibits sterol synthesis
Echinocandin/ pneumocandins	LY303,366 L 743,872	Inhibits cell wall synthesis of 1-3 β-glucan
Peptidyl nucleoside	Nikkomycin Z	Inhibits cell wall synthesis of chitin

triazole ring with *N*-carbon substitution that allows interaction with primary target sites within the fungal cell. At low concentrations, these compounds inhibit cytochrome P-450 enzymes, which leads to the accumulation of 14-γ-methylsterols and reduced biosynthesis of ergosterol. At higher concentrations, some azoles can cause direct cell membrane damage. The fluorinated pyrimidine, 5-fluorocytosine, is deaminated once inside the susceptible yeast cell: A cytosine deaminase converts it to 5-fluorouracil for incorporation into fungal RNA and thus disruption of protein synthesis.

In vitro testing of antifungal susceptibility and its correlation with in vivo response historically have been difficult because minimum inhibitory concentrations vary greatly under different test conditions.[53] The broth or agar dilution methods of testing can be affected by inoculum size, medium composition and pH, incubation temperature, duration of incubation, incubation atmosphere composition, and method of end-point determination.[54–56] Ongoing efforts to standardize in vitro antifungal testing involve comparing direct antifungal activity, pharmacokinetics of the agents, and prior clinical experience on treatment of certain fungal infections. Susceptibility testing of yeasts has shown progress,[57, 58] but a standardized protocol is not yet available for molds. Despite the concerns about clinical validation, our opinion is that yeasts and possibly molds from serious oculomycoses should be evaluated comparatively by in vitro susceptibility testing with available antifungal agents. This can allow detection of possibly drug-resistant fungi and can provide the grounds for clinical judgment of the best antifungal regimen.

Response to therapy depends on several factors. Host factors include the integrity of the immune defense mechanisms (especially cell-mediated functions) and the location and extent of infection. Pharmacokinetic factors include penetration and tissue distribution of the antifungal agent as well as predilection for tissue binding. Antimicrobial factors include the observable effect on the fungal organisms and the response in growth characteristics of the fungus in the presence of the antifungal agent. A further clinical problem in treatment is that when the organism encounters adverse conditions (elevated temperature, anaerobiosis, chemotherapeutic agents), it may revert to a dormant or slow growth state that is more difficult to eradicate with cell wall– or cell membrane–active antifungals and thus requires longer treatments. Finally, clinical experience—both that of the attending clinician and that gleaned from references in the literature—can be a helpful guiding factor. The following discussion summarizes specific therapeutic concepts in management of oculomycoses.

The single most important factor in the success of treatment for oculomycosis is early diagnosis and treatment. Fungal infections can have an indolent course, and the longer these infections remain untreated, the more difficult they are to eradicate. For this discussion, infections are divided into three categories: (1) keratomycosis, (2) endophthalmitis, and (3) orbital infection.

KERATOMYCOSIS

Fungal keratitis is usually caused by environmentally widespread molds such as *Aspergillus* species, *Fusarium* species, *Paecilomyces* species, and *Curvularia* species, but other fungi, such as *Candida* species and *C. neoformans,* also can cause keratitis in immunocompromised hosts. Identification of the fungus and comparative in vitro susceptibility testing to available antifungal drugs is usually important. For fungal corneal ulcers, pimaricin remains the most reliable topical antifungal agent in a 5% suspension or as a 1% ointment for treatment of superficial ocular injuries or prophylaxis with high-risk injuries for oculomycosis. It also is not as irritating to the eye as the other polyenes, such as amphotericin B. Unfortunately, pimaricin therapy has two drawbacks. First, although it has broad-spectrum antifungal activity across many species, isolates may be relatively resistant to its antifungal activity, with only half the strains studied being inhibited by 3 μg/mL or less.[59] Second, it has limited ability to penetrate the cornea. Nystatin is less active in vitro than the other polyenes but is reasonably well tolerated in a 3% ointment. Amphotericin B can be irritating to the eye, and in high concentrations (5%) can lead to punctate epithelial erosions. Even so, it is frequently used in a topical solution for serious infections. Topical antifungals are likely to be most successful early in the infection, before it has extended into deeper layers of the cornea. It is emphasized that proper cultures for isolation and identification of the fungus should be taken before beginning therapy.

The second approach to therapy of keratomycosis is the use of systemic antifungal agents. For superficial fungal ulcers, this second line of therapy may not be necessary, but deeper corneal infections may require it. The azole compounds have become attractive candidates for systemic administration. They are safe and relatively broad-spectrum. The ocular pharmacology of these azole compounds (miconazole, ketoconazole, fluconazole, and itraconazole) has been examined in both humans and animals.[60, 61] The rank of penetration into eye structures such as vitreous body and aqueous humor, from highest to lowest, is fluconazole, ketoconazole, miconazole, and itraconazole. The azoles' penetration into the eye appears to be improved by inflammation, as is the case with other drugs. Azoles have been shown to penetrate into corneal tissue of rabbits and can be found in corneal tissue even when the eyes are not inflamed.[61, 62] Therefore, it is reasonable to anticipate that future reports will show the success of these agents in the management of fungal keratitis and scleritis. Flucytosine is another agent with excellent penetration into eye structures and has shown some success in *Candida* keratitis. Its major limitation is its narrow spectrum of activity. It inhibits only a portion of *Candida* species, *C. neoformans,* and some dematiaceous molds. For corneal infections, systemic amphotericin B therapy has not been widely used. It has been used, however, as a topical preparation and in fungal scleral infections as a subconjunctival injection. The success of subconjunctival injection of amphotericin B remains unclear, and it can be extremely painful and sometimes produces tissue necrosis and nodules.[63, 64] Its limited eye penetration and toxicity have reduced enthusiasm for its use in infection at this site except for the most difficult cases.

In addition to antifungal therapy, some eyes require excisional keratoplasty, particularly in cases of impending perforation. Even in these cases, however, aggressive antifungal chemotherapy before and after surgery may improve the final level of visual acuity.

There is no strong evidence that topical or systemic steroids help in the management of fungal eye infections. In fact, they are often the major risk factor for these infections and their progression. Prevention of inflammation and resultant tissue destruction and the preservation of visual acuity are vital objectives, but there are no guidelines to balance the positive effects of steroids on inflammation versus the negative effects of stimulating fungal growth. Therefore, adjunctive corticosteroid therapy should not routinely be used in fungal eye infections.

ENDOPHTHALMITIS

There are two types of fungal endophthalmitis. Exogenous endophthalmitis is associated with trauma or surgery in which the organism is introduced directly into the ocular structures. Endogenous endophthalmitis is generally produced by *Candida* species or *Aspergillus* species from a chorioretinal lesion, and extension into the vitreous body accompanies systemic dissemination of the fungus. It may also occur with the endemic mycoses, such as blastomycosis, after the initial pulmonary infection. The need to manage these infections has significantly intensified over the last decade because of expanding immunocompromised populations, complex surgical procedures, and increasing use of antibiotics and intravenous catheters. The most important therapeutic principle in endophthalmitis is early diagnosis and correct identification of the fungus.[65] For instance, in patients with candidemia who are not neutropenic, a prospective evaluation of the eye may identify an early ocular infection in a third of the patients.[32] Early treatment is more likely to yield a better visual outcome. Animal models of endogenous *C. albicans* endophthalmitis suggest that early treatment with either azoles or amphotericin B is more successful than delaying treatment for a week despite similar numbers of yeasts at each time period.[61, 66] Correct identification of the organism by blood or ocular fluid cultures and determination of in vitro susceptibility to various antifungal agents helps identify the most promising antifungal agents for successful treatment.

Candida endophthalmitis remains the most common invasive ocular pathogen. Because there are no comparative studies on therapeutic regimens, it remains reasonable to select the antifungal agent with the most successful experience, amphotericin B. Systemic amphotericin B in doses of 0.5 to 1 mg/kg/day has been used to control *Candida* endophthalmitis. Amphotericin B has very low levels as measured in the vitreous body and aqueous humor, but these measurements do not account for drug that is bound to tissue.[67, 68] Because the penetration of amphotericin B is poor, however, intraocular therapy has been used. In a primate model, up to 3 mg of intravitreal amphotericin B was tolerated without permanent retinal toxicity, and a human took 50 mg of amphotericin B over a 6-month period without serious retinal toxicity.[69] A slowly given 1- to 5-mg intravitreal injection is probably not toxic to the retina. Now that liposomal amphotericin B is available, it may be possible to deliver even more drug to this site of infection.[70, 71] The value of intravitreal amphotericin B is not proved and toxicity questions do remain, but it may be of particular benefit when the vitreous body is significantly involved, as in cases requiring vitrectomy and in *Aspergillus* infections extending into the vitreous body.[72]

Flucytosine remains a possible agent for ocular *Candida* infections with its high penetration into the vitreous body and aqueous humor.[73] There has been little experience with its use alone, and concern over primary resistance in a portion of *Candida* isolates remains.[74] An attractive regimen for *Candida* endophthalmitis would be combination chemotherapy with amphotericin B and flucytosine.[75] This combination regimen has been successful in prospective studies in the treatment of cryptococcal meningitis, and its in vitro synergy against *Candida* by virtue of different mechanisms of antifungal action theoretically could eradicate the fungus more rapidly and improve visual outcome. However, no prospective studies have proved this hypothesis.

With the advent of the azole compounds, clinicians have another treatment avenue. The early azoles (ketoconazole and miconazole) had some successes and failures. The newer azole (fluconazole) has excellent ocular pharmacokinetics and may be helpful in managing ocular fungal infections. The only comparative data regarding the efficacy of these compounds are from animals.[61, 66] These models suggest that amphotericin B may still be more potent in eradicating *Candida* from the eye than the azole compounds are. There have also been case reports of *Candida* and *Coccidioides* infections in which miconazole was not effective but patients improved after receiving amphotericin B therapy.[76] Such results, however, should not necessarily dissuade clinicians from carefully using these newer azole compounds in fungal endophthalmitis, because more clinical experience with these compounds in ocular infections is needed. For example, one report on ocular candidiasis in drug addicts cited an excellent response to ketoconazole treatment.[34] Although amphotericin B and flucytosine remain the most attractive combination regimen for *Candida*, a polyene-azole combination might be useful in certain eye infections, particularly if both antifungals have in vitro activity against the fungus. The concern about polyene-azole antagonism in vitro has not been proved in vivo. Another combination regimen that may be considered is fluconazole plus flucytosine. These two oral agents reach high drug levels within ocular tissue. Finally, the regimen of amphotericin B plus rifampin has been used successfully both in animals and in humans.[77, 78] The point of this discussion is that combination antifungal chemotherapy can be considered rational treatment if proper identification and comparative in vitro susceptibility testing on the fungus are performed.

Therapeutic vitrectomy may be helpful in certain patients and likely clears the eye of inflammatory debris.[79, 80] For this treatment, our current understanding makes it reasonable to select patients with extensive vitreous involvement and likely visual impairment from scarring, with progressive inflammation despite antifungal agents, and patients with extensive vitreal involvement but an unclear underlying pathogen.

ORBITAL INFECTION

Fungal infections in the orbit that do not initially invade ocular structures are generally caused by a member of Zygomycetes such as *Rhizopus* species or by *Aspergillus* species.[8, 13, 81] The rhinocerebral form of zygomycosis is a characteristic acute progression of infection into the orbit, causing orbital swelling and eventual paralysis of orbital structures.[13, 82] Generally caused by *Rhizopus arrhizus*, this infection primarily affects diabetics, particularly if acidosis has occurred; cancer patients; or patients receiving chelation or steroid therapy. The infection starts in the nasal or sinus cavities and invades the regional arterial vessels by direct extension, causing thrombosis and leading to ischemic necrosis. Extension through the orbital apex into the brain occurs as infection progresses. A black eschar in the nasal area or drainage of "black pus" from the eye suggests this diagnosis.[13] Identifying the patient at risk and performing an early examination of the nasal and sinus areas for signs of disease often leads to diagnosis before the orbit becomes involved. *Aspergillus* infections of the sinus have eroded through bone or invaded local vessels and entered the orbit, producing proptosis. Therefore, evaluation of recent proptosis of ocular structures should include a careful examination of the sinuses.

Early débridement of infarcted tissue is essential to a successful outcome and may obviate the need for subsequent orbital exenteration. The goal of treatment remains the prevention of extension into the brain. The immediate control of the underlying disease, such as acidosis, is also important; finally, amphotericin B at 0.7 to 1 mg/kg/day or a lipid formulation of amphotericin B is usually given. The length of therapy should be tailored to the patient's response and extent of infection.

Conclusion

Fungal infection in the eye is most often of exogenous origin in an immunocompetent host whose local tissue defenses have been damaged. The growth characteristics of the fungus can result in superficial infection or invasion into deep tissues, where it may alter its growth pattern in response to the local milieu. Effective therapy of such infections must be selected from the small number of antifungal agents and requires recognition of the limitations of susceptibility testing, the importance of tissue penetration and absorption, and the need for protracted treatment. Because of these limitations, success of therapy primarily depends on early diagnosis of the fungal infection and correct identification of the particular fungus.

REFERENCES

1. Leber T: Keratomycosis aspergillina als Ursache von hypopyonkeratitis. Graefes Arch Clin Exp Ophthalmol 25:285, 1979.
2. Chick EW, Conant NF: Mycotic ulcerative keratitis: A review of 148 cases from the literature. Invest Ophthalmol Vis Sci 1:419, 1962.
3. Blake J: Ocular hazards in agriculture. Ophthalmologica 158:125, 1969.
4. Devoe AG, Silva-Hutner M: Fungal infections of the eye. *In* Locatcher-Khorazo D, Seegal BC (eds): Microbiology of the Eye. St. Louis, CV Mosby, 1972, pp 208–239.
5. Jones DB: Fungal keratitis. *In* Duane T (ed): Clinical Ophthalmology. Philadelphia, Harper & Row, 1986.
6. Schell WA: Oculomycosis caused by dematiaceous fungi. Proceedings of the VIth International Conference on the Mycoses. Pan American Health Organization 879:105–109, 1986.
7. Scholz R, Green WR, Kutys R, et al: *Histoplasma capsulatum* in the eye. Ophthalmology 91:1100–1104, 1984.
8. Agarwal LP, Malik SRK, Mohan M, Mahopatra LN: Orbital aspergillosis. Br J Ophthalmol 46:559–562, 1962.
9. Okun E, Butler WT: Ophthalmologic complications of cryptococcal meningitis. Arch Ophthalmol 71:52–57, 1964.
10. Font RL, Spaulding AB, Green WR: Endogenous mycotic panophthalmitis caused by *Blastomyces dermatitidis*. Arch Ophthalmol 77:217, 1967.
11. Blumenkranz MS, Stevens DS: Endogenous coccidioidal endophthalmitis. Ophthalmology 87:974, 1980.
12. Cassady JR, Foerster HC: *Sporotrichum schenckii* endophthalmitis. Arch Ophthalmol 85:71, 1977.
13. Rinaldi MG: Zygomycosis. Infect Dis Clin North Am 3:19–41, 1989.
14. Edwards JE, Foos RY, Montgomerie JZ: Ocular manifestation of *Candida septicemia*. Review of 76 cases of hematogenous *Candida* endophthalmitis. Medicine 53:47–75, 1974.
15. Griffin JR, Pettit TH, Fishman LS: Blood-borne *Candida* endophthalmitis: A clinical and pathologic study of 21 cases. Arch Ophthalmol 89:450–456, 1973.
16. Ando N, Takator K: Fungal flora of the conjunctival sac. Am J Ophthalmol 94:67, 1982.
17. Wilson LA, Ahearn DG, Jones DB, Sexton RR: Fungi from the outer eye. Am J Ophthalmol 67:52, 1969.
18. Mitsui Y, Hanabusa J: Corneal infections after cortisone therapy. Br J Opthalmol 39:244, 1955.
19. Nema HV, Ahuja OP, Bal A, Mohapatra LN: Mycotic flora of the conjunctiva. Am J Ophthalmol 62:968, 1966.
20. Kobayashi GS: Fungi. *In* Davis BD (ed): Microbiology. Philadelphia, JB Lippincott, 1990.
21. Beyt BE, Waltman SR: Cryptococcal endophthalmitis after corneal transplantation. N Engl J Med 298:825–826, 1978.
22. Gordon MA, Norton SW: Corneal transplant infection by *Paecilomyces lilacinus*. Sabouraudia 23:295–301, 1985.
23. Perry HD, Donnenfeld ED: Cryptococcal keratitis after keratoplasty. Am J Ophthalmol 110:320–321, 1990.
24. McCray E, Rampell N, Solomon SL, et al: Outbreak of *Candida parapsilosis* endophthalmitis after cataract extraction and intraocular lens implantation. J Clin Microbiol 24:625–628, 1986.
25. Miller GR, Rebell G, Magoon RC, et al: Intravitreal antimycotic therapy and the cure of mycotic endophthalmitis caused by a *Paecilomyces lilacinus* contaminated pseudophakos. Ophthalmic Surg 9:54–63, 1978.
26. O'Day DM: Fungal endophthalmitis caused by *Paecilomyces lilacinus* after intraocular lens implantation. Am J Ophthalmol 83:130–131, 1977.
27. Pettit TH, Olson RJ, Foss RY, Martin WJ: Fungal endophthalmitis following intraocular lens implantation: A surgical epidemic. Arch Ophthalmol 98:1025–1039, 1980.
28. Wilson LA, Ahearn DG: Association of fungi with extended-wear soft contact lenses. Am J Ophthalmol 101:434–436, 1986.
29. Henderson DK, Hockey LJ, Vukakic LJ, Edwards JE Jr: Effect of immunosuppression on the development of experimental hematogenous *Candida* endophthalmitis. Infect Immun 27:628–631, 1980.
30. Freeman JB, Davis PL, Maclean LD: *Candida* endophthalmitis associated with intravenous hyperalimentation. Arch Surg 108:237–240, 1974.
31. Cantrill HS, Rodman WP, Ramsey RC, Knobloch WH: Post-partum *Candida* endophthalmitis. JAMA 243:1163–1165, 1980.
32. Brooks RG: Prospective study of *Candida* endophthalmitis in hospitalized patients with candidemia. Arch Intern Med 149:2226–2228, 1989.
33. Edwards JE Jr: Candida endophthalmitis. *In* Bodey GP, Fainstein V (eds): Candidiasis. New York, Raven Press, 1985, pp 211–227.
34. Dupont B, Drouhet E: Cutaneous, ocular and osteoarticular candidiasis in heroin addicts. New clinical and therapeutic aspects in 38 patients. J Infect Dis 152:577–591, 1985.
35. Blachie JD, Danta G, Sorrell T, Collignon P: Ophthalmological complications of cryptococcal meningitis. Clin Exp Neurol 21:263–270, 1985.
36. Crump JR, Elner SG, Elner VM, Kauffman CA: Cryptococcal endophthalmitis: Case report and review. Clin Infect Dis 14:1069–1073, 1992.
37. Doft BH, Curtin VT: Combined ocular infection with cytomegalovirus and cryptococcosis. Arch Ophthalmol 100:1800–1803, 1982.
38. Denning DW, Armstrong RW, Fishman M, Stevens DA: Endophthalmitis in a patient with disseminated cryptococcosis and AIDS who was treated with itraconazole. Rev Infect Dis 13:1126–1130, 1991.
39. Johnston SR, Corbett EL, Foster O, et al: Raised intracranial pressure and visual complications in AIDs patients with cryptococcal meningitis. J Infect 24:185–189, 1992.
40. Rex JH, Larsen RA, Dismukes WE, et al: Catastrophic visceral loss due to *Cryptococcus neoformans* meningitis. Medicine 72:207–224, 1993.
41. Macular Photocoagulation Study Group: Argon laser photocoagulation for ocular histoplasmosis. Results of a randomized trial. Arch Ophthalmol 101:1347, 1983.

42. Kwon-Chung KJ, Lehman D, Good C, Magee PT: Genetic evidence for role of extracellular proteinase in virulence of *Candida albicans*. Infect Immun 49:571–575, 1985.
43. Kathary MH, Chase T Jr, MacMillan JD: Correlation of elastase production by some strains of *Aspergillus fumigatus* with ability to cause pulmonary invasive *Aspergillus* in mice. Infect Immun 43:320–325, 1984.
44. Edwards JE, Montgomerie JZ, Ishida K, et al: Experimental hematogenous endophthalmitis due to *Candida*: Species variation in ocular pathogenicity. J Infect Dis 135:294–297, 1977.
45. Lance SE, Friberg TR, Kowalski RP: *Aspergillus flavus* endophthalmitis and retinitis in an intravenous drug abuser. A therapeutic success. Ophthalmology 95:947–949, 1988.
46. Roney P, Barr CC, Chun CH, Raff MJ: Endogenous aspergillus endophthalmitis. Rev Infect Dis 8:955–958, 1986.
47. O'Day DM, Akrabawi PL, Head WS, Ratner HB: Laboratory isolation techniques in human and experimental fungal infections. Am J Ophthalmol 87:688, 1979.
48. Robin JB, Arffa RC, Avni I, Rao NA: Rapid visualization of three common fungi using fluorescein-conjugated lectins. Invest Ophthalmol Vis Sci 27:500, 1986.
49. Liu K, Howell DN, Perfect JR, Schell WA: Morphologic criteria for the preliminary identification of *Fusarium, Paecilomyces*, and *Acremonium* species by histopathology. Am J Clin Pathol 109:45–54, 1998.
50. Wilson LA, Sexton RR: Laboratory diagnosis in fungal keratitis. Am J Ophthalmol 66:646, 1969.
51. Robin JB, Chan R, Rao NA, et al: Fluorescein-conjugated lectin visualization of fungi and acanthamoeba in infectious keratitis. Ophthalmology 96:1198, 1989.
52. Pierce AM, Pierce HD, Unrau AM, Oehlschlager AC: Lipid composition and polyene antibiotic resistance of *Candida albicans* mutants. Biochem Cell Biol 56:135, 1978.
53. Warnock DW: Antifungal drug susceptibility testing. *In* McGinnis MR, Borgers M (eds): Current Topics in Medical Mycology. New York, Springer Verlag, 1989, p 403.
54. Ericksson HM, Sherris JC: Antibiotic sensitivity testing: Report of an international collaborative study. APMIS 217:1, 1971.
55. Drutz DJ: *In vitro* antifungal susceptibility testing and measurement of levels in body fluids. Rev Infect Dis 9:392–397, 1987.
56. Pfaller MA, Rinaldi MG, Galgiani JN, et al: Collaborative investigation of variables in susceptibility testing of yeasts. Antimicrob Agents Chemother 34:1648–1654, 1990.
57. National Committee for Laboratory Standards: Reference methods for broth dilution antifungal susceptibility testing for yeasts: Approved standard 17-9. Villanova, PA, National Committee for Clinical Laboratory Standards, 1997, pp 1–29.
58. Rex JH, Pfaller MA, Galgiani JN, et al: Development of interpretive breakpoints for antifungal susceptibility testing: Conceptual framework and analysis of in vitro–in vivo correlation data for fluconazole, itraconazole, and *Candida* infections. Clin Infect Dis 24:235–247, 1997.
59. Jones BR: Principles in the management of oculomycosis. Am J Ophthalmol 79:719–751, 1975.
60. Foster CS, Stefanygzyn M: Intraocular penetration of miconazole in rabbits. Arch Ophthalmol 97:1703–1706, 1979.
61. Savani DV, Perfect JR, Cobo LM, Durack DT: Penetration of new azole compounds into the eye and efficacy in experimental *Candida* endophthalmitis. Antimicrob Agents Chemother 31:6–10, 1987.
62. Ishibashi Y, Matsumoto T: Oral ketoconazole therapy for experimental *Candida albicans* keratitis in rabbits. Sabouraudia 22:323–330, 1984.
63. Foster CS: Ocular toxicity of topical antifungal agents. Arch Ophthalmol 99:1081–1084, 1980.
64. Bell RN, Ritchey JP: Subconjunctival nodules after amphotericin B injection. Arch Ophthalmol 90:402–404, 1973.
65. Jones DB: Therapy of postsurgical fungal endophthalmitis. Ophthalmology 85:357–373, 1978.
66. Jones DB, Green MT, Osato MS, et al: Endogenous *Candida albicans* endophthalmitis in the rabbit. Arch Ophthalmol 99:2182–2187, 1981.
67. Green WR, Bennett JE, Goos RD: Ocular penetration of amphotericin B: A report of laboratory studies and a case report of postsurgical cephalosporium endophthalmitis. Arch Ophthalmol 73:769–775, 1965.
68. Fisher JF: Penetration of amphotericin B into the human eye. J Infect Dis 147:164–165, 1983.
69. Denning DW, Stevens DA: Antifungal and surgical treatment of invasive aspergillosis: Review of 2,121 published cases. Rev Infect Dis 12:1147–1201, 1990.
70. Perraut LE Jr, Perraut LE, Bleiman B, Lyons J: Successful treatment of *Candida albicans* endophthalmitis with intravitreal amphotericin B. Arch Ophthalmol 99:1565–1567, 1981.
71. Stern GA, Fetkenhour CL, O'Grady RB: Intravitreal amphotericin B treatment of *Candida* endophthalmitis. Arch Ophthalmol 95:89–93, 1977.
72. Axelrod AJ, Peyman GA, Apple DJ: Toxicity of intravitreal injection of amphotericin B. Am J Ophthalmol 76:578–583, 1973.
73. Walsh JA, Halft MH, Miller MH, et al: Ocular penetration of 5-flucytosine. Invest Ophthalmol Vis Sci 17:691–694, 1978.
74. Robertson DM, Riley FC, Hermans PE: Endogenous *Candida oculomycosis*: Report of two patients treated with flucytosine. Arch Ophthalmol 91:33, 1974.
75. Medoff G, Comfort M, Kobayashi GS: Synergistic action of amphotericin B and 5-flurocytosine against yeast-like organisms (35943). Proc Soc Exp Biol Med 138:571–574, 1971.
76. Blumenkranz MS, Stevens DA: Therapy of endogenous fungal endophthalmitis: Miconazole or amphotericin B for coccidioidal and candidal infection. Arch Ophthalmol 98:1216–1220, 1980.
77. Stern GA, Okumoto M, Smolin G: Combined amphotericin B and rifampin treatment of experimental *C. albicans* keratitis. Arch Ophthalmol 79:721–722, 1979.
78. Lou P, Kazdan J, Bannatyne RM, Cheung R: Successful treatment of *Candida* endophthalmitis with a synergistic combination of amphotericin B and rifampin. Am J Ophthalmol 83:12–15, 1977.
79. Snip RC, Michels RG: Pars plana vitrectomy in the management of endogenous *Candida* endophthalmitis. Am J Ophthalmol 82:699, 1976.
80. Huang K, Peyman GA, McGetrick J: Vitrectomy in experimental endophthalmitis. Part I. Fungal infection. Ophthalmic Surg 10:84, 1979.
81. Sacho H, Stead KJ, Klugman KP, Lawrence A: Infection of the human orbit by *Aspergillus stromatoides*. Mycopathologia 97:97–99, 1987.
82. Gass JDM: Ocular manifestations of acute mucormycosis. Arch Ophthalmol 65:226, 1961.
83. Rinaldi MG, Seidenfeld SM, Fothergill AW, McGough DA: *Pythium insidiosum* as an agent of a devastating orbital/facial mycosis: Mycological and management aspects. [Abstract] ASM Abstract F-111989.
84. Imwidthaya P: Mycotic keratitis in Thailand. J Med Vet Mycol 33:81, 1995.
85. Arora R, Venkateswarlu K, Mahajan VM: Keratomycosis—A retrospective histopathologic and microbiologic analysis. Ann Ophthalmol 20:306–315, 1988.
86. Specht CS, Mitchell KT, Bauman AE, Gupta M: Ocular histoplasmosis with retinitis in a patient with acquired immune deficiency syndrome. Ophthalmology 98:1356, 1991.
87. Sukumarank: Ulcerative keratomycosis: Case reports on three different species of fungi. Med J Malasia 46:388, 1991.
88. Liesegang TJ, Forster RK: Spectrum of microbial keratitis in south Florida. Am J Ophthalmol 90:38–47, 1980.
89. Shadomy HJ, Dixon DM: A new Papulaspora species from the infected eye of a horse: *Papulaspora equi*. Mycopathologia 106:35–39, 1989.
90. Resnikoff S, Nolard N, Tsouria-Belaid A, et al: Les ulceres corneens d'origine fongique au Mali. J Mycol Med 3:235, 1993.
91. Poira VC, Bharad VR, Dongre DS, Kulkarni MV: Study of mycotic keratitis. Indian J Ophthalmol 33:229–231, 1985.
92. Pflugfelder SC, Flynn HW, Zwickey TA, et al: Exogenous fungal endophthalmitis. Ophthalmology 95:19–30, 1988.
93. Margo CE, Fitzgerald CR: Postoperative endophthalmitis caused by *Wangiella dermatitidis*. Am J Ophthalmol 110:322, 1990.
94. Sachs SW, Baum J, Mies C: *Beaveria bassiana* keratitis. Br J Opthalmol 69:548–550, 1985.
95. McDonnell PJ, Werblin TP, Sigler L, Green WR: Mycotic keratitis due to *Beauveria alba*. Cornea 3:213–216, 1985.
96. Thomas PA, Kuviakose T: Keratitis due to *Arthrobotrys oligospora* Fres. 1850. J Med Vet Mycol 28:47–50, 1990.
97. Mathews MS, Kuriakose T: Keratitis due to *Cephallophora irregularis thaxter*. J Med Vet Mycol 33:359, 1995.
98. Guarro J, de Vroey C, Gene J: Concerning the implication of *Arthrobotrys oligospora* in a case of keratitis. J Med Vet Mycol 29:349, 1991.
99. Ormerod LD: Causation and management of microbial keratitis in subtropical Africa. Ophthalmology 94:1662–1668, 1987.
100. Wright ED, Clayton YM, Howlader A, et al: Keratomycosis caused by *Dichotomophthoropsis nymphaearum*. Mycoses 33:477, 1990.

101. Shukla PK, Jain M, Lal B, et al: Mycotic keratitis caused by *Phacotrichoconis crotalariae*. Mycoses 32:230–232, 1986.
102. Cordeiro MF, Graham EM: Retinal infections. Br J Hosp Med 51:402, 1994.
103. Neumayr TG: Bilateral rhinosporidiosis of the conjunctiva. Arch Ophthalmol 71:379–381, 1964.
104. Dago-Akribi A, Ette M, Miomande MI, et al: Aspects anatomocliniques de la rhinosporidiose en Cote d'Ivoire. A propos de 9 cas observes en 18 ans. Ann Pathol 13:97, 1993.
105. Al-Rajihi AA, Awad AH, Al-Hedaithy SSA, et al: *Scytalidium dimidiatum* fungal endophthalmitis. Br J Ophthalmol 77:388, 1993.
106. Kirkness CM, Seal DV, Clayton YM, Punithalingam E: *Sphaeropsis subglobosa* keratomycosis—First reported case. Cornea 10:85, 1991.

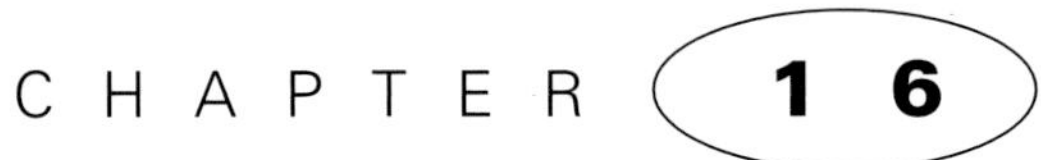

Ocular Virology

Thomas J. Liesegang

General Properties of Viruses

Viruses are obligate intracellular pathogens. Unlike bacteria and protozoa, viruses contain only RNA or DNA central cores and lack the metabolic machinery necessary for replication. Viruses exploit the host cell's metabolic machinery for nucleic acid transcription, translation, and the production of infectious progeny virions. Viruses can infect bacteria, plants, animals, and, in certain instances, other viruses. Many viruses cause clinically evident diseases that are debilitating or chronic, but usually not life-threatening to the host. In rare instances, viruses can cause encephalitis and other life-threatening illnesses. This viral adaptivity has ensured not only the survival of the virus but also transmission to noninfected hosts and retention within the hosts as a latent infection. This chapter focuses on human and animal viruses, specifically those that are responsible for direct ocular infections or those that induce ocular pathology as a manifestation of systemic viral infection (Fig. 16–1).[1–6]

STRUCTURE AND CLASSIFICATION

Viruses are the smallest and simplest structures of any known infectious agents (18 to 400 nm). Structurally, virions have a protein coat (the capsid) that surrounds the nucleic acid core. This viral core can be single- or double-stranded RNA or DNA. The nucleocapsid, the term for the viral core and capsid unit, may be surrounded by a lipoprotein membrane, the envelope. The viral envelope is composed of both host cell membrane and virus-specific protein subunits. The mixed host cell–virus composition of the envelope confers initial immunologic immunity to the virus and is of major importance during initial infectious events.[2] Most viruses have a defined symmetry of the protein coat subunits. The parsimonious use of structural proteins in a repetitive motif minimizes the amount of the viral genome that must be committed to encode the capsid components. The three types of symmetry of animal viruses include icosahedral, helical, and complex symmetry. The helically symmetric viruses have repeating subunits of capsids that are bound periodically along the helical spiral formed by the viral nucleic acid. The icosahedral symmetry has a nearly spherical shape, with several axes of rotational symmetry.

Many morphologic and functional properties of viruses are used for classification. The first classification of viruses as a group distinct from other microorganisms was based almost exclusively on their ability to pass through filters of a

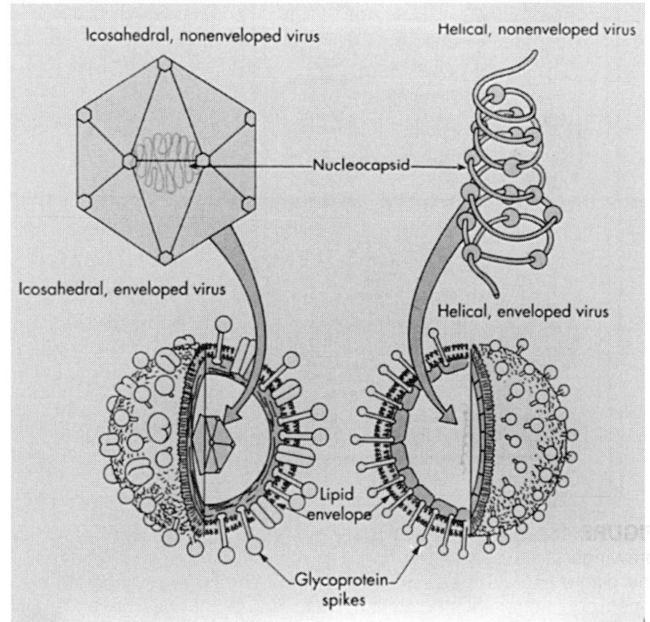

FIGURE 16–1. Schematic diagram of viral particles. Enveloped and nonenveloped virions have a helical or icosahedral shape. (Modified from Murray PR, Drew WL, Kobayashi GS, et al: Medical Microbiology. *In* Weissfeld AS, Sahm DF, Forbes BA: Bailey and Scott's Diagnostic Microbiology, 10th ed. St. Louis, CV Mosby, 1998.)

small pore size. Other classifications were based on the diseases they caused, including the clinical symptoms associated with the overt or recurrent infection. The three criteria now employed to classify viruses are: (1) the type of nucleic acid contained in the core and whether the core contains single- or double-stranded DNA or RNA, (2) the type of capsid symmetry (icosahedral, helical, or complex), including the configuration of the capsomers, and (3) the presence or absence of a viral envelope (Fig. 16–2).[2] Since 1966, the classification and nomenclature of viruses at the higher taxonomic levels (families and genera) have been systematically organized by the International Committee on Taxonomy of Viruses.[1, 7] The highest taxon used is the order, named with the suffix *-virales.* Families are named with the suffix *-viridae,* subfamilies with the suffix *-virinae,* and genera with the suffix *-virus.* Currently, viral species are also designated by vernacular terms—for example, measles virus. More recent attempts have been to reorganize classification along lines of genetic relatedness. Electron micrographs of negatively stained viral particles (virions) and thin-section electron micrographs of virus-infected tissues and cultured cells allow rapid identification of such essential characteristics of virions as their size, shape, symmetry, surface features, presence or absence of an envelope, and information about site and method of assembly (Table 16–1). The use of high-resolution x-ray crystallographic techniques has provided views of viral structure at the atomic level. Viruses are important pathogens not only for patients; health care workers are at occupational risk for a vast array of viral infections that cause significant illness and transmission to other patients. These include especially adenovirus, but also varicella, measles, rubella, and mumps, which may be treated by the ophthalmologist.[8]

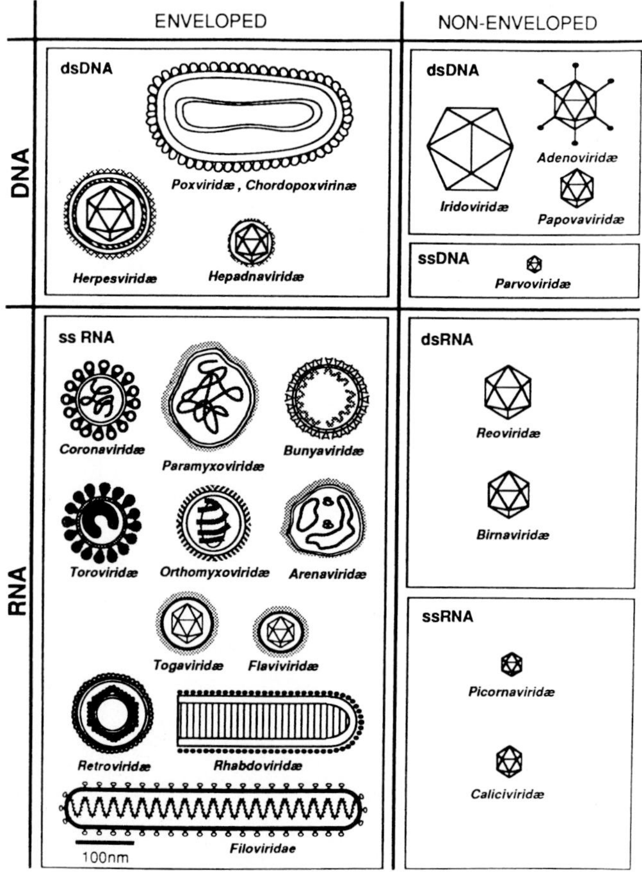

FIGURE 16–2. The International Committee on Taxonomy of Viruses drawings of viruses in the common virus families of vertebrates. All the diagrams have been drawn similarly: Vertical lines separate enveloped and nonenveloped viruses, and horizontal lines separate DNA and RNA viruses. Within each of the resulting four sections, single-stranded (ss) and double-stranded (ds) genomes are indicated. The relative sizes of the viruses vary somewhat within each class. (From Francki RI, et al: Classification and nomenclature of viruses: Fifth report of the International Committee on Taxonomy of Viruses. Arch Virol 2[Suppl]:61, 1991.)

Some of the current problems for viral taxonomists are those presented by recently discovered forms of life that have properties differing from those of any other known biologic entities. These include viroids and prions and the recognition of satellites, hybrids of unrelated viruses, and pseudotypes and pseudovirions, as well as the introduction of synthetic recombinant DNA genes and viral vectors.[7]

LIFE CYCLE

Replication

The initial step in the infection replication process occurs with the attachment of the virus to the host cell via viral-cell receptor interactions initiated by a random collision. Attachment may involve the interaction between specific proteins on the viral surface (virion attachment protein) and specific receptors in the target cell membrane. An example of host-virus receptors is the $CD4^+$ marker on T lymphocytes and the fibroblast growth factor β receptor that mediates attachment of herpes simplex virus (HSV) 1.[2, 9, 10] The presence of host cell receptors specific for viral attachment is the major determinant of cell tropism. Cells that lack the necessary receptors are ordinarily resistant to viral infection. The host-viral receptor interaction is influenced by temperature, pH, receptor affinity, and the concentration of viral and host receptors, similar to a receptor-ligand reaction.

After attachment, the virion penetrates the host cell. The nature of this penetration is poorly understood but includes receptor-mediated endocytosis with uptake of the virion via host endosomes or direct injection of the virus core through the membrane. Fusion with the plasma membrane of the cell is an alternative entry for enveloped viruses. Uncoating of the virus is the third step in the host cell–virus interaction and involves physical separation of the nucleic acid from the surrounding capsid. At this stage, viral infectivity to other host cells is lost, but viral nucleic acid is available for translocation to the cell nucleus.[2]

Regardless of whether the infecting viral nucleic acid is single- or double-stranded DNA or RNA, translation depends on the production of messenger RNA (mRNA). There is no enzymatic mechanism in host cells to replicate RNA from an RNA template. The host cell enzymes for making mRNA from DNA are all located in the nucleus and are therefore not accessible to DNA viruses, whose replication is exclusively cytoplasmic. The genome in positive-strand RNA viruses serves as its own mRNA template. In negative-strand RNA viruses, an RNA polymerase reverse transcriptase allows the production of a positive strand of mRNA prior to replication. DNA viruses subdivide mRNA synthesis

TABLE 16–1. **Properties of Important Viruses Causing Ocular Disease**

Nucleic Acid Core	Shape of Virus	Capsid Symmetry	Virion: Enveloped or Naked	Physical Type of Nucleic Acid	Polarity of Single-Stranded Nucleic Acid	No. of Genes (approx.)	No. of Capsomers	Viral Particle Size (nm)	Molecular Weight of Nucleic Acid in Virion (× 10^6)	Site of Capsid Assembly	Site of Nucleocapsid Envelopment	Viral Family
DNA	Icosahedral	Icosahedral	Non-enveloped	Single-stranded	+ or −	3–4	32	18–26	1.5–2.2	Nucleus	Nucleus	Parvoviridae
				Double-stranded circular		5–8	72	45–55	3–5	Nucleus	Nucleus	Papovaviridae
				Double-stranded		30	252	70–90	20–30	Nucleus	Nucleus	Adenoviridae
	Spherical	Icosahedral	Enveloped	Double-stranded		160	162	150–200	90–130	Nucleus	Nuclear membrane	Herpesviridae
	Brick-shaped	Complex	Complex coats	Double-stranded		300		230 × 400	130–200	Cytoplasm	Cytoplasm	Poxviridae
	Icosahedral	Complex	Complex coats	Double-stranded circular		4		42	1.6	Nucleus	Cytoplasm	Hepadnaviridae
RNA	Icosahedral	Icosahedral	Non-enveloped	Single-stranded	+	4–6	32	20–30	2.3–2.8	Cytoplasm	Cytoplasm	Picornaviridae
	Icosahedral			Single-stranded	+	4–6	32	35–39	2.6	Cytoplasm	Cytoplasm	Caliciviridae
	Spherical			Double-stranded segmented		10–12		60–80	12–15	Cytoplasm	Cytoplasm	Reoviridae
	Spherical	Icosahedral	Enveloped	Single-stranded	+	10	32	50–70	4	Cytoplasm	Surface membrane	Togaviridae
	Spherical	Unknown or complex	Enveloped	Single-stranded	+	10		45–50	4	Cytoplasm	Intracytoplasmic membrane	Flaviviridae
				Single-stranded segmented	−	10		50–300	3–5	Cytoplasm	Surface membrane	Arenaviridae
				Single-stranded	+	30		80–160	7	Cytoplasm	Intracytoplasmic membrane	Coronaviridae
				Single-stranded diploid	+	4		~100	7–10	Cytoplasm	Surface membrane	Retroviridae
	Spherical	Helical	Enveloped	Single-stranded segmented	−	>3		90–100	6–15	Cytoplasm	Intracytoplasmic membrane	Bunyaviridae
	Spherical			Single-stranded segmented	−	10		80–120	5	Cytoplasm	Surface membrane	Orthomyxoviridae
	Spherical			Single-stranded	−	>10		150–300	5–7	Cytoplasm	Surface membrane	Paramyxoviridae
	Bullet-shaped			Single-stranded	−	5		75 × 180	4	Cytoplasm	Surface membrane	Rhabdoviridae

and protein production into several sequentially ordered gene classes: immediate early, early, and late gene expression. RNA viruses tend to synthesize all products simultaneously. The number and diversity of viral enzymes vary, depending on the complexity of the virus. The genomes of small viruses probably encode for only three or four unique proteins, whereas those of the largest viruses may encode for several hundred proteins. Due to their multiple enzymes, the herpesviruses are among the most sensitive viruses amenable to antiviral therapeutic intervention, because antiviral agents can be targeted against virus-specific enzymes with minimal toxicity to uninfected host cells.[11]

Release of progeny viruses depends on whether the virus is enveloped or nonenveloped. Infection with nonenveloped viruses tends to result in the lysis of the host cell after virion assembly. Enveloped viruses, on the other hand, insert virus-encoded glycoproteins into the host cell membrane; the nucleocapsid then buds through the altered cell membrane and obtains its envelope by exocytosis (Fig. 16–3). The envelope of the herpesviruses is acquired by budding through the inner lamella of the nuclear membrane; the enveloped virions then pass directly from the space between the two lamellae of the nuclear membrane to the exterior of the cell via the cisternae of the endoplasmic reticulum.

In addition to host cell lysis and viral release, many viruses can establish a persistent infection in which the virus is continuously replicated or, alternatively, a latent infection in which the virus is intermittently replicated. Examples of persistent viral infections include congenital rubella or congenital cytomegaloviral infection.[2, 12] Latent viral infection, on the other hand, is the occult infection of the host cell without the presence of detectable virus and clinically evident disease. This stage of viral infection can exist for the life of the host. Periodically, latent viral infections can reactivate and reestablish disease in the host, usually at or near the initial infection site.[13–16] Herpes simplex and herpes zoster are examples of viruses that include latency life-cycle stages. Other latent viruses, called slow viruses, require a prolonged incubation period prior to the appearance of clinical disease in the host. The survival mechanisms of these slow viruses are poorly understood (e.g., kuru and Creutzfeldt-Jakob disease).

Pathogenesis

To induce clinically evident disease, a virus must successfully contact the host, encounter and infect cells, replicate, and induce cell injury and cell death. The majority of viruses gain entry to the host via host mucosal surfaces such as the respiratory, gastrointestinal, conjunctival, or genital epithelium. Other routes of host entry include bloodborne viral transmission (encountered in hepatitis or human immunodeficiency virus [HIV] infections) and insect vector transmission (rickettsial infections).[3] The capacity of a virus to produce illness or death is called virulence, and it is often measured in terms of the amount of virus required to kill or cause infection in 50% of a cohort of mice infected under defined conditions.

Viruses replicate and cause disease localized usually to the site of entry. After primary replication, the viral infection can become disseminated to other locations distant from the site of viral entry. Mechanisms by which viruses are disseminated throughout the host include: (1) hematogenous spread (mumps and measles), (2) neuronal spread (herpes simplex and varicella-zoster), and probably (3) lymphatic spread. Despite various routes of dissemination, viruses are limited to infecting only those cells with receptors that permit viral adherence and penetration.[9, 10]

Clinically evident viral disease is the result of cell damage at replication sites. Replication and host cell destruction result in changes to the tissues such as the cutaneous lesions of viral exanthems, corneal epithelial dendritic lesions, or physiologic alterations to the target organs. Clinical illness, however, is an inadequate criterion to characterize viral infections, because the viral infection is sometimes inapparent.

The determinants of viral virulence and of host susceptibility/resistance are multifactorial. Within a susceptible species, the resistance of individual animals varies not only with the genetic composition of the host but also with age, nutritional status, stress, and many other factors. These genetic and physiologic factors determine the "nonspecific," "natural," or "innate" resistance of the host, in contrast with the "acquired," immunologically "specific" resistance to reinfection that results from the operation of the immune response.[17]

The establishment and maintenance of a persistent infection imply two requisites: avoidance of elimination by the immune system and limitation of expression of the genome. The several alternative routes to persistence may be subdivided into four categories: (1) acute infections with late complications (e.g., subacute sclerosing panencephalitis), (2) latent infections (herpesviruses), (3) chronic infections (hepatitis, rubella, acquired immunodeficiency syndrome [AIDS]), and (4) slow infections (AIDS, subacute spongiform encephalopathies). Oncogenic viruses are involved in about 15% of human cancers because of genetic alterations caused by these viruses that involve certain common intracellular molecular pathways.[18, 19]

HOST IMMUNE RESPONSE

A wide variety of host factors can dramatically affect the ultimate tropism of a virus, including the age, immune status, genetic composition, and nutritional state of the host.[20] The host response to viral infection takes numerous forms. The host immune system responds to viral infection with both nonspecific and specific defenses. Nonspecific and specific responses are not either/or phenomena but involve interactions of a complex host network that eliminate the viruses and provide protection against reinfection of the host.[10, 21] Nonspecific mechanisms, which include interferon, the complement system, and phagocytic cells, do not require prior exposure to viral antigens. These nonspecific mechanisms constitute the initial host defense against primary viral infection. The interferons are evolutionarily conserved molecules that retard viral penetration, uncoating, transcription, translation, and assembly, representing an important factor of host resistance to viral infection. Although interferons can protect host cells from viral infection, some viruses have developed resistance. Furthermore, the inflammatory response initiated by interferons sometimes causes damage to tissue and constitutes a pathogenic mechanism for viral disease.[22]

Specific host immune responses are directed toward virus-

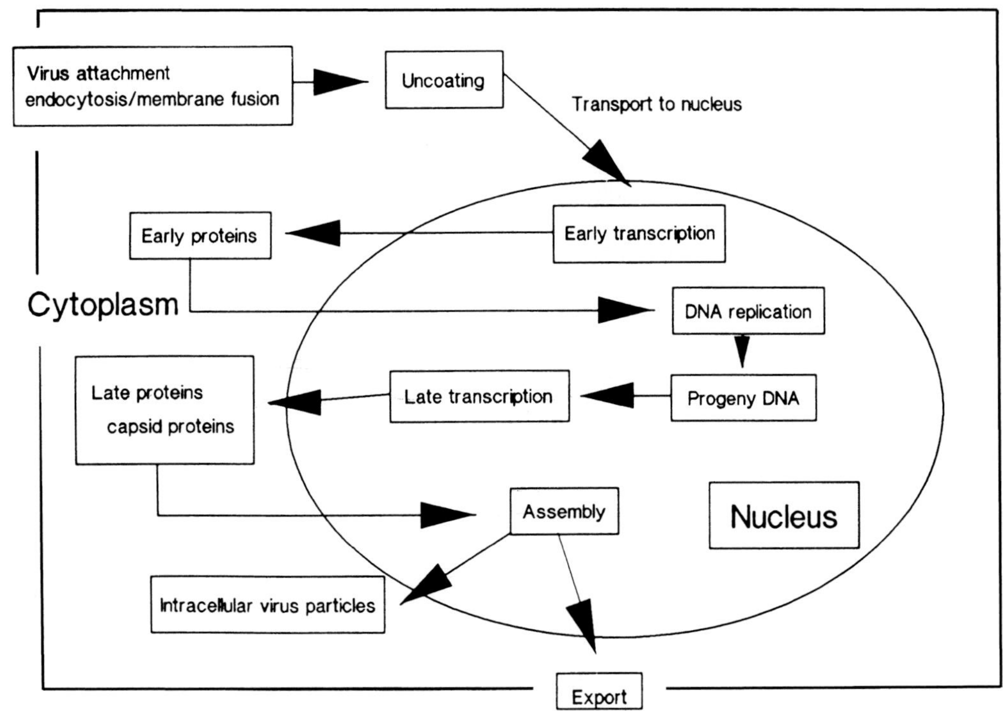

A **DNA Virus Replication**

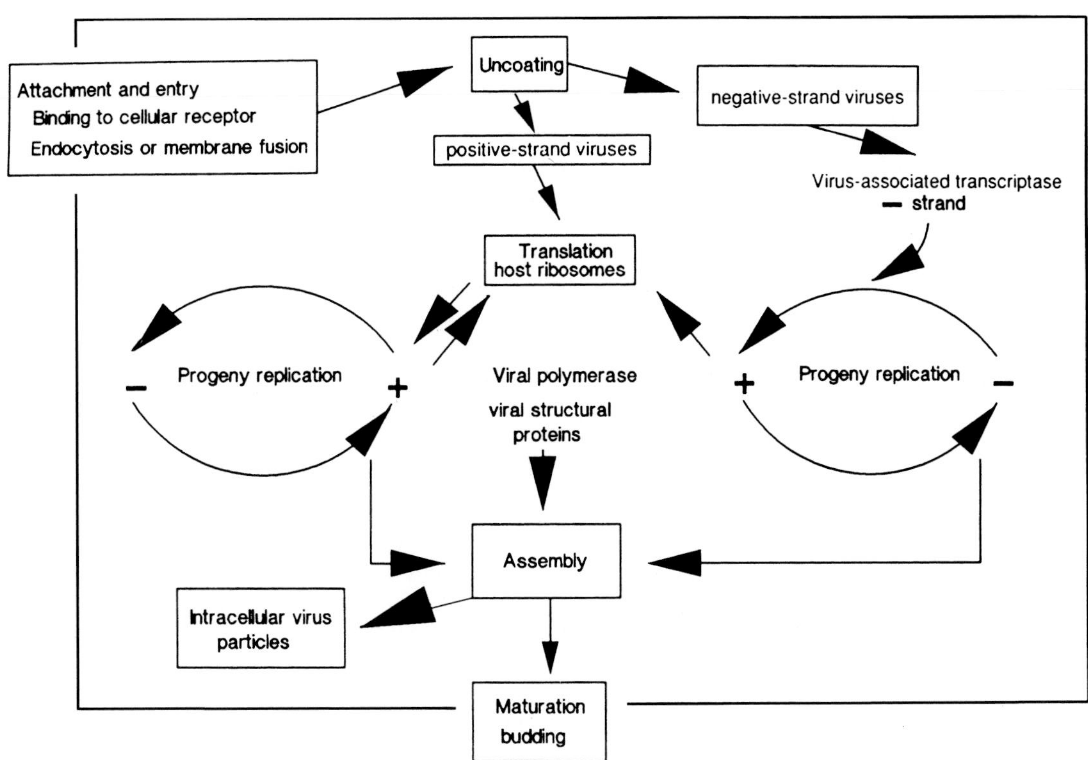

B **RNA Virus Replication**

FIGURE 16–3. Summary of the replication process for DNA *(A)* and RNA *(B)* viruses. (From Volk WA, et al [eds]: Essentials of Medical Microbiology. Philadelphia, JB Lippincott, 1991.)

encoded proteins stimulating B- or T-lymphocyte responses; these are generally not detectable until several days after primary infection. Specific immunity constitutes the second-line host defense and is complex. In essence, viral proteins, either as part of virus particles or expressed on the surfaces of infected cells, interact with macrophages that bear type II histocompatibility antigens on their surfaces, thus initiating a cascade that results in the development of both cellular and humoral immunity. Potential viral antigens in B-cell mediated humoral immunity include whole or subparts of the virion that are exposed to the host during viremia. T cell–regulated cell-mediated immunity recognizes virus-specific proteins that are presented on the host cell surface either as unique viral antigens in combination with host antigens or as virus-induced alterations in host antigens. The most potent antigens are proteins of 100,000 Da or larger.

Because each protein can have multiple antigenic sites, numerous antibodies can be induced by a single viral antigen. Antibodies with many specificities are made against virus particles; most viruses have several proteins on their surfaces, each with several epitopes distributed in several functional domains. Host antibodies may interact with the viral proteins in a variety of ways. Neutralizing antibodies bind to the virus and render it noninfectious. Other antibodies may bind with the virus in ways that do not influence infectivity but stimulate phagocytosis or the complement system, resulting in effective elimination of the virus. As a result, the spectrum of antibodies formed against any particular virus particle is highly complex. Individuals with only humoral antibody deficiency are able to cope normally with many common viral infections such as those caused by HSV, cytomegalovirus (CMV), varicella, and measles. However, the inability to limit the replication of poliovirus and other enteroviruses in the central nervous system (CNS) is recognized as a consequence of antibody deficiency.

The cellular limb of the immune system is also activated during viral infection. Its salient features include activation of cytotoxic T lymphocytes, natural killer cells, and macrophages. T cell–mediated immunity is stimulated not by soluble antigens but rather by viral proteins on the host cell membrane. The categories of T cells involved in cellular immunity include cytotoxic T cells (that destroy cells presenting viral antigen), delayed-type hypersensitivity T cells (that secrete lymphokines and are chemotactic for macrophages and polymorphonuclear leukocytes), helper T cells (that mediate both B- and T-lymphocyte responses), and suppressor T cells (that downregulate the host immune response to viral infections).[23, 24] The complement system also plays a role in the pathogenesis. Complement may initiate lysis of free virus and of virus-infected cells in the presence of antibody.

Although common to all viral infections, the exact nature of the immune response mounted varies for each particular virus. Ironically, in many cases, the host immune response may not be entirely beneficial. Some ocular viral infections, such as herpes simplex stromal keratitis and herpes zoster ophthalmicus, induce an immune response vigorous enough to cause as much structural and functional damage as the viral infection.[25, 26]

Diagnostic Virology

Laboratory confirmation of ocular viral infections depends on the ability of the clinician to obtain specimens at appropriate times in the course of infection and on the proper specimen handling after collection.[27–29] Communication between the physician and virology laboratory staff regarding the clinical syndrome and suspected etiologic viruses allows for meaningful and timely interpretation of laboratory results. For most viral cultures, swabs are used and then rinsed in a broth medium; calcium alginate swabs are known to adversely affect recovery of herpes simplex virus.[30] Specimens should be transported on ice or refrigerated. Although exciting, the newer molecular diagnostic assays are not yet standardized, and results should be interpreted cautiously. Serologic tests have drawbacks, including cross-reactivity, delay, and inability to distinguish acute and past exposure on the basis of a single assay.

Several approaches are taken to obtain laboratory confirmation of a clinical diagnosis (Table 16–2). The most rapid diagnostic approach is direct examination of the clinical specimen by light microscopy. Other direct observation techniques include electron microscopy (EM), cytology, and the direct detection of viral antigens by fluorescence, immunoassays, or nucleic acid probes.[31–34] The use of monoclonal antibodies has increased the specificity and reproducibility of these tests and made the commercial development of immunoassays possible. Because of problems associated with the use and disposal of radioisotopes, radioimmunoassays have been replaced in clinical laboratories by other methods. All of these rapid techniques yield results on viral diagnosis early in the course of infection, usually within 24 to 48 hours. Drawbacks to the use of some of these techniques are the need for specific viral antibodies or nucleic acid probes that may not be available for all clinical viruses. Cytology and EM are easily performed, but in general these techniques are not specific.[35, 36]

Another diagnostic approach is viral isolation, followed by identification. Isolation of an infectious virus is used to confirm both direct clinical examination and serologic findings. The isolation of an infectious virus is considered the gold standard in diagnostic virology. Isolation of a virus does not necessarily prove causality of disease, however. In cases of latent viral infection with intermittent virus shedding or in cases of multiple viral infections, the isolated agent may not be directly responsible for the clinical disease.[35–37]

Another diagnostic approach is serologic examination. This approach typically involves obtaining patient sera during both the acute and convalescent periods (2 weeks after the onset of clinical disease). The major disadvantage of viral identification and confirmation by serologic methods is that these techniques can involve up to a 2-week delay to obtain a final diagnosis. Frequently, by the time a diagnosis based on serology is made, the information is no longer therapeutically useful. The same techniques that are used to detect antigens in clinical specimens can be used to detect antibodies. Antigen is immobilized on a solid phase and used to capture free antibody from a serum sample. A radioactive label or the action of an enzyme label on a chromogen (for enzyme immunoassay [EIA]), fluorochrome (for fluorescence immunoassays), or a chemiluminescent substrate is used as an indicator of the antigen-antibody complex.

DIRECT OBSERVATION TECHNIQUES

Cytology and Histopathology

Even though they provide few specific diagnoses, cytology often allows the initial, early recognition of viral infections.

TABLE 16–2. **Various Viral Diagnostic Methods**

Morphologic
- Tzanck's smears
- Papanicolaou's, Giemsa's, Wright's smears
- Biopsy (H & E stains)
- Electron microscopy
  - Visualization of virion or envelope by negative staining
  - Thin sections
  - Pseudoreplication

Immunomorphologic
- Immunofluorescence techniques
- Immunoperoxidase techniques
- Immunoelectron microscopy—antibodies, colloidal gold

Serology
- Nonspecific
  - Complement fixation
  - Anticomplement immunofluorescence
  - Latex particle agglutination
  - Hemagglutination inhibition
  - Gel immunodiffusion
  - Radioimmunoassay
  - Enzyme-linked immunosorbent assay
  - Immunofluorescence
  - Time-resolved fluoroimmunoassay
- Specific
  - Virus neutralization
  - Western immunoblotting
  - Protein-specific assays

Viral culture
- Conventional cell cultures
  - Detection of cytopathic effects
- Centrifugation-enhanced cultures (shell vial cultures)
- Pre-cytopathic effect (CPE) detection immunomorphologic techniques
  - Immunofluorescence, immunoperoxidase
- Pre-CPE detection immunologic techniques
  - Enzyme immunoassays
  - Latex agglutination
  - Monoclonal antibody systems
- Viral serotyping
  - Enzyme-linked immunoassay (ELISA), neutralization, DNA hybridization

Immunologic virology
- ELISA
- Agar gel diffusion
- Countercurrent immunoelectrophoresis

Molecular virology
- DNA hybridization
  - Detection by radioactive, fluorescence, peroxidase, biotin, digoxigenin, or chromogenic labels
- DNA restriction endonuclease analysis
- PCR, isothermal amplification
  - Detection of amplification products by gel electrophoresis and by filter hybridizations (Southern blots, dot blots, slot blots, and sandwich hybridization) or by in situ hybridization

Cytologic testing is readily available in most hospital settings and physicians' offices. Scrapings from the clinical lesions (skin or ocular tissues) are streaked onto a glass microscope slide. The slide is fixed in Bouin's solution for 1 hour and subsequently stained with H & E, Tzanck's, Giemsa's, or Papanicolaou's stain and examined by light microscopy. Although this technique is far less specific and sensitive than isolation of virus in cell culture or by immunologic staining, it may be helpful in rapidly diagnosing HSV, varicella-zoster virus, CMV, measles, and rabies infection. Cytology during herpesviral infections typically shows distinctive inclusions that represent abnormal accumulations of host cellular material caused by the virus-induced disruption of host cell metabolic activity. Multinucleated giant cells and ballooning cytoplasm may also be observed in herpes simplex, varicella-zoster, and cytomegaloviral infections and are characteristic of these viral infections (Table 16–3).[6] Specific features or inclusions are found for only a few viruses. The Cowdry type A inclusions are brilliant, more specific intranuclear inclusion that virtually fills the nucleus with a clear halo separating the inclusion from the nuclear membrane.[38] Other features that help increase specificity are cytoplasmic inclusions, cell size, and multinucleation.[29] Immunoperoxidase and immunofluorescence staining can be used to increase the sensitivity and specificity as well as to detect other viral agents not causing cytologic changes.

Electron Microscopy

Viral particles in a tissue specimen or lesion fluid are beyond the limits of light microscopy but may be directly visualized by EM.[39] This technique is most reliable during acute, clinically active viral infections, when the numbers of viral particles are high (10^6 to 10^7 particles/mL). The specimen must be fixed or processed immediately. If viral particles are observed, a presumptive diagnosis regarding the category of the causative viral agent may be made on the basis of distinctive morphology. A definitive diagnosis cannot be made, however, because many viruses, such as HSV and varicella-zoster virus, are indistinguishable by EM.

Two electron microscopic techniques can be used. Electron-dense substances such as phosphotungstic acid and uranyl acetate negatively stain viruses against a darkly contrasting background. This technique is simple with regard to specimen preparation time, but because ophthalmic preparations are frequently cellular, distinguishing viral particles

TABLE 16–3. **Differential Features of Viral Infections and Inclusions**

Nuclear inclusions
- Herpes simplex, varicella-zoster
  - Eosinophilic with clear chromatin halo (Cowdry A)
- Adenovirus
  - Smudgy eosinophilic
- Molluscum contagiosum
  - Eosinophilic cytoplasmic

Cytoplasmic inclusions
- Pox viruses
  - Large eosinophilic bodies and granular subparticles are individual viruses

Combined nuclear and cytoplasmic inclusions
- Cytomegalovirus
  - Large cell size
  - Nuclear inclusions fill nucleus, inclusions can be smudgy
  - Cytoplasmic inclusions
- Measles
  - Red nuclear inclusions can be small, have large halo
  - Cytoplasmic inclusions relatively large

Multinucleation
- Herpes simplex, varicella-zoster
  - Molding of nuclei prominent
- Measles
  - Nuclei do not mold, large cytoplasmic inclusions

Classic histopathologic pattern
- Human papilloma virus
  - Verruciform warts, koilocytic squamous cells
  - Squamous intraepithelial lesion

from tissue debris may be difficult. Thin-section specimen preparation is much more labor-intensive. The fine structure of the virus and surrounding host cells, however, is preserved, allowing for localization of virus in situ.[40, 41] Several modifications have increased the sensitivity for specific agents. In immunoelectron microscopy (IEM), virus-specific antibody is added to the liquid specimen to aggregate viral particles, enabling easier detection. Solid-phase IEM uses staphylococcal protein A to capture the aggregates, further increasing the sensitivity.[32] Other techniques have been devised to enhance the sensitivity of EM for detecting viruses, including pseudoreplication (transferring viral particles from an agar surface onto a collodion film in the form of a pseudoreplica) and agar gel diffusion (viral particles are concentrated on an agar surface and transferred onto a grid, while salts and debris diffuse into the agar). The use of virus-specific antibodies and colloidal gold in IEM has allowed the enhanced visualization of both viral particles and soluble viral antigen in clinical specimens.[42] EM has been largely replaced by other methods for identification of many viral infections.

Immunofluorescence

Direct, indirect, and anticomplement fluorescent staining methods are available for detecting viral antigen associated with infected cells; characteristic fluorescent cytoplasmic or nuclear staining patterns are seen.[43] Specimens for immunostaining may be obtained from lesions by scraping or aspirate centrifugation. The clinical isolate is obtained, then smeared onto a clean glass slide, and treated with fluorescein-conjugated virus-specific antiserum. The slide is incubated at 36°C for 30 to 60 minutes, washed in phosphate-buffered saline, and observed under fluorescent microscopy. The direct method, using virus-specific antibody conjugated with a fluorescent label, is more specific and rapid because there is only one incubation step; this is less sensitive than the indirect method. The indirect staining, using unlabeled virus-specific antibody in the first step and an antiimmunoglobulin conjugate in the second step, is more sensitive because more label can be bound to the antigen; however, nonspecific background fluorescence may reduce the overall usefulness of the assay.[32] Antibodies can react nonspecifically with leukocytes in the specimen. To decrease nonspecific binding, the specimen may be treated with normal serum prior to incubation with specific antiviral antibodies in an attempt to block nonspecific binding. Although this test is specific, viral isolation is recommended to confirm the diagnosis. The experience required and the subjectivity of these tests are a drawback. Immunofluorescence is a rapid and specific technique routinely used to detect adenoviral, rabies, herpes simplex, respiratory syncytial viral, mumps, measles, varicella-zoster, and cytomegaloviral infections.[44, 45]

Immunoperoxidase

Immunoperoxidase is a widely used diagnostic immunostaining technique that uses antibody conjugated with enzymes, such as horseradish peroxidase, rather than fluorescence as the indicator. Observation of the immunoperoxidase staining involves light, rather than fluorescent, microscopy; thus, the surrounding tissue can be observed simultaneously for histopathology. Immunoperoxidase reactions use the peroxidase enzyme to produce an orange-brown precipitate localized at the binding sites in the specimen. The technique is similar to immunofluorescent staining in that the specimen is overlaid with normal serum to decrease nonspecific binding and then overlaid with peroxidase-conjugated antibody followed by incubation and washing. Peroxidase substrate is then added, and detectable color changes in areas of specific antiviral antibody binding are produced. In certain situations, immunoperoxidase staining is preferable to immunofluorescence techniques. Immunofluorescence fades over time, and photography is necessary for permanent documentation. The immunoperoxidase technique is particularly useful in laboratories without access to a fluorescent microscope.[31, 35, 46] A modification of the immunoperoxidase technique is the peroxidase-antiperoxidase (PAP) method, which uses unconjugated antiviral antibody and soluble complexes of PAP as an enzyme label to provide increased sensitivity compared with the standard immunoperoxidase assay.[42] The avidin–biotinylated peroxidase complex technique begins like the PAP technique; it relies on the affinity of avidin for biotin and may amplify binding because of the multiple sites for biotin.

Enzyme Immunoassays

Enzyme-linked immunosorbent assays (ELISAs) are available in a variety of formats for detection of several viral agents by solid-phase or membrane-phase techniques. In solid-phase tests, the antigen is captured by virus-specific antibody bound to a solid surface, usually a plastic microtiter well or tube. In membrane tests, a membrane replaces the solid support. With either technique, the captured antigen is detected by binding of an enzyme-linked antibody to the antigen. After washing unbound antibody out, a colorimetric substrate for the enzyme is added. There are many variations of this technique. The solid-phase format is most suitable for batch testing and can be automated; commercial kits are available for adenovirus, HSV, and other viruses. The membrane technique is available in single-test formats for some viruses, is simple to perform, and can be performed with little equipment in physicians' offices.[32]

Agglutination

Agglutination tests to detect viral antigens are based on visible agglutination of particles, such as latex, red blood cells, or polystyrene, to which virus-specific antibody has been absorbed. Although agglutination methods are less sensitive than EIA or fluorescence, they are easily performed.[32] Few commercially available kits detect ocular viral pathogens.

Nucleic Acid Hybridization and Gene Amplification

Recombinant DNA technology has provided another highly specific technique of viral identification based on detection of viral nucleic acids rather than on antibody-antigen interactions and visualization. The principle of nucleic acid hybridization is that single-stranded DNA hybridizes by hydrogen-bonded base pairing to another single stand of DNA (or

RNA) of complementary base sequence. A major factor determining the specifity of the test is the nature of the probe itself—that is, whether it corresponds in length with the whole viral genome, a single gene, or a much shorter nucleotide sequence deliberately chosen to represent either a variable or a conserved region of the genome. Traditionally, radioisotopes have been used to label nucleic acids, with the signal being read by counting in a spectrometer or by autoradiography. The trend now is toward nonradioactive labels. Some of these produce a signal directly (fluorescein or peroxidase), whereas others act indirectly by binding to another labeled compound that emits the signal (biotin or digoxigenin). Biotinylated probes can be combined with various types of readouts—for example, an avidin-based enzyme immunoassay. These techniques not only are useful in the confirmation of acute infections but also are increasingly used as a clinical research tool for investigating various chronic diseases in which a viral etiology is suspected.[47, 48] Chemiluminescent substrates, such as luminol, are being exploited.[3]

Several amplification techniques have been developed for detection of nucleic acids. The best known is the polymerase chain reaction (PCR), which enables a single copy of any gene sequence to be amplified in vitro at least a millionfold within a few hours.[43] The journal *Science* selected the PCR as the major scientific development of 1989 and DNA polymerase as the molecule of the year. Dr. Kary Mullis, inventor of the PCR, was awarded the Nobel Prize for Medicine in 1993.[49] Viral DNA extracts from a very small number of virions or infected cells can be amplified to the point at which they can be readily identified using labeled probes in a hybridization assay. Moreover, the PCR can be modified for the detection of viral RNA by incorporating a preliminary step in which reverse transcriptase is used to convert the RNA to DNA. It is not necessary to amplify the whole genome, but it is necessary to know at least part of the nucleotide sequence in order to synthesize two oligonucleotide primers representing the extremities of the region one chooses to amplify. Isothermal amplification is a technique that does not require the temperature cycling and accompanying equipment of the PCR. In the research laboratory, detection of amplification products has often relied on methods such as gel electrophoresis, in situ hybridization, Southern blot hybridization, or dot-blot hybridization. These methods are difficult for the clinical laboratory. Other detection techniques, such as EIA-like techniques, are being evaluated.[32]

The sensitivity and versatility of nucleic acid hybridization for a viral genome may overtake probing for antigen as the diagnostic method of choice in many laboratories. These procedures are invaluable when dealing with viruses that cannot be cultured satisfactorily, that contain inactivated virus, or that are latent infections. The occurrence of false-positive results due to amplicon contamination continues to be a concern; to help ensure the reliability of these assays, the National Committee for Clinical Laboratory Standards is developing guidelines for the use of molecular methods in the diagnosis of infectious diseases.[32] The added sensitivity provided by gene amplification can create new concerns, because the medical relevance of finding the viral genome in tissues is still in its infancy and can raise undue concern, as demonstrated by studies reporting carcinogenic types of papillomavirus in high percentages of healthy women. The PCR has been applied to almost all the viral infections included in this chapter.[50–54] The current end-points are difficult to measure, too cumbersome, time-consuming, and impractical for widespread clinical diagnostic use. In the future, however, PCR analysis of nucleotides extracted from ocular biopsy samples may become the new gold standard of viral identification.[49, 55]

Viral Isolation

Viral isolation remains the gold standard against which newer methods must be compared. Culture is the only method that can identify a new virus or produce a supply of live virus for further examination or drug sensitivity testing. The yield of virus is optimized by collection of samples during the acute phase of infection. Conjunctival or corneal scrapings are transferred onto a moistened swab and placed into viral culture media. Calcium alginate swabs should be avoided, because these swabs may bind and inactivate viruses. The culture is transported to the laboratory as soon as possible. If the specimen cannot be transferred within 12 hours, it should be maintained at 4°C. Freezing, particularly in the case of enveloped viruses, causes a significant decrease in the viral titer. In the laboratory, culture medium is expressed from the swab, and the inoculum is transferred onto the appropriate cell line. It is imperative that the clinician inform laboratory personnel of the clinical symptoms of the suspected viruses.

The choice of the most suitable host cell system depends on the virus one predicts. Primary cultures, established directly from tissue, contain a variety of types of differentiated cells and hence support the growth of a broad spectrum of viruses. Continuous heteroploid cell lines from human cancers or monkey kidney have the great advantage of immortality. Any given cell line is generally capable of supporting the growth of only a limited range of viruses. Diploid strains of human embryonic fibroblasts offer a useful compromise in that they can be successfully passaged for a year or so in vitro and yet are susceptible to a wide range of different human viruses. Monolayer cultures for viral diagnostic purposes are generally grown in screw-capped glass tubes or vials, sometimes containing a removable coverslip for subsequent staining. The inoculated cultures are held at the temperature and pH of the human body and are slowly rotated on a roller drum or kept stationary.

When the virus is inoculated onto a susceptible cell line, it produces a characteristic change in the host cell. This alteration is called cytopathologic effect (CPE) and allows a presumptive identification of the virus.[42] The cultures are inspected two or three times a week for the development of specific CPE. Although rapidly growing viruses such as HSV can produce a detectable CPE within a day or two, some slow agents, such as CMV, rubella, and some adenoviruses, take 1 to 4 weeks.[56] Factors that affect the sensitivity of conventional cell cultures and the time to detection of CPE include selection of the cell line, passage number, age and condition of the monolayer, growth medium, temperature of incubation, blind passages, and use of roller drums versus stationary incubation. The virus is identified definitively with virus-specific antisera that inhibits viral growth or interacts with viral antigens, thereby neutralizing the infectious virions.[57, 58]

Although optimizing all of these techniques provided incremental improvements in recovery, major improvements were not observed until the introduction of centrifugation-enhanced or shell vial culture and pre-CPE detection techniques using specific fluorescent antibody, immunoperoxidase staining, or EIAs of the cell monolayer. This is similar to those techniques used for detecting viral antigens in clinical samples.[32] A novel approach to cell cultures uses a cell line genetically engineered to express β-galactosidase when infected with HSV.[59] The EIA technique is probably the most commonly used, although neutralization remains the gold standard for defining and distinguishing serotypes. For most diagnostic purposes, it is not necessary to "type" the isolate antigenically. In certain situations, epidemiologic information is important to the public health, and it may be necessary to characterize subtle differences between variants, strains, or subtypes within a given serotype. The PCR technique holds promise in this evaluation.

SEROLOGIC TECHNIQUES

All serologic methods depend on quantitative and qualitative evaluations of humoral immunity and antibody production.[2, 60] Serologic techniques can be employed in two ways. First, specific viral antibody may be used to identify unknown viral isolates or antigens, as discussed earlier (viral typing). Serology can be used the other way around—that is, to identify antibody using panels of known antigens or to quantitate antibody in sera from infected patients. In the case of humoral immunity, immunoglobulin (Ig) M antibodies appear early in the course of infection and are followed by IgG antibody induction. The IgM antibodies typically disappear within the first few weeks after infection, whereas IgG antibodies persist for many years following acute infection. Quantitative serologic techniques are based on documentation of a significant rise in antibody titer to the virus. The patient's serum is collected as soon as possible after the onset of infection (acute or primary serum); convalescent serum is collected in the period 2 to 3 weeks after the onset of the viral infection. A fourfold increase in the titer of antibody from the acute to convalescent period is generally considered to be diagnostic of a viral infection. In a number of situations, finding antibody in a single specimen of serum can be diagnostic, such as when a specific antibody of the IgM class is found or when a seriously ill patient is found to have antibodies against an exotic virus (e.g., Ebola), or when an ongoing infection (e.g., HIV) causes a marker of the continued infection. Evaluation of a single serum allows for only a presumptive diagnosis. Detection of specific IgM has been used with success in the diagnosis of infections due to varicella-zoster virus, Epstein-Barr virus, CMV, and measles, rubella, and coxsackieviruses and is currently the procedure of choice to establish a recent or active infection due to hepatitis A virus.[42] Elevated IgM titers may also reflect reactivation of latent viral infection rather than a response to a primary infection. In congenital infections, IgM is uniquely diagnostic. Unlike IgG, IgM does not cross the placental barrier, and in a neonate, the finding of IgM antibodies indicates congenital infection.[61]

Commonly used techniques for quantitating antibodies include virus neutralization, complement fixation, hemagglutination inhibition, radioimmunoassay, the ELISA, Western immunoblotting, latex particle agglutination, immunofluorescence, and gel immunodiffusion. These assays are methods of evaluating populations of different antibodies to the various viral antigens. The antibodies detected in the complement-fixation tests are only transiently present in the host during the acute and convalescent periods, but antibodies detected by the neutralization test are typically present for years following viral infection.

Viral Neutralization

The neutralization test is based on the ability of specific antibodies to neutralize viral infectivity. Neutralizing antibodies are specific and their presence can be demonstrated by adding serum containing the antibody to a suspension of virus and subsequent inoculation of the combination onto susceptible cell monolayers. If neutralizing antibodies are present, these antibodies bind to the virus and the virus is unable to infect the cell monolayer. The titer of neutralizing antibodies may be determined either by using a constant amount of serum and varying the concentration of virus or, conversely, the viral concentration may be kept constant and a serial dilution of the serum performed. The numeric value assessed to the titer of neutralizing antibody in the serum is the reciprocal of the highest dilution at which the serum prevents development of viral CPE. A single positive test result, without assessing the concentration of neutralizing antibody in convalescent serum, is beneficial only if the neutralizing antibody is IgM. Because neutralizing antibodies may persist in the host serum for many years, documentation of their presence does not confirm causality in acute disease.

Complement Fixation

The complement system is a complex of multiple plasma proteins that interact sequentially to induce cell lysis. The complement fixation test is based on the principle that complement combines with viral antigen only in the presence of specific antibody. A known concentration of viral antigen and complement is mixed with the patient's serum. If complement fixing–specific antibody-antigen complexes are present, the available complement is bound. The antigen-antibody and complement mixture is incubated with hemolysin-sensitized sheep red blood cells. If complement is present that has not been fixed by the antigen-antibody complex, it hemolyzes the red blood cells. Conversely, if the antigen-antibody complexes are present, they fix the available complement and the red blood cells remain unlysed. The effective use of the complement fixation test depends on the availability of stable, specific viral antigens. The test requires many manipulations and at least 48 hours for both stages of the test to be completed, and it often yields nonspecific results. It is used with only a few suspected viral infections.

Hemagglutination Inhibition

Viruses, including rubella, mumps, measles, Newcastle disease, vaccinia, and adenovirus, agglutinate erythrocytes from different species. Host serum is introduced to a suspension of erythrocytes with a predetermined standardized concentration of viral antigen. When antibody is present in the serum, the agglutination of red blood cells is prevented. The lack of agglutination is determined by the formation of a diffuse red granular lining at the bottom of the reaction tube. A diagnosis of primary viral infection by hemagglutination requires serum samples from acute and convalescent disease stages. These specimens are serially diluted, exposed to viral antigen, and then mixed with red blood cells. The highest dilution of serum that results in the complete inhibition of hemagglutination is considered the hemagglutination inhibition titer. A fourfold or greater increase in the titer from the acute to the convalescent phase is diagnostic of a viral infection.[62] The hemagglutination inhibition tests for most viral agents are performed only at reference laboratories.

Enzyme-Linked Immunosorbent Assay

The ELISA is used in diagnostic virology for the detection of both viral antigen (as shown earlier) and antibody, as well as other biologic products, including hormones, peptides, and toxins. The ELISA technique is similar to that of tissue immunoperoxidase staining. The initial step in the solid-bound ELISA is binding of viral antigen to a solid phase, typically a polystyrene well. Patient serum is added, and, if specific antiviral antibody is present, it binds to the solid phase antigen. The well is rinsed, and peroxidase-conjugated antiantibody (antihuman IgG or IgM) is added to the well. Peroxidase substrate is then added to the assay. Detection of antibody in the serum is indicated by a color change in the wells. A standardized assay, using previously determined concentrations of viral antibody, is performed along with test serum. The amount of antibody in test serum can thus be rapidly correlated with known standards, and titers of the antibody in the serum can be determined. By reversing the sequence, ELISAs may also be used to detect viral antigen. In this case, the antibody is bound to the solid phase, and the viral infected suspension is added to the plates. The well is washed and peroxidase-conjugated antiviral antigen is introduced. When the substrate is added, if the result is positive, a color change is observed.[36, 46, 63–66] The introduction of membrane-bound ELISA components has improved sensitivity and ease of use dramatically. Several commercially available ELISA or modified ELISA viral diagnostic tests are available, including those for HSV-1 and -2, CMV, and rubella. These kits are beneficial in the diagnosis of herpes simplex ocular infections because of their ease of handling, the rapid availability of results (usually within 4 to 6 hours), and the selectivity in differentiating between HSV and varicella-zoster virus ocular infections.[64] Antibody-capture ELISAs are particularly valuable for detecting IgM in the presence of IgG. Anti-IgM antibodies are fixed to the solid phase, and thus only IgM antibodies, if present in the patient's serum, are bound. Rubella is diagnosed using this technology, usually in research settings. The advances in ELISA methods, including membrane-fixed antibodies, fluorescent and enzymatic labels, antibody-capture formats, and monoclonal antibodies, have brought ELISA methodology to the forefront of routine serologic assay techniques.

Flow Cytometry

Flow cytometry is the measurement of the physical or chemical characteristics of cells while they pass single-file in a fluid stream through a measuring apparatus. Originally used in the fields of immunology and oncology, it is now being applied to molecular biology and diagnostic microbiology. Multiparameter flow cytometers use a single laser beam to allow the simultaneous quantitative measurement of a number of cellular properties, including cell number, cell size, cellular granularity, and up to three different fluorochrome-labeled cells.[67] Blood, bronchoalveolar savage, and urine specimens are ideal, but soft organs, lymph nodes, and other tissues can be mechanically manipulated to release single cells. Surface or intracellular antigens from virus-infected cells can be detected rapidly by this technique. The technique has been applied to the papovavirus, the lentivirus (HIV-1 and -2), and the herpesviruses. This technique holds promise for rapid detection of virus once antibodies against specific surface or intracellular antigens are available, after amplification in cell culture, or both. It may also represent a means of monitoring the effects of antiviral therapy as well as distinguishing cells that may be latently infected.

Herpesviruses

Family: Herpesviridae
Subfamilies
Alphaherpesvirinae
Genus: Simplexvirus (herpes simplex–like viruses)
Type 1
Type 2
Genus: Varicellovirus (varicella-zoster virus)
Betaherpesvirinae
Genus: Cytomegalovirus (cytomegalovirus)
Genus: Roseolovirus (human herpesvirus 6)
Genus: Human herpesvirus 7
Gammaherpesvirinae (lymphoproliferative herpesviruses)
Genus: Lymphocryptovirus (Epstein-Barr virus)
Genus: Human herpesvirus 8 (Kaposi's sarcoma herpesvirus)

The herpesviruses are large DNA viruses that cause lifelong infections with intermittent clinical manifestations. These viruses can reactivate spontaneously throughout the life of the host and can reestablish clinical disease at the site of the initial, primary infection. Although there are many types of herpesviruses within the animal kingdom, only eight are human herpesviruses, five of which cause recognizable ocular disease.[2] Although most herpes DNA is similarly organized, most show little homology of nucleic acid sequence. The relatedness is best recognized by similarities in location of selected genes or clusters of genes and by stretches of amino acids that are conserved in critical protein domains. The herpesviruses are icosahedral enveloped viruses that derive their envelope from the host cell membrane (Fig. 16–4). The envelope is required for the infectivity of the virus. Ordinarily, infection requires direct inoculation or, in the case of varicella-zoster virus, infection can be established by airborne droplet contamination. Herpesviruses vary widely in their abilities to infect different types of cells, a

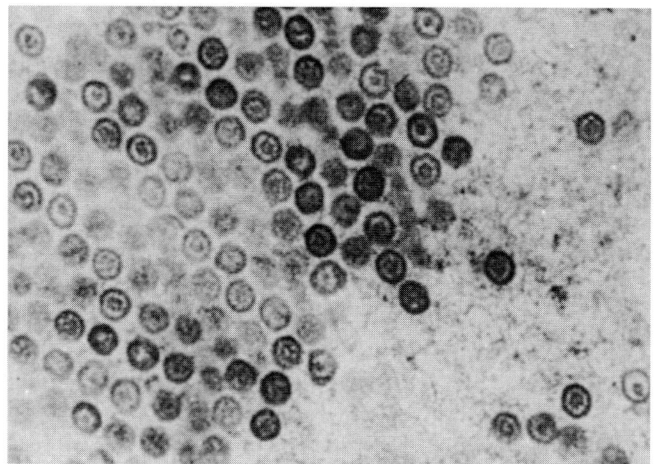

FIGURE 16–4. Electron micrograph showing crystalline array of herpes simplex virus.

feature that is considered in classifying the virus into subfamilies. Another biologic attribute of most herpesviruses is the ability to transform cells; to date, however, only lymphotropic herpesviruses have proved to be tumorigenic (leading to lymphoproliferative malignancies). Herpesviruses induce disease in three ways: (1) by direct destruction of tissues, (2) by provoking immunopathologic responses, and (3) by facilitating neoplastic transformation.

Herpes Simplex Virus Types 1 and 2

The HSV genome is a linear double-stranded DNA. Important characteristics of this subfamily include a short replication cycle, production of lytic infection in tissue culture, and establishment of latency in neural ganglia.[68–70] These viruses have a unique DNA sequence organization composed of a long unique region and a short unique region flanked by repeating sequences. The HSV can be isolated from the associated sensory nerve ganglia within 6 to 24 hours after primary infection. Recovery of virus from the ganglion does not require HSV replication in the ganglion. Latency has been demonstrated in humans within trigeminal, sacral, and vagal ganglia. The presumed route of access to the ganglion is by retrograde axonal transport of the HSV virion to the neuronal soma. In the neurosoma, HSV can induce a productive infection that results in ganglion neuron death, or the virus may establish a latent infection in the cell body. The neuron appears to be unique in that production of fully infectious virus does not always result in cell lysis. During latent infection, the state of the HSV genome remains controversial.[13, 14] The HSV can exist in a dynamic state of continuous low-level production of virus or in a static state with no production of infectious virus.[71] Most evidence to date supports the static-state theory of HSV latency.[72] In situ nucleic acid hybridization and immunofluorescence analysis of latently infected ganglia demonstrate the presence of latency-associated transcripts (RNA) and early nonstructural protein, VP175, respectively.[73–76] Late structural viral products and RNA transcripts from these gene regions are not detected. In addition to neuronal herpesviral latency, there is considerable evidence for a role of extraneuronal latency in herpetic keratitis. Sabbaga and coworkers[77] detected the continued presence of HSV nucleic acid sequences in corneal tissues after resolution of stromal disease in the rabbit.[77–79] In human keratoplasty samples, Rong and associates demonstrated the presence of HSV thymidine kinase and latency-associated transcript sequences by PCR amplifications.[80] Contributions of extraneuronal latent or persistent HSV infections to the HSV ocular disease pattern remain unclear. The fact that HSV can be detected in these nonneuronal cell types between periods of active clinical disease affords new possibilities for intervention and therapy of ocular HSV-induced disease.

The prevalence of HSV-1 infections increases gradually from childhood, reaching 80 to 90% by later adult years, whereas HSV-2 infection is typically acquired as a sexually transmitted disease. Transmission can result from direct contact with infected secretions from either a symptomatic or asymptomatic (but shedding) host. Preexisting infection with HSV-1 may modify the severity of HSV-2 infection. The classic presentation of primary HSV-1 is herpes gingivostomatitis with recurrences as orolabial infections. The most serious infection caused by HSV-1 is encephalitis. Other manifestations include the herpetic whitlow as well as conjunctivitis and epithelial and stromal keratitis. The classic presentation of a primary HSV-2 infection is herpes genitalis, which can subsequently lead to neonatal herpes. Asymptomatic shedding of these viruses occurs. HSV infections in the immunosuppressed can be severe, although HSV keratitis does not seem to be more severe or frequent.[81]

Triggers for reactivation of HSV are poorly understood. In the rabbit model of latent infection, neurosurgical manipulation, iontophoresis, intrastromal injection, and corneal trauma[82] are all mechanisms that have been demonstrated to induce reactivation of HSV. The reactivation mechanism common to all of these manipulations is unknown. Ocular pathology resulting from reactivation of HSV can cause the most severe ocular morbidity. Not all patients with HSV infections follow a similar clinical course. Two hypotheses have been advanced to explain the documented clinical differences. These include genetic viral strain differences, resulting in alterations in neurovirulence and pathogenicity, and variability in the host immune system response to the viral infection.

Support for the primary role of host immunogenetics and its containment of latent virus and response to reactivation is based on the observation that different inbred strains of mice had varied susceptibilities to ocular HSV-1 infection.[82] Also, the induction of cell-mediated immune tolerance to HSV-1 antigen in A/J mice prevented host T-cell hyperresponsiveness as the etiology of stromal keratitis in the murine model.[83] A variety of humoral and cell-mediated immune mechanisms are recruited in response to primary and recurrent HSV infections, including the production of various types of antibodies, the production of interferon, the activation of macrophages, the induction of T lymphocyte–mediated reactivity, and the development of both natural killer cell–dependent and antibody-dependent lymphocyte cytotoxicity.

The second hypothesis concerning the genetic properties proposes that the infecting virus strain can determine the reactivation rates and the clinical disease pattern. The patterns of reactivation of three different HSV-1 strains in inbred mice and the rate of HSV recurrence and clinical ocular disease severity depended on the virus strain.[84] In A/J mice infected with RE strain HSV-1, CD4 cells were preferentially activated in stromal disease states, whereas the KOS strain preferentially activated CD8 cells.[25] This work suggests that a complex interaction between viral genetics and the host immune system influences the clinical patterns of reactivated disease.

HSV grows rapidly and may be isolated in a wide variety of primate cell lines.[70, 85] Conventional cell culture is relatively rapid, with the majority of isolates detected within 1 to 3 days, and it is the most specific and sensitive diagnostic test available. Numerous methods to speed detection in cell culture or to facilitate detection of positive cultures include latex agglutination, fluorescence, immunoperoxidase, solid-phase and membrane ELISA, probe kits, and genetically engineered cell lines.[32, 34] Final viral identification after isolation may be made by neutralization testing, immunofluorescence, immunoperoxidase, or the ELISA.

Morphologic tests for the laboratory diagnosis of HSV include the Tzanck smear and EM.[34] The Tzanck smear is prepared by scraping the base of a vesicle and inoculating a microscopic slide. Syncytial giant cells may be detected with either Wright's or Giemsa's stain. Cowdry type A intranuclear inclusions stain poorly with Giemsa's but may be readily observed with Bouin's, Zenker's, H & E, or Papanicolaou's stain. These inclusions may also be observed during varicella-zoster ocular infection. Methods of direct examination of clinical material include immunoperoxidase, immunofluorescence staining, the ELISA (Surecell and Herpchek), and avidin-biotin enzyme conjugate assays;[86] reported sensitivities range from 50% to 100%. The combination of culture with the direct antigen EIA, Herpchek, yields the most rapid and sensitive diagnosis.[87] Direct test results are more likely to be positive in young, vesicular lesions. EM may be performed but does not distinguish between the various herpesviruses. The use of labels such as enzyme- or ferritin-tagged antibodies along with EM may allow the process to differentiate the various viruses. DNA hybridization techniques are available and allow for detection of HSV-1 and HSV-2 separately from varicella-zoster virus. The PCR is useful in the diagnosis of HSV encephalitis as well as ocular lesions.[51, 88]

A diagnosis of HSV on the basis of serology depends on the standard fourfold increase in antibody titers between acute and convalescent sera. Hemagglutination inhibition, complement-fixation, and neutralizing-antibody tests are routinely used. The recurrence of HSV disease often does not result in an increase in antibody titers. Titers may increase, however, during varicella-zoster viral reactivation. Acyclovir, valacyclovir, and famciclovir are available for systemic use against various clinical forms of HSV. For local ophthalmic use, trifluorothymidine is preferred, with alternatives being vidarabine or idoxuridine. Pharmaceutical companies are becoming resistant to producing the latter two ophthalmic preparations because of a limited market.

VARICELLA-ZOSTER VIRUS

Varicella-zoster virus (VZV), herpesvirus 3, is 150 to 200 nm in size with icosahedral symmetry and a nuclear membrane–derived envelope. Unlike in HSV, there is no documented antigenic variation among VZV strains; nonepidemiologically related strains may be differentiated with only one or two restriction enzymes.[89–91] VZV shares minor antigens with the HSV and major antigens with the other Herpesviridae that induce varicella-zoster–like syndromes in simian species.

Two human clinical syndromes, chickenpox and shingles (herpes zoster), are caused by VZV infection.[92, 93] Varicella-zoster infection typically occurs in childhood, but secondary herpes zoster is more commonly a disease of the sixth or seventh decade of life or in immunocompromised patients.[94, 95] Immunocompromised persons have a higher incidence of both chickenpox and shingles. The upper respiratory tract infection is initiated by droplet transmission of the virus. Local replication of VZV occurs in the respiratory epithelium, followed by a generalized viremia. During viremia, an exanthem called chickenpox results. It is also presumed that during viremia, sensory ganglia are seeded with VZV and a latent infection is established. Unlike HSV, VZV most probably reactivates sporadically throughout the life of the host based on the increases of circulating IgM levels against VZV in the absence of clinical disease. The second clinical syndrome caused by VZV, herpes zoster or shingles, is a reactivation of the initial latent viral infection. The fifth cranial nerve is the most frequently affected of the sensory nerve ganglia, with 7 to 21% of cases affecting the ophthalmic distribution. Ocular complications (herpes zoster ophthalmicus) are numerous because of the spread of the virus through the cranial sinus and adnexal tissues. Complications include blepharitis, conjunctivitis, scleritis, keratitis, uveitis, retinitis, and optic neuritis. It is currently accepted that cell-mediated immunity is responsible for maintaining VZV in a latent state, with antibodies to VZV persisting for life.[94] Herpes zoster is a frequent infection in persons with HIV infection. Although the occurrence of cutaneous dissemination is infrequent, complications such as VZV retinitis, acute retinal necrosis, and chronic progressive encephalitis have been reported, probably via the hematogenous route.[96] Unlike HSV, VZV cannot be cultured from explants of ganglia, although it can be demonstrated by EM and other antigenic or DNA detection modes, including the PCR.[97]

VZV isolates from ocular samples or lesion fluid are usually identified and verified as VZV by immunofluorescence or by viral neutralization. The Tzanck test with the Giemsa stain, Papanicolaou stain, or other techniques detects typical multinucleated giant cells and inclusions.[34] VZV is difficult to recover from clinical samples but can be isolated occasionally on human fibroblastic cell lines. Isolation of VZV is a relatively slow method and is often less sensitive than immunofluorescent staining of lesion material or EM, because infectious virus persists for a short time in vesicles and is more labile than viral particles and antigens. Specific identification of isolates can be accomplished by immunofluorescent staining and other methods of antigen detection such as the ELISA. The detection of VZV is always significant because, unlike the case with HSV, asymptomatic shedding of VZV does not appear to occur. VZV is more readily isolated from vesicular fluid aspirated from lesions located around the eye or on dermatome V-1. VZV-induced CPE is usually evident within 5 to 7 days post inoculation but may require up to 28 days. The shell vial assay reduces detection time to 48 hours and significantly increases sensitivity, identifying virus that fails to produce CPE in conventional cell culture. A comparison of fluorescent antibody of vesicle cells, conventional cell culture, and shell vial shows fluorescent antibody to be the most sensitive method for diagnosis.[98] Hybridization detection and PCR amplification techniques are being used to detect VZV.[99, 100]

Serologic techniques may also be used to detect rises in serum antibodies. Useful antibody assays include immune adherence hemagglutination, fluorescence antibody to membrane antigen, or the ELISA. The ELISA is capable of detecting IgG and IgM responses, is reliable for determining immune status, and is readily automated.[101] The presence of neutralizing antibodies is not protective against VZV reactivation or against clinical herpes zoster disease. A fourfold or greater increase in antibody titer to VZV in the absence of a similar rise to HSV antigen is diagnostic of a current VZV infection.[89] The demonstration of VZV IgM in serum is highly suggestive of acute VZV infection.

Three oral drugs are currently approved in the United States for treatment of herpes zoster in the normal host: acyclovir,[102] valacyclovir (prodrug of acyclovir),[103] and famciclovir (a prodrug of penciclovir).[104] Corticosteroids reduce the duration of acute neuritis but do not reduce the incidence or duration of post-herpetic neuralgia.[105, 106] Immunocompromised patients who develop herpes zoster should be treated with intravenous acyclovir. Despite the lack of data from large-scale controlled trials, the safety and efficacy of intravenous acyclovir have led to its acceptance as the drug of choice for varicella in immunocompromised patients. For immunocompetent children, supportive care alone is recommended by most infectious disease experts.[93] A live, attenuated varicella vaccine was approved for use in the United States in 1995, the long-term results of which are awaited.[107]

CYTOMEGALOVIRUS

CMV is a large DNA member of the family Herpesviridae. Infection with CMV results in a variety of disorders that depend largely on the immune status of the host. CMV persists in the body of the host, resulting in latency. Little is known about the localization of latent CMV.[108] It is a ubiquitous herpesvirus that usually results in asymptomatic infection but can cause a variety of diseases ranging from congenital, perinatal, acquired, disseminated CMV infection to severe chronic infection in immunocompromised persons.[61, 109, 110] It is a recognized cause of CMV mononucleosis in normal immunocompetent subjects. The prevalence of antibodies to CMV varies and is related to socioeconomic status. CMV can be transmitted from an infected maternal carrier, from donor organs to organ transplant recipients, from exposure to infected saliva or urine, and via sexual activity in adulthood.[61]

The sites of latency of CMV are not precisely known, but they probably include the circulating peripheral mononuclear cells and possibly polymorphonuclear leukocytes. Until the explosive rise in iatrogenically immunosuppressed transplant organ recipients and the epidemic due to infection with HIV, the major complication associated with CMV infection was intrauterine infection that resulted in severe and usually fatal congenital abnormalities. More recently, CMV retinitis, an ocular sign of disseminated CMV infection, has become a major problem and is the most common cause of blindness among patients with AIDS[109, 111, 112]; the CD4 lymphocyte count is usually less than 50 per mm^3. The virus has been cultured from the aqueous or vitreous humor, although this is not essential for the diagnosis. It is also seen in transplant patients and in cancer patients receiving immunosuppressive drugs. Laboratory investigations of CMV infections have been severely hindered by the lack of an animal model of human CMV infection. Current models of CMV infection use species-specific strains of CMV, either murine or guinea pig, that induce different pathologies and have different antiviral sensitivity profiles.[113, 114] A reproducible model of human CMV retinitis in the rabbit was developed that successfully evaluated anti-CMV therapeutic agents.[115]

Symptomatic clinical infection with CMV in immunocompromised patients may result in decreased cell-mediated immunity, pneumonitis, hepatitis, and adrenalitis as well as retinitis. CMV infection results in necrotizing retinitis with severe visual loss. Several investigators have found concurrent infection with CMV and HIV in the same cell. The atypical and aggressive nature of CMV infection in patients with HIV infection suggests that HIV may potentiate CMV infection. Histologically, CMV retinitis destroys all layers of the retina, and both intranuclear and intracytoplasmic inclusions can be observed.

Increased recognition of the clinical importance of CMV infection has led to a demand for rapid, reliable methods for detection of current and previous CMV infection.[116] Diagnostic methods have increased exponentially.[117] CMV infection is diagnosed by virus recovery from tissue or fluid samples on susceptible human fibroblast cell monolayers. CMV produces CPE in diploid fibroblast cells in 3 to 28 days, with an average of 7 days. Shell vial for CMV has a sensitivity equivalent to conventional cell culture but takes only 16 hours to complete.[118] During infection with CMV, the virus can be present in the urine, oropharynx, peripheral leukocytes, and tear film. Cytopathic effect is characterized by large, swollen, rounded cells, occasionally clumped with intranuclear inclusions. More rapid diagnostic techniques, such as diagnostic cytology and EM, may be more clinically useful. Serology, including neutralization tests, complement fixation tests, and ELISA detection, is useful in diagnosing CMV infection and can be used in the analysis of acute and convalescent sera. The presence of virus-specific IgM or a fourfold increase in IgG antibodies may indicate disease. PCR methods have been used as well as labeled, cloned, viral nucleic acid probes.[119–121] An antigenemia immunoassay uses monoclonal antibody to detect CMV protein in peripheral blood leukocytes.[122, 123] This assay requires only 3 to 5 hours to complete; its clinical utility must be further established.[124]

Interpretation of the results of specimens containing CMV is most difficult. Primary CMV infection is usually asymptomatic and is commonly followed by silent reactivation of the latent virus throughout the patient's life. On the other hand, CMV disease in immunocompromised patients can be life-threatening. Detection of CMV in urine or respiratory secretions, however, is not diagnostic of significant disease. Detection of CMV in uncontaminated tissue, such as the lung or the eyes, or in blood collected by venipuncture suggests an active role in disease.

Antivirals such as ganciclovir, cidofovir, and foscarnet are useful in the treatment of CMV retinitis but require lifetime treatment. Local treatment includes intravitreal ganciclovir injections and implants, intravitreal foscarnet, or intravitreal cidofovir.[125] CMV immunoglobulin is protective against primary infection when administered to transplant patients who receive organs from infected donors.[126, 127] Live attenuated CMV vaccines that do not induce a chronic or latent CMV infection have been developed and are currently being evaluated.

EPSTEIN-BARR VIRUS

The Epstein-Barr virus (EBV), human herpesvirus 4, is an icosahedral double-stranded DNA virus. In vivo infection of lymphocytes by EBV leads to their transformation into lymphoblastoid cell lines capable of continuous growth in culture.[128–130] EBV is distinguished from other herpesviruses by its ability to immortalize these B lymphocytes. These immortalized B cells contain the EBV genome as an episome in a latent state and persistently express EBV nuclear antigen. Immortalization of B lymphocytes is a complex process that involves a coordinated interplay among a number of viral and host gene products.[131] The infection can reactivate throughout the life of the host, usually in response to immunosuppression. Latent virus can be activated by stimulation of host B cells by chemicals or by antibodies to surface immunoglobulin.[131] There are two strains of EBV, and coinfection with both strains is possible. The fate of EBV following infection of human cells depends on the particular type of cell infected and the pattern of gene transcription used by the virus.[130]

There are two major consequences of EBV infection of B lymphocytes, depending on whether the active or passive latent transcriptional program is activated. If the active latent transcription program is used, B cells are growth-transformed into lymphoblasts. The passive transcriptional program is used by the virus after infecting small resting B cells. This sets the stage for lifelong persistence in immunocompetent hosts. In contrast with that of B cells, EBV infection of epithelial cells is a more complicated issue.[130] Depending on the type of epithelial cell infected and the state of cellular differentiation, either a latent persistent infection may ensue or a lytic infection may occur with release of infectious viral particles. The EBV is a ubiquitous virus, with 90% of adults demonstrating antibodies to EBV by the third decade of life following a subclinical infection.[2] In lower socioeconomic groups, infection typically occurs in childhood; in higher socioeconomic groups, infection occurs in adolescents and young adults. EBV manifests low contagiousness, and most cases of infectious mononucleosis are probably contracted by intimate contact between susceptible individuals and asymptomatic shedders of EBV. Infection with EBV is typically asymptomatic. Infectious mononucleosis is most commonly caused by EBV; about 10 to 20% of cases are caused by CMV. EBV usually initiates infection in the oropharyngeal epithelium. An active infection ensues that can persist for years in mucosa-associated lymphoid tissue.[132] No shedding into the tears has been detected.

The ocular complications of EBV include conjunctivitis, epithelial (including dendritic) and stromal (nummular) keratitis, optic neuritis, retinitis, and uveitis. Accumulating evidence suggests that EBV plays a significant role in Sjögren's syndrome and possibly in the iridocorneal endothelial syndrome.[132, 133] This virus is also associated with 90 to 95% of endemic Burkitt's lymphoma and with nasopharyngeal carcinoma. EBV has also been implicated in other tumors, including oral hairy leukoplakia, a subset of Hodgkin's lymphoma, a subset of large cell lymphoma, a subset of peripheral T-cell lymphoma, and a subset of gastric carcinomas.[134]

Serum antibodies to EBV viral capsid antigen and nuclear antigen are produced for the life of the host (Table 16–4).[129] Among the most sensitive methods of detecting EBV infection is immunofluorescent staining of peripheral lymphocytes and detection of the Epstein-Barr nuclear antigen (EBNA) or the Epstein-Barr viral capsid antigen (EBVCA). Patients with acute infectious mononucleosis have elevated IgG and IgM antibodies against EBVCA. Persistent antibodies against EBNA become detectable several weeks or months after the onset of clinical disease and remain detectable for life. The presence of elevated EBVCA IgG or IgM antibodies in association with rising EBNA antibodies is diagnostic of recent EBV infection. Elevated EBVCA IgM antibodies with nondetectable EBNA antibodies is also consistent with a primary EBV infection. An increase in VCA antibodies is a sensitive marker of ongoing infection. From the titers and profile of antibodies to EBVCA, EBNA, and early antigen in the acute phase serum, the patient can be classified as susceptible, immune (with past infection), or having a primary infection (see Table 16–4).[128] In the presence of EBNA antibodies, early-antigen antibodies suggest a reactivated past infection. Activation of corneal disease from EBV is not correlated with a rise in EBV antibody titers. The heterophile agglutination test is less specific and less reliable; these are IgM antibodies that react with antigenic horse and sheep blood cells. Most EBV-infected patients with clinical mononucleosis develop antibodies that agglutinate sheep red blood cells (monospot test). A rapid immunochromato-

TABLE 16–4. **Serologic Responses of Patients With Epstein-Barr Virus–Associated Diseases**

Antibody to Antigen	Susceptible (Nonimmune)	Primary Infection	Reactivation Infection	Past Infection	Burkett's Lymphoma	Nasopharyngeal Cancer
IgG VCA	−	+	+	+	+ + +	+ + +
IgM VCA	−	+	−	−	−	−
IgA VCA	−	+	?	−	−	−
IgG EA/D	−	(+)	(+)	−	−	+ + +
IgA EA/D	−	?	?	−	−	+ + +
IgG EA/R	−	−	(±)	−	+ + +	(±)
Anti-EBNA (Raji)	−	−	+	+	+	+ + +

+, Detectable at ≥1 : 5; −, not detectable at <1 : 5; + + +, detectable at high titer; (+), present in ~80% of patients; ±, detectable at low titer; (±), present in ~30% of patients; ?, unknown.

graphic test has been shown to accurately detect infectious mononucleosis-associated heterophile antibodies.[135] Isolation of EBV (in cultured B lymphocytes) is not routinely performed in clinical laboratories. EBV DNA has been detected by the PCR method in various ocular tissues (10% of normal corneal epithelium and 32% of normal lacrimal gland);[136] the significance remains unknown.

Treatment of EBV infections is largely supportive. Acyclovir has not been demonstrated to be of sufficient clinical benefit in uncomplicated infections.[131, 137] A vaccine is being studied.[138]

HUMAN HERPESVIRUS TYPE 8

Kaposi's sarcoma is a previously rare, tumor-like lesion of controversial biologic nature. It has since the early 1980s become frequent in patients with AIDS, particularly homosexuals. Kaposi's sarcoma is also endemic in Central Africa, predominantly in otherwise healthy men but also in women and children. Herpesvirus DNA sequences have been noted in more than 95% of AIDS Kaposi lesions by PCR techniques and Southern blot analysis. The same herpesvirus-like DNA sequences are present in AIDS-associated Kaposi's sarcoma, classic Kaposi's sarcoma, and the Kaposi's sarcoma that occurs in HIV-negative homosexual men, suggesting the virus is a causal agent and not merely an opportunistic infection.[139] These same DNA sequences occur in an unusual subgroup of AIDS-related B-cell lymphomas, but not in any other lymphoid neoplasm, suggesting a pathogenic role in AIDS-related body-cavity lymphomas.[140, 141] These Kaposi-associated herpesvirus-like sequences appear to define a new human herpesvirus (human herpesvirus type 8).[142] The virus has also been isolated and propagated.[143, 144] The virus has also been demonstrated in peripheral blood mononuclear cells of HIV-infected patients.[145]

Adenoviruses

Family: Adenoviridae
Genus: Mastadenovirus
Human Adenovirus

Adenoviruses are nonenveloped, double-stranded DNA viruses with an icosahedral shape, capable of constructing 10 structural proteins. They replicate in the cell nucleus and tend to be host-specific.[146, 147] They produce a characteristic CPE that is accompanied by accumulation of antigenic components in the host cell culture fluids. In each virion there are 252 capsomeres, 240 hexons, and 12 pentons. Each penton has a rodlike fiber that projects outward a variable length with a terminal knob.[146] The fibers are responsible for hemagglutination and are used in the classification of the various adenoviral types. There are 47 known human serotypes, divided into seven groups based on genome homology. Within an adenoviral type there is 90% genomic homology compared with 20% interadenoviral type homology. Adenoviruses constitute two genera: the Aviadenovirus that infects birds, and the Mastadenovirus that infects mammals. Human adenoviruses have the ability to transform cells in culture, and some of the serotypes, particularly type A adenoviruses, are capable of inducing tumors in neonatal hamsters. The oncogenic potential of adenoviruses in humans has not been demonstrated. Adenovirus has become one of the preferred vectors for DNA transfer into mammalian cells and is being intensively studied for gene therapy into several different human organs.[148]

Replication is initiated by adenoviral fiber-mediated attachment to the host cell surface. The virion penetrates the cell and is uncoated in the cell nucleus. Like many DNA viruses, adenoviral replication is divided into early and late transcription and protein synthesis. Early transcription occurs at seven regions of the genome, involving both strands of the DNA. These transcripts are translated into 20 primary nonstructural proteins. At the conclusion of early replication events, there is simultaneous replication of viral DNA in the nucleus and late transcription of structural proteins. Assembly of the virion occurs in the cytoplasm, where hexon and penton capsomers are formed. Capsid formation and insertion of DNA occur in the nucleus. Viral particles lyse the cell.[149]

Adenoviruses are highly epitheliotropic and have a narrow host range; they have been recovered from virtually every organ system. Adenovirus illnesses are endemic throughout the year and occur in all age groups. They cause localized outbreaks of respiratory disease in the winter and spring, outbreaks of swimming pool–associated pharyngoconjunctival fever in the summer, and epidemics of keratoconjunctivitis associated with industrial eye trauma or ophthalmologic procedures. Adenovirus causes gastroenteritis in young children and epidemics of acute respiratory disease in new military recruits and is also an increasing problem in the immunocompromised host.[150]

In ocular disease, transmission is mainly through direct contact with infected material. In children, adenovirus appears most frequently as pharyngoconjunctival fever characterized by conjunctivitis, pharyngitis, rhinitis, cervical adenitis, and temperatures to 38°C.[151] It is common in children's summer camps; contaminated swimming pools are implicated in spread of this disease, with most studies showing type 3 or 7 as the causative agents. It begins as a monocular infection followed by binocular involvement. Some limited serotype differences have been demonstrated in infectivity titers and clinical course.[152] Keratoconjunctivitis occurring in an epidemic form in adult populations has been associated with types 8, 19, and 37 most frequently.[151] This conjunctivitis may be insidious in onset. Keratitis begins as the conjunctivitis wanes, and the cornea may remain involved for several months, producing a visual disturbance. Secondary spread occurs in household contacts and in ophthalmologists' offices. The virus can be isolated readily for at least 9 days after the onset of symptoms. The virus can survive in a desiccated state for many days, potentially contributing to its spread.[153] Adenovirus can cause a form of acute hemorrhagic conjunctivitis (type 11 or 21).

Immunity to adenovirus is lifelong with type-specific immunity; maternal antibodies confer protective immunity for the first 6 months of life. Adenoviruses may be isolated in cell culture on human embryonic kidney, HeLa (human cervical carcinoma), or HEp-2 (human laryngeal tumor) cell lines. The typical cytopathologic effect of adenoviral infection includes rounded and swollen cells with acidification of the cell culture. Adenoviruses can be detected directly in clinical specimens by rapid tests that measure their common, group-specific hexon antigen. Fluorescent antibody tests are fast, convenient, and qualitative. The ELISA (Adenoclone), radioimmunoassays, and time-resolved fluoroimmunoassays are somewhat less convenient and vary in their specificity.[146, 154] For serotyping, the virus must be grown out in cell culture and typed by hemagglutination inhibition and neutralization tests with hyperimmune type-specific antisera. Restriction enzyme analysis is used to measure adenovirus interrelationships.[150] Serology of acute and convalescent sera with complement fixation, neutralization testing, and hemagglutination inhibition can be performed. A diagnosis of adenoviral infection is based on a fourfold increase in antibody titer from acute to convalescent sera.

No specific treatment for adenovirus infection is available, although cidovovir holds promise. Many natural and synthetic products have been tried, including thymic humoral factors, pooled IgG, and vaccines. The best strategies are those of prevention and containment of outbreaks in ophthalmology clinics.[155]

Human Immunodeficiency Virus

Family: Retroviridae
  Subfamily: Lentivirinae
    Genus: Lentivirus
      Human immunodeficiency virus types 1 and 2
    Genus: HTLV-BLV group
      Human T-cell lymphocyte virus types 1 and 2

The HIVs are classified in the family Retroviridae and genus Lentivirinae. As may be assumed by their name, they are characterized by long incubation and latency times.[156] HIV has a positive-sense RNA genome and, by EM, a cylindrically shaped core. The virion is 80 to 130 nm in diameter and has a unique three-layered structure. Like other retroviruses, HIV contains a virus capsid, the single-stranded RNA genome, and the viral enzyme protease, reverse transcriptase, and integrase. HIV isolates show genetic variability, resulting from the relatively low fidelity of reverse transcripts in conjunction with the extremely high turnover of virions in vivo.[157, 158] In 1986, a subcommittee of the International Committee on Taxonomy of Viruses recommended that this new subfamily of viruses variously called lymphadenopathy-associated virus, HTLV-III, or AIDS-associated retrovirus be named human immunodeficiency virus.

The lentiviruses are characterized by tropism for cells of hematopoietic or neurologic origin and by the ability to induce immune system suppression.[159–161] There are two genetically distinct forms of HIV: HIV-1 is the viral type most frequently encountered in the United States and Europe and results in severe clinical disease; HIV-2 has approximately 55% homology with HIV-1 and appears to be prevalent only in western Africa and has a much less virulent clinical course.[162–164] Interestingly, HIV-2 is more closely related to the macaque simian immunodeficiency virus than HIV-1 is. These two viruses share 75% nucleic acid homology.[165] All genomes contain the three genes common to all retroviruses: *gag*, *pol*, and *env* genes. HIV-2 is less efficient at being transmitted sexually and at being transmitted vertically. The viral load in persons infected with this virus is much lower than that found in persons infected with HIV-1.

The HIV envelope is cell membrane–derived and contains transmembrane glycoproteins gp41 and gp120, which are important in HIV adherence and penetration.[166–168] The viral gp120 binds to the CD4 receptors on human T lymphocytes, and gp41 is required for fusion.[169] There is a poorly defined host cell fusion receptor that is required for entry of the HIV into the host cell. Therefore, some human T cells express CD4 but presumably not the fusion receptor. After penetration of the virus into the host cell, the virus uncoats, and viral RNA is transcribed to DNA via reverse transcriptase. The HIV DNA integrates itself into the host cell genome and begins virus-encoded protein production. Assembly of virions occurs in the host cell cytoplasm, and complete virions escape the host cell by budding through the cell membrane. The HIV may also remain latent within the cell, integrated into the host genome. In this state, the viral nucleic acid produces little or no messenger RNA.[170] There is evidence that the virus evades immune pressure by the continuous production of new mutants resistant to current immunologic attack, resulting in the accumulation of antigenic diversity during the asymptomatic period.[171]

The World Health Organization estimates that 30 million adults and 10 million children throughout the world will be HIV-infected by the year 2000, the majority being in developing countries. HIV is transmitted by three routes: intimate sexual contact, exchange of contaminated blood, and from mother to fetus or to infant. The cell-free titer in saliva, urine, and milk is at least 10-fold less than that in plasma. The largest group of persons infected with HIV are exposed through unprotected sexual contact, with differences depending on sexual preferences. Intravenous drug users have experienced an explosive increase in numbers; transmission through accidental needle sticks remains very low because of the volume of virus involved. Newborns of infected mothers are at risk, as are blood transfusion recipients. At present there is no vaccine to protect a person from HIV infection, and there are no curative therapies.

There is great heterogeneity within HIV-1, and this heterogeneity makes the synthesis of a vaccine problematic.[172, 173] Diversity among HIV isolates may account for differences in the clinical expression of AIDS. The time from infection with HIV to onset of clinical disease varies from several months to 10 or more years, and the stimulus for activation of HIV from a latent to productive state is unknown. There is also evidence that a single strain of HIV may, over the course of infection, mutate toward greater virulence. This may account, in part, for the gradually progressive nature of the clinical disease.[174, 175] The consequences of the CD4 receptor for HIV adherence are selective infection of helper T cells and the development of severe immunodeficiency.

HIV infects a wide variety of tissues in humans, including bone marrow, lymph node, blood, brain, skin, and bowel and is associated with persistent infections in some tissues.[176] The outcome of this infection depends on the particular viral strain, and the susceptibility can vary depending on the target cell. Lentiviruses in general are associated with a number of diseases that have long incubation periods and involve the hematopoietic and CNS. HIV infection in humans can lead to a variety of disease states, including an acute mononucleosis-like syndrome, prolonged asymptomatic infection, a symptomatic state, and AIDS. The distinctive symptoms of acute infection include lymphadenopathy, macular rash, fever, myalgia, arthralgia, headache, fatigue, diarrhea, sore throat, and neurologic manifestations. Progression from HIV infection to AIDS differs among different populations. It appears that in the absence of treatment, an estimated 50% of infected persons will progress to AIDS within 10 years after infection. The most common reported clinical symptoms predictive for progression to AIDS are persistent herpes zoster infections, oral candidiasis, oral hairy leukoplakia, and constitutional symptoms such as sustained weight loss, fatigue, night sweats, and persistent diarrhea (AIDS-related complex). Other AIDS-predicting symptoms include vulvovaginal candidiasis, moderate or severe cervical dysplasia, and pelvic inflammatory disease. AIDS-defining diseases and symptoms include Kaposi's sarcoma, *Pneumocystis carinii* pneumonia, chronic diarrhea often caused by cryptosporidia, cryptococcal meningitis, toxoplasmosis, encephalopathies and dementia, CMV retinitis, esophageal candidiasis, anal-rectal carcinomas, B-lymphocytic lymphomas, pulmonary tuberculosis, recurrent pneumonia, and invasive cervical cancer (Table 16–5). Other classifications include $CD4^+$ T-lymphocyte percentages of less than 14.

HIV has been isolated from the aqueous as well as from tears, conjunctiva, cornea, iris, and retina.[177] In addition to multiple opportunistic infections with various pathogens, including herpesvirus, *P. carinii,* and *Treponema pallidum,* neurologic abnormalities are found in 60% or more of patients with AIDS.[111, 178–181] Forty to 95% of patients with AIDS develop ocular manifestations.[112] HIV may occasionally contribute to nonspecific intraocular inflammation (e.g., iridocyclitis) or serve as a contributing factor in the pathogenesis of secondary disorders. The microvasculopathy in HIV-infected patients results in cotton-wool spots and retinal hemorrhages. The virus may act as a cofactor in CMV retinopathy, being found in the same retinal cells at autopsy. The secondary infections of the eye tend to be severe and associated with significant morbidity and mortality. The spectrum of opportunistic infections is shown in Table 16–5. CMV is by far the most common severe infection. Dual infection of the retina with HIV and CMV has been reported by several investigators, and a possible potentiating interaction between the viruses that influences the clinical course of retinal disease has been raised.[182] The frequency of varicella-zoster retinopathy is increasing. Toxoplasmic retinochoroiditis is common in Europe and South America. The remaining infections usually occur only with overwhelming disseminated infections late in the syndrome and signal further waning of immune defenses.[183] External ocular infections are less common, perhaps because of the natural defenses locally. Any anatomic defect or contact lens wear presents risk factors. Kaposi's sarcoma appears to be a herpesvirus-induced neoplasm common in AIDS patients.

TABLE 16–5. **Spectrum of Ocular Infections in HIV-Infected Patients**

External ocular infections
Staphylococcus species
Pseudomonas species
Capnocytophaga species
Herpes simplex virus
Varicella-zoster virus
Molluscum contagiosum
Microsporidia
Candida albicans
Chlamydia trachomatis (lymphogranuloma venereum)
Intraocular infections
Endogenous bacteria
Nocardia species
Cytomegalovirus
Herpes simplex virus
Varicella-zoster virus
Toxoplasma gondii
Pneumocystis carinii
Candida albicans
Fusarium species
Histoplasma capsulatum
Sporotrichum schenckii
Cryptococcus neoformans
Bipolaris hawaiiensis
Treponema pallidum
Mycobacterium avium complex
M. tuberculosis

HIV infection can be diagnosed by viral isolation, nucleic acid detection, or serology. All of these tests have limitations.[184] Important caveats to HIV detection are (1) the time period between the time of infection with culture positivity and conversion to seropositivity, and (2) the fact that IgM detection is not reliable even in determining congenital HIV infection. Serodiagnosis is the primary means of detecting HIV infections, both for the screening of blood donors and in the evaluation of symptomatic persons. The serologic diagnosis of HIV infection relies on sensitive screening tests such as the enzyme immunoassay for IgG antibodies to HIV that uses viral lysate or recombinant proteins and the antigen material. Identification of antibody to HIV glycoproteins is also useful in the diagnosis. If a sample is reactive, the sample is repeated. Although the ELISA is extremely sensitive for HIV, positive results are confirmed by Western blot, immunoprecipitation assays, or indirect immunofluorescence. The current ELISAs have lower specificity, primarily because the viral antigen is contaminated with host cell antigens, and patients with a variety of autoimmune diseases may show reactivity. The Western blot confirmatory test is more specific because of the possible antigenic differentiation based on the size of the HIV proteins to which the serum reacts. The Western blot identifies antibody specific for several HIV antigens. Antibody to HIV p24 and either gp41 or gp160 also confirms HIV infection.[185] HIV-1 and HIV-2, and human T-cell lymphocyte virus 1 immune status tests (ELISA), are used to screen units of blood for donation. Units with a positive HIV-1 screening result are confirmed as positive with the Western blot test.

In patients in whom serologic results are inconclusive, viral isolation and detection of viral nucleic acid by the PCR may be the most reliable means of diagnosis.[186] The PCR is currently a sensitive method for detecting HIV antigen, although false-positive results are a laboratory dilemma. The PCR is useful for the newborn population, who may have maternal HIV antibody confounding interpretation of serology tests, and for all patients who may not produce detectable antibody for months following primary infection.[187] The definitive test for active infection is the recovery of HIV from cells or cell-free fluids. Primary viral isolation from patient material depends on the level of HIV expressed. Viral isolation can take up to 4 to 5 weeks and is somewhat demanding. Viral culture requires cocultivation of peripheral blood mononuclear cells with phytohemagglutin-stimulated peripheral blood mononuclear cells from cord blood of an uninfected adult. Growth may be determined by solid-phase assay (e.g., ELISA) of cell culture supernatant for HIV p24 antigen. There are currently no HIV serotypes, but there are numerous HIV genotypes.

Direct or indirect immunofluorescence tests of HIV-infected cells have all been successful; they are not sensitive enough to directly detect the low numbers of infected lymphocytes in the peripheral blood. The ELISA for p24 antigen has been useful for detecting viral protein in cell culture supernatant and for detecting p24 protein in serum from infected persons but is of limited diagnostic utility because of its low sensitivity and predictive value.[188] EM can show the infected lymphocytes with HIV budding from the cell membrane as well as revealing the condensed cylindrical core. Immune EM has not been useful.

Laboratory testing is also useful to predict the risk of developing AIDS among asymptomatic seropositive patients. The single most useful measure of prognosis is the number of $CD4^+$ helper T lymphocytes in the peripheral blood; it is useful in determining patient eligibility for antiretroviral therapy, predicting disease progression, and monitoring disease activity. Current serologic tests may not be able to detect HIV during the incubation phase. Antibodies to HIV can be detected within 2 to 6 weeks of exposure but may take longer.

Currently, the only form of prevention is the avoidance of high-risk behaviors. HIV is inactivated by 10-minute exposure to 10% bleach (sodium hypochlorite), 50% ethanol, 35% isopropanol, 0.5% Lysol, 0.5% paraformaldehyde, or 0.3% hydrogen peroxide. Therapy is recommended based on $CD4^+$ cell count, plasma HIV RNA level, or clinical status. Preferred initial drug regimens include nucleoside combinations; at present, protease inhibitors are best reserved for patients at higher progression risk. For treatment failures or drug intolerance, subsequent regimens are determined by multiple factors.[189, 190] Using the phenomenon of "resistance reversal," in which resistance mutations to one drug reverse the effect of resistance mutations to another drug, researchers have identified promising combinations of antiretrovirals for clinical use.[191]

Human Papillomaviruses

Family: Papovaviridae
Genus: Papillomavirus
Human papillomavirus

The human papillomavirus (HPV) is a 45- to 55-nm nonenveloped icosahedral structure. It has a double-stranded circular DNA genome complexed with low-molecular-weight histones of cellular origin. The viral DNA constitutes 12% of the virion weight and consists of approximately 8000 base pairs with a molecular weight of 5.2×10^6 Da. The major capsid protein is 57 kDa, and there is also at least one minor capsid protein of 70 kDa. The major capsid protein represents 80% of the total viral protein. Genomic structure is similar among the various genus-specific papillomaviruses.[192] The viral genome is divided into early, late, and regulatory regions. The early region is 4.5 kb and consists of eight open reading frames that are necessary for transformation. The late region is 2.5 kb and controls transcription and replication.[193] There are approximately 70 distinct types of HPVs.[194–196] The genus-specific antigen is on the major capsid protein; however, serologic reagents are not yet available to distinguish all 70 types of HPVs. Thus, HPV types are not true serotypes but are type distinctions based on viral genome relatedness. A virus that has less than 50% duplex formation with other known viral types by liquid phase hybridization analysis is considered to represent a unique type. It is important to recognize that percent homology is a relative figure that does not parallel nucleic acid homology. An example is HPV-6 and HPV-11, which have 82% nucleotide homology yet 25% duplex formation in liquid reassociation analysis.

Papillomaviruses are widespread throughout nature, are genus-specific, and are generally found among higher vertebrates. Replication is tightly linked to squamous epithelial cell differentiation, with viral capsids being produced only in terminally differentiated squamous cells; therefore, traditional techniques for culturing cannot be used.[197, 198] HPV is highly tropic for epithelial cells of the skin and mucous membranes. These viruses have been found in association with warts, dysplasias, and carcinomas of the male and female genital tracts and conjunctiva.[196, 199, 200] Cutaneous areas are commonly infected by HPVs 1, 2, 3, and 4, whereas mucosal sites are most frequently infected by HPVs 6, 11, 16, and 18. Because papillomaviruses have never been successfully propagated in cell culture, these viruses cannot be studied by standard virologic techniques. Most knowledge about papillomaviruses has been obtained from recent advances in molecular biologic analysis of this viral infection. These techniques have led to an understanding of the genomic organization of these viruses, the functions of different viral genes, and the multiplicity of HPV types.

Three types of cutaneous HPV infections are widespread throughout the general population: plantar warts, common warts, and juvenile (flat) warts. Condyloma acuminatum, or anogenital wart, is the most common viral sexually transmitted disease in the United States and is increasing in incidence. Transmission from mothers to children during childbirth can rarely result in laryngeal papillomatosis.[197] The majority of HPV infections are self-limited, but it is clear that malignant tumors develop in a subset of infections that involve oncogenic viruses.[201] Histologic findings associated with HPV infection include acanthosis, hyperplasma, and koilocytosis, a nuclear pyknosis with cytoplasmic clearing. Viral antigen has been detected in lesions ranging from papillomas to dysplasia and invasive carcinoma. Grouping of HPVs can be based on clinical behavior.[196] The largest body of clinical literature is in gynecology, where HPV-16 and HPV-18 have been associated with a high risk for malignant transformation, HPV-31 has been associated with an intermediate risk, and HPV-6 and HPV-11 have been associated with a low risk. More than 90% of cervical cancers contain HPV DNA; the same types are also found in the precursor lesions, cervical intraepithelial neoplasias, with the genome being expressed.[202] A direct epidemiologic link is difficult to establish, and other cofactors may be involved in cervical cancer as well as other genitourinary cancers or in oral, laryngeal, and esophageal cancers. It appears that HPV DNA in benign keratocytic lesions from low-risk types rarely inserts in the host genome but exists as a self-replicating extrachromosomal episomal plasmid, whereas in severe dysplasia and carcinoma associated with high-risk HPV types, the HPV DNA shifts from a normal monomeric to a multimeric state, and this is associated with host DNA aneuploidy.[203, 204] Moreover, neoplasia is the result not simply of viral DNA insertion or its site of insertion, but of insertion of the viral DNA into the host genome with concurrent disruption of the open reading frame.[205] HPV diseases occur more frequently and are often severe in patients with both primary and secondary immunodeficiencies.[206]

In the conjunctiva, HPV can induce papillomatous lesions and epithelial dysplastic lesions consistent with conjunctival intraepithelial neoplasia and squamous cell carcinoma. Conjunctival papillomas can be pedunculated or sessile and are typically shiny, flesh-colored, and papillomatous. The epithelial dysplastic lesions usually begin at the limbus and appear gelatinous, gray, or hazy. Eyelid papillomas have the typical appearance of skin warts with a flesh-colored, papillomatous surface. Hyperkeratotic scaling is common. Dysplastic and squamous cell carcinomas of the eyelids typically show elevated flesh-colored lesions with hyperkeratosis and abnormal vasculature. McDonnell and associates detected HPV antigens in 8.2% of unilateral dysplastic and malignant squamous conjunctival lesions.[207] Odrich and coworkers have described three cases of bilateral conjunctival dysplasia or carcinoma in which HPV DNA was detected.[208] The exact role of HPV in conjunctival squamous carcinoma has yet to be defined.[209–212]

The diagnosis of HPV infection depends on morphologic identification by EM and viral nucleic acid detection. Immunoperoxidase techniques can be performed; however, viral antigens present in benign HPV-associated lesions are notably absent in intraepithelial neoplasia and invasive carcinoma, so the correct antigen must be probed. Nucleic acid hybridization is generally performed by Southern blotting with a ^{32}P-labeled probe or by in situ hybridization.[213] The PCR is sensitive but may not be specific in the evaluation of genitourinary tumors. HPV infection may elicit a serologic response; this disappears with disease resolution, with the significance remaining unknown.[214] At present, with our limited understanding of the natural history, transmission, and risk of development of malignancy associated with HPV infection, the relevance of detecting HPV DNA is unclear.[197]

The treatment of periocular HPV-induced lesions is with surgical excision or local destruction, including cryotherapy, cautery, chemical agents, keratolysis, or radiation. Special surgical modalities include the argon and carbon dioxide laser. Chemotherapeutic efforts include 5-fluorouracil or mitomycin, or retinoic acid. Immunotherapy with interferon or dinitrochlorobenzene has been tried.[196]

Poxviruses

Family: Poxviridae
  Subfamily: Chordopoxvirinae
    Genus: Orthopoxvirus
      Vaccinia virus
      Smallpox virus (variola)
    Genus: Molluscipoxvirus
      Molluscum contagiosum virus

The poxviruses are the largest and most complex of all animal viruses.[215] Poxviral replication is unique in that it occurs entirely in the host cytoplasm, producing eosinophilic inclusions called Guarnieri bodies. Its composition of 3% DNA, 90% protein, and 5% lipid is more similar to that of bacteria than that of viruses. The viral genome is large and encodes more than 100 polypeptides.[216] The most important of the Poxviridae are the variola, vaccinia, and the molluscum contagiosum viruses.[217]

Replication begins with fusion into the cytoplasm via host phagocytic vacuoles.[218] Viral RNA polymerase is present and transcribes about one-half of the viral genome into early mRNA. Protein products of early mRNA include an enzyme that completes uncoating of the core, DNA polymerase, thymidine kinase, and various other enzymes.[219] After uncoating is completed, at 1.5 to 6 hours post infection, DNA synthesis occurs and host macromolecular synthesis is inhibited. The viral genome is then transcribed, but only late mRNAs are translated to structural proteins. Areas of nucleic acid replication within the cytoplasm are called inclusion bodies.

Assembly of the virion is a complex process. Poxviruses synthesize viral membranes de novo, although some viral particles bud through the host membrane. Infectivity depends on the viral, not the host-derived, membrane.[220]

VARIOLA VIRUS AND VACCINIA VIRUS

The variola virus is the poxvirus responsible for smallpox. A severe systemic infection with a 2 to 40% mortality rate, smallpox has the ophthalmic complication of corneal lesions with secondary bacterial infection and corneal scarring. The World Health Organization has declared that smallpox has been eradicated since 1977.

The vaccinia virus is an orthopoxvirus used for vaccination against smallpox infection. The origin of the vaccinia virus is unclear; it is thought to be either a mutation of the cowpox or smallpox virus or a viral descendent of a now-extinct genus. Smallpox vaccination with vaccinia virus is no longer performed in the United States. Autoinoculation of the eyelid and cornea may occur after vaccination and can result in pox lesions of the lid and vascularized corneal scarring.

Because of the close antigenic similarity between vaccinia and variola viruses, routine serologic testing is, in general, not useful. The ELISA technique and radioimmunoassay have provided more sensitive differentiation between these agents; the monoclonal antibody technique provides an even more specific differentiation.

Orthopoxvirus infection is confirmed by viral isolation. The clinical specimen is inoculated into the chorioallantoic membrane of the chick embryo. At 2 to 3 days post inoculation, the vaccinia virus induces large pocks with necrotic centers; variola virus induces large pocks with necrotic centers; and variola virus induces a much smaller pock.[218] The orthopoxviruses also grow in tissue culture. Serology and EM do not reliably distinguish between different orthopoxviruses.

MOLLUSCUM CONTAGIOSUM VIRUS

Humans are the only known natural hosts for molluscum contagiosum virus (MCV) infection.[221] The virus potentially encodes 163 proteins, with many homologs with the smallpox virus. There are three genetic subtypes.[196] Special strategies seem to be used for coexistence with the human host.[222] MCV cannot be grown in tissue culture and must be identified on the basis of morphology or histopathology.[223] Its appearance on EM closely resembles the brick-shaped morphology of the vaccinia virus, but there is no antigenic cross-reactivity with any of the Poxviridae. By scanning EM, the MCV can also exist as a spherical, ellipsoid, or immature smaller spheroidal form.

MCV was once a disease of children but its prevalence increased, initially in association with sexually transmitted diseases and now with compromised immunity, iatrogenic immunosuppression, and patients with AIDS. In AIDS, the disease may be unremitting with increasing severity; in some cases, giant hyperkeratotic mollusca develop. MCV infection correlates with low $CD4^+$ counts, although immunodeficiency does not favor infection by specific subtypes. Clinically, molluscum infection occurs more frequently in children than adults and results in small umbilicated lesions. Transmission is by direct contact. The incubation period of molluscum infection may be as long as 6 months. The disease is self-limiting and may persist for up to 2 years. In ocular infections, one or more lesions of the eyelid may be encountered. Multiple lesions are usually the result of autoinoculation. Viral shedding from the lesions causes chronic follicular conjunctivitis. Molluscum is a poor immunogen, with as many as one-third of patients with clinical infection failing to develop antimolluscum antibodies. Second episodes of infection are well documented.

The diagnosis of molluscum may be made either on the basis of EM identification of poxvirus or by characteristic light-microscopic histopathology (Fig. 16–5). In EM, molluscum usually has a 230 × 330 nm brick-shaped morphology, but morphology is variable. Light-microscopic findings are characterized by hyaline acidophilic cytoplasmic accumulations commonly called molluscum bodies.

There is no specific antiviral therapy, and appropriate treatment is surgical excision. Local therapy with CO_2 laser, cryotherapy with liquid nitrogen, electrodesiccation, or incision and curettage is beneficial in some patients.[196, 224]

Paramyxoviruses

Family: Paramyxoviridae
- **Genus:** Paramyxovirus
  - Mumps virus
  - Newcastle disease virus
- **Genus:** Morbillivirus
  - Measles virus

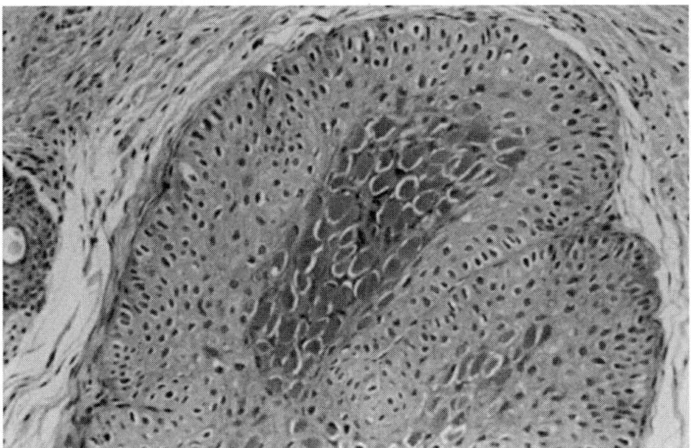

FIGURE 16–5. Photomicrograph of molluscum contagiosum histopathology. Eosinophilic bodies represent viral inclusions.

The Paramyxoviridae is a family of viruses that are antigenically stable but environmentally labile, secondary to their fragile envelope. They are composed of 1% RNA, 73% protein, and 20% lipid. These viruses have six structural proteins, including three that are complexed to RNA, one major protein that is found in association with the underside of the envelope, and two viral polymerases. There are also two transenvelope glycoproteins. There is also a hemagglutination protein that not only mediates hemagglutination but also interacts with host cell receptors for viral attachment and determines tropism. The F transenvelope protein allows penetration via membrane fusion.[225] The Paramyxoviridae comprises two genera: Paramyxovirus, which includes the mumps and Newcastle disease virus, and Morbillivirus, which includes the measles (rubeola) virus.

Paramyxoviral replication is initiated by hemagglutination protein attachment to the cell surface. The cleaved F protein is critical for penetration. Cleavage of this protein depends on extracellular enzymes; cells lacking the enzyme do not permit viral replication. After fusion, viral RNA polymerase transcribes the negative-strand RNA viral genome. Transcription and translation both occur in the cytoplasm. The nucleocapsid assembles and aligns along the cell membrane at sites of hemagglutination protein and F viral protein insertion. The particle exits the cell by budding and acquiring a lipid envelope.[226]

MEASLES (RUBEOLA) VIRUS

Humans are the only natural host for the measles virus, although other animals may be infected under experimental conditions. The enveloped virion is pleomorphic and very labile with chemical and heat.[227, 228] There is only one antigenic type of measles virus, but this virus is antigenically related to the canine distemper virus. The entire genome has been sequenced.

Measles is highly infectious with transmission via respiratory droplets. During the prodromal phase of the disease, which lasts 9 to 11 days, local replication in the respiratory tract precedes viremia. Measles virus has been isolated from the leukocytes of patients with clinical measles. Replication in the reticuloendothelial system is followed by secondary viremia that seeds epithelial surfaces, including the conjunctiva. Clinical disease is characterized by a maculopapular rash, fever, and respiratory symptoms of coryza and cough. At the onset of the disease, a Koplik spot appears typically as a blue spot-like ulceration on an erythematous buccal mucosa. Koplik's spots are pathognomonic and may sometimes involve the caruncle or conjunctiva. Other ocular manifestations of acute infection include mild catarrhal conjunctivitis and epithelial keratitis.[229] In immunocompromised patients or vitamin A–deficient children, measles keratitis may be followed by a secondary bacterial infection and corneal scarring or even perforation.[230] In the immunocompetent host, the conjunctivitis and keratitis resolve without sequelae within the first several days to weeks following infection. It has been postulated that the skin and mucous-membrane manifestations of measles actually represent hypersensitivity of the host to the virus, because the rash occurs simultaneously with the onset of the effector phase of the antiviral immune response and substantial evidence of immune activation.[231] Viral antigen has been demonstrated in the involved skin and mucous membranes, although it remains controversial whether endothelial or epithelial cells are involved.

A rare late complication of measles infection is subacute sclerosing panencephalitis. Typically, this infection usually occurs years following the acute infection in an infant or small child. It is characterized by the presence of latent measles virus found in the brain tissue and the replication of a measles virus defective in the production of one or more virus-encoded proteins. An inadequate immune response to primary infection is the presumed etiology, but the specific mechanism of this disease is not understood.[232] Immunologic abnormalities during measles infection may contribute to increased susceptibility to other infections.[233] Measles has been dramatically controlled since the introduction of live attenuated measles vaccine in 1963, but it remains a serious problem in developing countries and is imported into the United States from other countries, causing periodic outbreaks.[234, 235]

The diagnosis of measles is based on clinical findings; however, isolation of virus may be performed on specimens obtained during the febrile period of infection. Measles virus grows preferentially in monkey or human kidney cells and produces a characteristic CPE of multinucleated giant cells and inclusions visible on light microscopy. The measles virus is a slow-growing virus, and CPE is usually not apparent until 7 to 10 days post inoculation. A centrifugation-enhanced shell vial assay detects most measles isolates within 48 hours of inoculation.[236] Reverse transcription PCR has been described for the detection of measles virus RNA in nasal aspirates from acute measles and brain tissue in subacute sclerosing panencephalitis.[237] Paired serology testing may also be performed, with a fourfold increase in antibody titer between acute and convalescent considered to be diagnostic. Therapy is mainly supportive, although vitamin A can decrease the severity of measles in children.

NEWCASTLE DISEASE VIRUS

Newcastle disease virus is a pleomorphic, helically symmetric virus that contains nonsegmented negative-stranded RNA within a lipoprotein envelope that bears hemagglutinin, neuraminidase, and fusion glycoprotein spikes. The virus is resistant to extremes of temperature.

Newcastle disease virus is primarily a pathogen of the respiratory tract of chickens, with accidental infections in humans. Human infections are almost exclusively zoonoses of workers exposed to the virus in the poultry industry or in the laboratory by means of aerosols or autoinoculation.[238] After an incubation period of 1 to 2 days, mild to severe conjunctivitis develops, usually in one eye. There is periocular swelling and conjunctival infection. There is no corneal involvement. It can appear clinically like an adenoviral conjunctivitis. Rarely, systemic symptoms are present, but sequelae have not been recognized. The only viable method for diagnosis is viral culture. Requests are infrequent.[238]

MUMPS VIRUS

Mumps virus is a pleomorphic, enveloped virus that is destroyed by organic solvents, detergents, and heating and is relatively unstable. Humans are the only known natural host for the mumps virus. Transmission is person-to-person via respiratory droplets. The incubation period ranges from 7 to 25 days with an average of 8 days. Primary replication occurs in the upper respiratory tract at the site of inoculation followed by viremia with transmission of the virus to various organ systems, including the parotid gland. Of symptomatic cases, 95% have nonsuppurative parotid gland swelling; however, pancreatic, testicular, ovarian, and CNS involvement is common. One in 1000 symptomatic infected persons develops aseptic meningitis. Mumps in the postpubertal person is usually a more severe illness than in children and more commonly leads to extrasalivary gland involvement. Epidemiologic control of this infection is difficult in that viral shedding occurs 1 week prior to clinical symptoms, and, even during infection, one-third of infected persons do not display clinical disease.[121, 239]

Dacryoadenitis is a common ocular manifestation of mumps. Less frequently, keratitis, episcleritis, iridocyclitis, choroiditis, or optic neuritis is encountered.[240] Permanent immunity follows a single infection with the mumps virus. The presence of antibody to the HM protein confers immunity. Infants have passive immunity for the first 6 months of life, because neutralizing antibodies pass the placental barrier.

The diagnosis of mumps may be based on fluorescent antibody staining from conjunctival scrapings. Viral isolation is not a standard technique for mumps diagnosis, because the virus envelope is fragile. In clinically ambiguous cases, however, virus may be isolated from the saliva and cerebrospinal fluid for the first 1 to 5 days following the onset of clinical symptoms or from the urine for up to 2 weeks after the onset of clinical disease. The cell line of preference for isolation is monkey kidney cells in which characteristic CPE develops. Paired acute and convalescent sera may also be used to document mumps infection; neutralization, complement fixation, and hemagglutination inhibition testing may be used. There is some cross-reactivity with the parainfluenza virus.[241] The ELISA for IgM and IgG may be more specific than other serologic tests.

There is currently no established role for antiviral chemotherapy. Mumps immunoglobulin does not protect against infection once a patient has been exposed to the virus. Ninety-five percent of the people who have been immunized develop antimumps antibodies. There has been a 95% decline in the annual U.S. incidence of mumps since the licensure of the mumps vaccine in 1967.

Rubella Virus

Family: Togaviridae
  Genus: Rubivirus
    Rubella virus

The rubella virus is the sole togaviris in the Rubivirus genus.[242, 243] It is an enveloped icosahedral virus with a size that varies from 50 to 70 nm. There is also only one recognized rubella virus serotype. Rubella infection, also called German measles, causes rash, acute febrile illness, and lymphadenopathy. It is the mildest of the frequently encountered viral exanthemas.[244–246] Rubella virus is spread in droplets that are shed from the respiratory secretions of infected persons.

Although many infections with the agent are subclinical,

this virus has the potential to cause fetal infection with resultant birth defects and, uncommonly in adults, various forms of arthritis. Age is the most important determinant of the severity of rubella. Postnatal acquired rubella is generally a mild infection. The seriousness of this infection results from the effects of maternal infection on fetal development.[247] The virus causes decreased growth and replication of fetal cells, resulting in hypoplastic organ systems as well as fine structural abnormalities. Fetal complications associated with congenital rubella infection include prematurity, mental retardation, neurosensory deafness, cardiac anomalies, growth retardation, and encephalitic symptoms. Ocular complications are numerous and include glaucoma, retinopathy that has the characteristic fine granular "salt-and-pepper" appearance, microcornea, microphthalmos, iris hypoplasia, and cataract formation.[248] The development of fetal anomalies is directly related to fetal gestational age at the time of infection. With infection during the first month of gestation, fetuses display teratogenic effects. At 2 months of gestation, the rate of abnormalities decreases to 20% at 3 months of gestation, and only 4% of fetuses display abnormalities. Abnormalities are rare when infection occurs after 18 weeks of gestation. Intrauterine infection may result in chronic persistent infection of the newborn. Virus is shed in pharyngeal secretions, cerebrospinal fluid, and urine and may be detected as long as 12 to 18 months after birth. The level of viral shedding decreases with age; however, there have been reports of live virus isolated in cataracts of 4-year-old children with the congenital rubella syndrome.[248]

The clinical findings in children with congenital rubella may be divided into three categories. First, transient effects that resolve; second, permanent manifestations that are stable; and third, progressive lesions that may appear as late as adolescence. One such progressive manifestation is the increased rate of keratoconus that is found among patients with the congenital rubella syndrome during the second decade of life.[249]

A diagnosis of congenital rubella may be based on viral isolation or detection of specific antirubella antibodies.[250] Viral isolation is possible up to 18 months of age from pharyngeal, urine, or rectal swabbing. The cell line of choice for culture is monkey or rabbit kidney cells, although no CPE is produced and detection of infection has depended on interference testing with enterovirus.[32] The use of centrifugation-enhanced culture together with fluorescent antibody staining can shorten the detection time to 48 to 96 hours.[32] Reverse-transcription PCR detection has also been described.[251] The laboratory diagnosis of rubella may also be based on demonstration of rubella IgM antibodies in infants. The presence of IgG is nonspecific, because maternal IgG may cross the placental barrier. Immunoglobulin is synthesized by the infant and is diagnostic for infection.[252]

There is no specific treatment for rubella, and management is supportive. The vaccine for rubella may be given alone or with mumps and measles vaccine. Since introduction of the vaccine in 1969, there have been no subsequent large rubella epidemics in countries where the vaccine is widely used.

Coxsackieviruses

Family: Picornaviridae
Genus: Enterovirus
Coxsackieviruses
Human enteroviruses

The enteroviruses comprise 67 distinct serotypes within the family Picornaviridae, consisting of small viruses with a simple viral capsid and a single strand of positive-sense RNA. They are stable in liquid environments.

The enteroviruses are responsible for a wide array of clinical disease affecting many organ systems; enteric disease (despite the name of the virus) is not a prominent component. No disease is uniquely associated with any specific serotype, and no serotype is uniquely associated with any one disease.[253, 254] The enteroviruses are the most common cause of meningitis in the United States (and frequently mistreated with antiherpetic and antibiotic treatment). Additional acute clinical syndromes include poliomyelitis (now absent in developed countries), encephalitis, myocarditis, pleurodynia, neonatal sepsis, and hand-foot-mouth syndrome.

Acute hemorrhagic conjunctivitis has been associated with serotypes coxsackievirus A24 and enterovirus type 70. Adenovirus may be a major contributor to this disease or included in outbreaks of this enteroviral infection.[146, 151] Characteristically, the infection has a short incubation period, affects both eyes, causes swelling of the eyelids and chemosis, is associated with pain, and causes a serous discharge. It then resolves without sequelae in 7 to 10 days. The subconjunctival hemorrhages have been present in almost all cases. Although the presentation is impressive, the condition is benign in almost all cases. Rarely, radiculomyelitis follows in several weeks. Enterovirus has been implicated in several chronic illnesses, including juvenile-onset diabetes mellitus, chronic fatigue syndrome, dermatomyositis and polymyositis, congenital hydrocephalus, and amyotropic lateral sclerosis.

Isolation in tissue culture remains the gold standard with good susceptibility in numerous continuous cell lines, although it is labor-intensive. EM has little application, and immunoassays and serologic testing are difficult because of the absence of a widely shared antigen. PCR has been applied for universal, serotype-specific, and strain-specific detection with increasing success.[253]

Hepatitis C Virus

Family: Flaviviridae
Genus: Flavirus
Hepatitis C virus

Hepatitis C virus (HCV) is a small enveloped RNA virus that has been identified as the agent other than hepatitis A and B to be responsible for transfusion-associated hepatitis. Despite extensive efforts, virologists have failed to isolate the virus in cell culture. HCV is present in 0.2% of blood donors and up to 80% of intravenous drug users.[255] HCV establishes a chronic infection in 50 to 80% of cases, leading to liver damage, cirrhosis, and hepatocellular carcinoma. Other patients may develop essential mixed cryoglobulinemia, porphyria cutanea tarda, and membranoproliferative glomerulonephritis. In several (but not all) patients with classic Mooren's corneal ulcer, anti-HCV antibodies and HCV genomic RNA have been detected by PCR in the serum.[256, 257] Some of these patients have had hepatitis, and some patients have undergone systemic interferon therapy with improvement in their hepatitis and corneal ulceration.[256] Some patients have had an accompanying skin condition, hidradenitis suppurativa. More research is being performed on this recently recognized association.

Acknowledgments

The author wishes to acknowledge Lisa D. Kelly, M.D., and Edmund C. Dunkel, Ph.D., for their work as authors of this chapter in the first edition of this book.

REFERENCES

1. Brown F: The classification and nomenclature of viruses: Summary of results of meeting of the ICTV in Sendai, September 1984. Intervirology 25:141–143, 1986.
2. Fields BN, Knipe DM, Howley PM (eds): Virology, 3rd ed, vols 1 and 2. Philadelphia, Lippincott-Raven, 1996.
3. Laboratory diagnosis of viral diseases. *In* White DO, Fenner FJ (eds): Medical Virology, 4th ed. San Diego, Academic Press, 1994, pp 191–218.
4. Laboratory methods in basic virology. *In* Baron EJ, Peterson LR, Finegold SM (eds): Bailey and Scott's Diagnostic Microbiology, 9th ed. St. Louis, Mosby-Year Book, 1994, pp 634–688.
5. Darrell RW: Viral Diseases of the Eye. Philadelphia, Lea & Febiger, 1985.
6. Easty DL: Viral Diseases of the Eye. Chicago, Year Book, 1985.
7. Melnick JL: Taxonomy of viruses. *In* Lennette EH, Lennette DA, Lennette ET (eds): Diagnostic Procedures for Viral, Rickettsial, and Chlamydial Infections, 7th ed. Washington, D.C., American Public Health Association, 1995, pp 161–167.
8. Sepkowitz KA: Occupationally acquired infections in health care workers. Part I. Ann Intern Med 125(10):826–834, 1996.
9. Gospodarowicz D, Ferrara N, Schweigerer L, et al: Structural characterization and biological functions of fibroblast growth factor. Endocr Rev 8(2):95–114, 1987.
10. Dalgleish AG, Beverley PC, Clapham PR, et al: The CD4 (T4) antigen is an essential component of the receptor for the AIDS retrovirus. Nature 312(5996):763–767, 1984.
11. Menage MJ, de Clercq E, van Lierde A, et al: Antiviral drug sensitivity in ocular herpes simplex virus infection. Br J Ophthalmol 74(9):532–535, 1990.
12. Hara J, Fujimoto F, Ishibashi T, et al: Ocular manifestations of the 1976 rubella epidemic in Japan. Am J Ophthalmol 87(5):642–645, 1979.
13. Cook ML, Bastone VB, Stevens JG: Evidence that neurons harbor latent herpes simplex virus. Infect Immun 9(5):946–951, 1974.
14. Hill TJ, Harbour DA, Blyth WA: Isolation of herpes simplex virus from the skin of clinically normal mice during latent infection. J Gen Virol 47(1):205–207, 1980.
15. Stevens JG, Cook ML: Latent herpes simplex virus in sensory ganglia. *In* Plard M (ed): Perspectives in Virology, vol 8. New York, Academic Press, 1973, pp 171–188.
16. Rock DL, Fraser NW: Detection of HSV-1 genome in central nervous system of latently infected mice. Nature 302(5908):523–525, 1983.
17. Determinants of viral virulence and host resistance. *In* White DO, Fenner FJ (eds): Medical Virology, 4th ed. San Diego, Academic Press, 1994, pp 103–118.
18. Mechanisms of viral oncogenesis. *In* White DO, Fenner FJ (eds): Medical Virology, 4th ed. San Diego, Academic Press, 1994, pp 170–190.
19. Mueller N: Overview: Viral agents and cancer. Environ Health Perspect 103(Suppl 8):259–261, 1995.
20. Tyler KL, Fields BN: Introduction to viruses and viral diseases. *In* Mandell GL, Bennett JE, Dolin R (eds): Mandell, Douglas and Bennett's Principles and Practice of Infectious Diseases, 4th ed. New York, Churchill Livingstone, 1995, pp 1314–1325.
21. Chandler JW: Host defenses and immunology of viral infections involving the eye. *In* Tasman W, Jaeger EA (eds): Duane's Foundations of Clinical Ophthalmology, vol 2. Philadelphia, Lippincott-Raven, 1986, pp 1–12.
22. Sen GC, Lengyel P: The interferon system: A bird's eye view of its biochemistry. J Biol Chem 267(8):5017–5020, 1992.
23. Buimovici-Klein E, Cooper LZ: Cell-mediated immune response in rubella infections. Rev Infect Dis 7(Suppl 1):S123–S128, 1985.
24. Newell CK, Martin S, Sendele D, et al: Herpes simplex virus–induced stromal keratitis: Role of T-lymphocyte subsets in immunopathology. J Virol 63(2):769–775, 1989.
25. Hendricks RL, Tumpey TM: Contribution of virus and immune factors to herpes simplex virus type I–induced corneal pathology. Invest Ophthalmol Vis Sci 31(10):1929–1939, 1990.
26. Pavan-Langston D: Ocular viral diseases. *In* Galasso GJ, Merigan TC, Buchanan RA (eds): Antiviral Agents and Viral Diseases of Man, 3rd ed. New York, Raven Press, 1990.
27. Wilson ML: General principles of specimen collection and transport. Clin Infect Dis 22(5):766–777, 1996.
28. Lennette DA: Collection and preparation of specimens for virological examination. *In* Baron EJ, Pfaller MA, Tenover FC, Yolken RH (eds): Manual of Clinical Microbiology, 6th ed. Washington, D.C., ASM Press, 1995, pp 868–875.
29. Schwab IR: Diagnostic techniques for ocular viral infections. *In* Tasman W, Jaeger EA (eds): Duane's Foundations of Clinical Ophthalmology, vol 2. Philadelphia, Lippincott-Raven, 1990, pp 1–10.
30. Woods GL, Washington JA: The clinician and the microbiology laboratory. *In* Mandell GL, Bennett JE, Dolin R (eds): Mandell, Douglas and Bennett's Principles and Practice of Infectious Diseases, 4th ed. New York, Churchill Livingstone, 1995, pp 169–199.
31. Catalano RA, Webb RM, Smith RS, et al: A modified immunoperoxidase method for rapid diagnosis of herpes simplex I keratitis. Am J Clin Pathol 86(1):102–104, 1986.
32. Mann LM, Woods GL: Rapid diagnosis of viral pathogens. Clin Lab Med 15(2):389–405, 1995.
33. Clementi M, Menzo S, Manzin A, et al: Quantitative molecular methods in virology. Arch Virol 140(9):1523–1539, 1995.
34. Cohen PR: Tests for detecting herpes simplex virus and varicella-zoster virus infections. Dermatol Clin 12(1):51–68, 1994.
35. Collum LM, Mullaney J, Hillery M, et al: Two laboratory methods for diagnosis of herpes simplex keratitis. Br J Ophthalmol 71(10):742–745, 1987.
36. Crosby M: Immunologic tests for ocular herpes simplex virus. Ophthalmology 97(6):694–695, 1990.
37. Shibata D, Fu YS, Gupta JW, et al: Detection of human papillomavirus in normal and dysplastic tissue by the polymerase chain reaction. Lab Invest 59(4):555–559, 1988.
38. Garcia-Kennedy R: Cytology and surgical pathology of viral infections. *In* Lennette EH, Lennette DA, Lennette ET (eds): Diagnostic Procedures for Viral, Rickettsial, and Chlamydial Infections, 7th ed. Washington, D.C., American Public Health Association, 1995, pp 27–35.
39. Miller SE: Diagnosis of viral infections by electron microscopy. *In* Lennette EH, Lennette DA, Lennette ET (eds): Diagnostic Procedures for Viral, Rickettsial, and Chlamydial Infections, 7th ed. Washington, D.C., American Public Health Association, 1995, pp 37–78.
40. Boerner CF, Lee FK, Wickliffe CL, et al: Electron microscopy for the diagnosis of ocular viral infections. Ophthalmology 88(12):1377–1381, 1981.
41. Morgan C, Rosenkranz HS, Mednis B: Structure and development of viruses as observed in the electron microscope. V: Entry and uncoating of adenovirus. J Virol 4(5):777–796, 1969.
42. Gleaves CA, Hodinka RL, Johnston SLG, et al: Cumtech 15A. *In* Baron EJ (ed): Laboratory Diagnosis of Viral Infections. Washington, D.C., American Society for Microbiology, 1994.
43. Forghani B, Hagens S: Diagnosis of viral infections by antigen detection. *In* Lennette EH, Lennette DH, Lennette ET (eds): Diagnostic Procedures for Viral, Rickettsial, and Chlamydial Infections, 7th ed. Washington, D.C., American Public Health Association, 1995, pp 79–96.
44. Schwab IR, Raju VK, McClung J: Indirect immunofluorescent antibody diagnosis of herpes simplex with upper tarsal and corneal scrapings. Ophthalmology 93(6):752–756, 1986.
45. Walpita P, Darougar S: Double-label immunofluorescence method for simultaneous detection of adenovirus and herpes simplex virus from the eye. J Clin Microbiol 27(7):1623–1625, 1989.
46. Kowalski RP, Gordon YJ: Evaluation of immunologic tests for the detection of ocular herpes simplex virus. Ophthalmology 96(11):1583–1586, 1989.
47. Chou S, Merigan TC: Rapid detection and quantitation of human cytomegalovirus in urine through DNA hybridization. N Engl J Med 308(16):921–925, 1983.

48. Demmler GJ, Buffone GJ, Schimbor CM, et al: Detection of cytomegalovirus in urine from newborns by using polymerase chain reaction DNA amplification. J Infect Dis 158(6):1177–1184, 1988.
49. Mullis KB, Faloona FA: Specific synthesis of DNA in vitro via a polymerase-catalyzed chain reaction. Methods Enzymol 155:335–350, 1987.
50. Forghani B, Erdman DD: Amplification and detection of viral nucleic acids. *In* Lennette EH, Lennette DA, Lennette ET (eds): Diagnostic Procedures for Viral, Rickettsial, and Chlamydial Infections, 7th ed. Washington, D.C., American Public Health Association, 1995, pp 97–120.
51. Kowalski RP, Gordon YJ, Romanowski EG, et al: A comparison of enzyme immunoassay and polymerase chain reaction with the clinical examination for diagnosing ocular herpetic disease. Ophthalmology 100(4):530–533, 1993.
52. Fox GM, Crouse CA, Chuang EL, et al: Detection of herpesvirus DNA in vitreous and aqueous specimens by the polymerase chain reaction. Arch Ophthalmol 109(2):266–271, 1991.
53. Bobo L, Munoz B, Viscidi R, et al: Diagnosis of *Chlamydia trachomatis* eye infection in Tanzania by polymerase chain reaction/enzyme immunoassay. Lancet 338(8771):847–850, 1991.
54. Clementi M, Menzo S, Bagnarelli P, et al: Quantitative PCR and RT-PCR in virology. PCR Methods Appl 2(3):191–196, 1993.
55. Saiki RK, Gelfand DH, Stoffel S, et al: Primer-directed enzymatic amplification of DNA with a thermostable DNA polymerase. Science 239(4839):487–491, 1988.
56. White DO, Fenner FJ (eds): Medical Virology, 4th ed. San Diego, Academic Press, 1994.
57. Jackson JB, Coombs RW, Sannerud K, et al: Rapid and sensitive viral culture method for human immunodeficiency virus type 1. J Clin Microbiol 26(7):1416–1418, 1988.
58. Van Rij G, Klepper L, Peperkamp E, et al: Immune electron microscopy and a cultural test in the diagnosis of adenovirus ocular infection. Br J Ophthalmol 66(5):317–319, 1982.
59. Stabell EC, Olivo PD: Isolation of a cell line for rapid and sensitive histochemical assay for the detection of herpes simplex virus. J Virol Methods 38(2):195–204, 1992.
60. Herrmann KL, Erdman DD: Diagnosis by serologic assays. *In* Lennette EH, Lennette DA, Lennette ET (eds): Diagnostic Procedures for Viral, Rickettsial, and Chlamydial Infections, 7th ed. Washington, D.C., American Public Health Association, 1995, pp 121–138.
61. Griffiths PD, Stagno S, Pass RF, et al: Congenital cytomegalovirus infection: Diagnostic and prognostic significance of the detection of specific immunoglobulin M antibodies in cord serum. Pediatrics 69(5):544–549, 1982.
62. Hierholzer JC: Further subgrouping of the human adenoviruses by differential hemagglutination. J Infect Dis 128(4):541–550, 1973.
63. Coleman RM, Pereira L, Bailey PD, et al: Determination of herpes simplex virus type–specific antibodies by enzyme-linked immunosorbent assay. J Clin Microbiol 18(2):287–291, 1983.
64. Pavan-Langston D, Dunkel EC: A rapid clinical diagnostic test for herpes simplex infectious keratitis. Am J Ophthalmol 107(6):675–677, 1989.
65. Popow-Kraupp T: Enzyme-linked immunosorbent assay (ELISA) for mumps virus antibodies. J Med Virol 8(2):79–88, 1981.
66. Ziegelmaier R, Behrens F, Enders G: [ELISA (demonstration of IgG and IgM antibodies in cytomegaly and rubella virus infections)]. Ric Clin Lab 10(Suppl 2):83–92, 1980.
67. McSharry JJ: Uses of flow cytometry in virology. Clin Microbiol Rev 7(4):576–604, 1994.
68. Liesegang TJ: Biology and molecular aspects of herpes simplex and varicella-zoster virus infections. Ophthalmology 99(5):781–799, 1992.
69. Pereira FA: Herpes simplex: Evolving concepts. J Am Acad Dermatol 35(4):503–520, 1996.
70. Ashley RL: Herpes simplex viruses. *In* Lennette EH, Lennette DA, Lennette ET (eds): Diagnostic Procedures for Viral, Rickettsial, and Chlamydial Infections, 7th ed. Washington, D.C., American Public Health Association, 1995, pp 375–395.
71. Wagner EK, Guzowski JF, Singh J: Transcription of the herpes simplex virus genome during productive and latent infection. Prog Nucleic Acid Res Mol Biol 51:123–165, 1995.
72. Fraser NW, Valyi-Nagy T: Viral, neuronal and immune factors which may influence herpes simplex virus (HSV) latency and reactivation. Microb Pathog 15(2):83–91, 1993.
73. Rock DL, Nesburn AB, Ghiasi H, et al: Detection of latency-related viral RNAs in trigeminal ganglia of rabbits latently infected with herpes simplex virus type 1. J Virol 61(12):3820–3826, 1987.
74. Stevens JG, Wagner EK, Devi-Rao GB, et al: RNA complementary to a herpesvirus alpha gene mRNA is prominent in latently infected neurons. Science 235(4792):1056–1059, 1987.
75. Green MT, Courtney RJ, Dunkel EC: Detection of an immediate early herpes simplex virus type 1 polypeptide in trigeminal ganglia from latently infected animals. Infect Immun 34(3):987–992, 1981.
76. Green MT, Dunkel EC, Courtney RJ: Detection of herpes simplex virus induced polypeptides in rabbit trigeminal ganglia. Invest Ophthalmol Vis Sci 25(12):1436–1440, 1984.
77. Sabbaga EM, Pavan-Langston D, Bean KM, et al: Detection of HSV nucleic acid sequences in the cornea during acute and latent ocular disease. Exp Eye Res 47(4):545–553, 1988.
78. Pavan-Langston D, Rong BL, Dunkel EC: Extraneuronal herpetic latency: Animal and human corneal studies. Acta Ophthalmol Suppl 192:135–141, 1989.
79. Dunkel EC, Pepose J, Pavan-Langston D, et al: Molecular biology of ocular viral infections. *In* Piotigorsky J, Shinohara T (eds): Molecular Biology of the Eye: Genes, Vision & Ocular Disease. New York, Wiley, 1988, pp 397–483.
80. Rong BL, Pavan-Langston D, Weng QP, et al: Detection of herpes simplex virus thymidine kinase and latency-associated transcript gene sequences in human herpetic corneas by polymerase chain reaction amplification. Invest Ophthalmol Vis Sci 32(6):1808–1815, 1991.
81. Hodge WG, Margolis TP: Herpes simplex virus keratitis among patients who are positive or negative for human immunodeficiency virus: An epidemiologic study. Ophthalmology 104:120–124, 1997.
82. Dunkel EC, Pavan-Langston D: HSV-induced reactivation: Contribution of epinephrine after corneal iontophoresis. Curr Eye Res 6(1):75–84, 1987.
83. Morahan PS, Thomson TA, Kohl S, et al: Immune responses to labial infection of BALB/c mice with herpes simplex virus type 1. Infect Immun 32(1):180–187, 1981.
84. Meyers RL: Cell-mediated immunity: Relevance to ocular diseases. Invest Ophthalmol 14(9):635–639, 1975.
85. Arvin AM, Prober CG: Herpes simplex viruses. *In* Murray PR, Baron EJ, Pfaller MA, et al (eds): Manual of Clinical Microbiology, 6th ed. Washington, D.C., ASM Press, 1995, pp 876–883.
86. Lee SF, Storch GA, Reed CA, et al: Comparative laboratory diagnosis of experimental herpes simplex keratitis. Am J Ophthalmol 109(1):8–12, 1990.
87. Verano L, Michalski FJ: Comparison of a direct antigen enzyme immunoassay, Herpchek, with cell culture for detection of herpes simplex virus from clinical specimens. J Clin Microbiol 33(5):1378–1379, 1995.
88. Puchhammer-Stockl E, Heinz FX, Kundi M, et al: Evaluation of the polymerase chain reaction for diagnosis of herpes simplex virus encephalitis. J Clin Microbiol 31(1):146–148, 1993.
89. Gershon AA, LaRussa P, Steinberg SP: Varicella-zoster virus. *In* Murray PR, Baron EJ, Pfaller MA, et al (eds): Manual of Clinical Microbiology, 6th ed. Washington, D.C., ASM Press, 1995, pp 895–904.
90. Gershon AA, Forghani B: Varicella-zoster virus. *In* Lennette EH, Lennette DA, Lennette ET (eds): Diagnostic Procedures for Viral, Rickettsial, and Chlamydial Infections, 7th ed. Washington, D.C., American Public Health Association, 1995, pp 601–613.
91. Liesegang TJ: Varicella zoster viral disease. *In* Tasman W, Jaeger EA (eds): Duane's Foundations of Clinical Ophthalmology, vol 2. Philadelphia, Lippincott-Raven, 1991, pp 1–10.
92. Rockley PF, Tyring SK: Pathophysiology and clinical manifestations of varicella zoster virus infections. Int J Dermatol 33(4):227–232, 1994.
93. Balfour HH Jr: Clinical aspects of chickenpox and herpes zoster. J Int Med Res 22(Suppl 1):3A–12A, 1994.
94. Weller TH: Varicella and herpes zoster. Changing concepts of the natural history, control, and importance of a not-so-benign virus. N Engl J Med 309(22):1362–1368, 1983.
95. Pavan-Langston D, Dunkel EC: Herpes zoster ophthalmicus. Compr Ther 15(5):3–9, 1989.
96. Gnann JW, Whitley RJ: Natural history and treatment of varicella-zoster in high risk populations. J Hosp Infect 18:317–329, 1991.
97. Mahalingam R, Wellish M, Wolf W, et al: Latent varicella-zoster viral DNA in human trigeminal and thoracic ganglia. N Engl J Med 323(10):627–631, 1990.
98. Gleaves CA, Lee CF, Bustamante CI, et al: Use of murine monoclonal antibodies for laboratory diagnosis of varicella-zoster virus infection. J Clin Microbiol 26(9):1623–1625, 1988.

99. Koropchak CM, Graham G, Palmer J, et al: Investigation of varicella-zoster virus infection by polymerase chain reaction in the immunocompetent host with acute varicella. J Infect Dis 163(5):1016–1022, 1991.
100. Pavan-Langston D, Yamamoto S, Dunkel EC: Delayed herpes zoster pseudodendrites. Polymerase chain reaction detection of viral DNA and a role for antiviral therapy. Arch Ophthalmol 113(11):1381–1385, 1995.
101. Wasmuth EH, Miller WJ: Sensitive enzyme-linked immunosorbent assay for antibody to varicella-zoster virus using purified VZV glycoprotein antigen. J Med Virol 32(3):189–193, 1990.
102. Wood MJ, Kay R, Dworkin RH, et al: Oral acyclovir therapy accelerates pain resolution in patients with herpes zoster: A meta-analysis of placebo-controlled trials. Clin Infect Dis 22(2):341–347, 1996.
103. Beutner KR, Friedman DJ, Forszpaniak C, et al: Valacyclovir compared with acyclovir for improved therapy for herpes zoster in immunocompetent adults. Antimicrob Agents Chemother 39(7):1546–1553, 1995.
104. Vere Hodge RA: Famciclovir and penciclovir. The mode of action of famciclovir including its conversion to penciclovir. Antiviral Chem Chemother 42:67–84, 1993.
105. Wood MJ, Johnson RW, McKendrick MW, et al: A randomized trial of acyclovir for 7 days or 21 days with and without prednisolone for treatment of acute herpes zoster. N Engl J Med 330(13):896–900, 1994.
106. Whitley RJ, Weiss H, Gnann JW, et al and the NIAID Collaborative Study Group: Acyclovir with and without prednisone for the treatment of herpes zoster. A randomized, placebo-controlled trial of acyclovir with and without steroids for the treatment of herpes zoster in individuals over 50 years of age. Ann Intern Med 125(5):376–383, 1996.
107. Prevention of varicella: Recommendations of the advisory committee on immunization practices (ACIP). MMWR 45:1–36, 1996.
108. Bruggeman CA: Cytomegalovirus and latency: An overview. Virchows Arch B Cell Pathol Incl Mol Pathol 64(6):325–333, 1993.
109. Palestine AG, Stevens G Jr, Lane HC, et al: Treatment of cytomegalovirus retinitis with dihydroxy propoxymethyl guanine. Am J Ophthalmol 101(1):95–101, 1986.
110. Hanshaw JB: Cytomegalovirus infections. Pediatr Rev 16(2):43–48, 1995.
111. Palestine AG, Rodrigues MM, Macher AM, et al: Ophthalmic involvement in acquired immunodeficiency syndrome. Ophthalmology 91(9):1092–1099, 1984.
112. Rosenberg PR, Uliss AE, Friedland GH, et al: Acquired immunodeficiency syndrome. Ophthalmic manifestations in ambulatory patients. Ophthalmology 90(8):874–878, 1983.
113. Hayashi K, Kurihara I, Uchida Y: Studies of ocular murine cytomegalovirus infection. Invest Ophthalmol Vis Sci 26(4):486–493, 1985.
114. Aquino-de Jesus MJ, Griffith BP: Cytomegalovirus infection in immunocompromised guinea pigs: A model for testing antiviral agents in vivo. Antiviral Res 12(4):181–193, 1989.
115. Dunkel EC, de Freitas D, Scheer DI, et al: A rabbit model for human cytomegalovirus-induced chorioretinal disease. J Infect Dis 168(2):336–344, 1993.
116. Landini MP: New approaches and perspectives in cytomegalovirus diagnosis. Prog Med Virol 40:157–177, 1993.
117. Pass RF, Britt WJ, Stagno S: Cytomegalovirus. *In* Lennette EH, Lennette DA, Lennette ET (eds): Diagnostic Procedures for Viral, Rickettsial, and Chlamydial Infections, 7th ed. Washington, D.C., American Public Health Association, 1995, pp 253–277.
118. Gleaves CA, Smith TF, Shuster EA, et al: Rapid detection of cytomegalovirus in MRC-5 cells inoculated with urine specimens by using low-speed centrifugation and monoclonal antibody to an early antigen. J Clin Microbiol 19(6):917–919, 1984.
119. Stainer P, Kitchen AD, Taylor DL, et al: Detection of human cytomegalovirus in peripheral mononuclear cells and urine samples using PCR. Mol Cell Probes 6:51–58, 1992.
120. Miller MJ, Bovey S, Pado K, et al: Application of PCR to multiple specimen types for diagnosis of cytomegalovirus infection: Comparison with cell culture and shell vial assay. J Clin Microbiol 32(1):5–10, 1994.
121. Fenner TE, Garweg J, Hufert FT, et al: Diagnosis of human cytomegalovirus-induced retinitis in human immunodeficiency virus type 1–infected subjects by using the polymerase chain reaction. J Clin Microbiol 29(11):2621–2622, 1991.
122. The TH, van der Bij W, van den Berg AP, et al: Cytomegalovirus antigenemia. Rev Infect Dis 12(Suppl 7):S734–S744, 1990.
123. Landry ML, Ferguson D: Comparison of quantitative cytomegalovirus antigenemia assay with culture methods and correlation with clinical disease. J Clin Microbiol 31(11):2851–2856, 1993.
124. Erice A, Holm MA, Gill PC, et al: Cytomegalovirus (CMV) antigenemia assay is more sensitive than shell vial cultures for rapid detection of CMV in polymorphonuclear blood leukocytes. J Clin Microbiol 30(11):2822–2825, 1992.
125. Jabs DA: Treatment of cytomegalovirus retinitis in patients with AIDS. [Editorial] Ann Intern Med 125(2):144–145, 1996.
126. Snydman DR, Rubin RH, Werner BG: New developments in cytomegalovirus prevention and management. Am J Kidney Dis 21(2):217–228, 1993.
127. Boeckh M, Bowden R: Cytomegalovirus infection in marrow transplantation. Cancer Treat Res 76:97–136, 1995.
128. Lennette ET: Epstein-Barr virus. *In* Murray PR, Baron EJ, Pfaller MA, et al (eds): Manual of Clinical Microbiology, 6th ed. Washington, D.C., ASM Press, 1995, pp 905–910.
129. Lennette ET: Epstein-Barr virus (EBV). *In* Lennette EH, Lennette DA, Lennette ET (eds): Diagnostic Procedures for Viral, Rickettsial, and Chlamydial Infections, 7th ed. Washington, D.C., American Public Health Association, 1995, pp 299–312.
130. Pflugfelder SC, Chodosh J: The Epstein-Barr virus in ocular disease. *In* Tasman W, Jaeger EA (eds): Duane's Foundations of Clinical Ophthalmology, vol 2. Philadelphia, Lippincott-Raven, 1995, pp 1–14.
131. Straus SE, Cohen JI, Tosato G, et al: NIH conference. Epstein-Barr virus infections: Biology, pathogenesis, and management. Ann Intern Med 118(1):45–58, 1993.
132. Pflugfelder SC, Crouse CA, Atherton SS: Ophthalmic manifestations of Epstein-Barr virus infection. Int Ophthalmol Clin 33(1):95–101, 1993.
133. Miyasaka N, Saito I, Haruta J: Possible involvement of Epstein-Barr virus in the pathogenesis of Sjögren's syndrome. Clin Immunol Immunopathol 72(2):166–170, 1994.
134. Ambinder RF, Mann RB: Detection and characterization of Epstein-Barr virus in clinical specimens. Am J Pathol 145(2):239–252, 1994.
135. Farhat SE, Finn S, Chua R, et al: Rapid detection of infectious mononucleosis-associated heterophile antibodies by a novel immunochromatographic assay and a latex agglutination test. J Clin Microbiol 31(6):1597–1600, 1993.
136. Pflugfelder SC, Huang A, Crouse C: Epstein-Barr virus keratitis after a chemical facial peel. Am J Ophthalmol 110(5):571–573, 1990.
137. van der Horst C, Joncas J, Ahronheim G, et al: Lack of effect of peroral acyclovir for the treatment of acute infectious mononucleosis. J Infect Dis 164(4):788–792, 1991.
138. Morgan AJ: Epstein-Barr virus vaccines. Vaccine 10(9):563–571, 1992.
139. Moore PS, Chang Y: Detection of herpesvirus-like DNA sequences in Kaposi's sarcoma in patients with and without HIV infection. N Engl J Med 332(18):1181–1185, 1995.
140. Cesarman E, Chang Y, Moore PS, et al: Kaposi's sarcoma-associated herpesvirus-like DNA sequences in AIDS-related body-cavity–based lymphomas. N Engl J Med 332(18):1186–1191, 1995.
141. Otsuki T, Kumar S, Ensoli B, et al: Detection of HHV-8/KSHV DNA sequences in AIDS-associated extranodal lymphoid malignancies. Leukemia 10(8):1358–1362, 1996.
142. Chang Y, Cesarman E, Pessin MS, et al: Identification of herpesvirus-like DNA sequences in AIDS-associated Kaposi's sarcoma. Science 266(5192):1865–1869, 1994.
143. Mesri EA, Cesarman E, Arvanitakis L, et al: Human herpesvirus-8/Kaposi's sarcoma–associated herpesvirus is a new transmissible virus that infects B cells. J Exp Med 183(5):2385–2390, 1996.
144. Weiss RA: Human herpesvirus 8 in lymphoma and Kaposi's sarcoma: Now the virus can be propagated. Nature Medicine 2(3):277–278, 1996.
145. Humphrey RW, O'Brien TR, Newcomb FM, et al: Kaposi's sarcoma (KS)–associated herpesvirus-like DNA sequences in peripheral blood mononuclear cells: Association with KS and persistence in patients receiving anti-herpesvirus drugs. Blood 88(1):297–301, 1996.
146. Hierholzer JC: Adenoviruses. *In* Murray PR, Baron EJ, Pfaller MA, et al (eds): Manual of Clinical Microbiology, 6th ed. Washington, D.C., ASM Press, 1995, pp 947–955.
147. Hodge WG, Margolis T: Adenovirus. *In* Tasman W, Jaeger EA (eds): Duane's Foundations of Clinical Ophthalmology, vol 2. Philadelphia, Lippincott-Raven, 1994, pp 1–7.
148. Philipson L: Adenovirus—An eternal archetype. Curr Top Microbiol Immunol 199(Pt 1):1–24, 1995.

149. van Oostrum J, Smith PR, Mohraz M, et al: The structure of the adenovirus capsid. III: Hexon packing determined from electron micrographs of capsid fragments. J Mol Biol 198(1):73–89, 1987.
150. Hierholzer JC: Adenoviruses in the immunocompromised host. Clin Microbiol Rev 5(3):262–274, 1992.
151. Hierholzer JC: Adenoviruses. *In* Lennette EH, Lennette DA, Lennette ET (eds): Diagnostic Procedures for Viral, Rickettsial, and Chlamydial Infections, 7th ed. Washington, D.C., American Public Health Association, 1995, pp 169–188.
152. Roba LA, Kowalski RP, Gordon AT, et al: Adenoviral ocular isolates demonstrate serotype-dependent differences in in vitro infectivity titers and clinical course. Cornea 14(4):388–393, 1995.
153. Gordon YJ, Gordon RY, Romanowski E, et al: Prolonged recovery of desiccated adenoviral serotypes 5, 8, and 19 from plastic and metal surfaces in vitro. Ophthalmology 100(12):1835–1839, 1993.
154. Kinchington PR, Turse SE, Kowalski RP, et al: Use of polymerase chain amplification reaction for the detection of adenoviruses in ocular swab specimens. Invest Ophthalmol Vis Sci 35(12):4126–4134, 1994.
155. Gottsch JD: Surveillance and control of epidemic keratoconjunctivitis. Trans Am Ophthalmol Soc 94:539–586, 1996.
156. McCune JM: Viral latency in HIV disease. Cell 82(2):183–188, 1995.
157. Barre-Sinoussi F: HIV as the cause of AIDS. Lancet 348(9019):31–35, 1996.
158. Levy JA: Features of human immunodeficiency virus infection and disease. Pediatr Res 33(Suppl 1):S63–S69, 1993.
159. Barre-Sinoussi F, Chermann JC, Rey F, et al: Isolation of a T-lymphotropic retrovirus from a patient at risk for acquired immune deficiency syndrome (AIDS). Science 220(4599):868–871, 1983.
160. Fauci AS: AIDS: Newer concepts in the immunopathogenic mechanisms of human immunodeficiency virus disease. Proc Assoc Am Physicians 107(1):1–7, 1995.
161. Levy JA: Pathogenesis of human immunodeficiency virus infection. Microbiol Rev 57(1):183–289, 1993.
162. Clavel F, Guetard D, Brun-Vezinet F, et al: Isolation of a new human retrovirus from West African patients with AIDS. Science 233(4761):343–346, 1986.
163. Clavel F, Mansinho K, Chamaret S, et al: Human immunodeficiency virus type 2 infection associated with AIDS in West Africa. N Engl J Med 316(19):1180–1185, 1987.
164. Haseltine WA, Wong-Staal F: The molecular biology of the AIDS virus. Sci Am 259(4):52–62, 1988.
165. Franchini G, Gurgo C, Guo HG, et al: Sequence of simian immunodeficiency virus and its relationship to the human immunodeficiency viruses. Nature 328(6130):539–543, 1987.
166. Ho DD, Sarngadharan MG, Hirsch MS, et al: Human immunodeficiency virus neutralizing antibodies recognize several conserved domains on the envelope glycoproteins. J Virol 61(6):2024–2028, 1987.
167. Klatzmann D, Champagne E, Chamaret S, et al: T-lymphocyte T4 molecule behaves as the receptor for human retrovirus LAV. Nature 312(5996):767–768, 1984.
168. Landau NR, Warton M, Littman DR: The envelope glycoprotein of the human immunodeficiency virus binds to the immunoglobulin-like domain of CD4. Nature 334(6178):159–162, 1988.
169. Deen KC, McDougal JS, Inacker R, et al: A soluble form of CD4 (T4) protein inhibits AIDS virus infection. Nature 331(6151):82–84, 1988.
170. Fauci AS: The human immunodeficiency virus: Infectivity and mechanisms of pathogenesis. Science 239(4840):617–622, 1988.
171. Nowak MA: Variability of HIV infections. J Theor Biol 155(1):1–20, 1992.
172. Matthews TJ, Bolognesi DP: AIDS vaccines. Sci Am 259(4):120–127, 1988.
173. Emini EA, Putney SD: Human immunodeficiency virus. Biotechnology 20:309–326, 1992.
174. Fisher AG, Ensoli B, Looney D, et al: Biologically diverse molecular variants within a single HIV-1 isolate. Nature 334(6181):444–447, 1988.
175. Hahn BH, Shaw GM, Taylor ME, et al: Genetic variation in HTLV-III/LAV over time in patients with AIDS or at risk for AIDS. Science 232(4757):1548–1553, 1986.
176. Kaplan MH: Pathogenesis of HIV. Infect Dis Clin North Am 8(2):279–288, 1994.
177. Cantrill HL, Henry K, Jackson B, et al: Recovery of human immunodeficiency virus from ocular tissues in patients with acquired immune deficiency syndrome. Ophthalmology 95(10):1458–1462, 1988.
178. Holland GN, Pepose JS, Pettit TH, et al: Acquired immune deficiency syndrome. Ocular manifestations. Ophthalmology 90(8):859–873, 1983.
179. Holland GN, Sison RF, Jatulis DE, et al: Survival of patients with the acquired immune deficiency syndrome after development of cytomegalovirus retinopathy. UCLA CMV Retinopathy Study Group. Ophthalmology 97(2):204–211, 1990.
180. Khadem M, Kalish SB, Goldsmith J, et al: Ophthalmologic findings in acquired immune deficiency syndrome (AIDS). Arch Ophthalmol 102(2):201–206, 1984.
181. Pepose JS, Holland GN, Nestor MS, et al: Acquired immune deficiency syndrome. Pathogenic mechanisms of ocular disease. Ophthalmology 92(4):472–484, 1985.
182. Newman NM, Mandel MR, Gullett J, et al: Clinical and histologic findings in opportunistic ocular infections: Part of a new syndrome of acquired immunodeficiency. Arch Ophthalmol 101(3):396–401, 1983.
183. Holland GN, Levinson RD: Ocular infections associated with the acquired immunodeficiency syndrome. *In* Tasman W, Jaeger E (eds): Duane's Foundations of Clinical Ophthalmology, vol 2. Philadelphia, Lippincott-Raven, 1994, pp 1–14.
184. Proffitt MR, Yen-Lieberman B: Laboratory diagnosis of human immunodeficiency virus infection. Infect Dis Clin North Am 7(2):203–219, 1993.
185. Burgard M, Mayaux MJ, Blanche S, et al: The use of viral culture and p24 antigen testing to diagnose human immunodeficiency virus infection in neonates. The HIV Infection in Newborns French Collaborative Study Group. N Engl J Med 327(17):1192–1197, 1992.
186. Ou CY, Kwok S, Mitchell SW, et al: DNA amplification for direct detection of HIV-1 in DNA of peripheral blood mononuclear cells. Science 239(4837):295–297, 1988.
187. Muul LM: Current status of polymerase chain reaction assay in clinical research of human immunodeficiency virus infection. AIDS Updates 3:1, 1990.
188. McHugh TM, Vyas GN: Human immunodeficiency viruses. *In* Lennette EH, Lennette DA, Lennette ET (eds): Diagnostic Procedures for Viral, Rickettsial, and Chlamydial Infections, 7th ed. Washington, D.C., American Public Health Association, 1995, pp 407–421.
189. Carpenter CC, Fischl MA, Hammer SM, et al: Antiretroviral therapy for HIV infection in 1996. Recommendations of an international panel. International AIDS Society-USA. JAMA 276(2):146–154, 1996.
190. Saag MS, Hammer SM, Lange JM: Pathogenicity and diversity of HIV and implications for clinical management: A review. J Acquir Immune Defic Syndr 7(Suppl 2):S2–S10, 1994.
191. Vella S: HIV pathogenesis and treatment strategies. J Acquir Immune Defic Syndr Hum Retrovirol 10(Suppl 1):S20–S23, 1995.
192. Baker CC, Phelps WC, Lindgren V, et al: Structural and transcriptional analysis of human papillomavirus type 16 sequences in cervical carcinoma cell lines. J Virol 61(4):962–971, 1987.
193. Dartmann K, Schwarz E, Gissmann L, et al: The nucleotide sequence and genome organization of human papilloma virus type 11. Virology 151(1):124–130, 1986.
194. McCance DJ: Human papillomaviruses. Infect Dis Clin North Am 8(4):751–767, 1994.
195. Lorincz A: Human papillomaviruses. *In* Lennette EH, Lennette DA, Lennette ET (eds): Diagnostic Procedures for Viral, Rickettsial, and Chlamydial Infections, 7th ed. Washington, D.C., American Public Health Association, 1995, pp 465–480.
196. Bardenstein DS, Lass JH: Periocular involvement of papillomavirus and molluscum contagiosum virus. *In* Tasman W, Jaeger EA (eds): Duane's Foundations of Clinical Ophthalmology, vol 2. Philadelphia, Lippincott-Raven, 1996, pp 1–17.
197. Kiviat NB, Koutsky LA: Human papillomavirus. *In* Murray PR, Baron EJ, Pfaller MA, et al (eds): Manual of Clinical Microbiology, 6th ed. Washington, D.C., ASM Press, 1995, pp 1082–1089.
198. Prasad CJ: Pathobiology of human papillomavirus. Clin Lab Med 15(3):685–704, 1995.
199. Schiffman MH: Recent progress in defining the epidemiology of human papillomavirus infection and cervical neoplasia. J Natl Cancer Inst 84(6):394–398, 1992.
200. Syrjanen KJ: Human papillomavirus in genital carcinogenesis. Sex Transm Dis 21(Suppl 2):S86–S89, 1994.
201. Dyson N, Howley PM, Munger K, et al: The human papilloma virus-16 E7 oncoprotein is able to bind to the retinoblastoma gene product. Science 243(4893):934–937, 1989.
202. Anderson MC, Brown CL, Buckley CH, et al: Current views on cervical intraepithelial neoplasia. J Clin Pathol 44(12):969–978, 1991.

203. Choo KB, Pan CC, Liu MS, et al: Presence of episomal and integrated human papillomavirus DNA sequences in cervical carcinoma. J Med Virol 21(2):101–107, 1987.
204. Durst M, Kleinheinz A, Hotz M, et al: The physical state of human papillomavirus type 16 DNA in benign and malignant genital tumours. J Gen Virol 66(Pt 7):1515–1522, 1985.
205. zur Hausen H: Human papillomaviruses in the pathogenesis of anogenital cancer. Virology 184(1):9–13, 1991.
206. Palefsky J: Human papillomavirus-associated malignancies in HIV-positive men and women. Curr Opin Oncol 7(5):437–441, 1995.
207. McDonnell JM, Mayr AJ, Martin WJ: DNA of human papillomavirus type 16 in dysplastic and malignant lesions of the conjunctiva and cornea. N Engl J Med 320(22):1442–1446, 1989.
208. Odrich MG, Jakobiec FA, Lancaster WD, et al: A spectrum of bilateral squamous conjunctival tumors associated with human papillomavirus type 16. Ophthalmology 98(5):628–635, 1991.
209. Lass JH, Grove AS, Papale JJ, et al: Detection of human papillomavirus DNA sequences in conjunctival papilloma. Am J Ophthalmol 96(5):670–674, 1983.
210. Lass JH, Jenson AB, Papale JJ, et al: Papillomavirus in human conjunctival papillomas. Am J Ophthalmol 95(3):364–368, 1983.
211. McDonnell JM, McDonnell PJ, Stout WC, et al: Human papillomavirus DNA in a recurrent squamous carcinoma of the eyelid. Arch Ophthalmol 107(11):1631–1634, 1989.
212. McDonnell JM, McDonnell PJ, Mounts P, et al: Demonstration of papillomavirus capsid antigen in human conjunctival neoplasia. Arch Ophthalmol 104(12):1801–1805, 1986.
213. Gupta JW, Saito K, Saito A, et al: Human papillomaviruses and the pathogenesis of cervical neoplasia. A study by in situ hybridization. Cancer 64(10):2104–2110, 1989.
214. Viscidi RP, Sun Y, Tsuzaki B, et al: Serologic response in human papillomavirus–associated invasive cervical cancer. Int J Cancer 55(5):780–784, 1993.
215. Behbehani AM: Poxviruses. *In* Lennette EH, Lennette DA, Lennette ET (eds): Diagnostic Procedures for Viral, Rickettsial, and Chlamydial Infections, 7th ed. Washington, D.C., American Public Health Association, 1995, pp 511–520.
216. Shchelkunov SN: Functional organization of variola major and vaccinia virus genomes. Virus Genes 10(1):53–71, 1995.
217. Fenner F: Portraits of viruses: The poxviruses. Intervirology 11(3): 137–157, 1979.
218. Baxby D: Identification and interrelationships of the variola/vaccinia subgroup of poxviruses. Prog Med Virol 19:215–246, 1975.
219. Essani K, Dales S: Biogenesis of vaccinia: Evidence for more than 100 polypeptides in the virion. Virology 95(2):385–394, 1979.
220. Stern W, Dales S: Biogenesis of vaccinia: Relationship of the envelope to virus assembly. Virology 75(1):242–255, 1976.
221. Highet AS: Molluscum contagiosum. Arch Dis Child 67(10):1248–1249, 1992.
222. Senkevich TG, Bugert JJ, Sisler JR, et al: Genome sequence of a human tumorigenic poxvirus: Prediction of specific host response-evasion genes. Science 273(5276):813–816, 1996.
223. Buller RM, Burnett J, Chen W, et al: Replication of molluscum contagiosum virus. Virology 213(2):655–659, 1995.
224. Schwartz JJ, Myskowski PL: Molluscum contagiosum in patients with human immunodeficiency virus infection: A review of twenty-seven patients. J Am Acad Dermatol 27(4):583–588, 1992.
225. Orvell C: Structural polypeptides of mumps virus. J Gen Virol 41(3):527–539, 1978.
226. Matsumoto T: Assembly of paramyxoviruses. Microbiol Immunol 26(4):285–320, 1982.
227. Salmi AA: Measles virus. *In* Murray PR, Baron EJ, Pfaller MA, et al (eds): Manual of Clinical Microbiology, 6th ed. Washington, D.C., ASM Press, 1995, pp 956–962.
228. Bellini WJ, Rota PA: Measles (rubeola) virus. *In* Lennette EH, Lennette DA, Lennette ET (eds): Diagnostic Procedures for Viral, Rickettsial, and Chlamydial Infections, 7th ed. Washington, D.C., American Public Health Association, 1995, pp 447–454.
229. Dekkers NW: The cornea in measles. Doc Ophthalmol 52(1):1–119, 1981.
230. Sandford-Smith JH, Whittle HC: Corneal ulceration following measles in Nigerian children. Br J Ophthalmol 63(11):720–724, 1979.
231. Griffin DE, Ward BJ, Esolen LM: Pathogenesis of measles virus infection: An hypothesis for altered immune responses. J Infect Dis 170(Suppl 1):S24–S31, 1994.
232. Schneider-Schaulies J, Dunster LM, Schneider-Schaulies S, et al: Pathogenetic aspects of measles virus infections. Vet Microbiol 44(2–4):113–125, 1995.
233. Griffin DE: Immune responses during measles virus infection. Curr Top Microbiol Immunol 191:117–134, 1995.
234. Atkinson WL: Epidemiology and prevention of measles. Dermatol Clin 13(3):553–559, 1995.
235. Hutchins S, Markowitz L, Atkinson W, et al: Measles outbreaks in the United States, 1987 through 1990. Pediatr Infect Dis J 15(1):31–38, 1996.
236. Minnich LL, Goodenough F, Ray CG: Use of immunofluorescence to identify measles virus infections. J Clin Microbiol 29(6):1148–1150, 1991.
237. Shimizu H, McCarthy CA, Smaron MF, et al: Polymerase chain reaction for detection of measles virus in clinical samples. J Clin Microbiol 31(5):1034–1039, 1993.
238. Kleiman MB, Leland DS: Mumps virus and Newcastle disease virus. *In* Lennette EH, Lennette DA, Lennette ET (eds): Diagnostic Procedures for Viral, Rickettsial, and Chlamydial Infections, 7th ed. Washington, D.C., American Public Health Association, 1995, pp 455–463.
239. Librach IM: Ocular symptoms in glandular fever. Br J Ophthalmol 40:619, 1956.
240. Meyer RF, Sullivan JH, Oh JO: Mumps conjunctivitis. Am J Ophthalmol 78(6):1022–1024, 1974.
241. Swierkosz EM: Mumps virus. *In* Murray PR, Baron EJ, Pfaller MA, et al (eds): Manual of Clinical Microbiology, 6th ed. Washington, D.C., ASM Press, 1995, pp 963–967.
242. Chernesky MA, Mahony JB: Rubella virus. *In* Murray PR, Baron EJ, Pfaller MA, et al (eds): Manual of Clinical Microbiology, 6th ed. Washington, D.C., ASM Press, 1995, pp 968–973.
243. Best JM, O'Shea S: Rubella virus. *In* Lennette EH, Lennette DA, Lennette ET (eds): Diagnostic Procedures for Viral, Rickettsial, and Chlamydial Infections, 7th ed. Washington, D.C., American Public Health Association, 1995, pp 583–600.
244. Dorsett PH, Miller DC, Green KY, et al: Structure and function of the rubella virus proteins. Rev Infect Dis 7(Suppl 1):S150–S156, 1985.
245. Herrmann KL: Available rubella serologic tests. Rev Infect Dis 7(Suppl 1):S108–S112, 1985.
246. Waxham MN, Wolinsky JS: A model of the structural organization of rubella virions. Rev Infect Dis 7(Suppl 1):S133–S139, 1985.
247. Gregg NM: Congenital cataract following German measles in the mother. Trans Ophthalmol Soc 3:35–46, 1941.
248. Wolff SM: Rubella syndrome. *In* Darrell RW (ed): Viral Diseases of the Eye. Philadelphia, Lea & Febiger, 1985.
249. Boger WPD, Petersen RA, Robb RM: Keratoconus and acute hydrops in mentally retarded patients with congenital rubella syndrome. Am J Ophthalmol 91(2):231–233, 1981.
250. Skendzel LP: Rubella immunity. Defining the level of protective antibody. Am J Clin Pathol 106(2):170–174, 1996.
251. Eggerding FA, Peters J, Lee RK, et al: Detection of rubella virus gene sequences by enzymatic amplification and direct sequencing of amplified DNA. J Clin Microbiol 29(5):945–952, 1991.
252. de Mazancourt A, Waxham MN, Nicolas JC, et al: Antibody response to the rubella virus structural proteins in infants with the congenital rubella syndrome. J Med Virol 19(2):111–122, 1986.
253. Grandien M, Forsgren M, Ehrnst A: Enteroviruses. *In* Lennette EH, Lennette DA, Lennette ET (eds): Diagnostic Procedures for Viral, Rickettsial, and Chlamydial Infections, 7th ed. Washington, D.C., American Public Health Association, 1995, pp 279–297, 1995.
254. Rotbart HA: Enteroviruses. *In* Murray PR, Baron EJ, Pfaller MA, et al (eds): Manual of Clinical Microbiology, 6th ed. Washington, D.C., ASM Press, 1995, pp 1004–1011.
255. Wilber JC: Hepatitis C virus. *In* Murray PR, Baron EJ, Pfaller MA, et al (eds): Manual of Clinical Microbiology, 6th ed. Washington, D.C., ASM Press, 1995, pp 1050–1055.
256. Moazami G, Auran JD, Florakis GJ, et al: Interferon treatment of Mooren's ulcers associated with hepatitis C. Am J Ophthalmol 119(3):365–366, 1995.
257. Wilson SE, Lee WM, Murakami C, et al: Mooren-type hepatitis C virus–associated corneal ulceration. Ophthalmology 101(4):736–745, 1994.

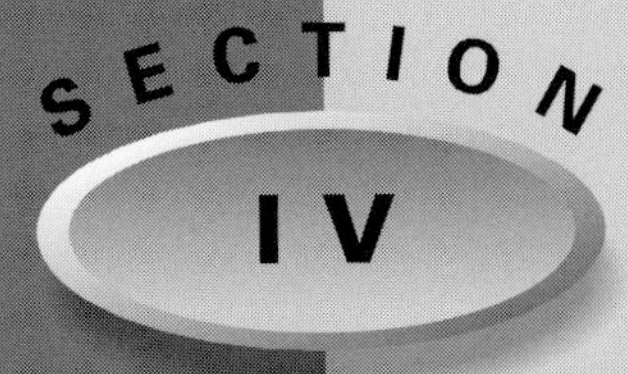

Pharmacology

Edited by

MARK B. ABELSON

ARTHUR H. NEUFELD

CHAPTER 17

Overview

Mark B. Abelson

The comprehension of normal ocular anatomy, physiology, and biochemistry is the necessary foundation for the recognition, classification, and understanding of clinical disease. The primary purpose of this exercise, however, is to apply the proper pharmacologic treatment for the relief of disease. It is toward this goal that efforts of basic scientists, clinicians, industry, and regulatory bodies are united. In this section our current knowledge of therapeutic alternatives is categorized. Readers must recognize that the progress in pharmacology is merely the bud at the tip of a rapidly growing tree into which all areas of ophthalmic science feed. To this end, they will find not only discussions of currently accepted therapy but also information on drugs now in development and concepts that may provide clues to new cures. Practically all ophthalmic agents have had their genesis in systemic pharmacology. As we understand more of the eye as a unique organ, however, this is changing. Botulinum toxin, first developed for the inhibition of ocular muscle spasm, is now being developed for torticollis. A potent new antihistamine first developed for use in the eye is now being administered nasally as well.

Although the past 50 years have brought us corticosteroids and antibiotics, and the past 20 years have presented α-adrenergic blocking agents, ancient drugs such as pilocarpine still have wide use and a valuable role in the treatment of glaucoma. The format of this section is intended to reflect this relationship in pharmacology—the use of drugs that have stood the test of time along with those whose mechanisms of action could not have been dreamed of even 10 years ago. In this approach, readers will find an integrated discussion of our knowledge of adrenergics with important reference to the role of these agents on blood flow (see Chap. 26, Adrenergic Agents). The modulation of blood flow is anticipated to play a significant role not only in glaucoma but also in the future treatment of macular degeneration and ischemic disorders.

Henry D. Perry and Eric D. Donnenfeld have contributed a comprehensive review of antibiotic agents to inform proper selection of therapy (see Chap. 20, Antibacterials). Eduardo Alfonso has reviewed available therapies, dosing regimens, and delivery routes for the treatment of fungal infections in the eye, in addition to providing suggestions for formulating ophthalmic compounds from available systemic agents (see Chap. 22, Antifungal Agents).

It is embarrassing to note that all current therapies used to treat dry-eye syndrome replace the aqueous phase of the tear film, with no regard for the multitude of other components of this film. Aside from increasing the viscosity of tear substitutes, therapy for this condition remains in the Dark Ages. Inflammation of the lacrimal gland or other contributing organ dysfunctions are allowed to proceed unchecked. However, newer therapies geared toward hormonal stimulation of the lacrimal gland and the use of peptides to facilitate reparation of the dehydrated epithelial surface are under investigation. Marshall D. Doane's analysis of the biophysical properties of the tear film and blink mechanism (see Chap. 29, Tear Film and Blink Dynamics) presents extremely useful understanding of the tear film as an organ; this understanding can be applied to the treatment of dry eye or for enhancing the effect of pharmacologic agents for other purposes. James D. Zieske and Ilene K. Gipson address epithelial wound healing with respect to epithelial growth factors, fibronectin, vitamin A, and the effect of various therapies on the normal corneal-healing processes (see Chap. 36, Agents That Affect Corneal Wound Healing: Modulation of Structure and Function).

The separation of side effects from drug activity has prompted the exploration of site-specific drugs, or prodrugs. Along this line, the search for steroids devoid of pressure-elevating effects is in progress, with loteprednol and rimexolone under evaluation. Steroid options currently available to the practitioner are discussed in Chapter 25, Corticosteroids in Ophthalmic Practice. The type, formulation, concentration, dosing regimens, delivery routes, tissue penetration, effects on specific disease processes, and potential side effects of steroids are considered in this chapter. Antiinflammatory agents, such as platelet-activating factor antagonists and leukotriene antagonists, are being developed concurrently for use in the eye and for systemic applications. Studies on newer, very potent antihistaminics reported by Gregg J. Berdy and myself in Chapter 28, Antihistamines and Mast Cell Stabilizers in Allergic Ocular Disease have revealed some apparent dual activity between H_1^- and H_2^- receptor types, and it is possible that both itching and hyperemia may be controlled without the addition of a vasoconstrictor. The search for effective mast cell stabilizers is ongoing, and the fruits of these labors are now being evaluated in the clinical setting. Through this research, olopatadine has been introduced. Olopatadine is an antihistiminic with mast cell–stabilizing properties. This dual activity provides relief from itching with a quick onset and a long (up to 8 hours) duration of action, allowing a b.i.d. dosing regimen.

Although practitioners have formulated and will continue to formulate their own ophthalmic preparations for topical and intraocular use, they will receive help from Joseph R. Robinson, Miguel F. Refojo, and myself with respect to pharmacokinetics and other considerations, such as pH and the effects of vehicles. I encourage students to pay particular attention to Chapter 18, Pharmacokinetics, as it provides the information necessary to maximize a drug's activity and its ability to reach the desired site of action. Drug delivery systems in the eye had an important beginning with pilocarpine inserts and with vehicles, such as those found in Betoptic S, Timoptic in Gelrite, and Pilopine. The goal of these systems was to enhance the dwell time, thus decreasing the necessary number of instillations, and ideally increasing the compliance of the patient. It is quite reasonable to suggest that future developments in pharmacology will be focused, in large part, on improving drug delivery systems and enhancing pharmacokinetics.

The last 5 years have seen a new class of glaucoma medications. Latanoprost (Zalatan) has been introduced as a prostaglandin analog using the well-known property of inflammatory agents to decrease intraocular pressure. Brimonidine is an α_2-adrenergic agonist providing an alternative to β-blockers for first-line therapy. Brimonidine lowers intraocular pressure by decreasing aqueous production and increasing uveoscleral outflow. Arthur H. Neufeld discusses these and many other advances in glaucoma therapy in Chapter 38.

In Chapter 27 King W. To, Arthur Neufeld, and myself discuss nonsteroidal antiinflammatory drugs, including the expanded claim that they reduce pain (ketorolac tromethamine [Acular]; diclofenac sodium [Voltaren]), and photophobia (diclofenac). Exciting studies are evaluating agents for neuroprotection and the regulation of blood flow. At this point, diseases like cystoid macular edema and cataracts have not been approached with a clear therapeutic answer.

The cost of agents, patent protection issues, and the general fiscal crisis surrounding health care figure large in how many dollars are available for future research and development. The effect of this on the pace and focus of research and development efforts is uncertain. Positive indicators are present, however. Improved concepts of the design of clinical studies and the availability of an increasing number of clinical research scientists, supported by increased patient acceptance of and participation in clinical trials, are important resources. The Food and Drug Administration regulatory agency for new ophthalmic drugs is now staffed by clinical research scientists who are ophthalmologists interested not only in the regulatory process but also in ophthalmic pharmacology, clinical science, and the needs of patients.

In time, few, if any, of the drugs discussed here will be in common use. We cannot help but wonder how these words and thoughts will appear to readers who consult these pages 50, or even 20, years from now for historical background—perhaps no different than historical records appear to us, who laugh inwardly at the prominent role played by cathartics, leeches, and bloodletting in times past. Nevertheless, it is the scientific method, the process, and the framework that we hope they will carry forward to achieve their own advances in pharmacology.

CHAPTER 18

Ocular Pharmacokinetics

Nimit Worakul, Nurşen Ünlü, and Joseph R. Robinson

The biologic activity of a drug, whether it be therapeutic or toxic, is proportional to the concentration of that drug at the receptor site or biophase. Moreover, the persistence of these effects is directly related to the residence time of this drug at the receptor. These statements can be paraphrased by saying that the toxic and therapeutic properties of a drug are a direct result of the absorption, distribution, metabolism, and elimination properties of the drug in the biophase.

Getting a particular drug to a receptor requires its administration at a site that is remote from the target, such as injection into the blood stream or perhaps in drop form to the front of the eye. The drug must then diffuse across several tissues (absorption), distribute into a variety of tissues and fluids (distribution), be subject to a wide array of metabolizing enzymes (metabolism), and then be eliminated from the area (elimination). Describing this time course of drug movement into and through tissues constitutes the field of *pharmacokinetics*. If instead of using the drug concentration in a particular tissue as a function of time, a biologic response, such as pupillary diameter, is employed, the field is known as *pharmacodynamics*. Pharmacokinetics assumes that the drug concentration is proportional to the biologic response, which is true most, but not all, of the time. Thus, quantitative descriptions of drug movement, using rate and equilibria constants, are more reliable when based on pharmacodynamic rather than pharmacokinetic analysis. Pharmacokinetics describes the quantitative relationship between the administered dose and dosing regimen and the observed plasma or tissue concentration of the drug, or both, whereas pharmacodynamics can be defined as the quantitative relationship between the observed plasma or tissue concentration, or both, of the active form of the drug and the pharmacologic effect.[1, 2] These terms may also be defined as what the body does to the drug (pharmacokinetics) and what the drug does to the body (pharmacodynamics).[3]

Progress in ophthalmic pharmaceuticals during the last decade has been impressive.[4, 5] Many products in this area have been or are being developed and include solutions,[6] suspensions,[7] ointments, gels,[8, 9] intravitreal injectables,[10] subconjunctival injectables,[11, 12] iontophoretic systems,[13] collagen shields,[13] and ocular inserts.[14] One of the most important tools to develop and assess these products is an accurate pharmacokinetic and pharmacodynamic model. The primary objective of a given pharmacokinetic and pharmacodynamic model must be to enhance the accuracy of estimates of the dynamic state of drug behavior in an actual clinical situation.[5] Many pharmacokinetic and pharmacodynamic models have been reported in the literature and represent varied levels of sophistication. Several excellent reviews on this subject are available.[15–23]

Clinical Utility

Following is a small sample of the applications of pharmacokinetics to clinical practice.

DOSING FREQUENCY

The frequency with which drugs are administered is typically governed by how rapidly the drugs are removed by metabolism or clearance of the unmetabolized drug. The loss of a drug is described by the half-life of the drug, i.e., the time for the tissue concentration to fall to one-half of its value. Redosing is commonly every half-life so that a series of peaks and valleys is established as shown in Figure 18–1.

TIME TO REACH STEADY STATE

Figure 18–1 shows that the tissue drug level rises because each subsequent dose adds to the quantity of drug left from the earlier dose. In most cases a steady-state level is reached within a finite number of doses, typically four to six doses.

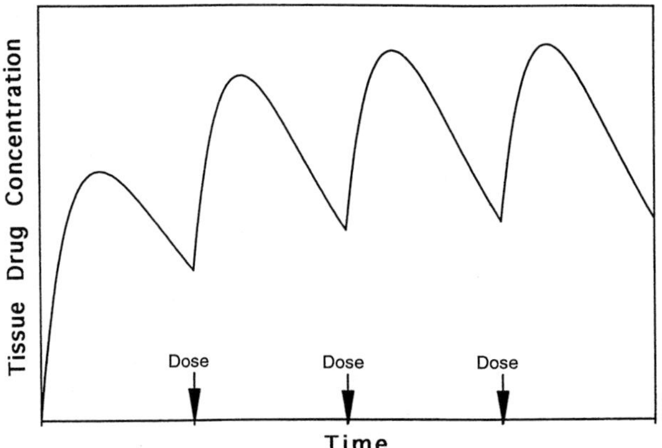

FIGURE 18–1. Hypothetical tissue drug concentration versus time for multiple doses of the same drug at set time intervals.

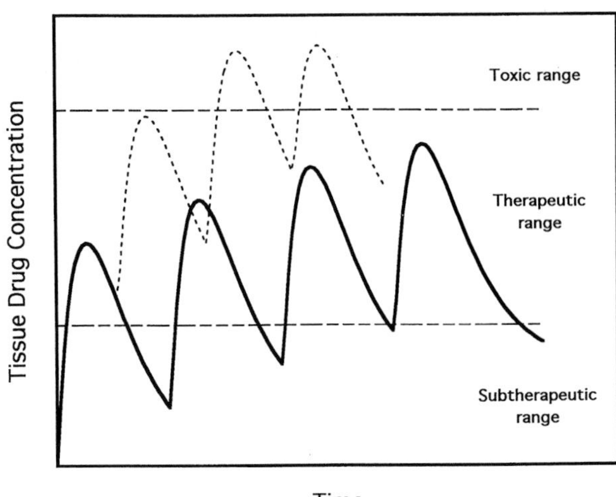

FIGURE 18–2. Hypothetical tissue drug concentration versus time for multiple doses of the same drug given time intervals either before or after the half-life of the drug. - - - - before the half-life; —— after the half-life.

STEADY-STATE MAXIMUMS AND STEADY-STATE MINIMUMS

Suppose the dosing interval is much earlier, or later, than the half-life of the drug. Figure 18–2 gives a few hypothetical examples of the impact of dosing interval. It is easy to see that dosing too soon can push the drug into the toxic range and dosing too late can give periods of time when the levels are subtherapeutic. The importance of the dosing interval cannot be underestimated to achieve therapeutic effectiveness and minimal toxicity.

METHODS OF DRUG APPLICATION

The eye is an extraordinarily protected organ that excludes foreign chemicals, such as drugs, through a variety of mechanisms. Understanding the various loss pathways from a topically applied drug can ensure that therapy is maximized and both local and systemic toxicity minimized. These loss pathways and potential remedies are discussed later.

Pharmacokinetic Parameters

A profile of drug concentration in ocular tissue can be dissected to provide important information. Figure 18–3 shows a typical profile.

C_{max}

The maximal level of drug in the tissue is C_{max}. The level that is reached dictates therapeutic and toxic responses and is directly related to the applied drug concentration and the absorption and elimination rate constants.

T_{max}

The time to reach a maximal level of drug in the tissue is T_{max}. This parameter is a function of only the absorption and elimination rate constants and is independent of the applied concentration.

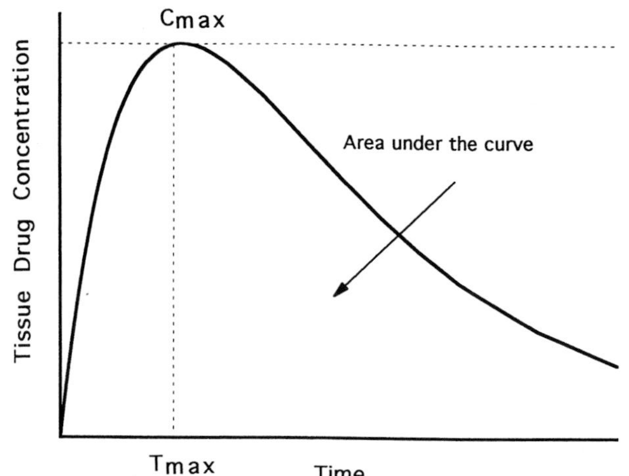

FIGURE 18–3. Typical profile of drug concentration versus time in an ocular tissue. C_{max}, maximal level of drug in tissue; T_{max}, time to reach maximal level of drug in tissue.

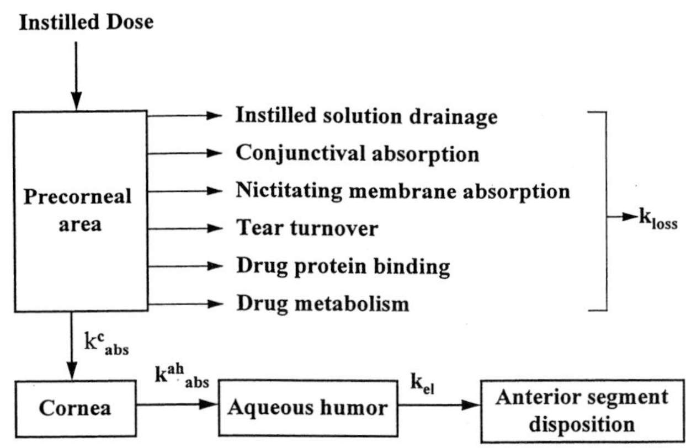

FIGURE 18–5. Model depicting precorneal and intraocular drug movement from topical dosing. k_{loss}, precorneal loss constant; k^{c}_{abs}, absorption rate constant from precorneal into cornea; k^{ah}_{abs}, absorption rate constant from cornea into aqueous humor; k_{el}, elimination rate constant from aqueous humor into anterior segment.

Area Under the Curve

The area under the curve yields the total amount of drug absorbed from an applied dose. The *bioavailability* of a drug, i.e., how much drug was instilled or injected versus how much actually got in, is computed from the area under the curve.

The dependency of the profile of the tissue concentration versus time on the magnitude of the absorption and elimination rate constant can be appreciated by inspection of Figure 18–4. A therapeutic response is expected only in the cross-hatched area.

Pharmacokinetic Models

The numerous pathways accounting for drug loss from the precorneal area in the rabbit can be described with a primitive model depicting precorneal and intraocular drug movement from topical dosing, as shown in Figure 18–5.[15, 24] The instilled dose drains away from the front of the eye of humans within 2 to 3 minutes, leaving a small amount of drug. This small quantity of drug left in the resident tear volume is further subject to loss through tear turnover, metabolism in the tear film, absorption into surrounding tissues, and perhaps binding to proteins in the tear film. Thus, there is extensive loss of drug from an instilled solution, and much of this loss is independent of the absorption, distribution, metabolism, and elimination properties of the drug.

A typical example of an aqueous humor drug concentration profile for a topically applied drug such as pilocarpine is shown in Figure 18–6. There are several important characteristics of this figure. First, the drug disappears from the aqueous humor in discrete steps and, in fact, the disappearance is triphasic. This probably represents the distribution

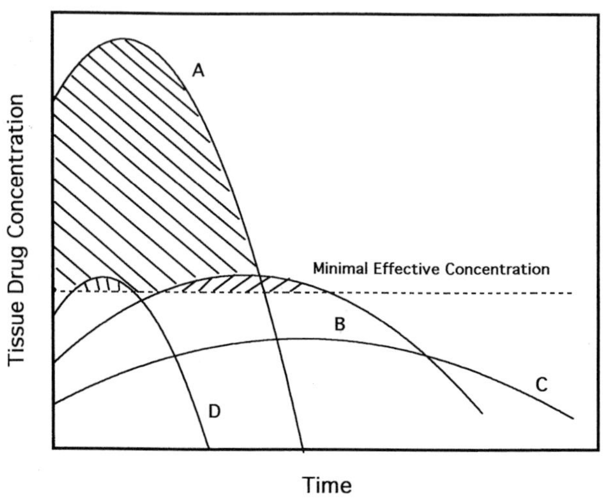

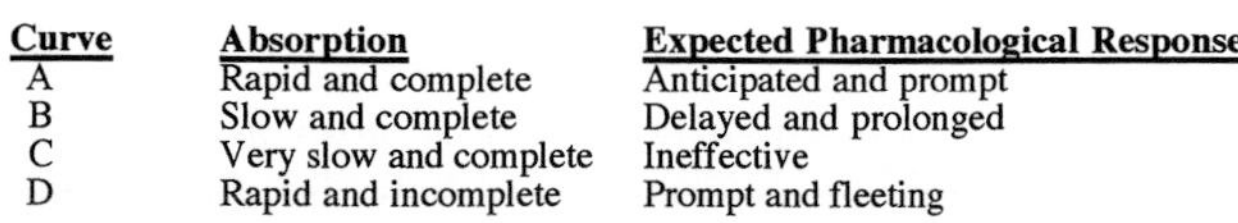

Curve	Absorption	Expected Pharmacological Response
A	Rapid and complete	Anticipated and prompt
B	Slow and complete	Delayed and prolonged
C	Very slow and complete	Ineffective
D	Rapid and incomplete	Prompt and fleeting

FIGURE 18–4. Various patterns of tissue drug concentration versus time with changing absorption and elimination rate constants.

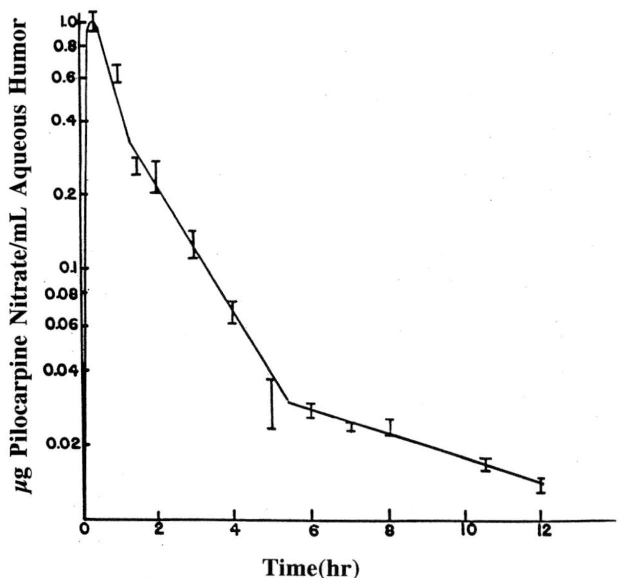

FIGURE 18–6. Aqueous humor concentration of pilocarpine versus time profile after institution of 25 μL of 1 × 10^{-2} M solution.

of the drug into various anterior segment tissues that become reservoirs of the drug. Hence as time proceeds, the loss of drug occurs with successively smaller elimination rate constants. Second, the drug achieves a C_{max} in a relatively short period of time—20 to 40 minutes is typical—giving the impression that the drug is rapidly absorbed across the cornea. In fact, the drug is typically not rapidly absorbed across the cornea, and the early peak drug level is due to an unusual constraint imposed by the kinetics of drug loss from the precorneal pocket.

The simplest pharmacokinetic model is to consider the eye as one compartment, as shown in Figure 18–7*A*.[24, 25] The equation describing drug concentration in this model is dependent on absorption and elimination rate constants. It is well known that for most drugs the true rate constant for absorption into the eye is much smaller than the elimination rate constant. This would normally lead to the classic "flip-flop" pharmacokinetic model in which the computed rate constant for the first portion of the pharmacokinetic profile would represent the elimination rate constant and the terminal line could be used to generate the absorption rate constant, exactly opposite to what intuition would suggest. What stops this from becoming a classic flip-flop model is a kinetic scheme known as a *parallel elimination pathway*. In this model, all rate constants describing loss of the instilled dose from the tear film are added together and the sum of these constants produces an apparent absorption rate constant that is larger than the elimination rate constant.

Figure 18–7*B* shows the nature of the model. In brief, summing all the loss rate constants depicted in Figure 18–5 yields an overall loss rate constant k_{loss}. The apparent absorption rate constant k_{abs} is described as

$$\text{Apparent } k_{abs} = k_{loss} + \text{true } k_{abs}$$

The magnitude of k_{loss} is typically in the range of 0.5 min^{-1}, whereas the true k_{abs} is two to three orders of magnitude smaller. It is for this reason that most topically applied drugs show an early peak drug level, and the time of this peak level is essentially independent of the properties of the drug.

These data suggest that to significantly improve ocular drug bioavailability, it is necessary to make the k_{loss} term smaller by one to two orders of magnitude or to increase the true k_{abs} by one to two orders of magnitude. Ocular delivery systems that decrease drainage loss, e.g., gels and inserts, can substantially decrease k_{loss}. Moreover, penetration enhancers would be needed to increase the true k_{abs} by one to two orders of magnitude.

Based on this short pharmacokinetic analysis, it is easy to understand why the typical bioavailability of a topically applied dose is only 1 to 10%. Clearly, the loss parameters have an enormous impact.

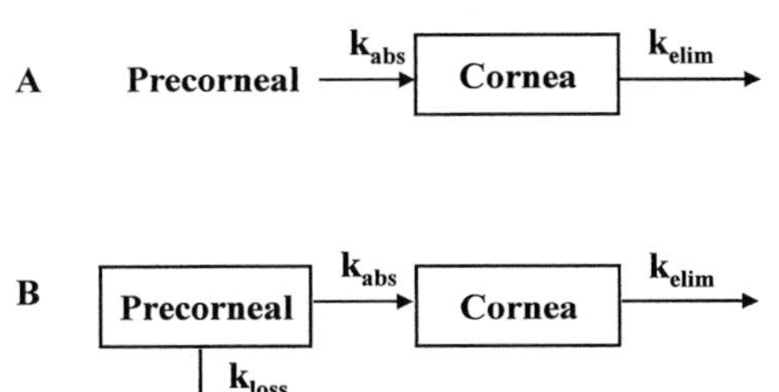

FIGURE 18–7. Schematic of two-compartment model without *(A)* and with *(B)* the precorneal loss constant. k_{loss}, precorneal loss constant; k_{abs}, absorption rate constant; k_{elim}, elimination rate constant.

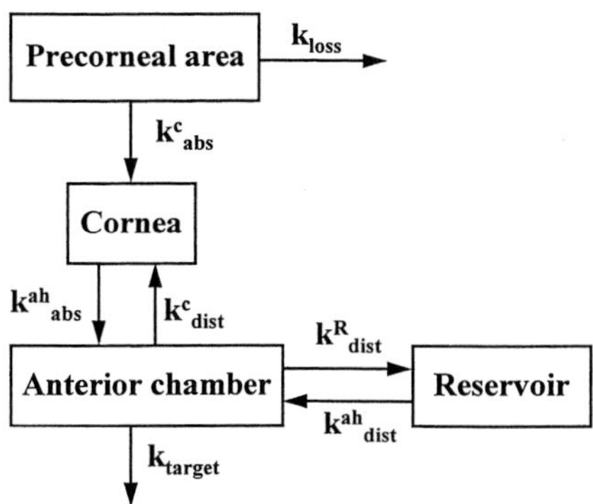

FIGURE 18–8. Schematic of four-compartment model in which the anterior chamber is in equilibrium with a reservoir. k, rate constant for drug transports into and out of various areas. K_{loss}, elimination rate constant from the precorneal area; $K^{ah}{}_{abs}$, the apparent absorption rate constants into the cornea and aqueous humor, respectively; $K^{c}{}_{dist}$, $K^{R}{}_{dist}$, and $k^{ah}{}_{dist}$, the distribution rate constants into the cornea, respectively and aqueous humor respectively; K_{target}, the absorption rate constant into the target area.

A much more complicated model is needed to adequately describe the pathway from precorneal application through the cornea and into the aqueous humor followed by distribution into the surrounding tissues. A four-compartment model, shown in Figure 18–8, was used to fit the data for both cornea and aqueous humor obtained after topical administration of pilocarpine to the albino rabbit eye. A mathematical derivation of this pharmacokinetic model was also reported.[25] However, the model treated the cornea as a simple semipermeable membrane. In fact, the cornea consists of an epithelium, stroma, and endothelium. The results from pharmacokinetic studies demonstrated that the lipophilic epithelium acts as a barrier to drug penetration by hydrophilic drugs and as a reservoir of pilocarpine. Movement of water-soluble drugs through the hydrophilic stroma is usually rapid. Therefore, the corneal stroma and endothelium are kinetically homogeneous with aqueous humor. A model that treats the cornea as three separate tissues corrects this deficiency as shown in Figure 18–9*A* and Table 18–1.[24, 25] The major assumptions for this model are that

1. There is instantaneous and complete mixing of instilled drug solution and tears.
2. Pilocarpine metabolism in the tear fluid is negligible.
3. The tissues constituting the compartments are homogeneous.
4. The iris, ciliary body, lens, and vitreous humor constitute the reservoir.

For the lipophilic drug fluorometholone, the corneal stroma-endothelium and aqueous humor are logically separated[26] as shown in Figure 18–9*B* and Table 18–1. Eller and colleagues[27] proposed a pharmacokinetic model in which a drug is administered at a constant rate to the corneal surface from a reservoir and then passively transported across the cornea into the aqueous humor. From the aqueous humor, drug may reversibly distribute to adjacent tissues, particularly the iris–ciliary body, or be eliminated from the eye into the body via the aqueous humor. The assumption of this model is that the cornea acts as a net barrier to absorption and not as a compartment, since the quantity of drug that resides in the cornea during the infusion time period is

TABLE 18–1. **Parameters of Models Described in Figure 18–9**

Parameter	Coefficient Associated With
P_p	Transfer of drug between precorneal area and corneal epithelium
P_n	Nonproductive loss
K_d	Drainage
$Q_T(t)$	Tear flow
P_a	1. Transfer of drug between corneal epithelium and corneal stroma–endothelium–aqueous humor 2. Transfer of drug between corneal epithelium and corneal stroma–endothelium
P_m	Drug loss via metabolism in or lateral diffusion from corneal epithelium
P_{ao}	Drug elimination from aqueous humor
P_r	1. Transfer of drug between corneal stroma–endothelium–aqueous humor and reservoir 2. Transfer of drug between aqueous humor and reservoir
P_{ro}	Drug elimination from reservoir
P_s	Transfer of drug between corneal stroma–endothelium and aqueous humor
P_{so}	Drug elimination from corneal stroma–endothelium

constant. This model was used for the lipophilic drugs ethoxzolamide,[27] ibuprofen, and ibufenac.[28]

Rao and coworkers[28] modified this model for use with hydroxyethoxy analogs of ibuprofen and ibufenac. This model represents the corneal epithelium and endothelium as barriers and the corneal stroma as a separate compartment.

A multicompartment model was developed to simulate the pharmacokinetic data obtained from the injection of cyclosporine into the anterior chamber.[29] The model described cyclosporine concentration in various ocular tissues and fluids by providing separate compartments for the aqueous humor, conjunctiva, sclera, lens, and iris–ciliary body

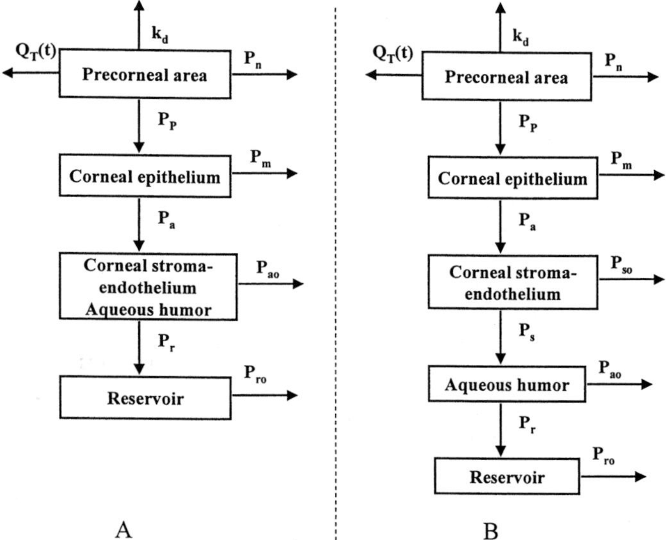

FIGURE 18–9. *A,* Schematic of four-compartment model that considers corneal stroma–endothelium and aqueous humor as one compartment. *B,* schematic of five-compartment model that considers the corneal stroma–endothelium and aqueous humor as separate compartments. See also Table 18–1.

and two subcompartments for the cornea (lipophilic cellular layers and hydrophilic stroma). The assumptions for this model are that

1. The concentration within each compartment is uniform.
2. The potential pathways for the elimination of cyclosporine from the aqueous humor to the vitreous and from the cornea, conjunctiva, and sclera to the systemic circulation were not included in this model.

Some reports have attempted to model the pharmacokinetics of drugs in the posterior segment of the eye. In the case of topical ophthalmic drug administration, the possibility of scleral absorption was evaluated by Ahmed and associates[30] for the lipophilic drugs propranolol, timolol, nadolol, and penbutolol, and the hydrophilic compounds sucrose and inulin. The results showed that resistance to penetration for all compounds tested in the outer layer of the sclera is much less than that of the corneal epithelium. The cornea offered substantially more resistance to inulin (a hydrophilic drug) than did the sclera.[31] However, the cornea and conjunctiva offered comparable resistance against timolol (a lipophilic drug).[30] In addition, Schoenwald and coworkers[32] have shown that the conjunctival-scleral route of entry produced higher iris–ciliary body concentrations of methazolamide analogs and 6-carboxyfluorescein, but not of rhodamine B (a lipophilic dye). The explanation of this phenomenon is that a hydrophilic drug is absorbed into the ciliary body through vessel uptake into the sclera and deposits within the ciliary body, whereas a lipophilic drug penetrates across the cornea and diffuses through the pupil against aqueous flow to enter the posterior chamber.

Drugs that are introduced into the vitreous humor by intravitreal injection spread through the vitreous humor and into the anterior chamber at the same rate that they diffuse in free solution.[17] Two pathways of exit from the vitreous chamber were predicted: (1) through the anterior hyaloid membrane into the posterior chamber and out of the eye with aqueous drainage and (2) directly across the retinal surface. The loss of drug from the vitreous chamber can be characterized by assuming that diffusion across the iris is negligible:

$$K_v = \left(\frac{f}{V_v}\right)\left(\frac{C_a}{C_v}\right)$$

where k_v is the transfer coefficient, f is the aqueous humor flow rate, V_v is the volume of vitreous humor, and C_a and C_v are drug concentrations in aqueous humor and vitreous humor, respectively.

A more recent study uses computer simulation to evaluate the in vivo and in vitro pharmacokinetic correlation of dexamethasone sodium after intravitreal injection of *m*-sulfobenzoate in rabbits[33]. The mathematical model was developed based on Fick's second law of diffusion by assuming that the vitreous body is a cylinder with three major pathways for elimination: the posterior aqueous chamber, the retinal–choroid–scleral membrane, and the lens, as shown in Figure 18–10. Results showed that the major route of elimination of the drug was through the posterior aqueous humor because of an absence of barrier membrane between the boundaries. By using the ratio of the product of the diffusion

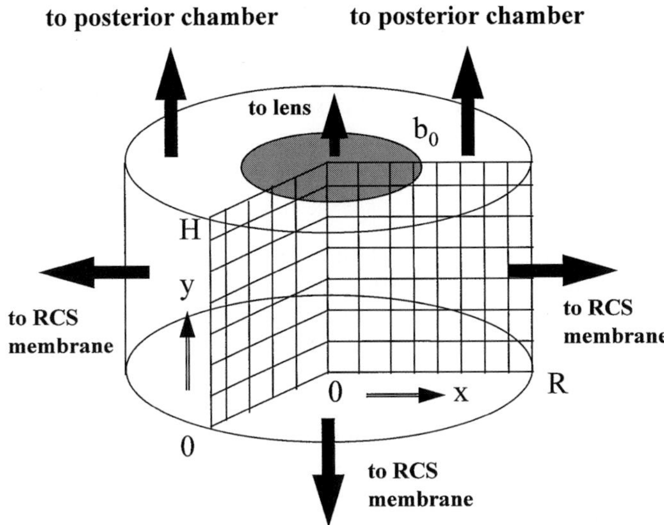

FIGURE 18–10. Cylindrical model of the vitreous body of rabbits for analyzing the pharmacokinetics of intravitreal drug delivery; the surface of the vitreous body is divided into three areas of elimination pathways: the posterior chamber, the retinal–choroid–scleral (RCS) membrane, and the lens. RCS, retina/choroid/sclera; H, effective height of vitreous body; R, b_0, effective radius of vitreous body and lens, respectively; x, y, horizontal and vertical axes, respectively.

coefficient and the effective area of the posterior chamber, the retinal–choroid–scleral membrane, and the lens (50:4:0.1), the authors concluded that after intravitreal injection, most hydrophilic drugs are eliminated by the annular gap between the lens and the ciliary body, and the retinal–choroid–scleral membrane may act as a major route of elimination of lipophilic drugs.

Models Derived from Drug Delivery

The five-compartment model shown in Figure 18–11 was developed to study the mechanism involved in transcorneal permeation of drugs from delivery devices.[34] The model consists of the tear film, epithelium, stroma, endothelium, and aqueous humor, which were assumed to be perfectly mixed and adequately represented by plane sheet barriers of known physical thickness with constant surface area. In this model, four routes of drug loss—lacrimal drainage, conjunctival absorption, aqueous drainage, and iris–ciliary body absorption—were included. By using simple mass balances and flux relationships, the investigators could convert the

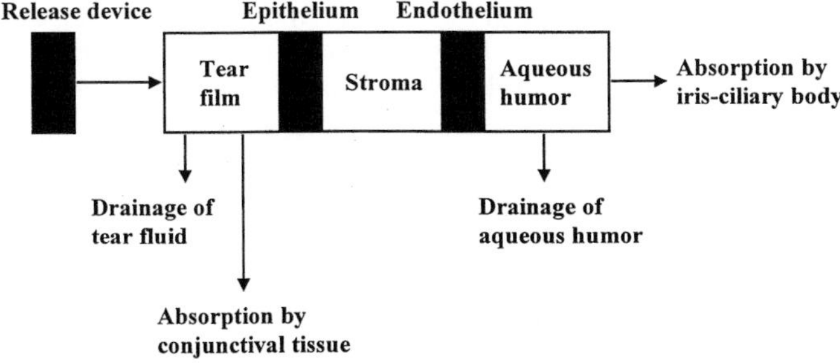

FIGURE 18–11. Schematic of five-compartment model that was developed for drug delivery devices.

compartment model to a series of mathematical expressions. More details about the mathematical equations and assumptions can be found in the original paper. The model was validated by using the experimental in vivo data compared with predicted aqueous humor drug concentrations from the model. The results showed an excellent correlation, and it was also possible to predict the amount of drug lost through each of the four elimination pathways. This model was modified by adding the compartments for the conjunctiva and the iris–ciliary body to compare pharmacokinetic differences between ocular inserts and eye drops of timolol.[35] Two other modifications of the model were added to account for conditions that occurred as a result of the experimental methods:

1. A reduction in tear flow, caused by the anesthetic during the period the devices were sutured in place
2. The unexpected corneal epithelial abrasion that occurred as a result of contact between the cornea and the suture

The results indicated that the model parameters required to predict ocular drug levels after administration by a controlled-release ocular insert are different from those of eye drop administration.

A multicompartment model was constructed to describe ophthalmic drug delivery with nanoparticle preparations.[36] This model was constructed from the data that showed that nanoparticle preparations might be able to create a precorneal depot.[37] This can enhance drug penetration directly to its site of action, the trabecular meshwork,[36] through the scleral or noncorneal pathway.[31, 38]

Grass and Lee[39] described and developed methods for constructing a pharmacokinetic model that can be used to predict the effect of increasing drug retention in the conjunctival sac, and varying the rate of release of the drug from a controlled drug delivery device, on the ratio of drug concentration in aqueous humor and plasma after topical dosing in rabbits. The pharmacokinetic model simulating timolol kinetics in both aqueous humor and plasma after topical dosing in the eye was constructed in separate segments and then linked in a stepwise manner. This model was validated in each segment by using previous published data on intravenous, nasal, and ocular dosing. The investigators concluded that this model may be useful in designing drug delivery strategies to improve the safety of topical eye medications by minimizing systemic absorption and maximizing drug delivery to ocular tissues. Moreover, it may be possible to scale the data obtained in rabbits to humans.

Pharmacodynamic Models

Ophthalmic pharmacologic responses such as miosis and mydriasis,[40, 41] light reflex inhibition,[12, 42–46] and intraocular pressure (IOP) have been used as parameters for investigating the effectiveness of ocular drug administration.

The miotic response of the eye was used to show the effect of cholinergic drugs.[17, 18, 36, 47] The general equation shows a linear relationship as

$$m_r = -k_{dm}t + m_0$$

where m_r describes the miotic response at time t, m_0 is a value for the theoretical miosis at time $t = 0$, and $k_{\rm dm}$ is the decrease of the miosis coefficient, i.e., pupil response coefficient, which is equivalent to the slope of the curve determined by linear regression.[36]

By using the curve of miotic response versus time, one can also calculate d_{max} and M_{max}, where d_{max} is the maximal duration of the miotic effect (the time axis intercept), M_{max} is the maximal miotic effect at t_{max}, and t_{max} is the time for maximal miotic effect.

Another mathematical model of the miotic response and the mydriasis response of the pupil from pilocarpine and carbachol, respectively,[17, 18] is

$$R_l = \frac{R}{R_{max} - R}$$

where R is the difference in pupil diameter before and after instillation, R_{max} is the difference between pupil diameter before instillation and maximum or minimum attainable pupil diameter with a large dose of the drug, and R_l is the response parameter. For a miotic response, $R = D_0 - D$ and $R_{max} = D_0 - D_{min}$, whereas for a mydriatic response, $R = D - D_0$ and $R_{max} = D_{max} - D_0$, where D_0 is the diameter of the pupil before use of the drug, D is the pupil diameter at the time of administration, and D_{max} and D_{min} are the maximum and minimum possible size of the pupil. D_{min} was induced by light reaction after pretreatment with 0.5% physostigmine. D_{max} was determined in the dark after topical administration of cyclopentolate or cocaine. The maximal and minimal diameter of the pupil was also defined as 8.5 and 1 mm, respectively. Therefore, the response parameter can be rewritten as follows:

$$\text{For miotic response, } R_l = \frac{D_0 - D}{D - 1}$$

$$\text{For mydriatic response, } R_l = \frac{D - D_0}{8.5 - D}$$

Plots of response and drug concentrations on a logarithmic scale show that a correlation slope of the regression line is very close to unity. Thus the relation can be expressed as

$$R_l = \frac{R}{R_{max} - R} = q'C$$

where C is the concentration of the drug and q' is the proportionality constant.

The linearized response R_l may be calculated for pupil diameter at various time intervals after instillation and plotted against the time after instillation. These plots were made for pilocarpine and tropicamide.[6, 18] The following equation describes the curves:

$$R_l = R_L\,[(e^{-A(t - t_0)} - e^{-B(t - t_0)})]$$

where R_L is the value of R_l at the intercept of the A and B components of the curves, t_0 is the lag time between instillation and the first response, and A and B are apparent elimination and absorption rate constants that are related to the rate of drug release from the cornea into the anterior chamber and to the rate of loss from the anterior chamber.

Chien and Schoenwald[41] showed another mathematical equation (an E_{max} model) for mydriatic activity of phenylephrine and its prodrug. The relation between drug concentration in aqueous humor corresponding to the mydriatic response was predicted by a Michaelis-Menten relationship:

$$\Delta E(t) = \frac{\Delta E_{max}\, C_a(t)}{K'_m + C_a(t)}$$

Where $\Delta E(t)$ is the mydriatic response at time t; ΔE_{max} is the maximal mydriatic response of the drug; K'_m is the drug concentration in aqueous humor required to produce half the maximal mydriatic response ($\frac{1}{2}\Delta E_{max}$), which is equal to the drug concentration in iris required to produce $\frac{1}{2}\,\Delta E_{max}$ divided by the partition coefficient of the drug between the iris and the aqueous humor; and $C_a(t)$ is the drug concentration in the aqueous humor at time t, which can be calculated by the equation

$$C_a(t) = M\,[e^{-A_1(t - t_0)} - e^{-B_1(t - t_0)}]$$

where M is the value of C_a at the intercept of the A_1 and B_1 components of the curve and depends on the initial dose of the drug, the fraction absorbed, and the kinetic parameters A_1 and B_1.

Since mydriatic tolerance was developed by phenylephrine, K'_m was changed and calculated at a set time interval by the following equation:

$$K'_m(t) = \left[\frac{\Delta E_{max}}{\Delta E(t)} - 1\right] C_a(t)$$

Another biologic response that can be assessed from a kinetic point of view is IOP versus time. The pharmacodynamic coefficients of the IOP response, area under the curve (AUC), t_{max}, I_{max}, and $\Delta\frac{1}{2}$, can be calculated; I_{max} is determined as the maximal IOP reduction at t_{max}, and $\Delta\frac{1}{2}$ is a value calculated from the width of the IOP response at half the height. The $\Delta\frac{1}{2}$ values show the duration of the IOP reduction response.[36]

An E_{max} model can be modified for the IOP reduction response as described by the same equation as for the mydriatic response:[48]

$$\Delta E = E - E_0 = \frac{(E_{max}\, C)}{(EC_{50} + C)}$$

where ΔE is a corresponding IOP reduction effect, E_0 is the baseline IOP, and EC_{50} is the aqueous humor concentration C that produces 50% of the maximal effect E_{max}.

The expression of IOP reduction in different ways was reviewed by using the relationship between the drug-induced IOP reduction and the control level of the IOP.[18] This relationship showed a linear relation that can be represented by

$$\frac{\Delta P_i}{P_i - 9} = X$$

where ΔP_i is the IOP reduction, P_i is the control level IOP, and X is the value that varies with changes in the drug concentration.

The results showed that the slope of the relation increased with increasing concentration of the drug without significantly altering the intercept. Therefore, X can be used to express the drug effect on the IOP response.

Zimmer[36] used this relative enhancement to compare the pharmacodynamic effects (miosis and IOP reduction) between aqueous solutions and nanoparticle preparations with different doses of pilocarpine. This value is useful to develop an appropriate drug delivery preparation. The relative enhancement was calculated by the following equation:

$$\text{Relative enhancement (\%)} = \frac{PD(NP)}{PD(AS)} \times 100$$

where PD(NP) is the pharmacodynamic effects of nanoparticle preparations and PD(AS) is the pharmacodynamic effects of aqueous solutions.

Light reflex inhibition (LRI), which is the amplitude of reflex responses to 0.5-second light flashes, can be calculated by the following equation:

$$LRI\ (\%) = \frac{(RAU_t - RAT_t) - (RAU_0 - RAT_0)}{RAU_t} \times 100$$

where RAT and RAU are the reflex amplitude of treated eye and untreated eye, respectively (each at time t or time $t = 0$).

When the LRI was used to investigate the relative bioavailability of pilocarpine, the results showed that it was inhibited in parallel with miosis.[12]

TABLE 18–2. **Comparison of Pharmacokinetic Factors Between Rabbit and Human Eye**

Pharmacokinetic Factors	Rabbit	Human
Tear volume (μL)	5–10	7–30*
Tear turnover rate (μL/min)	0.5–0.8	0.5–2.2
Spontaneous blinking rate†	4–5 times/hr	6–15 times/min
Lacrimal punctum or puncta	1	2
Nictitating membrane‡	Present	Absent
pH of lacrimal fluids	7.3–7.7	7.3–7.7
Turnover rate of lacrimal fluids (% min^{-1})	7	16
Buffering capacity of lacrimal fluids	Poor	Poor
Milliosmolarity of tear (mOsm/L)	305	305
Initial drainage rate constant (min^{-1})	0.55	1.6
Corneal thickness (mm)	0.35–0.45	0.52–0.54
Corneal diameter (mm)	15	11–12
Corneal surface area (cm^2)	1.5–2.0	1.04
pH of aqueous humor	8.2	7.1–7.3
Aqueous humor volume (mL)	0.25–0.3	0.1–0.25
Aqueous humor turnover rate (μL/min)	3–4.7	2–3
Protein content of tears (%)	0.5	0.7
Protein content of aqueous humor (μg/mL)	0.55	30
Ratio of conjunctival surface to corneal surface	9	17

Data from references 5, 15, 17, 20, 21, 23, 40, 49, 51 to 59.
*Range depends on blinking rate and conjunctival sac volume.
†Occurs during normal waking hours without apparent external stimuli.
‡Significance of nictitating membrane from precorneal area is small relative to overall loss rate.

RABBIT MODEL

Because many anatomic and physiologic factors of the rabbit and human eye are similar (Table 18–2) and the animal is relatively inexpensive and easy to handle, rabbits have been used as an animal model in most ocular experiments. However, some differences between the rabbit and human eye could affect drug kinetics. For example, the blinking rate in humans (6 to 15 times/min) is higher than in rabbits (4 to 5 times/hr) and could allow the penetration of drug through the cornea of the rabbits more than that of humans because of a high drug concentration at the corneal surface[49, 50] and low drug solution drainage in the New Zealand albino rabbit eye.[23] Moreover, rabbits appear to be less sensitive than humans to moderate increases of vehicle viscosity, especially for a suspension-type paraffin ointment that gave better results in humans, probably because shear effects facilitate drug release.[40] Therefore, clinical trials in humans must always be used to confirm data from rabbits.

Factors Influencing Ocular Bioavailability

As can be seen in Figure 18–12, a substantial portion of the drug winds up in the systemic circulation and only a fraction of the dose actually crosses eye tissue to reach the interior of the eye. A substantial number of factors can influence the ratio of ocular to systemic drug load.

SOLUTION OSMOTICITY

Tears are slightly hypertonic, i.e., approximately 330 mOsm. Hypertonic solutions above 400 mOsm are unpleasant to the eye and induce lacrimation, which in turn causes greater precorneal drainage loss. In contrast, hypotonic solutions as low as 100 mOsm are still comfortable in the eye and may actually lead to an increase in the bioavailability of water-soluble drugs, presumably through a solvent drag effect.

SOLUTION pH

The comfort zone of an ocular solution is rather narrow and typically in the pH 6 to 8 range. Outside this range, the

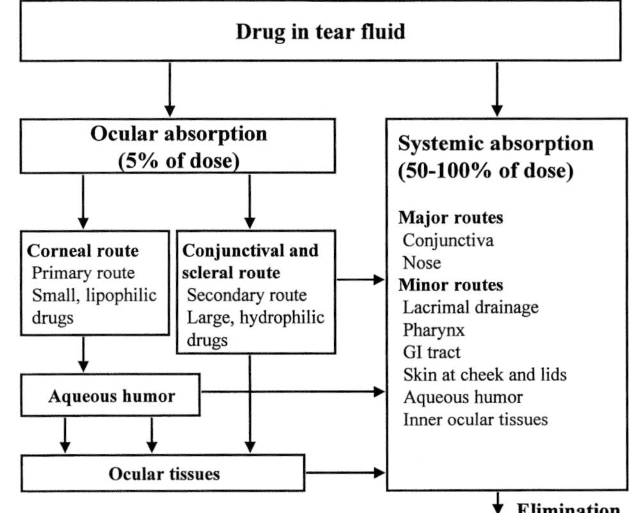

FIGURE 18–12. Typical profile of the fate of a topically applied drug.

solution can be uncomfortable and induce lacrimation. This causes drug loss. The pH boundaries outside of which actual tissue damage occurs rapidly are below pH 4 and above pH 10. The ability of the eye to restore physiologic pH is very good, and this occurs within a short time because of lacrimation and a high turnover rate of tears. Nevertheless, pH discomfort occurs outside the pH 6 to 8 range, and because of the tighter proximity of the lid to the globe, the eye of Asians experiences a greater discomfort than the eye of whites.

With an ionizable drug, it is sometimes tempting to adjust the pH either above or below the comfort range pH of 6 to 8 to convert the drug to a more favorable form for absorption, i.e., the undissociated form of the drug. It is common to see any gain in drug bioavailability through pH adjustment eliminated by precorneal loss owing to discomfort and lacrimation.

SUSPENSIONS

The driving force for drug absorption is drug concentration, so a 10% solution is absorbed at a rate that is 10 times that of a 1% solution. This is not so with a suspension. A 10% and a 1% suspension have exactly the same amount of drug in solution, and all additional drug is insoluble. Unless the excess solid dissolves within the residence time of the solid in the precorneal pocket (2 minutes), it is lost from the front of the eye and does not contribute to ocular tissue drug levels. Thus, a 10% suspension is rarely 10 times more bioavailable than a 1% suspension.

VISCOSITY

From the earlier discussion, it is clear that the factor contributing the most to precorneal drug loss is drainage. An increase in the viscosity of the solution would appear to remedy this problem. However, solution viscosities above 30 to 50 cp are often uncomfortable in the eye and, indeed, it is commonly necessary to go to a ringing gel, above 100,000 cp, before an appreciable difference in drug bioavailability is noted. These highly viscous products can leave an unpleasant film in the patient's eye on awakening and can feel uncomfortable in the eye. A better approach to the precorneal residence time problem is to employ a phase-change polymer. These systems are liquid in the bottle but when placed in the eye undergo solidification because of differences in temperature, pH, or specific ions. Such phase-change solutions are typically better accepted by the patient.

INSERTS

A solid insert containing drug minimizes drainage of the solution but is often not patient friendly. Systems that are insoluble and must therefore be put in, and subsequently removed, are the least patient friendly, whereas soluble inserts need only be put in and not removed. Although giving better ocular drug bioavailability, a sustained effect, these inserts have not found wide commercial success.

Conclusions

Quantitative understanding of the time course of drugs in the eye through pharmacokinetic analysis provides mechanistic insight into the fate of drug disposition in this organ. It also provides clinical strategies for how to optimize drug use in treatment as well as suggesting critical barriers that must be overcome to either improve therapy or reduce toxicity for a particular drug.

REFERENCES

1. Fleishaker JC, Ferry JJ: Pharmacokinetic-Pharmacodynamic Modeling in Drug Development: Concepts and Applications. *In* Derendorf H, Hochhaus G (eds): Handbook of Pharmacokinetic/Pharmacodynamic Correlation. Boca Raton, FL, CRC Press, 1995, pp 57–78.
2. Lima JJ: Pharmacokinetics and pharmacodynamics. *In* Swarbrick J, Boylan JC (eds): Encyclopedia of Pharmaceutical Technology, vol 12. New York, Marcel Dekker, 1995, pp 29–52.
3. Holford NH, Scheiner LB: Kinetics of pharmacologic response. *In* Rowland M, Tucker G (eds): Pharmacokinetics: Theory and Methodology. Elmsworth, NY, Pergamon Press, 1986, pp 189–212.
4. Hecht G: Ophthalmic preparations. *In* Gennaro AR (ed): Remington: The Science and Practice of Pharmacy, 19th ed, vol II. Easton, PA, Mack, 1995, pp 1563–1576.
5. Reddy IK, Ganesan MG: Ocular therapeutics and drug delivery: An overview: *In* Reddy IK (ed): Ocular Therapeutics and Drug Delivery: A Multi-disciplinary Approach. Lancaster, PA, Technomic, 1996, pp 3–29.
6. Nagataki S, Mishima S: Pharmacokinetics of instilled drugs in the human eye. Int Ophthalmol Clin 20(3):33–49, 1980.
7. Gurny R: Preliminary study of prolonged acting drug delivery system for the treatment of glaucoma. Pharm Acta Helv 56:130–132, 1981.
8. Lewis RA, Schoenwald RD, Barfknecht CF, et al: Aminozolamide gel: A trial of topical carbonic anhydrase inhibitor in ocular hypertension. Arch Ophthalmol 1986; 104:842–844.
9. Miyazaki S, Ishii K, Takada M: Use of fibrin film as a carrier for drug delivery: A long-acting delivery system for pilocarpine into the eye. Chem Pharm Bull 30:3405–3407, 1982.
10. Berthe P, Baudouin C, Garraffo R, et al: Toxicologic and pharmacokinetic analysis of intravitreal injections of foscarnet, either alone or in combination with ganciclovir. Invest Ophthalmol Vis Sci 35:1038–1045, 1994.
11. Barza M, Doft B, Lynch E: Ocular penetration of ceftriazone, ceftazidime, and vancomycin after suconjunctival injection in humans. Arch Ophthalmol 111:492–494, 1993.
12. Kelly JA, Molyneux PD, Smith SA, et al: Relative bioavailability of pilocarpine from a novel ophthalmic delivery system and conventional eyedrop formulations. Br J Ophthalmol 73:360–362, 1989.
13. Friedberg ML, Pleyer U, Mondino BJ: Device drug delivery to the eye: Collagen shields, iontophoresis, and pumps. Ophthalmology 98:725–732, 1991.
14. Grass GM, Cobby J, Makoid MC: Ocular delivery of pilocarpine from erodible matrices. J Pharm Sci 73:618–621, 1984.
15. Lee VH-L, Robinson JR: Review: Topical ocular drug delivery: Recent developments and future challenges. J Ocul Pharmacol 2:67–108, 1986.
16. Jarvinen K, Jarvinen T, Urtti A: Ocular absorption following topical delivery. Adv Drug Delivery Rev 16:3–19, 1995.
17. Maurice DM, Mashima S: Ocular pharmacokinetics. *In* Sear ML (ed): Handbook of Experimental Pharmacology: Pharmacology of the Eye, vol 69. New York, Springer-Verlag, 1984, pp 19–116.
18. Mishima S: Clinical pharmacokinetics of the eye. Invest Ophthalmol Vis Sci 21:504–541, 1981.
19. Frangie JP: Clinical pharmacokinetics of various topical ophthalmic delivery systems. Clin Pharmacokinet 29:130–138, 1995.
20. Schoenwald RD: Ocular pharmacokinetic/pharmacodynamic. *In* Mitra AK (ed): Ophthalmic Drug Delivery System. New York, Marcel Dekker, 1993, pp 83–110.
21. Schoenwald RD: Pharmacokinetics in ocular drug delivery. *In* Edman P (ed): Biopharmaceutics of Ocular Drug Delivery. Boca Raton, FL, CRC Press, 1993, pp 159–191.
22. Schoenwald RD: Ocular drug delivery: Pharmacokinetic considerations. Clin Pharmacokinet 18:255–269, 1990.
23. Urtti A, Salminen L: Minimizing systemic absorption of topically administered ophthalmic drugs. Surg Ophthalmol 37:435–456, 1993.
24. Lee VH-L, Robinson JR: Mechanistic and quantitative evaluation of precorneal pilocarpine disposition in albino rabbits. J Pharm Sci 68:673–684, 1979.

25. Makoid MC, Robinson JR: Pharmacokinetics of topically applied pilocarpine in the albino rabbit eye. J Pharm Sci 68:435–443, 1979.
26. Sieg JW, Robinson Jr: Mechanistic studies on transcorneal penetration of fluorometholone. J Pharm Sci 70:1026–1029, 1981.
27. Eller MG, Schoenwald RD, Dixson JA, et al: Topical carbonic anhydrase inhibitors IV: Relationship between excised corneal permeability and pharmacokinetic factors. J Pharm Sci 74:525–529, 1985.
28. Rao CS, Schoenwald RD, Barfknecht CF, et al: Biopharmaceutical evaluation of ibufenac, ibuprofen, and their hydroxyethoxy analogs in the rabbit eye. J Pharmacokinet Biopharmaceut 29:357–387, 1992.
29. Oh C, Saville BA, Cheng Y-L, et al: A compartment model for the ocular pharmacokinetics of cyclosporine in rabbits. Pharm Res 12:433–437, 1995.
30. Ahmed I, Gokhale RD, Shah MV, et al: Physicochemical determinants of drug diffusion across the conjunctiva, sclera, and cornea. J Pharm Sci 76:583–586, 1987.
31. Ahmed I, Patton TF. Disposition of timolol and inulin in the rabbit eye following corneal versus non-corneal absorption. Int J Pharm 38:9–21, 1987.
32. Schoenwald RD, Deshpande G, Rethwisch DG, et al: Penetration into the anterior chamber via the conjunctival/scleral pathway. J Ocul Pharmacol Therapeutics 13:41–59, 1997.
33. Ohtori A, Tojo K: In vivo/in vitro correlation of intravitreal delivery of drugs with the help of computer simulation. Biol Pharm Bull 17(2):283–290, 1994.
34. Friedrich SW, Cheng Y-L, Saville BA: Theoretical corneal permeation model for ionizable drugs. J Ocul Pharmacol 9:229–249, 1993.
35. Friendrich S, Saville BA, Cheng Y-L, et al: Pharmacokinetic differences between ocular inserts and eyedrops. J Ocul Pharmacol 12(1):5–18, 1996.
36. Zimmer A: Pharmacokinetics and pharmacodynamics of pilocarpine-loaded PBCA nanoparticles in the glaucomatous rabbit eye. Doctoral thesis. John W. Goethe, University of Frankfurt, Germany, 1993.
37. Zimmer A, Kreuter J, Robinson JR: Studies on transport pathway of PBCA nanoparticles in ocular tissues. J Microencapsul 8:497–504, 1991.
38. Ahmed I, Patton TF: Importance of the noncorneal absorption route in topical ophthalmic drug delivery. Invest Ophthalmol Vis Sci 26:584–587, 1985.
39. Grass GM, Lee VH-L: A model to predict aqueous humor and plasma pharmacokinetics of ocular applied drugs. Invest Ophthalmol Vis Sci 34:2251–2259, 1993.
40. Saettone MF, Giannaccini B, Barattini F, et al: The validity of rabbits for investigations on ophthalmic vehicles: A comparison of four different vehicles containing tropicamide in humans and rabbits. Pharm Acta Helv 57:47–55, 1982.
41. Chien D-S, Schoenwald RD: Ocular pharmacokinetics and pharmacodynamics of phenylephrine and phenylephrine oxazolidine in rabbit eyes. Pharm Res 7:476–483, 1990.
42. Putnam ML, Schoenwald RD, Duffel MW, et al: Ocular disposition of aminozolamide in the rabbit eye. Invest Ophthalmol Vis Sci 28:1373–1382, 1987.
43. Lee VH-L, Luo AM, Li S, et al: Pharmacokinetic basis for nonadditivity of intraocular pressure lowering in timolol combinations. Invest Ophthalmol Vis Sci 32:2948–2957, 1991.
44. Urtti A, Rouhiainen H, Kaila T, et al: Controlled ocular timolol delivery: Systemic absorption and intraocular pressure effects in humans. Pharm Res 11:1278–1282, 1994.
45. Brechue WF, Maren TH: pH and drug ionization affects ocular pressure lowering of topical carbonic anhydrase inhibitors. Invest Ophthalmol Vis Sci 34:2581–2587, 1993.
46. Sharir M, Pierce WM Jr, Chen D, et al: Pharmacokinetics, acid-base balance and intraocular pressure effects of ethyloxaloylazolamide: A novel topically active carbonic anhydrase inhibitor. Exp Eye Res 58:107–116, 1994.
47. Kreuter J: Particulates nanoparticles and microparticles. *In* Mitra AK (ed): Ophthalmic Drug Delivery System. New York, Marcel Dekker, 1993, 275–287.
48. Tang-Liu DD-S, Acheampong A, Chien D-S, et al: Pharmacokinetic and pharmacodynamic correlation of ophthalmic drugs. *In* Reddy IK (ed): Ocular therapeutics and drug delivery: A multi-disciplinary approach. Lancaster, PA, Technomic, 1996, pp 133–147.
49. Maurice DM: Prolonged-action drops. Int Ophthal Clin 33(4):81–91, 1993.
50. Maurice DM: The effect of the low blink rate in rabbits on topical drug penetration. J Ocul Pharmacol Therapeutics 11:297–304, 1995.
51. Zaki I, Fitzgerald P, Hardy JG, et al: A comparison of the effect of viscosity on the precorneal residence of solutions in rabbit and man. J Pharm Pharmacol 38:463–466, 1986.
52. Urtti A, Salminen L: Animal pharmacokinetic studies. *In* Mitra AK (ed): Ophthalmic Drug Delivery System. New York, Marcel Dekker, 1993, pp 121–136.
53. Chrai SS, Patton TF, Mehta A, et al: Lacrimal and instilled fluid dynamics in rabbit eye. J Pharm Sci 62:1112–1121, 1973.
54. Carney LG, Hill RM: Human tear buffering capacity. Arch Ophthalmol 97:951–952, 1979.
55. Olejnik O: Conventional systems in ophthalmic drug delivery. *In* Mitra AK (ed): Ophthalmic Drug Delivery System. New York, Marcel Dekker, 1993, pp 177–198.
56. Stjernschantz J, Astin M: Anatomy and physiology of the eye, physiological aspects of ocular drug therapy. *In* Edman P (ed): Biopharmaceutics of Ocular Drug Delivery. Boca Raton, FL, CRC Press, 1993, pp 1–25.
57. Watsky MA, Jablonski M, Edelhauser HF: Comparison of conjunctival and corneal surface areas in rabbit and human. Curr Eye Res 7:483–486, 1988.
58. Conrad JM, Robinson JR: Aqueous chamber distribution volume measurement in rabbits. J Pharm Sci 66:219–224, 1977.
59. Hutak CM, Jacaruso RB: Evaluation of primary ocular irritation: Alternatives to the Draize test. *In* Reddy IK (ed): Ocular Therapeutics and Drug Delivery: A Multidisciplinary Approach. Lancaster, PA, Technomic, 1996, pp 489–525.

CHAPTER 19

Anesthetics

Martin A. Acquadro, Joseph C. Kim, and Mohandas M. Kini

Premedication

Premedication for alleviation of anxiety is not a substitute for adequate preoperative discussion with the patient. A study comparing various techniques, including no preoperative visit or drug, preoperative discussion alone, premedications alone, and preoperative discussion with premedication, demonstrated interesting results. The group of patients who displayed the most anxiety were those who were premedicated without preoperative discussion or consultation. The patients with the least anxiety were those who had both preoperative discussion and preoperative medication. The patients who had only preoperative discussion, without any premedication, were not much more anxious, as a percentage of the population studied, than those who received both preoperative discussion and premedication.[1]

The goals of preanesthetic medication include decreased anxiety, analgesia if preoperative pain is evident, and, if necessary, diminished airway secretions and diminished gastric acidity and volume. All these goals should be accomplished without excessive sedation, which could compromise the cardiopulmonary system.[2–4]

PHARMACODYNAMICS

Benzodiazepines

Anxiolytics are usually used as preoperative medications. Benzodiazepines (Table 19–1) are the most common of the anxiolytic agents. When given in the usual doses, they produce the greatest relief of anxiety with the least cardiopulmonary depression. These drugs are rarely implicated as a cause of nausea and vomiting. They can raise the threshold for central nervous system (CNS) toxicity of local anesthetics[5] and are not analgesic, but they compound the anxiolytic effects of some analgesics in small to moderate doses. Diazepam is usually given orally. The solvent used in parenteral preparations can result in pain and phlebitis. Lorazepam can be given orally or parenterally and often produces amnesia. It can also result in prolonged sedation.[4]

Midazolam has become popular because of its water solubility, rapid onset and short duration of action, and reliability. It can be given intramuscularly or intravenously and often produces amnesia with few side effects. Mental function returns to normal within 4 hours, making midazolam a popular choice for ambulatory surgery and regional anesthesia. Diazepam is more likely to produce cumulative effects than lorazepam or midazolam.[4]

Barbiturates

Patients scheduled for surgery often benefit from taking a hypnotic agent the night before, to help them sleep. Used this way, barbiturates are effective and safe. Generally, pentobarbital or secobarbital, given in a dose of 100 to 200 mg orally at bedtime, is effective.[2] Associated nausea and vomiting are rare, and cardiopulmonary depression is minimal.[4]

If barbiturates are used in lieu of opioids and given preop-

TABLE 19–1. **Premedicants—Anxiolytics and Hypnotics[4, 8, 11]**

Agent	Dosage/ Metabolism	Effects
Benzodiazepines		
Midazolam IV	0.03–0.07 mg/kg tE: 1–4 hr M: Liver E: Kidney	CNS depression, amnesia, ↑ seizure threshold, BP and respiratory depression; may cause paradoxical CNS excitement
Diazepam	IV: 0.03–0.1 mg/kg PO: 0.05–0.15 mg/kg tE: 7–10 hr (2–8 days for active metabolites) M: Liver E: Kidney	
Lorazepam	IV: 0.05 mg/kg PO: 1–10 mg/kg tE: 14 hr M: Liver E: Kidney	
Barbiturates		
Secobarbital	IV: 50 mg q 15 min up to 250 mg IM: 100–200 mg PO: 100–200 mg tE: 20–28 hr M: Liver E: Kidney	CNS depression; may cause depression of BP, hiccoughs, laryngospasm, respiratory depression, exacerbation of porphyria; agents cross placenta; may antagonize oral anticoagulants
Pentobarbital	IV: 1 mg/kg up to 500 mg IM: 100–200 mg PO: 100–200 mg tE: 20–50 hr M: Liver E: Kidney (mostly), liver	

BP, blood pressure; CNS, central nervous system; E, route of excretion; IM, intramuscularly; IV, intravenously; M, site of metabolism; PO, per os; tE, elimination half-life.

TABLE 19–2. **Premedicants—Analgesics**[4, 8, 11]

Agent	Dosage/Metabolism	Opioid Effects
Meperidine	IV: 0.5–1.0 mg/kg IM/SC: 0.5–1.0 mg/kg PO: 1 mg/kg q 2–4 hr tE: 1.5–4 hr M: Liver E: Kidney	Analgesic, central nervous system depression, euphoria, respiratory depression, bronchospasm (rare), ↓ blood pressure, nausea, vomiting, dysphoria, ↓ biliary pressure, ↓ gastrointestinal/genitourinary motility. Agents cross placenta. Greater incidence of skeletal rigidity with fentanyl (accumulation with frequent dosing). Narcotics, particularly Demerol, should be avoided in patients taking MAO inhibitors.
Morphine	IV: 0.1 mg/kg IM: 0.1 mg/kg tE: 2–4 hr M: Liver E: Kidney	
Fentanyl	IV: 10–100 μg IM: 50–100 μg/kg t½: α: 1–2 min tE: 4 hr M: Liver E: Kidney	

E, route of excretion; IM, intramuscularly; IV, intravenously; M, site of metabolism; PO, per os; SC, subcutaneously; tE, elimination half-life; t½, half-life.

eratively, the clinician may expect the patient to awaken more quickly from general anesthesia, to experience pain earlier, and perhaps to be restless during emergence and as consciousness is regained. This is thought to be due to an antianalgesic action of barbiturates.[2] Patients who habitually use barbiturates or alcohol may exhibit tolerance to barbiturates.[2, 4]

Antihistamines

Antihistamines are used as anxiolytics as well as H_1 histamine receptor blockers. Hydroxyzine and diphenhydramine are common agents.[4]

Narcotics

If the patient experiences preoperative pain, morphine is an effective preoperative analgesic (Table 19–2). The choice of narcotic is usually governed by the desired duration of activity. Morphine's clinical effects persist 4 to 6 hours; fentanyl's action lasts approximately 1 to 2 hours. Urinary retention, wheezing, constipation, and nausea and vomiting are not uncommon with opioid analgesics. The respiratory depressant action of morphine may cause hypoventilation and increased carbon dioxide tension with resultant increased intracranial pressure. Advantages and disadvantages need to be considered in the decision to use opioids in preanesthetic medication.[2, 4]

Meperidine is used commonly as an intramuscular medication. There is some concern that the metabolite of meperidine, normeperidine, may result in confusion, agitation, and seizures, particularly in the elderly, in patients with renal failure, and in children. This is more often a problem with long-term repeated dosing.

Phenothiazines

Phenothiazines lack amnestic activity but do have anxiolytic, antihistaminic, and antiemetic properties. They are often combined with barbiturates and opioids. The incidence of postoperative respiratory depression is increased, and emergence can be delayed.[4]

Antiemetics

Ondansetron hydrochloride is a commonly used selective blocking agent of the serotonin 5-HT3 receptor, administered orally or intravenously. These serotonin 5-HT3 receptors are found centrally in the area postrema chemoreceptor trigger zone and peripherally on vagal nerve terminals. Although it is not certain whether ondansetron's effectiveness comes from antagonism of central, peripheral, or both receptor sites, the drug is effective against perioperative and chemotherapy-induced emesis. The incidence of side effects is low when the drug is given in normal doses to normal patients.[6]

Butyrophenones. The most common butyrophenone is droperidol (Table 19–3). In adults it is an antiemetic at very small doses, and cardiopulmonary stability is maintained. It should be noted that droperidol does have α_1-adrenergic-blocking activity and must be given with caution if hypotension is already evident. Restlessness and extrapyramidal dyskinesia may be noted. Atropine is an effective antidote. A patient may exhibit catatonia and appear outwardly calm though he or she is in fact experiencing panic secondary to dysphoria produced by the action of droperidol.[4]

TABLE 19–3. **Premedicants—Antiemetics**[4, 6, 8, 11]

Agent	Dosage/ Metabolism	Effects
Droperidol	IV: 0.625–2.5 mg IM: 2.5–10 mg tE: ? M: Liver E: Kidney, liver	Antiemetic, antipsychotic. May cause dysphoria, extrapyramidal effects, hypotension secondary to α-blockade.
Hydroxyzine	IM: 25–100 mg PO: 25–100 mg tE: 3 hr M: Liver E: Liver, kidney	Central nervous system depression, antiemetic effects, antagonism of histamine action on H_1 receptors. May cause dry mouth.
Ondansetron	IV: 4 mg slow PO: 8–16 mg, 1 hr before induction M: Liver E: Kidney, liver	Antiemetic—chemotherapy and post anesthesia N/V. Hypotension, bradycardia, tachycardia, angina, second-degree heart block, bronchospasm, extrapyramidal effects, seizures.

E, route of excretion; IM, intramuscularly; IV, intravascularly; M, site of metabolism; PO, per os; tE, elimination half-life.

H_2 Histamine Receptor Antagonists

Cimetidine and ranitidine block H_2 receptors and decrease gastric acid secretion. Ranitidine has become more popular, because it appears to cause fewer cardiovascular and CNS side effects than cimetidine.[4]

Antacids

Particulate and nonparticulate antacids effectively raise gastric acid pH. If aspiration is a concern, a nonparticulate antacid is preferred, because particulate antacids may cause more lung damage. Sodium citrate is a commonly used nonparticulate antacid.[4]

Gastrointestinal Transit Time

Metoclopramide, a dopaminergic antagonist, increases gastrointestinal motility and pyloric relaxation, thereby increasing the speed of gastric emptying. Sodium citrate or anticholinergic agents may interfere with the action of metoclopramide.[4]

TABLE 19–4. **Premedicants—Antagonists and Gastrokinetic Agents**[4, 8, 11]

Agent	Dosage/ Metabolism	Effects
Cimetidine	IV/IM/PO: 300 mg q 6–8 hr tE: 2 hr M: Liver E: Kidney	May increase blood levels of propranolol or benzodiazepines and potentiate oral anticoagulants; may cause confusion
Ranitidine	IV/IM: 50 mg q 6–8 hr PO: 150 mg q 12 hr tE: 2–3 hr M: Liver E: Kidney	Antagonizes histamine action on H_2 receptors with decreased gastric acid secretion
Metoclopramide	IV/IM: 10 mg PO: 10–15 mg tE: 2–6 hr M: Liver E: Kidney	↑ Gastrointestinal motility and ↓ esophageal sphincter tone; extrapyramidal symptoms (rare)

E, route of excretion; IM, intramuscularly; IV, intravenously; M, site of metabolism; PO, per os; tE, elimination half-life.

Anticholinergics

The antisialagogue action of anticholinergics was more helpful when ether was in common use.[2] Ether often caused an excessive amount of respiratory tract secretion. Concern now focuses on countering the vagal effects associated with administration of the newer inhalational anesthetics, manipulation of the airway, and traction of the eye muscles.[2, 4, 7] An anticholinergic is often unnecessary preoperatively. A common and effective treatment for bradydysrhythmia associated with traction of the ocular muscles is relieving the muscle traction stimulus.[7] If the vagal effect continues to be a problem, it can be treated with atropine or glycopyrrolate.[6] Atropine causes oral dryness and blurred vision.[2, 4] Atropine does not produce increased intraocular pressure when recommended doses are given for vagal blocking action and is not contraindicated in patients with glaucoma.[4] As an antisialagogue, scopolamine is far superior to atropine, but it is less effective in preventing the reflex bradycardia during general anesthesia.[4] Scopolamine produces more sedation than atropine, and dysphoria and restlessness following its administration are not uncommon. Glycopyrrolate is a quaternary amine and is longer acting than either atropine or scopolamine. It produces less sedation than scopolamine and is a less effective antisialagogue, but it is more effective than atropine.[4]

PHARMACOKINETICS

Among the benzodiazepines, diazepam is metabolized by the liver, with one-third of the metabolites being oxazepam. The active metabolites are excreted principally by the kidneys. In general, the benzodiazepines, barbiturates, and antihistamines are metabolized by the liver and excreted by the kidneys, though the amount of drug eliminated by the kidneys and liver varies somewhat.[4, 8] Ondansetron and the butyrophenones are also metabolized by the liver and excreted by the kidneys.[6] Ten percent of droperidol is excreted unchanged.[4, 8] Morphine is metabolized by the liver and excreted by the kidneys, as are the other opioids. Tables 19–2 through 19–5 list many of the drugs commonly used.[4, 8]

General Anesthetics

A patient under general anesthesia has no perception of any sensation. This state, which allows surgical procedures to be performed, can be induced with a wide variety of drugs, either singly or in combination. The objectives of a general anesthetic include analgesia, unconsciousness, and absence of movement.[9–12]

General anesthetics are commonly administered intravenously or inhalationally. These routes are preferred over the intramuscular or oral route because of greater drug predictability and reliability. Common inhalational and intravenous agents are reviewed in this section.[11]

TABLE 19–5. **Premedicants—Anticholinergics**[4, 8, 11]

Agent	Dosage/Metabolism	Effects
Atropine	IV/IM: 0.4–1.2 mg t½ α: 1 min tE: 2 hr M: Minimal E: Kidney (some by liver)	Tachydysrhythmias, dry mouth, urinary retention; crosses blood-brain barrier and placenta
Scopolamine	IV/IM: 0.3–0.6 mg tE: 3 hr E: Kidney	Crosses blood-brain barrier and placenta; may cause excitement or delirium; superior antisialogogue
Glycopyrrolate	IV/IM/SC: 0.1–0.2 mg PO: 1–2 mg E: Kidney	Does not cross blood-brain barrier or placenta; otherwise similar to atropine

E, route of excretion; IM, intramuscularly; IV, intravenously; M, site of metabolism; PO, per os; tE, elimination half-life.

INHALATIONAL AGENTS

The common inhalational general anesthetic agents include nitrous oxide and the halogenated agents halothane, enflurane, isoflurane, desflurane, and sevoflurane. To compare various inhalational agents and the concentrations in the alveoli during steady state that produce equivalent levels of anesthesia, the concept and definition of minimum alveolar concentration (MAC) are necessary. The MAC of anesthetic at one atmosphere that produces immobility in 50% of patients or animals exposed to a noxious stimulus is a useful measure of potency of inhalational agents.[5, 11, 13, 14]

Anesthetic potency is correlated with lipophilia. The more potent the general anesthetic, the more lipophilic it is.[11] Researchers cannot agree on one specific mechanism of action; many believe that general anesthetics work at many different levels and by a variety of mechanisms. This may explain why diverse inorganic and organic compounds can bring on the state of general anesthesia. The various theories of the mechanism of action of general anesthetics are reviewed in references 15 to 17.

Although general inhalational anesthesia can start with administration of oxygen, nitrous oxide, and an inhalation agent, the more common technique is to administer a hypnotic, such as propofol or thiopental sodium (Pentothal), intravenously.[18] General inhalational anesthesia is often maintained with oxygen, nitrous oxide, and a halogenated agent.[11] Additional agents may include opiates or muscle relaxants. The decisions to administer inhalational agents by mask or endotracheal intubation, and to allow the patient to breathe spontaneously or to control ventilation, are based on surgical and anesthetic requirements.

Pharmacodynamics

Figure 19–1 shows the chemical structures of the general inhalational halogenated anesthetic agents in common use.[11] Enflurane and isoflurane are ethers with a difluoromethyl group bonding to the 1 carbon via an ether bond. The newer halogenated agents, desflurane and sevoflurane, are also ethers. Desflurane is a fluorinated methyl ethyl ether, and sevoflurane is a fluorinated isopropyl ether. For children and adults, halothane and sevoflurane are far less irritating to breathe and have a lower incidence of coughing, laryngospasm, and excitation during ventilatory induction when compared with enflurane, isoflurane, or desflurane.[6, 11] The principal advantages of sevoflurane and desflurane over halothane, enflurane, and isoflurane are their low solubility in blood, which produces rapid induction of anesthesia, and low tissue solubility, which results in rapid elimination and awakening.[6]

The depth of anesthesia with the halogenated agents can be judged by observing blood pressure, because they produce dose-dependent reductions of arterial blood pressure principally through peripheral vasodilation.[6, 11, 18] There should be little change of pulse rate or blood pressure and no body movement in response to surgical stimulation. Following induction of anesthesia with the halogenated agents halothane or sevoflurane, or with hypnotic intravenous agents such as thiopental or propofol, the clinician should start with a high inspired concentration of the inhalational agent. As maintenance of anesthesia proceeds, the inspired concentration of anesthetic is lowered, because the alveolar concentration increases during maintenance.[18] As a steady state is approached, based on patient response to surgical stimulation, further appropriate concentration adjustments of the inhalational agents can be made rapidly.[11, 18]

Halothane, Enflurane, Isoflurane, Desflurane, and Sevoflurane

Cardiovascular System. With all five agents, blood pressure decreases by peripheral vasodilation as the depth of anesthesia increases. Cardiac output with halothane decreases 20 to 50% from the baseline value. The decrease in cardiac output is less with enflurane, desflurane, and sevoflurane. Cardiac output is well maintained with isoflurane. Heart rate decreases most with halothane, less with enflurane, desflurane, and sevoflurane, and may increase with isoflurane. This may explain why cardiac output is maintained by use of isoflurane. All five agents diminish baroreceptor reflex responses (tachycardia) to hypotension and vasomotor reflex responses (increased peripheral resistance) to hypovolemia, and they produce little change in the sympathoadrenal response and levels of catecholamines in the plasma.[6, 11] Inotropy and contractility diminish with all five agents, most notably with halothane. Negative inotropy is less obvious and similar at equipotent concentrations of isoflurane and sevoflurane. Desflurane produces the least negative inotropy. All five agents diminish sympathetic activ-

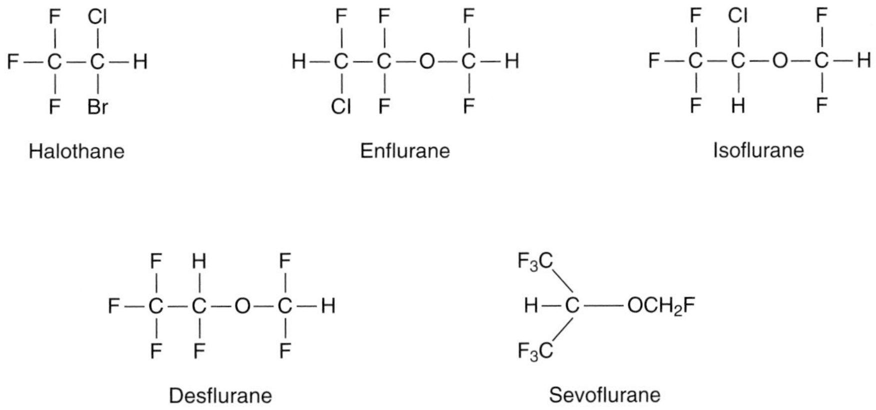

```
   F  Cl
   |  |
F—C—C—H
   |  |
   F  Br
```
Halothane

```
   F  F     F
   |  |     |
H—C—C—O—C—H
   |  |     |
   Cl F     F
```
Enflurane

```
   F  Cl    F
   |  |     |
F—C—C—O—C—H
   |  |     |
   F  H     F
```
Isoflurane

```
   F  H     F
   |  |     |
F—C—C—O—C—H
   |  |     |
   F  F     F
```
Desflurane

```
F3C
    \
 H—C——OCH2F
    /
F3C
```
Sevoflurane

FIGURE 19–1. Chemical structure of five commonly used inhalational agents.[6, 11]

ity and increase vagal predominance, particularly halothane. This is most common when halothane is given to a child, especially in association with manipulation of the airway.[6, 11]

Like isoflurane, desflurane in typical clinical settings does not sensitize the heart to catecholamines; in one study, however, the ventricular arrhythmogenic threshold of sevoflurane was between that of enflurane and isoflurane with submucosal injection of epinephrine.[6] Dysrhythmias are most common with halothane. Reentrant tachycardia is common, because the normal conduction pathway is slowed and the refractory period of the conductive tissue is increased. Increased automaticity also occurs with halothane, which is augmented by adrenergic agonists. Exogenous epinephrine should be limited in local anesthetics to a concentration of 1:100,000. No more than 0.1 mg of epinephrine in 10 minutes or 0.3 mg of epinephrine in 1 hour should be administered when halothane is used.[10] With enflurane, isoflurane, desflurane, or sevoflurane, three times this amount may be permissible. Unlike isoflurane, the other halogenated agents—halothane, enflurane, desflurane, and probably sevoflurane—do not cause coronary artery vasodilation that may lead to coronary artery steal syndrome. With the exception of isoflurane, the coronary circulation generally remains responsive to myocardial demands for oxygen. With isoflurane, coronary blood vessels are maximally dilated at about 1.5 MAC. Blood flow is maintained despite decreased myocardial oxygen demand. Some patients with ischemic heart disease have narrowed blood vessels in some regions of myocardium. These regions depend on collateral vessels for their blood supply. Dilation of normal coronary vessels by isoflurane may result in a steal of blood from the collateral vessels that exacerbates ischemia.[6, 19]

Pulmonary System. The halogenated agents all cause increasing respiratory depression as the concentration of the agent is increased. They all cause a moderate (approximately 20%) increase in $PaCO_2$ that reflects an increase in the rate of breathing insufficient to offset a decrease in tidal volume. Minute volume is reduced with all five agents. Depression of ventilation reflects a direct depressant effect on the medullary ventilatory center and perhaps peripheral effects on intercostal muscle function. Bronchial smooth muscle relaxation may be produced by a direct effect or indirectly by reductions in afferent nerve traffic or central medullary depression of bronchoconstriction reflexes.[6] With all five agents, respiratory depression is more evident when opioids are used; assisted or controlled ventilation is usually administered to avoid excessive hypercarbia. Hypercarbia in relation to dysrhythmia potential can be more problematic with halothane than with the other halogenated agents. With all five inhalational agents, pulmonary exchange of oxygen becomes less efficient, and an inspired oxygen concentration of 35% or more is indicated. All produce blunting of hypoxic pulmonary vasoconstriction, which can result in increased pulmonary shunt flow of blood.

All five agents produce increases in secretions, coughing, and laryngospasm, though halothane and sevoflurane are least often problematic. This is why sevoflurane and the less costly halothane are often employed in spontaneously ventilated children and adult patients for induction of anesthesia. For patients who tolerate an intravenous line at the start of anesthesia, and no anticipated problems with endotracheal intubation, intravenous induction is generally the method of choice.[6, 11, 20]

Nervous System. Of the five agents, enflurane is associated with a higher incidence of seizure activity. The seizures are short-lived and self-limited and generally can be prevented by avoiding deep anesthesia or hyperventilation. Interestingly, the drug does not appear to aggravate seizures in epileptic patients, but avoidance of enflurane is recommended for these patients. The halogenated agents have similar effects on the CNS. With the halogenated agents, cerebral oxygen consumption is decreased. There is also basal vasodilation, and cerebral blood flow is increased whereas perfusion pressure remains constant. As a result, intracranial pressure is increased. All effects are most marked with halothane. The cerebrovascular system remains responsive to carbon dioxide tension; with hyperventilation, cerebral blood flow, metabolism, and intracranial pressure are reduced.[11, 20]

Muscular System. All five halogenated agents reduce the response of skeletal muscle to nerve stimulation and enhance the neuromuscular blocking effects of depolarizing and nondepolarizing muscle agents. All five agents produce uterine vasodilation and a dose-dependent decrease in uterine blood flow. The halogenated agents have a direct muscle relaxing effect and appear to act centrally as well as peripherally at the neuromuscular junction. The halogenated agents potentiate muscle relaxants, and less neuromuscular blocking agent is required. The least potentiation occurs with halothane and nitrous oxide. Potentiation of neuromuscular blocking drugs may involve desensitization of the postjunctional membrane. Any of the three halogenated agents can trigger malignant hyperthermia.[6, 11]

Renal System. All five agents cause a dose-dependent reduction in renal blood flow and glomerular filtration rate. The effects can be somewhat attenuated by preoperative hydration and prevention of hypotension. The changes in renal function are rapidly reversed on conclusion of anesthesia and during recovery. The quantity of fluoride released by metabolism is least with desflurane, followed by isoflurane, and these agents are most frequently used for patients with renal disease. Sevoflurane undergoes oxidative metabolism in the liver with a serum fluoride concentration of approximately 22 μmol/L after a 1-MAC-hour exposure. The magnitude of sevoflurane metabolism resembles that of enflurane (peak plasma fluoride concentrations after a 2.5-MAC-hour exposure to enflurane are about 20 μmol/L).[6] When enflurane is used in the presence of renal failure, concentrations of fluoride ion decline rapidly after the anesthetic is discontinued. It is postulated that much of the fluoride enters bone. It is therefore probable that anesthesia with enflurane or sevoflurane is safe for patients with renal disease.[6, 11, 20]

Gastrointestinal System. With halothane, enflurane, and isoflurane, and probably with desflurane and sevoflurane, blood flow decreases with increasing depth of anesthesia as systemic arterial pressure declines. There is no evidence of direct ischemia. Hepatic necrosis has been reported with repeated administration of enflurane. Hepatic failure has not been reported with isoflurane. Isoflurane is less metabolized by the liver when compared with enflurane and halothane; this could be why isoflurane is not linked to hepatic failure. Halothane has been studied most extensively. The diagnosis of halothane hepatitis is one of exclusion. The pathologic appearance of hepatitis is similar whether the cause is sensitivity to halothane, damage by some other hepatotoxic drug, or transmission of hepatitis virus. The National Halothane Study of 1966, a retrospective analysis of more than 850,000 administrations of anesthetics, suggested a small incidence of hepatic necrosis in which there was no damage by some other hepatotoxic drug, no transfusion of blood, and no evidence of transmission of hepatitis virus or involvement of the liver by some other disease process.

The incidence of halothane hepatitis appears to be low: approximately 1 in 10,000 administrations for adults, and far less for children. It often occurs after repeated administrations of halothane over a short period. The unpredictable occurrence of this syndrome may be the principal reason that halothane use in adults has declined. More recent thinking indicates that the inherent risks of the surgery involved, along with such factors as major blood loss, major volume shifts, intraabdominal and intrathoracic operations, and periods in which prolonged hypotension may occur, may contribute to hepatic damage. Furthermore, if hepatitis is caused by a halogenated agent, that agent does not necessarily have to be halothane (enflurane and isoflurane may also be involved). It is postulated that the oxidative, and particularly the reductive, metabolites of these inhalational agents are responsible for the hepatitis. A chemically reactive or immunogenic product may result. This excess of toxic product or metabolite may be capable of inducing an immune response, which may be the main factor that leads to hepatitis.[6, 11, 20–23]

Pharmacokinetics

Some 60 to 80% of halothane is exhaled in the first 24 hours after it is administered. Smaller amounts continue to be exhaled for several days to weeks. Of the portion not exhaled, approximately 50% undergoes biotransformation. The remainder is eliminated unchanged via other routes. The cytochrome P-450 system of the endoplasmic reticulum of hepatocytes is responsible for the biotransformation. Little fluorine is removed, but chlorine, and to a lesser extent bromine, are removed. Analysis of the urine shows the fluorine-containing compounds in the form of trifluoroacetic acid.[11]

Approximately 80% of enflurane can be recovered unchanged in expired gas. Of the remaining enflurane, 2 to 10% is metabolized by the liver.[24] A number of factors make enflurane, an ether, different from halothane. The ether bond increases molecular stability. The carboflurane bond is a higher-energy bond than that between carbon and bromine or carbon and chlorine. With the absence of bromine, and the presence of chlorine and fluorine, the incorporation of the ether bond results in less biotransformation of enflurane. Furthermore, because it is less soluble than halothane in fatty tissue, enflurane leaves the fatty tissue more rapidly in the postoperative period. This allows less time for degradation of enflurane.[11]

Desflurane undergoes the least biotransformation, followed by isoflurane, with 0.2% being metabolized.[25] This is far less liver metabolism than for halothane, and less liver metabolism than for enflurane and sevoflurane. The magnitude of sevoflurane metabolism resembles that of enflurane. With less biotransformation by liver metabolism, smaller quantities of fluorine and trifluoroacetic acid are generated. This accounts for hepatic and renal toxicity being lowest with desflurane and isoflurane when compared with enflurane, possibly sevoflurane, or halothane.[6, 11]

Tables 19–6 and 19–7 summarize the advantages and disadvantages of the pharmacodynamic and pharmacokinetic properties of the three halogenated agents.[6, 11]

Nitrous Oxide

Nitrous oxide is a colorless and odorless gas with very low solubility in blood. Nitrous oxide alone can predictably cause surgical anesthesia only when given under hyperbaric conditions. The MAC value is 105%, but variability among patients is considerable. Analgesia can be induced with 20% nitrous oxide; some patients lose consciousness when breathing 30% nitrous oxide, and the majority do so with 80%. Using nitrous oxide as a single agent at 80% concentration risks hypoxia. Patients also often recall intraoperative events when nitrous oxide is used alone. Even with nitrous oxide plus a narcotic, intraoperative recall is not uncommon. If a combination of narcotic, nitrous oxide, and muscle relaxant is used, the patient is immobilized and unable to communicate, but unconsciousness cannot be ensured. Because this can be unsettling to the patient, frequently the clinician adds a potent inhalational agent or intravenous drug such as a hypnotic or anxiolytic. The main advantage of nitrous oxide is to reduce the needed concentration of inhalational anesthetic. Smaller doses of halogenated agents combined with nitrous oxide produce less circulatory and respiratory depression and more rapid recovery. The uptake of nitrous oxide is rapid, which has two beneficial effects during the administration of anesthesia: the concentration effect and the second-gas effect.

When a very high concentration of an anesthetic is inhaled, the partial pressure of the anesthetic in arterial blood increases faster than if a smaller concentration of the anesthetic were administered. As the anesthetic is rapidly taken up by the blood, the gas administered by the anesthesia machine is rapidly drawn into the alveoli, which continue to lose gas rapidly to the passing blood. This is the advantage of using a high percentage of nitrous oxide in the initial stage of anesthesia, and it makes use of the concentration effect. The second gas effect occurs when a potent inhalational agent is combined with nitrous oxide. As nitrous oxide is rapidly taken up by the blood from the alveoli, and nitrous oxide in the alveoli is rapidly being replaced by the anesthesia machine, the rate of delivery of halogenated agent to the alveoli increases. Thus, the rise in arterial tension of halogenated agents is more rapid.

To summarize, the concentration effect results from the capacity of a rapidly absorbed gas to facilitate its own uptake. In the second-gas effect, a rapidly absorbed gas increases the rate of uptake of the second anesthetic gas.[20, 26] During emergence from anesthesia, the process is reversed. The possibility of diffusional hypoxia is a concern because it can cause postoperative hypoxemia, particularly if this is accompanied by respiratory depression. As nitrous oxide rapidly comes out of blood into the alveoli, oxygen concentration can be diluted. If room air is used, nitrous oxide filling alveoli from the blood can bring the 21% oxygen concentration of room air down to much lower levels, and

TABLE 19–6. **Pharmacodynamics of Inhalational General Anesthetics**[6, 11]

Organ System Effects	Halothane	Enflurane	Isoflurane	Desflurane	Sevoflurane
Cardiovascular					
Peripheral vasodilation	+	+	+ +	+	+
Blood pressure	–	–	– –	–	–
Inotropy	– –	–	–	–	–
Heart rate	–	+	+ +	= +	=
Cardiac output	– –	–	=	–	–
Propensity for dysrhythmias	+ +	+ =	=	=	=
Catecholamines	=	=	=	+	=
Sympathoadrenal activity	=	=	=	=	=
Pulmonary					
Bronchodilation	+	+	+	+	+
Response to hypoxia	–	– –	–	–	–
End tidal CO_2	+	+ +	+	+	+
Shunt (Q/S)	+	+	+	+	+
Hypoxic pulmonary vasoconstriction	+	+	+	+	+
Airway irritation	+	+ +	+ +	+ +	=
Central Nervous System					
Seizure activity	=	+	=	=	=
Cerebral blood flow	+ + +	+ +	+	+	+
Cerebrospinal fluid pressure	+ +	+	=	=	=
Intracranial pressure	+ +	+	=	+	+
Cerebral metabolic rate	–	–	–	–	–
Muscle					
Relaxation	+	+ +	+	+	+
Synergism with relaxants	+	+	+	+	+
Malignant hyperthermia trigger	+	+	+	+	+
Renal					
Renal blood flow	–	–	–	–	–
Glomerular filtration rate	–	–	–	–	–
Fluoride ion	–	+ +	+ (minimal)	+ (min)	+ (min)
Hepatic/Gastrointestinal					
Splanchnic blood flow	–	–	Hepatic cell function	–	–
Trifluoroacetic acid	+ +	+	+	+	–

Key: =, no change; +, increase; –, decrease.

hypoxia can result. This is why 100% oxygen is administered during the emergence phase.[11, 20]

In general, nitrous oxide has a sympathomimetic effect when added to halogenated agents.[11, 27, 28] The combined use of nitrous oxide and halogenated anesthetic results in decreased amounts of halogenated agents required and less hypotension.[11] With nitrous oxide combined with enflurane, activation of the sympathetic nervous system is less marked than when nitrous oxide is combined with halothane.[28] When nitrous oxide is used alone with narcotics, it does not displace sympathomimetic activity but rather causes further cardiovascular depression. Nitrous oxide has little effect on respiration when used alone, but it further depresses respiration when combined with other inhalational agents.[11] Nitrous oxide has little effect on the CNS, but response to hypoxia is diminished. Little, if any, skeletal muscle relaxation occurs when nitrous oxide is used alone.[11] There is no evidence that nitrous oxide triggers malignant hyperthermia. The gastrointestinal, renal, and hepatic systems show no effect from administration of nitrous oxide.[11]

Of note, methionine synthetase, a vitamin B_{12}–dependent enzyme, is inactivated following prolonged administration of nitrous oxide, which results in interference with DNA synthesis. This can cause diminished bone marrow production of red and white blood cells. Also, oxidation of the cobalt atom in vitamin B_{12} by nitrous oxide can result in megalo-

TABLE 19–7. **Pharmacokinetics of Inhalational General Anesthetics**

	Halothane	Enflurane	Isoflurane	Desflurane	Sevoflurane
Metabolism	20% Liver	2% Liver	0.2% Liver	<0.02%	5%
Ion concentration	$CL^- > Br^- > F^-$	F^-	F^- (minimal)	F^- (minimal)	F^-
Elimination	60–80% via lung in first 24 hr	80% via lung	99% + via lung	99% + via lung	95%

blastic changes in the bone marrow, with neuropathy. These changes do not normally occur during clinical anesthesia for surgery.[11]

Nitrous oxide is excreted by the lungs, and there is little, if any, biotransformation. Table 19–8 summarizes the advantages and disadvantages of nitrous oxide.[11]

INTRAVENOUS AGENTS

Hypnotics

Barbiturates are not analgesics and may even increase sensitivity to pain.[2, 11] Their main uses are induction of anesthesia and induction of amnesia. The respiratory and cardiovascular systems are depressed, and excessive doses may cause marked hypotension and apnea. When barbiturates are used alone without analgesia, it is not unusual to see tachycardia and other sympathetic responses, including dilated pupils, tears, sweating, tachypnea, and even movement or vocalization in response to surgical stimulation.[11]

When a barbiturate is administered for induction of general anesthesia, coughing, laryngospasm, and bronchospasm can occur upon mask ventilation or early attempts at laryngoscopy without muscle paralysis. Saliva, insertion of an airway, obstruction by soft tissues, and airway manipulation may trigger these responses.[11]

Thiopental is the most common induction agent used, followed by methohexital sodium. Both cause a decrease in arterial blood pressure and reduction of cardiac output. The clinician must be careful when administering these agents in the presence of hypovolemia, sepsis, or any kind of cardiovascular instability, because a normal induction dose may result in cardiac arrest.[11]

Extravascular injection may result in severe pain and tissue necrosis. With intraarterial injection, the endothelium and deeper layers of the arterial blood vessels can be immediately damaged and endarteritis can follow. Associated thrombosis and arterial spasm are common, which can result in vascular ischemia and gangrene.[11] Propofol is chemically unrelated to the barbiturates. It is a propylphenol. The principal indication is amnesia and unconsciousness, and the emergence from anesthesia is more rapid with propofol than with thiopental. Emergence is characterized by minimal postoperative confusion.[11]

Propofol can cause a 30% decrease in systemic arterial pressure predominantly due to peripheral vasodilation. This can be of some concern in the elderly, and one must be careful when administering propofol in conjunction with opioids.[11] There is some pain at the site of injection, but phlebitis or thrombosis is rare.[11]

Benzodiazepines

Benzodiazepines can be used for induction, but they mainly function as anxiolytics and amnestics. Larger doses of benzo-

TABLE 19–8. **Advantages and Disadvantages of Inhalational Agents**[6, 11]

Agent	Advantages	Disadvantages
Nitrous oxide	Nonirritating, colorless, odorless Very rapid onset and recovery Little or no toxicity with ordinary use Excellent supplement with halogenated or opioid agents (smaller doses of all agents and fewer complications)	No muscle relaxant activity If used alone to achieve adequate anesthesia, can result in hypoxia Transient postanesthetic hypoxia may occur as large volume is exhaled Air pockets in closed spaces may expand in skull, chest, abdomen
Halothane	Causes laryngospasm but is least irritating to airway Bronchospasm uncommon Controlled hypotension decreases blood loss	For proper analgesia, nitrous oxide or opioids usually must be added Relaxant drugs added for enhanced muscle relaxation Visceral reflexes blunted with atropine Transient dysrhythmias Incidence of hepatic necrosis
Enflurane	More rapid changes in depth of anesthesia with little change of pulse and respirations compared with halothane Less dysrhythmia, postoperative shivering, nausea and vomiting than with halothane Good additive action with muscle relaxants Dysrhythmias less likely when used with epinephrine compared with halothane	Deep anesthesia is associated with cardiopulmonary depression Seizure activity associated with relatively high concentrations, aggravated by hypocarbia
Isoflurane	More rapid adjustment of anesthesia depth compared with halothane Cardiac output well maintained Dysrhythmias less likely when used with epinephrine compared with halothane Potentiates muscle relaxants (lower concentration suffices)	More pungent odor than halothane Increasing depression of cardiopulmonary function with increasing depths of anesthesia
Desflurane	More rapid induction and emergence than isoflurane, enflurane, or halothane Minimal liver metabolism No change in serum fluoride concentration No coronary steal Otherwise similar to isoflurane	Coughing and excitement Otherwise similar to isoflurane
Sevoflurane	Less of an airway irritant; good for mask induction More rapid induction and emergence than isoflurane, enflurane, or halothane No coronary steal	Serum fluoride concentration is similar to that of enflurane

diazepines can induce hypnosis and unconsciousness. Use of a benzodiazepine as a sole agent is helpful when no analgesia is required. The principal advantage of benzodiazepines is the minimal depression of the cardiovascular system. Very large doses, however, can cause a 20% decline in systemic arterial blood pressure and vascular resistance. The stability of the cardiovascular system with smaller doses has made these drugs particularly attractive for use in monitored anesthetic care and general anesthesia. One must be prepared for apnea, and ventilatory support should be readily available. Benzodiazepines generally have little effect on renal, hepatic, and gastrointestinal systems. They do not produce neuromuscular paralysis, but they can be used to induce relaxation of spastic muscles.

CNS depression can be antagonized by physostigmine. Physostigmine inhibits acetylcholinesterase. It crosses the blood-brain barrier more easily than other acetylcholinesterase agents. It is wise to consider administering atropine or glycopyrrolate with physostigmine to prevent excessive salivation, abdominal cramps, nausea and vomiting, and bradydysrhythmia.[11]

Opioids

Opioids are principally used for analgesia. In larger doses, opioids can induce unconsciousness, but the common technique of combining nitrous oxide and narcotic alone can result in insufficient amnesia in some patients. Some patients become hypertensive during surgical stimulation and may recall intraoperative events. Table 19–9 reviews narcotic agents.[8, 11, 29, 30]

Local Anesthetics

Local anesthetics are a class of similar compounds that reversibly block conduction in peripheral and central nervous tissue when applied in appropriate concentrations. Local anesthetics cause both sensory and motor paralysis in the innervated area.

The era of local anesthesia commenced in 1864, when Koller described the local anesthetic effect of cocaine and introduced it for use in ophthalmology. Because cocaine, the alkaloid isolated in 1860 from the leaves of an Andean mountain shrub, *Erythroxylon coca*, has serious CNS toxicity and causes sloughing of the corneal epithelium, its use in ophthalmology is limited. This prompted the German chemical industry to seek less toxic synthetic substitutes and resulted in the discovery in 1905 of procaine, which became the prototype for current local anesthetics. The most widely used agents in ophthalmology today are lidocaine, tetracaine, and bupivacaine.

All clinically useful agents are either aminoesters or aminoamides (Fig. 19–2). The amide or ester link contributes to the anesthetic potency. The typical local anesthetic

TABLE 19–9. **Intravenous General Anesthetics**[4, 6, 8, 11]

Agent	Induction Dose	Half-Life	Organ System Effects	Metabolism/Elimination
Thiopental	1–4 mg/kg	t½ α 3 min tE: 5–10 hr	↓ CNS ↓ CBF ↓ ICP ↓ BP ↑ HR ↓ RR ↑ Bronchospasm	Liver/kidneys
Methohexital	1–2 mg/kg	tE: 1–2 hr	↓ CNS ↓ RR ↓ CV	Liver/kidneys
Midazolam	0.25–0.35 mg/kg	tE: 1–4 hr	↓ CNS Amnesia ↑ Seizure threshold	Liver/kidneys
Diazepam	0.1–0.5 mg/kg	tE: 7–10 hr; (active metabolite: 2–8 days)	↓ CNS Amnesia ↑ Seizure threshold	Liver/kidneys
Morphine	1–3 mg/kg	tE: 2–4 hr	Analgesia ↓ CNS Euphoria ↑ Respiratory depression	Liver/kidneys
Fentanyl	50–100 μg/kg	t½ α: 1–2 min tE: 4 hr	Similar to morphine, but chest wall rigidity more common with fentanyl	Liver/kidneys
Ketamine	IV loading dose (LD): 1–3 mg/kg	t½ α: 10–18 min tE: 2.5 hr	Poor visceral analgesia; good somatic analgesia	
	Maintenance dose: ⅓–½ LD	↑ Airway reflexes ↑ HTN ↑ IOP ↑ CBF ↑ Cerebral metabolic rate	Liver/kidneys	
Propofol	IV induction 2.0–2.5 mg/kg IV maintenance 100–200 μg/kg/min	t½: 5–10 min tE: 1–3 days	↓ CNS ↓ RR ↓ BP	Liver

BP, blood pressure; CBF, cerebral blood flow; CNS, central nervous system; HR, heart rate; HTN, hypertension; ICP, intracranial pressure; IOP, intraocular pressure; RR, respiratory rate.

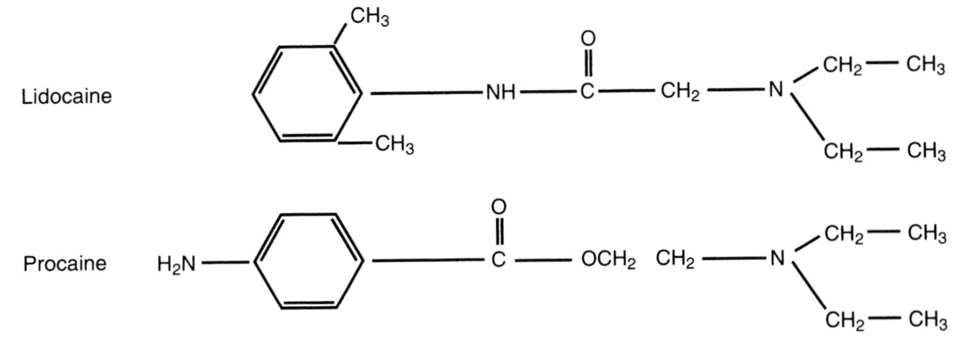

FIGURE 19–2. Chemical structure of lidocaine and procaine.

molecule, exemplified by procaine and lidocaine, consists of a lipophilic (hydrophobic) aromatic ring group joined to a more hydrophilic base, the tertiary amine, by an intermediate band (Fig. 19–3). Increasing the size of the alkyl substitution produces compounds that are more hydrophobic, thus increasing the duration and potency of the agent. Addition of a butyl group to the tertiary amine (bupivacaine) or to the aromatic region (tetracaine) increases the lipophilia of these compounds, resulting in increased potency and duration of action.

MECHANISM OF ACTION

Local anesthetics block the generation and conduction of nerve impulses. All excitable cells have ionic disequilibria across semipermeable membranes, providing the potential

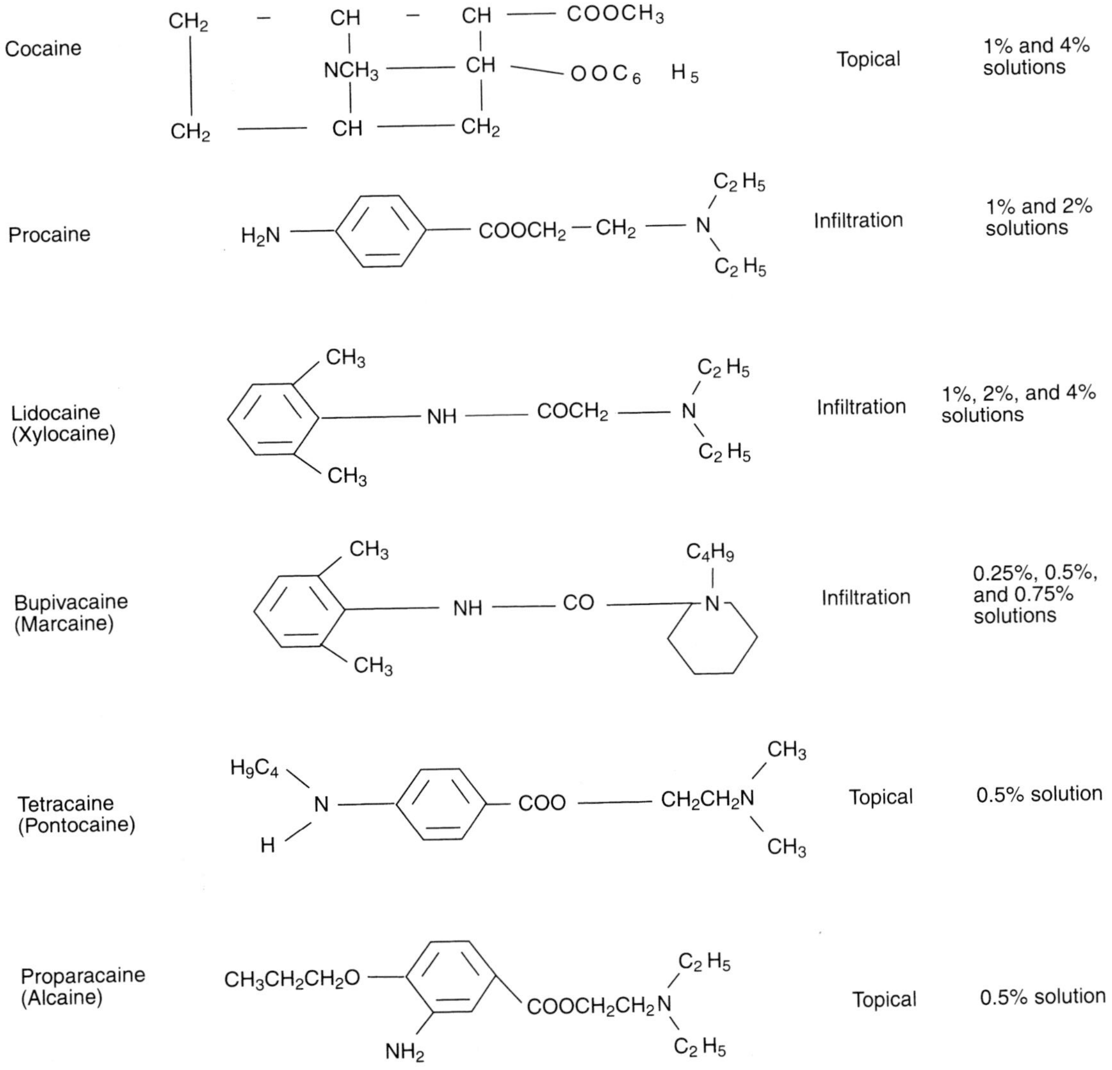

FIGURE 19–3. Commonly used local anesthetics in ophthalmology.

energy for impulse conduction. The Na^+,K^+-ATPase, the membrane-bound enzyme, maintains the ionic disequilibrium in nerve cells, pumping out three sodium (Na^+) ions for every two of potassium (K^+) that are absorbed. During an action potential, Na^+ channels open briefly, allowing a small quantity of Na^+ to flow into the cell, causing depolarization. Local anesthetics block impulses by inhibiting individual Na^+ channels, thereby reducing the aggregate Na^+ current, which may be modified by inhibition of the recently discovered K^+ channels.[31–33] The interplay between these competing channels determines the relative potency of the various local anesthetics, whose pharmacologic effects also depend on the temperature and pH of the medium.

Biochemical analysis of Na^+ channels shows the presence of one major glycoprotein with a molecular mass of approximately 200,000 Da, with differing numbers of subunits of 40,000 Da, depending on the tissue of origin. The Na^+ channel is oriented with its glycosylated groups of the glycoprotein on the outside surface of the cell membrane.

Similarly, voltage-gated K^+ channels make up a large molecular family of membrane proteins involved in the generation of nerve impulses. Like the proteins gating the Na^+ channels, these proteins span the cell membranes, forming K^+-selective pores that are rapidly switched open or closed, depending on the membrane voltage. Recent cloning of the first K^+ channel has resulted in recombinant DNA manipulation of the K^+-channel genes, leading to a molecular understanding of K^+-channel behavior, especially toward elucidation of functional domains responsible for channel gating and ionic selectivity. Local anesthetics act by several different mechanisms on ionic channels. They may decrease the fraction of active channels by interfering directly with activation; they may inhibit or alter the conformational steps whereby channels change from an open form; or they may reduce the ionic currents flowing through open channels. In spite of various methods of detecting currents through single-ion channels, the lack of general approaches for crystallizing membrane proteins has presented a direct view of the structural complexities of their mechanisms.

Recent work by Franks and Lieb[34] suggests a more precise theory of both local and general anesthetic action. Challenging the well-entrenched "lipid hypothesis," these authors suggest that anesthetics operate not indiscriminately on membrane lipids but precisely on certain sensitive membrane proteins regulating ionic channels that govern the responses of nerve cells. If the nerve cell's anesthetic-sensitive proteins are isolated, "designer anesthetics" could be synthesized to lock onto the sites specifically in order to enhance an anesthetic's sensitivity and minimize its toxicity.

The chronology of local anesthetic action can be summarized as follows:[35]

1. When local anesthetic molecules are deposited near the nerve, partial removal of the molecules occurs by circulation, tissue binding, and local hydrolysis of aminoester anesthetics. The remaining molecules penetrate the nerve sheath.
2. After equilibrium is achieved inside the nerve axon's membranes, depending on the lipophilia of base and cation species, Na^+ channels are prevented from opening by inhibition of conformational changes that occur with channel activation.
3. The rates and onset of recovery from block are governed by the slow diffusion of local anesthetic molecules in and out of the nerve, not by the much faster binding and dissociation from ionic channels.

CLINICAL PHARMACOLOGY

Successful ophthalmic anesthesia depends on knowledge of the pharmacologic properties of commonly used local agents. Aminoesters such as procaine are hydrolyzed in the plasma by cholinesterase enzymes. The aminoamides, lidocaine and bupivacaine, are extremely stable and undergo biotransformation and enzymatic degradation in the liver. Allergic reactions to aminoamides are extremely rare compared with reactions to aminoesters.

For a local anesthetic to be successfully and safely used in ophthalmic anesthesia, it must have potency, rapid onset of action, long duration of sensory and motor block, and minimal systemic toxicity. The individual profile of an agent is determined mainly by its physicochemical characteristics.

In addition to the physicochemical properties, latency also depends on the concentration. Lidocaine has a more rapid onset of action than bupivacaine, and 0.75% bupivacaine causes a more rapid anesthetic effect than 0.25% bupivacaine. Procaine has a short duration of action, lidocaine an intermediate duration, and bupivacaine the longest duration. Mixtures of local anesthetics, such as lidocaine and bupivacaine, have become popular for ophthalmic anesthesia, because they combine the advantages of rapid onset but short duration of action of lidocaine, and slow onset but long duration of action of bupivacaine. For example, a 2% solution of lidocaine mixed with equal parts of a 0.75% solution of bupivacaine produces anesthesia within 5 minutes that lasts 3 to 4 hours. At a concentration of 1:200,000, vasoconstrictors such as epinephrine, mixed into the local anesthetic, decrease the rate of vascular absorption and subsequent biotransformation. This allows more anesthetic agent to reach the membrane receptors and prolongs the depth and duration of anesthesia. With a judicious combination of lidocaine and bupivacaine and a dilute vasoconstrictor such as epinephrine, the duration of sensory and motor blockade is considerably enhanced; this permits the ophthalmologist to perform complicated intraocular procedures and minimize postoperative pain and discomfort.

TOXICITY

The effectiveness and safety of local anesthetics depend on proper dosage, correct administration, and preparedness for emergencies. Systemic side effects, such as neurologic and cardiac crises, are avoided by using the smallest effective anesthetic dose for a given procedure, thereby avoiding high plasma levels and their associated effects. Unintentional intravascular injection of local anesthetics can cause convulsions and respiratory depression, and possibly arrest. Cardiovascular stimulation or depression and cardiac arrest also may occur. Thus, clinicians must be well versed in basic life support techniques in order to manage toxic reactions due to local anesthetics. Ready availability of oxygen and of cardiopulmonary resuscitative drugs administered by a skilled anesthesiologist promote rapid and successful recovery.

Anesthetic solutions that contain epinephrine should be used with extreme caution in patients with cardiovascular disease such as hypertension, arteriosclerotic or cerebrovascular disease, diabetes, heart block, or thyrotoxicosis. Patients taking medication for systemic hypertension may also be more susceptible to alterations in blood pressure.

DRUG INTERACTIONS

Cardiovascular arrhythmia may occur when local anesthetic agents with epinephrine are used during general anesthesia with halothane. Patients receiving monoamine oxidase inhibitors or tricyclic antidepressants may experience severe and prolonged hypertension with local anesthetics containing epinephrine, thus vasoconstrictors are best avoided. CNS toxicity may occur when local anesthetics are used in conjunction with narcotic analgesics and phenothiazine-type compounds. In patients taking echothiophate for control of glaucoma, inhibition of plasma cholinesterases may result in increased plasma levels of local anesthetics and possibly cardiovascular and neurologic complications.

REFERENCES

1. Egbert LD, Battit GE, Turndorf H, et al: The value of the preoperative visit by an anesthetist. JAMA 185:553, 1963.
2. Dripps RD, Eckenhoff JE, Vandam LD: Premedication, transport to the operating room, and preparation for anesthesia. *In* Dripps RD, Eckenhoff JE, Vandam LD (eds): Introduction to Anesthesia: The Principles of Safe Practice, 6th ed. Philadelphia, WB Saunders, 1982, pp 34–44.
3. Firestone LL: General preanesthesic evaluation. *In* Firestone LL, et al (eds): Clinical Anesthesia Procedures of the Massachusetts General Hospital, 3rd ed. Boston, Little, Brown, 1988, pp 3–14.
4. Kennedy SK, Longnecker DE: History and principles of anesthesiology. *In* Gilman AG, et al (eds): The Pharmacological Basis of Therapeutics, 8th ed. New York, Pergamon, 1990, pp 269–284.
5. de Jong RH, Hearmer JE: Diazepam- and lidocaine-induced cardiovascular changes. Anesthesiology 39:633, 1973.
6. Omoigui S: The Anesthesia Drugs Handbook, 2nd ed. St. Louis, CV Mosby, 1995, pp 256, 296, 359–391.
7. Donlon JV Jr: Anesthesia and eye, ear, nose, and throat surgery. *In* Miller RD (ed): Anesthesia, 4th ed. New York, Churchill Livingstone, 1994, pp 2175–2196.
8. Kofke WA, Firestone LL: Commonly used drugs. *In* Firestone LL, et al (eds): Clinical Anesthesia Procedures of the Massachusetts General Hospital, 3rd ed. Boston, Little, Brown, 1988, pp 590–650.
9. Nunn JF, Utting JE, Brown BR Jr: Introduction. *In* Nunn JF, Utting JE, Brown BR Jr (eds): General Anesthesia, 5th ed. London, Butterworths, 1989, pp 1–6.
10. Calverley RK: Anesthesia as a specialty: Past, present, and future. *In* Barash PG, Cullen BF, Stoelting RK (eds): Clinical Anesthesia. Philadelphia, JB Lippincott, 1989, pp 3–34.
11. Marshall BE, Longnecker DE: General anesthetics. *In* Gilman AG, et al (eds): The Pharmacological Basis of Therapeutics, 8th ed. New York, Pergamon, 1990, pp 285–310.
12. Hickel RS: Administration of general anesthesia. *In* Firestone LL, et al (eds): Clinical Anesthesia Procedures of the Massachusetts General Hospital, 3rd ed. Boston, Little, Brown, 1988, pp 136–166.
13. Eger EI, Saidman LJ, Brandstater B: Minimum alveolar anesthetic concentration, a standard of anesthetic potency. Anesthesiology 26:756, 1965.
14. Eger EI: Anesthetic Uptake and Action. Baltimore, Williams & Wilkins, 1974.
15. Richter JJ: Mechanisms of general anesthesia. *In* Barash PG, Cullen BF, Stoelting RK (eds): Clinical Anesthesia. Philadelphia, JB Lippincott, 1989, pp 281–292.
16. Koblin DD: Mechanisms of action. *In* Miller RD (ed): Anesthesia. New York, Churchill Livingstone, 1990, pp 51–84.
17. Halsey MJ: Molecular mechanisms of anaesthesia. *In* Nunn JF, Utting JE, Brown BR Jr (eds): General Anesthesia, 5th ed. London, Butterworths, 1989, pp 19–29.
18. Dripps RD, Eckenhoff JE, Vandam LD: Fundamentals of inhalational anesthesia. *In* Dripps RD, Eckenhoff JE, Vandam LD (eds): Introduction to Anesthesia: The Principles of Safe Practice, 6th ed. Philadelphia, WB Saunders, 1982, pp 101–115.
19. Buffington CW, Davis KB, Gillispie S, Pettinger M: The prevalence of steal-prone coronary anatomy in patients with coronary artery disease: An analysis of the Coronary Artery Surgery Study Registry. Anesthesiology 69:721, 1988.
20. Dripps RD, Eckenhoff JE, Vandam LD: Inhalational anesthetics. *In* Dripps RD, Eckenhoff JE, Vandam LD (eds): Introduction to Anesthesia: The Principles of Safe Practice, 6th ed. Philadelphia, WB Saunders, 1982, pp 116–135.
21. Stock JG, Strunin L: Unexplained hepatitis following halothane. Anesthesiology 63:424, 1985.
22. Boden JM, Rice SA: Metabolism and toxicity. *In* Miller RD (ed): Anesthesia, 3rd ed. New York, Churchill Livingstone, 1990.
23. Berman LM, Holaday DA: Inhalation anesthetic metabolism and toxicity. *In* Barash PG, Cullen BF, Stoelting RK (eds): Clinical Anesthesia. Philadelphia, JB Lippincott, 1989.
24. Carpenter RL, Eger EI II, Johnson BH, et al: The extent of metabolism of inhaled anesthetics in humans. Anesthesiology 65:201, 1986.
25. Holaday DA, Fiserova-Bergerova V, Latto IP, Zumbiel MA: Resistance of isoflurane to biotransformation in man. Anesthesiology 43:325, 1975.
26. Epstein RM, Rackow H, Salanitre E, Wolf G: Influence of the concentration effect on the uptake of anesthetic mixtures: The second gas effect. Anesthesiology 25:364, 1964.
27. Hornbein TF, Martin WE, Bonica JJ, et al: Nitrous oxide effects on the circulatory and ventilatory responses to halothane. Anesthesiology 31:250, 1969.
28. Smith NT, Caverly RK, Prys-Roberts C, et al: Impact of nitrous oxide on the circulation during enflurane anesthesia in man. Anesthesiology 48:345, 1978.
29. Philbin DM, Rosow CE, Schneider RC, et al: Fentanyl and sufentanil anesthesia revisited: How much is enough? Anesthesiology 73:5, 1990.
30. Hug CC Jr: Does opioid anesthesia exist? Anesthesiology 73:1, 1990.
31. Strichartz GR, Ritchie JM: The action of local anesthetics on ion channels of excitable tissues. *In* Strichartz GR (ed): Handbook of Experimental Pharmacology, vol 81. Berlin, Springer-Verlag, 1987, pp 21–52.
32. Miller C: 1990: Annus mirabilis of potassium channels. Science 252:1092, 1991.
33. Butterworth JF, Strichartz GR: Molecular mechanisms of local anesthesia: A review. Anesthesiology 72:711, 1990.
34. Franks NP, Lieb WR: Stereospecific effects of inhalational general anesthetic optic isomers on nerve ion channels. Science 254:427, 1991.
35. Strichartz GR, Covino BG: Local anesthetics. *In* Miller RD (ed): Anesthesia, 3rd ed. New York, Churchill Livingstone, 1990.

CHAPTER 20

Antibacterials

Henry D. Perry and Eric D. Donnenfeld

Fluoroquinolones

OVERVIEW AND MECHANISM OF ACTION

The fluoroquinolone agents are the newest class available in the fight against microbes. Fluoroquinolone agents act by inhibiting the supercoiling of DNA by the enzyme DNA gyrase. This action is bactericidal and occurs during cell replication. Fluoroquinolones offer the advantage of low toxicity due to the lack of DNA gyrase in mammalian cells. The available topical agents include norfloxacin, ciprofloxacin, and ofloxacin, and there are a growing number of compounds soon to be approved by the U.S. Food and Drug Administration (FDA), including enoxacin, lomefloxacin, fleroxacin, perfloxacin, sparfloxacin, and tosufloxacin.[1]

SPECTRUM OF ACTIVITY

The quinolone agents are generally more active against gram-negative bacteria than gram-positives, although they have broad-spectrum activity. They are generally active against enteric gram-negative rods, such as *Haemophilus influenzae* and *Neisseria gonorrhoeae.* They are moderately active against *Staphylococcus aureus, Staphylococcus epidermidis,* and *Pseudomonas aeruginosa*; activity against *Streptococcus pneumoniae* is marginal. The beta-hemolytic streptococcal and the enterococcal sensitivity varies among the compounds. Resistance does not commonly develop during treatment for *Escherichia coli* (or other Enterobacteriaceae infections) but does occur in infections due to *P. aeruginosa* and *S. aureus.*[2] The currently available fluoroquinolones do not have activity against anaerobes, but some agents under development appear to have adequate anaerobic activity. Ciprofloxacin and ofloxacin are active against some atypical *Mycobacteria,* including *Mycobacterium avium-intracellulare, Mycobacterium marinum,* and *Mycobacterium chelonei.* Ofloxacin is active against chylamydial infections, including *Chlamydia trachomatis.* In general, ofloxacin and ciprofloxacin have a very comparable spectrum of activity against gram-positive and gram-negative organisms. Ciprofloxacin has minimally better activity against gram-negative bacteria, whereas ofloxacin has a minimally better spectrum of activity against gram-positive infections, including streptococcal species. Norfloxacin has a less broad spectrum of activity compared with both ciprofloxacin and ofloxacin.

PHARMACOLOGY

The quinolones are well absorbed after oral and nasogastric tube administration and have variable pathways of metabolism or excretion. The oral quinolones achieve systemic levels comparable to those of intravenous antibiotics because of their high absorption and intrinsic solubility. Ciprofloxacin, norfloxacin, and ofloxacin are all available in a 0.3% commercial solution as an eye drop.

Both ciprofloxacin and ofloxacin can be used to treat corneal ulcers and are particularly active against enteric gram-negative bacilli and *Pseudomonas.* In double-masked control clinical trials, ciprofloxacin and ofloxacin were shown to be equivalent to fortified tobramycin and cefazolin in the treatment of bacterial keratitis.[3, 4] These antibiotics have very high intrinsic solubility and achieved high levels in the cornea.[5, 6] Ofloxacin, which is the most soluble of the antibiotics, achieves high aqueous concentrations with topical treatment.[7, 8]

OPHTHALMIC INDICATIONS

The quinolones, especially ciprofloxacin and ofloxacin, can be used to treat corneal ulcers caused by enteric gram-negative bacilli and *Pseudomonas.* This class of antibiotics is also effective for the treatment of bacterial conjunctivitis. Ofloxacin (Ocuflox) is slightly more efficacious than ciprofloxacin (Ciloxan) for preoperative cataract prophylaxis. To limit the spread of resistant organisms, use should be short term in the prophylaxis of cataract patients (1 week).

TOXICITY

Toxicity, fever, rash, and nausea have occurred in about 4% of patients given oral quinolone therapy. Occasionally patients have elevation of levels of liver enzymes. The drugs can crystallize in the urine, especially in patients who are dehydrated. Interstitial nephritis has been reported after high doses of ciprofloxacin. Insomnia and restlessness have occurred in elderly patients taking fluoroquinolones. Children should not be given quinolones because of animal studies that have shown crystal deposits in cartilage in a dog model, and for this reason, the topical fluoroquinolones are not recommended for children younger than 2 years. There is no evidence in humans for ocular toxicity with the new fluoroquinolones, despite the fact that cataracts occurred in cats after months of perfloxacin therapy, and macular bulla formation occurred in patients with renal failure on flumequine (a quinolone used in Europe). The topical administration of ciprofloxacin has been associated with crystal deposits in the cornea.[9, 10] This occurs in approximately 20% of patients treated with ciprofloxacin for bacterial keratitis. This crystallization has not been seen with norfloxacin or ofloxcin, presumably due to their high solubility. It is not known whether the crystal formation delays epithelial healing or retards penetration of antibiotic into the corneal stroma.

Tetracyclines

OVERVIEW AND MECHANISM OF ACTION

Tetracyclines are among the broadest-spectrum agents available. Tetracycline antibiotics inhibit bacterial protein synthesis by binding to the 30-S ribosomes. They are bacteriostatic for most organisms. Various forms of tetracycline are available, including chlortetracycline (topical), oxytetracycline, doxycycline, minocycline, and tetracycline. Tetracyclines also inhibit collagenase and polymorphonuclear leukocyte migration. They also have an antilipase action, fostering the production of long-chain fatty acids.[11]

SPECTRUM OF ACTION

Tetracyclines are active against gram-positive organisms, Enterobacteriaceae, *Vibrio* species, *Rickettsia, M. marinum,* and malarial parasites. They are not usually effective against *P. aeruginosa, Bacteroides* species, or group B streptococci. Organisms commonly acquire resistance to tetracycline via plasmids, and resistance to *S. aureus* has climbed to about 40% in the United States. In vitro susceptibility testing is necessary to confirm the activity of tetracycline against most organisms.

PHARMACOLOGY

Of the available tetracyclines, doxycycline has the best penetration into the eye. These drugs should be avoided in patients with renal failure, as they are antianabolic and can speed the decline of renal function in persons with chronic renal failure. Doxycycline is highly protein bound, with a long half-life, so that it can be given once a day. Doxycycline and minocycline can also be given intravenously.

OPHTHALMIC INDICATION

Tetracycline is indicated in the treatment of ocular trachoma. It is also effective in Lyme disease and nocardial infections. Minocycline has been used to treat *M. marinum* infections. Tetracyclines have been shown to be active in treating noninfectious corneal ulceration and acne rosacea.[12]

REFERENCES

1. Hooper D, Wolfson J: Fluoroquinolone antimicrobial agents. N Engl J Med 324–384, 1991.
2. Trucksis M, Hooper D, Wolfson J: Emerging resistance to fluoroquinolones in staphylococci: An alert. Ann Intern Med 114:424, 1991.
3. Hyndiuk RA, Eiferman RA, Delmar RC, et al: Comparison of ciprofloxacin ophthalmic solution 0.3% (Ciloxacan) to fortified tobramycin/cefazolin in the treatment of bacterial corneal ulcers. Ophthalmology 103:1854–1863, 1996.
4. O'Brien TP, Maguire MG, Fink NE, et al: Efficacy of ofloxacin versus cefazolin and tobramycin in the therapy for bacterial keratitis. Arch Ophthalmol 113:1257–1265, 1995.
5. Donnenfeld ED, Perry HD, Snyder RW, et al: Intracorneal, aqueous humor, and vitreous humor penetration of topical and oral ofloxacin. Arch Ophthalmol 115:173–176, 1997.
6. McDermott ML, Tran TD, Cowden JW, Bugge CJL: Corneal stromal penetration of topical ciprofloxacin in humans. Ophthalmology 100:197–200, 1993.
7. Jackson WB, Kirsch IS, Goldstein DA, Discepola M: A clinical trial of perioperative ofloxacin combined with tobramycin to evaluate external ocular adnexal sterilization and anterior chamber penetration. Invest Ophthalmol Vis Sci 34:858, 1993.
8. Donnenfeld ED, Schrier A, Perry HD, et al: Penetration of topically applied ciprofloxacin, norfloxacin, and ofloxacin into the aqueous humor. Ophthalmology 101:902–905, 1994.
9. Leibowitz HM: Clinical evaluation of ciprofloxacin 0.3% ophthalmic solution for treatment of bacterial keratitis. Am J Ophthalmol 112:34S–47S, 1991.
10. Bower KS, Kowalski RP, Gordon YJ: Fluoroquinolones in the treatment of bacterial keratitis. Am J Ophthalmol 121:712–715, 1996.
11. Dougherty JM, McCulley JP, Silvany RE, Meyer DR: The role of tetracycline in chronic blepharitis inhibition of lipase production in staphylococci. Invest Ophthalmol Vis Sci 32(11):2970–2975, 1991.
12. Perry HD, Hodes LW, Seedor JA, et al: Effects of doxycycline hyclate on corneal epithelial wound healing in the rabbit alkali burn model. Cornea 12:379–382, 1993.

CHAPTER 21

Antivirals

Thomas John

Antiviral research appears to have gained momentum and has entered a new productive phase with the challenges of medical management of acquired immunodeficiency syndrome (AIDS). However, progress in the chemotherapy of viral diseases has continued to fall behind compared with that made in antibacterial treatment over the last several decades. As a result, fewer antiviral agents are currently available to treat specific viral infections compared with the broad range of antibiotics available to treat various bacterial infections. This is partly owing to the fact that viruses are obligate intracellular parasites that use the metabolic processes of the invaded host cell. Hence, the major barrier in antiviral therapy is formulating antiviral drugs that do not interfere with the normal host-cell metabolism by causing toxic side effects in the uninfected host cells. However, efforts to find new, effective, and clinically safe antiviral drugs have been intensive. Adding to this challenge is the emergence of new or more recently described human viral infections such as AIDS that can involve the eye.

Theoretically, antiviral drugs may be effective by interacting directly with the virus, a virus-encoded enzyme or other protein, or a cellular receptor or factor required for viral replication or pathogenesis.[1] To date, the most effective molecular targets of antiviral treatment have been the viral enzymes and proteins that play a role in the assembly of the virus.[1] The continuing search for new antiviral agents may result in the development of drugs that are effective at one or more stages of viral infection of the host cell, namely, the initial adherence or adsorption of the virus to the host cells by electrostatic interaction and receptors, viral penetration into the host cell (e.g., by pinocytosis), release of viral nucleic acid by uncoating, and replication, transcription, and translation of viral genome within the infected host cell. The development of antiviral drugs that are licensed currently for clinical use has resulted from an increased understanding of the molecular biology of viral structures, enzymes, and replicative mechanisms and virus-host-cell interactions. Although newer antiviral agents are being introduced into the marketplace, continued research in this field is required to provide better and safer antiviral drugs in the future.

Classification of Viruses

Viruses are made up of a nucleic acid core that contains either ribonucleic acid (RNA) or deoxyribonucleic acid (DNA) and is surrounded by a protein-containing outer coat. The classification of a virus is based on the type of nucleic acid core (RNA or DNA). Viruses can also be subdivided based on their morphology (whether the virus shell has an envelope), the site of viral multiplication (in the nucleus or cytoplasm of the host cell), and serologic type.

Descriptions of some viral infections (RNA and DNA viruses) of ocular importance follow.

RNA VIRUSES

Togaviridae. Rubella virus (rubella, German measles).

Paramyxoviridae. Measles virus (rubeola, measles); mumps virus (mumps, epidemic parotitis); Newcastle virus (Newcastle disease).

Orthomyxoviridae. Influenza virus (influenza).

Picornaviridae. Enterovirus type 70 (acute hemorrhagic conjunctivitis, picornaviral hemorrhagic conjunctivitis); coxsackie A24 virus (acute hemorrhagic conjunctivitis, picornaviral hemorrhagic conjunctivitis).

Rhabdoviridae. Rabies virus (rabies, hydrophobia).

Retroviridae. Human immunodeficiency virus types 1 and 2 (HIV-1, HIV-2) (AIDS).

DNA VIRUSES

Herpesviridae. Herpes simplex virus (HSV) types 1 and 2 (herpes simplex infection, "cold" sores, keratitis, genital infections, encephalitis); varicella-zoster virus (VZV) herpesvirus 3 (chickenpox and shingles); Epstein-Barr virus (EBV) or herpesvirus 4 (infectious mononucleosis, association with Burkitt's lymphoma); cytomegalovirus (CMV) or herpesvirus 5 (CMV disease, cytomegalic inclusion disease).

Adenoviridae. Adenovirus types 3 and 7 (pharyngoconjunctival fever, acute follicular conjunctivitis); adenovirus types 8, 19, and 37 (epidemic keratoconjunctivitis).

Poxviridae. Molluscum contagiosum virus (molluscum contagiosum); vaccinia virus (ocular vaccinia); variola virus (smallpox).

United States Food and Drug Administration–Approved Antiviral Drugs for Ophthalmic Use

The eye and adnexal structures may be directly infected by RNA and DNA viruses or involved secondarily as part of a systemic viral infection. Since the last publication of this chapter there has been a significant increase in the number of Food and Drug Administration (FDA)–approved antiviral drugs from eight to approximately 18, for clinical use. Of these 18 drugs, only three are approved for ocular use: idoxuridine (Stoxil, Herplex), trifluridine (Viroptic) (both pyrimidine nucleosides), and vidarabine (Vira-A) (purine nucleoside). The remaining antiviral drugs for systemic use include acyclovir (Zovirax) (purine nucleoside), ganciclovir (Cytovene), foscarnet (Foscavir), cidofovir (Vistide), didanosine (Videx), famciclovir (Famvir), indinavir (Crixivan), lamivudine (Epivir), nevirapine (Viramune), rimantadine (Flumadine), ritonavir (Norvir), saquinavir (Invirase), stavudine (Zerit), valacyclovir (Valtrex), zalcitabine (Hivid), zidovudine (Retrovir), amantadine (Symmetrel), and ribavirin (Virazole). This chapter describes the ophthalmic antiviral drugs and other systemic antiviral agents such as acyclovir, ganciclovir, foscarnet, cidofovir, and zidovudine.

IDOXURIDINE (STOXIL, HERPLEX)

Idoxuridine (5-iodo-2′-deoxyuridine, IDU), a nucleoside analog of thymidine, was the first clinically effective antiviral drug used as a topical ophthalmic preparation.[2–5] Thymidine, a nucleoside found in DNA, has a methyl group at the 5 position of the pyrimidine ring, which in IDU is replaced by a single iodide substituent (Fig. 21–1). This chemical substitution provides IDU with its antiviral property.

Prusoff, who first synthesized IDU at Yale University,[6] noted that the drug has an inhibitory effect on DNA polym-

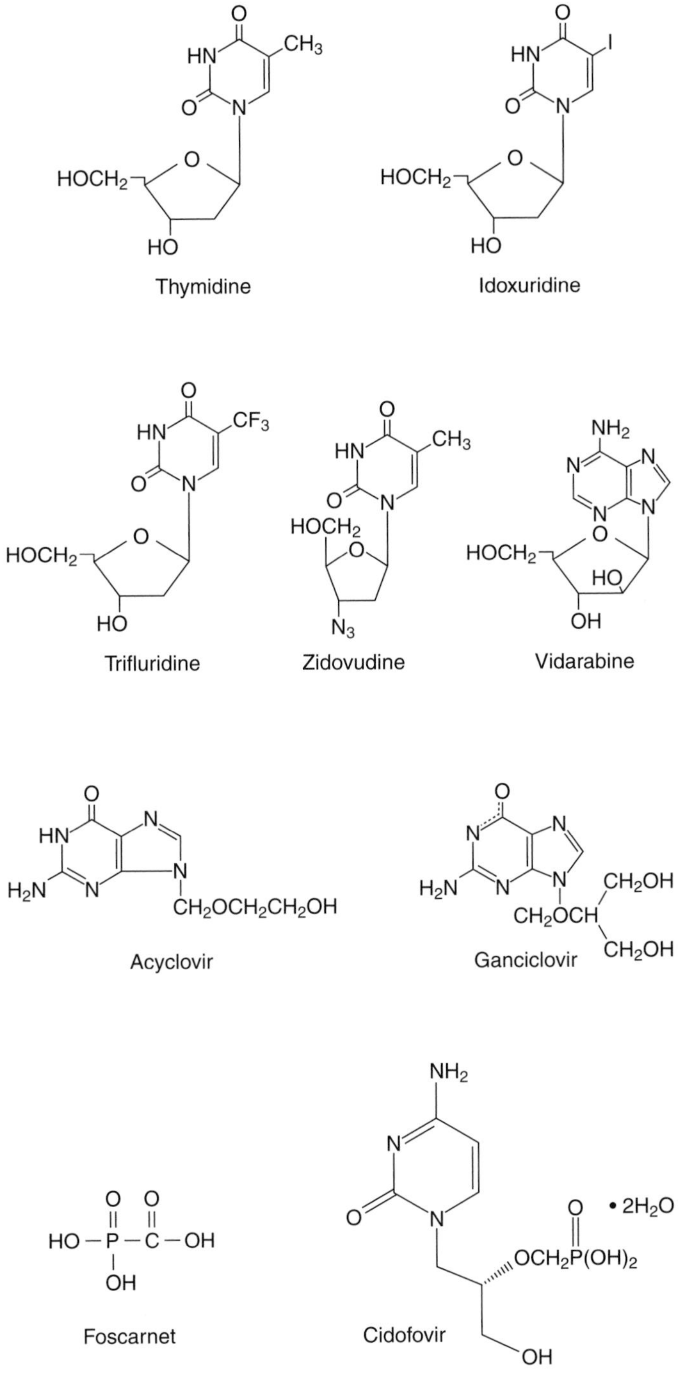

Thymidine

Idoxuridine

Trifluridine

Zidovudine

Vidarabine

Acyclovir

Ganciclovir

Foscarnet

Cidofovir

FIGURE 21–1. Structures of thymidine and antivirals.

erase in Ehrlich ascites tumor cells.[7] In 1961, Hermann reported IDU had antiviral properties against HSV in tissue culture.[8] Another study showed IDU to be effective in treating herpes simplex keratitis in rabbits.[4] The next step was the application of the laboratory data to the clinical setting. In 1962, Kaufman and associates[5] reported the ocular efficacy of IDU as an antiviral agent in the treatment of herpes simplex keratitis.

Because IDU is similar to thymidine, it replaces thymidine in the enzymatic step of viral replication. Thus, IDU irreversibly inhibits the incorporation of thymidine into viral DNA. This incorporation of the thymidine analog, namely, IDU, into viral DNA[9] renders the newly formed viral particles noninfective.[10] This substituted nucleoside is also incorporated into the normal host cell DNA, which possibly accounts for the toxicity that may occur during IDU treatment. However, the virus-infected cells preferentially take up IDU, delaying the onset of toxicity. The activity of IDU is limited primarily to DNA viruses, mainly the herpesvirus group; the drug is active in vitro against HSV, vaccinia virus, varicella virus, and CMV.[11, 12]

IDU is poorly soluble in water, and only a 0.1% solution can be formulated. The ophthalmic ointment is available as a 0.5% preparation. It is recommended that the IDU solution be stored in a refrigerator (45°F to 50°F) and the ophthalmic ointment at controlled room temperature (59°F to 86°F). Because it is light-sensitive, IDU should be protected in dark bottles. Outdated IDU solutions are known to cause ocular irritation and punctate corneal epithelial staining.[13]

The corneal epithelial toxicity that results from IDU therapy may cause difficulty in management. It is important to ascertain clinically if a nonhealing dendritic or ameboid corneal ulcer is the result of IDU toxicity or HSV that is resistant to the medication. If the corneal findings result from drug toxicity, discontinuation of IDU is indicated; if the toxicity results from viral drug resistance, an alternative antiviral drug with or without débridement of the corneal epithelium is necessary. The clinical features of IDU toxicity are listed in Table 21–1. Punctal stenosis and occlusion have been reported to occur as early as 1 or 2 weeks after IDU therapy was instituted.[14] Other adverse reactions include occasional irritation, pain, pruritus, and photophobia. IDU does not retard healing of the corneal epithelium;[15] however, it inhibits corneal stromal healing,[16] causing decreased tensile strength of corneal wounds in eyes treated with IDU.[17] Hence, it may be advisable not to use IDU in the immediate postoperative period following penetrating keratoplasty for herpes keratitis or other corneal stromal incisions.

TABLE 21–1. **IDU Toxicity on Ocular and Adnexal Structures**

Site	Toxicity
Cornea	Fine punctate epithelial keratopathy
	Filamentary keratitis
	Indolent corneal ulceration
	Perilimbal edema
	Late superficial vascularization
	Superficial stromal opacification
Conjunctiva	Punctate staining with rose bengal or fluorescein
	Follicular conjunctivitis
	Chemosis, congestion
	Perilimbal edema
	Conjunctival scarring
Lid margins	Edema of meibomian gland orifices
	Punctal edema and occlusion[14]
Lids	Ptosis
	Allergic contact blepharodermatitis
Other	Preauricular lymphadenopathy

IDU drops are used frequently to treat herpes simplex corneal infection. However, even if the medication was absorbed systemically, the frequent topical application should cause no toxic side effect, because IDU is rapidly inactivated by nucleotidases. After intravenous administration of IDU, most of the active form of the drug disappears from the blood in about 30 minutes.[18]

The main clinical use of IDU is in the treatment of herpes simplex keratitis, but it may also be used for ocular vaccinia infection. However, it is not recommended for treating other corneal viral infections. Because topical IDU has poor intraocular penetration,[19] it is used primarily for epithelial herpes simplex infection. Idoxuridine may be used for both primary and recurrent corneal epithelial herpes simplex infections and as corneal prophylaxis against herpes simplex infection in the case of primary herpes simplex infection involving the eyelid margins.

Experimentally, it has been shown that IDU, 0.1%, applied topically to rabbit eyes before HSV inoculation prevented herpes keratitis.[20] In 1963, Maxwell[21] reported that in 1500 cases of herpes keratitis treated with IDU, the epithelial lesions responded best to treatment compared with stromal keratitis. In another study,[5] 75 of 76 cases of herpes simplex dendritic keratitis responded well to treatment with IDU. The drug's poor intracorneal and intraocular penetration may account for the less favorable response of herpes simplex keratitis and uveitis. In these cases, topical corticosteroid should be combined with topical antiviral therapy to prevent steroid activation of herpes keratitis. Experimentally, it has been shown that IDU protected the rabbit cornea against steroid activation of herpes simplex keratitis.[22]

TRIFLURIDINE (VIROPTIC)

Trifluridine (5-trifluoromethyl-2′-deoxyuridine, trifluorothymidine, F_3T, Viroptic) is a fluorinated nucleoside analog of thymidine. The methyl group at the 5′ position of the pyrimidine ring of thymidine (see Fig. 21–1) is changed in F_3T such that each hydrogen of the methyl group is replaced by a fluoride substituent (see Fig. 21–1). This chemical change provides F_3T with its antiviral properties.

Heidelberger and associates[23] first synthesized F_3T for the treatment of cancer. Its efficacy as an antiviral agent was soon detected.[24] It is the current drug of choice for the treatment of epithelial herpes simplex keratitis.

Trifluridine is a potent inhibitor of thymidylate synthetase and therefore inhibits DNA synthesis. Trifluridine is incorporated into viral DNA directly, rendering the viral particle noninfectious.[11] However, its antiviral mechanism of action is not fully known. In addition, F_3T is also incorporated into mammalian cells. It has exerted mutagenic, DNA-damaging, and cell-transforming activities in various standard in vitro test systems. From a clinical standpoint, the significance of these test results has yet to be fully understood. Trifluridine is active against HSV types 1 and 2 and vaccinia virus both in vitro and in vivo. It also has an in vitro inhibitory effect against some strains of adenovirus.

TABLE 21–2. **Preservatives in Ophthalmic Antiviral Medications**

Preparation	Preservatives	Manufacturer
Idoxuridine		
Ointment 0.5% (Stoxil)	None	SmithKline Beecham
Solution 0.1% (Dendrid)	EDTA, benzalkonium chloride 0.01%	Alcon
Iodoxuridine 0.1% (Herplex)	EDTA, benzalkonium chloride	Allergan
Iodoxuridine (Stoxil)	Thimerosal 1 : 50,000	SmithKline Beecham
Trifluridine		
Solution 10 mg/mL (Viroptic)	Thimerosal 0.001%	Burroughs Wellcome
Vidarabine Ointment 3% (Vira-A)	None	Parke-Davis

Trifluridine in a 1% solution is twice as potent and 10 times more soluble than IDU.[17, 25, 26] It is also lipid-soluble. The drug's biphasic solubility enhances corneal penetration, which was shown to be by simple diffusion.[27] Trifluridine penetrates the intact cornea into the aqueous humor, and if the corneal epithelium is disrupted by ocular surface disease or abrasion, corneal penetration is further enhanced.[27] Experimentally, F_3T is partly metabolized to 5-carboxy-2′-deoxyuridine as the drug passes through the cornea, as evidenced by the presence of both F_3T and 5-carboxy-2′-deoxyuridine on the endothelial side.[27] In a rabbit model of herpetic uveitis, topical F_3T was shown to be effective because of its penetration into the anterior chamber.[28] In another study of rabbit herpes simplex keratouveitis, 1% F_3T and 0.1% IDU had almost similar control of uveitis, keratitis, and conjunctivitis.[29] The efficacy of topical 1% F_3T was also demonstrated in rabbits with herpes simplex keratitis[30] and may also be due to its intracorneal penetration property.

As in the experimental studies, intraocular penetration of topical F_3T has been shown to occur in humans.[31] This penetration of F_3T into the aqueous humor may be enhanced in the presence of compromised corneal integrity and corneal stromal or uveal inflammation. However, unlike the in vitro results of ocular penetration of F_3T, 5-carboxy-2′-deoxyuridine was not found in detectable concentrations within the aqueous humor at the time of penetrating keratoplasty in patients who received F_3T preoperatively.[31] The passage of F_3T through the human cornea without any significant metabolic degradation is therapeutically helpful in the treatment of herpes keratouveitis compared with other antiviral drugs such as IDU or vidarabine.

Systemic absorption of F_3T following therapeutic dosing appears to be negligible. The half-life of F_3T in serum is only 12 minutes, rendering it ineffective as a systemic antiviral agent. The drug should not be used during pregnancy unless the potential benefits outweigh the potential hazards to the fetus. Although it is unlikely that F_3T is excreted in human milk after ophthalmic use, it should not be prescribed for nursing mothers unless the potential benefits outweigh the potential risks.

Trifluridine is supplied as a 1% sterile ophthalmic solution that should be refrigerated (2°C to 8°C; 36°F to 46°F). The preservative in F_3T 1% solution is thimerosal 0.001% (Table 21–2). The recommended dosage is initially one drop every 2 hours while awake (maximum, nine drops daily). When healing is complete, F_3T should be continued for 7 days, one drop every 4 hours while awake. It should not be used for more than 3 weeks. The most frequent adverse reactions of F_3T are transient burning or stinging upon ocular instillation and palpebral edema. Other side effects of F_3T include punctate epithelial keratopathy,[32, 33] contact blepharodermatitis, filamentary keratitis,[32] corneal stromal edema, ocular irritation, hypersensitivity reaction, keratitis sicca, and increased intraocular pressure.

Trifluridine is an effective antiviral drug and the drug of choice for topical treatment of human epithelial herpetic keratitis.[24–36]

VIDARABINE (VIRA-A)

Vidarabine (9-β-D-arabinofuranosyladenine) is a substituted purine nucleoside known previously as adenine arabinoside (Ara-A) (see Fig. 21–1).

Vidarabine is the second antiviral drug developed for human use.[37] Lee and colleagues[38] and Reist and coworkers[39] first synthesized the compound in the early 1960s as a potential anticancer agent. It has subsequently been obtained from fermentation cultures of *Streptomyces* antibiotics.[40]

The mechanism of action of vidarabine, although not fully established, appears to interfere with the early steps of viral DNA synthesis and arrests the growth of the viral deoxynucleotide chain. Thus, the mechanism of action of vidarabine differs from IDU in that IDU is incorporated into the viral DNA, which results in a fraudulent DNA or noninfective viral particles. This difference permits vidarabine to act against IDU-resistant herpetic strains and in those patients who are allergic to IDU. Vidarabine is less toxic than IDU, and, like IDU, is not a completely selective antiviral agent. Although vidarabine can affect normal cells, it is thought to be sufficiently safe for systemic use. Vidarabine is rapidly deaminated to hypoxanthine arabinoside (Ara-Hx). The principal metabolite, Ara-Hx, possesses antiviral activity that is less potent than the parent drug, vidarabine. Vidarabine is effective against herpes simplex, varicella-zoster, and vaccinia (DNA viruses).[41–43] It has a limited range of activity against RNA viruses[42] and no antiviral action against adenovirus keratoconjunctivitis.[44] Subepithelial corneal infiltrates developed in both vidarabine-treated patients and controls.[44]

Because vidarabine is insoluble, it is formulated as a 3% ophthalmic ointment. The recommended dosage is five times a day at 3-hour intervals. Clinicians should consider other forms of treatment if there is no clinical improvement after 1 week or if complete corneal reepithelialization fails to occur in 3 weeks. Following reepithelialization, an additional week of treatment at a reduced dosage of twice daily should be continued to prevent recurrence of infection. Vidarabine treatment should not be continued for more than 3 weeks.

Vidarabine penetrates the aqueous humor better than IDU. Two hours after topical application of 3% vidarabine in petrolatum to rabbit eyes, aqueous levels of 6 mg/mL of the drug were detected; 0.5% IDU failed to produce any detectable aqueous levels.[45] This is compatible with the clinical impression that vidarabine treatment may be useful in herpetic uveitis.[45] Although vidarabine has been used intravenously in humans for herpetic uveitis,[46] this is not a popular mode of treatment. Vidarabine was also the first drug shown to be effective systemically in the treatment of herpetic encephalitis.[47]

Like other antiviral agents, vidarabine is not free from side effects, especially corneal epithelial punctate keratopathy.[48, 49] Other possible adverse reactions include foreign body sensation, lacrimation, conjunctival hyperemia, burning, irritation, pain, photophobia, sensitivity, and punctal occlusion.

Significant systemic absorption of vidarabine is not expected to occur after topical ocular use. In experimental animals, vidarabine is rapidly deaminated to its principal metabolite, Ara-Hx, in the gastrointestinal tract.

Although the chance of fetal damage with ocular use of vidarabine during pregnancy is remote, it is best avoided unless the potential benefit of therapy justifies the potential risk to the fetus. Similarly, because it is unknown whether vidarabine is excreted in breast milk, it is best to avoid prescribing it to nursing mothers. Excretion in breast milk appears unlikely with ocular use, because even if the drug was absorbed, it would be rapidly deaminated in the gastrointestinal tract.

Topical use of vidarabine for herpes simplex keratoconjunctivitis was found to be as effective as IDU and less irritating.[49] Similarly, no significant difference was noted between vidarabine and trifluridine in the treatment of herpes simplex dendritic corneal ulcers.[35, 36] However, trifluridine was more effective than vidarabine in the treatment of herpes simplex geographic corneal ulcers.[35] In another multicenter study comparing the overall efficacy of 3% vidarabine ointment with 3% acyclovir ointment in the treatment of dendritic or geographic herpetic keratitis in 66 patients, no statistically significant difference existed between the two medications in healing rate, the final visual acuity, the frequency of selected complications such as punctate epithelial keratitis, or the development of stromal keratitis.[50] This is contrary to the earlier in vitro and animal experiments, the results of which suggested that acyclovir might be a more effective antiviral agent than vidarabine.[51, 52]

Experimentally, vidarabine was compared with IDU to evaluate which drug was less toxic to the corneal epithelium.[53] The rate of rabbit corneal epithelial wound closure of 5- and 10-mm epithelial defects was not significantly different among the eyes treated with 3% vidarabine, 0.5% IDU, and placebo antibiotics,[53] indicating that neither 3% vidarabine nor 0.5% IDU retarded corneal epithelial wound healing. The quality of the regenerated corneal epithelium as evaluated by slit lamp was significantly better with vidarabine than with IDU.[41, 53] However, 3% vidarabine and 0.5% IDU interfere with stromal healing to the same degree.[41, 53]

Vidarabine therapy may be useful in cases of IDU resistance. In one study in which vidarabine 3% ointment was used to treat 56 cases of IDU-resistant herpes simplex keratitis,[54] 80% of epithelial herpes keratitis and 52% of herpes stromal keratitis healed within 2 weeks of treatment being initiated.[54] Others have also shown vidarabine to be effective in many patients intolerant of or resistant to IDU.[49]

FDA-Approved Antiviral Drugs for Systemic Use

ACYCLOVIR (ZOVIRAX)

Acyclovir, [9-(2-hydroxyethoxymethyl) guanine], is a synthetic purine nucleoside analog derived from guanine, but it differs from guanine by the presence of an acyclic side chain. Although acyclovir is available commercially for parenteral use as the sodium salt and for oral use as the base, it is not currently available as an ophthalmic preparation in the United States.

Acyclovir is a highly effective antiviral agent.[55] When used to treat HSV and VZV, acyclovir interferes with DNA synthesis, thus inhibiting virus replication. However, the exact mechanisms of action against other susceptible viruses are not fully understood.

In herpesvirus-infected cells in vitro, the antiviral activity of acyclovir appears to be dependent primarily on the intracellular conversion of acyclovir to acyclovir triphosphate. The conversion of acyclovir to acyclovir monophosphate occurs mainly via virus-coded thymidine kinase. Acyclovir monophosphate is phosphorylated to the diphosphate via cellular guanylate kinase and to the triphosphate via other cellular enzymes (e.g., phosphoglycerate kinase, pyruvate kinase, phosphoenolpyruvate carboxykinase). In contrast, in uninfected cells in vitro, acyclovir is only phosphorylated minimally by host cell enzymes. It appears that acyclovir is also converted to acyclovir triphosphate by other mechanisms, because acyclovir has antiviral activity against, for example, EBV and CMV that apparently do not code for viral thymidine kinase. It appears that acyclovir triphosphate is produced to some extent within EBV- and CMV-infected cells via unidentified cellular phosphorylating enzymes.

Acyclovir takes advantage of the subtle differences between viral and cellular enzyme function in DNA synthesis. A slight difference exists between the viral and cellular thymidine kinase. Because acyclovir is a nucleoside analog, it can function as a substrate for viral thymidine kinase but not for cellular thymidine kinase. Hence, acyclovir can enter the sequence of DNA formation primarily in virus-infected cells. The viral DNA polymerase more effectively utilizes the acyclovir triphosphate than does the cellular DNA polymerase. The viral DNA polymerase has a 10- to 30-fold or greater affinity in vitro for the acyclovir triphosphate than does the cellular α-DNA polymerase. When the acyclovir analog enters the DNA chain, DNA synthesis is terminated. Thus, viral DNA growth is more susceptible to acyclovir than the uninfected host cells.[56–59] Acyclovir has minimal pharmacologic effects in vitro on the uninfected host cells, because of its poor uptake into these cells; phosphorylation and intracellular conversion to acyclovir triphosphate are minimal; and the cellular α-DNA polymerase has a low affinity for acyclovir triphosphate.

Acyclovir has antiviral activity against HSV types 1 and 2 (HSV-1 and HSV-2), VZV, EBV, herpes simiae (B virus), and CMV.

Acyclovir is a crystalline white powder with a solubility of 1.3 mg/mL in water at 25°C. Commercially available acyclovir sodium is a sterile, white, crystalline, lyophilized powder. At a pH of 7.4 and 37°C, it is almost completely un-ionized and has a maximum solubility of 2.5 mg/mL.

Acyclovir capsules, suspension, and the commercially available acyclovir sodium sterile powder should be stored in tight, light-resistant containers at 15°C to 25°C. Reconstituted acyclovir sodium solution (50 mg acyclovir/mL) is stable for 12 hours at 15°C to 30°C. Upon refrigeration, a precipitate may form that redissolves at room temperature. This precipitation and subsequent redissolution do not appear to affect drug potency. Bacteriostatic water that contains parabens should not be used for injection, because this diluent is incompatible with the drug and may cause precipitation.

Acyclovir has been detected in the brain, kidney, saliva, lung, liver, muscle, spleen, uterus, vaginal mucosa and secretions, semen, cerebrospinal fluid, and herpetic vesicular fluid. Acyclovir diffuses into cerebrospinal fluid and crosses the placenta. Evidence indicates that the drug is distributed into milk via an active transport mechanism. Acyclovir is metabolized to 9-carboxymethoxymethylguanine (CMMG) and 8-hydroxy-9-(2-hydroxyethoxymethyl) guanine. In in vitro herpesvirus-infected cells, acyclovir is metabolized to acyclovir mono-, di-, and triphosphate. Acyclovir is excreted mainly in urine via glomerular filtration and tubular secretion.

Piorier and associates[60] evaluated the intraocular penetration of 3% acyclovir ointment, vidarabine monophosphate, and 1% F_3T drops following their administration to patients with normal corneas before cataract extraction. The authors detected substantial levels of acyclovir in the aqueous humor, even though only meager levels of vidarabine monophosphate and no F_3T were detected. Hence, 3% acyclovir may be superior to other antiviral agents with regard to corneal penetration and in the treatment of deep herpetic keratitis and uveitis. However, acyclovir topical treatment did not significantly reduce the incidence of stromal keratitis that developed with herpes simplex epithelial keratitis.[61]

In experimental herpes simplex corneal infections in three groups of rabbits treated five times a day with either 0.5% IDU, 3% vidarabine, or 3% acyclovir ointment, there was 50% less severe iritis, epithelial loss, and conjunctivitis in the acyclovir group compared with the other groups.[51] Also, recoverable virus on day 6 was much less in the acyclovir-treated rabbits' eyes compared with the other two groups.[51] Acyclovir does not interfere with corneal epithelial or stromal healing in rabbit eyes.[62]

Topical or oral acyclovir is useful in treating herpes simplex epithelial keratitis.[59, 63–73] Pavan-Langston and associates[59] compared the efficacy of acyclovir 3% ointment with vidarabine 3% ointment in the treatment of patients with dendritic or geographic herpes keratitis. Within 2 weeks, more than 90% of the patients healed with no significant difference between the two drugs.[59] However, herpes dendritic corneal ulcers healed more rapidly when 3% acyclovir was combined with débridement compared with 3% acyclovir alone, 2 and 5 days, respectively.[63] In its antiherpetic effect, acyclovir is comparable with topical F_3T.[64]

In a study[65] comparing oral acyclovir (400 mg five times daily) to 3% acyclovir ointment (five times daily) in the treatment of herpes simplex dendritic corneal ulceration, the authors found that healing occurred in 5 days in 89% of patients on oral acyclovir and 97% of patients on topical acyclovir ointment. Thus, oral acyclovir may be an alternative to topical acyclovir ointment for the treatment of herpes simplex dendritic lesions.[65] In a controlled trial[66] of oral acyclovir or placebo for 7 days with minimal wiping, débridement in herpes simplex dendritic corneal ulcers was carried out in 31 patients. At the end of treatment, the corneal lesions had healed in 67% of patients receiving acyclovir and 43% of patients given a placebo. Although there was no significant difference in the proportion of corneal lesions that healed in the two groups at 7 days, the rate of healing was significantly faster in the acyclovir group.[66] Jensen and colleagues[71] found that 3% topical acyclovir ointment was useful both in epithelial and stromal herpes simplex corneal infections. However, they also found that acyclovir ointment was equally effective in herpetic keratitis in patients either receiving débridement or no débridement.[71] Also, 3% acyclovir ointment (five times daily) in combination with (-interferon eye drops (30,000,000 IU/mL), once daily) has been found useful in the treatment of herpes simplex dendritic keratitis.[73]

Systemic acyclovir is useful in the treatment of genital herpes simplex infections, herpes simplex encephalitis, acute treatment of herpes zoster (shingles), VZV (chickenpox) infections in immunocompromised adults and children, and in mucosal or cutaneous herpes simplex (HSV-1 and HSV-2) infections in immunocompromised adults and children. Acyclovir is useful to treat acute stages of herpes zoster infection.[74–76] Acyclovir was effective in reducing the incidence and severity of common complications of herpes zoster ophthalmicus.[74] It may promote resolution of signs and symptoms and shorten the duration of virus shedding, especially if treatment is begun within 72 hours of the onset of skin lesions.[77] The dosage of acyclovir in the treatment of herpes zoster is 800 mg (four 200-mg capsules) every 4 hours orally five times daily for 7 to 10 days. When topical acyclovir was compared with topical steroids in the treatment of herpes zoster keratouveitis in 40 patients, topical acyclovir was found to be superior in duration of treatment and absence of recurrences after discontinuation. Patients in the group receiving steroid treatment experienced a 63% recurrence rate.[78]

McGill[79] reported that 15 of 18 patients with ocular herpes zoster infections were controlled with topical acyclovir therapy alone. These patients were treated with 3% acyclovir ophthalmic ointment five times daily until healing occurred, followed by three times daily for another 2 to 6 weeks. Cobo[80] also showed the beneficial effects of oral acyclovir in reducing the complications of herpes zoster ophthalmicus. Seiff and associates[81] recommended intravenous acyclovir (30 mg/kg/day) in immunocompromised patients with herpes zoster ophthalmicus.

Acyclovir has also been used intravitreally experimentally[82, 83] and clinically.[84] Two patients with acute retinal necrosis were treated with intravitreal infusion of acyclovir, vitrectomy, and prophylactic scleral buckles; both patients had an uneventful postoperative course and recovered visual acuity.[84]

Topical use of acyclovir is well tolerated. Morgan and colleagues[72] reported that no significant toxicity was noted in patients following topical treatment of herpetic ocular infections with 3% acyclovir ophthalmic ointment for 14 days. Systemic side effects of oral acyclovir include nausea, vomiting, and headache. Less common adverse reactions include diarrhea, dizziness, anorexia, fatigue, edema, skin rash, leg pain, inguinal adenopathy, medication taste, and sore throat.

GANCICLOVIR (CYTOVENE)

Ganciclovir, a synthetic purine nucleoside analog of guanine, is structurally and pharmacologically related to acyclovir. It differs from acyclovir only by a second terminal hydroxymethyl group at C-2 of the acyclic side chain on the ribose ring. This structural difference contributes to the substantially increased antiviral activity of ganciclovir against CMV and in less selectivity for viral DNA.

The exact mechanism of action of ganciclovir is not fully known, but it appears to exert its antiviral effect on human CMV and other human herpesviruses by interfering with DNA synthesis via competition with deoxyguanosine for incorporation into viral DNA and by incorporation into growing viral DNA chains. The phosphorylated form of ganciclovir that is active can competitively inhibit viral DNA polymerase and can also be incorporated into growing DNA chains as a false nucleotide, resulting in the termination of DNA synthesis and in the formation of a mutant DNA chain and thus inhibition of viral replication. Although the drug inhibits cellular a-DNA polymerase, it requires a higher concentration than that required to inhibit viral DNA polymerase.

The antiviral effect is primarily dependent on the intracellular conversion of the drug to ganciclovir triphosphate. The formation of ganciclovir monophosphate appears to be the rate-limiting step in the formation of ganciclovir triphosphate. In contrast to acyclovir, which is only minimally phosphorylated by cellular (host cell) enzymes, ganciclovir seems to be more susceptible to phosphorylation by enzymes in uninfected cells, especially in rapidly dividing cells, such as bone marrow. This phosphorylation in uninfected cells can range from less than 10% to being equal to that in virus-infected cells. The increased antiviral effect of ganciclovir against CMV compared with acyclovir has been attributed to slower catabolism of ganciclovir triphosphate by intracellular phosphatases.

Ganciclovir is virustatic rather than virucidal. Clinically, ganciclovir seems primarily to suppress virus activity and not eradicate the virus. Hence, the disease reactivates on discontinuation of the drug. Also, experimentally, when the drug is removed from culture medium in vitro, previously inhibited viral DNA synthesis resumes, with restored viral replication. Additional data supporting the view that ganciclovir is virustatic come from histopathologic studies of enucleated globes from patients who died while receiving ganciclovir therapy.[85, 86] These studies showed that ganciclovir does not eliminate CMV from the retina[85, 86] nor does it suppress expression of all viral genes.[85]

Although ganciclovir has antiviral activity both in vitro and in vivo against various Herpesviridae (herpes simplex types 1 and 2, human herpesvirus type 6, EBV, and VZV), its main clinical use has been against human CMV.

Ganciclovir sodium sterile powder (commercial preparation) is a white to off-white, crystalline, lyophilized powder with a solubility of 3 mg/mL in water at 25°C and neutral pH. Following reconstitution with sterile water for injection, the ganciclovir sodium solution is colorless and a solution containing ganciclovir 50 mg/mL has a pH of about 11.

Ganciclovir sodium sterile powder has an expiration date of 3 years from the date of manufacture. The drug should be stored at room temperature and should not be exposed to temperatures greater than 40°C. Reconstituted ganciclovir sodium solution with sterile water for injection (ganciclovir 50 mg/mL) is stable for 12 hours at 15°C to 30°C and should not be refrigerated, otherwise a precipitate may form. To avoid precipitation, bacteriostatic water for injection containing parabens should not be used to reconstitute ganciclovir sodium. Because ganciclovir is poorly absorbed from the gastrointestinal tract, intravenous administration is preferred. Ganciclovir is 1 to 2% bound to plasma proteins. Although the tissue distribution of ganciclovir is not fully known, autopsy studies on patients who received intravenous ganciclovir suggest that the drug concentrates mainly in the kidneys with lower concentrations in the liver, lung, brain, and testes.[87] Ganciclovir appears to have good ocular distribution following intravenous administration; concentrations in the aqueous and vitreous humors 2.5 hours after intravenous administration were, respectively, 0.4 and 0.6 times the simultaneous plasma concentration of the drug.[88] Ganciclovir crosses the blood-brain barrier. It is unknown whether ganciclovir is distributed into human milk; however, no drug is present in animal milk. It also crosses the placenta in animals. The primary route of excretion is in urine, and it appears to be mainly via glomerular filtration. Except for intracellular phosphorylation of the drug, it is not significantly metabolized in humans and is mainly excreted unchanged in the urine.

The primary clinical use of ganciclovir is in the treatment of CMV retinitis in immunocompromised patients, including those with AIDS. The safety and efficacy of the drug have not been established for congenital or neonatal CMV disease; for the treatment of other cytomegaloviral infections, such as pneumonitis or colitis; or for use in nonimmunocompromised individuals.

The intravenous route of ganciclovir therapy has been shown to be effective in the treatment of cytomegaloviral retinitis in immunocompromised patients.[89–95] However, ganciclovir is only suppressive against CMV; without improvement in immunocompetence, the retinitis will recur or progress following cessation. After induction therapy with ganciclovir for CMV retinitis and discontinuation of the drug, relapse of CMV usually occurs within 4 weeks in immunosuppressed patients. Hence, for the duration of the patient's immunosuppression, long-term maintenance therapy and intermittent induction therapy seem to be necessary.

Ganciclovir has also been administered intravitreally in patients with CMV retinitis.[96–101] It was found to be effective and safe both as an alternative to intravenous ganciclovir therapy in myelosuppressed patients and as a supplement to intravenous therapy in uncontrolled CMV retinitis.

GANCICLOVIR IMPLANT (VITRASERT)

The ganciclovir implant reflects a new direction in treating CMV retinitis in patients with AIDS by providing local concentrated therapy to the infected retina without the risks of systemic toxicity associated with other routes of administration. Additionally, the sustained intravitreal release of ganciclovir negates the need for repeated injections. The implant is placed surgically in the vitreous cavity, which can provide therapeutic levels of up to 8 months depending on the rate of drug release.[102, 103] Although the ganciclovir implant has been shown to be effective in treating CMV retinitis, there was the increased risk of CMV retinitis developing in the fellow eye and of systemic involvement in the patients who received implants compared with patients who received the drug intravenously.[102] To decrease this risk, these patients may be given oral ganciclovir.[104]

The most common dose-limiting adverse effect of ganciclovir is neutropenia (absolute neutrophil count $< 1000/mm^3$), which is potentially fatal. Usually, interruption of ganciclovir therapy or a decrease in dosage results in increased neutrophil counts. Thrombocytopenia (platelet count $< 50{,}000/mm^3$) can also result from a direct, dose-dependent effect of the drug. Less commonly, anemia and eosinophilia can occur less frequently. Ocular side effects include rhegmatogenous retinal detachment as a result of ganciclovir-induced resolution of retinitis. For the most part, intravitreal therapy has been well tolerated, and local reactions, such as foreign-body sensation, small conjunctival or vitreous hemorrhage, conjunctival scarring, and scleral induration, have been noted occasionally in patients receiving multiple intravitreal injections. Because of the high pH of the ganciclovir infusion solution, inflammation, phlebitis, and pain at the site of intravenous infusion can occur.

FOSCARNET (FOSCAVIR)

Foscarnet (phosphonoformic acid trisodium), an organic analog of inorganic pyrophosphate, is structurally unrelated to other available antiviral drugs. Following intravenous administration of foscarnet, it is not metabolized to any significant extent, and, therefore, does not cause any major interference with the host cellular processes. The drug is excreted renally.[105] It is active against herpesviruses (CMV, HSV, EBV, VZV), and HIV. It inhibits herpesvirus DNA polymerases and HIV-1 reverse transcriptase. Foscarnet directly affects the pyrophosphate binding site of DNA polymerase and, therefore, does not require phosphorylation to activate.[106] It has been shown to be useful in the treatment of HIV-infected patients with acyclovir-resistant HSV and VZV infections and in CMV retinitis.[107] Like ganciclovir, foscarnet is virustatic. It may be administered intravenously or intravitreally (Table 21–3) to treat CMV retinitis. Foscarnet is poorly absorbed orally and because gastrointestinal side effects are common, it is not used orally. Foscarnet should not be administered by rapid or bolus intravenous injection because the toxicity may be increased by excessive plasma levels. An infusion pump must be used.

Foscarnet, like ganciclovir, is considered a drug of choice to treat CMV retinitis in patients with AIDS. It is especially useful in those patients who are intolerant to or unresponsive to ganciclovir therapy. Because foscarnet does not cause myelosuppression, it can be used in conjunction with zidovudine. Foscarnet can be administered intravenously in combination with ganciclovir in patients with CMV retinitis that is resistant to one drug. This combination therapy reduces the dosage of the individual drug, appears to be fairly well tolerated, and has prolonged sight in patients with CMV retinitis.[108]

TABLE 21–3. **Intravitreal Antivirals**

Drug	Dosage
Ganciclovir (Cytovene)	200–400 μg/0.1 mL
Foscarnet (Foscavir)	1200 μg/0.05 mL
Cidofovir (Vistide)	20 μg/0.1 mL

In the initial treatment of CMV retinitis in patients with AIDS, foscarnet seems to be as equally effective as ganciclovir.[109, 110] However, to prevent recurrent CMV retinitis, chronic maintenance therapy is required with foscarnet, the same as with ganciclovir.[111] Foscarnet is more effective than ganciclovir in prolonging life in patients with AIDS, which may be the result of the anti-HIV effect and because it can be used with zidovudine.[112]

Foscarnet is not as well tolerated as ganciclovir by patients because of the side effects, i.e., fever and gastrointestinal effects including nausea, vomiting, diarrhea, anorexia, and abdominal pain. The most significant side effect with foscarnet is renal impairment, and, therefore, it is necessary to monitor the serum creatinine levels and adjust the drug dosage accordingly.[113] Because foscarnet can alter the plasma electrolyte levels[107, 114, 115] and cause seizures, patients treated with foscarnet should be monitored for any alterations in the plasma electrolyte levels.

The current foscarnet induction dose recommendations are either 60 mg/kg three times a day or 90 mg/kg twice a day for 2- to 3-week period.[116] As with ganciclovir, maintenance therapy is required with foscarnet, and the dosage range suggested is 90 to 120 mg/kg/day.[116] Some authors recommend the higher dosage of 120 mg/kg/day to obtain a better response when treating CMV retinitis without significantly increasing toxicity.[117, 118]

Intravitreal foscarnet has been used to treat CMV retinitis in patients with AIDS.[119] This route is especially useful for patients in whom ganciclovir is contraindicated as a result of acyclovir allergy, and intravenous foscarnet is contraindicated because of renal failure. Foscarnet is passed through a 0.22-μm filter, and 1200 μg (0.05 mL) is injected intravitreally.[119] The recommended dose is two injections of foscarnet as induction therapy per week for 3 weeks followed by a maintainance dose of one injection per week (see Table 21–3).[119]

CIDOFOVIR (VISTIDE)

Cidofovir (Vistide) was approved by the FDA in June 1996. It is an acyclic nucleotide analog that inhibits CMV DNA polymerase and thus inhibits CMV replication. It has been used intravitreally to treat CMV retinitis in patients with AIDS (see Table 21–3). Ocular side effects include decreased intraocular pressure and mild uveitis.[120]

ZIDOVUDINE (RETROVIR)

Zidovudine is a thymidine analog that differs from thymidine in its structure; i.e., zidovudine has a 3′-azido group rather than a 3′-hydroxyl group.

Zidovudine is effective against HIV and appears to prolong survival and decrease the frequency of opportunistic infections in patients with AIDS or AIDS-related complex (ARC).[121]

The exact mechanism of antiviral activity of zidovudine is not fully understood. It appears to inhibit in vitro replication of retroviruses, including HIV, by interfering with viral RNA-directed DNA polymerase (reverse transcriptase). It has a virustatic effect against retroviruses. The antiviral effect of zidovudine appears to be dependent on the intracellular drug conversion to zidovudine triphosphate. Because phosphorylation of zidovudine is dependent on cellular rather than viral enzymes, conversion of zidovudine to its active triphosphate derivative occurs in both virus-infected and uninfected cells.

Zidovudine is active in vitro against many human and animal retroviruses, including HIV (formerly HTLV-III/LAV). It has also some in vitro activity against EBV.

Zidovudine occurs as a white to off-white, odorless, crystalline solid. The oral solution of the drug containing zidovudine 50 mg/5 mL is colorless to pale yellow with a pH of 3 to 4. Zidovudine injection for intravenous infusion is a sterile solution that contains zidovudine 10 mg/mL of water for injection.

Zidovudine capsules should be stored at 15°C to 25°C and protected from light, heat, and moisture. The oral solution and the intravenous infusion should also be stored at 15°C to 25°C and protected from light.

Zidovudine is absorbed rapidly from the gastrointestinal tract, with peak serum concentrations usually occurring within 0.4 to 1.5 hours. Tissue absorption of the drug shows considerable inter-individual variation (range of 42 to 95%). Zidovudine appears to be widely distributed in body tissues or fluids, including cerebrospinal fluid and semen. It is 34 to 38% bound to plasma proteins. Zidovudine crosses the human placenta. It is unknown whether zidovudine is distributed into human milk, but it is present in milk in mice. Zidovudine is rapidly metabolized via glucuronidation in the liver and is eliminated mainly in urine via both glomerular filtration and tubular secretion.

Zidovudine is currently labeled by the FDA for the management of HIV infections in certain asymptomatic adults who have an absolute helper/inducer ($CD4^+$, $T4^+$) T-cell count from peripheral blood of 500/mm^3 or less at the time drug therapy is initiated, early symptomatic HIV infection, or advanced symptomatic infections (e.g., AIDS or advanced ARC). Although zidovudine is not a cure for HIV infections, it may ameliorate some manifestations of infection. The long-term efficacy of the drug has yet to be determined. Zidovudine has an in vivo virustatic effect against HIV and, thus, cannot eliminate HIV from infected patients. Whereas ganciclovir remains the treatment of choice for CMV retinitis, zidovudine may have a beneficial effect on CMV retinitis in some patients.[122] However, it must be emphasized that zidovudine is not effective in most cases of CMV retinitis with AIDS.[123] It has also been shown that HIV may be the cause of uveitis that may be responsive to systemic zidovudine therapy.[124]

The most common adverse effects of zidovudine therapy are anemia, granulocytopenia, nausea, and headache.

REFERENCES

1. Crumpacker CS: Molecular targets of antiviral therapy. N Engl J Med 321:163, 1989.
2. Robins RK: Nucleosides and nucleotides: Past, present, and future. Ann N Y Acad Sci 255:597, 1975.
3. Prusoff WH, Chen MS, Fischer PG, et al: Role of nucleosides in virus and cancer chemotherapy. Adv Ophthalmol 38:3, 1979.
4. Kaufman HE: Clinical cure of herpes simplex keratitis by 5-iodo-2′-deoxyuridine. Proc Soc Exp Biol Med 109:251, 1962.
5. Kaufman HE, Martola EL, Dohlman CH: Use of 5-iodo-2′-deoxyuridine (IDU) in the treatment of herpes simplex keratitis. Arch Ophthalmol 68:235, 1962.
6. Prusoff WH: Synthesis and biological activities of iododeoxyuridine: An analog of thymidine. Biochem Biophys Acta 32:295, 1959.
7. Welch AD, Prusoff WH: A synopsis of recent investigations of 5-iodo-2′-deoxyuridine. Cancer Chemother Rep 6:29, 1960.
8. Hermann EC Jr: Plaque inhibition test for detection of specific inhibitors of DNA containing viruses. Proc Soc Exp Biol Med 107:142, 1961.
9. Prusoff WH, Bakhle YS, McCrea JF: Incorporation of 5-iodo-2′-deoxyuridine into the deoxyribonucleic acid of vaccinia virus. Nature 199:1310, 1963.
10. Jones BR: Prospects in treating viral diseases of the eye. Trans Ophthalmol Soc UK 87:537, 1967.
11. Prusoff WH, Goz B: Potential mechanisms of action of antiviral agents. Fed Proc 32:1679, 1973.
12. Prusoff WH, Ward DC: Nucleoside analogs with antiviral activity. Biochem Pharmacol 25:1233, 1976.
13. Maloney ED, Kaufman HE: Antagonism and toxicity of IDU by its degradation products. Invest Ophthalmol 2:55, 1963.
14. Patterson A, Jones BR: The management of ocular herpes. Trans Ophthalmol Soc UK 87:59, 1967.
15. Laibson PR, Sery TW, Leopold IH: The treatment of herpetic keratitis with 5-iodo-2′-deoxyuridine (IDU). Arch Ophthalmol 70:52, 1963.
16. Polack FM, Rose J: The effect of 5-iodo-2′-deoxyuridine (IDU) in corneal healing. Arch Ophthalmol 71:520, 1964.
17. Payrau P, Dohlman CH: IDU in corneal wound healing. Am J Ophthalmol 57:999, 1964.
18. Sande MA, Mandell GL: Antimicrobial agents. *In* Gilman AG, Goodman LS, Gilman A (eds): The Pharmacological Basis of Therapeutics, 6th ed. New York, Macmillan, 1980, p 1240.
19. Kaufman HE: Chemotherapy of herpes keratitis. Invest Ophthalmol 2:504, 1963.
20. Kaufman HE, Nesburn AB, Maloney ED: IDU therapy of herpes simplex. Arch Ophthalmol 67:583, 1962.
21. Maxwell E: Treatment of herpes keratitis with 5-iodo-2′-deoxyuridine (IDU): A clinical evaluation of 1,500 cases. Am J Ophthalmol 56:571, 1963.
22. Kaufman HE, Maloney ED: IDU and hydrocortisone in experimental herpes simplex keratitis. Arch Ophthalmol 68:396, 1962.
23. Heidelberger C, Parsons DG, Remy DC: Synthesis of 5-trifluoromethyluracil and 5-trifluoromethyl-2′-deoxyuridine. J Med Chem 7:1, 1964.
24. Kaufman HE, Heidelberger C: Therapeutic antiviral action of 5-trifluoromethyl-2′-deoxyuridine in herpes simplex keratitis. Science 145:585, 1964.
25. McGill JI, Holt-Wilson AD, McKinnon JR, et al: Some aspects of the clinical use of trifluorothymidine in the treatment of herpetic ulceration of the cornea. Trans Ophthalmol Soc UK 94:342, 1974.
26. McGill J, Fraunfelder FT, Jones BR: Current and proposed management of ocular herpes simplex. Surv Ophthalmol 20:358, 1976.
27. O'Brien WJ, Edelhauser HF: The corneal penetration of trifluorothymidine, adenine arabinoside, and idoxuridine: A comparative study. Invest Ophthalmol Vis Sci 16:1093, 1977.
28. Sugar J, Varnell E, Centifanto Y, Kaufman HE: Trifluorothymidine treatment of herpetic iritis in rabbits and ocular penetration. Invest Ophthalmol 12:532, 1973.
29. Pavan-Langston D, Lass J, Campbell R: Antiviral drops: Comparative therapy of experimental herpes simplex keratouveitis. Arch Ophthalmol 97:1132, 1979.
30. McNeill JI, Kaufman HE: Local antivirals in a herpes simplex stromal keratitis model. Arch Ophthalmol 97:727, 1979.
31. Pavan-Langston D, Nelson DJ: Intraocular penetration of trifluridine. Am J Ophthalmol 87:814, 1979.
32. Coster DJ, McKinnon JR, McGill JI, et al: Clinical evaluation of adenine arabinoside and trifluorothymidine in the treatment of corneal ulcers caused by herpes simplex virus. J Infect Dis 133:A17, 1966.
33. Hyndiuk RA, Charlin RE, Alpren TV, Schultz RO: Trifluridine in resistant human herpetic keratitis. Arch Ophthalmol 96:1839, 1978.
34. Laibson PR, Arentsen JJ, Mazzanti WD, Eiferman RA: Double controlled comparison of IDU and trifluorothymidine in thirty-three patients with superficial herpetic keratitis. Trans Am Ophthalmol Soc 75:316, 1977.
35. Coster DJ, Jones BR, McGill JI: Treatment of amoeboid herpetic ulcers with adenine arabinoside or trifluorothymidine. Br J Ophthalmol 63:418, 1979.
36. Van Bijsterveld OP, Post H: Trifluorothymidine versus adenine arabinoside in the treatment of herpes simplex keratitis. Br J Ophthalmol 64:33, 1980.
37. Pavan-Langston D, Dohlman CH: A double-blind clinical study of

adenosine arabinoside therapy of viral keratoconjunctivitis. Am J Ophthalmol 74:81, 1972.

38. Lee WW, Benitez A, Goodman L, Baker BR: Potential anticancer agents. XL: Synthesis of the b-anomer of 9-(D-arabinofuranosyl)-adenine. J Am Chem Soc 82:2648, 1960.
39. Reist EJ, Benitez A, Goodman L, et al: Potential anticancer agents. LXXVI: Synthesis of purine nucleosides of b-D-arabinofuranose. Organic Chem 27:3274, 1962.
40. Parke, Davis, and Company: British Patent 1,159,290 (1969). Chem Abstr 71:797572, 1969.
41. Pavan-Langston D: Use of vidarabine in ophthalmology: A review. Ann Ophthalmol 9:835, 1977.
42. Schabel FM Jr: The antiviral activity of 9-beta-D-arabinofuranosyladenine (ARA-A). Chemotherapy 13:321, 1968.
43. Keeney RE, Buchanan RA: Clinical application of adenine arabinoside. Ann N Y Acad Sci 255:185, 1975.
44. Waring GO III, Laibson PR, Satz JE, Joseph NH: Use of vidarabine in epidemic keratoconjunctivitis due to adenovirus types 3, 7, 8 and 19. Am J Ophthalmol 82:781, 1976.
45. Pavan-Langston D, Dohlman CH, Geary P, Sulzewski D: Intraocular penetration of Ara A and IDU therapeutic implications in clinical herpetic uveitis. Trans Am Acad Ophthalmol Otolaryngol 77:op455, 1973.
46. Abel R Jr, Kaufman HE, Sugar J: Intravenous adenine arabinoside against herpes simplex keratouveitis in humans. Am J Ophthalmol 79:659, 1975.
47. Whitley RJ, Soong SJ, Dolin R, et al: Adenine arabinoside therapy of biopsy-proved herpes simplex encephalitis. National Institute of Allergy and Infectious Diseases collaborative antiviral study. N Engl J Med 297:289, 1977.
48. Jones BR: Rational regimen of administration of antivirals. Trans Am Acad Ophthalmol Otolaryngol 79:104, 1975.
49. Pavan-Langston D, Buchanan RA: Vidarabine therapy of simple and IDU-complicated herpetic keratitis. Trans Am Acad Ophthalmol Otolaryngol 81:op813, 1976.
50. Jackson WB, Breslin CW, Lorenzetti DW, et al: Treatment of herpes simplex keratitis: Comparison of acyclovir and vidarabine. Can J Ophthalmol 19:107, 1984.
51. Pavan-Langston D, Campbell R, Lass J: Acyclic antimetabolite therapy of experimental herpes simplex keratitis. Am J Ophthalmol 86:618, 1978.
52. Bauer DJ, Collins P, Tucker WE Jr, Macklin AW: Treatment of experimental herpes simplex keratitis with acycloguanosine. Br J Ophthalmol 63:429, 1979.
53. Langston RH, Pavan-Langston D, Dohlman CH: Antiviral medication and corneal wound healing. Arch Ophthalmol 92:509, 1974.
54. O'Day DM, Poirier RH, Jones DB, Elliott JH: Vidarabine therapy of complicated herpes simplex keratitis. Am J Ophthalmol 81:642, 1976.
55. Schaefer HJ, Beauchamp L, de Miranda P, Elion GB: 9-(2-Hydroxyethoxymethyl) guanine activity against viruses of the herpes group. Nature 272:583, 1978.
56. Miller WH, Miller RL: Phosphorylation of acyclovir (acycloguanosine) monophosphate by GMP kinase. J Biol Chem 255:7204, 1980.
57. Derse D, Cheng YC, Furman PA, et al: Inhibition of purified human and herpes simplex virus-induced DNA polymerase by 9-(2-hydroxyethoxymethyl) guanine triphosphate. J Biol Chem 265:11447, 1981.
58. Furman PA, St. Clair MH, Fyfe JA, et al: Inhibition of herpes simplex virus-induced DNA polymerase activity and viral DNA replication by 9-(2-hydroxyethoxymethyl) guanine and its triphosphate. J Virol 32:72, 1979.
59. Pavan-Langston D, Lass J, Hettinger M, Udell I: Acyclovir and vidarabine in the treatment of ulcerative herpes simplex keratitis. Am J Ophthalmol 92:829, 1981.
60. Piorier RH, Kingham JD, de Miranda P, Annel M: Intraocular antiviral penetration. Arch Ophthalmol 100:1964, 1982.
61. Collum LM, Logan P, McAuliffe-Curtin D, et al: Randomised double-blind trial of acyclovir (Zovirax) and adenine arabinoside in herpes simplex amoeboid corneal ulceration. Br J Ophthalmol 69:847, 1985.
62. Lass JH, Pavan-Langston D, Park NH: Aciclovir and corneal wound healing. Am J Ophthalmol 88:102, 1979.
63. Wilhelmus KR, Coster DJ, Jones BR: Acyclovir and débridement in the treatment of ulcerative herpetic keratitis. Am J Ophthalmol 91:323, 1981.
64. La Lau C, Oosterhuis JA, Versteeg J, et al: Acyclovir and trifluorothymidine in herpetic keratitis. Preliminary report of a multicenter trial. Doc Ophthalmol 50:287, 1981.
65. Collum LMT, McGettrick P, Akhtar J, et al: Oral acyclovir (Zovirax) in herpes simplex dendritic corneal ulceration. Br J Ophthalmol 70:435, 1986.
66. Hung SO, Patterson A, Clark DI, Rees PJ: Oral acyclovir in the management of dendritic herptic corneal ulcerations. Br J Ophthalmol 68:398, 1984.
67. Charpentier B, Lefevre JJ, Verneau A, Fries D: Severe herpetic keratoconjunctivitis following kidney transplantation cured by acycloguanosine. Nouv Press Med 9:255, 1980.
68. Collum LMT, Logan P, Hillary IB, Ravenscoft T: Acyclovir in herpes keratitis. Am J Med 73:290, 1982.
69. Young B, Patterson A, Ravenscroft T: Double-blind clinical trial of acyclovir and adenine arabinoside in herpetic corneal ulceration. Am J Med 73:311, 1982.
70. Jones BR, Coster DJ, Fison PN, et al: Efficacy of acycloguanosine (Wellcome 248U) against herpes simplex corneal ulcers. Lancet 1:243, 1979.
71. Jensen KB, Nissen SH, Jessen F: Acyclovir in the treatment of herpetic keratitis. Acta Ophthalmol 60:557, 1982.
72. Morgan KS, Wander AH, Kaufman HE, et al: Toxicity and tolerance of 9-(2-hydroxyethoxymethyl) guanine. Chemotherapy 26:405, 1980.
73. de Koning EWJ, van Bijsterveld OP, Cantell K: Combination therapy for dendritic keratitis with acyclovir and alpha-interferon. Arch Ophthalmol 101:1866, 1983.
74. Cobo LM, Foulks GN, Liesegang T, et al: Oral acyclovir in the treatment of acute herpes zoster ophthalmicus. Ophthalmology 93:763, 1976.
75. Huff JC, Bean B, Balfour HH, et al: Therapy of herpes zoster with oral acyclovir. Am J Med 85:84, 1988.
76. Morton P, Thompson AN: Oral acyclovir in the treatment of herpes zoster in general practice. N Z Med J 102:93, 1989.
77. Cobo LM, Foulks GN, Liesegang T, et al: Oral acyclovir in the therapy of acute herpes zoster ophthalmicus: An interim report. Ophthalmology 92:1574, 1985.
78. McGill J, Chapman C: A comparison of topical acyclovir with steroids in the treatment of herpes zoster keratouveitis. Br J Ophthalmol 67:746, 1983.
79. McGill J: Topical acyclovir in herpes zoster ocular involvement. Br J Ophthalmol 65:542, 1981.
80. Cobo LM: Reduction of the ocular complications of herpes zoster ophthalmicus by oral acyclovir. Am J Med 85(Suppl):90, 1988.
81. Seiff SR, Margolis T, Graham SH, O'Donnell JJ: Use of intravenous acyclovir for treatment of herpes zoster ophthalmicus in patients at risk for AIDS. Ann Ophthalmol 20:480, 1988.
82. Pulido JS, Palacio M, Peyman GA, et al: Toxicity of intravitreal antiviral drugs. Ophthalmic Surg 15:666, 1984.
83. Small GH, Peyman GA, Srinivasan A, et al: Retinal toxicity of combination antiviral drugs in an animal model. Can J Ophthalmol 22:300, 1987.
84. Peyman GA, Goldberg MF, Uninsky E, et al: Vitrectomy and intravitreal antiviral drug therapy in acute retinal necrosis syndrome: Report of two cases. Arch Ophthalmol 102:1618, 1984.
85. Pepose JS, Newman C, Bach MC, et al: Pathologic features of cytomegalovirus retinopathy after treatment with the antiviral agent ganciclovir. Ophthalmology 94:414, 1987.
86. Teich SA, Castle J, Friedman AH, et al: Active cytomegalovirus particles in the eyes of an AIDS patient being treated with 9-[2-hydroxy-1-(hydroxymethyl) ethoxymethyl] guanine (ganciclovir). Br J Ophthalmol 72:293, 1988.
87. Shepp DH, Dandliker PS, de Miranda P, et al: Activity of 9-[2-hydroxy-1-(hydroxymethyl) ethoxymethyl] guanine in the treatment of cytomegalovirus pneumonia. Ann Intern Med 103:368, 1985.
88. MacArthur RB: Ganciclovir: Approved and investigational uses for the treatment of cytomegalovirus retinitis. Mt Sinai J Med 57:378, 1990.
89. Felsenstein D, D'Amico DJ, Hirsch MS, et al: Treatment of cytomegalovirus retinitis with 9-[2-hydroxy-1-(hydroxymethyl)-ethoxymethyl] guanine. Ann Intern Med 103:377, 1985.
90. D'Amico DJ, Talamo JH, Felsenstein D, et al: Ophthalmoscopic and histologic findings in cytomegalovirus retinitis treated with BW-B759U. Arch Ophthalmol 104:1788, 1986.
91. MacDonald EA: Treatment of cytomegalovirus retinitis in a patient with AIDS with 9-(1,3-dihydroxy-2-propoxymethyl) guanine. Can J Ophthalmol 22:48, 1987.
92. Holland GN, Sakamoto MJ, Hardy D, et al and the UCLA CMV Retinopathy Study Group: Treatment of cytomegalovirus retinopathy

in patients with acquired immunodeficiency syndrome. Arch Ophthalmol 104:1794, 1986.

93. Holland GN, Sidikaro Y, Kreiger AE, et al: Treatment of cytomegalovirus retinopathy with ganciclovir. Ophthalmology 94:815, 1987.
94. Jabs DA, Newman C, Bustros SD, Polk BF: Treatment of cytomegalovirus retinitis with ganciclovir. Ophthalmology 94:824, 1987.
95. Orellana J, Teich SA, Winterkorn JS, et al: Treatment of cytomegalovirus retinitis with ganciclovir (9-[2-hydroxy-1-(hydroxymethyl) ethoxymethyl) guanine (BW B759U)]. Br J Ophthalmol 72:525, 1988.
96. Henry K, Cantrill H, Fletcher C, et al: Use of intravitreal ganciclovir (dihydroxy propoxymethyl guanine) for cytomegalovirus retinitis in patients with AIDS. Am J Ophthalmol 103:17, 1987.
97. Ussery FM, Gibson SR, Conklin RH, et al: Intravitreal ganciclovir in the treatment of AIDS-associated cytomegalovirus retinitis. Ophthalmology 95:640, 1988.
98. Heery S, Hollows F: High-dose intravitreal ganciclovir for cytomegaloviral (CMV) retinitis. Aust N Z J Ophthalmol 17:405, 1989.
99. Harris ML, Mathalone MBR: Intravitreal ganciclovir in CMV retinitis: Case report. Br J Ophthalmol 73:382, 1989.
100. Cantrill HL, Henry K, Melroe NH, et al: Treatment of cytomegalovirus retinitis with intravitreal ganciclovir: Long-term results. Ophthalmology 96:367, 1989.
101. Heinemann MH: Long-term intravitreal ganciclovir therapy for cytomegalovirus retinopathy. Arch Ophthalmol 107:1767, 1989.
102. Martin DF, Parks DJ, Mellow SD, et al: Treatment of cytomegalovirus retinitis with an intraocular sustained-release ganciclovir implant. Arch Ophthalmol 112:1531, 1994.
103. Sanborn GE, Anand R, Torti R, et al: Sustained release ganciclovir therapy for treatment of cytomegalovirus retinitis: Use of an intravitreal device. Arch Ophthalmol 110:188, 1992.
104. Schwartz DM: New therapies for cytomegalovirus retinitis. *In* Smolin G (Ed): New drugs in ophthalmology. Int Ophthalmol Clin 36 (2):1–9, 1996.
105. Paul AA, Leeper HF, Friberg TR: CMV retinitis and the use of FK506. Transplant Proc 23:3042, 1991.
106. Osberg B: Antiviral effects of phosphonoformate (PFA foscarnet sodium). Pharmacol Ther 19:387, 1983.
107. Rickman LS, Freeman WR: Medical and virological aspects of ocular HIV infection for the ophthalmologist. Semin Ophthalmol 10:91, 1995.
108. Weinberg DV, Murphy R, Naughton K: Combined daily therapy with intravenous ganciclovir and foscarnet for patients with recurrent cytomegalovirus retinitis. Am J Ophthalmol 117:776, 1994.
109. Palestine AG, Polis MA, DeSmet MD, et al: A randomized controlled trial of foscarnet in the treatment of cytomegalovirus retinitis in patients with AIDS. Ann Intern Med 115:665, 1991.
110. Studies of Ocular Complications of AIDS Research Group in Collaboration with the AIDS Clinical Trial Group: Foscarnet-ganciclovir cytomegalovirus retinitis trial: 4. Visual outcomes. Ophthalmology 101:1250, 1994.
111. Jacobson MA, O'Donnell JJ, Mills J: Foscarnet treatment of cytomegalovirus retinitis in patients with acquired immunodeficiency syndrome. Antimicrob Agents Chemother 33:736, 1989.
112. Studies of Ocular Complications of AIDS Research Group, in Collaboration with the AIDS Clinical Trial Group: Mortality in patients with the acquired immunodeficiency syndrome treated with either foscarnet or ganciclovir for cytomegalovirus retinitis. N Engl J Med 326:213, 1992.
113. LeHoang P, Girard B, Robinet M, et al: Foscarnet in the treatment of cytomegalovirus retinitis in acquired immune deficiency syndrome. Ophthalmology 96:865, 1989.
114. Colucciello M: Phosphonoformate (foscarnet) for CMV retinitis in AIDS. Am J Ophthalmol 98:317, 1995.
115. Friedberg DN: Cytomegaloving retinitis. *In* Stenson SM, Friedberg DN (eds): Aids and the Eye. New Orleans, Contact Lens Association of Ophthalmologists, 1995, pp 65–83.
116. Ahmed I, Everett A: Medical management of cytomegalovirus retinitis. *In* Everett A, Ahmed I (eds): AIDS and ophthalmology: New solutions. Ophthalmol Clin North Am 10:15, 1997.
117. Holland GN, Levinson RD, Jacobson MA, et al: Dose-related differences in progression rates of cytomegalovirus retinopathy during foscarnet maintenance therapy. Am J Ophthalmol 119:576, 1995.
118. Jacobsen MA, Causey D, Polsky B, et al: A dose-ranging study for daily maintenance intravenous foscarnet therapy for cytomegalovirus retinitis in AIDS. J Infect Dis 168:444, 1993.
119. Diaz-Llopis M, Chipont E, Sanchez S, et al: Intravitreal foscarnet for cytomegalovirus retinitis in a patient with acquired immunodeficiency syndrome. Am J Ophthalmol 114:742, 1992.
120. Kirsch LS, Arevalo JF, Chavez de la Paz E, et al: Intravitreal cidofovir (HPMPC) treatment cytomegalovirus retinitis in patients with acquired immune deficiency syndrome. Ophthalmology 102:533, 1995.
121. Fischl MA, Richman DD, Grieco MH, et al and the AZT Collaborative Working Group: The efficacy of 3′-azido-3′-deoxythymidine (azidothymidine) in the treatment of patients with AIDS and AIDS-related complex: A double blind placebo-controlled trial. N Engl J Med 317:185, 1987.
122. Guyer DR, Jabs DA, Brant AM, et al: Regression of cytomegalovirus retinitis with zidovudine: A clinicopathologic correlation. Arch Ophthalmol 107:868, 1989.
123. Jabs DA, Enger C, Bartlett JD: Cytomegalovirus retinitis and acquired immunodeficiency syndrome. Arch Ophthalmol 107:75, 1989.
124. Farrell PL, Heinemann MH, Roberts CW, et al: Response of human immunodeficiency virus-associated uveitis to zidovudine. Am J Ophthalmol 106:7, 1988.

CHAPTER 22

Antifungal Agents

Eduardo C. Alfonso

The choice of an antifungal agent in ophthalmology depends on several variables, including the primary site of infection, the route of administration, the organism involved, and the sensitivity data available.[1–5] The major classes of antifungals used in ophthalmology are polyenes, imidazoles, and pyrimidines (Table 22–1).[6] Other compounds have been tried as antifungals, but the clinical experience is very limited.[7, 8] These include rose bengal, salicylic acid, benzoic acid, thimerosal, gentian violet, silver nitrate, zinc, copper sulfate, boric acid, potassium, iodide, and iodine. A great number of experimental compounds are described in the literature.[9–12] For most of these, sufficient data on the treatment of human mycoses are lacking.[13–16]

Polyene Antibiotics

Polyene antibiotics are produced from a *Streptomyces* species.[17, 18] Their chemical configuration gives them their basic classification based on the number of double bonds as well as the number of carbon atoms (group I <30 atoms; group II >30 atoms).[19] They interact with cell membrane sterols, primarily ergosterol, which causes increased permeability that leads to cell lysis.[20] It is the binding to mammalian cell membrane cholesterol that accounts for their toxicity. Two mechanisms of action of the polyene antibiotics are known and depend on the size of the antifungal molecule.[21] Small molecules such as natamycin work by an all-or-none mechanism of action. They bind to the esterols in the fungal cell wall, forming "blisters" and causing lysis of the cell. This action is not concentration dependent. The larger molecules, such as amphotericin, work by creating "pores" in the cell wall, allowing small ions such as potassium to leak out and causing imbalances in the osmotic gradient and eventual cell lysis. This mechanism of action is concentration dependent and may be altered by changes in the osmotic environment.[22] Other factors have been implicated in the interaction of the polyenes with cell membranes.[23] The most widely used of the polyenes are amphotericin B and natamycin.[24]

AMPHOTERICIN B

Amphotericin B is most commonly used in ophthalmology as a topical preparation for keratitis and scleritis, intraocularly for endophthalmitis, and systemically for these conditions and for scleritis, dacryocystitis, and cellulitis.[25–29] The spectrum of organisms and in vitro sensitivities identified in the published literature and in our laboratory is presented in Tables 22–2 and 22–3, respectively.[30–33] Dosages for antifungal agents are given in Table 22–4.

For the treatment of keratitis and scleritis, a topical concentration of 2.5 to 10 mg/mL given every 30 to 60 minutes for the first 48 to 72 hours appears to deliver the optimal dose.[34, 35] Higher concentrations may cause surface toxicity.[36, 37] This concentration is achieved by mixing the powdered amphotericin with sterile water.[38] The mixture should be stored in a dark bottle and refrigerated to maintain drug stability. Subconjunctival injection of amphotericin is not recommended because of severe toxicity.[7, 39]

For endophthalmitis, intravitreal injection of 5 μg of amphotericin in 0.1 mL appears to be safe and effective in humans.[1, 40–44] Concurrent surgical management of the vitreous is often necessary to control the infection.[45, 46]

TABLE 22–1. **Classification of Antifungals**

Polyenes	Imidazoles	Triazoles	Pyrimidines	Others
Amphotericin B†§	Clotrimazole§	Fluconazole*†	Flucytosine*	Pradicimicins‖
Amphotericin B methyl ester†	Miconazole†§	Itraconazole*†		Cispentacin‖
Natamycin‡	Econazole§	Terconazole§		Jasplakinolide‖
	Ketoconazole*§	Vibunazole*§		Terbinafine‖
	Thiabendazole*	Alteconazole*§		Nystatin§
	Bifonazole§			
	Butoconazole§			
	Croconazole§			
	Fenticonazole§			

*Oral.
†Intravenous.
‡Ocular.
§Dermatologic.
‖Not available.

TABLE 22–2. **Antimicrobial Activity of Antifungal Agents Based on Published Reports**

Antifungal Agent	*Alternaria*	*Aspergillus*	*Candida*	*Cephalo-sporium*	*Clado-sporium*	*Curvularia*	*Fusarium*	*Paecilomyces*	*Penicillium*
Polyenes									
Amphotericin	S	S	S		S	S	S	R	S
Nystatin		S	S						S
Natamycin		S	S	S	S		S	R	
Imidazoles									
Clotrimazole	S	S	S		S	S	I	S	
Miconazole		S	S		S		I	I	
Econazole		S	I		S		S	I	
Ketoconazole		I	S		S		S		S
Triazoles									
Itraconazole		S	S				R	S	
Fluconazole		S	S				S		S
Pyrimidines									
Flucytosine		R	S		S		R	R	I

Abbreviations: S, susceptible; I, variable susceptibility; R, resistant.

For intravenous use, a test dose of 1 mg of amphotericin in 150 mL of 5% dextrose in water is given.[47, 48] Once this test dose is tolerated, 1 to 5 mg is given over 4 to 6 hours. The dose is increased by 5 mg daily until the desired dose of 0.5 to 1 mg/kg/day is reached. If chills, fever, nausea, or hypertension develops with the test dose, the patient may require concomitant use of 25 to 30 mg of hydrocortisone intravenously.[49] Also, aspirin, diphenhydramine, or prochlorperazine may be required. Other potential side effects are a decrease in the glomerular filtration rate to 20 to 60% of normal, which may be restored to normal after cessation of therapy for approximately 5 days.[50] Hypokalemia may require potassium supplements. A drop in the platelet count and hematocrit may also be observed during therapy. Hepatic damage occurs rarely. The water-soluble semisynthetic methyl ester derivative of amphotericin B has been shown in animal models to carry fewer side effects than the parent compound.[51–53]

TABLE 22–3. **Ten-Year Summary of Sensitivity Testing of Clinical Isolates at the Microbiology Laboratory of the Bascom Palmer Eye Institute***

Antifungal	*Fusarium* (*n* = 40)	*Candida* (*n* = 10)	*Aspergillus* (*n* = 15)	*Curvularia* (*n* = 6)
Amphotericin				
Range	0.078–5.0	0.08–5.0	0.01–2.5	0.04–0.31
Mean	1.2 (S)	2.7 (S)	1 (S)	0.16 (S)
Natamycin				
Range	0.15–5.0	0.31–5.0	0.62–25.0	0.62–2.50
Mean	1.5 (S)	2.5 (S)	2 (S)	1.4 (S)
Ketoconazole				
Range	0.78–50.0	0.10–1.6	0.78–250	0.20–12.50
Mean	10.9 (I)	0.71 (S)	4 (S)	2.7 (S)
Miconazole				
Range	0.78–50.0	0.78–62.0	0.20–3.10	0.05–3.1
Mean	14.21 (I)	2 (S)	1.2 (S)	1.3 (S)
Flucytosine				
Range	0.05–100.0	0.05–3.10		25–100
Mean	921 (R)	1.2 (S)		68 (R)

Abbreviations: S, susceptible; I, variable susceptibility; R, resistant.
*Ranges and means in micrograms per milliliter.

NATAMYCIN

Natamycin (pimaricin) is a small semisynthetic tetraene and is considered the least toxic, the least irritating, and the most stable of the polyenes.[23] It has been available for topical use as a 5% suspension since its approval by the U.S. Food and Drug Administration in the late 1970s.[54, 55] It has a broad spectrum of sensitivities, especially to *Fusarium* species, as shown in Table 22–3.[56, 57] It has decreased penetration through an intact epithelium, and surface débridement may be desirable during therapy.[58, 59] Since natamycin is used as a suspension, it can dry on the ocular surface and cause irritation.[56] Lavage with a saline solution of the lid margins is often necessary. Natamycin can be toxic to the corneal and conjunctival epithelium, causing hyperemia and epithelial defects.[59] As with amphotericin, topical therapy is given every 30 to 60 minutes for the first 48 to 72 hours, and treatment is usually continued on a tapering fashion for 3 to 6 weeks depending on the activity of the keratitis.[6]

Subconjunctival and intravitreal administration are not recommended because of significant toxicity.[61, 62] Systemic intravenous use of natamycin does not render significant levels in the eye, and oral preparations are not well absorbed.[63, 64]

NYSTATIN

Nystatin has been studied experimentally in ophthalmology, and cases have been reported in which it has been used in external ocular infections caused by *Candida*.[40, 65] It has been used as the dermatologic ointment, which has a concentration of 100,000 U/g, and at a frequency of application every 4 to 6 hours. Subconjunctival injections show marked toxicity, and experimental intravitreal injection of 0.1 mL of a concentration of 2000 U/mL did not cause a significant reaction and cured an experimental case of *Aspergillus* endophthalmitis.[18, 66]

Azoles

IMIDAZOLES

The imidazoles possess a broad spectrum of antifungal activity, but in contrast to the polyenes, they are relatively resis-

TABLE 22–4. **Antifungal Dosages**

Antifungal Agent	Topical	Subconjunctival	Intravitreal	Intravenous	Oral
Amphotericin B	2.5–10.9 mg/mL	750 μg/mL every other day	5–10 μg	Maintenance dose 1 mg/kg/day refrigerated	
Clotrimazole	1% suspension 1% solution	5–10 mg (0.5–1 mL)			60–150 mg/kg/day (adults)
Econazole	1% suspension 1% ointment			30 mg/kg/day	200 mg t.i.d.
Fluconazole	2% suspension 1% solution				400 mg/day initial dose 200 mg/day maintenance dose
Itraconazole	2% suspension				200 mg/day
Ketoconazole	1% suspension				200–400 mg/day
Miconazole	1% suspension 1% solution (10 mg/mL)	5–10 mg (0.5–1 mL)	0.25 mg	600–3600 mg/day divided into three doses	
Natamycin	50 mg/mL				
Nystatin	Ointment 100,000 U/g				
Thiabendazole	4% suspension				25 mg/kg/day
Flucytosine	10 mg/mL				50–150 mg/kg/day at 6-hr intervals

tant to light, hydrolysis, and pH changes and are soluble in organic substances.[67] A number of compounds are available as approved preparations for systemic use.

The imidazoles have a combination of mechanisms for antimycotic activity.[68–70] At low concentrations, miconazole, econazole, and ketoconazole affect the formation of ergosterol needed by the cell membranes.[71] At high concentrations, clotrimazole and miconazole can disrupt lysosomes, causing direct cell membrane damage. In addition, most imidazoles inhibit catalase and cytochrome C peroxidase intracellulary, causing accumulation of hydrogen peroxide and leading to cell death. There also appears to be a triggering mechanism of host defense cells by the imidazoles. When ketoconazole is added in vitro to polymorphonuclear leukocytes and macrophages, it has the ability to eradicate both the yeast and the mycelial forms of *Candida*, in the absence of polymorphonuclear leukocytes and macrophages.[72] One can see that because of these combined mechanisms of action, most of the imidazoles can be fungistatic and fungicidal.[73, 74]

Clotrimazole

Clotrimazole has a wide spectrum of activity against numerous fungi, but poor results have been obtained with *Fusarium*. Most strains are inhibited at concentrations of 2 to 4 mg/mL, which can be readily achieved with topical and oral administration (see Table 22–3).[75, 76] It is poorly absorbed parenterally.[77]

The topical preparation of clotrimazole is made by dilution in arachis oil to a 1% solution. It has been applied hourly for 2 to 3 days, then tapered over 8 to 12 weeks.[78] Oral administration in a dosage range of 60 to 150 mg/kg/day can be given with an achievable serum concentration of 0.4 to 5.5 mg/mL. No commercial oral dosage forms are available in the United States. Clotrimazole has been recommended by several authors as the drug of choice for *Aspergillus* infections of the eye.[78–80] Side effects of the systemic administration of clotrimazole may include anorexia, nausea, hallucinations, confusion, and epigastric pain. It should not be given in the first 3 months of pregnancy or to patients with a history of hypersensitivity, adrenal, or liver problems. Liver enzyme level elevations are normal with the use of clotrimazole, and these tend to return to normal once the drug is withdrawn.[81]

Miconazole

Miconazole is a phenethylimidazole that is very stable in solution.[82] Its mechanism of action is similar to that of the other imidazoles.[70] It has a broad spectrum of activity against *Cryptococcus, Aspergillus, Curvularia, Candida, Microsporum, Paecilomyces*, and *Trichophyton* (see Table 22–3).[83–86]

Miconazole may be given intravenously in dosages ranging from 200 to 3600 mg/day in three divided doses. In children, a dose of 15 mg/kg per infusion should not be exceeded.[82] It may also be used as a topical, subconjunctival, or intravitreal preparation.[87] For topical use, a 1% solution in arachis oil or a 10 mg/mL commercial solution (Monistat IV) is well tolerated. It is also available as a 2% dermatologic ointment, but this may cause some irritation to the eye.[88] For subconjunctival injections, 10 mg/day may be used. For intravitreal injections, 0.25 to 0.50 mg may be used.[86, 89, 90]

After intravenous administration of miconazole, reported side effects may be a rash with pruritis, chills, nausea, and vomiting. These side effects may be minimized by the concomitant administration of antihistamines and antiemetics.[91, 92] Reports also mention a possible decrease in sodium levels and the hematocrit, with aggregation of erythrocytes and thrombocytosis.[85] Topical use of miconazole may cause surface toxicity after prolonged use.[90, 93, 94]

Ketoconazole

Ketoconazole is a synthetic acetylchichlorophenyl imidazole. It dissolves in water with a resultant pH of about 3.[95] Its mechanism of action is similar to that of the other imidazoles.[68, 96] This drug has a broad spectrum of activity in vitro (see Table 22–3).[97]

Ketoconazole is available for oral administration. It is well absorbed from the gastrointestinal tract and bound to albumin, and high therapeutic blood levels are maintained.[68] Ninety percent of the drug is excreted by the liver and the remainder by the kidneys.[95] Ketoconazole is available in 200-mg tablets with a recommended daily dose of 200 to 400 mg. A topical preparation may be formulated in a 1 to 5% concentration by dissolving in arachis oil.[98, 99] Ketoconazole may also be dissolved in polyethooxylated castor oil[67] or in 4.5% boric acid.[7, 100]

Systemic side effects associated with the use of ketoconazole have been minor and usually reversible. Pruritus, nausea, vomiting, diarrhea, cramps, gynecomastia,[101] and elevations in liver enzyme levels have been reported after oral administration.[101] Topical use of ketoconazole shows minimal reversible toxicity in animals.[102] Ketoconazole can affect the efficacy and concentration of cyclosporine, warfarin, phenytoin, and theophylline.[103]

In ophthalmology, topical ketoconazole has been used clinically and experimentally for the treatment of keratitis.[99, 104, 105] Oral ketoconazole has been used in both experimental[35] and human keratitis.[106] In experimental endophthalmitis, ketoconazole was effective if started 24 hours after injection.[107] It has been suggested that oral ketoconazole may augment topical natamycin therapy.[25, 108]

Thiabendazole

Thiabendazole is a thiazolyl benzimidazole. Its primary clinical use for many years has been in the treatment of roundworm infections.[108] Its mechanism of action is similar to that of the other imidazoles.[68] It has been shown to be active against ocular isolates of fungi, but poor results have been obtained against *Candida* and *Aspergillus* species (see Table 22–3).[85, 99]

Oral thiabendazole may be given at a dose of 25 mg/kg two times per day with a maximal daily dose of 3 g. Its peak serum concentration is in 1 to 2 hours, and 90% is excreted in the urine.[68] Topical application of a 4% thiabendazole suspension has been reported in the treatment of *Aspergillus flavus* keratitis.[109] Side effects have been few, the major ocular side effects being surface irritation and dryness and mild reversible hepatic disease.[18]

Clinical experience with thiabendazole in ophthalmology is limited, and this drug has been reserved for cases unresponsive to conventional treatment.[110]

Econazole

Econazole is a deschlorophenethylimidazole.[23] Its mechanism of action is similar to that of the other imidazoles.[68] The spectrum of activity is similar to that of the other imidazoles, with increased activity against *Aspergillus, Fusarium*, and *Penicillium*. It has less activity aginst *Candida*.[111]

Econazole is available as a dermatologic ointment. For topical use, a 1% suspension may be prepared in arachis oil.[112] For oral use, 200 mg of econazole three times a day may be used. For intravenous use, 30 mg/kg/day is recommended.[112] The systemic preparation is not commercially available in the United States.

The clinical use of econazole in ophthalmology is very limited.[112]

TRIAZOLES

The triazoles—fluconazole, itraconazole, terconazole, and others (see Table 22–1) were developed in order to increase the spectrum of activity and reduce the side effects of their predecessors, the imidazoles.

Fluconazole

Fluconazole is perhaps the most widely used member of the triazoles because of in vitro studies that have shown a very wide spectrum of activity against many pathogens.[113] The in vivo activity has not followed its laboratory spectrum of activity. It has been used for the treatment of *Candida* species.[114] It has also been used for the treatment of experimental endophthalmitis in its oral form[16] and in the treatment of experimental *Candida albicans* keratitis in a topical solution.[16, 115]

Oral fluconazole can be given in a dose of 50 to 40 mg/day, with the usual adult dose being 200 mg/day. A topical 1% solution in sterile water can be made. The 2 mg/L aqueous solution for intravenous use can also be applied topically.[116]

Systemic side effects of fluconazole include gastrointestinal upset, headaches, rash, hepatotoxicity, anaphylaxis, Stevens-Johnson syndrome, and thrombocytopenia. Fluconazole can increase cyclosporine's serum concentration and decrease the metabolism of warfarin. Rifampin can increase the metabolism of fluconazole.[117]

Itraconazole

Itraconazole also has, like fluconazole, a wider spectrum of activity than the imidazoles. Its spectrum of activity includes excellent in vitro activity against *Aspergillus*. Its broad spectrum of antifungal activity includes *Candida* species, *Paecilomyces, Paracoccidioides*, and *Coccidioides*.[118] It has not been very effective against *Fusarium*.[119]

It has had a very limited use in clinical ophthalmology. In an experimental model of *Candida* endophthalmitis, it was shown to be as effective as fluconazole and ketoconazole.[16] There is a published report of successful treatment of *Aspergillus* scleritis with oral itraconazole after cataract surgery.[120] The oral administration of itraconazole appears to have less penetration than other triazoles into the cornea, aqueous, and vitreous.[16]

Itraconazole has been used in its oral preparation as an adult dose of 200 mg/day. Side effects include gastrointestinal upset, hypertriglyceridemia, and hypokalemia.[121]

Pyrimidines

The pyrimidines are a group of antimetabolites with known antifungal activity. The main drug in this group is flucytosine.[122]

FLUCYTOSINE

Flucytosine (5-FC) is a fluorinated pyrimidine that is soluble in water and alcohol. Several mechanisms of action have been described.[123] It may alter fungal RNA and DNA synthesis. It enters the cytoplasm by the action of cytosine permease and it is then deaminated by cytosine deaminase into 5-fluorouracil. It is then phosphorylated and incorporated into RNA. In the nucleus, 5-FC forms 5-fluoro-2′-deoxyuridylic acid (FdUMP), which inhibits thymidilate synthetase and thus DNA synthesis.[124]

Flucytosine has a limited spectrum of activity, and resistance may be acquired at low doses (see Table 22–2).[48, 125] The limited activity and resistance of 5-FC are due to the fungal cell's inability to transport the drug into its cytoplasm and incorporate it into its RNA or insufficient FdUMP synthesis to inhibit DNA formation.[123] The spectrum of activity may be enhanced and the emergence of resistance may be reduced by concomitant administration of amphotericin B.[2, 32, 125, 126]

Both topical and oral preparations of 5-FC may be used.[127] It is available for oral administration in 250- and 500-mg capsules. It is water soluble and rapidly absorbed from the gastrointestinal tract. The recommended dose of 5-FC is 50 to 150 mg/kg/day at 6-hour intervals. The drug is excreted unchanged in the urine, and thus the dosage should be adjusted according to the creatinine clearance.[128]

A topical preparation of 1% 5-FC may be formulated; it has limited penetration and thus is primarily effective for surface infections (conjunctivitis, blepharitis, and canaliculitis) and anterior stromal keratitis.[129]

Most side effects reported with 5-FC have been minimal and reversible.[126] Reversible elevations in levels of liver enzymes, aspartate aminotransferase, and alkaline phosphatase may be seen. Anemia, leukopenia, and thrombocytopenia have been reported in patients with other severe underlying disorders who are taking 5-FC. Two patients with intestinal perforations have been reported.

In ophthalmology, 5-FC has been used to treat primarily surface infections such as blepharitis, conjunctivitis, canaliculitis, and anterior keratitis.[108] The topical preparation of 5-FC is preferred, since subconjunctival injections offer little enhancement of penetration and are associated with toxicity and discomfort.[127] Its primary use has been in cases of *Candida* keratitis that have not responded clinically to amphotericin B, in which 5-FC is added to the topical regimen.[130]

REFERENCES

1. Axelrod AJ, Peyman GA, Apple DJ: Toxicity of intravitreal injection of amphotericin B. Am J Ophthalmol 76:578, 1973.
2. Beggs WH: Mechanisms of synergistic interactions between amphotericin B and flucytosine. J Antimicrob Chemother 17:402, 1986.
3. Harris DJ Jr, Stulting RD, Waring GO III, Wilson LA: Late bacterial and fungal keratitis after corneal transplantation. Spectrum of pathogens, graft survival and visual prognosis. Ophthalmology 95:1450, 1988.
4. Jones DB, Sexton R, Rebell G: Mycotic keratitis in south Florida: A review of 39 cases. Trans Ophthalmol Soc UK 89:781, 1969.
5. O'Day DM: Selection of appropriate antifungal therapy. Cornea 6:238, 1987.
6. Cohen J: Antifungal chemotherapy. Lancet 2:532, 1982.
7. Duane TD (ed): Clinical Ophthalmology, vol 4. Hagerstown, MD, Harper & Row, 1990.
8. Jones DB: Fungal keratitis. *In* Duane T (ed): Clinical Ophthalmology, vol 4. Hagerstown, MD, Harper & Row, 1985.
9. Cruciani M, Di Perri G, Concia E, et al: Fluconazole and fungal ocular infection. [Letter] J Antimicrob Chemother 25:718, 1990.
10. Davey PG: New antiviral and antifungal drugs. BMJ 300:793, 1990. [Published erratum appears in BMJ 300:1378, 1990.]
11. Delescluse J: Itraconazole in tinea versicolor: A review. J Am Acad Dermatol 23:551, 1990.
12. Odds FC, Cheesman SL, Abbott AB: Antifungal effects of fluconazole (UK 49858), a new triazole antifungal, in vitro. J Antimicrob Chemother 18:473, 1986.
13. de Lomas JG, Fons MA, Nogueira JM, et al: Chemotherapy of *Aspergillus fumigatus* keratitis: An experimental study. Mycopathologia 89:135, 1985.
14. Depont B, Drouhet E: Early experience with itraconazole in vitro and in patients: Pharmacokinetic studies and clinical results. Rev Infect Dis 9:571, 1987.
15. Ringel SM: New antifungal agents for the systemic mycoses. Mycopathologia 109:75, 1990.
16. Savani DV, Perfect JR, Cobo LM, Durack DT: Penetration of new azole compounds into the eye and efficacy in experimental *Candida* endophthalmitis. Antimicrob Agents Chemother 31:6, 1987.
17. Gold W, Stoud HA, Pagano JF, Donovick R: Amphotericins A and B, antifungal antibiotics produced by a streptomycete. I: In vitro studies. Antibiotics Annu 3:579, 1995–1956.
18. Havener WH: Ocular Pharmacology, 5th ed. St. Louis, CV Mosby, 1983.
19. Kotler-Brajtburg J, Medoff G, Kobayashi GS, et al: Classification of polyene antibiotics according to chemical structure and biological effects. Antimicrob Agents Chemother 15:716, 1979.
20. O'Day DM, Ray WA, Robinson RD, et al: In vitro and in vivo susceptibility of *Candida* keratitis to topical polyenes. Invest Ophthalmol Vis Sci 28:874, 1987.
21. Kuroda S, Uno J, Arai T: Target substances of some antifungal agents in the cell membrane. Antimicrob Agents Chemother 13:454, 1978.
22. Hamilton-Miller JMT: Chemistry and biology of the polyene macrolide antibiotics. Bacteriol Rev 37:1266, 1973.
23. Lorian V: Antibiotics in Laboratory Medicine, 4th ed. Baltimore, Williams & Wilkins, 1996, p 202.
24. Goodman LS, Gilman AG, Gilman A: The Pharmacological Basis of Therapeutics. New York, Macmillan, 1990.
25. Grayson M: Diseases of the Cornea, 2nd ed. St. Louis, CV Mosby, 1983.
26. Jones DB, Green MT, Osato MS, et al: Endogenous *Candida albicans* endophthalmitis in the rabbit. Chemotherapy for systemic effect. Arch Ophthalmol 99:2182, 1981.
27. Jones DB: Therapy of postsurgical fungal endophthalmitis. Ophthalmology 85:357, 1978.
28. Stern GA, Fetkenhour CL: Intravitreal amphotericin B treatment of *Candida* endophthalmitis. Arch Ophthalmol 95:89, 1977.
29. Stern GA, Okumoto M, Smolin G: Combined amphotericin B and rifampin treatment of experimental *Candida albicans* keratitis. Arch Ophthalmol 97:721, 1979.
30. Brajtburg J, Elberg S, Medoff G, Kobayashi GS: Increase in colony-forming units of *C. albicans* after treatment with polyene antibiotics. Antimicrob Agents Chemother 19:199, 1981.
31. Brajtburg J, Kobayashi D, Medoff G, Kobayashi GS: Antifungal action of amphotericin B in combination with other polyene and imidazole antibiotics. J Infect Dis 146:138, 1982.
32. Edwards IE, Morrison J, Henderson DK, Montgomerie JZ: Combined effect of amphotericin B and rifampin on *Candida* sp. Antimicrob Agents Chemother 17:484, 1980.
33. Eilard T, Beskow D, Norrby R, et al: Combined treatment with amphotericin B and flucytosine in severe fungal infections. J Antimicrob Chemother 2:239, 1976.
34. Chin GN, Hyndiuk RA, Kwasny GP, Schultz RO: Keratomycosis in Wisconsin. Am J Ophthalmol 79:121, 1975.
35. Green WR, Bennett JE, Goos RD: Ocular penetration of amphotericin B. Arch Ophthalmol 73:769, 1964.
36. Foster JBT, Almeda E, Littman ML: Some intraocular and conjunctival effects of amphotericin B in man and in the rabbit. Arch Ophthalmol 60:555, 1958.
37. Wood TO, Williford W: Treatment of keratomycosis with amphotericin B 0.15%. Am J Ophthalmol 81:847, 1976.
38. O'Day DM, Head WS, Robinson RD, Clanton JA: Bioavailability and penetration of topical amphotericin B in the anterior segment of the rabbit eye. J Ocul Pharmacol 2:371, 1986.
39. Bell R, Ritchey JP: Subconjunctival nodules after amphotericin B injection: Medical therapy for *Aspergillus* corneal ulcer. Arch Ophthalmol 90:402, 1973.
40. Axelrod AJ, Peyman GA: Intravitreal amphotericin B treatment of experimental fungal endophthalmitis. Am J Ophthalmol 76:584, 1973.

41. Axelrod AJ, Peyman GA, Apple DJ: Toxicity of intravitreal injection of amphotericin B. Am J Ophthalmol 78:875, 1974.
42. Fine BS, Zimmerman LE: Therapy of experimental intraocular *Aspergillus* infection. Arch Ophthalmol 64:69, 1960.
43. Jerraut LZE Jr, Perraut LE, Bleiman B, Lyons J: Successful treatment of *Candida albicans* endophthalmitis with intravitreal amphotericin B. Arch Ophthalmol 99:1565, 1981.
44. Lou P, Kazdan J, Bannatyne RM, Cheung R: Successful treatment of *Candida* endophthalmitis with a synergistic combination of amphotericin B and rifampin. Am J Ophthalmol 83:12, 1977.
45. Brod RD, Flynn HW Jr, Clarkson JG, et al: Endogenous *Candida* endophthalmitis. Management without intravenous amphotericin B. Ophthalmology 97:662, 1990.
46. Huang K, Peyman GA, McGetrick J: Vitrectomy in experimental endophthalmitis. 1: Fungal infection. Ophthalmic Surg 10:84, 1979.
47. Medoff G, Disnukes EE, Meade RH III, Moses JM: A new therapeutic approach to *Candida* infections. Arch Intern Med 130:241, 1972.
48. Medoff G, Kobayashi GS: Medical progress. Strategies in the treatment of systemic fungal infections. N Engl J Med 302:145, 1980.
49. Bennett JE, Dismukes WE, Duma RJ, et al: A comparison of amphotericin B alone and combined with flucytosine in the treatment of cryptococcal meningitis. N Engl J Med 301:126, 1979.
50. Butler WT, Bennet JE, Alling DW, et al: Nephrotoxicity of amphotericin B: Early and late effects in 81 patients. Ann Intern Med 61:175, 1964.
51. Bannatyne RM, Cheung R: Comparative susceptibility of *Candida albicans* to amphotericin B and amphotericin B methyl ester. Antimicrob Agents Chemother 12:449, 1977.
52. McGetrick JJ, Peyman GA, Nyberg MA: Amphotericin B methyl ester: Evaluation for intravitreous use in experimental fungal endophthalmitis. Ophthalmic Surg 10:25, 1979.
53. O'Day DM, Ray WA, Head WS, Robinson RD: Efficacy of antifungal agents in the cornea. IV: Amphotericin B methyl ester. Invest Ophthalmol Vis Sci 25:851, 1984.
54. Jones DB: Decision-making in the management of microbial keratitis. Ophthalmology 88:814, 1981.
55. Natamycin for keratomycosis. Med Lett Drugs Ther 21:79, 1979.
56. Jones DB, Forster RK, Rebell G: *Fusarium solani* keratitis treated with natamycin (pimaricin). Arch Ophthalmol 88:147, 1972.
57. O'Day DM, Ray WA, Robinson RD, Head WS: Correlation of in vitro and in vivo susceptibility of *Candida albicans* to amphotericin B and natamycin. Invest Ophthalmol Vis Sci 28:596, 1987.
58. Newmark E, Ellison AC, Kaufman HE: Pimaricin therapy of *Cephalosporium* and *Fusarium* keratitis. Am J Ophthalmol 69:458, 1970.
59. Newmark E, Kaufman HE, Polack RM, Ellison AC: Clinical experience with pimaricin therapy in fungal keratitis. South Med J 64:935, 1971.
60. O'Day DM, Head WS, Robinson RD, Clanton JA: Corneal penetration of topical amphotericin B and natamycin. Curr Eye Res 5:877, 1986.
61. Ellison AC: Intravitreal effects of pimaricin in experimental fungal endophthalmitis. Am J Ophthalmol 81:157, 1976.
62. Ellison AC, Newmark E: Intraocular effects of pimaricin. Ann Ophthalmol 8:98, 1976.
63. Ellison AC: Intravenous effects of pimaricin on mycotic endophthalmitis. Ann Ophthalmol 11:157, 1979.
64. Ellison AC, Newmark E, Kaufman HE: Chemotherapy of experimental keratomycosis. Am J Ophthalmol 68:812, 1969.
65. Mangiaracine AB, Liebman SD: Fungus keratitis (*Aspergillus fumigatus*). Treatment with nystatin. Arch Ophthalmol 58:695, 1957.
66. Tabbara KF, Hyndiuk RA: Infections of the Eye. Boston, Little, Brown, 1986.
67. Plempel M: Pharmacokinetics of imidazole antimycotics. Postgrad Med J 55:662, 1979.
68. Borgers M: Mechanism of action of antifungal drugs, with special reference to the imidazole derivatives. Rev Infect Dis 2:520, 1980.
69. Iwata K, Kanda Y, Yamaguchi H, Osumi M: Electron microscopic studies on the mechanism of action of clotrimazole on *Candida albicans*. Sabouraudia 11:205, 1973.
70. Sud IJ, Feingold DS: Heterogeneity of action mechanisms among antimycotic imidazoles. Antimicrob Agents Chemother 20:71, 1981.
71. DeNollin S, Borger M: The ultrastructure of *Candida albicans* after in vitro treatment with miconazole. Sabouraudia 12:341, 1974.
72. Stern GA: In vitro antibiotic synergism against ocular fungal isolates. Am J Ophthalmol 86:359, 1978.
73. Moody MR, Young VM, Morris MJ, Schimpff SC: In vitro activities of miconazole, miconazole nitrate, and ketoconazole alone and combined with rifampin against *Candida* sp. and *Torulopsis glabrata* recovered from cancer patient. Antimicrob Agents Chemother 17:871, 1980.
74. Schacter LP, Owellen RJ, Rathbun HK, Buchanan B: Antagonism between miconazole and amphotericin B. Lancet 2:318, 1976.
75. Beggs WH, Sarosi GA, Steele NM: Inhibition of potentially pathogenic yeast-like fungi by clotrimazole in combination with 5-fluorocytosine or amphotericin B. Antimicrob Agents Chemother 9:863, 1976.
76. Plempel M, Buchel KH, Bartmann K, Regel E: Antimycotic properties of clotrimazole. Postgrad Med J 50(Suppl 1):11, 1974.
77. Duhm B, Medenwald H, Puetter J, et al: The pharmacokinetics of clotrimazole ^{14}C. Postgrad Med J (Suppl):13, 1974.
78. Jones BR: Principles in the management of oculomycosis. Trans Am Acad Ophthalmol Otolaryngol 79:15, 1975.
79. Jones BR: Principles in the management of ocular mycoses. Am J Ophthalmol 79:719, 1975.
80. Jones BR, Richards AB: Clotrimazole in the treatment of ocular infection by *Aspergillus fumigatus*. Postgrad Med J 50 (Suppl 1):39, 1974.
81. Tettenborn D: Toxicity of clotrimazole. Postgrad Med J (Suppl):17, 1974.
82. Van Cutsem JM, Tienpont D: Miconazole, a broad-spectrum antimycotic agent with antibacterial activity. Chemotherapy 17:392, 1972.
83. Corrado ML, Kramer M, Cummings M, Eng RH: Susceptibility of dematiaceous fungi to amphotericin B, miconazole, ketoconazole, flucytosine and rifampin alone and in combination. Sabouraudia 20:109, 1982.
84. Cosgrove RF, Beezer AE, Miles RJ: In vitro studies of amphotericin B in combination with the imidazole antifungal compounds clotrimazole and miconazole. J Infect Dis 138:681, 1978.
85. Dixon D, Shadomy S, Shadomy HJ, et al: Comparison of the in vitro antifungal activities of miconazole and a new imidazole, R41,400. J Infect Dis 138:245, 1978.
86. Fitzsimons RB, Nicholls MD, Billson FA, et al: Fungal retinitis: A case of *Torulopsis glabrata* infection treated with miconazole. Br J Ophthalmol 64:672, 1980.
87. Foster CS: Miconazole therapy for keratomycosis. Am J Ophthalmol 91:622, 1981.
88. Foster CS, Lass JH, Moran-Wallace K, Giovanoni R: Ocular toxicity of topical antifungal agents. Arch Ophthalmol 99:1081, 1981.
89. Foster CS, Stefanyszyn M: Intraocular penetration of miconazole in rabbits. Arch Ophthalmol 97:1703, 1979.
90. Fowler BJ: Treatment of fungal endophthalmitis with vitrectomy and intraocular injection of miconazole. J Ocul Ther Surg 3:43, 1984.
91. Fitsimons R, Peters AL: Miconazole and ketoconazole as a satisfactory first-line treatment for keratomycosis. Am J Ophthalmol 101:605, 1986.
92. Ishibashi Y, Matsumoto Y, Takei K: The effects of intravenous miconazole on fungal keratitis. Am J Ophthalmol 98:433, 1984.
93. Gallo J, Grunstein H, Clifton-Bligh P, et al: Miconazole in fungal endophthalmitis. Lancet 1:53, 1982.
94. Jaben SL, Forster RK: Intraocular miconazole therapy in fungal endophthalmitis. Invest Ophthalmol Vis Sci 20(Suppl):109, 1981.
95. Bisschop MP, Merkus JM, Scheygrond H, et al: Treatment of vaginal candidiasis with ketoconazole, a new, orally active antimycotic. Eur J Obstet Gynaecol Reprod Biol 9:253, 1979.
96. Van Den Bossche H, Willemsens G, Cools W, Cornelissen F: Inhibition of ergosterol synthesis in *Candida albicans* by ketoconazole. Arch Int Physiol Biochim 87:849, 1979.
97. Borelli D, Fuentes J, Leiderman E, et al: Ketoconazole, an oral antifungal: Laboratory and clinical assessment of imidazole drugs. Postgrad Med J 55:657, 1979.
98. Oji EO: Ketoconazole: A new imidazole antifungal agent has both prophylactic potential and therapeutic efficacy in keratomycosis of rabbits. Int Ophthalmol 5:163, 1982.
99. Oji EO: Study of ketoconazole toxicity in rabbit cornea and conjunctiva. Int Ophthalmol 5:169, 1982.
100. Torres MA, Mohamed J, Cavazos-Adame H, Martinez LA: Topical keratoconazole for fungal keratitis. Am J Ophthalmol 100:293, 1985.
101. DeFelice R, Johnson DG, Galgiani JN: Gynecomastia with ketoconazole. Antimicrob Agents Chemother 19:1073, 1981.
102. Komadina TG, Wilkes TDI, Shock JP, et al: Treatment of *Aspergillus fumigatus* keratitis in rabbits with oral and topical ketoconazole. Am J Ophthalmol 99:476, 1985.
103. Bodey JT: Azole antifungal agents. Clin Infect Dis 14(Suppl 1):161, 1992.

104. Maichuk IF, Karimov MK, Lapshina NA: Ketoconazole in the treatment of ocular mycoses. Vestn Oftalmol 106:44, 1990.
105. Rajasekaran J, Thomas PA, Srinivasan R: Ketoconazole in keratomycosis. *In* Blodi F, Brancato R, Cristini G, et al: Proceedings of the XXV International Congress of Ophthalmology, Rome, May 4–10, 1986, pp 2462–2467.
106. Ishibashi Y: Oral ketoconazole therapy for keratomycosis. Am J Ophthalmol 95:342, 1983.
107. Chu W, Foster CS, Moran K, Giovanoni R: Intraocular penetration of ketoconazole. Invest Ophthalmol Vis Sci 18(Suppl):133, 1979.
108. Smolin G, Thoft RA: The Cornea. Boston, Little, Brown, 1987.
109. Upadhyay MP, West EP, Sharma AP: Keratitis due to *Aspergillus flavus* successfully treated with thiabendazole. Br J Ophthalmol 64:30, 1980.
110. Smolin G, Okumoto M (eds): Antimicrobial Agents in Ophthalmology. New York, Masson, 1983.
111. Rysselaere M: The effect of econazole in experimental oculomycosis in rabbits. Mykosen 24:238, 1981.
112. Oji EO, Clayton YM: The role of econazole in the management of oculomycosis. Int Ophthalmol 4:137, 1981.
113. Richardson K, Cooper K, Marriott MS, et al: Design and evaluation of a systemically active agent, fluconazole. Ann N Y Acad Sci 544:4, 1988.
114. Isulka B, Stambridge T: Fluconazole in the treatment of candidal prosthetic valve endocarditis. BMJ 297:178, 1988.
115. Brooks JH, O'Brien TP, Wilhelmus KR, et al: Comparative topical triazole therapy of experimental *Candida albicans* keratitis. Invest Ophthalmol Vis Sci 31(Suppl):2793, 1990.
116. Brammer KW, Farrow PR, Faulkner JK: Pharmacokinetics and tissue penetration of fluconazole in humans. Rev Infect Dis 12(Suppl 3):S318, 1990.
117. Rhee P, O'Brien TP: Pharmacotherapy of fungus infections of the eye. *In* Zimmerman TJ (ed): Textbook of Ocular Pharmacology. Philadelphia, Lippincott-Raven, 1997, pp 587–607.
118. Sugar AM: Fluconazole and itraconazole: Current status and prospects for antifungal therapy. Curr Clin Top Infect Dis 13:74, 1998.
119. Bloom PA, Laidlaw DA, Easty DL, Warnoch DW: Treatment failure in a case of fungal keratitis caused by *Pseudallescheria boydii*. Br J Ophthalmol 76:367, 1992.
120. Carlson AN, Foulks J, Perfect J, Kim J: Fungal scleritis after cataract surgery. Cornea 11:151, 1992.
121. Heykants J, Van Peer A, Lavrijsen K, et al: Pharmacokinetics of oral antifungals and their clinical implications. Br J Clin Pract 71(Suppl): 50, 1990.
122. Shadomy S, Kirchoff CB, Ingroff AE: In vitro activity of 5-fluorocytosine against *Candida* and *Torulopsis* species. Antimicrob Agents Chemother 3:9, 1973.
123. Wagner GE, Shadomy S: Studies on the mode of action of 5-fluorocytosine in *Aspergillus* species. Chemotherapy 25:61, 1979.
124. Diasio RB, Bennett JE, Myers CE: Mode of action of 5-fluorocytosine. Biochem Pharmacol 27:703, 1978.
125. Firkin FC: Therapy of deep-seated fungal infections with 5-fluorocytosine. Aust N Z J Med 4:462, 1974.
126. Hardel EJ, Hermans PE: Treatment of fungal infections with flucytosine. Arch Intern Med 135:231, 1975.
127. Walsh JA, Haft DA, Miller MM HG, et al: Ocular penetration of 5-fluorocytosine. Invest Ophthalmol 17:691, 1978.
128. Polak A: Pharmacokinetics of amphotericin B and flucytosine. Postgrad Med J 55:667, 1979.
129. Romano A, Segal E, Eyelan E, Stein R: Treatment of external ocular *Candida* infections with 5-fluorocytosine. Ophthalmologica 172:282, 1976.
130. Montgomerie JZ, Edwards JE Jr, Guze LB: Synergism of amphotericin B and 5-fluorocytosine for *Candida* species. J Infect Dis 132:82, 1975.

CHAPTER 23

Antiparasitics

Nalini A. Madiwale

Parasitic infections are a major public health problem throughout the world. Onchocerciasis is one of the leading causes of blindness across the African continent and causes a major socioeconomic burden on patients. Acanthamebiasis is one of the most frustrating causes of keratitis in the developed nations.

The control and eradication of parasitic infections require a multifaceted approach that includes vector control, health education, and improved sanitation. Nevertheless, chemotherapy remains the most efficient and effective means of control of parasitic diseases. There is cause for optimism in many areas. Medical cures of *Acanthamoeba* keratitis are becoming more common. Control of onchocerciasis is now considered feasible. Ocular cysticercosis, previously amenable to surgical treatment only, can now be managed medically.

Improved methods of maintaining parasites in vitro, assessment of in vivo and in vitro activity of antiparasitic agents, and the development of animal models for ocular parasitic infections have all been very encouraging.[1–3] The emergence of resistant strains is frustrating but spurs ongoing basic and clinical research into the development of newer and safer drugs.

Only those parasitic infections of ocular importance that are amenable to chemotherapy are discussed in this chapter. A brief account of the life cycle and ocular manifestations of the relevant parasitic infections is followed by a detailed account of the chemotherapeutic regimens for their treatment. The pharmacology of the systemic and topical antiparasitic agents is discussed in alphabetic order. The therapeutic regimens and ocular side effects of the medications are summarized in Tables 23–1 and 23–2, respectively.

TABLE 23–1. **Chemotherapeutic Options in Parasitic Infections**

Infection	Chemotherapeutic Agents	Comments
Acanthamoeba keratitis	Topical PHMB, propamidine isethionate, neomycin	Protocol not established. Propamidine not freely available in United States
Extraocular cysticercosis	Albendazole	
Giardiasis	Metronidazole, quinacrine	
Leishmaniasis	Pentostam,* Amphotericin B†	
Loiasis	DEC	
Malaria	Chloroquine	
Microsporidiosis	Topical fumagillin	
Onchocerciasis	Ivermectin,* Amocarzine, DEC + suramin†	
Toxoplasmosis	Pyrimethamine and sulfadiazine + prednisone	Triple therapy
	Clindamycin and sulfadiazine	
	Trimethoprim-sulfamethoxazole (Bactrim) alone or with clindamycin	
	Pyrimethamine + clindamycin + SD + adjuvant oral steroids	Quadruple therapy

Abbreviations: PHMB, polyhexamethylene biguanide; DEC, diethylcarbamazine citrate.
*First choice.
†Second choice.

TABLE 23–2. **Drugs Used in Chemotherapy of Parasitic Infections**

Drug	Indications and Dosage	Ocular Side Effects
Chloroquine	Malaria	Visual disturbances, unusual at antimalarial dose
DEC	Loiasis: Test dose 0.5 mg/kg then 2 mg/kg t.i.d. PO × 3–4 wk Onchocerciasis: 0.5 mg/kg t.i.d. × 3 days; 1 mg/kg t.i.d. × 3 days; 2–3 mg/kg t.i.d. × 12 days	Increase in corneal microfilariae, globular limbitis, exacerbation of eye lesions, RPE changes
Albendazole	15 mg/kg/day for 30 days	
Ivermectin	Onchocerciasis: 150 μg/kg, single dose, annually	
Metronidazole	Giardiasis: 250 mg t.i.d. × 5 days	
Pentostam	Leishmaniasis: 20 mg/kg IM or IV × 30 days	
Pyrimethamine	Toxoplasmosis: 100 mg/kg × 1 day PO loading dose; 25 mg/kg b.i.d × 2–6 wk	
Quinine	Malaria	Cinchonism*
Sulfadiazine	Toxoplasmosis: 500 mg q.i.d. PO 2–6 wk	Stevens-Johnson syndrome in sensitive patients
Suramin	Test dose: 100 mg IV, then 1 g/wk for 5 wk	Worsening of eye lesions, papillitis, optic atrophy

Abbreviations: DEC, diethylcarbamazine citrate; RPE, retinal pigment epithelial changes.
*Blurred vision, dyschromatopsia, photophobia, night blindness, constricted visual fields, retinal vascular spasm, optic atrophy.

Chemotherapy of Protozoal Infections

ACANTHAMOEBA KERATITIS

Acanthamoeba is a free-living ubiquitous ameba responsible for a keratitis that has become clinically and epidemiologically important in America and Europe since the 1970s. The life cycle of these organisms consists of an active trophozoite and a dormant cystic phase.

Keratitis is by far the most common mode of presentation of *Acanthamoeba* infection.[4] The wearing of contact lenses, especially in association with the use of homemade saline and cold disinfection methods is a prominent risk factor. Exposure to organic material, dust, and water may play a role in contacting the infection in non–contact lens wearers. Clinical features include gradually worsening keratitis, perineuritis, central or paracentral ring infiltrate, pain disproportionate to the extent of keratitis, recurrent breakdown and healing, scleritis, uveitis, hypopyon, secondary glaucoma, and cataract. Posterior segment involvement is rare.[4]

The prognosis of this potentially blinding condition has improved considerably in the last few years. Increased awareness, improved diagnostic techniques such as confocal microscopy, and the availability of new therapeutic agents have made early diagnosis and medical cure a frequent occurrence. Therapy is now predominantly topical, and therapeutic keratoplasty is less frequent. The use of topical steroids is controversial. In vitro activity of currently used antiamebic agents is summarized in Table 23–3. In vitro drug-sensitivity testing correlates poorly with clinical treatment but is of value in the development of new therapeutic agents. There is no consensus on the optimal medical treatment for *Acanthamoeba* keratitis, and there is a lack of controlled clinical data. No national protocol is in place. Nevertheless, a combination of propamidine isethionate (Brolene) and polyhexamethylene biguanide (PHMB), appears to be emerging as the first line of treatment.[5] In vitro studies support the value of combination therapy over monotherapy. Chlorhexidine 0.02% has shown in vitro cysticidal activity. Its efficacy has been reported in isolated cases.

The following are published reports of treatment regimens that led to the successful management of *Acanthamoeba* keratitis. They are all uncontrolled case studies of small groups of patients treated at single institutions. The results should be interpreted with appropriate caution.

TABLE 23–3. **In Vitro Activity of Antiamebic Drugs**

Drug	Mean TMAC (μg/mL)	Mean MCC (μg/mL)
Propamidine	0.6	46.0
PHMB	1.3	2.2
Neomycin	12.0	>500
Chlorhexidine	0.71	2.77

Abbreviations: TMAC, minimal concentration for 100% amebicidal activity for trophozoites; MCC, minimal concentration for 100% cysticidal activity; PHMB, polyhexamethylene biguanide.

1. Elder[6] and colleagues reported 23 cases of culture-positive *Acanthamoeba* keratitis. Of these, 19 cases were managed with neomycin and propamidine isethionate as the first line of treatment. A medical cure was obtained in 9 (47%) cases. The medical failures were then treated with PHMB and propamidine isethionate. Eight (80%) of these patients were medically cured with the second line of treatment. The lack of response to therapy in 2 cases was not related to drug resistance. One patient was cured surgically, and the other was refractory to all treatment and progressed to pthysis. All 4 patients treated initially with PHMB and propamidine isethionate were cured.
2. Larkin[7] and coworkers obtained a medical cure in five of six cases of confirmed *Acanthamoeba* keratitis refractory to therapy with multiple antiamebic agents. Three patients received PHMB alone and three a combination of PHMB and propamidine isethionate. Topical steroids and surgical management were used adjunctively. The intensive treatment consisted of PHMB 0.02% every 1 to 3 hours with gradual tapering concurrent with clinical improvement.
3. Varga[8] and associates reported a medical cure in six eyes of five patients with combination therapy consisting of neomycin, propamidine isethionate, and PHMB. The regimen consisted of a loading dose of all three agents, treatment every hour for 1 to 3 days, intensive treatment every 2 hours while awake for 4 to 7 days, and maintenance therapy every 4 hours for 7 to 21 days. After this the medications were gradually tapered to continue at 1 drop per day for 1 year.
4. Moore and McCulley[9] reported five cases of the successful management of *Acanthamoeba* keratitis. Four cases were managed by intensive inpatient treatment with topical propamidine isethionate and neomycin-polymyxin-gramicidin (Neosporin) drops every 15 minutes round the clock for 3 days followed by administration four times a day for a year. A clinical cure and excellent vision were achieved in all four patients. One patient, treated with propamidine isethionate and neomycin-polymyxin-gramicidin drops four times a day for 15 months achieved a clinical cure and good visual outcome with keratoplasty. None of these patients received concurrent topical steroids. The average length of follow-up was 32 months.

The rationale for intensive treatment is to saturate the cornea with the drug to kill trophozoites, encourage encystment, and kill the excysting trophozoites by maintaining high levels of the drug for a prolonged period of time.

GIARDIASIS

Giardiasis is a waterborne infection caused by *Giardia lamblia*, a binuclear flagellate protozoan that affects the upper part of the gastrointestinal tract. A water supply contaminated with cysts is the usual source of infection. An increased prevalence among homosexual males has been documented, suggesting that sexual practices may play a role in transmission.

Iridocyclitis,[10] choroiditis, and a hemorrhagic retinopathy can coexist with both latent and overt systemic infections. The basis of the ocular involvement is thought to be immunologic.

Metronidazole, 250 mg three times a day for 5 days, provides effective treatment. Quinacrine is equally effective, but it is no longer available in the United States. Concurrent ocular steroids are needed to control the exacerbation of inflammation that occurs after initiation of treatment.

LEISHMANIASIS

Mucocutaneous leishmaniasis[11] is caused by *Leishmania braziliensis*. About 10 to 20% of the patients show ocular involvement. The extracellular, flagellate, and promastigote forms are injected into the skin through the bite of the *Phlebotomus* mosquito. The parasites proliferate as aflagellate amastigotes within macrophages and endothelial cells of capillaries. Lysis of the amastigotes by host macrophages and lymphocytes causes an open ulcer. During a mosquito bite, the amastigotes enter the vector and transform into promastigotes that are transmitted to the next human through the saliva of the infected vector.[12]

Ocular manifestations include granular or nodular conjunctivitis, interstitial keratitis, nodular keratitis with heavy pannus formation, and ulcerative keratitis.[12]

Sodium stibogluconate (Pentostam) is the drug of choice for the treatment of leishmaniasis. The recommended dose is 20 mg/kg IM or IV for 30 days. However, amphotericin B, 0.25 to 1 mg/kg/day IV for up to 8 weeks, is used when antimonials are ineffective or contraindicated.

MICROSPORIDIOSIS

Human microsporidiosis was very rare until its emergence as an opportunistic infection in acquired immunodeficiency disease (AIDS).[13] Microsporidia are obligate intracellular spore-forming protozoans. They are transmitted by highly resistant spores. The sporoplasm is injected into the host cell and replication (merogony) occurs before further spore formation (sporogony). To date, three genera have been implicated in ocular infections. They are *Encephalitozoon*, *Nosema*, and *Septata*. Nosema causes corneal stromal ulceration in immunocompetent individuals. *Encephalitozoon* and *Septata* cause an intractable keratoconjunctivitis in patients with disseminated AIDS.[14, 15] The keratoconjunctivitis responds well to intensive hourly treatment with topical fumagillin. Maintenance therapy is necessary to prevent recurrence.

TOXOPLASMOSIS

Toxoplasmosis is caused by *Toxoplasma gondii*, an obligate intracellular protozoan of cosmopolitan distribution. The domestic cat is the definitive host. Oocysts excreted in cat feces have been shown to survive in soil for long periods of time. Human infection can occur after ingestion of either tissue cysts (bradyzoites) or oocysts (sporozoites). Transmission occurs by contact with contaminated feces; ingestion or handling of infected meat; or drinking of contaminated water. Transplacental spread causes a congenital infection. On entry into the host, the cyst wall is disrupted, releasing actively replicating, invasive tachyzoites. The host's immune response then transforms the tachyzoites into slowly dividing bradyzoites in tissue cysts. The tissue cysts remain dormant for prolonged periods of time. Their rupture causes reactivation of disease. The life cycle is completed only when the cat ingests infected uncooked meat.[16]

Acute focal retinochoroiditis, papillitis, papilledema, vitritis, and recurrent retinitis are commonly seen ocular manifestations. A granulomatous anterior uveitis is sometimes seen. In the immunocompetent host, toxoplasmosis is a self-limiting disease. In the immunocompromised host the retinochoroiditis takes on a severe necrotizing form and occurs in conjunction with life-threatening systemic infection.

Treatment is indicated only in vision-threatening, active lesions in immunocompetent patients, and in all active lesions in immunosuppressed patients. No cysticidal agent is available, although azithromycin is being investigated as such. All the currently used drugs are active against tachyzoites. Systemic steroids are used only in conjunction with the antiparasitic agents. Topical steroids and cycloplegics are used as needed. The use of systemic steroids alone is strongly contraindicated. The duration of treatment is usually 3 to 4 weeks for immunocompetent patients. Patients with AIDS may need continued treatment with at least one antiparasitic agent. There is no true consensus regarding the treatment.

The following are accepted regimens of treatment:

1. The classic triple-drug combination.[16] Pyrimethamine, loading dose of 75 mg/day followed by 25 mg twice a day, plus sulfadiazine, loading dose of 2 g followed by 1 g four times a day, plus prednisone, 60 to 100 mg/day. Supplemental folinic acid is given in a dose of 3 to 5 mg two to three times per week orally, to counteract the leukopenia and thrombocytopenia caused by pyrimethamine. Trisulfapyrimidine can be substituted for sulfadiazine.
2. Clindamycin 150 to 300 mg four times a day with sulfadiazine.[17] Treatment with clindamycin should be approached with extreme caution because of the possibility of a potentially fatal pseudomembranous colitis that can occur with its use.
3. Trimethoprim-sulfamethoxazole, alone or in conjunction with clindamycin.[18] Trimethoprim-sulfamethoxazole (Bactrim DS, a fixed-combination antibiotic consisting of 160 mg of trimethoprim and 800 mg of sulfamethoxazole) is given twice a day for 4 to 6 weeks. Better patient compliance and tolerance are the main advantages of this regimen.
4. Quadruple therapy.[19] A retrospective study conducted by Lam and Tessler points to the merits of quadruple therapy. The agents used were pyrimethamine, loading dose 75 mg then 25 mg/day, plus sulfadiazine, loading dose 2 g, then 1 g four times per day, plus clindamycin, 300 mg four times per day, plus prednisone, 60 to 80 mg on alternate days. The pyrimethamine was discontinued after 1 week if there was clinical improvement and after 2 weeks regardless of the clinical course. The entire treatment lasted 3 weeks. In the first week 54% of patients showed improvement, and within the second week 81% responded. There were no serious side effects, and the treatment was well tolerated.

A prospective multicenter trial compared patients receiving the following treatment regimens with an untreated group of patients with peripheral foci of retinochoroiditis: (1) pyrimethamine, sulfadiazine, and prednisone; (2) clindamycin, sulfadiazine, and prednisone; and (3) trimethoprim-sulfamethoxazole (Bactrim DS) and prednisone. Group 1 showed the greatest decrease in the size of the lesion and the best improvement in visual acuity. There was no difference in the duration of inflammatory activity between treated and untreated groups.

MALARIA AND BABESIOSIS

Malaria and babesiosis (Nantucket fever) are two other diseases caused by protozoans that are associated with significant morbidity and mortality. The clinical features of malaria are essentially secondary to hemolytic anemia, vasoocclusive phenomena caused by infected red cells, and immunologic responses of the host. Ocular manifestations include conjunctival hemorrhage, lid edema, acute dacryoadenitis, uveitis, retinal vascular occlusions, proliferative retinopathy, papilledema, optic neuritis, and oculomotor palsies.[12] Retinal nerve fiber layer infarcts have been described in babesiosis.[20] The treatment of these conditions is outside the domain of the ophthalmologist and hence not within the scope of this chapter. Of the various drugs used in the treatment of malaria and babesiosis, only chloroquine and quinine have ocular side effects, and these are summarized in Table 23–2.

Chemotherapy of Helminthic Infections

CYSTICERCOSIS

Cysticercosis is commonly caused by the encystment of the larvae of the cestode *Taenia solium*. It is endemic to Africa, East Europe, Southeast Asia, and South America.[21]

Humans are the definitive host in taeniasis and the intermediate host in cysticercosis. The latter occurs by the ingestion of eggs of *T. solium* through fecal contamination of food and water. Ocular involvement occurs in the form of cysts in the subretinal space, vitreous, anterior segment, subconjunctival space, extraocular muscles, and orbit. It presents with symptoms including a decrease in vision, diplopia, flashes of light, proptosis, and restriction of extraocular movements.

Extraocular cysticercosis has been primarily treated by surgery.[22] Sihota and Honavar report a prospective randomized controlled clinical trial of 24 patients with a definitive diagnosis of cysticercosis made by ultrasonography and enzyme-linked immunosorbent assay. This study establishes the efficacy of oral albendazole. Patients treated with albendazole, 15 mg/kg for 1 month, showed clinical and ultrasonographic improvement. There was no change in the control group. Considering the fact that any surgical intervention for extraocular cysticercosis is prone to intraoperative complications due to adhesions to important structures and to significant postoperative scarring, medical therapy merits consideration as the first line of treatment.

LOIASIS

Loa loa, the African eye worm native to West Africa, the Congo basin, and Sudan, is the causative organism of loiasis.

The microfilariae circulate in the blood stream with a

diurnal periodicity and are ingested by the mango fly (genus *Chrysops*), the vector and intermediate host. The microfilariae migrate to the thoracic musculature of the fly and undergo a 10- to 12-day developmental cycle producing infective larvae. These are then transmitted to a fresh host through a fly bite. The microfilariae develop into adult worms that release fresh microfilariae.[11]

The migration of adult worms is dramatically symptomatic with intense itching and chemosis when the worm presents in the subconjunctival space. Immobilization and extraction of the worm constitutes the immediate treatment.

Diethylcarbamazine citrate (DEC), 200 mg twice a day for 3 days once a month, is used for chemoprophylaxis.

Treatment in symptomatic individuals consists of DEC, 25 to 50 mg as a test dose on the first day, then 2 mg/kg three times a day after meals for 3 to 4 weeks. Intense inflammatory reactions due to dead microfilariae sometimes necessitate the concurrent use of antihistamines and steroids.[1]

ONCHOCERCIASIS

Onchocerciasis is caused by the nematode *Onchocerca volvulus*. It is widely distributed across the African continent and South America. Humans are the only known reservoir of onchocerciasis. The female *Simulium* fly is the intermediate host and vector. The simuliid ingests the microfilariae when it bites an infected person during a blood meal. The larvae then transform into infective forms that may enter a new host when the simuliid takes another blood meal. The larvae migrate in the body for approximately 1 year before they settle in a nodule, which is most frequently subcutaneous. Here, the male and female mate and produce numerous microfilariae that migrate to various parts of the body.[11]

Ocular manifestations of onchocerciasis include punctate keratitis surrounding dead microfilariae; sclerosing keratitis; anterior uveitis with secondary cataract and glaucoma; chorioretinitis; and papillitis with severe constriction of the visual fields.[23]

For several years DEC and suramin were the only two drugs available for the treatment of onchocerciasis. DEC is effective against microfilariae but causes an initial aggravation of the ocular disease and has several troublesome side effects. Suramin is active against adult worms but has a very high intrinsic toxicity. These two drugs were at best suboptimal for mass treatment and prophylaxis of onchocerciasis and are at the present time reserved for the treatment of selected severe cases. The treatment regimen consisted of decreasing doses of DEC over 18 days followed by suramin IV, 1 g/wk for 5 weeks.[24]

Ivermectin[25–28] has revolutionized the treatment of onchocerciasis and has largely replaced DEC and suramin. Numerous double-blind placebo-controlled studies have demonstrated the efficacy and safety of ivermectin, its suitability for mass therapy, and its superiority over DEC.[29] Community-based treatment with ivermectin has been shown to reduce the transmission of onchocerciasis. Ivermectin is usually given in a single, annual, oral dose of 150 μg/kg. This dosage seems to be adequate for all except the intensely infested patients with severe ocular involvement in hyperendemic areas.[30–33] Increasing experience and further trials with repeated ivermectin treatment in hyperendemic areas without vector control have shown side effects requiring therapy in 32% after the first dose, 18% after the second dose, and 11% after the third dose. Severe side effects were only seen in 9% after the initial dose, within 48 hours. Therefore, ivermectin cannot be freely dispensed without supervision.[34] In contrast to DEC, ivermectin does not exacerbate or precipitate optic neuritis.[35] Long-term studies in holoendemic areas with vector control show that annual treatment is adequate for control. It resulted in improvement of early and advanced anterior segment lesions, reduction in microfilarial loads, and no worsening of posterior segment lesions.

Amocarzine is an oral antifilarial agent that has macro- and microfilaricidal activity.[36, 37] Field trials conducted in Ecuador and Guatemala show that it is efficacious and well tolerated. The addition of this macrofilaricidal drug to the armamentarium should greatly improve the possibilities of control.

Pharmacology of the Antiparasitic Agents

SYSTEMIC AGENTS

Amocarzine

Amocarzine[36, 37] is an isothiocyanate derivative with macro- and microfilaricidal properties. It is a red-colored agent. Absorption is regular and sustained, and bioavailability is better after postprandial administration. Sixty-four percent of the administered dose is excreted as *N*-oxide metabolite and can be measured by urine colorimetry. The optimal dose is 3 mg/kg b.i.d. for 3 days. Field trials with amocarzine have shown rapid and sustained reduction of skin microfilariae counts. Ophthalmic tolerance was very good, with improvement of anterior segment lesions and stability of postsegment lesions. Systemic tolerance was also very good. Mild pruritus and skin rash on day 4 or 6 were common. Dizziness and mild reversible disorientation occurred rarely. There was a slow decrease in eosinophils, and liver function tests remained normal.

Albendazole

Albendazole is a benzamidazole with broad-spectrum antihelmintic activity. It is the drug of choice for cysticercosis. Its primary mode of action is thought to be inhibition of microtubule polymerization. The gastrointestinal absorption is increased when the drug is given with a fatty meal. It is rapidly converted into an active sulfoxide metabolite, which is then well distributed in the various tissues and achieves penetration into cysts. The dosage used for extraocular cysticercosis is 15 mg/kg/day for 30 days. Albendazole is well tolerated. It occasionally causes gastrointestinal symptoms, headache, and dizziness. It rarely causes jaundice. It is contraindicated in pregnant women due to its teratogenic properties.

Diethylcarbamazine

DEC is a piperazine derivative. It is no longer the drug of choice for treatment of onchocerciasis but is mainly used in the treatment of loiasis. The mechanism of action of DEC is twofold, consisting of: (1) a decrease in the muscular activity of the microfilariae and their immobilization, probably by virtue of the hyperpolarizing effect of the piperazine moiety; and (2) a change in the surface membranes of the microfilariae, rendering them more susceptible to the host defense mechanisms. DEC is effective against adult worms and microfilariae of *L. loa* and only microfilariae of *O. volvulus*.

DEC is well absorbed from the gastrointestinal tract, rapidly equilibrates with all tissues except fat, and does not have a cumulative effect. Over 50% of the drug is excreted unchanged in acidic urine.

DEC has low intrinsic toxicity. Anorexia, nausea, headache, and less frequently vomiting and skin rash occur and subside in a few days despite the continuation of treatment. Leukocytosis peaks in 4 to 5 days and subsides in a few weeks. Reversible proteinuria can occur. The drug appears to be safe in pregnancy. The major adverse effects of DEC are a direct or indirect result of the host response to the death of the microfilariae. A severe encephalitis may be induced in patients heavily infected with *L. loa*. Patients with onchocerciasis typically manifest the Mazzotti reaction, which occurs in a few hours after the first dose and lasts 3 to 7 days. It consists of itching, skin rash, painful lymphadenopathy, fever, tachycardia, arthralgia, and headache. Higher doses can be tolerated after this reaction subsides. In the eye, it produces migration of microfilariae into the cornea, straightening and immobility of the microfilariae, punctate keratitis, limbitis, and uveitis. Atrophy of the retinal pigment epithelium and worsening of posterior segment lesions also occur.

Ivermectin

Ivermectin is a member of a new class of semisynthetic macrocyclic lactones called avermectins. It has a broad spectrum of antiparasitic activity. Ivermectin is now the drug of choice for onchocerciasis.

Ivermectin is absorbed through the gastrointestinal tract and is mainly concentrated in the liver and adipose tissue. Peak plasma levels are achieved 4 hours after oral administration. Its half-life is about 10 hours. Animal studies indicate nearly all of the drug is excreted in the feces unchanged. Extremely low levels of the drug are found in the brain. Not much is known about the pharmacokinetics of ivermectin in the eye. It can be speculated that because the drug is a macrocyclic lactone, it has poor ocular penetration and therefore does not achieve microfilaricidal concentrations in the eye. This would cause microfilarial movement out of the eye along a concentration gradient.

The exact mode of action of ivermectin is unknown. It modifies the release of the neurotransmitter γ-aminobutyric (GABA), but the relationship of this property to the microfilaricidal activity is unclear. The microfilaricidal action of ivermectin is slow, unlike that of DEC, and hence there is no exacerbation of ocular inflammation. Ivermectin is neither macrofilaricidal nor embryotoxic. It causes an initial increase followed by a decrease in embryogenesis. There is a sequestration of normally developed embryonic forms in the uterus of the adult female worms. The failure of microfilariae to be released explains the lack of build-up of microfilariae after single-dose treatment. It is also possible that an annual single-dose treatment with ivermectin continued for the life span of the adult worm (10 to 15 years) can interrupt transmission and provide clinical prophylaxis and treatment of ocular onchocerciasis. It is used in a single dose of 150 μg/kg.

Systemic side effects of ivermectin are mild and transient, consisting of headache, muscle ache, and painful glands lasting a few hours; a skin rash lasting a few days; an asymptomatic and intermittent increase in the pulse rate, a decrease in the blood pressure, an increase in temperature, and electrocardiographic changes. Severe systemic side effects requiring medical attention occur only after the first dose in about 9% of patients.

Ivermectin therapy is not associated with the exacerbation of ocular inflammation, and this is an overwhelming advantage over medications previously used in the treatment of onchocerciasis.

The hematologic changes associated with the administration of ivermectin are a transient decrease in hemoglobin levels; neutrophil leukocytosis; lymphocytopenia; and an initial fall followed by a steady rise in the eosinophil count.[38, 39]

Metronidazole

Metronidazole is a nitroimidazole with a broad spectrum of antiprotozoal and antimicrobial activity. The mechanism of action is linked to the ability of the nitro group to trap electrons from electron transport proteins and divert them from normal energy-yielding pathways. Studies with mammalian DNA reveal that reduced metronidazole levels can cause the loss of helical structure and strand breakage of DNA.

Metronidazole is completely and promptly absorbed from the gastrointestinal tract, and therapeutic plasma levels are observed 1 hour after oral administration of a single dose of 500 mg. The half-life of the drug is 8 hours. Ten percent of the drug is bound to plasma proteins. It shows good penetration into body tissues and fluids. Metronidazole crosses the blood-brain barrier. Greater than 50% of the systemic clearance occurs in the liver. Phase I biotransformation by oxidation yields active metabolites. Conjugation with glucuronides also occurs.

The most common side effects associated with metronidazole are headache, nausea, dry mouth, and a metallic taste. Occasionally, vomiting, diarrhea, and abdominal pain occur. Neurotoxicity in the form of dizziness, ataxia, convulsions, encephalopathy, and sensory neuropathies occur. These necessitate prompt withdrawal of the drug. Temporary and reversible leukopenia can occur. Metronidazole has a well-documented disulfiram-like effect. Patients should therefore be cautioned against using alcohol. Active central nervous system disease is a contraindication, and severe hepatic or renal dysfunction necessitate a reduction in dosage. Metronidazole and its metabolites have mutagenic activity and hence should not be used in the first trimester of pregnancy.

Sodium Stibogluconate

Sodium stibogluconate (Pentostam) is a pentavalent antimonial agent that is used in the therapy of leishmaniasis. It interferes with the glycolysis and oxidation of fatty acids in the organelles called *glycosomes* within the amastigotes.

Nonspecific binding of antimony to the sulfhydryl groups in the amastigote protein may be another mechanism of action.

Sodium stibogluconate is rapidly absorbed when given intramuscularly or intravenously and is eliminated in two phases. The first rapid phase has a half-life of 2 hours, and a second slow phase has a half-life of 33 to 76 hours.

Pain at the site of intramuscular injection, gastrointestinal disturbance, muscle pain, joint stiffness, and a reversible increase in hepatic transaminases are relatively mild side effects of pentostam administration. However, reversible T-wave flattening and an increase in the QT interval may precede serious arrhythmias.

Pyrimethamine

Pyrimethamine is a diaminopyrimidine with the following structural formula:

Pyrimethamine is a competitive antagonist of folic acid by virtue of its preferential inhibition of dihydrofolate reductase of the parasites. This prevents the reduction of dihydrofolate to tetrahydrofolate that is necessary for the synthesis of purines and pyrimidines. Pyrimethamine is synergistic to sulfas by virtue of this sequential inhibition and hence is almost always used with sulfonamide. It is only active against actively proliferating *Toxoplasma* organisms.[23] Pyrimethamine is slowly and completely absorbed after oral administration. It accumulates in the kidney, lung, liver, and spleen. Elimination is slow, with a half-life of 80 to 95 hours.

An occasional skin rash and decreased hematopoiesis are associated with the use of pyrimethamine. Large doses of pyrimethamine for a long period of time can cause a megaloblastic anemia that is readily reversible by discontinuing the drug or administering folinic acid. A severe reversible thrombocytopenia as a result of hematologic depression is an important side effect of pyrimethamine therapy and necessitates discontinuation of the drug.

Quinacrine

Quinacrine is an acridine derivative previously used as an antimalarial but currently used only for the treatment of giardiasis. Its production has been discontinued, and it is no longer available in the United States.[1]

Sulfonamides

Sulfonamides are structural analogs and competitive antagonists of *para*-aminobenzoic acid (PABA). They act by the inhibition of dihydropteroate synthetase, which is the enzyme responsible for the incorporation of PABA into dihydropteroic acid, the immediate precursor of folic acid. Sulfonamides are synergistic to other antifolates such as pyrimethamine and trimethoprim. Sulfadiazine in combination with pyrimethamine is the treatment of choice for toxoplasmosis. Sulfonamides are rapidly absorbed from the gastrointestinal tract. After a single dose, peak plasma levels are reached in 3 to 6 hours, and therapeutic concentrations occur in the cerebrospinal fluid in 4 hours. They readily cross the placental barrier. Sulfonamides are metabolized in the liver and excreted mainly by the kidneys in the acetylated and the free form. The excretion of both forms is accelerated by the administration of alkali, which decreases tubular reabsorption. The acetylated form of sulfonamides loses the antimicrobial activity while retaining the toxicity of the parent compound.

The most common side effects associated with the use of sulfonamides are fever, urticaria, and gastrointestinal disturbances. Urinary tract disturbances such as crystalluria and hematuria are associated with deficient hydration and acidic or neutral urinary pH. Hemolytic anemia, especially in patients with a glucose-6-phosphate dehydrogenase deficiency; reversible agranulocytosis; and an irreversible aplastic anemia are rarely seen. The Stevens-Johnson syndrome, exfoliative dermatitis, serum sickness, and a sometimes fatal acute necrosis of the liver can occur on the basis of hypersensitivity to the sulfonamides.

Suramin

Suramin is the only drug effective against adult *Onchocerca volvulus*. It is microfilaricidal to a lesser extent. Suramin is an organic urea compound with high intrinsic toxicity and hence needs to be administered under close supervision. It has been largely replaced by ivermectin in the treatment of onchocerciasis. It is now used with DEC only in the treatment of very severe cases of onchocerciasis.

TOPICAL AGENTS

All the following topical agents except fumagillin are antimicrobial agents used in the treatment of *Acanthamoeba* keratitis. They are discussed in alphabetic order.

Dibromopropamidine and Propamidine Isethionate

Dibromopropamidine isethionate and propamidine isethionate are both aromatic diamidines with a broad spectrum of antibacterial and antifungal activity. They are marketed in England as Brolene ointment (0.15%) and drops (0.1%), respectively. They are not available in the United States.

Intensive use of the ointment causes local irritation, and the similar use of drops causes increased conjunctival injection, chemosis, follicular conjunctivitis, punctate corneal erosions, and a linear keratopathy. All these changes are reversible and do not necessitate discontinuation of medication.[40, 41]

Fumagillin

Fumagillin is a water-insoluble antibiotic secreted by *Aspergillus fumigatus*. Fumagillin bicyclohexylammonium salt (Fumidil B) is the water-soluble form of fumagillin. Fumagillin can be formulated for topical use in the strength of 70 μg/mL. It is approved by the Food and Drug Administration as an investigational drug. The mechanism of action is not clearly defined. It is possible that fumagillin inhibits microsporidial proliferation by altering the DNA content or inhibiting RNA synthesis. It is used in the treatment of microsporidial keratitis and is well tolerated on topical administration.[14]

Neomycin

Neomycin is an aminoglycoside antibiotic available commercially in combination with polymyxin B and gramicidin. It is used in conjunction with propamidine isesthionate and polyhexamethylene biguanide in the treatment of *Acanthamoeba* keratitis. Topical neomycin has a high incidence of ocular surface toxicity and allergic blepharoconjunctivitis.

Polyhexamethylene Biguanide

Polyhexamethylene biguanide is a polymeric biguanide used in contact lens disinfection. It is used as a 0.02% solution. Intensive treatment with PHMB is well tolerated and does not result in ocular surface toxicity.[6]

$$-\left[-(CH_2)_3-\overset{H}{\underset{|}{N}}-\underset{\underset{NH}{\|}}{C}-\overset{H}{\underset{|}{N}}-\underset{\underset{NH.\ HCl}{\|}}{\overset{H}{\underset{|}{C}}}-(CH_2)_3-\right]_n-$$

where $n = 2$ to 40

REFERENCES

1. Hardman JG, Limbird LE (eds): Goodman and Gilman's The Pharmacological Basis of Therapeutics, 9th ed. New York, McGraw-Hill, 1995.
2. Cote MA, Irvine JA, Rao NA, et al: Evaluation of the rabbit as a model of *Acanthamoeba keratitis*: RID 13(Suppl 5):S443, 1991.
3. Badenoch PR, Johnson AM, Christy PE, et al: A model of *Acanthamoeba keratitis* in the rat: RID 13(Suppl 5):S445, 1991.
4. Auran JD, Starr MB, Jakobiec FA: *Acanthamoeba* keratitis: A review of literature. Cornea 6:2, 1987.
5. Hay J, Kirkness CM, Seal DV, et al: Drug resistance and *Acanthamoeba* keratitis: The quest for alternative antiprotozoal chemotherapy. Eye 8:555, 1994.
6. Elder J, Kilvington. S, Dart JKG: Clinicopathologic study of in vitro sensitivity testing and *Acanthamoeba* keratitis: Invest Ophthalmol Vis Sci 35:1059, 1994.
7. Larkin DFP, Kilvington S, Dart JKG: Treatment of *Acanthamoeba* keratitis with polyhexamethylene biguanide. Ophthalmology 99:185, 1992.
8. Varga JH, MC, Wolf TC, et al: Combined treatment of *Acanthameba* keratitis with propamidine, neomycin and polyhexamethylene biguanide. Am J Ophthalmol 115:466, 1993.
9. Moore MB, McCulley JP: *Acanthamoeba* keratitis associated with contact lenses: Six consecutive cases of successful management. Br J Ophthalmol 109:121, 1990.
10. Anderson ML, Griffith DG: Intestinal giardiasis associated with ocular inflammation. J Clin Gastroenterol 7:169, 1985.
11. Markell EK, Voge M, John DT: Medical Parasitology, 6th ed. Philadelphia, WB Saunders, 1986.
12. Duke Elder S: System of Ophthalmology, XV: Summary of Systemic Ophthalmology. St. Louis, CV Mosby, 1976.
13. Curry A, Canning EU: Human microsporidiosis. J Infec 27:229, 1993.
14. Diesenhouse MC, Wilson LA, Corrent GF, et al: Treatment of microsporidial keratoconjunctivitis with topical fumagillin. Am J Ophthalmol 115:293, 1993.
15. Lowder CY, McMahon JT, Meisler DM, et al: Microsporidial keratoconjunctivitis cause by *Septata intestinalis* in a patient with acquired immunodeficiency syndrome. Am J Ophthalmol 121:715, 1996.
16. Jabs DA: Ocular toxoplasmosis. Int Ophthalmol Clin 30:264, 1990.
17. Nussenblatt RB, Palestine AG: Uveitis: Fundamentals and Clinical Practice. Chicago, Year Book Medical, 1989.
18. Opremcak EM, Scales DK, Sharpe MR: Trimethoprim-sulfamethoxazole therapy for ocular toxoplasmosis. Ophthalmology 99:920, 1992.
19. Lam S, Tessler HH: Quadruple therapy for ocular toxoplasmosis. Can J Ophthalmol 28:58, 1993.
20. Oritz JM, Eagle RC: Ocular findings in human babesiosis (Nantucket fever). Am J Ophthalmol 93:307, 1982.
21. Kean BH, Sun T, Ellsworth RM: Color Atlas/Text of Ophthalmic Parasitology, 1st ed. New York, Igaku-Shoin, 1991.
22. Sihota R, Honavar SG: Oral albendazole in the management of extraocular cysticercosis. Br J Ophthalmol 78:621, 1994.
23. Thylefors B: Onchocerciasis in review. Int Ophthalmol Clin 30:21, 1990.
24. Anderson J, Fuglsang H: Further studies on the treatment of ocular onchocerciasis with diethylcarbamazine and suramin. Br J Ophthalmol 62:450, 1978.
25. Greene BM, Taylor HR, Cupp EW, et al: Comparison of ivermectin and diethylcarbamazine in the treatment of onchocerciasis. N Engl J Med 313:133, 1985.
26. Albiez EJ, Newland HS, White AT, et al: Chemotherapy of onchocerciasis with high doses of diethylcarbamazine or a single dose of ivermectin: Microfilaria levels and side effects. Trop Med Parasitol 39:19, 1988.
27. Diallo S, Aziz MA, Larviere M, et al: A double-blind comparison of the efficacy and safety of ivermectin and diethylcarbamazine in a placebo controlled study of Senegalese patients with onchocerciasis. Trans R Soc Trop Med Hyg 80:927, 1986.
28. Dadzie KY, Bird AC, Schulz-Key H, et al: Ocular findings in a double-blind study of ivermectin versus diethylcarbamazine versus placebo in the treatment of onchocerciasis. Br J Ophthalmol 71:78, 1987.
29. Taylor HR, Pacqúe M, Munoz B, et al: Impact of mass treatment of onchocerciasis with ivermectin on the transmission of infection. Science 250:116, 1990.
30. Rothova A, Van Der Lelij A, Stilma JS, et al: Ocular involvement in patients with onchocerciasis after repeated treatment with ivermectin. Am J Ophthalmol 110:6, 1990.
31. Stilma JS, Rothova A, Van Der Lelij G, et al: Ocular and systemic side effects following ivermectin treatment in onchocerciasis patients from Sierra Leone. Acta Leidensia 59:207, 1990.
32. Van Der Lelij A, Rohtova A, Klaassen-Broekema, et al: Decrease in adverse reactions after repeated ivermectin treatment in onchocerciasis. Doc Ophthalmol 75:215, 1990.
33. Taylor HR: Onchocerciasis. Int Ophthalmol 14:189, 1990.
34. Murdoch A, Abiose O, Babalola A, et al: Ivermectin and onchocercal optic neuritis: Short-term effects. Eye 8:456, 1994.
35. Dadzie KY, Remme J, De Sole G: Changes in ocular onchocerciasis after two rounds of community based ivermectin in a holo-endemic onchocerciasis focus Trans R Soc Trop Med Hyg 85:267, 1991.
36. Zea-Flore G, Beltranena F, Poltera AA, et al: Amocarzine investigated as oral onchocercacidal drug in 272 adult male patients from Guatemala. Results from three dose regimens spread over three days. Trop Med Parasitol 42:240, 1991.
37. Guderian RH, Anselmi M, Proano R, et al: Onchocercacidal effect of three drug regimens of amocarzine in 148 patients of two races and both sexes from Esmeraldas, Ecuador Trop Med Parasitol 42:263, 1991.
38. Awadzi K, Dadzie KY, Schulz-Key H, et al: The chemotherapy of onchocerciasis X. An assessment of four single dose treatment regimes of MK-933 (ivermectin) in human onchocerciasis. Ann Trop Med Parasitol 79:63, 1985.
39. Njoo FL, Stilma JS, Van Der Lelij A: Effects of repeated ivermectin treatment in onchocerciasis. Doc Ophthalmol 79:261, 1992.
40. Wright P, Warhurst D, Jones BR: *Acanthamoeba* keratitis successfully treated medically. Br J Ophthalmol 69:778, 1985.
41. Johns KJ, Head WS, O'Day DM: Corneal toxicity of propamidine. Arch Ophthalmol 106:68, 1988.

CHAPTER 24

Cholinergic Agents

John H.K. Liu and Kristine Erickson

Cholinergic agents play an important role in ocular pharmacology and toxicology.[1–5] Cholinergic agonists applied topically are widely used in the treatment of glaucoma and accommodative esotropia. Topical cholinergic antagonists are useful in producing mydriasis and cycloplegia for intraocular diagnosis, surgery, and treatment. The pharmacology of cholinergic agents is based on their actions upon neural synapses and neuroeffectors in which the endogenous neurotransmitter is acetylcholine; agonists mimic the action of acetylcholine, and antagonists impair the action of acetylcholine and other cholinergic agonists. A brief review of the acetylcholine life cycle would help explain the rationales of using cholinergic agonists and antagonists.

Synthesis, Action, and Degradation of Acetylcholine

Normally, acetylcholine is synthesized from choline and acetyl coenzyme A by the enzyme choline acetyltransferase in the cytoplasm of specific nerves and stored in the synaptic vesicles located at the axonal terminal.[6] There is a wide distribution of cholinergic neurons, identified by localization of choline acetyltransferase, in both the central nervous system (CNS) and the peripheral nervous system. The network of cholinergic nerves in the CNS is not as well characterized as in the periphery. However, the synthesis, action, and degradation of acetylcholine are thought to be similar in both central and peripheral nervous systems. Among the peripheral locations, all of the preganglionic fibers and the parasympathetic postganglionic fibers of the autonomic nervous system are cholinergic.[7] Somatic motor nerves are also cholinergic (they do not have ganglia in the periphery). Associated with the cholinergic innervation, there are membrane receptors at postganglionic nerve fibers, postjunctional neuroeffectors, and neuromuscular junctions that respond to acetylcholine during neural transmission. On the proximal side of synaptic and junction clefts, prejunctional cholinergic receptors may also modulate specific neural activities. Some acetylcholine-containing cells and cholinergic receptors are not associated with innervation. For instance, the corneal epithelium has one of the highest concentrations of acetylcholine molecules, most of which do not reside in the neurons.[8, 9] The physiologic role of these nonneural acetylcholines in the cornea has not been clarified. The blood vessel contains a significant number of nonneural cholinergic receptors, and their impact on the pharmacology of exogenous cholinergic agents is significant.

During the resting stage in neural transmission, a continuous small release of acetylcholine in quanta (approximately 1000 molecules) into the junctional cleft occurs. It produces a small depolarization in electrical potential across the postjunctional membrane, called miniature end-plate potentials (MEPPs). It is believed that MEPPs serve as a continuous stimulation in maintaining a cholinergic tone of the neuroeffector, which is important in certain tissues such as the skeletal muscle.[10] During an active neural transmission, the arrival of an action potential at the axonal terminal causes an influx of Ca^{2+} ions that rapidly depolarizes the membrane potential. Axonal and vesicular membranes fuse, and exocytosis of acetylcholine from synaptic vesicles follows. One action potential may cause the release of several hundred quanta of acetylcholine into the synaptic or junctional clefts. These acetylcholine molecules bind with receptors, located mainly on the postsynaptic site, around the clefts. When enough acetylcholine molecules react with postsynaptic receptors, an excitatory postsynaptic potential (EPSP) occurs owing to membrane depolarization by an increase of Na^+ permeability. Similarly, an inhibitory postsynaptic potential (IPSP) may occur owing to hyperpolarization by an increase of K^+ or anion permeability. When the EPSP exceeds the threshold potential, an action potential generates in the postsynaptic neuron. In motor end-plates of muscle fibers, a similar action potential is called the end-plate potential (EPP). On the other hand, an IPSP opposes an excitatory potential generated by subsequent stimuli on the same neuron. In the neuroeffectors, the stimulation of receptors by acetylcholine activates membrane-bound G proteins. The activation of G proteins may directly modulate ion channels or may initiate specific intracellular signal transductions and consequently affect ion channels. Together, these cellular events eventually create a variety of biologic responses.

Acetylcholine is a flexible molecule that binds with various membrane receptors to form unique conformations. Cholinergic receptors traditionally are divided into two classes, muscarinic and nicotinic, based on the similarity in reactions caused by two prototype stimulants, muscarine and nicotine.[11] Although acetylcholine is the common neurotransmitter for both the muscarinic and nicotinic receptors, the concentrations of exogenous acetylcholine needed to cause muscarinic and nicotinic responses are different. In general, a 1000-fold higher dose of acetylcholine is needed to produce nicotinic responses rather than muscarinic responses.

In recent years, a more diversified classification of cholinergic receptors emerged after the discovery of more selective agents for different muscarinic receptors and by the results from molecular cloning of various cholinergic receptors.[10, 12] Presently, five subtypes of muscarinic receptors and two subtypes of nicotinic receptors, which have distinct anatomic localizations and biochemical specificities, have been identified. Stimulations of muscarinic receptor 1, 3, and 5 subtypes activate a cell membrane enzyme, phospholipase C, through a pertussis toxin-insensitive "G protein". This consequently changes the cellular utility of inositol phosphates (mainly inositol-1,4,5-trisphosphate), diacylglycerol, calcium ion, and protein kinase C. Stimulation of these muscarinic receptor subtypes also causes the release of arachidonic acid. These cellular changes lead to a variety of physiologic responses in various neuroeffectors. Stimulation of muscarinic receptor 2 and 4 subtypes activates specific G proteins that are pertussis toxin–sensitive. This activates potassium channels and inhibits adenylate cyclase-mediated cellular events. In most tissues studied, several muscarinic receptor subtypes coexist. There are two subtypes of nicotinic receptors. The neuronal nicotinic receptors are located at the autonomic ganglia, at the adrenal medulla, and in the CNS. The muscular nicotinic receptors are located at the neuromuscular junctions in skeletal muscles. Stimulation of these nicotinic receptors opens cationic channels in the postsynaptic neurons to propagate action potentials and in the postjunctional muscular endplates to contract muscles.

Muscarinic receptors may coexist with nicotinic receptors. In sympathetic ganglia, in addition to the normal EPSP (which has a latency of 1 msec and a duration of 10 to 50 msec) generated by the stimulation of nicotinic receptors, stimulation of postsynaptic muscarinic receptor subtype 1 generates a slow EPSP that has a longer latency and a duration of 10 seconds.[13] This slow EPSP probably participates in a long-lasting modulation of synaptic excitability.[14]

Endogenously released acetylcholine is hydrolyzed rapidly by acetylcholinesterase located in cholinergic nerves, synapses, and neuroeffectors. This enzyme has an anionic site that binds with the quaternary nitrogen group of acetylcholine and an esteratic site that binds with the ester linkage of acetylcholine. The ester linkage is broken down first to form acyl acetylcholinesterase and choline. Choline moves away from the enzyme, and a water molecule moves in and reacts with the acyl acetylcholinesterase to free the acetate. The enzyme is then ready to react with another acetylcholine molecule. The hydrolysis process is very fast (less than 1 msec in the neuromuscular junction) in order to maintain the readiness of neurons and neuroeffectors for the next wave of acetylcholine molecules. The hydrolyzed products, choline and acetate, have little activity on the cholinergic receptor. Choline can be taken up by presynaptic terminals by active transport mechanisms for the synthesis of acetylcholine. Under normal physiologic conditions, termination of endogenous acetylcholine by diffusion away from the synaptic or junctional clefts is unimportant. Acetylcholine can also be hydrolyzed by butyrylcholinesterase found in the plasma, liver, and other organs. This nonspecific enzyme can be significant in degrading exogenous acetylcholine.

Along this life cycle of acetylcholine, several sites may be manipulated pharmacologically to produce either a cholinergic or an anticholinergic (cholinolytic) action. The first site is the nerve terminal where synthesis and release of acetylcholine takes place. Several agents belong to this category: hemicholinium blocks the transport of choline across the cell membrane of the nerve terminal, vesamicol blocks the transport of acetylcholine into the synaptic vesicle, botulinus toxin prevents the release of acetylcholine, and venom of black widow spider causes a transient release of acetylcholine before a permanent blockade. Botulinus toxin has an interesting ophthalmic application. Injection of botulinus toxin into the extraocular muscle weakens muscle contraction for a long time by blocking neural acetylcholine release. Therefore, bolulinus toxin can be used as an alternative for strabismus surgery.[15]

Important sites for pharmacologic application are membrane receptors. Cholinergic agonists stimulate receptors and mimic the action of acetylcholine, and cholinergic antagonists react with receptors and block reactions with acetylcholine and other cholinergic agonists. The prototypes of cholinergic agonists are muscarine and nicotine. The prototype muscarinic antagonist is atropine, which reacts with all muscarinic receptor subtypes. Among the five distinct muscarinic receptor subtypes, relatively selective antagonists for muscarinic receptor 1, 2, and 3 subtypes have been developed.[16] Neuromuscular and ganglionic blockers react specifically with nicotinic receptors at neuromuscular junctions and autonomic ganglia.

Another important site for pharmacologic manipulation of the cholinergic system is acetylcholinesterase. By inhibiting or slowing the degradation of acetylcholine, the quantity of endogenous acetylcholine at the neuroeffectors (muscarinic receptors) and at neuromuscular junctions and synapses (nicotinic receptors) can be increased. The potency and duration of cholinergic action is therefore enhanced and prolonged.

A very large number of cholinergic agents acting on all three sites have been developed. However, only a limited number of agents, aimed mainly at the latter two sites, have practical clinical applications. Cholinergic agents are currently classified into four groups: (1) agents directly stimulating the muscarinic receptor, (2) acetylcholinesterase inhibitors, (3) antimuscarinic agents, and (4) agents reacting with nicotinic receptors at neuromuscular junctions and autonomic ganglia.

Direct-Acting Muscarinic Agonists

The direct-acting muscarinic agonists stimulate the receptors at neuroeffectors, autonomic ganglia, and other muscarinic receptors not associated with innervation. These muscarinic agonists (parasympathomimetics) are divided into two groups based on their chemical structures (Fig. 24–1). The first group consists of acetylcholine and structurally related choline esters such as carbachol, methacholine, and bethanechol. The second group consists of natural alkaloids and synthetic analogs, including pilocarpine, muscarine, arecoline, and aceclidine (synthetic), which do not possess a structural similarity with acetylcholine and are not degraded by cholinesterases.

Owing to the wide distribution of muscarinic receptors, the systemic administration of muscarinic agonists causes broad reactions throughout the body.[17] When applied to the eye, muscarinic agonists cause miosis by contraction of the pupillary sphincter muscle. Stimulation of muscarinic receptors in the ciliary muscle causes accommodative myopia. Intraocular pressure (IOP) falls owing to the facilitation of aqueous humor outflow. This is probably a result of the ciliary muscle contraction causing traction of the scleral spur and widening of the spaces in the trabecular meshwork.[3, 18]

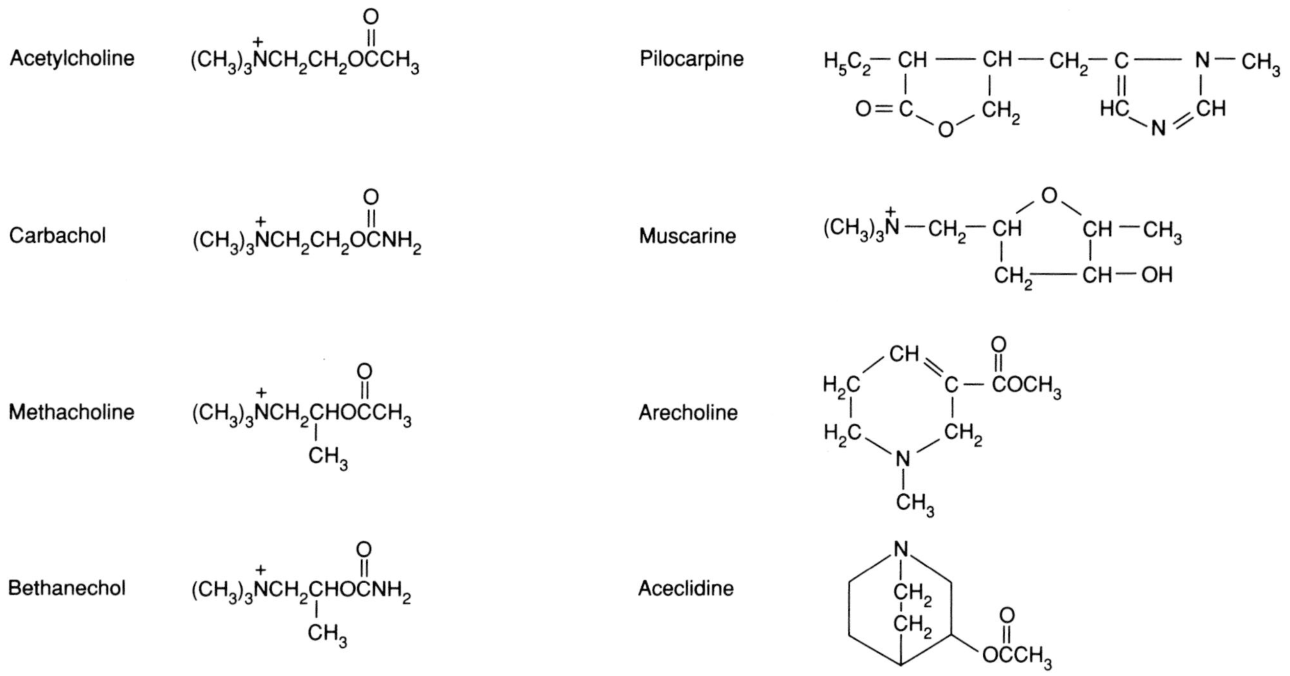

Acetylcholine $(CH_3)_3\overset{+}{N}CH_2CH_2OCCH_3$ (C=O)

Carbachol $(CH_3)_3\overset{+}{N}CH_2CH_2OCNH_2$ (C=O)

Methacholine $(CH_3)_3\overset{+}{N}CH_2CH(CH_3)OCCH_3$ (C=O)

Bethanechol $(CH_3)_3\overset{+}{N}CH_2CH(CH_3)OCNH_2$ (C=O)

Pilocarpine

Muscarine

Arecholine

Aceclidine

FIGURE 24–1. Structural formulas of direct-acting muscarinic agents.

It appears that muscarinic stimulation has no significant effect on the production of aqueous humor. Lacrimal secretion increases as a result of the stimulation of muscarinic receptors.[19, 20]

Acetylcholine causes limited CNS actions after systemic administration owing to its quaternary ammonium structure that does not penetrate the blood-brain barrier readily. Systemic administration of acetylcholine has little therapeutic utility because of its short duration of action and its diffused spectrum of biologic responses. Intraocularly administered acetylcholine, however, is useful during cataract extraction and in certain anterior segment surgeries when a quick action is needed and the action can be localized inside the eye.[21, 22] For extending the duration of action, structural changes of the acetylcholine molecule have produced therapeutically useful compounds. Having changed the acetyl group into a carbamyl group, compounds such as carbachol and bethanechol are resistant to acetylcholinesterase and nonspecific esterases. The duration of action is prolonged. Therefore, topical application of carbachol can be used to control glaucoma and accommodative esotropia. When a relatively longer duration of action is needed during intraocular surgery, carbachol can replace acetylcholine. Owing to the structural modification, carbachol acquires significant nicotinic activity at the autonomic ganglia; it may also release acetylcholine from the cholinergic nerves.

The nicotinic activity of acetylcholine can be reduced by the addition of a methyl group at the β-carbon. Methacholine and bethanechol, both having a methyl group at their β-carbon, produce primarily muscarinic action. A selectivity toward muscarinic action is desired clinically because with these agents only the parasympathetic neuroeffectors, not skeletal muscles and autonomic ganglia, are stimulated. Muscarine, the prototype muscarinic agonist, is structurally somewhat similar to methacholine but is not readily hydrolyzed by esterases because it has no ester linkage. The effect of acetylcholine and methacholine can be significantly enhanced by the administration of anticholinesterases that slow down the degradation of these compounds. By the same rationale, the effect of carbachol and bethanechol is only additive with the effect of anticholinesterases.

Among the three major cholinergic alkaloids, muscarine acts only at the muscarinic receptors. Arecoline has an additional effect at nicotinic receptors. Pilocarpine works predominantly at muscarinic receptors but has substantial nicotinic activity. Because these alkaloids administered systemically cause long and broad cholinergic activities, systemic use of these alkaloids is also limited. These natural alkaloids, however, have an important ophthalmic use. Pilocarpine is one of the oldest and most widely used antiglaucoma medicines. When applied to the eye, pilocarpine causes typical cholinergic responses: miosis, spasm of accommodation, and transient ocular hypertension followed by a prolonged decrease in IOP. It appears that muscarinic receptors in the iris sphincter muscle are more sensitive than receptors in the ciliary muscle. Miosis occurs before the effect on accommodation, and the duration of miosis is longer than the change in accommodation. Interestingly, laboratory data indicate that the effects of aceclidine, an analog of arecoline, on the outflow facility of aqueous humor and on accommodation can further be dissociated, although both actions occur via muscarinic receptors in the ciliary muscle.[23] Contraction of the ciliary muscle may cause rare precipitation of retinal detachment.[24] Owing to its long-term effect on IOP, pilocarpine in various preparations is used in the treatment of glaucoma.[25] In heavily pigmented eyes, a higher concentration of pilocarpine may be needed to lower IOP than is needed in lightly pigmented eyes.[26]

Anticholinesterase Agents

Acetylcholinesterase hydrolyzes acetylcholine at neuroeffector junctions and neural synapses. The application of anticholinesterase agents allows the accumulation of endogenous acetylcholine in the junctional and synaptic clefts to induce muscarinic and nicotinic responses. Therefore, the pharmacologic actions of anticholinesterases are similar to those of acetylcholine, except the mechanism is indirect. In general, the ophthalmic effects of anticholinesterases are similar to those of direct-acting cholinergic agonists. Physostigmine, a natural anticholinesterase, has been used to treat glaucoma for over a century. In the earlier years of World War II, synthetic anticholinesterases, the organophosphates, were developed. The organophosphates are widely used as agricultural insecticides as well as in chemical warfare. According to the mode and duration of action, anticholinesterases can be classified into three classes (for their structural formulas, see Fig. 24–2).

ULTRA–SHORT-ACTING, REVERSIBLE ANTICHOLINESTERASES

Edrophonium inhibits acetylcholinesterase by an interaction between its quaternary nitrogen and the anionic site of acetylcholinesterase. The inhibition of acetylcholinesterase is short and reversible because of the formation of only an ionic bond and the rapid renal elimination of edrophonium. This agent is used in the diagnosis of myasthenia gravis. The test is performed in a patient with manifest skeletal muscle palsy. It consists of an intravenous injection of edrophonium. If edrophonium improves or eliminates the muscle palsy, the etiology is presumed to be myasthenia gravis.

SHORT-ACTING, REVERSIBLE ANTICHOLINESTERASES

Agents such as demecarium, physostigmine, and neostigmine have carbamyl ester linkages that form a covalent bond with the esteratic site of acetylcholinesterase. These agents serve as an alternate substrate for acetylcholinesterase. The alcohol moiety of these agents is cleaved away by the enzyme to form a carbamoyl acetylcholinesterase complex that is more stable than the acyl acetylcholinesterase complex when the substrate is acetylcholine. The formation of a carbamoyl acetylcholinesterase complex lasts for hours. Therefore, after treatment with these anticholinesterases, less free acetylcholinesterase is available, and endogenous acetylcholine is hydrolyzed at a much slower rate for several hours.

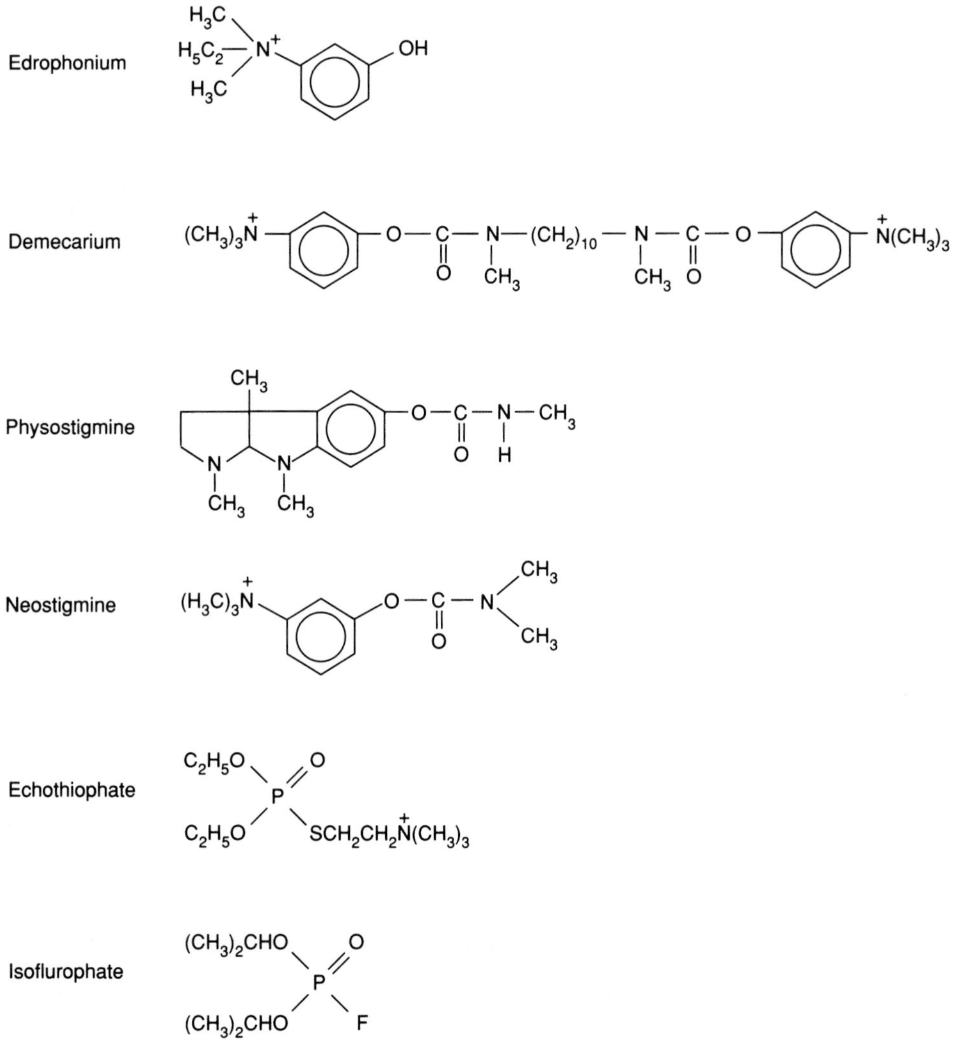

Edrophonium

Demecarium

Physostigmine

Neostigmine

Echothiophate

Isoflurophate

FIGURE 24–2. Structural formulas of anticholinesterases.

LONG-ACTING, IRREVERSIBLE ANTICHOLINESTERASES

These are organophosphorus compounds that bind with the esteratic site of acetylcholinesterase irreversibly. The substrate-enzyme complex is extremely stable and lasts for days to weeks. Return of the enzyme activity depends on the synthesis of new acetylcholinesterase. Echothiophate and isoflurophate are useful long-acting anticholinesterases in clinical ophthalmology.

In addition to their effects on acetylcholinesterase, physostigmine and quaternary ammonium anticholinesterases have direct actions at some cholinergic receptors, either as agonists or as antagonists. The pharmacologic basis of anticholinesterase agents is, nevertheless, the prevention of the hydrolysis of acetylcholine. Preparations of anticholinesterases are used in clinical conditions in the eye, gastrointestinal tract, and skeletal muscle. Elevated IOP in glaucoma patients can be reduced with physostigmine, demecarium, echothiophate, or isoflurophate. When applied to the eye, anticholinesterases cause conjunctival hyperemia, miosis, and a block of accommodation. Long-term therapy with long-acting anticholinesterases may result in cataract development[27, 28] owing to the inhibition of cholinesterase in the lens.[29] Long-acting anticholinesterases are also frequently misused for homicidal and suicidal purposes.

An overdose of anticholinesterase may produce excessive stimulation of cholinergic receptors throughout the body. Symptoms include muscle weakness, hypersalivation, sweating, nausea, vomiting, abdominal pain, urinary incontinence, diarrhea, bradycardia, severe hypotension, and bronchospasm. Muscarinic antagonists, such as atropine, can be used for symptomatic treatment. Intoxication by organophosphorus compounds is long-lasting and should be treated immediately with pralidoxime. Pralidoxime reactivates the bound acetylcholinesterase and inactivates free organophosphorus compounds in the plasma. Organophosphorus compounds also produce chronic axonal degeneration and demyelination owing to the inhibition of neurotoxic esterase, which is difficult to treat.[30]

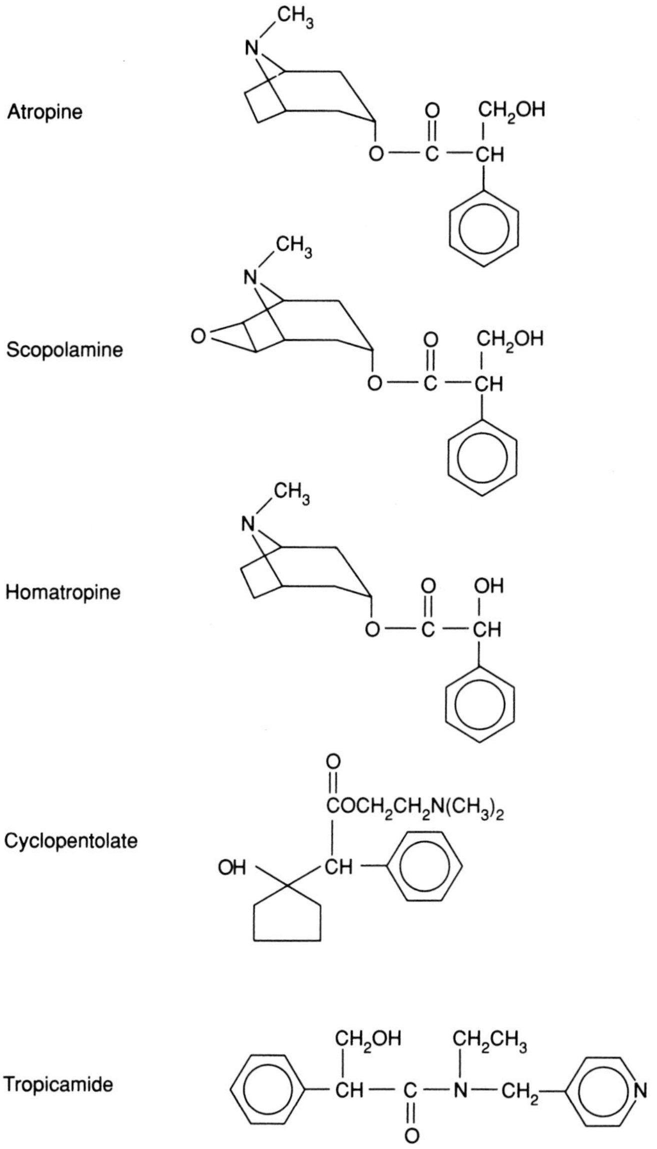

Atropine

Scopolamine

Homatropine

Cyclopentolate

Tropicamide

FIGURE 24–3. Structural formulas of muscarinic antagonists.

Muscarinic Cholinergic Antagonists

Cholinergic antagonists work at receptors to counteract the effect of acetylcholine or other cholinergic agonists. The antagonism may occur at the muscarinic receptors of neuroeffectors or nicotinic receptors of neuromuscular junctions and autonomic ganglia. The effects of cholinergic antagonists can be overcome by increasing the concentration of acetylcholine or agonists at the receptors. In practice, the term *cholinergic antagonist* generally refers to muscarinic antagonists only, because antinicotinic agents can be called neuromuscular blockers or ganglionic blockers. Except in very high concentrations, antimuscarinic (parasympatholytic) agents have little action at the neuromuscular junction. In sympathetic ganglia, which contain muscarinic subtype 1 receptors, antimuscarinic actions might cause significant effects.

Certain natural belladonna alkaloids, atropine and scopolamine (Fig. 24–3), are antimuscarinic agents. These agents are tertiary ammonium compounds that penetrate the blood-brain barrier well and can cause significant CNS actions. In therapeutic doses, atropine causes fewer CNS effects than scopolamine. Adding a methyl group to the nitrogen of these compounds creates quaternary ammonium compounds (methylatropine and methylscopolamine) with reduced permeability across the blood-brain barrier and, therefore, causes fewer CNS effects. However, these quaternary ammonium compounds have significant nicotinic-blocking activity. Homatropine is a semisynthetic antimuscarinic agent. Synthetic antimuscarinic agents, cyclopentolate and tropicamide, are structurally very different from belladonna alkaloids (see Fig. 24–3). These antimuscarinic agents have a short duration of action, which makes them ideal for pupillary dilation in ophthalmic diagnosis.

Antimuscarinic agents have been used in a wide variety of clinical conditions. Because these agents are not specific for selective muscarinic receptor subtypes, the systemic use of antimuscarinic agents is always accompanied by side effects. Patient compliance is poor during long-term therapy. Antimuscarinic agents are used topically as an aid in refraction, internal eye examination, and other diagnostic procedures; to produce mydriasis and cycloplegia before, during, and after intraocular surgery; and to treat anterior uveitis and some secondary glaucomas. Antimuscarinic agents cause mydriasis owing to the paralysis of the sphincter muscle of the iris. The pupillary light reflex disappears. The wide pupillary dilation may cause photophobia. Cycloplegia occurs owing to the paralysis of the ciliary muscle. Mydriasis generally occurs more rapidly than cycloplegia, persists longer, and can be obtained with lower drug concentrations. The mydriatic effect of atropine differs from the mydriasis caused by sympathetic agonists, which do not cause cycloplegia.

The normal systemic dose of atropine (0.6 mg) has little or no ocular effect. An equal dose of scopolamine causes miosis and cycloplegia. Atropine and scopolamine applied topically cause mydriasis and cycloplegia for a long period of time. Accommodation and pupillary reflex may not recover for several days up to 2 weeks. Homatropine, cyclopentolate, and tropicamide cause a shorter mydriasis and cycloplegia. If a complete, prolonged cycloplegia is needed, atropine and scopolamine are preferred rather than the synthetic compounds. When only mydriasis is desired, weaker compounds, such as cyclopentolate and tropicamide, are preferred. Mydriasis by the short-acting antimuscarinic agents can be counteracted by pilocarpine. Mydriasis due to atropine and scopolamine can be only partially reversed by pilocarpine or by anticholinesterases. After a short-term systemic treatment of antimuscarinic agents in glaucoma patients, an interference of aqueous humor outflow and an increase of IOP rarely occur owing to the relaxation of the ciliary muscle.[31] However, topical treatment or long-term systemic treatment may increase IOP in certain patients with open-angle glaucoma.[32] In patients with narrow-angle glaucoma treated with topical antimuscarinic agents, relaxation of the sphincter muscle may further decrease the angle and cause an acute glaucoma attack.

The belladonna alkaloids are easily absorbed through the gastrointestinal tract. Topical application of these alkaloids for ophthalmic examination can also cause significant systemic absorption via the nasolacrimal duct. Infants and children are more vulnerable to atropine intoxication after topical application. The quaternary ammonium derivatives of belladonna alkaloids are poorly absorbed through the gastrointestinal route but are still significantly absorbed after ocular applications. Some antihistamine agents may cause a similar intoxication owing to their antimuscarinic activities.

Cholinergic Agents Working at Neuromuscular Junctions and Ganglia

Nicotinic receptor subtypes at the neuromuscular junctions and autonomic ganglia can be distinguished by selective pharmacologic agents. Neuromuscular blockers (Fig. 24–4) react with nicotinic receptors at the neuromuscular junction and are classified into two categories: (1) Nondepolarizing blockers such as d-tubocurarine. These agents compete with endogenous acetylcholine for receptors. The normal neuromuscular transmission by acetylcholine is blocked without membrane depolarization. (2) Depolarizing blockers such as succinylcholine and decamethonium. These agents bind with nicotinic receptors and then open Na^+ channels, which

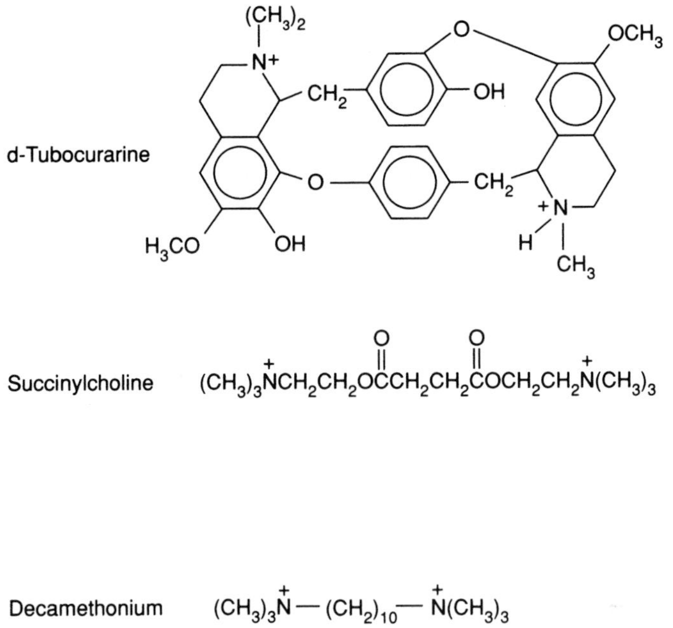

d-Tubocurarine

Succinylcholine $(CH_3)_3\overset{+}{N}CH_2CH_2OCCH_2CH_2COCH_2CH_2\overset{+}{N}(CH_3)_3$

Decamethonium $(CH_3)_3\overset{+}{N}-(CH_2)_{10}-\overset{+}{N}(CH_3)_3$

FIGURE 24–4. Structural formulas of neuromuscular blockers.

causes a membrane depolarization and a desensitization of membrane to neural transmission. The mechanism of action of neuromuscular blockers is different from that of botulinus toxin. Injection of botulinus toxin into the extraocular muscles to treat strabismus is based on the blockade of acetylcholine release at neuromuscular junctions.

The major clinical application of neuromuscular blockers is as an adjuvant in surgical anesthesia. Neuromuscular blockers relax skeletal muscles, including the extraocular muscles.[33] Rapidly moving muscle with a high degree of innervation is more easily affected by these agents. Therefore, the effect of systemic neuromuscular blockers would be observed in this sequence: eyelids, facial muscles, neck muscles, extremities, trunk, and diaphragm. The toxic symptoms produced by neuromuscular blockers are general muscle paralysis and respiratory failure. If intoxication occurs after the administration of the nondepolarizing neuromuscular blockers, anticholinesterase (such as neostigmine) can be used as an effective antidote. It should be noted that serum cholinesterases are responsible for the degradation of another neuromuscular blocker, succinylcholine. The effect of succinylcholine in paralyzing skeletal muscles may be enhanced with a topical administration of anticholinesterases.[34]

Two types of agents can stimulate cholinergic receptors at the autonomic ganglia. The first type of agents stimulate the muscarinic receptors at autonomic ganglia, and their effects can be blocked by atropine-like antimuscarinic agents. The second type of agents, such as nicotine (Fig. 24–5), stimulate nicotinic receptors at the ganglia. Their effects can be blocked by nondepolarizing ganglionic blockers that compete with stimulators for the nicotinic receptors. Ganglionic nicotinic stimulators are useful tools in research but have no clinical application. There are two types of clinically useful ganglionic blockers. The first type of blockers, such as hexamethonium and trimethaphan (see Fig. 24–5), cause no ganglionic stimulation and no membrane potential change.

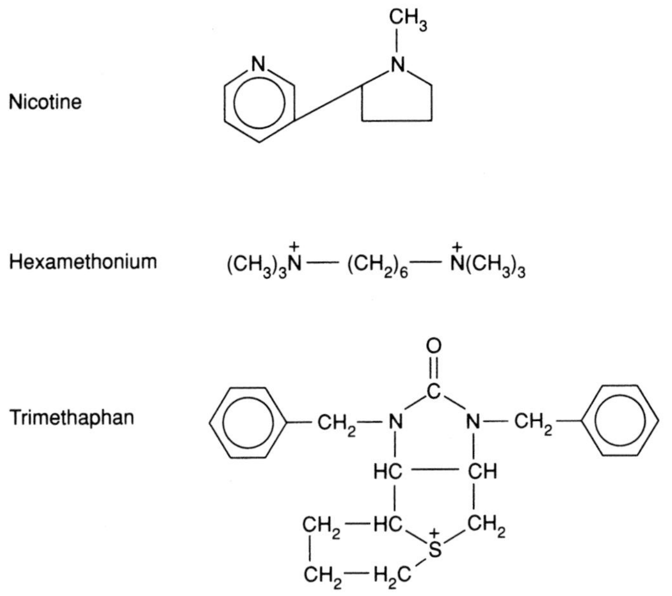

Nicotine

Hexamethonium $(CH_3)_3\overset{+}{N}—(CH_2)_6—\overset{+}{N}(CH_3)_3$

Trimethaphan

FIGURE 24–5. Structural formulas of ganglionic stimulator and blockers.

They either compete with acetylcholine for nicotinic receptors or block the opened ion channels. The second type of blockers impair neural transmission with initial stimulation of the nicotinic receptors and then blockade by persistent depolarization. A prolonged application of nicotine may result in desensitization of the nicotinic receptors by this mechanism.

The major clinical use of ganglionic blockers is in the control of certain systemic hypertensions and autonomic hyperreflexia. This therapy may be accompanied by serious side effects, because a large number of autonomic ganglia are affected. After systemic administration of ganglionic blockers, mydriasis and cycloplegia may appear, because the predominant autonomic tone at the iris and ciliary muscle is parasympathetic. Ganglionic blockers have no specific application in clinical ophthalmology.

REFERENCES

1. Shaffer RN: Autonomic ocular drugs: Desirable and undesirable effects. Invest Ophthalmol 3:498, 1964.
2. Grant WM: Toxicology of the Eye, 2nd ed. Springfield, IL, Charles C Thomas, 1974.
3. Kaufman PL, Wiedman T, Robinson JR: Cholinergics. *In* Sears ML (ed): Pharmacology of the Eye. Handbook of Experimental Pharmacology, vol 69. Berlin, Springer-Verlag, 1984, pp 149–191.
4. AMA Drug Evaluations, 6th ed. Chicago, American Medical Association, 1986, pp 327–368.
5. Leopold IH, Duzman E: Observations on the pharmacology of glaucoma. Annu Rev Pharmacol Toxicol 26:401, 1986.
6. Tucek S: Choline acetyltransferase and the synthesis of acetylcholine. *In* Whittaker VP (ed): The Cholinergic Synapse. Handbook of Experimental Pharmacology, vol 86. Berlin, Springer-Verlag, 1988, pp 125–165.
7. Guyton AC: The autonomic nervous system; the adrenal medulla. *In* Guyton AC (ed): Textbook of Medical Physiology, 8th ed. Philadelphia, WB Saunders, 1991, pp 667–678.
8. Mindel JS, Mittag TW: Choline acetyltransferase in ocular tissues of rabbits, cats, cattle, and man. Invest Ophthalmol 15:808, 1976.
9. Mindel JS, Mittag TW: Variability of choline acetyltransferase in ocular tissues of rabbits, cats, cattle and humans. Exp Eye Res 24:25, 1977.
10. Lefkowitz RJ, Hoffman BB, Taylor P: Drugs actions at synaptic and neuroeffector junctional sites. *In* Gilman AG, Rall TW, Nies AS, Taylor P (eds): Goodman and Gilman's The Pharmacological Basis of Therapeutics, 8th ed. New York, Pergamon, 1990, pp 84–121.
11. Dale HH: The beginnings and the prospects of neurohumoral transmission. Pharmacol Rev 6:7, 1954.
12. Bonner TI: New subtypes of muscarinic acetylcholine receptors. *In* Levine RR, Birdsall NJM (eds): Subtypes of Muscarinic Receptors IV. Cambridge, Elsevier, 1989, pp 11–15.
13. Libet B: Generation of slow inhibitory and excitatory postsynaptic potentials. Fed Proc 29:1945, 1970.
14. Weight FF, Schulman JA, Smith PA, et al: Long-lasting synaptic potentials and the modulation of synaptic transmission. Fed Proc 38:2084, 1979.
15. Scott AB: Botulinum toxin injection into extraocular muscles as an alternative to strabismus surgery. Ophthalmology 87:1044, 1980.
16. Watson S, Abbott A: Receptor nomenclature supplement. *In* Trends in Pharmacological Sciences. Cambridge, Elsevier, 1990, p 18.
17. Taylor P: Cholinergic agonists. *In* Gilman AG, Rall TW, Nies AS, Taylor P (eds): Goodman and Gilman's The Pharmacological Basis of Therapeutics, 8th ed. New York, Pergamon, 1990, pp 122–130.
18. Van Buskirk EM, Grant WM: Lens depression and aqueous outflow in enucleated primate eyes. Am J Ophthalmol 76:632, 1973.
19. Dartt DA: Signal transduction and control of lacrimal gland protein secretion: A review. Curr Eye Res 8:619, 1989.
20. Mircheff AK: Lacrimal fluid and electrolyte secretion: A review. Curr Eye Res 8:607, 1989.
21. Rizzuti AB: Acetylcholine in surgery of the lens, iris and cornea. Am J Ophthalmol 63:484, 1967.
22. Beasley H: Miotics in cataract surgery. Trans Am Ophthalmol Soc 69:237, 1971.
23. Erickson-Lamy K, Schroeder A: Dissociation between the effect of aceclidine on outflow facility and accommodation. Exp Eye Res 50:143, 1990.
24. Beasley H, Fraunfelder FT: Retinal detachments and topical ocular miotics. Ophthalmology 86:95, 1979.
25. Nardin GF, Zimmerman TJ, Zalta AH, et al: Ocular cholinergic agents. *In* Ritch R, Shields MB, Krupin T (eds): The Glaucomas. St Louis, CV Mosby, 1989, pp 515–521.
26. Harris LS, Galin MA: Effect of ocular pigmentation on hypotensive response to pilocarpine. Am J Ophthalmol 72:923, 1971.
27. de Roetth A: Lens opacities in glaucoma patients on phospholine iodide therapy. Am J Ophthalmol 62:619, 1966.
28. Van Buskirk EM: Hazards of medical glaucoma therapy in the cataract patient. Ophthalmology 89:238, 1982.
29. Michon J Jr, Kinoshita JH: Cholinesterase in the lens. Arch Ophthalmol 77:804, 1967.
30. Abou-Donia MB: Organophosphorus ester-induced delayed neurotoxicity. Annu Rev Pharmacol Toxicol 21:511, 1981.
31. Lazenby GW, Reed JW, Grant WM: Short-term tests of anticholinergic medication in open-angle glaucoma. Arch Ophthalmol 80:443, 1968.
32. Lazenby GW, Reed JW, Grant WM: Anticholinergic medication in open-angle glaucoma: Long term tests. Arch Ophthalmol 84:719, 1970.
33. Burde RM. The extraocular muscles: Anatomy, physiology, and pharmacology. *In* Moses RA (ed): Adler's Physiology of the Eye. St Louis, CV Mosby, 1981, pp 84–121.
34. Gerber SL, Cantor LB, Brater DC: Systemic drug interactions with topical glaucoma medications. Surv Ophthalmol 35:205, 1990.

CHAPTER 25

Corticosteroids in Ophthalmic Practice

Mark B. Abelson and Salim Butrus

Corticosteroids (glucocorticoids and mineralocorticoids) are 21-carbon structures that are synthesized by adrenocorticotropic hormone (ACTH)-controlled conversion of cholesterol in the adrenal cortex. They can take the form of cortisol, cortisone, corticosterone, or aldosterone. They can also exist in synthetic forms such as prednisone, methylprednisolone, dexamethasone, triamcinolone, betamethasone, medrysone, fluorometholone (FML), and others.

Historically, in 1930 Swingle, Pfiffner, Hartman, and coworkers prepared adrenocortical extracts that had a reasonable degree of activity. In 1935, Kendall first isolated and characterized cortisone in the laboratory. In 1942, Reichstein and Shoppee identified the chemical and crystalline structure of steroids.[1] The first advantageous clinical result of steroids was reported by Hench and coworkers in 1949.[2] They observed the dramatic effects of cortisone and ACTH in the treatment of rheumatoid arthritis and subsequently provoked the interest of many investigators with remarkable therapeutic applications that extended to other diseases.

In 1954, Stone and Hechter established that ACTH actually controls the enzymatic conversion of cholesterol to steroids in the adrenal cortex through cleavage of the side chain of the cholesterol molecule.[3] Later, Haynes took a further step by demonstrating that this conversion is mediated by adenosine 3′,5′-cyclic monophosphate (cAMP).[4, 5]

Corticosteroids and ACTH were first introduced into ocular therapy by Gordon and McLean in 1950. It was not until 1951, with the introduction of topical and systemic use of cortisone, that cortisone acetate was prepared as drops; ointment; and subconjunctival, retrobulbar, and anterior chamber injection formulations. In 1952, ocular penetration studies of steroids started to surface. By that time, modification of chemical structures of cortisone and hydrocortisone led to a series of compounds with better penetration and bioavailability and more potent antiinflammatory effects. In 1959, 0.1% Decadron eye drops were introduced for treating ocular inflammation.[6] In 1956, it became clear that inflammation in anterior ocular structures is best treated with steroid drops and posterior uveitis by oral therapy. It was quickly recognized that topical therapy minimized systemic side effects, but its ocular side effects began to be appreciated.

Chemical Properties and Structure-Activity Relationships

Cortisone, the first steroid used therapeutically for antiinflammatory effect, is a 21-carbon four-ringed structure (Fig. 25–1). Modification of this structure at different sites changes its biologic potency, transcorneal penetration, and, thus, effectiveness and side effects.[5]

Different sites of alterations (see Fig. 25–1) result in different antiinflammatory potency and duration of action of these different compounds (Table 25–1). These modifications and alterations can be summarized as follows:

1. Prednisone and prednisolone have, in addition to the basic nucleus, a 1,2 double bond in ring A (see Fig. 25–1*B*). This modification increases their carbohydrate-regulating potency and prolongs their metabolism compared with cortisol.
2. Methylation of carbon 6 in ring B leads to 6 α-methyl prednisolone. This compound has slightly greater antiinflammatory effect than prednisolone.
3. Fluorination at a 9 α position in ring B, as in fluorocortisone (9 α-fluorocortisol) enhances its antiinflammatory property.
4. 11-Desoxycortisol has an oxygen function at the c-11 site of ring C, augmenting its antiinflammatory activity.
5. Methylation or hydroxylation at site 16 in ring D eliminates the sodium-retaining effects and has only a slight effect on the antiinflammatory potency.
6. In ring D, 17α-hydroxylation is present in most of the antiinflammatory steroids.

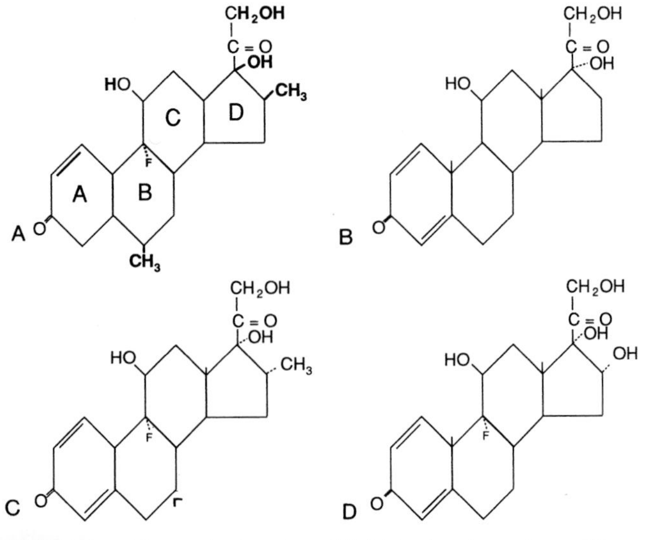

FIGURE 25–1. The cortisol nucleus *(A)*. Note the sites where different chemical groups are added to form compounds with different antiinflammatory potency. Prednisolone *(B)*; dexamethasone *(C)*; triamcinolone *(D)*.

TABLE 25–1. **Classification of Glucocorticoids**

Natural Steroids	Biologic Half-Life (hr)	Antiinflammatory Effect
Cortisol	8–12	1
Cortisone	8–12	0.8
Corticosterone	8–12	0.3
Synthetic steroids		
Prednisone	12–36	4
Prednisolone	12–36	4
6-Methylprednisolone	12–36	5
Triamcinolone	12–36	5
9-Fluorocortisol	12–36	10
Paramethasone	36–72	10
Betamethasone	36–72	25
Dexamethasone	36–72	25

7. Most of the active synthetic analogs and all natural corticosteroids have the hydroxyl group attached to carbon 21 in ring D.

Mechanism of Action, Site of Activity, and Ophthalmic Indications

Corticosteroids have numerous effects on many stages of inflammation and arms of the immune response. Despite widespread use, their precise mechanism of action is not well understood. There is consensus that they work at two levels: molecular and cellular. At the molecular level corticosteroids freely penetrate cell membranes and bind to a specific steroid-binding protein receptor in the cytoplasm, forming a steroid-receptor complex. [7–18] This complex then moves into the nucleus and binds to chromatin, signaling the production of messenger RNA and coding for enzymes and proteins that determine the response of that particular cell to the hormone (Fig. 25–2).[5, 19] The cytoplasmic steroid-binding receptor has binding sites that exhibit high affinity for glucocorticoids, such as natural occurring cortisol and corticosterone, and synthetic corticosteroids, such as prednisolone, dexamethasone, and triamcinolone.[20] In contrast, these receptors have a low affinity for estrogens, androgens, cortisone, and prednisone. Hence, cortisone and prednisone are inactive compounds that are activated when transformed to cortisol and prednisolone. Glucocorticoid receptors have been identified in the iris, ciliary body, cornea, sclera, trabecular meshwork, and Schlemm's canal.[21–23]

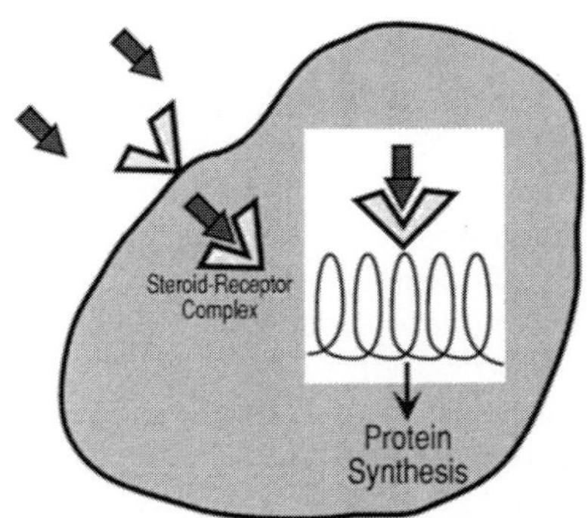

FIGURE 25–2. Binding of corticosteroid to a receptor and subsequent entry into the cell cytoplasm and nucleus. This leads to the synthesis of specific proteins and specific target cell responses.

These molecular and cellular changes result in steroid-induced inhibition of all the cardinal signs of inflammation, such as pain, heat, redness, and edema.[13, 24] This is achieved through inhibition of: (1) leukocyte chemotaxis, (2) production of potent chemical mediators, and (3) function of immunocompetent cells. Corticosteroids have the dual characteristics of being both antiinflammatory and immunosuppressant.[25] They accomplish their antiinflammatory activity through the following mechanisms:

1. Constriction of blood vessels and reduction of vascular permeability induced by acute inflammation. This minimizes leakage into the target site of fluid, proteins, and inflammatory cells.[26]
2. Stabilization of intracellular lysosomal membranes and inhibition of the expression of various damaging enzymes; inhibition of polymorphonuclear (PMN) cell degranulation is also significantly inhibited.
3. Stabilization of mast cell and basophil membranes is important in inhibiting the process of degranulation and subsequent release of histamine (vasoactive amines), bradykinin, platelet-activating factor (PAF), proteases, and eosinophilic chemotactic factors (ECF).
4. Mobilization of PMNs from the bone marrow results in neutrophilic leukocytosis (Fig. 25–3).[27] Corticosteroids simultaneously prevent adherence of PMNs to the vascular endothelium, making them less mobile and less accessible to the site of inflammation.[28]
5. Suppression of lymphocyte proliferation and lymphopenia. In small- to moderate-sized doses, corticoste-

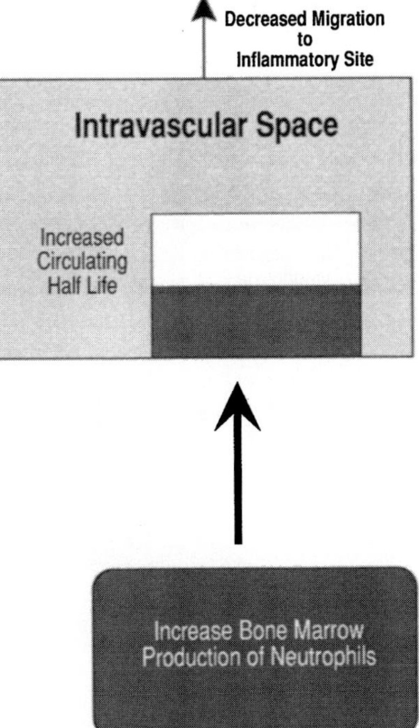

FIGURE 25–3. Schematic effects of corticosteroids on bone marrow and circulating neutrophils. (Adapted from Nussenblatt RB, Palestine AG: Uveitis: Fundamentals and Clinical Practice. Chicago, Year Book, 1989.)

roids more significantly affect T lymphocytes. In larger doses, B lymphocytes are affected as well, and, thus, antibody production. Corticosteroids do not destroy T lymphocytes but rather affect their redistribution into circulation, concentrating them in the bone marrow (Fig. 25–4).[29–31]

6. Reduction of circulating eosinophils and monocytes.
7. Inhibition of macrophage recruitment and migration.[32, 33] Steroids also interfere with the ability of macrophages to process antigens.
8. Suppression of fibroplasia.[34]
9. Depression of the bactericidal activity of monocytes and macrophages.
10. Via a protein called macrocortin, steroids inhibit phospholipase A_2, resulting in inhibition of arachidonic acid degradation and subsequent synthesis of prostaglandins and leukotrienes by cyclooxygenase and lipoxygenase pathways (Fig. 25–5).[35–39]

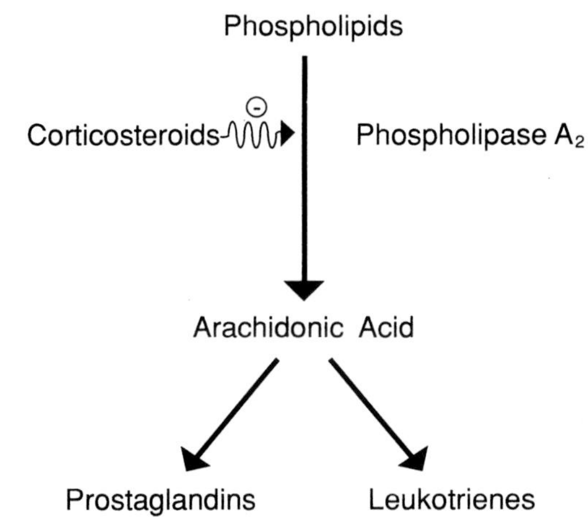

FIGURE 25–5. Corticosteroids prevent formation of prostaglandins and leukotrienes through inhibition of phospholipase A_2 and release of arachidonic acid.

Absorption, Rate, and Excretion After Ophthalmic Delivery

Corticosteroids are readily absorbed by the cornea, conjunctiva, and sclera. Corneal penetration is a limiting factor for their antiinflammatory effect. The penetration of corticosteroids through the normal cornea is a complex process in which multiple factors determine the rate of penetration. In general, these factors are similar to those governing penetration (i.e., relative water- and lipid solubility).[40, 41] Other factors include viscosity, concentration, hydrogen ion concentration (pH), tonicity, condition of the corneal epithelium, size of particles in suspension, and addition of other compounds or vehicles, such as preservatives or methylcellulose. Part of the topically applied corticosteroid can go through the upper and lower puncti and then through the nasal mucosal blood vessels into the circulation, where it binds to globulin and albumin. Eighty percent of circulating cortisol is bound to α-globulin as transcortin (corticosteroid-binding globulin), an inactive transport complex. A smaller portion is bound to albumin, and this portion can diffuse into the extravascular fluid and bathe tissue cells. Synthetic analogs of cortisol do not compete with it for binding to transcortin. In addition, synthetic analogs are less bound to albumin, enabling them to diffuse more completely into the extravascular tissue than cortisol.[25]

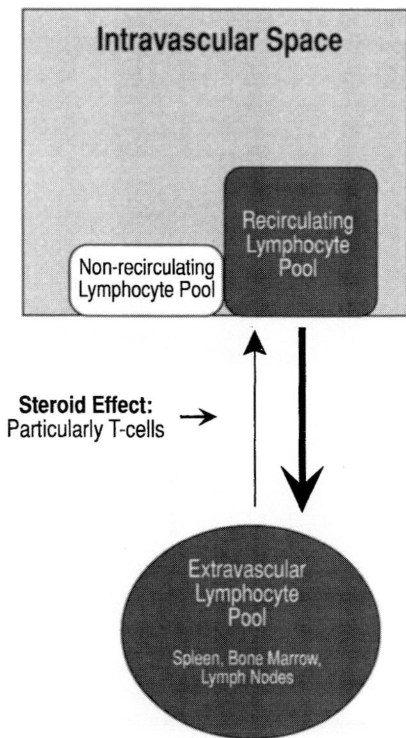

FIGURE 25–4. Schematic effects of corticosteroids on lymphocytes. (Adapted from Nussenblatt RB, Palestine AG: Uveitis: Fundamentals and Clinical Practice. Chicago, Year Book, 1989.)

Tritiated dexamethasone applied topically to rabbit eyes was traced and found in plasma, kidneys, urine, and liver. Systemic absorption of topical dexamethasone phosphate is considerable: as much as 20 to 35% of the drug was found systemically in rabbits 24 hours after instillation.[42, 43] Reduction of the double bond in the 1,5 position in the liver and kidney renders the corticosteroid inactive. All synthetic analogs of cortisol are metabolized more slowly by the liver, owing to chemical modifications of the steroid molecule (see Fig. 25–1) and the rapid equilibration in blood and peripheral tissues.

Pharmacokinetics

Four factors regarding ophthalmic corticosteroids must be considered[20]: (1) ocular penetration of the corticosteroid through the cornea; (2) antiinflammatory potency, topically and once in the aqueous humor; (3) duration of action; and (4) side effects. Different routes by which corticosteroids are delivered into the eye include topical, periocular, oral, parenteral, and intravitreal.

The penetration of corticosteroids is dependent on the cornea and on the physical and chemical properties of the corticosteroid. The ideal steroid should be biphasic in polarity, because the cornea contains both hydrophobic and hydrophilic layers.[44] Removal of the corneal epithelium reduces the hydrophobic properties and allows greater penetration by hydrophilic preparations. Particle size may also affect the bioavailability of corticosteroids.[45, 46] Results suggest that ophthalmic dexamethasone suspensions can be optimized for bioavailability by using suspensions with the smallest particle possible. Particle size for prednisolone acetate (<5 μm and 5 to 10 μm in diameter), however, did not affect the degree of corneal penetration. Both fractions of prednisolone acetate achieved comparable levels in the aqueous humor.

Topical preparations can take the form of solutions, suspensions, or ointments. Phosphate and hydrochloride preparations are relatively hydrophilic and thus are water soluble. Acetate and alcohol derivatives are hydrophobic and fat soluble. Alcohol preparations possess intermediate hydrophobicity between phosphates and acetates.[47] Owing to the respective polarities, phosphates are generally formulated as solutions, whereas acetates are generally formulated as suspensions and ointments. Acetates, owing to their hydrophobic nature, appear to penetrate the cornea to a greater extent than do phosphates.[48–51]

Corticosteroids can also be released from a drug depot placed on the ocular surface or by iontophoresis. Examples of drug depots are cotton pledgets[52] and collagen shields.[53] One advantage of drug depots is the steady, sustained, and slow release of the corticosteroid over the ocular surface.

Dexamethasone phosphate penetrates into the cornea and aqueous humor within 10 minutes. It reaches a peak within 30 to 60 minutes and remains inside the eye from several hours to 24 hours.[42] The corneal tissue concentration of tritiated dexamethasone alcohol (Maxidex) reaches 14.79 μg/g of cornea 7.5 minutes after instillation, then declines to 1.86 μg/g at 4 hours.[54]

One-percent prednisolone phosphate (Inflamase) is a highly soluble compound with limited lipid solubility. Thus, it traditionally was thought that this compound had limited solubility through an intact cornea. Its corneal level, however, reaches 10 μg/g, while the aqueous humor concentration reaches 0.5 μg/g 30 minutes after instillation. When the corneal epithelium is removed, the corneal concentration reaches 235 μg/g and in aqueous humor 17 μg/g.[55]

It has been shown that 1.1% tritiated dexamethasone phosphate instilled into rabbit eyes reaches the aqueous humor. Its major metabolite in the anterior chamber is 9α-fluoro-11β-hydroxy-16α-methyl-1,4-androstadiene-3,17-dione. Ocular penetration of corticosteroids is better when they are injected subconjunctivally than when they are instilled. Hydroxycortisone is found in the anterior chamber almost immediately after subconjunctival injection. Its degree of penetration is not related to external factors such as lid movements or tear volume. It is usually injected near the site of inflammation to obtain maximal antiinflammatory benefits.

Antiinflammatory Effects of Topical Ophthalmic Corticosteroids

Any attempt to compare the inflammatory potency of different ophthalmic corticosteroids should take into account these following considerations: (1) type of corticosteroid, (2) formulation, (3) concentration, and (4) what model of inflammation is used. Models of ocular inflammation in animals and humans are difficult to design and standardize, and some do not reflect clinical action in humans. Furthermore, some current data on corticosteroids have been extrapolated from previous studies conducted on organ systems other than the eye.[56]

Studies by Leibowitz, Kupferman, and Cox involved measuring decreased radioactivity of radiolabeled neutrophils in a rabbit keratitis model induced by injection of clove oil.[57–67] This research focused on the comparison of the sodium phosphate, alcohol, and acetate derivatives of dexamethasone and prednisolone (Table 25–2). Data indicated that after a given period, corneal drug concentration administered with the corneal epithelium intact was highest with prednisolone acetate, followed by prednisolone sodium phosphate and dexamethasone alcohol suspension; no dexamethasone sodium phosphate was absorbed. With a denuded epithelium the highest concentration was achieved with the prednisolone sodium phosphate solution, followed by the dexamethasone sodium phosphate solution, prednisolone acetate, and last, the dexamethasone alcohol suspension. With intact and denuded epithelium, the drug concentrations in the aqueous humor followed the same pattern. The results with denuded epithelium may more accurately represent the clinical situation in keratitis.[57–60]

With an intact epithelium but in the presence of intraocular inflammation (i.e., experimentally induced anterior or posterior uveitis), prednisolone acetate concentration *in the cornea* was highest with the sodium phosphate solutions of prednisolone and dexamethasone equivalent, and was least with the dexamethasone acetate and alcohol. Concentrations of prednisolone acetate suspension and the sodium phosphate solution were equivalent in the aqueous humor in the eye inflamed with uveitis, followed by the dexamethasone solution, and last, the dexamethasone alcohol suspension. Thus, with *intraocular* inflammation, for which the highest concentration of drug is most desirable in the aqueous humor, it is interesting that there was no difference between the prednisolone acetate suspension and the sodium phosphate solution.[64]

Leibowitz and Kupferman also evaluated these steroid derivatives for antiinflammatory potency in a model of corneal inflammation. A significant increase in antiinflammatory effect was noted with prednisolone acetate compared with

TABLE 25–2. **Comparison of Different Topical Corticosteroids in Suppressing Rabbit Corneal Inflammation**

Corneal Epithelium Intact	% Decrease	Corneal Epithelium Absent	% Decrease
Prednisolone acetate 1%	51	Prednisolone acetate 1%	53
Dexamethasone alcohol 0.1%	40	Dexamethasone alcohol 0.1%	42
Prednisolone sodium phosphate 1%	28	Prednisolone sodium phosphate 1%	47
Fluoromethalone alcohol 0.1%	31	Fluorometholone alcohol 0.1%	37
Dexamethasone sodium phosphate 0.1%	19	Dexamethasone sodium phosphate 0.1%	22
Dexamethasone sodium phosphate ointment 0.05%	13		

the sodium phosphate solution when evaluated with the corneal epithelium intact. When the corneal epithelium was absent there was no significant difference between the two[64, 66] or dexamethasone alcohol. Thus, when a break in the corneal epithelium is associated with corneal inflammation, the greater absorption of the sodium phosphate solution equilibrates their relative potency. The dexamethasone sodium phosphate solution was clearly significantly inferior with the epithelium intact or absent.[64, 66]

Changing the concentration and dosing frequency of a particular steroid obviously changes its antiinflammatory potency. Increasing the concentration of prednisolone acetate from 0.125 to 1% produces a significant increase in its corneal concentration[58] and antiinflammatory effectiveness.[63, 64] However, if the concentration of prednisolone acetate is increased from 1% to 2 or 3%, the corneal concentration is elevated but antiinflammatory potency is not affected.[67]

The concentrations in the cornea and aqueous humor of the corticosteroid, and thus their antiinflammatory potency, depend to a large extent on the frequency of instillation. For example, hourly instillation of 1% prednisolone acetate produces much more effective suppression of corneal inflammation than does instillation every 4 hours.[65] Maximum suppression is obtained if the drug is instilled every 5 minutes (Table 25–3).[65]

The ocular bioavailability of topical prednisolone preparations has been further investigated. One criticism of the clove oil model used by Leibowitz and others is that the oil alters the absorption of water-soluble drugs in favor of water-insoluble drugs because of the oil barrier in the stroma after injection. A pharmacokinetic model of absorption of water-insoluble drugs, such as prednisolone acetate, and water-soluble drugs, such as prednisolone phosphate, was used to compare the drug elimination rate in the precornea and anterior chamber, the rate of drug dissolution, the rate of drug penetration in the cornea, and the rate of drug transport into the aqueous humor. In this mathematical model the two forms of prednisolone had similar absorption capacity.[55] Similar bioavailability was also found in a rabbit eye model in vivo when prednisolone phosphate, acetate, and their metabolite, prednisolone, were directly quantitated in aqueous humor by reverse-phase high-performance liquid chromatography (HPLC).[68, 69]

In light of the fact that the acetate and phosphate forms may actually be equivalent under optimal conditions of dissolution, the drawbacks of using a suspension in clinical practice may be the deciding factor in determining which is superior. Suspensions need to be shaken, and if particles are not evenly distributed, incorrect doses may be removed from the bottle. Patient compliance for shaking suspension eyedrops has been reported to be poor.[70] The risks of incorrect dosing and sudden cessation of steroid administration are well known.[71, 72] The difficulty of predicting a steroid concentration in suspension drops suggests that the consistent dosing provided by solutions may be superior.

TABLE 25–3. **Dosage Schedules and Antiinflammatory Effectiveness of Topical Prednisolone Acetate 1%**

Regimen	Total Doses Delivered (No.)	Decrease in Corneal Inflammation (%)
1 drop q 4 hr	6	11
1 drop q 2 hr	10	30
1 drop q 1 hr	18	51
1 drop q 30 min	34	61
1 drop q 15 min	66	68
1 drop each eye for 5 min every hr	90	72

Two weaker topical corticosteroids are also available for ocular use. FML, 0.1 and 0.25% suspensions, has much less corneal penetration[73] than prednisolone but does have moderate antiinflammatory effects.[74] Surprisingly, the lower concentration of 0.1% FML acetate has a therapeutic effect comparable to 1% prednisolone in alleviating corneal (but not intraocular) inflammation. Lower ocular levels are required to produce a substantial therapeutic effect in the cornea. FML has mildly hydrophilic properties, concentrating in the corneal epithelial layer and reaching saturation levels before passing on through the hydrophilic layers of the stroma. This may explain why FML penetrates the cornea in comparatively low concentrations, yet produces moderate but effective suppression of corneal inflammation.[74]

Medrysone (HMS) is another relatively weak corticosteroid. It comes in a 1% suspension and, owing to its weak effect on the cornea, is used only for minor conjunctival inflammation.

Loteprednol etabonate is a newly formulated steroid that may offer the therapeutic benefits of the existing steroid agents, but with minimum side effects. Hence, it is called a "soft drug." Its molecular structure is a modification of prednisolone (see Fig. 25–1*B*), where a labile ester function occupies the 17-position and a stable carbonate group occupies the 17-position. The "soft drug" undergoes rapid hydrolysis in the anterior chamber to the inactive 17-carboxylic acid derivative after it penetrates the cornea.[75] In animals it was shown to retain its antiinflammatory effects in the cornea,[76] and in one study in humans it was shown to be useful in treating giant papillary conjunctivitis.[77]

Rimexolone is another "soft steroid" with decreased propensity to raise IOP.[78] The corticosteroid is indicated for the treatment of postoperative inflammation following cataract surgery and for treatment of anterior uveitis, and is commercially available as a 1% ophthalmic suspension (Vexol). In a study consisting of 197 patients who had undergone cataract extraction, rimexolone 1% was significantly more effective than placebo in reducing postoperative inflammation.[79] The degree of improvement with rimexolone was comparable to that of bethamethasone.[80] Rimexolone did not induce any clinically significant side effects. Rimexolone has also been shown to reduce the signs and symptoms associated with allergic conjunctivitis.[81] The ocular hypotensive effect of rimexolone 1% has been shown to be comparable to that of FML alcohol 0.1%, but less than that of dexamethasone phosphate 0.1% and prednisolone acetate 1%.

Corticosteroids are also available as ointment. Although ointments increase contact time between the drug and the ocular surface, it has been shown that dexamethasone phosphate ointment allows less drug absorption in the cornea and anterior chamber than the solution form. This may be because the ointment forms a barrier, preventing rapid release of the drug into the tears.[66] In the case of FML, it was shown that FML crystals suspended in water or ointment both produced similar concentrations of drug in the aqueous humor, possibly because the tear film is oversaturated by microcrystals of the dissolved drug.[82] Corticosteroids may also be injected into parts of the eye. Supratarsal injection of corticosteroids has been investigated to treat refractory vernal keratoconjunctivitis.[83] All patients experienced dramatic symptomatic relief within 1 to 5 days, regardless of type of corticosteroid injected.

Ophthalmic Indications for Corticosteroid Therapy[84]

Since corticosteroids were first reported effective in the treatment of rheumatoid arthritis 40 years ago, they have become the most widely used antiinflammatory and immunosuppressant agents in medicine and ophthalmology. It is estimated that more than 5 million patients are treated with corticosteroids yearly. The antiinflammatory and antiallergic activity of corticosteroids are the most important reason for their clinical use in ocular disease. Table 25–4 lists the ophthalmic indications for corticosteroid treatment as primary or adjunctive therapy. Some of these indications are isolated inflammatory conditions and some are part of a multisystem process. It must be remembered that the antiinflammatory and immunosuppressive qualities of corticosteroids are nonspecific, palliative, and never curative.

The use of steroids in clinical ophthalmic practice may be divided into three classes of therapy: (1) posttraumatic control of inflammation after surgery; (2) abnormalities of excessive immunoreactivity; and (3) for diseases that have combined immune and infectious processes. Control of postoperative inflammation is certainly the indication for which steroids are used most. While the effect is clinically appreciated, it is interesting to note that no well-controlled double-blind study has actually shown the efficacy of steroids postoperatively. For this reason, the optimal dosing regimen has not been established.

The second group of conditions for which steroids are used is disorders of immune hyperreactivity. The immune system can cause damage with overzealous defense mechanisms which can lead to permanent tissue impairment. These disorders include iritis, posterior uveitis, immune infiltrates, allergic disorders, such as allergic conjunctivitis, atopic and vernal keratoconjunctivitis, and graft rejection.

The third class of disorders treated with steroids may originate with an infectious process. Disorders such as disciform herpes and bacterial corneal ulcers are treated very cautiously and judiciously with steroids, whereas the infection is treated or controlled with antibiotics. It must be recognized that even in the absence of an infectious agent, whenever complete immunosuppression is established by the use of steroids, prophylactic antimicrobial therapy should be considered. The sensitivity of treating such serious problems with steroids must be emphasized, because often only certain phases of these diseases respond to steroids, and in other phases steroids may be contraindicated. For a complete discussion of medical treatments the reader should refer to specific diseases.

In general, steroids are at first administered in medium-size or large doses to adequately suppress inflammation. The dose is then tapered gradually to prevent rebound inflammation. Often the physician can gain insight into the amount and severity of inflammation by observing the patient's response to steroids.

The potential usefulness of prophylactic therapy with steroids or of a loading, pretreatment period needs to be established. These are commonly recommended courses of treatment with systemic steroids. We have shown in the allergen challenge model that a 48-hour loading period was needed to achieve efficacy in inhibiting the signs and symptoms of ocular allergy.[85] Loading periods are considered the standard for nonsteroidal antiinflammatory agents, yet steroids are not commonly used like this in the perioperative period. Further investigation is needed to clarify this issue.

TABLE 25–4. **Some Indications for the Use of Corticosteroids in Ocular Disease**

Conjunctivitis	*Uvea*
Allergic (hay fever, vernal, atopic GPC)	Iridocyclitis
	Posterior uveitis
Viral (EKC, herpes zoster)	Sympathetic ophthalmia
Chemical burns	Vogt-Koyanagi-Harada syndrome
Cicatricial pemphigoid	
Mucocutaneous inflammation	Pars planitis
(Stevens-Johnson, graft vs. host disease, toxic epidermal necrosis)	Endophthalmitis
Keratitis	*Retina*
Herpes zoster	Vasculitides
Disciform herpes simplex	Choroiditis
Interstitial keratitis (syphilis, herpes simplex)	Retinitis
	Cystoid macular edema
	Acute retinal necrosis
Immune infiltrates (*Staphylococcus,* herpes, varicella, contact lens, EKC, leukemia)	
Peripheral ulcerative (connective tissue disease, e.g., Wegener's granulomatosis, polyarteritis nodosa)	*Optic Nerve*
	Optic neuritis
	Temporal arteritis
Mooren's ulcer	*Orbit*
Reiter's, Lyme disease, sarcoid	Graves' orbitopathy
Corneal graft rejection	Pseudotumor
Trauma and Postsurgery	*Extraocular Muscles*
Neoplasm	Myositis
Juvenile xanthogranuloma	Myasthenia gravis
Hemangioma	
Lids	*Sclera*
Blepharitis	Epscleritis
Atopic dermatitis	Scleritis
Discoid lupus	
Chalazion	

Side Effects of Topical Corticosteroid Therapy

Corticosteroid-induced side effects are either systemic or ocular, or both. Systemic side effects are most often associated with oral or parenteral corticosteroid therapy. It has been shown that 6 weeks of treatment with topical 0.1% dexamethasone sodium phosphate caused suppression of the adrenal cortex, reflected in a decrease in serum cortisol levels. Systemic absorption of steroids after topical treatment is actually considerable, and, if given to a patient with hay fever, it may improve systemic symptoms and decrease the blood eosinophil count. Potential systemic complications of corticosteroid therapy[85] are included in Table 25–5.

Since topical corticosteroids are the most widely used in treating many ocular conditions, their ocular toxicity and

TABLE 25–5. **Systemic Complications of Corticosteroid Therapy**

Musculoskeletal	*Metabolic*
Myopathy Osteoporosis, vertebral compression fractures Aseptic necrosis of bone	Precipitation of clinical manifestations, including ketoacidosis, diabetes mellitus Hyperosmolar nonketotic coma Hyperlipidemia Centripetal obesity
Gastrointestinal	*Endocrine*
Peptic ulcer (often gastric) Gastric hemorrhage Intestinal perforation Pancreatitis	Growth failure Secondary amenorrhea Suppression of hypothalamic-pituitary-adrenal system
Central nervous system	*Inhibition of fibroplasia*
Psychiatric disorders Pseudotumor cerebri	Impaired wound healing Subcutaneous tissue atrophy
Ophthalmic	*Suppression of the immune response*
Glaucoma Posterior subcapsular cataracts	Superimposition of a variety of bacterial, fungus, and viral infections in steroid-treated patients
Cardiovascular and renal	
Hypertension Sodium and water retention edema Hypokalemic alkalosis	

side effects should always be recognized. The patient must be aware of these side effects, particularly if corticosteroids are to be used for an extended period. Ocular side effects involve mainly the anterior segment, including the cornea, conjunctiva, trabecular meshwork, anterior chamber, and iris (Table 25–6). Topical corticosteroids may cause glaucoma or cataracts, enhance secondary herpetic or bacterial infections of the ocular surface, or inhibit corneal epithelial and stromal healing, resulting in further corneal melting and perforation. All of these potential ocular complications of prolonged corticosteroid therapy can be devastating and threaten vision.

The generalized effect of steroids on the delay of wound healing is important to consider, both in postoperative therapy and in association with epithelial and stromal defects. The steroid's effect on the fibroblast results in delayed collagen synthesis, which can cause or exacerbate corneal melting.[34, 72]

CATARACT INDUCTION BY CORTICOSTEROIDS

Several years after corticosteroids became widely used for rheumatoid arthritis, Black and coworkers[87, 88] reported the development of cataracts in patients receiving long-term systemic therapy. The dosage and duration of steroid therapy correlated with the incidence of posterior subcapsular cataract (PSC) formation. Seventy-five percent of patients who receive more than 16 mg/day of prednisone develop cataracts. If the dose is decreased to 10 mg/day for 1 year the chance of PSC formation is minimal. Individuals who have undergone prolonged topical corticosteroid therapy, such as for vernal or atopic keratoconjunctivitis or those who received corneal transplantation for keratoconus, are under the threat of developing PSCs. Donshik and coworkers have shown that 28 eyes of 86 transplanted for keratoconus developed PSCs after 1 year of 0.1% dexamethasone therapy.[89] It seems that PSC formation is significantly related to the total cumulative steroid dose and the total time that steroids were administered. Once PSCs have developed, cessation of corticosteroids does not resolve the opacity. It is also important to consider the overall status of the patient, because factors such as diabetes appear to increase susceptibility to these complications of topical steroid administration. The pathogenesis of corticosteroid-induced cataract formation has not been fully explained. One theory holds that corticosteroids enter the lens and bind to its fibers, leading to biochemical changes and protein aggregation in the cells.

TABLE 25–6. **Ocular Side Effects of Corticosteroid Therapy**

Cataracts	Mydriasis
Glaucoma	Ptosis
Secondary infection	Exophthalmos
Retardation of wound healing	Pseudotumor cerebri
Uveitis	

STEROIDS AND GLAUCOMA

Corticosteroids have been shown to produce increased intraocular pressure when applied topically to the eye[90–97] or given systemically.[98, 99] This elevation in intraocular pressure is usually reversible but can lead to optic nerve damage and visual field changes similar to those seen in patients with chronic open-angle glaucoma. The genetic basis for this predisposition is probably a recessive homozygous gene. Although the exact mechanism of corticosteroid-induced glaucoma is not clear, there is evidence of mucopolysaccharide deposition in the trabecular meshwork.[101] Identifying the effects of topical application of 0.1% dexamethasone has no predictive value.[100]

Steroids such as FML, which has limited intraocular bioavailability, have been shown to have less tendency toward induction of ocular hypertension.[102–106] A corticosteroid provocative test, Akingbehin found that 15 of 24 eyes treated with 0.1% dexamethasone showed a rise in intraocular pressure of more than 5 mm Hg, whereas only two of the 24 eyes treated with 0.1% FML showed such an increase.[102] In a study of 14 steroid responders to 0.1% dexamethasone, 13 were not affected by subsequent treatment with 0.1% FML.[103] Also, the time to an evoked ocular hypertension in known steroid responders was significantly longer (4 weeks) for 0.1% FML actetate than for 0.1% dexamethasone sodium phosphate.[104] Cantrill and associates showed that 0.1% dexamethasone had more than three times the ocular hypertensive effect of 0.1% in corticosteroid responders.[105] Mean intraocular pressure increases were also significantly lower with twice the concentration of FML (0.25%) compared with 0.1% dexamethasone sodium phosphate–treated eyes in known steroid responders who took the drugs four times daily for as long as 6 weeks.[106]

There has been much investigation into the development of steroids that do not elicit ocular hypertension and glaucoma. Lodoprednenolol, a steroid developed using the soft drug concept, is an inactive compound that is activated locally in the eye and is degraded in the blood stream, thus limiting systemic activity.[76, 77] It has been proposed that the side chain responsible for the steroid ocular hypertensive response is absent from this compound; however, most research into the structure-activity relationships of steroids has shown that a steroid's antiinflammatory activity is closely related to its ocular hypertensive activity.[107]

INFECTIONS ENHANCED BY CORTICOSTEROIDS

For bacterial, viral, and protozoal ocular infections, use of corticosteroids should always be given careful consideration. Corticosteroids substantially suppress the activation and migration of leukocytes, which is a major part of the cellular host defense against invading microorganisms and infection. Secondary infections caused by corticosteroids can take the form of bacterial conjunctivitis and keratitis, viral keratitis, or more serious vision-threatening infections, such as fungal keratitis, fungal endophthalmitis, and toxoplasmic chorioretinitis. Management of these complications involves tapering, and eventually stopping, the corticosteroid and initiating therapy with appropriate antiinfective agents. Prophylactic coverage with appropriate antiviral or antibacterial agents should be considered.[108]

REFERENCES

1. Reichstein T, Shoppee CW: The hormone of the adrenal cortex. Vitam Horm 1:346, 1943.
2. Hench PS, Kendall EC, Slocumb CH, et al: The effect of a hormone of the adrenal cortex (17-hydroxy-11-dehydrocorticosterone; compound E) and of pituitary adrenocorticotropic hormone on rheumatoid arthritis. Proc Staff Meet Mayo Clin 24:181, 1949.
3. Stone D, Hechter O: Studies on ACTH action in perfused bovine adrenals: The site of action of ACTH in corticosteroidogenesis. Arch Biochem Biophys 51:457, 1954.
4. Haynes RC Jr, Koritz SB, Peron FG: Influence of adenosine 3',5'-monophosphate on corticoid production by rat adrenal glands. J Biol Chem 234:1421, 1959.
5. Haynes RC Jr, Murad F: Adrenocorticotropic hormone: Adrenocortical steroids and their synthetic analogs. Inhibitors of adrenocortical steroid biosynthesis. *In* Gilman AG, Goodman LS, Rall TW, Murad F (eds): Goodman and Gilman's The Pharmacological Basis of Therapeutics. New York, MacMillan, 1970.
6. Gordon DM: Use of dexamethasone in eye disease. JAMA 172:311, 1960.
7. Ballard PL, Baxter JD, Higgins SJ, et al: General presence of glucocorticoid receptors in mammalian tissues. Endocrinology 94:998, 1974.
8. Baxter JD, Rousseau GG (eds): Glucocorticosteroid Hormone Action. Berlin, Springer-Verlag, 1979.
9. Cake MH, Litwack G: The glucocorticoid receptor in biochemical action of hormones. *In* Litwack G (ed): Biochemical Actions of Hormones, vol 3. New York, Academic Press, 1975.
10. Feldman D: The role of hormone receptors in the action of adrenal steroids. Annu Rev Med 26:83, 1975.
11. Higgins SJ, Gehring U: Molecular mechanisms of steroid hormone action. Adv Cancer Res 28:313, 1978.
12. Wicks WD: The mode of action of glucocorticoids. *In* Rickenberg HV (ed): Biochemistry of Hormones, vol 8. Baltimore, University Park Press, 1974.
13. Fahey JV, Guyre PM, Munck A: Mechanisms of anti-inflammatory actions of glucocorticoids. *In* Weissmann G: Advances in Inflammation Research, vol 2. New York, Raven Press, 1981.
14. Parrillo JE, Fauci AS: Mechanisms of glucocorticoid action on immune processes. Annu Rev Pharmacol Toxicol 19:179, 1979.
15. Fauci AS: Mechanisms of the immunosuppressive and antiinflammatory effects of glucorticosteroids. Immunopharmacology 1:1, 1978.
16. O'Malley BW: Mechanisms of action of steroid hormones. N Engl J Med 84:304, 1976.
17. Baxter JD, Forshaim PH: Tissue effects of glucocorticoids. Am J Med 53:573, 1972.
18. Thompson EB, Lippman ME: Mechanism of action of glucocorticoids. Metabolism 23:159, 1974.
19. Hallahan C, Young DA, Munck A: Time course of early events in the action of glucocorticoids on rat thymus cells in vitro. J Biol Chem 248:2922, 1973.
20. Leopold IH, Gaster RN: Ocular inflammation and anti-inflammatory drugs. *In* Kaufman HE, Barron BA, McDonald MB, Waltman SR (eds): The Cornea. New York, Churchill Livingstone, 1988.
21. Hernandez MR, Wenk EJ, Weinstein BI, et al: Glucocorticoid target cells in human outflow pathway: Autopsy and surgical specimens. Invest Ophthalmol Vis Sci 24:1612, 1983.
22. Southren AL, Dominguez MO, Gordon GG, et al: Nuclear translocation of cytoplasm glucocorticoid receptor in the iris-ciliary body and adjacent corneoscleral tissue of the rabbit following topical administration of various glucocorticoids. Invest Ophthalmol Vis Sci 24:147, 1983.
23. Mondino BJ, Aizuss DH, Farley MK: Steroids. *In* Lamberts DW, Potter DE (eds): Clinical Ophthalmic Pharmacology. Boston, Little, Brown, 1987.
24. Jasami MK: Anti-inflammatory steroids: Mode of action in rheumatoid arthritis and homograft rejection. *In* Vane JR, Ferriera SH (eds): Antiinflammatory Drugs. Berlin, Springer-Verlag, 1979.
25. Melby JC: Systemic corticosteroid therapy: Pharmacology and endocrinologic considerations. Ann Intern Med 8:505, 1974.
26. Greeson TP, Levan NE, Freedman RI, et al: Corticosteroid-induced vasoconstriction studied by xenon clearance. Invest Dermatol 61:242, 1973.
27. Bishop CR, Athens JW, Boggs DR, et al: Leukokinetic studies. XIII: A now steady-state kinetic evaluation of the mechanism of cortisone-induced granulocytosis. J Clin Invest 47:249, 1967.
28. Friedlaender MH: Corticosteroid therapy of ocular inflammation. Int Ophthalmol Clin 23:175, 1983.
29. Cohen JJ: Thymus-derived lymphocytes sequestered in the bone marrow of hydrocortisone treated mice. J Immunol 108:841, 1972.
30. Smolin G: Immunology. *In* Smolin G, Thoft RA (eds): The Cornea. Scientific Foundations and Clinical Practice. Boston, Little, Brown, 1983.
31. Claman HN: Corticosteroids and lymphoid cells. N Engl J Med 287:388, 1972.
32. Werb Z: Biochemical actions of glucocorticoids on macrophages in culture. J Exp Med 147:1695, 1978.
33. Dannenberg AM Jr: The antiinflammatory effects of corticosteroids. Inflammation 3:329, 1979.
34. Ashton N, Cook C: Effect of cortisone on healing of corneal wounds. Br J Ophthalmol 35:708, 1951.
35. Vane J, Botting R: Inflammation and the mechanism of action of antiinflammatory drugs. Endocr Rev 5:89, 1984.
36. Floman N, Zor U: Mechanism of steroid action in ocular inflammation. Invest Ophthalmol Vis Sci 16:69, 1977.
37. Kanrowitz F, Robinson DR, McGuire MB, et al: Corticosteroids inhibit prostaglandin production by rheumatoid synovia. Nature 258:737, 1975.
38. Gryglewski RJ: Steroid hormones, antiinflammatory steroids and prostaglandins. Pharmacol Res Commun 8:337, 1976.
39. Blackwell GJ, Carnuccio R, DiRosa M, et al: Macrocortin in polypeptide causing the antiphospholipase effect of glucocorticoids. Nature 287:147, 1980.
40. Gardner SK: Ocular drug penetration and pharmacokinetic principles. *In* Lamberts DW, Potter DE (eds): Clinical Ophthalmic Pharmacology. Boston, Little, Brown, 1987.
41. Maurice DM: Factors influencing the penetration of topically applied drugs. *In* Holly FJ (ed): Clinical Pharmacology of the Anterior Segment. Boston, Little, Brown, 1980.
42. Rosenblum C, Dengler RE, Geoffroy RF: Ocular absorption of dexamethasone phosphate disodium by the rabbit. Arch Ophthalmol 77:234, 1967.
43. Roters S, Aspacher F, Diestelhorst M: The influence of dexamethasone 0.1% eye drops on plasma cortisol and ACTH concentrations after cataract surgery. Ophthalmologica 210(4):211–214, 1996.
44. Kupferman A, Pratt MV, Camon EJ: Topically applied steroids in corneal disease. III: The role of drug derivative in stromal absorption of dexamethasone. Arch Ophthalmol 91:373–376, 1974.
45. Bisrat M, Glazer M: Effect of particle size on ocular permeability of prednisolone acetate in rabbits. Acta Pharm Nord 4(1):5, 1992.
46. Schoenwald RD, Stewart P: Effect of particle size on ophthalmic bioavailability of dexamethasone suspensions in rabbits. J Pharm Sci 69(4):391–394, 1980.

47. Gardner S: Comparison of topical ophthalmic corticosteroid drops. Ocular Ther Man 3(2):1–14, 1992.
48. Leibowitz HM, Kupferman A: Bioavailability and therapeutic effectiveness of topically administered corticosteroids. Trans Am Acad Ophthalmol Otolaryngol 79:78–88, 1975.
49. Leibowitz HM, Kupferman A: Antiinflammatory effectiveness in the cornea of topically administered prednisolone. Invest Ophthalmol 13:757–766, 1974.
50. Leibowitz HM, Kupferman A: Use of corticosterioids in the treatment of corneal inflammation. *In* Leibowitz HM (ed): Corneal Disorders: Clinical Diagnosis and Management. Philadelphia, WB Saunders, 1984.
51. McGhee CNS, Watson DG, Midgeley JM, et al: Penetration of synthetic corticosteroids in human aqueous humor. Eye 4:526, 1990.
52. Katz IM, Blackman WM: A soluble sustained-release artificial ophthalmic delivery unit. Am J Ophthalmol 83:728, 1977.
53. Hwang DG, Stern WH, Hwang PH, et al: Collagen shield enhancement of topical dexamethasone penetration. Arch Ophthalmol 107:137, 1989.
54. Short C, Keates RH, Donovan EF, et al: Ocular penetration studies. I: Topical administration of dexamethasone. Arch Ophthalmol 75:689, 1966.
55. Olejnick O, Weisbecker CA: Ocular bioavailability of topical prednisolone preparations. Clin Ther 12:2, 1990.
56. Havener WH: Corticosteroid Therapy in Ocular Pharmacology, 5th ed. St Louis, CV Mosby, 1983.
57. Cox WV, Kupferman A, Leibowitz HM: Topically applied steroids in corneal disease. I: The role of inflammation in stromal absorption of dexamethasone. Arch Ophthalmol 88:308, 1972.
58. Kupferman A, Leibowitz HM: Topically applied steroids in corneal disease. IV: The role of drug concentration in stromal absorption of prednisolone acetate. Arch Ophthalmol 91:377, 1974.
59. Kupferman A, Leibowitz HM: Topically applied steroids in corneal disease. V: Dexamethasone alcohol. Arch Ophthalmol 92:329, 1974.
60. Kupferman A, Leibowitz HM: Topically applied steroids in corneal disease. VI: Kinetics of prednisolone phosphate. Arch Ophthalmol 92:331, 1974.
61. Leibowitz HM, Less JH, Kupferman A: Quantitation of inflammation in the cornea. Arch Ophthalmol 92:427, 1974.
62. Leibowitz HM, Stewart RH, Kupferman A, et al: Evaluation of dexamethasone acetate as a topical ophthalmic formulation. Am J Ophthalmol 86:418, 1978.
63. Leibowitz HM, Kupferman A: Antiinflammatory effectiveness in the cornea of topically administered prednisolone. Invest Ophthalmol Vis Sci 13:757, 1974.
64. Kupferman A, Leibowitz HM: Antiinflammatory effectiveness of topically administered corticosteroid in the cornea without epithelium. Invest Ophthalmol 14:352, 1975.
65. Leibowitz HM: Management of inflammation in the cornea and conjunctiva. Ophthalmology 87:753, 1980.
66. Leibowitz HM, Kupferman A: Bioavailability and therapeutic effectiveness of topically administered corticosteroids. Trans Am Acad Ophthalmol 79:78, 1975.
67. Leibowitz HM, Kupferman A: Kinetics of topically administered prednisolone acetate optimal concentration for treatment of inflammatory keratitis. Arch Ophthalmol 94:1387, 1976.
68. Musson DG, Bidgood AM, Olejnick O: Assay methodology for prednisolone, prednisolone acetate and prednisolone sodium phosphate in rabbit aqueous humor and ocular physiological solutions. J Chromatogr 565:89, 1991.
69. Musson DG, Bidgood AM, Olejnick O: An in vitro comparison of the permeability of prednisolone, prednisolone sodium phosphate, and prednisolone acetate across the NZW rabbit cornea. J Ocul Pharmacol 8:139, 1992.
70. Apt L, Henrick A, Silverman LM: Patient compliance with the use of topical ophthalmic corticosteroid suspensions. Am J Ophthalmol 87:210, 1979.
71. Burch PG, Migeon CJ: Systemic absorption of topical steroids. Arch Ophthalmol 79:174, 1968.
72. Aronson SB, Moore TE Jr: Corticosteroid therapy in central stromal keratitis. Am J Ophthalmol 67:873, 1969.
73. Leibowitz HM, Kupferman A: Penetration of fluorometholone into the cornea and aqueous humor. Arch Ophthalmol 93:425, 1975.
74. Kupferman A, Leibowitz HM: Therapeutic effectiveness of fluorometholone in inflammatory keratitis. Arch Ophthalmol 93:1011, 1975.
75. Druzgala PD, Wu WM, Winwood D, et al: Ocular absorption and distribution of loteprednol etabonate: A "soft" steroid. Invest Ophthalmol Vis Sci 32 (Suppl):735, 1991.
76. Leibowitz HM, Kupferman A, Ryan WJ, et al: Corneal antiinflammatory steroidal "soft drug." Invest Ophthalmol Vis Sci 32 (Suppl):735, 1991.
77. Leibowitz RA, Ghormley NR, Insler MS, et al: Treatment of giant papillary conjunctivitis with loteprednol etabonate: A novel corticosteroid. Invest Ophthalmol Vis Sci 32 (Suppl):734, 1991.
78. Leibowitz HM, Rich R, Crabb JL, et al: Intraocular pressure raising potential of rimexolone 1.0% in steroid responders. Invest Ophthalmol Vis Sci 35 (Suppl):735, 1991.
79. Lehmann R, Sil K, Stewart R, et al: Comparison of rimexolone 1% ophthalmic suspension to placebo in control of postcataract surgery inflammation. Invest Ophthalmol Vis Sci 36 (Suppl):S793, 1995.
80. Corboy JM: Corticosteroid therapy for the reduction of postoperative inflammation after cataract extraction. Am J Ophthalmol 82:923, 1976.
81. Abelson MB, George M, Drake M, et al: Evaluation of rimexolone ophthalmic suspension in the antigen challenge model of allergic conjunctivitis. Invest Ophthalmol Vis Sci 33 (Suppl):2094, 1994.
82. Holsclaw DS, Whitcher JP, Wong IG, et al: Supratarsal injection of corticosteroid in the treatment of refractory vernal keratoconjunctivitis. Am J Ophthalmol 121(3):243–249, 1996
83. Sieg J, Robinson J: Vehicle effects on ocular drug bioavailability. I: Evaluation of fluorometholone. J Pharm Sci 64:931, 1975.
84. Jaanus SD: Anti-inflammatory drugs. *In* Bartett JD, Jaanus SD (eds): Clinical Ocular Pharmacology, 2nd ed. Boston, Butterworths, 1989.
85. George MA, Smith LM, Abelson MB: Efficacy of 1.0% prednisolone sodium phosphate in alleviating the signs and symptoms of allergic conjunctivitis induced by allergen challenge. Invest Ophthalmol Vis Sci 32 (Suppl):736, 1991.
86. Melby JC: Systemic corticosteroid therapy: Pharmacology and endocrinologic considerations. Ann Intern Med 81:505, 1974.
87. Black RL, Oglesby RB, Von Sallman L, et al: Posterior subcapsular cataracts induced by corticosteroids in patients with rheumatoid arthritis. JAMA 174:166, 1960.
88. Spaeth GI, Von Sallman L: Corticosteroids and cataracts. Int Ophthalmol Clin 6:915, 1966.
89. Donshik PC, Cavanaugh HD, Boruchoff DA, et al: Posterior subcapsular cataracts induced by topical corticosteroids following keratoplasty for keratoconus. Ann Ophthalmol 13:29, 1981.
90. Francois J: Cortisone et tension oculaire. Ann Ocul 187:805, 1954.
91. Stern JJ: Acute glaucoma during cortisone therapy. Am J Ophthalmol 36:389, 1953.
92. Armaly M: Effect on intraocular pressure corticosteroids and fluid dynamics. I: The effect of dexamethasone in the normal eye. Arch Ophthalmol 70:482, 1963.
93. Armaly M: Effect of corticosteroids on intraocular pressure and fluid dynamics. II: The effect of dexamethasone in the glaucomatous eye. Arch Ophthalmol 70:492, 1963.
94. Armaly M: Statistical attributes of the steroid hypertensive response in the clinically normal eye. Invest Ophthalmol Vis Sci 4:187, 1965.
95. Armaly M: Heritable nature of dexamethasone-induced ocular hypertension. Arch Ophthalmol 75:32, 1966.
96. Becker B, Mill SW: Corticosteroids and intraocular pressure. Arch Ophthalmol 70:500, 1963.
97. Becker B, Hahn KA: Topical corticosteroids and heredity in primary open-angle glaucoma. Am J Ophthalmol 57:544, 1964.
98. Bernstein HN, Schwartz B: Effects of long term systemic steroids on ocular pressure and tonographic values. Arch Ophthalmol 68:742, 1962.
99. Covell LL: Glaucoma induced by systemic steroid therapy. Am J Ophthalmol 45:108, 1954.
100. Johnson DH, Bradley JV, Acott TS: The effect of dexamethasone on glycosaminoglycans of human trabecular meshwork in perfusion organ culture. Invest Ophthalmol Vis Sci 31:2568, 1990.
101. Hodapp EA, Kass MA: Corticosteroid-induced glaucoma. *In* Ritch R, Shields MB (eds): The Secondary Glaucomas. St Louis, CV Mosby, 1982.
102. Akingbehin AO: Comparative study of the intraocular pressure effects of fluorometholone 0.1% versus dexamethasone 0.1%. Br J Ophthalmol 67:661, 1983.

103. Morrison E, Archer DB: Effect of fluorometholone (FML) on the intraocular pressure of corticosteroid responders. Br J Ophthalmol 68:581, 1984.
104. Stewart RH, Smith JP, Rosenthal AL: Ocular response to fluorometholone acetate and dexamethasone sodium phosphate. Curr Eye Res 3:835, 1984.
105. Cantrill HL, Palmberg PF, Zink HA, et al: Comparison of in vitro potency of corticosteroids with ability to raise intraocular pressure. Am J Ophthalmol 79:1012, 1975.
106. Kass M, Cheetham J, Duzman E, et al: The ocular hypertensive effect of 0.25% fluorometholone in corticosteroid responders. Am J Ophthalmol 102:159, 1986.
107. McLean JM: Discussion of Woods AC: Clinical and experimental observation on the use of ACTH and cortisone in ocular inflammatory disease. Trans Am Ophthalmol 48:293, 1959.
108. Stern GA, Buitross M: Use of corticosteroids in combination with antimicrobial drugs in the treatment of infectious corneal disease. Ophthalmology 98:847, 1991.

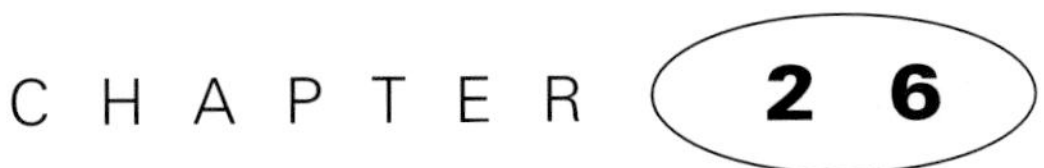

Adrenergic Agents

Martin B. Wax, Gary D. Novack, and Alan L. Robin

The past century has witnessed considerable progress in the use of adrenergic agents to treat glaucoma. The oldest member of this family, epinephrine, was initially used in 1900,[1, 2] whereas the newest, brimonidine tartrate, was approved by the Food and Drug Administration (FDA) in 1996. Although both of these drugs are pharmacologic agonists, the past quarter century has also been remarkable for the clinical development of numerous adrenergic receptor (adrenoceptor) antagonists that have become the current mainstay of intraocular pressure (IOP)-lowering drugs used to treat glaucoma. The development of these drugs for ocular use has paralleled the widespread medical use of similar drugs that cause either the blockade of the sympathetic neurotransmitter norepinephrine and the neurohormone epinephrine at α- and β-adrenoceptors, or conversely, agonist activation of α- and β-adrenoceptors. Common examples include the use of β-adrenoceptor antagonists for the treatment of hypertension and angina and the secondary prevention of acute myocardial infarction; selective β_2-adrenoceptor agonists such as bronchodilators for asthma; and α_2-adrenoceptor agonists and α_1-adrenoceptor antagonists for hypertension. Because these drugs have been important in drug therapy for decades, extensive research has enabled a keen understanding of the specific cellular perturbations induced by these drugs. The extent and degree to which these cellular events are known have been fortuitous for ocular investigators, who until recently have always understood the clinical effects of these drugs on IOP better than the underlying biochemical pharmacology and physiology that mediate the actions of these drugs.

Preclinical Studies

RECEPTOR/G PROTEIN/EFFECTOR SYSTEMS

Cells communicate with each other and with their extracellular environment through molecules such as hormones, growth factors, and neurotransmitters. Some information is transmitted by cell-specific transmembrane receptors that are coupled directly to an effector system generating intracellular signals. Examples of this group of receptors include ligand-gated ion channels (e.g., nicotinic acetylcholine and ionotropic glutamate) and enzyme-linked receptors (e.g., tyrosine kinases and phosphatases, and particulate guanylyl cyclase).[3] The majority of intracellular signals, however, occur via a three-protein transmembrane signaling system that consists of (1) a specific receptor that increases the probability of interaction with (2) one or more guanine nucleotide–binding proteins (G proteins) that act as transducers and signal amplifiers, which modulate the activity of (3) one of more effector systems.[4]

The G protein–coupled receptor superfamily is one of the largest and most diverse protein families.[5] Some 50 to 60% of all clinically relevant drugs exert their actions via G protein–coupled receptors. In addition to adrenergic agents, these receptors recognize a vast array of substances as diverse as light, protein and peptide hormones, odorants, eicosanoids, nucleotides, calcium ions, and lipid autacoids. More than 300 G-protein receptors have been cloned, and there are as many as 1000 members of this family.[4, 5] By resolving the primary structures of various G protein–coupled receptors including the light receptor, rhodopsin, it has become clear that all of these receptors, including the β-adrenergic receptor, share a common structural motif characterized by seven hydrophobic stretches of 20 to 25 amino acids that form transmembrane helices connected by alternating extracellular and intracellular loops (Fig. 26–1). The N-terminal is located extracellularly, and the C-terminal extends into the cytoplasm. The seven-transmembrane span architecture of the various receptors in this family activates one or more G proteins and thus transduces the signal of an extracellular ligand-receptor interaction to various intracellular effectors.[5]

The G proteins, which bind and hydrolyze guanosine

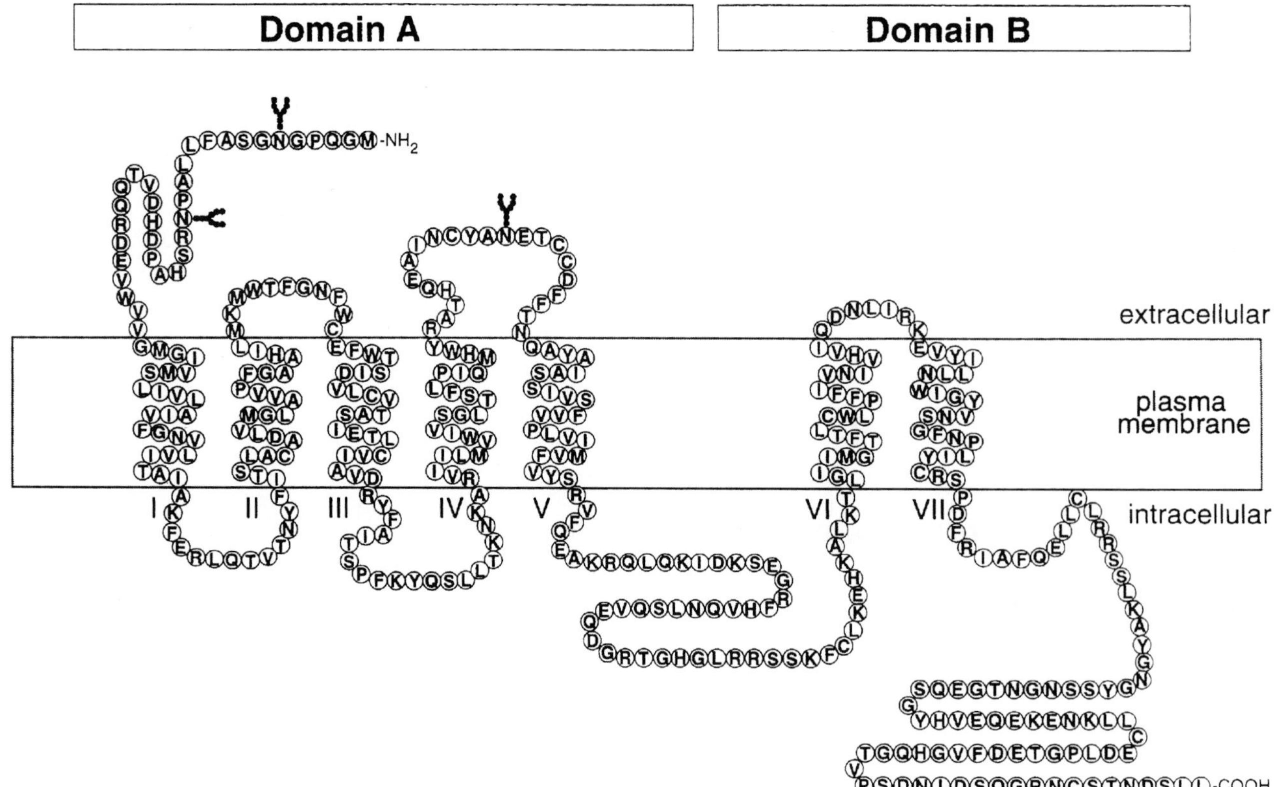

FIGURE 26–1. Diagram of the predicted structure and membrane topology of the human β_2-adrenergic receptor. (Reprinted from Hein L, Kobilke BK: Review: Neurotransmitter receptor IV. Neuropharmacology 34:357–366, 1995. Copyright 1995, with permission from Elsevier Science.)

triphosphate (GTP), are physically and functionally interposed between the receptor and the effector system.[6] G proteins are heterotrimeric with subunits designated α, β, and γ. Agonist binding to an adrenoceptor activates a G protein by catalyzing the release of guanosine diphosphate from the α subunit and its replacement by GTP. Following separation of the β and γ subunits, the α subunit hydrolyzes the bound GTP.[7] When the free α-GTP subunit comes into contact with an effector, it activates the latter to perform its biochemical function. Each of the G-protein subunits is structurally diverse, leading to a large number of distinct G proteins. The adrenoceptors interact preferentially with three classes of G proteins: G_s (β-adrenoceptor) mediating activation of adenylyl cyclase, G_i (α_2-adrenoceptors) mediating inhibition of adenylyl cyclase, and G_q (α_1-adrenoceptors) mediating activation of phospholipase C-β.[8] Adrenergic receptors can also be coupled to other effector systems such as ion channels.[9, 10] The original paradigm that a receptor activates a single effector within a particular cell has given way to the current concept of great promiscuity among individual receptors, G proteins, and effectors.[11] Although the major adrenoceptor subtypes usually couple preferentially to a particular G protein, a receptor can sometimes interact with different G proteins or effector systems depending on either agonist concentration or the characteristics of the particular cell in which it is expressed.[12–15] For example, although most α_2-adrenoceptors interact with G_i, the α_{2C} adrenoceptor acts preferentially with G_o.[15] A second tier of heterogeneity is also exemplified by β-adrenoceptors, which stimulate two second messenger pathways (adenylyl cyclase and calcium channels), both through activation of $G_s\alpha$.[16]

ADRENERGIC RECEPTOR SUBTYPE CLASSIFICATION

The initial subclassification of adrenoceptors into α and β types was based on their pharmacologic rather than their functional characteristics. Adrenergic receptors were first divided into the subtypes α and β by Ahlquist in 1948[17] based on the development of potent antagonists that were highly selective for each of the adrenoceptor subtypes. β-Adrenoceptors were further divided into the subtypes β_1 and β_2 by Lands and associates in 1967[18] based on the differences in the order of potency of the agonists epinephrine (adrenaline) and norepinephrine (noradrenaline). In the 1970s, α-adrenoceptors were further subdivided functionally into α_1 and α_2 subtypes[19, 20] based on the concept that α_2-adrenoceptors mediated inhibitory responses, whereas α_1-adrenoceptors mediated excitatory responses. However, this classification system was soon deemed as unreliable as that which based α-adrenoceptor classification on anatomic localization (i.e., prejunctional versus postjunctional receptors).[21, 22]

In the late 1980s, the development of more selective drugs and molecular cloning technology demonstrated the existence of distinct genes for additional adrenoceptor subtypes. At least nine distinct genomic or cDNA clones have been obtained for subtypes of adrenoceptors in several different species (three α_1-adrenoceptor subtypes,[23–25] three α_2-

adrenoceptor subtypes,[26–32] and three β-adrenoceptor subtypes[33–35]). Although the nomenclature of the β-adrenergic subtypes is clear, the nomenclature for the subtypes of different α-adrenoceptors has unfortunately been confusing. This is largely due to the inability to reconcile the pharmacologic classification with the functional data on the known cloned receptors. There are four pharmacologically defined subtypes of α_2-adrenoceptors (A, B, C, D), yet only three genes have been cloned.[36, 37] There is good evidence that α_{2A} and α_{2D} subtypes merely represent species differences in pharmacology.[31, 38] Because different functions are likely to be mediated by different subtypes, considerable effort has been directed toward understanding the physiologic roles of the various subtypes, of which little is currently known.

It is still useful, however, to consider adrenoceptors as belonging to one of three major types: α_1, α_2, and β.[39] This pharmacologic classification is based on three observations. First, selective agonists were identified that have high affinity for one of the three major types, but a 1000- to 10,000-fold lower affinity for the other two types. Second, each of the three major types of adrenoceptors couples to its second messenger system through a distinct family of G proteins (α_1-adrenoceptors are coupled through G_q, α_2-adrenoceptors are coupled through G_i, and β-receptors are coupled through G_s). Thus, all members within a particular family generally appear to activate the same, or similar, signal transduction mechanisms. Third, from a structural perspective, the amino-acid sequence of both β- and α_1-adrenoceptors have short third intracellular loops and a long COOH-terminal tail, whereas the α_2-adrenoceptors has a long third intracellular loop and a short COOH-terminal tail. Furthermore, α_1, α_2, and β types all have similarly predicted amino-acid sequence identities. Thus, there is no molecular reason to consider α_1 and α_2 types more closely related to each other than either type is to the β-adrenoceptor type.[40]

STRUCTURE AND FUNCTION RELATIONSHIP OF ADRENERGIC RECEPTORS

The three distinct but closely related subtypes of adrenoceptor families (α_1, α_2, β) are divided according to sequence homology, drug specificity, and mechanism of signal transduction. The sequence homology among families is about 40%, whereas the subtypes within a family have about 70 to 75% sequence homology.[41] Each family has a characteristic pharmacologic profile, although each subtype is the product of a separate gene and has a unique drug specificity and tissue distribution. The existence of so many subtypes suggests that additional highly selective drugs with possible therapeutic advantages could be developed. Because sequence homology is high among adrenoceptor families and higher among family subtypes, it is not surprising that molecular biology technology has revealed that certain critical regions of the adrenoceptor confer the specific pharmacologic properties to its family members.

Site-directed mutagenesis[42–45] and chimeric receptor studies[46–48] have identified the domains involved in ligand binding and G-protein coupling of adrenoceptors. In this approach, chimeras are synthesized between two related G protein–coupled receptors by splicing together two complementary helical regions from the two receptors to form a hybrid that contains, for example, the N-terminal to the helix 3 region of one receptor subtype with the helix 4 to the C-terminal region of another subtype. By moving the "splice junction" to different positions in the receptor sequence, it is possible to obtain information about which domains are critical for binding specific ligands or conferring specific pharmacologic properties to the receptor. Once general regions of the ligand-binding domains have been identified, specific point mutations in those regions may be made to further characterize the properties conferred by a given region of the receptor. These studies demonstrated that the ligand-binding pocket is made up of several hydrophilic membrane spanning domains of the adrenoceptor.[49, 50] Construction of a series of chimeric receptors in which increasingly long N-terminal stretches of the β_1-receptor were replaced by the analogous regions of the β_2-receptor showed that the relative potencies of epinephrine and norepinephrine switched from the β_1 to the β_2 phenotype as the helix 4 region was replaced.[51] Subsequent construction of more specific chimeras confirmed that replacement of helices 4 to 5 of the β_2-receptor with those from the β_1-receptor was sufficient to cause an increased affinity for norepinephrine and a decreased affinity for epinephrine.[52] However, no single residue replacement in this region accounted for the reversal of subtype specificity observed with the chimeric receptor. Thus, the binding pocket for the N-methyl substituent of epinephrine appears to involve either direct or conformational effects of multiple residues in the helix 4 to 5 region of the receptor.

Some studies have identified single amino acids involved in binding specific classes of ligands. For example, there is evidence for the specific interaction between the secondary amine of both agonists and antagonists with Asp113 in the third hydrophobic domain[45] as well as evidence for interactions between the hydroxyls on the aromatic ring of isoproterenol and serines 204 and 207 in the fifth hydrophobic segment.[43] Important regions for antagonist interaction, however, appear to involve the third and seventh hydrophobic domains.[47, 53]

The specificity of the receptor–G protein interaction appears to be localized to the second and third cytoplasmic domains[46, 54] and the carboxyl terminal. An exceptionally conserved sequence shared by many G protein–coupled receptors is an Asp-Arg-Tyr triplet that is located in the N-terminal of the second cytoplasmic loop. The Arg of this triplet is the only residue conserved among all rhodopsin-like G protein–coupled receptors and is thought to be central in the interaction between receptors and G proteins. Substitution of the conserved Arg by Asn in the α_2-adrenoceptor eliminated high-affinity guanine nucleotide–sensitive agonist binding and produced a rightward shift in the dose-response curves for agonist-mediated inhibition of forskolin-stimulated cyclic adenosine monophosphate (cAMP) production.[55] When Arg was mutated to Asn in the muscarinic M_1-receptor, antagonist or partial agonist binding was unaffected, whereas the full agonist carbachol bound to a single low-affinity site.[56]

Evidence also exists that the third cytoplasmic domain is involved in receptor–G protein specificity. For example, when 12 amino acids from the amino terminal segment of the third cytoplasmic domain of the muscarinic M_1-receptor were exchanged with the homologous domain of the turkey β-receptor, the chimeric receptor could activate phospholipase C as well as adenylyl cyclase only when bound to the muscarinic agonist acetylcholine, but not when bound to adrenoceptor agonists.[56a]

AGONIST/ANTAGONIST SPECIFICITY

Agonists

The original observation by Rodbell and coworkers in 1971 that specific binding of glucagon to liver membranes is regulated by GTP[57] has led to one of the central paradigms of molecular pharmacology—namely, agonists, but not antagonists, stabilize an activated high-affinity conformation of the receptor, thereby promoting biologic activation. In the case of G protein–coupled receptors, the ternary complex model defines the active form of the receptor as a complex involving the agonist, the receptor, and the G protein.[58] Once the ligand binds to the receptor/G-protein complex, the G protein induces a conformational shift of the receptor—for example, by moving the side chain of the conserved Arg out of the hydrophilic pocket toward the cytoplasm. This triggers a chain of events leading to a modified affinity of the complex for the ligand.[59] Thus, the current allosteric model of ternary complex activation[60] proposes that "agonist-specific" ligand binding to receptors "activates" receptors to a state that frees a structural constraint of the receptor so that it may then effectively interact with G proteins.

Antagonists

If agonist specificity implies that a structural alteration of the receptor/G-protein complex results from ligand activation, what then occurs when antagonist drugs occupy adrenoceptor sites? The traditional view has always been that antagonists simply occupy the receptor site, thus making it impossible for agonists to interact with receptors as long as the competitive principles of Michaelis-Menten binding kinetics are obeyed. Although less is known about the residues involved in antagonist binding of adrenoceptors, recent evidence suggests that such a view may be overly simplistic and that conformational changes of receptors may indeed occur in the presence of antagonists. Although receptors are often thought to be homodimers, it has been shown experimentally that the β_2-adrenoceptor can function as a heterodimer having two major domains: domain A from the N-terminal through the center of the third intracellular loop (located between the fifth and sixth transmembrane domains) and domain B from the middle of the third intracellular loop through the carboxyl terminal.[46] When synthesized as separate proteins, domains A and B can associate noncovalently to form a functional receptor. It has been suggested that these domains are relatively mobile with respect to each other and that agonists and antagonists stabilize the relative positions of the two domains by interacting with specific amino acids in both domains. Thus, agonist activation may involve movement of domain A relative to domain B[61] (Fig. 26–2).

Agonists stabilize a specific arrangement of these domains that can be recognized by G proteins, whereas antagonists stabilize an arrangement that cannot be recognized by G proteins. In the absence of ligand, the receptor may fluctuate between active and inactive conformational states as pre-

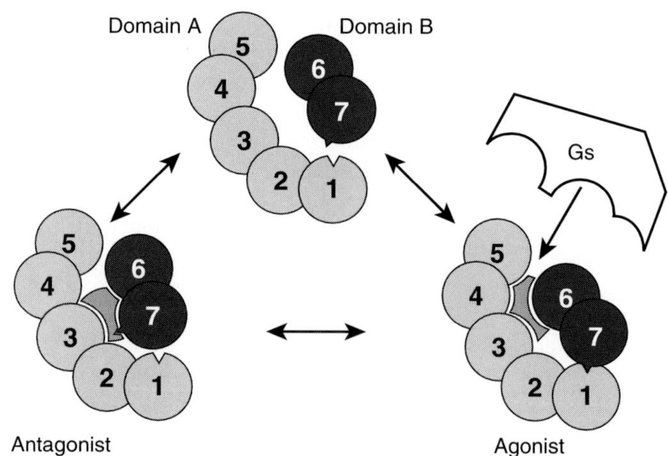

FIGURE 26–2. Model of a possible mechanism by which agonists and antagonists modify the structure of the β_2-adrenergic receptor. The model is viewed from the cytoplasmic side of the membrane. (Reprinted from Hein L, Kobilke BK: Review: Neurotransmitter receptor IV. Neuropharmacology 34:357–366, 1995. Copyright 1995, with permission from Elsevier Science.)

dicted by the allosteric ternary complex model, with the inactive conformation being more stable. It has been shown that wild type β_2-adrenoceptors have constitutive activity and can activate G_s (hence adenylyl cyclase) in the absence of agonists, particularly when the receptor is expressed at high levels.[60, 62] This constitutive activity can be inhibited by some antagonists (called inverse agonists or negative antagonists) but not by other "true" antagonists. In normal tissues, the constitutive activity of unoccupied β-adrenoceptors has been revealed by β-adrenoceptor antagonist inhibition of adenylyl cyclase activity and calcium channel activation.[63, 64] This observation supports the notion that both agonists and antagonists can induce conformational changes.[61] Pure antagonists may act to block access to agonists but not alter receptor conformation, thereby permitting low-level basal activation of G protein by receptor. In contrast, negative antagonists not only block access to agonists but induce a conformational change that prevents basal activation of G proteins.

Partial Agonists

A third class of compounds that interact with adrenoceptors are the so-called partial agonists. A partial agonist ligand binds to adrenoceptors with high affinity and, like antagonists, blocks agonist stimulation of the receptor. Unlike an antagonist, however, it can elicit some activation of the receptor. These compounds are also called antagonists with intrinsic sympathomimetic activity (ISA). In the β-adrenoceptor system, the efficacy of an agonist or partial agonist is typically defined in biochemical terms by the ability of a ligand to stimulate the second messenger cAMP by adenylyl cyclase. Because partial agonists stimulate cAMP only minimally, their efficacy is often determined by measuring signal amplification of already stimulated cAMP activity. Thus, differences in efficacy among partial agonists represent the differing abilities of individual compounds to activate G_s.[65] In addition, certain partial agonists at β-adrenoceptors demonstrate subtype selectivity for blockade or agonism.[66]

Partial agonists are traditionally used for the treatment of hypertension and congestive heart failure and include compounds such as pindolol, acebutolol, alprenolol, and carteolol.[65] Among these agents, carteolol is available for topical use as an ocular hypotensive agent (Ocupress). Advantages of partial agonists in the settings of patients with hypertension, a low heart rate, congestive heart failure, peripheral vascular disease, or obstructive airway disease may be the blockade of response to ambient levels of neurotransmitter and the absence of withdrawal syndromes or other side effects associated with the use of conventional antagonists. They also may offer some advantage in their effect on plasma lipoprotein concentrations during long-term treatment.[22, 67–69]

Analysis of the structure-activity relationship that may account for the unique properties of partial agonists includes the possibility that they are likely intermediate (between full agonists or complete antagonists) in their ability to interact with crucial serine residues (Ser204 and Ser207) on the β-adrenoceptor; these interactions allow either incomplete stimulation of the entire receptor population or full stimulation of only a portion of the entire receptor population.[65] In addition, as analysis of chimeric receptors expressed in transfected systems has shown, domains of the receptor that bind agonists may be different from those that interact with antagonists. Thus, the ability of a partial agonist to interact with two different domains may be a determinant of efficacy.[65]

β-ADRENERGIC RECEPTOR PHARMACOLOGY

Three distinct genes encoding β-adrenoceptors have been cloned to date.[34, 35, 70, 71] The cloned β_1-adrenoceptor has a high affinity for the endogenous catecholamines norepinephrine and epinephrine, a high affinity for the β_1-selective antagonists betaxolol and CGP 20,712A, and a low affinity for the β_2-selective antagonist ICI 118,551.[34, 72] At the cloned β_2-adrenoceptor, epinephrine is more potent than norepinephrine, and the β_2-selective antagonist ICI 118,551 occupies receptors with high potency. The confusion that has long surrounded "atypical" β-adrenoceptors was exacerbated by the isolation of a human gene that encodes for a receptor protein having about 40 to 50% homology with β_1- or β_2-adrenoceptors, and it has become known as the β_3-adrenoceptor. The β_3-adrenoceptor has since been cloned in rat adipose tissue and mice.[73, 74] When β_3-adrenoceptors were transfected in Chinese hamster ovary (CHO) cells to study their pharmacology, the product of this gene activated adenylyl cyclase with a higher affinity for norepinephrine than epinephrine (about a 20-fold difference); in general, however, catecholamines have a higher affinity for β_1- or β_2-adrenoceptors than for the β_3-adrenoceptor.[75, 76] More important is the finding that β_3-adrenoceptors mediate functional catecholamine-induced lipolysis to the selective β_3-adrenergic agonists such as BRL 37344[76] and have very low affinity for all known β-adrenoceptor antagonists.[35, 77]

β-Adrenergic Effector Systems

The effector systems that mediate the effects of β-adrenoceptor agonists are well established. Occupancy of the β-adrenoceptor results in a conformational change that leads to the activation of a subunit of the stimulatory G protein, G_s, that in turn activates the cell surface-associated enzyme adenylyl cyclase. This results in the conversion of adenosine triphosphate (ATP) to the second messenger cAMP. cAMP activates protein kinase A (PKA), which then phosphorylates certain key proteins in the cell that lead to particular cell responses.[78] Some of the consequences of PKA activation include the inhibition of myosin light chain phosphorylation, the inhibition of phosphoinositide hydrolysis, and the promotion of Ca^+/Na^+ exchange. Although β-adrenoceptor occupancy activates adenylyl cyclase, there is some evidence that independent activation of G_s that accompanies increased cAMP may also lead to activation of large-conductance potassium channels.[79] cAMP may also lead to the activation of protein kinase G, which facilitates relaxation of certain smooth muscles by inhibiting calcium mobilization.[80]

α_2-ADRENERGIC RECEPTOR PHARMACOLOGY

Many laboratories noted heterogeneity of α_2-adrenoceptors on the basis of both functional and radioligand binding studies. Most evidence for α_2-adrenoceptor studies originally came from radioligand binding studies in various tissues, functional studies in cell lines, and more recently in cells transfected with the genes or cDNA for the receptors.[39, 81] These studies have defined four pharmacologic and three molecular α_2-receptor subtypes.[82] In general, α_2-adrenoceptors are defined[83] as those that are sensitive to both the physiologic catecholamine agonists norepinephrine and epinephrine and the selective agonists such as B-HT 933 and UK-14,304, and they are antagonized by agents such as rauwolscine, yohimbine, and idazoxan. However, some α_2 subtypes also have high affinity for prazosin (previously thought to interact only with α_2-adrenoceptors), and others have relatively low affinity for yohimbine and rauwolscine compared with other α_2-adrenoceptors. Pharmacologically, the alignment of cloned α_2-adrenoceptors is better defined than that of α_1-adrenoceptor subtypes, with oxymetazoline and guanfacine being α_{2A}-selective and prazosin and ARC 239 being α_{2B}-selective.[77] Some evidence suggests that additional subtypes, or heterogeneity, or both exists. For example, two new α_2-adrenoceptor antagonists, SK&F 104978 and SK&F 104856, appear to functionally discriminate among α_2-adrenoceptors in a way that is not easily explained by their binding affinities at the known subtypes.[82] The affinities of several α_2-adrenoceptor antagonists for the expressed α_2-adrenoceptor clones are shown in Table 26–1.

α_2-Adrenergic Effector Systems

It has been postulated that the inhibition of adenylyl cyclase is a component of the signal transduction mechanism in most, if not all, cells that possess functional α_2-adrenoceptors.[84] The inhibition of adenylyl cyclase mediated by α_2-adrenoceptors is regulated by the G protein, G_i, that couples α_2-adrenoceptor occupancy to a reduction in the catalytic activity of adenylyl cyclase. Although the precise mechanism for this interaction is unknown, it has been shown that pertussis toxin inactivates G_i via ribosylation of the 41-kDa α-subunit of the G_i protein.[85] Inhibition of an adrenoceptor response by pertussis toxin has therefore been used as evidence for the critical role of inhibition of adenylyl cyclase in

TABLE 26–1. **Comparison of the Affinity (nM) of α_2-Adrenoceptor Antagonists for Expressed α_2-Adrenoceptor Clones**

Compound	Clone K_i (Expressed in Human CHO Cells)		
	α_{2A}	α_{2B}	α_{2C}
Rauwolscine	3.5	4.6	0.6
Yohimbine	1.6	7.2	1.1
SK&F 86466	9.4	15.8	19.8
SK&F 104078	114	142	64
Phentolamine	2.6	7.6	8.4
Prazosin	2133	365	95
Doxazosin	729	>5000	280
5-Methylurapidil	612	406	131
WB-4101	3.5	28	0.8
Indoramin	2240	528	476

Adapted from Hieble JP, Bondinell WE, Ruffolo RR: α- and β-adrenoreceptors: From the gene to the clinic. 1. Molecular biology and adrenoreceptor subclassification. J Med Chem 38:3415–3444, 1995. Copyright 1995 American Chemical Society.

the transduction of those responses. Additional, cell-specific, intracellular second-messenger systems may also be activated by α_2-adrenoceptors. These include stimulation of a plasma membrane–bound Na^+/H^+ exchange (antiporter) system in platelets that leads to an increase in intracellular pH resulting from enhanced extrusion of intracellular H^+, and to a concomitant release of membrane-bound calcium into the cell.[86, 87] In addition, in certain postjunctional vascular tissue receptors such as veins, α_2-adrenoceptors may mediate an influx of extracellular calcium that accompanies vasoconstriction, whereas in certain prejunctional receptors, the opposite—namely, a reduction of intracellular calcium—occurs.[88] The mechanism by which these calcium alterations occur is unknown, however.

α_1-ADRENERGIC RECEPTOR PHARMACOLOGY

In the mid-1980s, an unexpectedly complex analysis of the inhibition curves for the competitive antagonists WB-4101 and phentolamine used to displace ^{3}H-prazosin binding sites suggested the presence of two pharmacologically distinct α_1-adrenoceptor subtypes.[89] Presently, investigators have not agreed on the number or signaling mechanisms of the α_1-adrenoceptor subtypes. However, two native subtypes (α_{1A} and α_{1B}) can be distinguished pharmacologically, and three cDNAs encoding α_1 subtypes have been cloned.[41, 90] The α_{1A} subtype has a high affinity for the agonists methoxamine and oxymetazoline and the antagonists WB-4101, phentolamine, 5-methylurapidil, and (+) niguldipine but is resistant to alkylation by chloroethylclonidine. The α_{1B} subtype has considerably lower affinity for these agonists and antagonists but is insensitive to alkylation and inactivation by chloroethylclonidine. The two most selective agents currently available to distinguish among these subtypes are 5-methylurapidil and (+) niguldipine, both of which are at least 50 to 100 times more selective for the α_{1A} than for the α_{1B} subtypes. The profile of an increasing number of subtype-selective compounds at cloned and endogenous receptors has facilitated alignment between cloned and pharmacologically defined α_1-adrenoceptor subtypes. Thus, α_{1A}-adrenoceptors (previously designated α_{1C}), α_{1B}-adrenoceptors, and α_{1D} adrenoceptors (previously designated α_{1A}, α_{1D}, or $\alpha_{1A/D}$) are now recognized.[90] Table 26–2, however, reveals that although three clones have been isolated and expressed, none of them can account for the pharmacologically defined α_{1A} subtype. Most investigators agree that this unique subtype has not yet been cloned, despite extensive searches in tissues enriched in this pharmacologic subtype.[41]

α_1-Adrenergic Effector Systems

In most cells, the primary functional consequence of α_1-adrenoceptor activation is an increase in intracellular calcium.[91] This increase appears to result from the release of calcium from internal stores, from the influx of extracellular calcium into the cell, or both. Although there has been some evidence that α_{1A} and α_{1B} subtypes increase intracellular calcium by different mechanisms (α_{1A} by gating calcium influx through voltage gated channels, α_{1B} by mobilization of intracellular calcium via inositol phosphate production), these distinctions do not appear to be uniform or widely accepted.[41, 92] In addition, other signaling pathways known to be mediated by α_1-adrenoceptors, such as activation of phospholipases A_2 and D and potentiation of adenylyl cyclase activity, may also be potential regulatory mechanisms involved in the regulation of intracellular calcium by α_1-adrenoceptors.[93–96]

ADENYLYL CYCLASE AND REGULATION OF INTRAOCULAR PRESSURE—A UNIFYING HYPOTHESIS

The molecular changes that affect the production of cAMP by adenylyl cyclase are central to the regulation of aqueous humor inflow and outflow.[97, 98] In general, adrenergic agents increase outflow facility in primates; this is largely mediated by occupancy of α-adrenoceptor agonists. The effects of adrenergic agents on inflow, however, are mediated largely by occupancy of β-adrenoceptors and, concomitantly, the activity of adenylyl cyclase in the ciliary epithelium. A direct causal relationship of adenylyl cyclase activity and the production of aqueous humor is by no means clear, however. Compelling evidence garnered from a combination of in vitro studies of drug-mediated adenylyl cyclase activity and in vivo studies that assess the ability of various adrenergic drugs to lower IOP suggests a relationship by which a *net inhibition* of adenylyl cyclase activity underlies the apparent reduction of aqueous humor production by the ciliary processes.[99]

A net decrease of adenylyl cyclase activity may therefore result from either active, receptor-mediated blockade (as occurs with topical β-adrenergic antagonists such as timolol) or inhibition of adenylyl cyclase (as occurs with α_2-adrenergic agonists such as apraclonidine). In addition (Fig. 26–3), decreased adenylyl cyclase activity may result from desensitization of the stimulatory hormone/G protein/adenylyl cyclase cascade in the ciliary epithelium (as occurs with topical agonists such as epinephrine or isoproterenol).[100] Thus, the initial effect of β-adrenergic agonists such as isoproterenol or salbutamol (a selective β_2-adrenoceptor agonist) initially results in increased aqueous production, whereas prolonged stimulation results in desensitization of adenylyl cyclase activity in the ciliary epithelium and hence decreased aqueous

TABLE 26–2. **Comparison of the K_i (nM) Values of Native α_1-Adrenoceptor Subtypes from Rat Tissues with Those of Various cDNA Clones**

	Membranes		Clones		
Antagonist	***Rat*** α_{1A}	***Rat*** α_{1B}	***Rat*** α_{1D}	***Rat/Hamster*** α_{1B}	***Bovine*** α_{1A}
WB-4101	0.3	34	2	30	0.5
(+) Niguldipine	0.4	165	225	854	80
5-Methylurapidil	1	101	70	190	7
Oxymetazoline	3	193	2100	560	42

Adapted from Minneman KP, Esbenshade TA: α_1-Adrenergic receptor subtypes. Annu Rev Pharmacol Toxicol 34:117–133, 1994. With permission, from the Annual Review of Pharmacology and Toxicology, Volume 34 © 1994 by Annual Reviews.

production. The net functional effect that occurs in response to prolonged β-adrenoceptor occupancy by agonists therefore appears, similar to that which occurs from β-adrenoceptor blockade caused by drugs such as timolol. In both cases, decreased aqueous secretion results in reduced IOP.[99] Such an explanation is attractive in resolving the anomaly that both agonists and antagonists of β-adrenergic receptors lower IOP in primates and is supported experimentally.

Desensitization of rabbit iris/ciliary body membrane homogenates to stimulation of adenylyl cyclase activity has been documented after repeated topical administration of epinephrine in rabbit eyes for hours[100] and days.[101] In addition, according to ultrastructural evidence, within 30 minutes after topical treatment with 2% isoproterenol, sequestration of surface β-adrenergic receptors occurs in the nonpigmented epithelium of rabbit ciliary processes.[102] These findings thus substantiate the initial cellular events that occur in the process of desensitization of the β-adrenergic receptor/adenylyl cyclase system in this tissue.

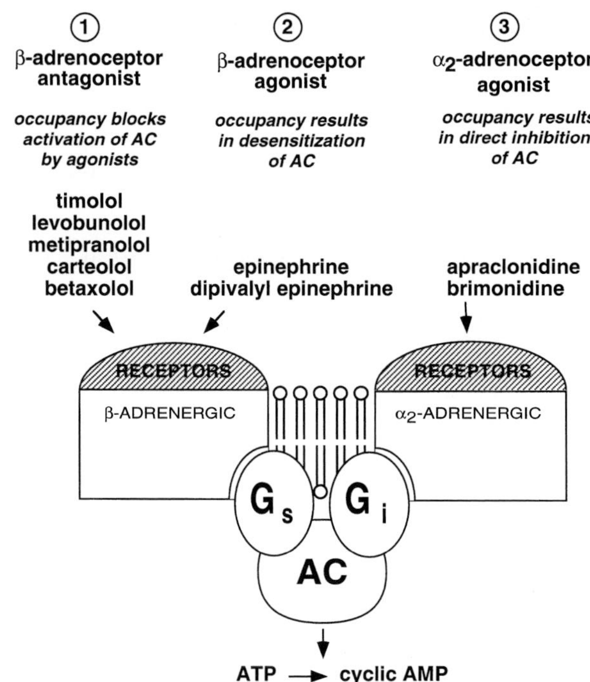

FIGURE 26–3. A schematic representation of the nonpigmented ciliary epithelial membrane containing β-adrenergic receptors, which activate adenylyl cyclase (AC) via the stimulatory guanine nucleotide binding protein (G_s), and α_2-adrenergic receptors, which attenuate AC activity via the inhibitory guanine nucleotide binding protein (G_i). AMP, adenosine monophosphate; ATP, adenosine triphosphate.

Studies of hydrostatically driven volume flow across the isolated rabbit ciliary epithelium have demonstrated that desensitization of β-adrenergic receptors achieved by successive in vivo daily treatments (3 days) with adrenergic agonists result in a diminished in vitro ability of adrenergic agonists to facilitate hydraulic conductivity.[103] Furthermore, studies that report a net reduction of IOP with both agonists and antagonists are consistent with fluorophotometric studies of adrenergic agonists that show varied effects (either increases or decreases in aqueous flow), depending largely on the time between topical drop instillation and measurements. Brubaker and colleagues[104] demonstrated that epinephrine produced a transient increase in aqueous humor formation initially, lasting several hours, followed by a prolonged phase (24 hours) during which aqueous humor is suppressed. It has been further postulated that endogenous adrenergic activity during the day serves to stimulate aqueous formation, and that this stimulation diminishes during sleep.[105, 106]

ADENYLYL CYCLASE AND ION TRANSPORT

Since Friedenwald's description (1933) of the ciliary body's "irreciprocal permeability to water," there has been substantial evidence that the active transport of solutes across ciliary epithelial layers creates an osmotic pressure gradient that results in the passive movement of water and hence, aqueous humor secretion.[107, 108] In current models of aqueous production, solute entry into the dual-layer ciliary epithelium occurs at the basolateral surface of the pigmented epithelial (PE) cells through several sodium-dependent cotransporters, including Na^+, H^+ exchange, Na^+-dependent $NaHCO_3^-$ exchange, electroneutral Na^+Cl^- cotransport, and others.[109–115] The nonpigmented ciliary epithelium (NPE) is thought to provide the main ion motive force for sodium-dependent cotransporters,[116] because physiologic and immunocytochemical evidence indicates that Na^+,K^+-ATPase resides in the basolateral membrane of the NPE.[117–121] Electroneutrality is thought to be maintained by anion channels in the NPE basolateral membrane.

β-Adrenoceptor antagonists such as timolol maleate lower IOP by inhibiting aqueous humor production.[122–124] These observations suggested that the regulation of adenylyl cyclase by adrenergic agents was not only pivotal to aqueous inflow, as discussed earlier, but presumably closely associated with the active ion transport processes that underlie aqueous production. In fact, it has recently been demonstrated that the β-adrenergic antagonist timolol, which reduces aqueous humor formation, inhibits cAMP-dependent, 4-4′-diisothiocyanatostilbene 2,2′disulfonic acid (DIDS)-sensitive chloride efflux;[125] this appears to be the basis for the hypotensive effect that occurs in response to virtually all topical β-adrenergic antagonists applied to the eye.

β-adrenoceptor antagonists appear to alter ion transport in the ciliary epithelium by at least two other significant mechanisms. An important contribution toward understanding their effect on active ion transport is the observation that protein kinase A activation reduced the activity of Na^+,K^+-ATPase in rabbit iris–ciliary body preparations.[126] These studies have been further extended to preparations of pure rabbit ciliary epithelium,[127] which demonstrate the attenuation of ouabain-sensitive Na^+,K^+-ATPase activity by dibutryl cAMP and forskolin. Although these studies identify a direct effect of cAMP on the sodium transport system in the ciliary epithelium, they are, curiously, almost directly opposite from the effects of cAMP on the chloride transport system in which activation of cAMP facilitates chloride ion transport. Thus, our understanding of the precise role of cAMP on these two transport systems, and their relationship with other important transport systems such as K^+ and HCO_3^-, remains incomplete. In addition to altering ion transport activity directly, β-adrenergic antagonists appear to alter the regional and subcellular distribution of yet another primary ion motive force in the ciliary epithelium, membrane-bound vacuolar H^+-ATPase, thus suggesting that changes in the intracellular distribution of the proton pump is another mechanism by which β-adrenergic antagonists regulate aqueous humor production.[128]

Clinical Studies

β-ADRENERGIC ANTAGONISTS

Prior to the introduction of topical β-adrenoceptor antagonists into ophthalmology, the most commonly used topical medications in the treatment of glaucoma were pilocarpine and epinephrine. These two classic medications have been used for more than 100 years. The introduction of the β-adrenoceptor antagonists completely changed the drug preference in glaucoma drug therapy in most countries (Table 26–3).

Propranolol was the first β-adrenoceptor antagonist that caused an ocular hypotensive effect in glaucoma patients following intravenous administration.[129, 130] In addition, it was found to be an effective hypotensive agent when administered topically[131] and orally.[132–136] Its main mechanism of action is to decrease aqueous humor formation,[137] although it has also been reported to both increase[138, 139] and decrease[140] outflow facility. Concerns over corneal anesthesia following topical propranolol limited its general acceptance.[141] Practolol, a β_1-selective adrenoceptor antagonist, was another effective topical ocular hypotensive that was recognized early,[142] but its clinical utility was limited because of serious adverse events such as oculomucocutaneous syndrome that occurred in approximately 5% of patients.[143] The chemical structures of key β-adrenoceptor antagonists currently in clinical use are shown in Figure 26–4.

Indications for Use

Timolol

Introduced for clinical use in America in 1978, topical timolol maleate (Timoptic, Timoptol) has been rapidly adopted as a standard treatment for open-angle glaucoma. Similar to propranolol, timolol is a nonselective β-adrenoceptor antagonist without intrinsic sympathomimetic activity. Timolol is apparently not metabolized in the eye, and its systemic metabolites have no significant pharmacologic activity.[144] Within the first hour after topical instillation in humans, the concentration of timolol in the anterior chamber is 1 to 2 μM (8 to 100 ng/mL),[145] which is approximately 1000 times the dissociation constant (K_d—i.e., the amount of drug that occupies 50% of the receptor binding sites at equilibrium) for timolol at the ocular β_2-adrenoceptor.[146] Most investigators think that antagonism of the β_2-adrenoceptor at the ciliary body is primarily responsible for the ocular hypotensive efficacy of timolol.[147, 148]

Given topically to humans with elevated IOP, timolol induces profound and long-lasting ocular hypotension. In the first published dose-response, time-response study of timolol in patients, mean decreases in IOP were over 30% (Table 26–4).[149] The maximal efficacy of 0.1%, 0.25%, and 0.5% timolol were similar, although after 12 and 24 hours after dosing, only 0.25% and 0.5% timolol appeared to pro-

TABLE 26–3. **Ophthalmic β-Adrenoceptor Antagonists Available in the United States**

	Timolol	Betaxolol	Levobunolol	Metipranolol	Carteolol
Strengths (in the United States)	0.25%, 0.5%	0.25% (Suspension); 0.5% (Solution)	0.25%, 0.5%	0.3%	1%
Brand names	Timoptic, Timoptic-XE, Timoptol	Betoptic, Betoptic-S	Betagan, Vistagan	Optipranolol	Ocupress
Property:					
Selectivity	NS	β_1	NS	NS	NS
Inflammation	N	N	N	Y	N
Active metabolite	N	N	Y	Y	N
Water-soluble	Y	Y	Y	Y	Very
ISA	N	N	N	N	Y
Combination	Y	N	N	N	N
Lipid benefit	N	N	N	N	Maybe
Vascular benefit	N	Maybe	N	N	N
Off-patent in United States	Y	N	Y	N	N

Abbreviations: N, no; Y, yes; NS, nonselective; ISA, intrinsic sympathomimetic activity.

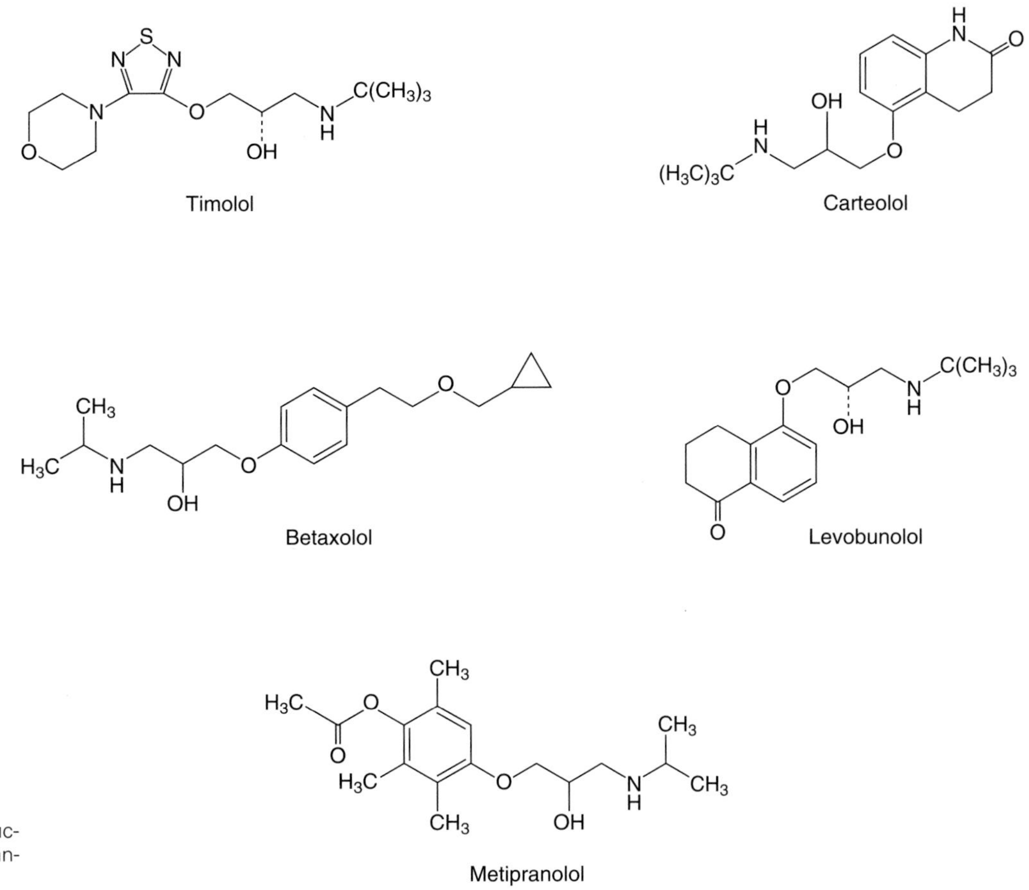

FIGURE 26–4. Chemical structures of key β-adrenoreceptor antagonists in clinical use.

duce an effect greater than vehicle. The ocular hypotensive efficacy of timolol was superior to that of pilocarpine, then the standard for ocular hypotensive efficacy, in a double-masked, randomized study in 28 patients (Table 26–5).[150] The timolol group showed a decrease of approximately 10 beats/min in heart rate versus a slight heart rate increase in the pilocarpine group. This was the first of many subsequent and related findings by which we have come to appreciate the numerous potential cardiovascular side effects of this class of glaucoma medications. In one long-term controlled study of 0.5% timolol given twice daily, the ocular hypotensive efficacy of timolol was approximately 7 mm Hg, or a 26% reduction. In a subset of these patients, chronic therapy with twice-daily timolol provided a consistent ocular hypotensive effect throughout the day.[151]

Early in the development of timolol, there was a report of a relatively rapidly developing tolerance, or "escape," to the ocular hypotensive effects of timolol.[150, 152, 153] Oksala and Salminen reported that approximately one-third of patients initially treated with timolol exhibited this escape.[154] Steinert and associates also described a longer-term "drift," or tolerance, in which approximately 30 to 40% of patients treated with timolol for 1 year required additional ocular hypotensive therapy.[150, 152, 155] As viewed now, nearly two decades later, the observation might also be explained as a change in disease state or compliance in those patients, rather than a tolerance to timolol per se. The failure rate with timolol in a controlled 4-year study was less than 15% per year.[156]

Krupin and associates[163] investigated several aspects of timolol efficacy in a paired-comparison study in 25 ocular

TABLE 26–4. **Acute Ocular Hypotensive Effects of Timolol (mm Hg)***

			Dose					
	Vehicle		*0.1%*		*0.25%*		*0.5%*	
Time (hr)	*Mean*	*%*	*Mean*	*%*	*Mean*	*%*	*Mean*	*%*
0	22.0		26.2		23.7		28.0	
2	1.0	4.5	8.5	32.4	7.8	32.9	8.7	31.1
12	6.1	27.7	6.5	24.8	9.0	38.0	11.0	39.3
24	2.0	9.1	6.6	25.2	6.6	27.8	11.1	39.6

*Treated eye only, selected times and doses.
Adapted from Zimmerman TJ, Kaufman HE: Timolol: Dose response and duration of action. Arch Ophthalmol 95:605–607, 1977.

TABLE 26–5. **Chronic Ocular Hypotensive Effect of Timolol: Mean and Percentage Change from Baseline (mm Hg)***

	Dose			
	Timolol		*Pilocarpine*	
Time (wk)	*Mean*	*%*	*Mean*	*%*
0	34.0		28.0	
2	−13.0	38	−7.5	27
6	−13.5	40	−7.0	25
10	−13.0	38	−7.0	25

*This was a titration study with thrice-a-day dosing. Values are as estimated from a graph.

Adapted from Boger WP, Steinert RF, Puliafito CA, Pavan-Langston D: Clinical trial comparing timolol ophthalmic solution to pilocarpine in open-angle glaucoma. Am J Ophthalmol 86:8–18, 1978. Copyright 1978, with permission from Elsevier Science.

hypotensive patients and found that the IOP was lower acutely with 0.25% timolol than chronically with either 0.25% or 0.5% timolol, and that both strengths of chronic administration were similar in their efficacy (Table 26–6). They also found that the fellow, untreated control eye showed decreases in IOP, thus identifying the potential for contralateral hypotensive effects via systemic absorption via topical drop delivery.[157–159] The contralateral effects of timolol may be relatively small in normal volunteers.[160] In rabbits, the aqueous humor level of timolol in the contralateral eye to treatment was 19.5 mg/mL, whereas the level in the ipsilateral eye was 328 mg/mL. Thus, even the timolol level in the contralateral rabbit eye is considerably more than that required for adenylyl cyclase inhibition (~ 0.8 mg/mL),[161, 162] which underscores the possibility that significant systemic levels of timolol, with correspondingly effective levels in the contralateral eye, may occur after topical eye drop delivery. The potential to elicit harmful systemic side effects due to systemic absorption of topical timolol prompted several investigators to consider whether a lower dose, or once-daily delivery of timolol, would retain hypotensive efficacy yet minimize these adverse effects. The efficacy of 0.25% timolol has been reported in both short-term[163] and long-term studies.[164] The chronic efficacy of even lower concentrations of timolol has been evaluated. In an open-label study, 0.1% timolol elicited a mean decrease in IOP of approximately 24%.[165] In another study, treatment with twice-daily 0.125% timolol resulted in a mean reduction in IOP of approximately 26%.[166]

With regard to dosing frequency, once-daily therapy with timolol, generally in the morning, has been reported to be an effective ocular hypotensive regimen. This finding is consistent with the observation that aqueous flow shows diurnal variation, and the ability of timolol to reduce this flow is greatest during the day.[167] It was found that the ocular hypotensive effect of once-daily 0.25% or 0.5% timolol ranged from 17 to 28%, which overlaps with that of twice-daily timolol. The most recent effort to develop an efficacious preparation of once-daily timolol that minimizes systemic side effects has resulted in a formulation of timolol in a gel-forming solution (Timoptic-XE). Given once daily in either 0.25% or 0.5% strengths, this formulation has been reported equivalent to the twice-daily solution.[168–170]

TABLE 26–6. **Ocular Hypotensive Effect of Timolol (mm Hg)**

	Baseline	0.25% Timolol, 1 hr	0.25% Timolol, 3–4 wk	0.5% Timolol, 3–4 wk
Treated eye	28.1 ± 5.3	18.5 ± 4.5	21.1 ± 4.2	20.4 ± 3.5
Control eye	26.7 ± 4.8	23.8 ± 4.9	25.0 ± 5.1	24.0 ± 3.9

Adapted from Krupin T, Singer PR, Perlmutter J, et al: One-hour intraocular pressure response to timolol: Lack of correlation with long-term response. Arch Ophthalmol 99:840–841, 1981.

The popularity of timolol is largely due to its ocular hypotensive efficacy, relative lack of untoward ocular symptoms, and duration of action, which required only once- or twice-daily instillation. For patients without contraindications, which are generally systemic, timolol is indicated for the treatment of primary open-angle glaucoma. Timolol is also useful in many cases of secondary glaucoma, aphakic glaucoma, and ocular hypertension.[171–173] Other uses include the prophylactic treatment of elevations in IOP after laser iridotomy or capsulotomy.[174–177] Timolol is also effective as a prophylactic treatment for elevations in IOP after cataract surgery.[178–180] An alternate salt, timolol hemihydrate, has been reported to be as efficacious as timolol maleate.[181] Timolol maleate is also available in a unit-of-use, nonpreserved form for patients with allergies to the preservative. Timolol 0.1% is available for general use in Europe.

Levobunolol

Levobunolol is a nonselective β-adrenoceptor antagonist without intrinsic sympathomimetic activity. Like timolol, it is more potent than propranolol when used orally as a treatment for systemic hypertension.[182] Levobunolol is metabolized to dihydrobunolol, a compound with equipotent β-adrenoceptor antagonistic effects in systemic and ocular animal models.[183–185] Topically applied, levobunolol readily penetrates the cornea in rabbits and is metabolized to dihydrobunolol.[186] In human iris–ciliary body tissue, the affinity of dihydrolevobunolol and levobunolol for the β-adrenoceptor is 6.7 nM and 3.9 nM, respectively, which is similar to the high potency achieved by timolol (1.4 nM) in the same tissue.[146] Levobunolol was introduced in the United States in 1985.

Given topically to humans with elevated IOP, levobunolol induces profound and long-lasting ocular hypotension. In concentrations of 0.03 to 2%, levobunolol caused mean decreases in IOP of 5 to 11 mm Hg (vehicle was 4 mm Hg), and the duration of activity with the higher concentrations was at least 24 hours. Given twice daily for 3 months, 0.5% and 1% levobunolol reduced mean IOP 9 mm Hg from an unmedicated baseline of 27 mm Hg.[187] The long-term efficacy of levobunolol was investigated in a large, double-masked comparison in which the mean reduction in IOP over 4 years with twice-daily 0.5% and 1% levobunolol was 7 mm Hg and was equivalent to that of timolol.[156] The rate of inadequate ocular hypotensive effect, as judged by the need to add additional ocular hypotensive therapy, was approximately 5 to 10% per year in patients receiving levobunolol, as is likely similar to that found in patients taking other β-blockers such as timolol.[156] Levobunolol was similar to timolol in controlling IOP throughout the day as measured in a subset of patients given diurnal examinations.[151] Levobunolol had no significant local anesthetic, mydriatic, or dry eye–inducing properties.[188–192]

In controlled studies, once-daily therapy of levobunolol was also found to be an effective ocular hypotensive regimen. The ocular hypotensive effect of once-daily 0.25% or 0.5% levobunolol is similar to that reported for twice-daily dosing.[193–196] Indeed, one double-masked study directly comparing the regimens of once-daily and twice-daily 0.5% levobunolol found them equivalent.[197] Chronic therapy apparently increases the potency of levobunolol.[156, 187, 192, 195, 198] Thus, as with timolol, one may consider using lower concentrations less frequently.

Similar to timolol, levobunolol has been reported effective for prophylactic treatment of elevations in IOP after cataract surgery and Nd:YAG laser capsulotomy.[199] As a prophylactic agent for post-cataract surgery elevations in IOP after cataract surgery, levobunolol was found the most effective, followed by timolol, whereas betaxolol was ineffective.[200] In a separate study of the same indication, carbachol was the most effective in controlling postoperative IOP, followed by timolol, oral acetazolamide, pilocarpine gel (Pilopine), and levobunolol. Betaxolol was somewhat less effective, and apraclonidine was not significantly better than the control.[180]

Ophthalmic levobunolol is supplied as a sterile solution of the levo-isomer of the hydrochloride salt with the viscosity agent polyvinyl alcohol 1.4%. Brand names include Betagan and Vistagan; generic preparations are also available. Multiuse containers of levobunolol are preserved with benzalkonium chloride 0.004%. In the United States, levobunolol is available in 0.25% and 0.5% strengths.

Metipranolol

Metipranolol is a nonselective β-adrenoceptor antagonist without intrinsic sympathomimetic activity. Metipranolol has an active metabolite, desacetyl-metipranolol, which is as effective as metipranolol in vitro.[201, 202] Metipranolol has been used for over 15 years worldwide as an oral treatment for systemic hypertension and topically for the treatment of elevated IOP.[201, 203–205] Metipranolol was approved for topical use in the United States in 1989, and its ophthalmic use has been reviewed.[203]

Given topically in a single dose in a vehicle-controlled study, metipranolol significantly reduced IOP.[206] On a more chronic basis, metipranolol has been used in concentrations ranging from 0.1% to 0.6%, and it has shown ocular hypotensive efficacy similar to that of other nonselective agents.[206–214] Germany has a combination product containing metipranolol and pilocarpine, and adjunctive therapy has been reported effective.[215–217]

Metipranolol has been used for the chronic treatment of elevated IOP in ocular hypertension and glaucoma. Its utility in IOP elevations after laser or cataract surgery, as well as its additivity with other ocular hypotensive agents, needs to be evaluated in future research. Ophthalmic metipranolol is supplied in the United States as Optipranolol, a sterile ophthalmic solution of 0.3% racemic metipranolol, preserved with 0.004% benzalkonium chloride, and labeled for twice-daily use.

Carteolol

Carteolol is a nonselective β-adrenoceptor antagonist similar to timolol, levobunolol, and metipranolol. Also similar to levobunolol and metipranolol, a primary metabolite of carteolol, 8-hydroxycarteolol, has ocular β-blocking properties, although unlike the other agents, its potency is much less than the parent compound.[218, 219] In contrast with these agents, as well as betaxolol, carteolol possesses intrinsic sympathomimetic activity (ISA), discussed later. The ocular hypotensive efficacy and ocular safety of topical carteolol has recently been reviewed.[220, 221] Topical carteolol has been marketed in the United States since 1990 and is available in Europe and Japan.

Several studies have reported the ocular hypotensive efficacy of carteolol. In an acute dose-response study, an increasing ocular hypotensive effect occurred in response to concentrations of carteolol ranging from 0.5 to 2%, each of which was more effective than vehicle.[222] In an 8-week study, 2% carteolol was found similar in ocular hypotensive efficacy to 0.75% carbachol.[223] In a vehicle-controlled crossover study of 2% carteolol in 12 patients for 2 weeks, carteolol significantly reduced IOP by 11% and 14% at 1 and 2 weeks, respectively.[224]

The ocular hypotensive efficacy of carteolol has been compared with that of timolol in several controlled studies. Overall, some studies have reported carteolol to be equivalent to timolol, whereas others have found timolol either more effective or longer lasting.[225–227] The two large studies reporting equivalency include a double-masked, parallel study in which 1% carteolol given twice daily was compared with 0.25% timolol given twice daily over 1 month. Carteolol was as effective as timolol in reducing IOP, and fewer patients reported adverse events, including eye irritation, in the group treated with carteolol.[226] In the second study reporting equivalency, 1% and 2% carteolol given twice daily were compared with 0.5% timolol given twice daily in 105 patients over a 3-month period. All three treatments were similarly effective and without significant ocular or systemic effects.[227] In two separate postmarketing studies involving more than 900 patients, carteolol was well tolerated and judged effective and safe in patients who switched from other β-adrenoceptor antagonists.[205, 228]

Carteolol is unique among ophthalmic β-adrenoceptor antagonists in having ISA, but it is unclear whether this confers a more favorable effect on serum lipids associated with its topical use. Given systematically, in contrast with traditional agents such as propranolol, carteolol has been found to have no effect on lipids and lipoproteins.[229] However, in controlled studies on healthy normal volunteers, topical carteolol eye drop treatment decreased high-density lipoprotein cholesterol levels by 3.3% and raised the ratio of total to high-density lipoprotein cholesterol levels by 4.0%; in comparison, timolol treatment decreased high-density lipoprotein cholesterol levels by 8% and raised the ratio of total to high-density lipoprotein cholesterol levels by 10.0%.[230, 231] Carteolol and timolol produced similar effects on lipids in a multicenter, double-blind comparison study in patients with primary open-angle glaucoma or ocular hypertension. Timolol increased mean cholesterol levels by 6 to 26 mg/dL, whereas carteolol decreased cholesterol levels by 6 to 15 mg/dL.[232]

Similar to the other β-adrenoceptor antagonists, carteolol has been used for the chronic treatment of elevated IOP in ocular hypertension and glaucoma. Its utility in IOP elevations following laser or cataract surgery, as well as its additivity with other ocular hypotensive agents, needs to be evaluated in future research. The current U.S. labeling for carteolol lists the same contraindications as for timolol. Ophthalmic carteolol is supplied in the United States as Ocupress, a sterile ophthalmic solution of 1% racemic carteolol, preserved with 0.005% benzalkonium chloride, and labeled for twice-daily use.

Betaxolol

Betaxolol is a β-adrenoceptor antagonist with relative selectivity for the β_1-adrenoceptor. Its apparent K_d at the ocular β_2-adrenoceptors in human iris–ciliary body is approximately 90 nM, which is nearly two orders of magnitude less potent than timolol (1.4 nM).[146] However, it is clear that the effective concentration of betaxolol in the aqueous humor following topical delivery is high enough to occupy β_2-adrenoceptors of the ciliary process epithelium, thus allowing it to be an effective ocular hypotensive agent by inhibiting aqueous production in a manner similar to that of other β-adrenoceptor antagonists.[233, 234] Although clinical doses of oral betaxolol result in plasma levels of 10 to 40 ng/mL,[235, 236] topical betaxolol generally results in plasma levels below the limit of detection.[37] Given orally, the half-life of oral betaxolol is 12 hours.[237] Betaxolol, systematically administered, appears to be metabolized to inactive compounds.[238, 239]

Initial studies reported that betaxolol solution had ocular hypotensive efficacy in concentrations of 0.25%, twice daily.[240–244] However, most subsequent studies evaluated the hypotensive efficacy of 0.5% betaxolol. Twice-daily 0.5% betaxolol was reported similar to 0.5% timolol in studies of 46 patients,[245] 41 patients,[246] 40 patients,[247] and 29 patients.[248] A study of similar size, 38 patients, reported that timolol was a more effective ocular hypotensive agent than betaxolol by approximately 2 mm Hg.[249] In a larger controlled, double-masked, 3-month study of approximately 30 patients per treatment group, mean reductions in IOP in the groups given 0.25% levobunolol, 0.5% levobunolol, and 0.5% betaxolol solutions, twice-daily, were 6.2, 6, and 3.7 mm Hg, respectively. This difference in efficacy between levobunolol and betaxolol was statistically significant, although systemic safety measures showed no statistically significant intergroup differences. There was also some suggestion that the duration of action of betaxolol was less than that of levobunolol.[250]

In a large (353-patient) study, patients whose conditions were successfully controlled by timolol therapy were switched to betaxolol therapy, or they remained on timolol therapy, and were evaluated for 3 months. Patients switched to the betaxolol ophthalmic solution experienced a significant increase in both ocular side effects (burning/stinging and tearing) and IOP when compared with patients who continued to receive timolol.[251] Betaxolol has been reported less effective that timolol or levobunolol in preventing post–cataract surgery elevations in IOP, especially when a viscoelastic agent is used.[180, 200, 252] Thus, it is probably not the agent of choice for this indication.

Several studies have evaluated the effect of betaxolol on the ocular vasculature. In rabbits receiving single, topical doses of phenylephrine, timolol, or betaxolol, all three agents caused substantial, localized constriction in the arterioles that supply the ciliary processes but did not affect the downstream bore of the same vessels. After 7 weeks, tolerance reduced the response to betaxolol to insignificant levels and that to phenylephrine substantially, whereas timolol maleate continued to produce levels of vasoconstriction identical to those of single-dose administration.[253] These findings suggest that tolerance-resistant relaxation of peripheral vascular beds may be a potential benefit of betaxolol therapy because it does not appear to occur after treatment with other β-adrenoceptor antagonists.

Two studies compared the effect of long-term betaxolol treatment on visual fields with timolol treatment. In a randomized, double-masked study with observations up to 30 months in 40 patients, timolol was more effective than betaxolol in decreasing IOP. Mean sensitivity increased in both groups by approximately 1 to 2 dB throughout the first 9 to 12 months of the study. After the first year of the study, mean sensitivity gradually decreased in both treatment groups, although the mean value in the betaxolol group was significantly greater than the mean value in the timolol group.[254] In a second, open-label, parallel study, timolol and betaxolol were compared for 2 years in 20 patients. As in the previous study, timolol was more effective than betaxolol as an ocular hypotensive agent throughout the 2 years. As measured by automated visual fields, retinal sensitivity decreased in the first 6 months in the timolol and betaxolol treatment groups by 0.5 to 0.6 dB and 0.2 to 0.3 dB, respectively. However, at the 1- and 2-year visits, retinal sensitivity increased 0.8 to 0.9 dB in the betaxolol treatment group only.[255] In an additional study in normal volunteers, neither betaxolol, epinephrine, pilocarpine, nor timolol had any influence on visual function as determined by high-pass, resolution perimetry.[256]

Ophthalmic betaxolol is supplied in the United States in two formulations. One product, Betoptic, is a sterile solution of 0.5% betaxolol HCl. The second product, Betoptic S, is a sterile ophthalmic suspension of 0.25% betaxolol HCl. The suspension is a unique formulation containing a polyacrylic acid polymer (carbomer 934P) and a cationic exchange resin, which is believed to increase the residence time in the human eye.[257] Both products are the racemic compound, preserved with 0.01% benzalkonium chloride and labeled for twice-daily use. The 0.25% suspension was as efficacious as the 0.5% solution in a large (352-patient), controlled, 3-month study. In addition, the prevalence of ocular discomfort upon topical instillation was significantly lower for 0.25% betaxolol suspension than for 0.5% betaxolol solution.[258]

Other β-Adrenoceptor Antagonists

Nadolol. Nadolol (Corgard), used clinically to treat angina and hypertension, is a nonselective β-adrenoceptor antagonist with no local anesthetic properties and a β-blocking potency equivalent to that of propranolol. However, its markedly fewer direct myocardial depressant effects are clinically interesting. The unique pharmacologic aspect of nadolol is that it is not metabolized; it is primarily excreted unchanged by the kidney.[259] Nadolol significantly reduced IOP in glaucomatous patients.[260–262] The reduction was maximal at 4 hours and lasted 6 to 24 hours. Blood pressure, pulse rate, and pupil diameter were not significantly affected. However, with long-term use, nadolol appears to be a less effective ocular hypotensive agent than timolol.[260] Diacetyl nadolol, a lipophilic prodrug analog that can penetrate the corneal epithelium 10 times better than nadolol, has been tested. A 2% preparation decreased IOP about as well as 0.5% timolol during the first 8 hours following topical administration.[263, 264]

Oxprenolol. Oxprenolol has ISA and a membrane stabilizing effect. Its administration in 1% solution produced, in glaucomatous eyes, a maximum drop in ocular pressure of 28%. The decrease was most pronounced at the second and third hours, and recovery was complete 6 to 12 hours later.[265] Although the drug was well tolerated, transient and slight hyperemia and some miosis were reported. Oxprenolol does not trigger tachycardia, the limiting side effect of isoproterenol. Topical oxprenolol also can apparently lead to corneal epitheliopathy.[266]

Pindolol. Pindolol has ISA but no local anesthetic action at clinically useful levels. It has only one-third the antiarrhythmic property of propranolol.[267] Instilled into the conjunctival sac of normal and glaucomatous eyes, the drug significantly reduced IOP.[267] With prolonged treatment, facility of outflow apparently increased. No effect on either pupil motility or corneal sensitivity was detectable. Smith and coworkers[268] reported that pindolol lowered IOP in both treated and untreated eyes with only minimal reduction in resting pupil diameter and light reflex response. The authors reported a decrease in resting heart rate and a reduction in exercise tachycardia after topical administration. Pindolol 0.25%, administered topically twice daily to the eyes of patients with open-angle glaucoma, controlled IOP as effectively as timolol 0.5% twice daily.[269]

Bupranolol. Bupranolol is available for general use in Germany. It is chemically related to propranolol and is more potent in blocking β-adrenoceptor sites. Topical application of a 0.5% solution significantly lowers IOP in glaucomatous eyes. In one study, the maximum effect (68%) occurred within 4 hours and lasted more than 24 hours. No significant effect on outflow facility, blood pressure, or tear flow was detectable. However, bupranolol produced local anesthesia in the eye, and tachyphylaxis could be a problem.[270–274]

Atenolol and Metoprolol. Atenolol, a β_1-selective adrenoceptor antagonist with no sympathomimetic or membrane stabilizing activity, is currently used clinically for the treatment of mild to moderate systemic hypertension. Topical ocular application of atenolol, as 1%, 2%, and 4% drops, reduced IOP in patients with ocular hypertension.[275–277] However, the ocular effect of atenolol is relatively short-lived: drops may have to be instilled 4 to 6 times daily for 24-hour control of IOP.[136] In this regard, the ocular duration of action is shorter than its oral, antihypertensive action, in which once-daily oral therapy is the standard. A single oral 50-mg dose of atenolol decreases IOP in patients with ocular hypertension, open-angle glaucoma, and chronic angle-closure glaucoma.[278] However, long-term drift and short-term escape have been reported for atenolol. Atenolol was ineffective in lowering IOP in cats.[279] Metoprolol, pharmacologically similar to atenolol, is used clinically to treat mild to moderate systemic hypertension. Topically administered metoprolol can effectively reduce IOP.[280–283] Patients with ocular hypertension or glaucoma treated with 3% metoprolol for 4 months were able to maintain IOPs between 23% and 30% below pretreatment values.[284] Metoprolol has been reported to be comparable in reducing IOP to pilocarpine (2 to 4%) and timolol (0.5%). However, other studies have found metoprolol to be less effective than timolol in reducing IOP.[283–289] Oral metoprolol has also been shown to be able to reduce IOP.[284, 288, 289] Topical metoprolol has been reported to cause allergic reactions.

Safety and Adverse Effects of β-Adrenoceptor Antagonists

Timolol

Timolol use is associated with numerous ocular effects.[290–292] A topical allergic reaction, somewhat similar to that reported for topical adrenoceptor agonists,[293–295] has been reported for timolol.[296] This reaction is a blepharoconjunctivitis, with chemosis, injection, and edema of the lids. This reaction may occur as early as in the first month of therapy or may occur with prolonged use. Similar reactions have been reported to occur with nadolol,[263] levobunolol,[189] and metoprolol.[297] Because antigenic cross-reactivity among β-antagonists is not complete,[297] the allergic sensitivity is likely related to the specific chemical structure of a given β-antagonist. With several β-adrenoceptor antagonists available for general use, patients developing allergies often can be switched to an alternative agent[298] and remain free of sensitivity to the newer agent.

In high concentrations, β-adrenoceptor antagonists stabilize membrane excitability. Clinically, this may be observed as decreased corneal sensitivity. In an early clinical report, van Buskirk found significant decreases in corneal sensitivity in several patients.[299, 300] In comparative studies using a quantitative esthesiometer, however, timolol ranks low among β-adrenoceptor antagonists in its corneal anesthetic effects.[141] In a large controlled study, corneal sensitivity was not of major clinical significance for timolol.[190] In some patients, timolol has been reported to induce superficial punctate keratitis[300] which, if untreated, may lead to corneal epithelial erosions.[301] Topical timolol may reduce tear break-up time,[302] elicit some dry-eye symptoms,[303] or decrease tear flow,[304] but it does not appear to induce the severe ocular pemphigoid reported with practolol.[305] Rare reported adverse ocular reactions include macular edema in aphakics, macular hemorrhage, retinal detachment, uveitis, and progressive cataracts,[300, 306] although a causal relationship to timolol use is unclear in these reports.

Whenever timolol is given topically, side effects resulting from systemic β-blockade are possible. The mean plasma level of 0.5% timolol in the first few hours after administration is approximately 1 ng/mL. Plasma levels of topical timolol can be higher in newborns (up to 20 ng/mL)[307] and lower with punctal occlusion or eyelid closure (0.4 ng/mL).[308] The oral administration of timolol results in levels of 5 to 50 ng/mL, in which the cardiac β-blockade is log-linear dose-dependent.[309]

The blood levels achieved with topical timolol are much less than those seen with chronic, oral administration. That significant β-adrenoceptor blockade can occur with topical instillation is probably the result of many factors. First, unlike oral administration, ocularly instilled medications may reach the heart directly, via nasolacrimal and pharyngeal absorption, without exposure to hepatic metabolism or mixing and dilution.[310] Thus, mean plasma levels 1 hour after an eye drop may underrepresent the acute levels in the heart. The amount of drug available for interaction with receptors also depends on many additional factors, including plasma protein binding.[311] It also appears that even with systemic administration, plasma levels are not always indicative of systemic β-blockade.[312]

The presence of pharmacologically effective plasma levels of timolol after topical instillation dictates that the clinician consider the risk of systemic β-blockade when administering any β-adrenoceptor antagonist therapy for glaucoma. β-Adrenoceptors are involved in many physiologic processes. Thus, antagonism of β-adrenoceptors can result in bradycardia, systemic hypotension, congestive heart failure, heart block, bronchospasm, diarrhea, and amnesia.[259] All of these adverse effects have been reported with topical timolol therapy. In some cases, these adverse events have been serious, life-threatening, and even lethal. Systemic adverse events may be more frequent in the elderly because of greater variability in dosage, a greater propensity for co-existing systemic conditions and, because of flaccid lids, potentially greater storage of instilled volumes in the lower cul-de-sac.[313]

Mean resting heart rate may decrease 3 to 10 beats/min during use of timolol.[156] Other cardiovascular effects include palpitations, systemic hypotension, and syncope.[306] As with oral β-adrenoceptor antagonists, topical timolol may reduce exercise- or isoproterenol-induced tachycardia. This may be a problem not only in patients with compromised cardiovascular status but in patients who normally engage in strenuous exercise.[311, 314–317]

Wheezing, dyspnea, bronchospasm, and other signs and symptoms of decreased respiratory function have been reported following timolol use.[300] Acute bronchospasm has occurred in previously asymptomatic asthmatic patients following the topical use of timolol.[318, 319] Timolol elicited an average decrease in forced expiratory volume (FEV_1) of 25% in patients with chronic obstructive pulmonary disease.[320] Scharrer and Ober evaluated the safety of timolol in 26 patients with relative cardiovascular and pulmonary contraindications to timolol.[321] Although 58% of the patients showed untoward reactions to timolol, 42% did not. This study demonstrates that not all patients who are expected to have a negative response to timolol actually do when challenged.[322] Bronchospasm often goes unnoticed in patients. Cross-over studies of patients who were switched from timolol to an agent with less or no β-adrenoceptor antagonistic properties (betaxolol, dipivefrin, or pilocarpine) found cases of clinically significant increases in pulmonary function.[322, 323]

Topical β-blocking agents have been associated with adverse central nervous system (CNS) effects, including depression, emotional lability, and sexual dysfunction. Complaints of lethargy, lightheadedness, weakness, fatigue, mental depression, dissociative behavior, and memory loss are most common. The onset of symptoms varies from a few days to months following initiation of therapy. These symptoms usually are mild and transient. Timolol sometimes must be discontinued because of these CNS effects.[306, 324]

Topical β-adrenoceptor antagonists also may elicit dermatologic signs and symptoms, including rashes, alopecia, urticaria, and discoloration of nails.[195, 300, 325–327] Other systemic effects reported after topical β-adrenoceptor antagonists treatment include myasthenia gravis and retroperitoneal fibrosis.[326, 328, 329] When treating a nursing mother, clinicians should also be aware that topically applied timolol may find its way to breast milk.[330]

Current labeling for timolol states that it is contraindicated in patients with bronchial asthma or with a history of bronchial asthma or severe chronic obstructive pulmonary disease. It is similarly contraindicated in patients with bradycardia or severe heart block, overt cardiac failure, and hypersensitivity to any component. More broadly, timolol therapy should be considered with caution in patients with any significant sign, symptom, or history for which systemic β-blockade would be medically unwise. This includes disorders of cardiovascular or respiratory origin (e.g., chronic obstructive pulmonary disease, asthma, chronic bronchitis, and emphysema), as well as a host of other conditions.[331] Spirometric evaluation after institution of timolol therapy may help identify patients in whom bronchospasm develops following commencement of therapy.[320] In general, however, it is best to avoid timolol in patients with asthma and other obstructive pulmonary diseases. Sympathetic stimulation may be essential to supporting the circulation in patients with diminished myocardial contractility, and its inhibition by β-adrenergic receptor blockade may precipitate more severe failure. β-Adrenoceptor blockade, as may occur with topical timolol, may masks the signs and symptoms of thyrotoxicosis or acute hypoglycemia. Thus, timolol should be administered cautiously in patients prone to such disorders, including diabetics.[332, 333]

Because using two β-adrenoceptor antagonists does not increase ocular hypotensive efficacy, such a combination can only increase the possibility of an untoward event and is therefore not advised. Timolol may cause a relative systemic overdose in children and infants, and thus it should be used cautiously in these patients.

Levobunolol

Because levobunolol is pharmacologically similar to timolol, its profile of side effects is similar, although there are fewer actual reports with the newer compound.[290] In some studies, its ocular comfort is similar to that of timolol,[190] although there is one report of its being slightly less comfortable than timolol.[334] Corneal anesthesia is not a significant problem with levobunolol.[141, 188, 190] Although allergic blepharoconjunctivitis can occur with levobunolol, it may also be acceptable in patients in whom timolol elicits an allergic reaction.[298] Dendritic keratopathy, resolving after cessation of treatment, has been reported with levobunolol.[335]

Levobunolol is similar to timolol in producing plasma levels of approximately 1 ng/mL after topical instillation.[336] In a cross-over study of normal volunteers, 0.5% levobunolol, in either a single 20-, 35-, or 50-μL drop, reduced maximal exercise-induced heart rate by approximately 9 beats/min, with no difference in either efficacy or safety among these three drop sizes.[337] The reduction in exercise-induced heart rate was similar to that caused by timolol.[314] Mean resting heart rate may decrease 3 to 10 beats/min during use of levobunolol, and blood pressure may decrease mildly.[156]

The contraindication labeling for levobunolol in the United States is currently the same as that for timolol. Thus, levobunolol is contraindicated in patients with bronchial asthma or with a history of bronchial asthma or severe chronic obstructive pulmonary disease. It is similarly contraindicated in patients with bradycardia or severe heart block, overt cardiac failure, and hypersensitivity to any component. As with timolol, caution should be used when considering levobunolol therapy in patients with any significant sign, symptom, or history for which systemic β-blockade would be medically unwise.

Metipranolol

Metipranolol is a potent and effective β_1- and β_2-adrenoceptor antagonist, and thus it shares the same potential for systemic β-blockade as timolol and levobunolol. In one study, two groups of asthmatic patients received either carteolol (1% and 2%) or metipranolol (0.3% and 0.6%) eye drops and underwent pulmonary function testing 30 minutes later. Mean FEV_1 decreased slightly with both agents: 7% with carteolol and 15% with metipranolol.[338] In a trial in normal volunteers, systemic β-adrenoreceptor blockade was assessed by the increase in isoproterenol dose required to elevate heart rate. The mean dose of isoproterenol required after 0.6% metipranolol was 5.2 μg, only slightly greater than that required for vehicle, 3.1 μg. The mean dose required after 0.5% timolol was higher, 10.9 μg, and after 2% carteolol even greater, 39.6 μg.[316] In a trial in normal volunteers, mean maximal heart rates obtained with a standard exercise protocol were 156, 154, and 152 beats/min for vehicle, 0.1% metipranolol, and 0.3% timolol, respectively. The authors concluded that metipranolol elicited less systemic β-adrenoceptor blockade than timolol in these doses.[339] In another study in normal volunteers based on bronchodilation, heart rate, and finger tremor, the order of increasing β-blockade was betaxolol, metipranolol, and timolol.[340] In a study of the effect of topical β-adrenoceptor antagonists on resting heart rate in elderly patients, timolol (0.25% and 0.5%), carteolol (1% and 2%), and metipranolol (0.3% and 0.6%) all decreased mean heart rate, whereas betaxolol (0.5% solution) did not.[341] Thus, some studies suggest that metipranolol, especially in lower concentrations, may elicit less of a systemic β-adrenoceptor blockade than timolol or some other agents.

Allergic blepharoconjunctivitis and periorbital dermatitis, known untoward effects of ophthalmic β-adrenoceptor antagonists,[290, 291] have also been reported with metipranolol use.[342] Uveitis associated with topical metipranolol was reported in approximately 30 patients at one hospital in the United Kingdom[343–345] and in two patients in the United States,[346, 347] but not in Germany.[348] The concern over a significant association of uveitis with metipranolol use has been greatly attenuated, however, by a recent study that found no evidence of uveitis in nearly 2000 patients using metipranolol, nor a single episode of uveitis in 3900 patients using other β-adrenoceptor antagonists.[349] The contraindication labeling for metipranolol in America are the same as for timolol and levobunolol.

Carteolol

In a cross-over study in 10 normal volunteers, 1% carteolol caused moderate corneal anesthesia relative to timolol and betaxolol.[350] In an evaluation of twice-daily treatment for 2 months in rabbits, carteolol (1% and 2%) did not elicit any changes in corneal anatomy as determined by electron microscopy. This was in contrast with befunolol (0.5% and 1%) and timolol (0.25% and 0.5%), which elicited pronounced desquamation of the corneal epithelium and pronounced disappearance of microvilli. However, none of the three eye drops caused pathologic changes in the parenchyma or endothelium of the cornea.[351]

As a potent and effective β_1- and β_2-adrenoceptor antagonist, carteolol shares with other agents in this class the potential for systemic β-adrenoceptor blockade. Although some authors theorize that the ISA of carteolol provides a more advantageous systemic safety potential, this is not fully borne out by clinical studies. The magnitude of the decrease in heart rates as well as systolic blood pressure was similar to that previously reported for noncardioselective β-adrenoceptor antagonists.[156] Studies also have reported that systemic β-adrenoceptor blockade induced by topical carteolol is either similar to or greater than that of timolol.[316, 338, 341, 352] In a study assessing the inhibition of exercise-induced tachycardia, carteolol and timolol were similar in their systemic β-blockade.[352]

Betaxolol

In several controlled studies, the stinging elicited by betaxolol solution was significantly greater than any discomfort elicited with timolol or levobunolol.[245, 248, 353, 354] Some studies suggest that betaxolol reduces corneal sensitivity—in some cases more than timolol[355–357]—whereas other studies found no significant effect.[350] Within its first year of marketing in the United States, the FDA received 56 reports of adverse events associated betaxolol solution. Forty-seven of these reports were of stinging, burning, or irritation.[358]

A significant clinical advantage of topical betaxolol in the treatment of elevated IOP is its reduced potential to adversely effect pulmonary function. In one study, nine patients with reactive airway disease in whom topical timolol produced at least a 15% reduction of FEV_1 were enrolled in a double-masked, cross-over study of topical 0.5% timolol, 1.0% betaxolol, or vehicle. On the average, timolol reduced mean FEV_1 approximately 25%, whereas betaxolol and placebo had little effect on mean FEV_1.[320] A similarly designed study in eight patients compared betaxolol with its vehicle and found no differences.[359] Another study found timolol, levobunolol, pindolol, befunolol, and metipranolol similar in reducing mean pulmonary function, whereas betaxolol was similar to its vehicle.[360] Although most of these studies used 0.5% timolol and 0.5% or 1.0% betaxolol solution, a more recent study reported that 0.25% betaxolol suspension produced fewer cardiovascular and pulmonary effects than 0.25% timolol solution in healthy volunteers.[361]

Subsequent studies evaluated betaxolol in patients with co-existent pulmonary disease and glaucoma. In an open-label study in nine patients (four of whom who had previously experienced reduced pulmonary function with timolol), betaxolol was added to the glaucoma therapeutic regimen and caused no change in mean FEV_1 and a mean reduction in IOP of 3 mm Hg.[362] This finding was replicated in placebo-controlled, randomized, double-masked cross-over trials.[363–365] In a parallel study in 24 subjects with 6 months of treatment, mean FEV_1 was decreased approximately 10% in the timolol-treated group, whereas there was no effect in either the betaxolol or befunolol-treated group.[366] Pulmonary and ophthalmic measurements made prior to and during chronic betaxolol treatment revealed that patients were largely able to use betaxolol without exacerbation of pulmonary symptoms and without deterioration in measured pulmonary function tests, whereas IOP was reduced.[367, 368] In a one-way cross-over evaluation, 40 patients who had various adverse experiences with timolol (e.g., dyspnea, bradycardia) were switched to betaxolol. In the follow-up period (3 to 31 months), 32 of these patients (80%) became free from adverse experiences. However, there was a mean increase in IOP of 2.5 mm Hg.[369]

These studies by no means suggest that all patients with co-existent pulmonary disease and glaucoma will be free of pulmonary side effects with betaxolol use, because betaxolol clearly has elicited such adverse systemic side effects in many patients.[370] Some pulmonary physicians strongly caution against the use of any β-adrenoceptor antagonist, regardless of cardioselectivity or route, in patients with existing respiratory disease. Should such therapy be contemplated, the internist or pulmonary specialist should work hand-in-hand with the eye-care specialist to ensure patient freedom from adverse effects while attempting to achieve adequate glaucoma control.[371]

Several controlled studies have investigated the potential of betaxolol to elicit systemic β_1-adrenoceptor blockade. In a study on resting cardiovascular function in aged patients, topical instillation of timolol (0.25% and 0.5%), carteolol (1% and 2%), and metipranolol (0.3% and 0.6%) decreased mean heart rate 14 to 17%. However, topical betaxolol, 0.5%, did not have any significant effect, although some patients in all groups did exhibit a 15 to 20% reduction in systolic blood pressure.[341] In a study of exercise-induced tachycardia in normal volunteers, the maximal heart rate obtained upon exercise was decreased by 9 beats/min with topical timolol and 4 beats/min by betaxolol. The effect of betaxolol was not significantly different from that of its vehicle.[314] Another study of exercise tachycardia showed no significant changes in exercise-induced tachycardia with topical betaxolol, in contrast with the reduction in maximal heart rate observed with timolol and levobunolol.[315] In another report, systemic β-blockade was evaluated in 16 healthy volunteers by assessing displacement of the bronchodilator (specific airway conductance), positive chronotropic (heart rate), and tremorogenic (finger-tremor amplitude) dose-response curve for inhaled isoproterenol. Compared with placebo, all β-antagonists resulted in a significant systemic β-blockade; the increasing order of effect was betaxolol (0.5%), metipranolol (0.6%), and timolol (0.5%).[340]

Although betaxolol generally elicits less systemic β-blockade than timolol or levobunolol, it is not without effects in some patients. Plasma levels of betaxolol appear to be relatively low after topical instillation.[37, 372] CNS side effects (e.g., insomnia, depression) appear to be lower with betaxolol than other β-adrenoceptor antagonists.[324, 373] Although several factors influence β-adrenoceptor antagonist activity in the CNS, such as lipophilicity and the ability of drug to cross the blood-brain barrier, receptor subtype selectivity may be yet another factor to account for these favorable findings. In patients using topical betaxolol, case reports of adverse experiences include congestive heart failure,[374] myocardial infarction within 5 minutes after the first drop of betaxolol,[375] dendritic keratopathy (resolving after cessation of treatment),[335] respiratory difficulties strongly suggestive of obstructive airway disease,[376] weakness and severe sinus bradycardia,[377] clinical depression,[378] and wheezing and objective reduction in pulmonary function.[379] With the exception of the patient with myocardial infarction, most patients recovered without significant sequelae when betaxolol therapy was stopped.

The current U.S. labeling for betaxolol states that it is contraindicated in patients with sinus bradycardia, greater than first-degree atrioventricular block, cardiogenic shock, or overt cardiac failure. It is also contraindicated in patients with hypersensitivity to any of its components. As noted earlier, severe respiratory reactions have occurred with this class of agents. Also, minor changes in heart rate and blood pressure in controlled studies suggest caution when using this agent in patients with a history of cardiac failure or heart block. Overall, the selection of betaxolol as an antiglaucoma agent is generally based on relative benefit versus risk. In head-to-head studies against noncardioselective agents, betaxolol is generally a less effective ocular hypotensive agent than other β-adrenergic antagonists. From a safety perspective, however, betaxolol may induce less systemic β-blockade than these other agents, and it appears to have a reduced profile of adverse pulmonary side effects. Although there is some evidence that betaxolol may differ from timolol in its effects on visual fields and vasculature, the clinical relevance of such observations is not yet clear.

Functional Studies

Aqueous Humor Dynamics

In aqueous humor dynamic studies, timolol decreased the production of aqueous humor.[122, 123] In a separate study, timolol did not significantly alter facility of outflow as measured tonographically.[380] Thus, the predominant mechanism of the ocular hypotensive action of timolol appears to be a decrease in the production of aqueous humor. In a single-drop study of aqueous humor dynamics in 40 ocular hypertensive patients, timolol eye drops induced a greater decrease of the aqueous humor flow (39%), followed equally by betaxolol (24%) and carteolol (20%).[381] Betaxolol reduces IOP primarily by reducing aqueous humor production.[233, 234, 382] In controlled studies of aqueous humor dynamics, betaxolol, although effective in reducing aqueous humor production, was less effective than levobunolol or timolol and similar in efficacy to carteolol. Betaxolol is also less potent that levobunolol, requiring a higher concentration to achieve equieffective reductions in aqueous humor flow.[234, 381] Levobunolol,[383, 384] carteolol,[385, 386] and metipranolol[207] have also been reported to decrease aqueous humor production. As with timolol, levobunolol reportedly has no effect on uveoscleral flow, outflow facility, or episcleral venous pressure.[383, 387] Carteolol has no effect on total outflow facility.[381, 388] Fluorophotometry and outflow measurements must be used to determine whether all new β-adrenoceptor antagonists are similar to timolol in solely affecting aqueous humor production.

Blood Flow Studies

The importance of understanding the role of the ocular microcirculation and the relative role of ischemia as it applies to the health of the optic nerve in glaucoma is now a subject that elicits little debate. Classic β-adrenoceptor antagonists typically increase vascular resistance by inhibiting β-adrenoceptor–mediated vasorelaxation, thereby reducing peripheral blood flow, which may also be due to a reduction of cardiac output.[390] Concern that the use of these agents to lower IOP may result in adverse effects on the blood supply to the retina, choroid, or optic nerve has resulted in several studies that examined the effects of these drugs on the posterior ocular circulation. Although authors disagree on the effects of β-adrenoceptor antagonists on the human retinal circulation, most studies have suggested that these agents either increase or cause no change in blood flow. Studies using laser Doppler velocimetry have shown that timolol, betaxolol, and perhaps levobunolol, but not carteolol, increase retinal blood flow.[391–396] Two studies using similar techniques showed no effect of timolol or propranolol on retinal blood flow, however.[397, 398] Topical timolol was also found to increase choroidal blood flow in cats.[399] Studies using Doppler ultrasonography to determine the effects of these agents have been less conclusive. Timolol has been shown to increase the blood velocity in the central retinal artery[400, 401] and to reduce the central artery resistive index.[402] In contrast, Harris and colleagues did not find either of these effects with betaxolol or timolol treatment.[403]

Even though the functional effects of β-adrenoceptor antagonists on ocular blood flow are not clear, several possibilities account for the potential vasodilator activity of some of these agents. For example, some β_1-adrenoceptor antagonists with ISA, such as pindolol, may produce less of a reduction in cardiac output than similar agents without ISA, or they may possess partial β_2-agonist properties that reduce the vasoconstrictive effects typically caused by β-adrenoceptor antagonists.[404] Furthermore, some β-adrenoceptor antagonists, such as carvedilol, labetalol, and bucindolol, may have mild α-adrenoceptor blocking activity, thus facilitating vasodilation.

It has also been suggested that some selective β_1-adrenoceptor antagonists such as betaxolol may have direct vascular relaxing action due to calcium channel antagonism properties, and thus they may be of particular benefit in patients with glaucoma.[405] However, it is important to note that betaxolol's effects on the inhibition of calcium flux across cell membranes in this and other studies occur at concentrations that are several orders of magnitude higher than those for which β-adrenoceptor antagonism occurs. For example, the concentration of betaxolol that attenuated 50% of the effects (i.e., the IC_{50}) of evoked calcium channel current in smooth muscle cells of guinea pig arteries or potassium-induced contractions of bovine retinal arteries were about 45 μM and 30 μM, respectively.[406, 407] Because the concentration of betaxolol in aqueous humor is approximately 1 μM 1 hour after topical instillation,[405] it is difficult to ascertain precisely how the relatively weak calcium channel antagonist properties of betaxolol might favorably effect the retinal circulation, because the concentration of betaxolol required for this effect appears to be significantly greater than typical clinical use can achieve.

Additivity with Other Agents

The ocular hypotensive effect of timolol with most other therapies is additive. This includes outflow agents (e.g., pilocarpine) and inflow agents (e.g., acetazolamide, apraclonidine). The additivity of timolol with epinephrine or with dipivefrin is more problematic. Conceptually, one would question the rationale for combining a β-adrenoceptor antagonist, timolol, with a mixed α/β-adrenoceptor agonist, epinephrine. However, this was viewed as an effective combination therapy for many years. The twice-daily regimen of each agent, as well as the relative lack of untoward ocular symptoms, made this a relatively easy duo-therapy for patients to use. Separating the instillation of timolol and dipivefrin by 3 hours, rather than 10 minutes, while of theoretical benefit, did not seem to alter the efficacy of this combination. However, in some studies, the additivity is less than complete and relatively short-lived.[124, 408–418] Topical timolol administered to patients receiving oral β-blocking agents for the treatment of systemic hypertension may further significantly reduce IOP.[419–421] Combined treatment with timolol and acetazolamide can reduce IOP more than with either alone.[415] Treatment with timolol plus pilocarpine also reduces IOP more than that with each agent alone.[409, 422–424]

Schenker and coworkers investigated the aqueous humor dynamics of the additivity of timolol and epinephrine.[124] They confirmed earlier work that timolol reduced aqueous humor production. They also reported that by itself, epinephrine both slightly increased aqueous humor production and increased uveoscleral outflow. Because the increase in outflow was greater than the increase in production, there was a net decrease in IOP. When timolol and epinephrine were combined, the net effect was a decrease in IOP, a decrease in aqueous humor production, and an increase in uveoscleral outflow.[124] The variability in the additivity of epinephrine to various β-adrenoceptor antagonists[408, 425] has led to reevaluation of the mechanism of action of the interaction of these two agents. One report, in cats, suggests that epinephrine decreases aqueous production, decreases uveoscleral flow, but increases total outflow facility.[426] Clearly, additional research is required to understand the mechanism of action of epinephrine and its interaction with timolol.

The profile of levobunolol is similar to that of timolol in its adjunct use with dipivefrin, pilocarpine, or acetazolamide.[384, 387, 427–429] The aqueous humor dynamics of the additivity of levobunolol and pilocarpine were investigated by Hayashi and associates.[384] Levobunolol decreased aqueous humor flow (production), and pilocarpine increased trabecular outflow.

Added to betaxolol, dipivefrin or epinephrine provided a greater differential pressure reduction than when added to timolol.[425, 430] Critics of this study have pointed out that although of mechanistic interest, this observation is more related to the fact that timolol is a more effective ocular hypotensive agent than betaxolol. The overall efficacy of the two combinations was similar.[431] Another study observed the additivity of dipivefrin to either timolol or betaxolol only in some patients.[432] In an open-label, noncomparative trial in 39 patients already using dipivefrin, betaxolol provided additional ocular hypotensive effect.[433] Betaxolol may be combined with pilocarpine, dipivefrin, or acetazolamide.[434]

β-ADRENERGIC AGONISTS

Indications for Use

Dipivefrin

Dipivefrin HCl (Propine, Pivalephrine) is a prodrug of epinephrine formed by the diesterification of epinephrine and pivalic acid. The corneal epithelium retards penetration of instilled catecholamines, which are hydrophilic, polar compounds. The pivaloyl groups make epinephrine more lipophilic and facilitates its penetration into the anterior chamber, thus overcoming the poor ability of epinephrine to pass through the epithelial and endothelial layers of the cornea.[435–437] Dipivefrin becomes active when it is hydrolyzed to epinephrine in the iris–ciliary body, cornea, and anterior chamber by esterases.[436, 436, 438, 439]

In general, the ocular hypotensive effect of dipivefrin is less impressive than that of the most β-adrenoceptor antagonists; in one study, however, the ocular hypotensive efficacy of dipivefrin was within 1 mm Hg of that of betaxolol.[440] In a 6-month cross-over treatment study of 17 glaucoma patients with 0.1% dipivefrin or 2% epinephrine, IOP decreased an average of 23.7% with dipivefrin and 27.4% with epinephrine.[436] Burning and irritation were reported in 24% of the epinephrine-treated eyes but only 3% of dipivefrin-treated eyes. Burning and stinging was the most frequent side effect reported (6% of patients). Conjunctival injection occurred in 6.5% of patients.

Substitution of dipivefrin for epinephrine has been reported to reduce extraocular and systemic side effects associated with epinephrine use. Because the intraocular concentration of epinephrine from the hydrolyzed dipivefrin is approximately equivalent to that of topical epinephrine itself, the incidence of some side effects remains unchanged with dipivefrin. In particular, both drugs cause mydriasis and risk of angle-closure glaucoma in susceptible eyes. The risk of epinephrine maculopathy in aphakic eyes is apparently the same when either agent is used. Most other side effects, however, are markedly reduced in frequency and severity. Dipivefrin can be used in patients wearing soft contact lenses without significant risk of adrenochrome staining. Tearing, conjunctival hyperemia, corneal edema, and blurred vision are rare. Topical dipivefrin also causes fewer allergic reactions compared with epinephrine preparations. Consequently, the majority of patients intolerant of epinephrine may be placed on dipivefrin without any significant side effects,[294] although some authors have suggested that the differences in the incidence of allergies of these drugs has been overestimated.[441] Also, although dipivefrin has been reported to be effective when used concomitantly with topical β-adrenoceptor antagonists,[428] other studies report that its average additivity in these conditions is relatively small.[408]

Epinephrine

Epinephrine, the major hormone secreted by the adrenal medulla, is used predominantly as an ocular hypotensive agent in primary open-angle glaucoma. Acute administration of epinephrine results in conjunctival blanching, slight mydriasis, and reduction of IOP. Mydriasis may occur within a few minutes and may persist for several hours. However, epinephrine in a 0.1% solution is not a good mydriatic in the normal human eye, probably because of its rapid destruction and its poor permeability.[442] The effect on IOP outlasts the vasoconstrictor and mydriatic effects. Epinephrine is also used a clinical tool for diagnosis of sympathetic denervation in Horner's syndrome and Fuch's heterochromatic iritis. Epinephrine only slightly relaxes the ciliary muscle so that cycloplegia is minimal. Epinephrine also appears to extend and facilitate the efficacy of local anesthetics by constricting vascular beds, thus minimizing the rate at which a drug is absorbed into the systemic circulation from its injection site. Epinephrine-induced vasoconstriction is also useful in surgery to control bleeding from capillaries and small arterioles, usually occuring with 5 minutes after topical administration or intraocular injection of epinephrine and generally lasting less than 1 hour.

Epinephrine is available as hydrochloride, borate, and bitartrate salts. In solution, it is amphoteric. The levorotatory isomer is approximately 15 times more potent than the dextrorotatory form. It is used topically as a 0.5 to 2% solution. The propensity of epinephrine, as with any catecholamine, to readily oxidize and discolor requires an antioxidant included in commercial preparations.

Epinephrine, an agonist at both α- and β-adrenoceptors, lowers IOP for 12 to 24 hours when applied topically. Topically applied epinephrine lowers IOP in patients with open-angle glaucoma but has only a slight effect in normal eyes.[443] Concentrations as low as 0.125% can lower ocular pressure; however, a 1% solution proved substantially better.[444] In selected patients, the effects of epinephrine are additive to those of carbonic anhydrase inhibitors and miotics, as well as β-adrenoceptor antagonists.[445]

Topically applied epinephrine frequently causes ocular discomfort and conjunctival irritation, including transient burning or stinging, lacrimation, and pain or ache around or in the eye. Conjunctival allergy sometimes occurs. Adverse effects on the cornea include epithelial edema, endothelial cell toxicity, adrenochrome deposits, and staining of soft contact lenses.

Treatment with epinephrine occasionally causes dramatic diminution in visual acuity, especially in aphakic patients.[446] Macular edema occurs in 10 to 20% of aphakic patients treated with epinephrine but usually disappears after discontinuance of treatment.[447] Injections of epinephrine solution into the anterior chamber can cause increased corneal thickness and loss of corneal endothelial cells.[447] It might be expected that the shift from predominantly intracapsular to extracapsular cataract extractions, as well as the insertion of an intraocular lens, might afford some protection against epinephrine-induced macular edema; this possibility merits further study. Occasionally reported systemic effects of topical epinephrine include palpitation, faintness, tachycardia, extrasystoles, cardiac arrhythmia, hypertension, anxiety, fear, trembling, sweating, and pallor. However, many of the side effects of topical epinephrine can be prevented by punctal occlusion for 15 to 30 seconds after application. This prevents the drug from draining into the lacrimal sac and nasopharynx, where it may be systemically absorbed.[448] In general, punctal occlusion may be useful for any topically applied drug with systemic effects.[308]

α-ADRENERGIC ANTAGONISTS

Thymoxamine

Thymoxamine is an α-adrenergic blocking agent that works by competitive antagonism of norepinephrine. When used as a 0.5% solution, it consistently produces miosis without affecting the IOP or the ciliary muscle–controlled facility of outflow.[449] The only regularly reported side effects at this concentration are transient burning and conjunctival hyperemia. Potential applications of thymoxamine include reversal of phenylephrine mydriasis, treatment of angle-closure glaucoma, treatment of persistent mydriasis after penetrating keratoplasty for keratoconus, reversal of lid retraction in thyroid ophthalmopathy, testing to differentiate angle-closure glaucoma from open-angle glaucoma with narrow angles, aiding in repositioning and maintaining the position of intraocular lenses, and treatment of pigmentary glaucoma. Increased iris pigmentation has been reported to decreased the miotic effect of thymoxamine, however.[450] Thymoxamine has been demonstrated to have some minimal ocular hypotensive effect in rabbit eyes, presumably due to its additional occupancy of α_2-adrenoceptors despite its primary pharmacologic properties as an α_1-adrenoceptor antagonist.[451]

Dapiprazole

Dapiprazole is an α-adrenergic antagonist that has been shown to be effective in facilitating miosis and that has a minimal effect as an ocular hypotensive agent.[452, 453] Its effect as an ocular hypotensive agent is more effective at 0.5% than at 0.25%.[453] Its hypotensive properties also can be augmented when used as a combination drop with 0.5% timolol.[454] Pupillary mydriasis can be reversed by intraocular dapiprazole (0.25%) after extracapsular cataract extraction,[455] and this effect appears to last longer than that of 1% acetylcholine. In addition to reversal of mydriasis, topical dapiprazole effectively reversed tropicamide-induced cycloplegia.[456] Accommodation showed significant recovery, with comfortable reading ability returning after approximately 30 minutes.[457] In this study, however, all of the subjects exhibited conjunctival hyperemia after the administration of dapiprazole. This side effect persisted through the entire 180-minute observation period that followed dapiprazole administration. Consistent with this observation, studies have demonstrated that dapiprazole partially reverses apraclonidine protection of the blood-aqueous barrier from traumatic laser-induced breakdown.[458] A sixfold increase in protein content of the aqueous humor of rabbit eyes with argon laser treatment of the iris was effectively eliminated with apraclonidine pretreatment. This effect was abolished when 0.5% dapiprazole was added to apraclonidine pretreatment and resulted in a twofold increase in aqueous protein content compared with apraclonidine pretreatment alone.

α-ADRENERGIC AGONISTS

Indirect Agonists (Re-Uptake Blockers)

Diagnostic Use in Horner's Syndrome

Hydroxyamphetamine. Hydroxyamphetamine (1%) is a phenylisopropylamine and, like ephedrine, is an indirect-acting sympathomimetic. It is used as a mydriatic for ophthalmologic examination and as a diagnostic tool to detect preganglionic sympathetic innervation that interferes with pupil dilation. By releasing endogenous norepinephrine from the postganglionic nerve terminal that innervates the iris dilator muscle, hydroxyamphetamine effectively stimulates the dilator muscle of the iris to produce mydriasis. Maximum mydriasis occurs in approximately 40 minutes and lasts for a few hours.[459] Thus, hydroxyamphetamine is an ineffective mydriatic in patients with defective postganglionic sympathetic innervation (i.e., postganglionic Horner's syndrome). However, the ability of hydroxyamphetamine to differentiate postganglionic from preganglionic lesions has been questioned.[460] Because the effect of hydroxyamphetamine is due to a release of endogenous norepinephrine and not a direct action on the receptor, it can be reduced or abolished by pretreatment with agents that deplete or inhibit the release of norepinephrine (e.g., guanethidine, reserpine, 6-hydroxydopamine, and cocaine).

Hydroxyamphetamine is slow-acting and can be easily counteracted by miotics. Thus, it may be the safest mydriatic for patients with a shallow chamber angle.[461] Other than occasionally precipitating narrow-angle glaucoma through its mydriatic action, ocular side effects from topical ocular administration of hydroxyamphetamine are insignificant and reversible.[461] Hydroxyamphetamine does not cause cycloplegia. Because of its lower lipophilicity relative to amphetamine, hydroxyamphetamine penetrates the blood-brain barrier poorly, and thus it almost lacks a CNS-stimulating effect. Photophobia, blurring of vision, or both, as well as allergic reactions in the eyelids and conjunctiva, have been reported. Systemic side effects are apparently frequent.

Cocaine. Cocaine (benzoylmethylecgonine) is an indirect-acting sympathomimetic drug. It is a potent, highly toxic, and long-lived local anesthetic. Because of this indirect sympathomimetic action, cocaine is the only local anesthetic to cause vasoconstriction and mydriasis. Cocaine is unique among the local anesthetics in retarding its own absorption through its ability to cause vasoconstriction, which consequently prolongs its action. The mydriatic effect of cocaine occurs within 5 to 20 minutes, reaching a maximum in about 30 minutes.[462] Dilation of the pupil typically lasts 6 hours, although it may last as long as 20 hours. Now used only occasionally in ophthalmic surgery, cocaine prevents the re-uptake of catecholamines by adrenergic nerve terminals,[463] prolonging the effect of norepinephrine and epinephrine. Its only nonanesthetic use has been in the pharmacologic diagnosis of Horner's syndrome. By inhibiting re-uptake of norepinephrine from nerve terminals, it is effective in dilating a normal pupil but not an uninnervated pupil. Therefore, it does not diagnose the presence of either a preganglionic or a postganglionic lesion causing Horner's syndrome.

In addition to mydriasis, cocaine causes partial cycloplegia.[464] Its main adverse effect is its potential to cause significant corneal toxicity.[465] The corneal epithelium can become dry and pitted and may slough. Acute attacks of narrow-angle glaucoma have been precipitated by cocaine. The interaction between cocaine and catecholamines contraindicates the use of cocaine in patients taking adrenergic-modifying drugs, such as guanethidine, reserpine, tricyclic antidepressants, methyldopa, and monoamine oxidase inhibitors,[465, 466] or sympathomimetics such as phenylephrine.[466] Systemic absorption of the drug can result in hyperreflexia, restlessness, delirium, tachycardia, irregular respiration, chills, and fever, all of which are traceable to CNS stimulation.[467] Of course, cocaine has a serious potential for abuse, and its storage and use require adequate security measures.

Direct Agonists

The clinical use of α-adrenoceptor agonists in the treatment of various forms of glaucoma diminished markedly in the late 1970s because of the widespread availability of β-adrenoceptor antagonists, which were not only efficacious ocular hypotensive agents but were initially perceived to be associated with less local and systemic side effects than currently available α-agonist preparations. However, the use of the α-agonists as IOP-lowering agents has increased markedly since the 1980s with the introduction of newer selective agents such as apraclonidine and, more recently, brimonidine.

Indications for Short-Term Use of α_2-Adrenoceptor Agonists

Control of Intraocular Pressure Elevation Following Laser Procedures. In the late 1970s laser therapy for glaucoma had become common. However, a relatively common complication of laser procedures such as iridotomy, trabeculoplasty, and laser capsulotomy was an acute postoperative rise in IOP that could potentially cause visual loss. There was no way to prospectively predict which eyes would experience this complication, and no therapy to date was completely effective at reducing the frequency or magnitude of this problem. A safe and easily tolerated prophylaxis would help if the therapy was effective with minimal adverse side effects so that it could be used on all patients prophylactically. Although pilocarpine and β-adrenoceptor antagonists were known to decrease IOP elevation after both iridotomy and trabeculoplasty, this complication was not eradicated; thus, the search for other useful agents continued.[468–471]

The use of new α-adrenoceptor agonists was partly related to the emergence of new technology such as the Nd:YAG laser. This laser had mostly photodisruptive effects with minimal thermal effects on ocular tissues, and thus it often caused problems with iris bleeding during iridotomy. Clinicians felt that it would be advantageous to have a medication that would cause vasoconstriction without mydriasis, which might induce pupillary block in a susceptible eye and thus cause an acute attack of angle-closure glaucoma. Because mydriasis is mediated by activation of α_1-adrenoceptors on the iris dilator, attention shifted to the possibility that α_2-adrenoceptor agonists would be effective hypotensive agents that would not induce mydriasis. Initial research demonstrated that α_2-adrenoceptor agonists such as clonidine were indeed effective ocular hypotensive agents similar to other commonly used drugs such as pilocarpine.[472] However, concern for the systemic hypotension associated with topical concentrations of 0.25% and 0.5% clonidine diminished enthusiasm for these compounds. Apraclonidine, a less lipophilic derivative of clonidine because of the addition of a para-amino side chain (hence the structural name, para-aminoclonidine), was developed in an effort to decrease the systemic absorption and thus minimize these adverse systemic effects (Fig. 26–5).

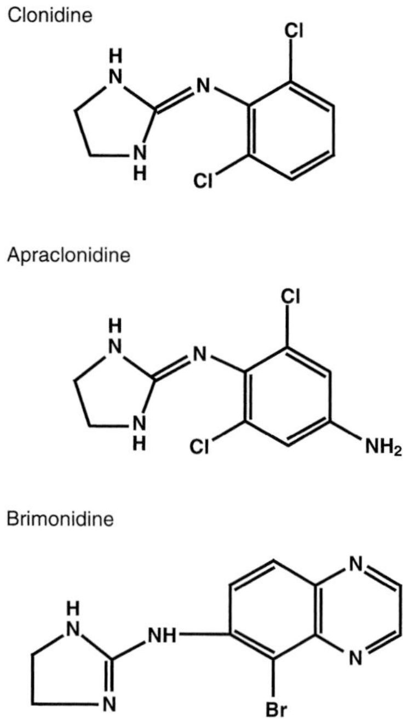

Although initial studies with apraclonidine demonstrated its effectiveness as an ocular hypotensive agent,[473] there was no evidence that pretreatment with apraclonidine decreased the potential complication of bleeding that occurred with Nd:YAG laser use. Furthermore, both apraclonidine and Nd:YAG laser iridotomy were investigational at this time, and U.S. regulatory laws restricted concomitant use of an investigational drug with an investigational procedure. It was noted, however, that the animals that were pretreated with

Clonidine

Apraclonidine

Brimonidine

FIGURE 26–5. Chemical structure of α_2-adrenoreceptor agonists.

apraclonidine prior to Nd:YAG laser iridotomy had lower IOPs than did animals not treated with apraclonidine, thus suggesting potential usefulness and prompting further studies. Initial single, multicentered studies compared the effectiveness of apraclonidine with placebo in diminishing the acute postoperative pressure elevations associated with argon and Q-switched Nd:YAG laser iridotomy, argon laser trabeculoplasty, and Q-switched Nd:YAG laser capsulotomy. Apraclonidine 1%, one drop 1 hour prior to therapy and then immediately after laser therapy, appeared to be effective[474] and is similar in effect to brimonidine.[475] Apraclonidine significantly decreased both the frequency (by 10 times) and the magnitude of this complication. Additionally, because of the adverse effects of high concentrations of topical clonidine on systemic blood pressure, blood pressure was measured at each time interval. Apraclonidine, even after two drops of 1% within 1 hour, had no adverse effects on systemic blood pressure.[476]

The efficacy of apraclonidine in preventing acute IOP elevations associated with argon laser trabeculoplasty was compared with that of timolol maleate, pilocarpine, acetazolamide, and dipivefrin. There appeared to be no significant difference among any of these four other medications.[473] However, apraclonidine was significantly better than the others in decreasing the magnitude and frequency of postoperative IOP elevations. Similarly, apraclonidine was more effective than timolol maleate in its ability to suppress the IOP elevation associated with argon laser iridotomy.[473] It is not clear why neither timolol nor acetazolamide, both aqueous humor suppressants, did not alter the postoperative IOP elevation as much as apraclonidine. One explanation that timolol may have had less effect than apraclonidine in one study was that 32 (91%) of the eyes in the group randomized to acute timolol treatment were already being treated with various chronic topical β-adrenoceptor antagonists.[477] Thus, chronic β-adrenoceptor antagonist therapy might have already maximally suppressed aqueous humor production so that additional β-adrenoceptor antagonist use following laser treatment had no further effect. Other authors have shown the additive effect of apraclonidine in both decreasing aqueous flow and decreasing IOP in eyes on chronic β-adrenoceptor antagonists.[478–480]

It is reasonable to assume that the ability of apraclonidine to further lower IOP in patients receiving concurrent β-adrenoceptor antagonists is due to the fact that apraclonidine actively inhibits aqueous production via α_2-adrenoceptor occupancy, thus resulting in adenylyl cyclase inhibition that is independent of and may be greater than that achieved by β-adrenoceptor antagonism only. Thus, apraclonidine and β-adrenoceptor antagonists in combination may be synergistic, because both medications lower IOP by attenuating adenylyl cyclase, a key regulatory enzyme in the formation of aqueous humor. Another possible explanation for the profound hypotension of these agents is that α_2-adrenoceptor activation produces vasoconstriction, which may decrease the passive ultrafiltration component of aqueous production as well as the active transport component. Lastly, brimonidine tartrate, another relatively selective α_2-adrenoceptor agonist, has been noted to not only decrease aqueous flow but to increase uveoscleral outflow.[481]

Control of Intraocular Pressure Elevation Following Surgery. Another procedure plagued afterward by acute IOP elevation is cataract surgery. The most effective pharmacologic agents in preventing this IOP elevation are muscarinics. Various studies show that both intracameral carbachol and acetylcholine, as well as postoperative pilocarpine gel, have been more effective than placebo in decreasing the frequency of this complication.[482, 483] However, despite the use of muscarinics, the rate of large postoperative IOP elevations remained relatively high. Other investigators have attempted to add nonselective β-adrenoceptor antagonists to prevent IOP elevation. This does not appear to consistently or adequately decrease the frequency of this complication.[199, 200, 484, 485] Following extracapsular cataract extraction, Fry demonstrated that carbachol was the most effective agent to minimize IOP elevation, whereas apraclonidine was ineffective when given at the end of the surgical procedure.[180] However, in a study in which apraclonidine 1% was instilled 1 hour preoperatively, the incidence of postoperative IOP elevation decreased.[486]

Apraclonidine 1% used immediately before and after cataract extraction by phacoemulsification with intraocular lens implantation also blunted postoperative IOP spikes.[487] Aqueous flare decreased in patients receiving the apraclonidine treatment compared with patients receiving a vehicle as a control. In a randomized, double-masked study of patients undergoing extracapsular cataract extraction combined with trabeculectomy, apraclonidine 1%, when instilled preoperatively and postoperatively, was more effective than placebo in decreasing postoperative IOP elevations. At 24 hours after surgery, 20% of the placebo-treated eyes and 2% (one patient) of the apraclonidine-treated eyes had IOPs greater than 40 mm Hg.[477] Other studies confirmed the efficacy of apraclonidine to decrease the frequency of postoperative IOP elevations, including those that arise after vitreoretinal surgery.[488, 489] Although the addition of apraclonidine does not eliminate this problem, it markedly decreases its frequency. It may be appropriate to add this medication routinely both prior to and immediately following cataract surgery (with or without concurrent trabeculectomy). Also, because this complication is much more common in eyes with preexisting glaucoma, prophylaxis appears to be especially important in these eyes.

Chronic Therapy

The initial success with the short-term use of α-agonists to control postoperative elevations of IOP led to interest in expanding the indications for their use for the long-term control of chronic glaucoma. Their use in chronic glaucoma was particularly attractive because selective α_2-adrenoceptor agonists were effective aqueous-flow suppressants that lower IOP during both waking hours and sleep,[478] and therefore they may offer a distinct advantage over other ocular hypotensive agents such as β-adrenoceptor antagonists, which do not appear to lower IOP at night.[167, 382]

Clonidine

Clonidine, given intravenously, was found to lower IOP in 1966.[490] More importantly, clonidine could also lower IOP when given topically.[491] Initial one-drop studies were encouraging, because this medication could be formulated for topical delivery yet cause no untoward side effects, despite knowledge of the central effects of this medication when given to subhuman primates. Multiple-drop studies demonstrated that clonidine, 0.125% and 0.25% given three times daily, could lower IOP as well as could topical pilocarpine.[472, 492, 493] The initial limited-drop studies involving clonidine suggested that IOP was lowered significantly with minimal side effects. Single-drop studies found no apparent systemic side effects associated with topical clonidine, although these studies eventually proved misleading.

IOP lowering with topical clonidine was soon associated with marked central systemic blood-pressure lowering and sedation.[472] Clonidine can produce systemic hypotension and bradycardia via the CNS. The mechanisms may involve inhibition of sympathetic outflow and enhancement of parasympathetic nervous activity.[494] The production of hypotension and sedation by α_2-adrenoceptor agonists has been shown to correlate well with their partition coefficient (their ability to penetrate the CNS). The greater the lipophilicity of the compound, the more likely it is to reach the systemic circulation and produce this effect. Both brimonidine and clonidine are more lipophilic than apraclonidine.[495]

Clonidine, administered to monkeys at a dose that reduced IOP 4 to 5 mm Hg, caused blood flow reduction of 19% in the choroid, 34% in the iris, and 42% in the ciliary body.[496] The authors hypothesized that clonidine-induced vasoconstriction and reduction of systemic blood pressure would have adverse effects on the arterioles supplying the optic nerve head and thus be undesirable. Furthermore, Heilmann demonstrated that ophthalmic artery pressure could be decreased in eyes with elevated IOP that received topical clonidine 0.5% and 0.25%.[497] These studies have severely curtailed the enthusiasm for continued use of clonidine for the treatment of chronic glaucoma.

Apraclonidine

Apraclonidine is an effective ocular hypotensive agent. Within 1 hour of drop instillation, apraclonidine 1% produces a rapid drop in IOP of at least 20% from baseline. The maximal effect is observed between 3 and 5 hours after dosing. At peak effect, apraclonidine 1% lowers IOP by 30 to 40% compared with baseline, and at trough it lowers it by 20 to 30%.[498–500] In dose-response studies comparing 0.125%, 0.25%, 0.5%, and 1.0%, either 0.25% or 0.5% appear to be at the top of the dose-response curve for the reduction of IOP.[501]

Apraclonidine is commercially available as Iopidine (Alcon, Inc., Fort Worth, TX) in concentrations of 0.5% in 5- and 10-mL bottles for chronic use and 1% in 0.1-mL dropperettes for short-term applications. For an anterior segment laser procedure, one drop of apraclonidine should be instilled in the target eye 1 hour prior to surgery, with a second drop given on completion of the procedure. Holmwood and coworkers demonstrated effectiveness with a single administration of apraclonidine after the laser procedure.[474] For chronic medical therapy, apraclonidine hydrochloride 0.5% should be instilled twice daily.

Apraclonidine has been evaluated in several studies as a primary ocular hypotensive agent. The first of these studies compared 0.25%, 0.5%, and 1% in a dose-response study lasting 8 days.[501] The first long-term study compared apraclonidine 0.25% and 0.5% three times a day with timolol 0.5% twice daily in a 3-month double-masked study. All three treatment groups exhibited similar IOP lowering. However, over the 90-day study period, 36% of patients on 0.5% apraclonidine and 9% of patients on 0.25% apraclonidine developed an ocular allergy and were withdrawn from the study. In contrast, none of the timolol-treated patients developed an allergy. Similar long-term studies have found that despite continued long-term lowering of IOP, local allergy seems to be the limiting factor in continued use of apraclonidine in approximately 25% of patients.[502] The risk of allergy, therefore, makes apraclonidine desirable as a first-line agent only when patients cannot tolerate other glaucoma medications.

There is presumptive evidence that the allergic reaction associated with apraclonidine is related to the amount and frequency of administration. Although there have been no well-controlled long-term or intermediate-term duration-of-action studies comparing twice-daily to thrice-daily administration of apraclonidine 0.5%, twice-daily administration might decrease the frequency of allergic responses while maintaining comparable IOP lowering. In October 1993, the FDA approved apraclonidine 0.5% for thrice-daily administration as an additive medication in eyes on maximally tolerated medications. In a double-masked, multicentered, parallel study, apraclonidine 0.5% three times a day was shown to lower IOP compared with the vehicle drug when added to maximally tolerated glaucoma medication.[503, 504] At 90 days, 61% of patients on apraclonidine avoided surgery compared with 33.9% in the control group. This study found an insignificant IOP-lowering effect in eyes already on two aqueous humor suppressants. Allergic reactions will likely prevent apraclonidine from becoming a first-line glaucoma therapy in most patients. However, its safety profile and continued efficacy should allow it to be an excellent candidate for second-line therapy following either a β-adrenoceptor antagonist or a prostaglandin. It is also a good choice when a β-adrenoceptor antagonist and prostaglandin are both contraindicated.

Brimonidine

Brimonidine, marketed as Alphagan (Allergan Pharmaceuticals, Irvine, CA), is another relatively selective α_2-agonist that is structurally similar to clonidine. Like clonidine, but in contrast with apraclonidine, brimonidine is a lipophilic drug. Because brimonidine is chemically related to clonidine and has affinity for the noradrenergic imidazoline receptor, its ocular hypotensive effects are thought to be mediated by ocular α_2-adrenoceptors. In preclinical studies, brimonidine appears to lower IOP in rabbits by α_2-adrenoceptor occupancy. However, in monkeys, activation of a CNS imidazoline receptor may mediates the ocular hypotensive effect in addition to the systemic effect on blood pressure and heart rate.[505] Brimonidine lowers IOP by decreasing aqueous humor production (up to 33%) without altering conventional outflow facility. In addition, brimonidine may increase uveoscleral outflow.[481] In primates, one drop in one eye also lowers the IOP in the fellow eye, suggesting that a contralateral effect occurs from systemic absorption, possible penetration into the central nervous system, or both,[506] similar to many other topical adrenergic agents.[505]

The first clinical trials with brimonidine evaluated its efficacy in the prevention of acute IOP rises after argon laser trabeculoplasty. Brimonidine 0.5%, like apraclonidine, was shown to be effective in decreasing elevations in IOP after argon laser trabeculoplasty.[475, 507, 508] In a vehicle-controlled, double-masked, multicenter study involving 232 patients who underwent 360-degree argon laser trabeculoplasty, brimonidine 0.5% was effective whether used prior to the procedure, after the procedure, or both prior to and following the trabeculoplasty. From this study, it appears that a single dose given before or after the laser procedure suffices to prevent postoperative pressure spikes, although the 0.5% concentration was associated with an undue amount of systemic hypotension. Likewise, sedation, another side effect related to α_2-adrenoceptors, appears to be dose-related and is associated with both the 0.5% and 0.2% solutions.[509] Presently, no data suggest that brimonidine suppresses the IOP elevations associated with cataract surgery, argon laser iridotomy, Nd:YAG laser iridotomy, or Nd:YAG laser posterior capsulotomy.

Brimonidine has been shown to lower IOP in various animal models over a dose range of 0.001 to 1.0%. In a 1-month dose-response study in humans, brimonidine in concentrations of 0.08%, 0.2%, and 0.5%, in a twice-daily dosing regimen, lowered IOP in open-angle glaucoma and ocular hypertensive patients, with a maximum IOP decrease between 20% and 30%.[509] The authors concluded that brimonidine 0.2% appeared to be the most effective dose because it was not only at the top of the dose-response curve but also had the fewer systemic and local side effects. However, there was a dose-response relationship among the 0.08%, 0.2%, and 0.5% solutions with regard to IOP lowering, a decrease in systolic blood pressure, and sedation. Some tolerance to the ocular hypotensive effect also occurred. On day 1 of therapy, the mean percent decrease in IOP from baseline was 16%, 22%, and 30% for the 0.08%, 0.2%, and 0.5% solutions, respectively. By day 28 of therapy, efficacy diminished significantly: 13%, 16%, and 14%, respectively. Furthermore, on day 1, 48% of the patients receiving the 0.2% solution and 79% of the patients receiving the 0.5% solution experienced a decrease of at least 20% in IOP. By day 28, only 31% of patients receiving the 0.2% solution and 21% of the patients receiving the 0.5% solution experienced a similar reduction. In addition, 29% of patients receiving the 0.5% solution and 10% of subjects receiving the 0.2% solution experienced fatigue.

Two clinical trials have compared brimonidine twice daily with both timolol maleate 0.5% and betaxolol 0.5% twice daily. IOP was measured 12 hours after the last administration of medications and then 3 hours after the first daily use. The 0.5% concentration of betaxolol was used as an active control, not the 0.25% suspension. This is important because the betaxolol suspension is much more comfortable and accounts for fewer adverse events than does the betaxolol solution. In the study comparing timolol with brimonidine, brimonidine was superior to timolol at putative peak (approximately 3 hours after dosing) but equivalent to or less effective than timolol at putative trough (approximately 12 hours after dosing).[510, 511] Some brimonidine-treated patients developed ocular allergic reactions similar to those reported for apraclonidine. Similar results were obtained when betaxolol was compared with brimonidine. The ocular hypotensive efficacy of brimonidine was superior to betaxolol only at the 3-hour time point. At all other time intervals, including a diurnal curve undergone by many patients, the two medications showed no significant difference. These results suggest that brimonidine may be a useful agent in patients in whom β-adrenoceptor antagonists are ineffective or a poor therapeutic choice because of adverse systemic side effects. The FDA also approved brimonidine 0.2% for chronic use in March of 1997, although with a frequency of three times daily rather than twice daily.

Adverse Effects of Selective α_2-Agonists

Apraclonidine

Many clinical studies have proved the safety of the long-term use of apraclonidine.[504, 512, 513] Patients receiving the drug may experience mild eyelid retraction and conjunctival blanching.[514] These effects are subtle and sometimes only detectable upon unilateral instillation. The eyelid retraction is likely due to α_1-adrenoceptor stimulation of Müller's muscle. The retraction, occurring in at least 50% of normal volunteers, begins within minutes of instillation and is maximal for 3 to 5 hours.[499] On average, the mean interpalpebral fissure increases 1.4 mm, but this does not occur with chronic therapy or bilateral instillation. Limited mydriasis occurs in about 45% of treated eyes. The increase in pupil size averages less than 1 mm and is usually not noticed by patients. The amount of mydriasis is less than that occurring with dipivefrin. Conjunctival blanching, occurring in up to 85% of patients, is probably caused by decreased blood flow to the limbal vessels. This phenomenon, and the report that apraclonidine 1% decreased conjunctival oxygen tension in normal volunteers, led to concern that the drug may decrease blood flow to the optic nerve. Studies indicate that the local effects on blood flow are restricted to the anterior segment, with the retina and optic nerve being unaffected.[499, 513–515]

The most troublesome side effect of chronic use of apraclonidine appears to be possible allergic blepharoconjunctivitis and dermatitis, similar to that occurring with topical epinephrine and dipivefrin. The periorbital region of affected patients becomes erythematous and edematous, and the skin often becomes scaly. Symptoms have been reported within 9 hours of starting apraclonidine therapy, but the reaction typically occurs weeks or months after initiation. The typical presenting complaint of apraclonidine allergy is red, itchy eyes. The follicular conjunctivitis clears 3 to 5 days after cessation of the medication without the need of additional treatment. The percentage of persons developing the allergy varies, averaging about 20% and increasing to nearly 50% with longer drug use. In one 3-month study, the incidence of ocular allergy was higher with apraclonidine 0.5% (36% of patients) than with apraclonidine 0.25% (9% of patients). With a twice-daily rather than a three-times-daily dosing schedule, the number of patients developing the allergy decreased to 9%.[504, 512, 513]

The most common systemic side effect of apraclonidine is a sensation of dry mouth or dry nose. This is not surprising when one recalls that clonidine was first introduced as a nasal decongestant. The dryness results from the direct absorption of apraclonidine through the nasolacrimal system, which causes vasoconstriction of the nasal and oral mucosa. These symptoms appear in approximately 20% of patients using apraclonidine 0.5%. They appear to be dose-related, decrease in severity over time, and may be minimized by nasolacrimal occlusion. Mild sedation may also occur with apraclonidine use. In a dose-response study of apraclonidine 0.125%, 0.25%, and 0.5%, the occurrence of fatigue in patients ranged from 0% to 10%. However, in double-masked studies, the frequency of fatigue was not any greater when compared with placebo.[498–501]

Apraclonidine has minimal adverse cardiovascular side effects.[476] It does not affect either the mean resting heart rate or the mean arterial blood pressure and, like brimonidine, has minimal effect on exercise-induced heart rate in normal healthy volunteers.[516] Additional adverse systemic effects of α_2-adrenoceptor agonists may include the potentiation of growth hormone secretion, inhibition of insulin release by a direct action on pancreatic beta cells, and increased platelet aggregation. None of these has been considered clinically significant in patients receiving topical α_2-adrenoceptor agonist eye-drop therapy.

Brimonidine

Brimonidine, like clonidine, is a highly lipophilic drug that can pass through the blood-brain barrier and cause potential CNS effects such as systemic hypotension. The most frequent side effects reported with brimonidine are dry mouth, conjunctival blanching, systemic hypotension, and drowsiness. These side effects appear to be dose-related.[509, 517] The dry mouth and conjunctival blanching appear to be α_1-adrenoceptor–mediated side effects, similar to those experienced with apraclonidine. Fatigue and drowsiness appear to be higher with brimonidine than apraclonidine, ranging from 4% to 29%.[509] Therefore, on the continuum of traditional α_1-adrenoceptor agonist adverse effects (e.g., dry mouth, lid retraction) and α_2-adrenoceptor agonist adverse effects (e.g., sedation and hypotension), brimonidine lies between apraclonidine and clonidine. In summary, dry mouth has been reported, but sedation is probably the more common adverse effect of brimonidine, especially with the 0.5% concentration as used for prevention of postlaser IOP elevation. Note that the 0.2% concentration is approved for chronic use in the United States.

Nordlund and colleagues have found that in normal humans, brimonidine does not affect pulmonary function as assessed by spirometry (FEV_1).[517] The same study found that neither betaxolol nor brimonidine affected heart rate, compared with a vehicle, during a 15-minute stress test. In contrast, timolol lowered the baseline heart rate and decreased the rate of response to exercise. In this study, both betaxolol and brimonidine were possibly safer in this regard than timolol.

Single-dose studies of brimonidine both in young, healthy male volunteers and in patients undergoing laser trabeculoplasty showed minimal effects on systolic and diastolic blood pressure.[517] However, in the 1-month dose-response study, brimonidine significantly lowered blood pressure, although without clinical adverse effects.[509] Therefore, with multiple dosing, it appears that brimonidine causes less hypotension than clonidine but possibly more than that observed with apraclonidine.

In short-term studies with brimonidine lasting less than 1 month, patients rarely developed allergic follicular conjunctivitis.[509] This appears to be a more frequent side effect with apraclonidine use. However, long-term studies comparing brimonidine twice daily to both timolol maleate and betaxolol have suggested that 10% of eyes develop an allergy to brimonidine and 30% must discontinue the use of brimonidine because of adverse events.[511, 518]

Selectivity of Topical α_2-Agonists

The affinity of topical α_2-agonists for the α_2-adrenoceptor assessed from radioligand binding studies has been used to characterize the selectivity of all three medications. All three medications are *relatively* selective α_2-agonists. By measuring the observed dissociation constants (K_d) of these drugs for both the α_2- and α_1-adrenoceptor, the α_2/α_1 selectivity of apraclonidine is approximately 528 times and that of brimonidine is approximately 759 times.[505] α_2 Selectivity therefore appears to be high enough for both drugs that their primary ocular effect is mediated by α_2-adrenoceptor activation at equimolar tissue concentrations. Thus, α_1 activation, either locally or systemically, occurs far less frequently at the usual ophthalmic doses of these drugs. For example, published data show the EC_{50} of apraclonidine to be 216 nM for causing α_1-receptor–mediated contraction of the rabbit iris dilator muscle (mydriasis) in vitro, whereas the EC_{50} for apraclonidine in activating α_2-receptors is 1.9 nM.[519] In some animal models, brimonidine is a more selective α_2-adrenoceptor agonist than either clonidine or apraclonidine,[519] but it too may elicit α_1-adrenoceptor agonism in humans. In human eyes receiving this medication prior to or after argon laser trabeculoplasty, many patients experienced lid retraction and conjunctival blanching,[475, 507, 508] effects attributed to α_1 agonism.

NEUROPROTECTION OF ADRENERGIC AGENTS

It is well recognized that IOP is an important risk factor in the progression of glaucomatous optic neuropathy. Efforts in future drug development for glaucoma, however, will likely be directed toward ascertaining whether new compounds facilitate nerve function independently from their ability to lower IOP. Interestingly, studies using two adrenergic agents have suggested they may be useful in this regard in addition to their well-known ability to lower IOP. In an animal model in which the rat optic nerve was subjected to a crush injury, treatment with the α_2-adrenoceptor agonist brimonidine appeared to protect the rat optic nerve from secondary damage.[519] Additional evidence that members of this class of agents are capable of neuroprotection arose in a rabbit model in which the α_2-agonist dexmedetomidine protected against ischemic brain damage.[520]

Provocative findings also suggest that the selective β_1-adrenoceptor antagonist, betaxolol, may have utility as a neuroprotective agent to attenuate the retinal degenerative changes normally seen in response to ischemia or excitotoxic glutamate-related compounds.[521] It is unclear, however, that the intraperitoneal delivery of drug used in the in vivo experiments, or the effects observed in the in vitro experiments of this report, are directly relevant to the common clinical use of topical betaxolol to lower IOP. Although the potential neuroprotectant properties of these adrenergic compounds are appealing, it is premature to suggest these compounds have clinical applicability in humans with glaucoma.

REFERENCES

1. Darier A: Leçons de thérapeutique oculaire. La huitième présentation. Bur Clin Opthalmol 1901.
2. Spengler E: Kritisches sammel-referat über die verwendung einiger neurer arneimittel. Der Augenheilkdunde Zeitschr Augenhielk 13:33–36, 1905.
3. Barnard EA: Receptor classes and the transmitter-gated ion channels. Trends Pharmacol Sci 17:368–374, 1992.
4. Gudermann T, Nurnberg B, Schultz G: Receptors and G proteins as primary components of transmembrane signal transduction. Part 1. G-protein-coupled receptors: Structure and function. J Mol Med 73:51–63, 1995.
5. Premont RT, Inglese J, Lefkowitz RJ: Protein kinases that phosphorylate activated G protein-coupled receptors. FASEB J 9:175–182, 1995.
6. Dohlman HG, Caron MG, Lefkowitz RJ: A family of receptors coupled to guanine nucleotide regulatory proteins. Biochemistry 26:2657–2664, 1987.
7. Conklin BR, Chabre O, Wong YH, et al: Recombinant Gqα. Mutational activation and coupling to receptors and phospholipase C. J Biol Chem 267:31–34, 1992.
8. Hieble JP, Bondinell WE, Ruffolo RR: α- and β-adrenoceptors: From the gene to the clinic. 1. Molecular biology and adrenoceptor subclassification. J Med Chem 38:3415–3444, 1995.
9. Barber DL, Ganz MB, Bongiorno PB, Strader CD: Mutant constructs of the β-adrenergic receptor that are uncoupled from adenylyl cyclase retain functional activation of Na-H exchange. Mol Pharmacol 41:1056–1060, 1992.
10. Surprenant A, Horstman DA, Akbarali H, Limbird LE: A point mutation of the α_2-adrenoceptor that blocks coupling to potassium but not calcium currents. Science 257:977–980, 1992.
11. Nichols AJ: α-Adrenoceptor signal transduction mechanisms. Prog Basic Clin Pharmacol 7:44–74, 1991.
12. Eason MG, Kurose H, Holt BD, et al: Simultaneous coupling of α_2-adrenergic receptors to two G-proteins with opposing effects. J Biol Chem 267:15795–15801, 1992.
13. Duzic E, Lanier SM: Factors determining the specificity of signal transduction by guanine nucleotide-binding protein-coupled receptors. J Biol Chem 267:24045–24052, 1992.
14. Green SA, Holt BD, Liggett SB: β_1- and β_2-adrenergic receptors display subtype-selective coupling to Gs. Mol Pharmacol 41:889–893, 1992.

15. Coupry J, Duzic E, Lanier SM: Factors determining the specificity of signal transduction by guanine nucleotide-binding protein-coupled receptors. J Biol Chem 267:9852–9857, 1992.
16. Birnbaumer L, Abramowitz J, Brown AM: Receptor-effector coupling by G proteins. Biochim Biophys Acta 1031:163–224, 1990.
17. Ahlquist RP: A study of the adrenotropic receptors. Am J Physiol 153:586–600, 1948.
18. Lands AM, Arnold A, McAuliff JP, et al: Differentiation of receptor systems activated by sympathetic amines. Nature 214:597–598, 1967.
19. Delbarre B, Schmitt H: A further attempt to characterize sedative receptors activated by clonidine in chickens and mice. Eur J Pharmacol 22:355–359, 1973.
20. Berthelsen S, Pettinger WA: A functional basis for classification of alpha-adrenergic receptors. Life Sci 21:595–606, 1977.
21. Langer SZ: Presynaptic regulation of catecholamine release. Biochem Pharmacol 23:1793–1800, 1974.
22. Starke K, Montel H, Gayk W, Merker R: Comparison of the effects of clonidine on pre- and postsynaptic adrenoceptors in the rabbit pulmonary artery. Arch Pharmacol 285:133–150, 1974.
23. Cotecchia S, Schwinn DA, Randall RR, et al: Molecular cloning and expression of the cDNA for the hamster α_1-adrenergic receptor. Proc Natl Acad Sci U S A 85:7159–7163, 1988.
24. Schwinn DA, Lomasney JW, Lorenz W, et al: Molecular cloning and expression of the cDNA for a novel α_1-adrenergic receptor subtype. J Biol Chem 265:5183–5189, 1990.
25. Lomasney JW, Cotecchia S, Lorenz W, et al: Molecular cloning and expression of the cDNA for the alpha 1 A-adrenergic receptor. J Biol Chem 266:6365–6369, 1991.
26. Kobilka BK, Matsui H, Kobilka TS, et al: Cloning, sequencing, and expression of the gene coding for the human platelet α_2-adrenergic receptor. Science 238:650–656, 1987.
27. Regan JW, Kobilka TS, Yang-Feng TL, et al: Cloning and expression of a human kidney cDNA for an α_2-adrenergic receptor subtype. Proc Natl Acad Sci U S A 85:6301–6305, 1988.
28. Lomasney JW, Lorenz W, Allen LF, et al: Expansion of the α-adrenergic receptor family: Cloning and characterization of a human α_2-adrenergic receptor subtype, the gene for which is located on chromosome 2. Proc Natl Acad Sci U S A 87:5094–5098, 1990.
29. Weinshank RL, Zgombick JM, Macchi M, et al: Cloning expression, and pharmacological characterization of a human α_{2B}-adrenergic receptor. Mol Pharmacol 38:681–688, 1990.
30. Lanier SM, Downing S, Duzie E, Homcy CJ: Isolation of rat genomic clones encoding subtypes of the α_2-adrenergic receptor. Identification of a unique receptor subtype. J Biol Chem 266:10470–10478, 1991.
31. Link R, Daunt D, Barsh G, et al: Cloning of two mouse genes encoding α_2-adrenergic receptor subtypes and identification of a single amino acid in the mouse α_2-C10 homolog responsible for an interspecies variation in antagonist binding. Mol Pharmacol 42:16–27, 1992.
32. Blaxall HS, Cerutis DR, Hass NA, et al: Cloning and expression of the α_{2C}-adrenergic receptor from the OK cell line. Mol Pharmacol 45:176–181, 1994.
33. Dixon RAF, Kobilka BK, Strader DJ, et al: Cloning of the gene and cDNA for mammalian beta-2-adrenergic receptor and homology with rhodopsin. Nature 321:75–79, 1986.
34. Frielle T, Collins S, Daniel KW, et al: Cloning of the cDNA for the human beta-1-adrenergic receptor. Proc Natl Acad Sci U S A 84:7920–7924, 1987.
35. Emorine LJ, Marullo S, Briend-Sutren MM, et al: Molecular characterization of the human β_3-adrenergic receptor. Science 245:1118–1121, 1989.
36. Novack GD, Leopold IH: Aqueous humor and cerebrospinal fluid: A new hormonal twist. Am J Ophthalmol 104:297–300, 1987.
37. Bloom G, Richmond C, Alvarado JA, Polansky J: Betaxolol vs timolol: Plasma radio-receptor assays to evaluate systemic complications of beta-blocker therapy for glaucoma. Invest Ophthalmol Vis Sci Suppl 26(3):125, 1985.
38. MacKinnon AC, Spedding M, Brown CM: Alpha 2-adrenoceptors: More subtypes but fewer functional differences. Trends Pharmacol Sci 15:119–123, 1994.
39. Bylund DB: Subtypes of α_2-adrenoceptors: Pharmacological and molecular biological evidence converge. Trends Pharmacol Sci 9:356–361, 1988.
40. Bylund DB: Pharmacological characteristics of alpha-2 adrenergic receptor subtypes. Ann N Y Acad Sci 763:1–7, 1995.
41. Minneman KP, Esbenshade TA: α_1-Adrenergic receptor subtypes. Annu Rev Pharmacol Toxicol 34:117–133, 1994.
42. O'Dowd BF, Hnatowich M, Regan J, et al: Site-directed mutagenesis of the cytoplasmic domains of the human beta 2 adrenergic receptor. J Biol Chem 263:15985–15992, 1988.
43. Strader CD, Candelore MR, Hill WS, et al: Identification of two serine residues involved in agonist activation of the beta adrenergic receptor. J Biol Chem 264:13572–13578, 1989.
44. Strader CD, Sigal IS, Dixon RA: Structural basis of beta adrenergic receptor function. FASEB J 3:1825–1832, 1989.
45. Strader CD, Gaffney T, Sugg EE, et al: Allele-specific activation of genetically engineered receptors. J Biol Chem 266:5–8, 1991.
46. Kobilka BK, Kobilka TS, Regan JW, et al: Chimeric alpha-2-beta-2-adrenergic receptors: Delineation of domains involved in effector coupling and ligand binding specificity. Science 240:1310–1316, 1988.
47. Suryanarayana S, Daunt DA, vonZastrow M, Kobilka BK: A point mutation in the seventh hydrophobic domain of the alpha 2 adrenergic receptor increases its affinity for a family of beta receptor antagonists. J Biol Chem 266:15488–15492, 1991.
48. Guan XM, Peroutka SJ, Kobilka BK: Identification of a single amino acid residue responsible for binding of a class of beta receptor antagonists to 5HT1A receptors. Mol Pharmacol 41:695–698, 1992.
49. Dohlman HG, Caron MG, Strader CD, et al: Identification and sequence of a binding site peptide of the beta 2 adrenergic receptor. Biochemistry 27:1813–1817, 1988.
50. Matsui H, Lefkowitz RJ, Caron MG, Regan JW: Localization of the fourth membrane spanning domain as a ligand binding site in the human alpha 2 adrenergic receptor. Biochemistry 28:4125–4130, 1989.
51. Frielle T, Daniel KW, Caron MG, Lefkowitz RJ: Structural basis of β-adrenergic receptor subtype specificity studied with chimeric β_1/β_2-adrenergic receptors. Proc Natl Acad Sci U S A 85:9494–9498, 1988.
52. Dixon RAF, Hill WS, Candelore MR, et al: Genetic analysis of the molecular basis for β-adrenergic receptor subtype specificity. Proteins 6:267–274, 1989.
53. Suryanarayana S, Kobilka BK: Amino acid substitutions at position 312 in the seventh hydrophobic segment of the $\beta 2$ adrenergic receptor modify ligand binding specificity. Mol Pharmacol 44:111–114, 1993.
54. Wong SK, Parker EM, Ross EM: Chimeric muscarinic cholinergic: β-Adrenergic receptors that activate Gs in response to muscarinic agonists. J Biol Chem 265:6219–6224, 1990.
55. Chung FZ, Wang CD, Potter PC, et al: Site-directed mutagenesis and continuous expression of human β-adrenergic receptors. J Biol Chem 263:4052–4055, 1988.
56. Zhu SZ, Wang SZ, Hu J, El-Fakahany EE: An arginine residue conserved in most G protein-coupled receptors is essential for the function of the M_1 muscarinic receptor. Mol Pharmacol 45:517–523, 1994.
56a. Cotecchia S, Ostrowski J, Khelsberg MA, et al: Discrete amino acid sequences of the α_1-adrenergic receptor determine the selectivity of coupling to phosphatidylinositol hydrolysis. J Biol Chem 267:1633–1639, 1992.
57. Rodbell M, Krans HMJ, Pohl SL, Birnbaumer L: The glucagon-sensitive adenyl cyclase system in plasma membranes of rat liver. IV. Binding of glucagon: Effect of guanyl nucleotides. J Biol Chem 246:1872–1876, 1971.
58. Lefkowitz RJ, Cotecchia S, Samana P, Costa T: Constitutive activity of receptors coupled to guanine nucleotide regulatory proteins. Trends Pharmacol Sci 14:303–307, 1993.
59. Oliveira L, Paiva ACM, Sander C, Vriend G: A common step for signal transduction in G protein-coupled receptors. Trends Pharmacol Sci 15:170–172, 1994.
60. Chidiac P, Hebert TE, Valiquette M, et al: Inverse agonist activity of beta-adrenergic antagonists. Mol Pharmacol 45:490–499, 1994.
61. Hein L, Kobilka BK: Review: Neurotransmitter receptors IV. Adrenergic receptor signal transduction and regulation. Neuropharmacology 34:357–366, 1995.
62. Samama P, Pei G, Costa T, et al: Negative antagonists promote an inactive conformation of the beta 2-adrenergic receptor. Mol Pharmacol 45:390–394, 1994.
63. Mewes T, Dutz S, Ravens U, Jakobs KH: Activation of calcium currents in cardiac myocytes by empty beta-adrenoceptors. Circulation 88:2916–2922, 1993.
64. Gotze K, Jakobs KH: Unoccupied β-adrenoceptor-induced adenylyl cyclase stimulation in turkey erythrocyte membranes. Eur J Pharmacol 268:151–158, 1994.
65. Jasper JR, Insel PA: Evolving concepts of partial agonism: The β-adrenergic receptor as a paradigm. Biochem Pharmacol 43:119–130, 1992.

66. Waller DG: A renaissance in cardiovascular therapy? Br J Clin Pharmacol 30:157–171, 1990.
67. Frishman WH: Clinical significance of beta-1-selectivity and intrinsic sympathomimetic activity in a beta-adrenergic blocking drug. Am J Cardiol 59:33–37F, 1987.
68. Boissel JP, Leizorovicz A, Picolet H, Peyrieux J-C: Secondary prevention after high-risk acute myocardial infarction with low-dose acebutolol. Am J Cardiol 66:251–260, 1990.
69. Prichard BNC: Pharmacologic aspects of intrinsic sympathomimetic activity in beta-blocking drugs. Am J Cardiol 59:13F–17F, 1987.
70. Dixon RAR, Kobilka BK, Strader DJ, et al: Cloning of the gene and cDNA for mammalian β-adrenergic receptor and homology with rhodopsin. Nature 321:75–79, 1986.
71. Kobilka BK, Dixon RAF, Frielle T, et al: cDNA for the human beta-2 adrenergic receptor: A protein with multiple membrane-spanning domains and encoded by a gene whose chromosomal location is shared with that of the receptor for platelet-derived growth factor. Proc Natl Acad Sci U S A 84:46–50, 1987.
72. Marullo S, Emorine LJ, Strosberg AD, Delavier-Klutchko C: Selective binding of ligands to β1, β2 or chimeric β1/β2-adrenergic receptors involves multiple subsites. EMBO J 9:1471–1476, 1990.
73. Muzzin P, Revelli J, Kuhne F, et al: An adipose tissue-specific β-adrenergic receptor. J Biol Chem 266:24053–24058, 1991.
74. Nahimas C, Blin N, Elalouf J, et al: Molecular characterization of the mouse β_3-adrenergic receptor: Relationship with the atypical receptor of adipocytes. EMBO J 10:3721–3727, 1991.
75. Tate KM, Briend-Sutren MM, Emorine LJ, et al: Expression of three human beta-adrenergic-receptor subtypes in transfected Chinese hamster ovary cells. Eur J Biochem 196:357–361, 1991.
76. Galitzky J, Carpene C, Bousquet-Melou A, et al: Differential activation of β_1-, β_2- and β_3-adrenoceptors by catecholamines in white and brown adipocytes. Fundam Clin Pharmacol 9:324–331, 1995.
77. Michel MC, Philipp T, Brodde O-E: α- and β-Adrenoceptors in hypertension: Molecular biology and pharmacological studies. Pharmacol Toxicol 70(Suppl II):1–10, 1992.
78. Ross EM: Pharmacodynamics: Mechanisms of drug action and the relationship between drug concentration and effect. *In* Hardman JG, Limbird LE, Molinoff PB, et al (eds): Goodman and Gilman's The Pharmacological Basis of Therapeutics, 9th ed. New York, McGraw-Hill, 1996, pp 29–41.
79. Kume H, Hall IP, Washabau RJ, et al: Beta-adrenergic agonists regulate KCa channels in airway smooth muscle by cAMP-dependent and -independent mechanisms. J Clin Invest 93:371–379, 1994.
80. Torphy TJ: β-Adrenoceptors, cAMP and airway smooth muscle relaxation: Challenges to the dogma. Trends Pharmacol Sci 15:370–374, 1994.
81. Bylund DB: Subtypes of alpha-1 and alpha-2 adrenergic receptors. FASEB J 6:832–839, 1992.
82. Bylund DB, Eikenberg DC, Hieble JP, et al: IV. International union of pharmacology nomenclature of adrenoceptors. Pharmacol Rev 46:121–136, 1994.
83. Ruffolo RR Jr, Nichols AJ, Stadel JM, Hieble JP: Pharmacologic and therapeutic applications of a_2-adrenoceptor subtypes. Annu Rev Pharmacol Toxicol 32:243–279, 1993.
84. Fain JN, Garcia-Sainz JA: Role of phosphatidylinositol turnover in α_1- and of adenylate cyclase inhibition in α_2-effects of catecholamines. Life Sci 26:1183–1194, 1980.
85. Murayama T, Ui M: Loss of the inhibitory function of the guanine nucleotide regulatory component of adenylate cyclase due to its ADP ribosylation by islet-activating protein, pertussis toxin, in adipocyte membranes. J Biol Chem 258:3319–3326, 1983.
86. Limbird LE: GTP and Na^+ modulate receptor-adenyl cyclase coupling and receptor-mediated function. Am J Physiol 247:E59–E68, 1984.
87. Sweatt JD, Johnson SL, Cragoe EJ, Limbird LE: Inhibitors of Na^+/H^+ exchange block stimulus-provoked arachidonic acid release in human platelets. J Biol Chem 260:12910–12918, 1985.
88. Ruffolo RR Jr, Hieble JP: α-Adrenoceptors. Pharmacol Ther 61:1–64, 1994.
89. Morrow AL, Creese I: Characterization of α_1-adrenergic receptor subtypes in rat brain: A reevaluation of [^{3}H]-WB 4101 and [^{3}H]-prazosin binding. Mol Pharmacol 29:321–330, 1986.
90. Michel MC, Kenny B, Schwinn DA: Classification of α_1-adrenoceptor subtypes. Naunyn-Schmiedebergs Arch Pharmacol 352:1–10, 1995.
91. Harrison JK, Pearson WR, Lynch KR: Molecular characterization of α_1 and α_2-adrenoceptors. Trends Pharmacol Sci 12:62–67, 1991.
92. Han C, Abel PW, Minneman KP: α_1-Adrenoceptor subtypes linked to different mechanisms for increasing intracellular Ca^{2+} in smooth muscle. Nature 329:333–335, 1987.
93. Burch RM, Luini A, Axelrod J: Phospholipase A_2 and phospholipase C are activated by distinct GTP binding proteins in response to α_1-adrenergic stimulation in FRTL-5 thyroid cells. Proc Natl Acad Sci U S A 83:7201–7205, 1986.
94. Llahi S, Fain JN: α_1-Adrenergic receptor-mediated activation of phospholipase D in rat cerebral cortex. J Biol Chem 267:3679–3685, 1992.
95. Robinson JP, Kendall DA: Niguldipine discriminates between α_1-adrenoceptor mediated second messenger responses in rat cerebral cortex slices. Br J Pharmacol 100:3–4, 1990.
96. Minneman KP, Atkinson BA: Interaction of subtype-selective antagonists with α_1-adrenergic receptor mediated second messenger responses in rat brain. Mol Pharmacol 40:523–530, 1991.
97. Neufeld AH: Mechanism of action of adrenergic drugs in the eye. *In* Drance SM, Neufeld AH (eds): Glaucoma: Applied Pharmacology in Medical Treatment. Orlando, FL, Grune & Stratton, 1984, pp 277–324.
98. Sears ML: Regulation of aqueous flow by the adenylate cyclase receptor complex in the ciliary epithelium. Am J Ophthalmol 100:194–198, 1985.
99. Wax MB: Signal transduction in ciliary epithelial cells. *In* Drance S, VanBuskirk M, Neufeld A (eds): Pharmacology of Glaucoma. Baltimore, Williams & Wilkins, 1992, pp 184–210.
100. Mittag T, Tormay A: Desensitization of the beta-adrenergic receptor-adenylate cyclase complex in rabbit iris-ciliary body induced by topical epinephrine. Exp Eye Res 33:497–503, 1981.
101. Bartels SP, Liu JHK, Neufeld AH: Decreased beta-adrenergic responsiveness in cornea and iris-ciliary body following topical timolol or epinephrine in albino and pigmented rabbits. Invest Ophthalmol Vis Sci 24:718–724, 1983.
102. Brandt JD, Bartels SP, Neufeld AH: Adrenergic stimulation of ciliary process epithelium causes surface membrane internalization. Invest Ophthalmol Vis Sci 28:431–444, 1987.
103. Green K, Mayberry L: Drug effects on the hydraulic conductivity of the isolated rabbit ciliary epithelium. Q J Exp Physiol 70:271–281, 1985.
104. Townsend OJ, Brubaker RF: Immediate effect of epinephrine on aqueous formation in the normal human eye as measured by fluorophotometry. Invest Ophthalmol Vis Sci 19:256–266, 1980.
105. Brubaker RF, Gaasterland D: The effect of isoproterenol on aqueous humor formation in humans. Invest Ophthalmol Vis Sci 25:357–359, 1984.
106. Larson RS, Brubaker RF: Isoproterenol stimulates aqueous flow in humans with Horner's syndrome. Invest Ophthalmol Vis Sci 29:621–625, 1988.
107. Cole DF: Ocular fluids. *In* Davson H (ed): The Eye, 3rd ed. New York, Academic Press, 1984, pp 269–390.
108. Cole DF: Secretion of the aqueous humor. Exp Eye Res 25:161–176, 1977.
109. Civan MM, Peterson-Yantorno K, Coca-Prados M, Yantorno RE: Regulatory volume decrease by cultured non-pigmented ciliary epithelial cells. Exp Eye Res 54:181–191, 1992.
110. Yantorno RE, Carre DA, Coca-Prados M, et al: Whole cell patch clamping of ciliary epithelial cells during anisosmotic swelling. Am J Physiol 262:C501–C509, 1992.
111. Wolosin JM, Bonanno JA, Hanzel D, Machen T: Bicarbonate transport mechanisms in rabbit ciliary body epithelium. Exp Eye Res 52:397–407, 1991.
112. Carre DA, Tang C-SR, Krupin T, Civan MM: Effect of bicarbonate on intracellular potential of rabbit ciliary epithelium. Curr Eye Res 11:609–624, 1992.
113. Edelman JL, Sachs G, Adorante JS: Ion transport asymmetry and functional coupling in bovine pigmented and nonpigmented ciliary epithelial cells. Am J Physiol 266:C1210–C1221, 1994.
114. Mitchell CH, Jacob TJC: A nonselective high conductance channel in bovine pigmented ciliary epithelial cells. J Memb Biol 150:105–111, 1996.
115. Jacob TJC, Civan MM: Role of ion channels in aqueous humor formation. Am J Physiol 271:C703–C720, 1996.
116. Bartels SP: Aqueous humor formation: Fluid production by a sodium pump. *In* Ritch R, Shields MB, Krupin T (eds): The Glaucomas, vol 1. St. Louis, CV Mosby, 1989, pp 199–218.
117. Okami T, Yamamoto A, Omori K, et al: Quantitative immunocyto-

chemical localization of Na+, K+-ATPase in rat ciliary epithelial cells. J Histochem Cytochem 37:1353–1361, 1989.
118. Usukura J, Fain GL, Bok D: [3H] ouabain localization of Na-K ATPase in the epithelium of rabbit ciliary body pars plicata. Invest Ophthalmol Vis Sci 29:606–614, 1988.
119. Flugel C, Lutjen-Drecoll E: Presence and distribution of Na+/K+-ATPase in the ciliary epithelium of the rabbit. Histochemistry 88:613–621, 1988.
120. Ghosh S, Freitag AC, Martin-Vasallo P, Coca-Prados M: Cellular distribution and differential gene expression of the three alpha subunit isoforms of the Na, K-ATPase in the ocular ciliary epithelium. J Biol Chem 265:2935–2940, 1990.
121. Coca-Prados M, Lopez-Briones L: Evidence that the alpha and alpha (+) isoforms of the catalytic subunit of (Na+, K+)-ATPase reside in distinct ciliary epithelial cells of the mammalian eye. Biochem Biophys Res Comm 145:460–466, 1987.
122. Coakes RL, Brubaker RF: The mechanism of timolol in lowering intraocular pressure. Arch Ophthalmol 96:2045–2048, 1978.
123. Yablonski ME, Zimmerman TJ, Waltman SR, Becker B: A fluorophotometric study of the effect of topical timolol on aqueous humor dynamics. Exp Eye Res 27:135–142, 1978.
124. Schenker HW, Yablonski ME, Podos SM, et al: Fluorophotometric study of epinephrine and timolol in human subjects. Arch Ophthalmol 99:1212–1226, 1981.
125. Chen S, Inoue R, Inomata H, Ito Y: Role of cyclic AMP-induced C1 conductance in aqueous humour formation by the dog ciliary epithelium. Br J Pharmacol 112:1137–1145, 1994.
126. Delamere NA, Socci RR, King KL: Alteration of sodium, potassium-adenosine triphosphatase activity in rabbit ciliary processes by cyclic adenosine monophosphate-dependent protein kinase. Invest Ophthalmol Vis Sci 31:2164–2170, 1990.
127. Delamere NA, King KL: The influence of cyclic AMP upon NA+, K+-ATPase activity in rabbit ciliary epithelium. Invest Ophthalmol Vis Sci 33:430–435, 1992.
128. Wax MB, Saito I, Tenkova T, et al: Vacuolar H+ ATPase in the ocular ciliary epithelium. Proc Natl Acad Sci U S A 94:6752–6757, 1997.
129. Vale J, Phillips CI: Effect of DL- and D-propranolol on ocular tension in rabbits and patients. Exp Eye Res 9:82–90, 1970.
130. Phillips CI, Howitt G, Rowlands DJ: Propranolol as ocular hypotensive agent. Br J Ophthalmol 51:222–226, 1967.
131. Bucci MG, Missiroli A, Pecori-Giraldi J, et al: La somministrazione locale del propranolol nella terapia del glaucoma. Boll d'Ocul 47:51–60, 1968.
132. Watanabe K, Chiou GC: Action mechanism of timolol to lower the intraocular pressure in rabbits. Ophthalmic Res 15:160–167, 1983.
133. Ohrstrom A, Pandolfi M: Long-term treatment of glaucoma with systemic propranolol. Am J Ophthalmol 86:340–344, 1978.
134. Pandolfi M, Ohrstrom A: Treatment of ocular hypertension with oral beta-adrenergic blocking agents. Acta Ophthalmol 52:464–467, 1974.
135. Wettrell K, Pandolfi M: Propranolol vs acetazolamide. A long-term double-masked study of the effect on intraocular pressure and blood pressure. Arch Ophthalmol 97:280–283, 1979.
136. Wettrell K, Pandolfi M: Effect of topical atenolol on intraocular pressure. Br J Ophthalmol 61:334–338, 1977.
137. Takats I, Szilvassy I, Kerek A: [Intraocular pressure and circulation of aqueous humour in rabbit eyes following intravenous administration of propranolol (Inderal)]. Graefes Arch Clin Exp Ophthalmol 185:331–342, 1972.
138. Green K, Kim K: Interaction of adrenergic antagonists with prostaglandin E2 and tetrahydrocannabinol in the eye. Invest Ophthalmol 15:102–111, 1976.
139. Takase M, Araie M, Matsuo T: A single dose study of topical befunolol on intraocular pressure in man. Nippon Ganka Gakkai Zasshi 86:87–98, 1982.
140. Takats I, Tieri O, Polzella A: Emploi clinique et mechanisme d'action du propanololum. Ophthalmologica 170:36–42, 1975.
141. Draeger J: Corneal Sensitivity: Measurement and Clinical Importance. Wien/New York, Springer-Verlag, 1984.
142. Vale J, Phillips CI: Practolol (Eraldin) eye drops as an ocular hypotensive agent. Br J Ophthalmol 57:210–214, 1973.
143. Felix RH, Ive FA, Dahl MG: Cutaneous and ocular reactions to practolol. BMJ 4:321–324, 1974.
144. Novack GD: Ophthalmic beta-blockers since timolol. Surv Ophthalmol 31:307–327, 1987.
145. Phillips CI, Bartholomew RS, Levy AM, et al: Penetration of timolol eye drops in human aqueous humor: The first hour. Br J Ophthalmol 69:217–218, 1985.
146. Wax MB, Molinoff PB: Distribution and properties of beta-adrenergic receptors in human irs/ciliary body. Invest Ophthalmol Vis Sci 28:420–430, 1987.
147. Woodward DF, Chen J, Padillo E, Ruiz G: Pharmacological characterization of β-adrenoceptor subtype involvement in the ocular hypotensive response to β-adrenergic stimulation. Exp Eye Res 43:61–75, 1986.
148. Elena P-P, Kosina-Boix M, Moulin G, Lapalus P: Autoradiographic localization of beta-adrenergic receptors in rabbit eye. Invest Ophthalmol Vis Sci 28:1436–1441, 1987.
149. Zimmerman TJ, Kaufman HE: Timolol: Dose response and duration of action. Arch Ophthalmol 95:605–607, 1977.
150. Boger WP, Steinert RF, Puliafito CA, Pavan-Langston D: Clinical trial comparing timolol ophthalmic solution to pilocarpine in open-angle glaucoma. Am J Ophthalmol 86:8–18, 1978.
151. Silverstone DE, Arkfeld D, Cowan G, et al: Long-term diurnal control of intraocular pressure with levobunolol and with timolol. Glaucoma 7:138–140, 1985.
152. Boger WP: Timolol: Short term "escape" and long term "drift." Ann Ophthalmol 11:1239–1242, 1979.
153. Boger WP, Puliafito CA, Steinert RF, Langston EP: Long-term experience with timolol ophthalmic solution in patients with open-angle glaucoma. Ophthalmology 85:259–267, 1978.
154. Oksala A, Salminen L: Zur trachyphylaxie bei timololbehandlung des chronischen glaukoms. Klin Monatsbl Augenheilkd 177:451–454, 1980.
155. Steinert RF, Thomas JV, Boger WPI: Long-term drift and continued efficacy after multiyear timolol therapy. Arch Ophthalmol 99:100–103, 1981.
156. Levobunolol Study Group: Levobunolol: A four-year study of efficacy and safety in glaucoma treatment. Ophthalmology 96:642–645, 1989.
157. Spinelli D, Montanari P, Vigasio F, Cormanni V: Effects du maléate de timolol sur l'oeil controlatéral sans traitement. J Fr Ophthalmol 5:152–158, 1982.
158. Gibbens MV: Sympathetic influences on the consensual ophthalmotonic reaction. Br J Ophthalmol 72:750–753, 1988.
159. Gibbens MV: The consensual ophthalmotonic reaction. Br J Ophthalmol 72:746–749, 1988.
160. Martin XD, Rabineau PA: Intraocular pressure effects of timolol after unilateral instillation. Ophthalmology 95:1620–1623, 1988.
161. Urtti A, Salminen L: A comparison between iris-ciliary body concentration and receptor affinity of timolol. Acta Ophthalmol 63:16–18, 1985.
162. Salminen L, Urtti A: Kinetics of ophthalmic timolol in albino and pigmented rabbit eyes. Ophthalmic Res 16:200, 1984.
163. Krupin T, Singer PR, Perlmutter J, et al: One-hour intraocular pressure response to timolol: Lack of correlation with long-term response. Arch Ophthalmol 99:840–841, 1981.
164. Boozman FW, Foerster RJ, Allen RC, et al: The long-term efficacy of twice-daily 0.25% levobunolol and timolol. Arch Ophthalmol 106:614–618, 1988.
165. Dausch D, Schad K: Eignet sich 0.1% ige Timolol-maleate augentropflosung zur therapie des chronischen glaukoms? Klin Monatsbl Augenheilkd 180:141–145, 1982.
166. Long D, Zimmerman T, Spaeth G, et al: Minimum concentration of levobunolol required to control intraocular pressure in patients with primary open-angle glaucoma or ocular hypertension. Am J Ophthalmol 99:18–22, 1985.
167. Topper JE, Brubaker RF: Effects of timolol, epinephrine, and acetazolamide on aqueous flow during sleep. Invest Ophthalmol Vis Sci 26:1315–1319, 1985.
168. Shedden AH: Timolol maleate in gel-forming solution: A novel formulation of timolol maleate. Chibret Int J Ophthalmol 10:32–36, 1994.
169. Hommer A, Nowak A, Huber-Spitzy V: Multicenter double-blind study with 0.25% timolol in Gelrite (TG) once daily vs. 0.25% timolol solution (TS) twice daily. German Study Group. Ophthalmologe 92:546–549, 1995.
170. Laurence J, Holder D, Vogel R, et al: A double-masked, placebo-controlled evaluation of timolol in gel vehicle. J Glaucoma 1993:177–182, 1993.
171. Airaksinen PJ, Saari KM, Tiainen TJ, Jaanio EA: Management of acute closed-angle glaucoma with miotics and timolol. Br J Ophthalmol 63:822–825, 1979.

172. Wilson RP, Spaeth GL, Poryzees E: The place of timolol in the practice of ophthalmology. Ophthalmology 87:451–454, 1980.
173. Wilson RP, Kanal N, Spaeth GL: Timolol: Its effectiveness in different types of glaucoma. Ophthalmology 86:43–50, 1979.
174. Migliori ME, Beckman H, Channell MM: Intraocular pressure changes after neodymium-YAG laser capsulotomy in eyes pretreated with timolol. Arch Ophthalmol 105:473–475, 1987.
175. Liu PF, Hung PT: Effect of timolol on intraocular pressure elevation following argon laser iridotomy. J Ocular Pharmacol 3:249–255, 1987.
176. Richter CU, Arzeno G, Pappas HR, et al: Prevention of intraocular pressure elevation following neodymium-YAG laser posterior capsulotomy. Arch Ophthalmol 103:912–915, 1985.
177. Stilma JS, Boen-Tan TN: Timolol and intra-ocular pressure elevation following Neodymium:YAG laser surgery. Doc Ophthalmol 61:233–239, 1986.
178. Obstbaum SA, Galin MA: The effects of timolol on cataract extraction and intraocular pressure. Am J Ophthalmol 88:1017–1019, 1979.
179. Packer AJ, Fraioli AJ, Epstein DL: The effect of timolol and acetazolamide on transient intraocular pressure elevation following cataract extraction with alpha-chymotrypsin. Ophthalmology 88:239–243, 1981.
180. Fry LL: Comparison of the postoperative intraocular pressure with Betagan, Betoptic, Timoptic, Iopidine, Diamox, Pilopine Gel, and Miostat. J Cataract Refract Surg 18:14–19, 1992.
181. DuBiner HB, Hill R, Kaufman H, et al: Timolol hemihydrate vs timolol maleate to treat ocular hypertension and open-angle glaucoma. Am J Ophthalmol 121:522–528, 1996.
182. Novack GD: Minireview: Levobunolol for the long-term treatment of elevated intraocular pressure. Gen Pharmacol 17:373–377, 1986.
183. DiCarlo FJ, Leinweber F-J, Szpiech JM, Davidson IWF: Metabolism of L-bunolol. Clin Pharmacol Ther 22:858–863, 1977.
184. Quast U, Vollmer KO: Binding of beta-adrenoceptor antagonists to rat and rabbit lung: Special reference to levobunolol. Arzneimittelforschung 34:579–584, 1984.
185. Woodward DF, Novack GD, Williams LS, et al: The ocular beta-blocking activity of dihydrolevobunolol. J Ocular Pharmacol 3:11–15, 1987.
186. Tang-Liu D, Shackleton M, Richman JB: Ocular metabolism of levobunolol. J Ocular Pharmacol 4:269–278, 1988.
187. Bensinger R, Keates E, Gofman J, et al: Levobunolol: A three month efficacy study in the treatment of glaucoma and ocular hypertension. Arch Ophthalmol 103:375–378, 1985.
188. Cinotti A, Cinotti D, Grant W, et al: 0.5% and 1.0% levobunolol compared with 0.5% timolol for the long-term treatment of chronic open-angle glaucoma and ocular hypertension. Am J Ophthalmol 99:11–17, 1985.
189. Ober M, Scharrer A, David R, et al: Long-term ocular hypotensive effect of levobunolol: Results of a one-year study. Br J Ophthalmol 69:593–599, 1985.
190. Berson F, Cohen H, Foerster RJ, et al: Levobunolol compared with timolol: Ocular hypotensive efficacy and ocular and systemic safety. Arch Ophthalmol 103:379–382, 1985.
191. Geyer O, Lazar M, Novack GD, et al: Levobunolol compared with timolol for the control of elevated intraocular pressure. Ann Ophthalmol 18:289–292, 1987.
192. Geyer O, Lazar M, Novack GD, et al: Levobunolol compared with timolol: A four-year study. Br J Ophthalmol 72:892–896, 1988.
193. David R, Foerster RJ, Ober M, et al: Glaucoma treatment with once-daily levobunolol. Am J Ophthalmol 104:443–444, 1987.
194. Rakofsky S, Lazar M, Almog Y, et al: Once-daily levobunolol for glaucoma therapy. Can J Ophthalmol 24:2–6, 1989.
195. Wandel T, Lewis RA, Partamian L, et al: Glaucoma treatment with once-daily levobunolol. Am J Ophthalmol 101:298–304, 1986.
196. Wandel TA, Fishman D, Novack GD, et al: Ocular hypotensive efficacy of 0.25% levobunolol once-daily. Ophthalmology 95:252–254, 1988.
197. Rakofsky S, Melamed S, Cohen JS, et al: A comparison of the ocular hypotensive efficacy of once-daily and twice-daily levobunolol treatment. Ophthalmology 96:8–11, 1989.
198. Duzman E, Ober M, Scharrer A, Leopold IH: A clinical evaluation of the effects of topically applied levobunolol and timolol on increased intraocular pressure. Am J Ophthalmol 94:318–322, 1982.
199. Silverstone DE, Novack GD, Kelley EP, Chen KS: Prophylactic treatment of intraocular pressure elevations after Neodymium:YAG laser posterior capsulotomies and extracapsular cataract extractions with levobunolol. Ophthalmology 95:713–718, 1988.
200. West DR, Lischwe TD, Thompson VM, Ide CH: Comparative efficacy of the β-blockers for the prevention of increased intraocular pressure after cataract extraction. Am J Ophthalmol 106:168–173, 1988.
201. Sugrue MF, Armstrong JM, Gautheron P, et al: A study on the ocular and extraocular pharmacology of metipranolol. Graefes Arch Clin Exp Ophthalmol 22:123–127, 1985.
202. Noack E: Ocular hypotensive action of beta-adrenergic blockers, with special consideration of metipranolol (Beta-Ophthiole). Klin Monatsbl Augenheilkd 189:1–3, 1986.
203. Battershill PE, Sorkin EM: Ocular metipranolol: A preliminary review of its pharmacodynamic and pharmacokinetic properties, and therapeutic efficacy in glaucoma and ocular hypertension. Drugs 36:601–615, 1988.
204. Muller O, Knobel HR: Effectiveness and tolerance of metipranolol—Results of a multicenter long-term study in Switzerland. Klin Monatsbl Augenheilkd 188:62–63, 1986.
205. Schnarr K-D: Vergleichende multizentrische untersuchung von carteolol-augentropfen mit anderen betablockern bei 768 patienten unter alltagsbedingugen. Klin Monatsbl Augenheilkd 192:167–176, 1988.
206. Dausch D, Brewitt H, Edelhoff R: Metipranolol eye drops: Clinical suitability in the treatment of chronic open angle glaucoma. *In* Merte H-J (ed): Metipranolol: Pharmacology of Beta-Blocking Agents and Use of Metipranolol in Ophthalmology. Wien, Springer-Verlag, 1983, pp 132–147.
207. Serle JB, Lustgarten JS, Podos SM: A clinical trial of metipranolol, a noncardioselective beta-adrenergic antagonist, in ocular hypertension. Am J Ophthalmol 112:302–307, 1991.
208. Mertz M: Results of a 6 weeks' multicenter double-blind trial: Metipranolol vs Timolol. *In* Merte H-J (ed): Metipranolol: Pharmacology of Beta-Blocking Agents and Use of Metipranolol in Ophthalmology. Wien/New York, Springer-Verlag, 1984, pp 93–105.
209. Merkle W: Bericht über die ergebnisse mit neuen betarezeptorenblockern in der glakomtherapie. Fortschr Ophthalmol 79:413–414, 1983.
210. Krieglstein GK, Novack GD, Voepel E, et al: Levobunolol and metipranolol: Comparative ocular hypotensive efficacy, safety and comfort. Br J Ophthalmol 71:250–253, 1987.
211. Kruse W: Metipranolol—Ein neuer betarezeptorenblocker. Klin Monatsbl Augenheilkd 182:582–584, 1983.
212. Mills KB, Wright G: A blind randomized cross-over trial comparing metipranolol 0.3% with timolol 0.25% in open-angle glaucoma: A pilot study. Br J Ophthalmol 70:39–42, 1986.
213. Schmitz-Valkenberg P, Jonas J, Brambring DF: Reductions in pressure with metipranolol 0.1%. Z Prak Augenheilkdunde 5:171–175, 1984.
214. Demailly P, Lecherpie F: Metipranolol 0.1%: Effect of one single dose on the nycthemeral pressure curve in an eye with chronic open angle primitive glaucoma. J Fr Ophthalmol 10:447–449, 1987.
215. Schmitz-Valkenberg P, Kessler C: Low-dose combination or high-dose separate solutions in glaucoma [Abstract]. Invest Ophthalmol Vis Sci Suppl 33:1122, 1992.
216. Christ T, Kessler C: Single, combination or separate solutions in glaucoma treatment? [Abstract]. Invest Ophthalmol Vis Sci Suppl 33:1122, 1992.
217. Scharrer A, Ober M: Fixed combination of metipranolol 0.1% and pilocarpine 2% compared with the individual drugs in glaucoma therapy: A controlled randomized study for intraindividual comparison of efficacy and tolerance. Klin Monatsbl Augenheilkd 189:450–455, 1986.
218. Mori H, Kido M, Murakami N, et al: Metabolic fate of carteolol hydrochloride [5-(3-tert-butylamino-2-hydroxypropoxy)-3,4-dihydrocarbostyril hydrochloride, OPC-1085], a new beta-blocker. V. Identification of metabolites in rat, dog and human [Author's Translation]. Yakugaku Zasshi 97:305–308, 1977.
219. Sugiyama K, Enya T, Kitazawa Y: Ocular hypotensive effect of 8-hydroxycarteolol, a metabolite of carteolol. Int Ophthalmol Clin 13:85–89, 1989.
220. Chrisp P, Sorkin EM: Ocular carteolol: A review of its pharmacological properties, and therapeutic use in glaucoma and ocular hypertension. Drugs Aging 2:58–77, 1992.
221. Stewart WC: Carteolol, an ophthalmic β-adrenergic blocker with intrinsic sympathomimetic activity. J Glaucoma 3:339–345, 1994.
222. Kitazawa Y, Azuma I, Takase M, Koememushi S: Ocular hypotensive effects of carteolol hydrochloride in primary open-angle glaucoma and ocular hypertensive patients: A double-masked cross-over study for the determination of concentrations optimal for clinical use. Acta Soc Ophthalmol Jpn 85:798–804, 1981.

223. Ishikawa T, Okisaka S, Hiwatari S: Pilocarpine, carbachol and carteolol on open-angle glaucoma and ocular hypotension. Nippon Ganka Gakkai Zasshi 85:837–842, 1981.
224. Duff GR, Graham PA: A double-crossover trial comparing the effects of topical carteolol and placebo on intraocular pressure. Br J Ophthalmol 72:27–28, 1988.
225. Duff GR, Newcombe RG: The 12-hour control of intraocular pressure on carteolol 2% twice daily. Br J Ophthalmol 72:890–891, 1988.
226. Scoville B, Mueller B, White BG, Krieglstein GK: A double-masked comparison of carteolol and timolol in ocular hypertension. Am J Ophthalmol 105:150–154, 1988.
227. Stewart WC, Shields MB, Allen RC, et al: A 3-month comparison of 1% and 2% carteolol and 0.5% timolol in open-angle glaucoma. Graefes Arch Clin Exp Ophthalmol 229:258–261, 1991.
228. Schnaudigel O-E, Becker H, Fuchs H-B: Carteolol: Praxisgerechte prüfung von wirksamkeit und verträglichkeit eines neuen betablockers in der behandlung des glaukoms. Klin Monatsbl Augenheilkd 192:248–251, 1988.
229. Frishman WH, Covey S: Penbutolol and carteolol: Two new beta-adrenergic blockers with partial agonism. J Clin Pharmacol 30:412–421, 1990.
230. Freedman SF, Freedman NJ, Shields MB, et al: Effects of ocular carteolol and timolol on plasma high-density lipoprotein cholesterol level. Am J Ophthalmol 116:600–611, 1993.
231. Coleman AL: How beta blockers affect blood lipids. Rev Ophthalmol 82–83, 1995.
232. Kitazawa Y: Multicenter double-blind comparison of carteolol and timolol in primary open-angle glaucoma and ocular hypertension. Adv Ther 10:95–131, 1993.
233. Reiss GR, Brubaker RF: The mechanism of betaxolol, a new hypotensive agent. Ophthalmology 90:1369–1372, 1983.
234. Gaul GR, Will NJ, Brubaker RF: Comparison of a non-cardioselective beta adrenoceptor blocker and a cardioselective blocker in reducing aqueous flow in humans. Arch Ophthalmol 107:1308–1311, 1989.
235. Frisk-Holmberg M, Strom G: Exercise during therapeutic beta-blockade: A two-year study in hypertensive patients. Clin Pharmacol Ther 40:395–399, 1986.
236. Warrington SJ, Turner P, Kilborn JR, et al: Blood concentrations and pharmacodynamic effects of betaxolol (SL 75212) a new beta-adrenoceptor antagonist after oral and intravenous administration. Br J Clin Pharmacol 10:449–452, 1980.
237. Giudicelli JF, Richer C, Ganansia J, et al: Betaxolol: Beta-adrenoceptor blocking effects and pharmacokinetics in man. *In* Morselli PL, Cavero I, Kilborn JR, et al (eds): Betaxolol and Other β_1-Adrenoceptor Antagonists. LERS Monograph Series. New York, Raven Press, 1983, pp 89–99.
238. Morselli PL, Thiercelin JF, Padovani P, et al: Comparative pharmacokinetics of several beta-blockers in renal and hepatic insufficiency. *In* Morselli PL, Cavero I, Kilborn JR, et al (eds): Betaxolol and Other β_1-Adrenoceptor Antagonists. LERS Monograph Series. New York, Raven Press, 1983, pp 233–241.
239. Beresford R, Heel RC: Betaxolol: A review of its pharmacodynamic and pharmacokinetic properties, and therapeutic efficacy in hypertension. Drugs 31:6–28, 1986.
240. Caldwell DR, Salisbury CR, Guzek JP: Effects of topical betaxolol in ocular hypertensive patients. Arch Ophthalmol 102:539–540, 1984.
241. Feghali JG, Kaufman PL: Decreased intraocular pressure in the hypertensive human eye with betaxolol, a beta-1-adrenergic antagonist. Am J Ophthalmol 100:777–782, 1985.
242. Radius RL: Use of betaxolol in the reduction of elevated intraocular pressure. Arch Ophthalmol 101:898–900, 1983.
243. Levy NS, Boone L: Effect of 0.25% betaxolol v placebo. Glaucoma 5:230–232, 1983.
244. Berrospi AR, Leibowitz HM: Betaxolol: A new beta-adrenergic blocking agent for treatment of glaucoma. Arch Ophthalmol 100:943–946, 1982.
245. Berry DB, van Buskirk EM, Shields MB: Betaxolol and timolol: A comparison of efficacy and side effects. Arch Ophthalmol 102:42–45, 1984.
246. Feghali JG, Kaufman PL, Radius RL, Mandell AI: A comparison of betaxolol and timolol in open angle glaucoma and ocular hypertension. Acta Ophthalmol 66:180–186, 1988.
247. Levy NS, Boone L, Ellis E: A controlled comparison of betaxolol and timolol with long-term evaluation of safety and efficacy. Glaucoma 7:54–62, 1986.
248. Stewart RH, Kimbrough RL, Ward RL: Betaxolol vs. Timolol: A six-month double-blind comparison. Arch Ophthalmol 104:46–48, 1986.
249. Allen RC, Hertzmark E, Walker AM, Epstein DL: A double-masked comparison of betaxolol vs timolol in the treatment of open-angle glaucoma. Am J Ophthalmol 101:535–541, 1986.
250. Long DA, Johns GE, Mullen RS, et al: Levobunolol and betaxolol: A double-masked controlled comparison of efficacy and safety in patients with elevated intraocular pressure. Ophthalmology 95:735–741, 1988.
251. Vogel R, Tipping R, Kulaga SF, Clineschmidt CM: Changing therapy from timolol to betaxolol. Effect on intraocular pressure in selected patients with glaucoma. Timolol-Betaxolol Study Group. Arch Ophthalmol 107:1303–1307, 1989.
252. Gross JG, Meyer DR, Robin AL, et al: Increased intraocular pressure in the immediate postoperative period after extracapsular cataract extraction. Am J Ophthalmol 105:466–469, 1988.
253. van Buskirk EM, Bacon DR, Fahrenbach WH: Ciliary vasoconstriction after topical adrenergic drugs. Am J Ophthalmol 109:511–517, 1990.
254. Messmer C, Flammer J, Stumpfig D: Influence of betaxolol and timolol on the visual fields of patients with glaucoma. Am J Ophthalmol 112:678–681, 1991.
255. Collignon-Brach J: Long-term effect of ophthalmic β-adrenoceptor antagonists on intraocular pressure and retinal sensitivity in primary open-angle glaucoma. Curr Eye Res 11:1–3, 1992.
256. Martin-Boglind LM, Graves A, Wanger P: The effect of topical antiglaucoma drugs on the results of high-pass resolution perimetry. Am J Ophthalmol 111:711–714, 1991.
257. Weinreb RN, Jani R: A novel formulation of an ophthalmic beta-adrenoceptor antagonist. J Parenteral Sci Tech 46:51–53, 1992.
258. Weinreb RN, Caldwell DR, Goode SM, et al: A double-masked three-month comparison between 0.25% betaxolol suspension and 0.5% betaxolol ophthalmic solution. Am J Ophthalmol 110:189–192, 1990.
259. Hoffman BB, Lefkowitz RJ: Catecholamines and sympathomimetic drugs. *In* Gilman AG, Rall TW, Nies AS, Taylor P (eds): Goodman and Gilman's The Pharmacological Basis of Therapeutics, 8th ed. New York, Pergamon Press, 1990, pp 187–220.
260. Krieglstein GK, Mohamed J: The comparative multiple-dose intraocular pressure responses of nadolol and timolol in glaucoma and ocular hypertension. Acta Ophthalmol 60:284–292, 1982.
261. Krieglstein GK, Kontic D: Nadolol and labetalol: Comparative efficacy of two beta-blocking agents in glaucoma. Graefes Arch Clin Exp Ophthalmol 216:313–317, 1981.
262. Krieglstein GK: Nadolol eye drops in glaucoma and ocular hypertension: A controlled clinical study of dose response and duration of action. Graefes Arch Clin Exp Ophthalmol 217:309–314, 1981.
263. Duzman E, Rosen N, Lazar M: Di-acetyl nadolol: 3-Month ocular hypotensive effect in glaucomatous eyes. Br J Ophthalmol 67:668–673, 1983.
264. Duzman E, Chen CC, Anderson J, et al: Diacetyl derivative of nadolol. I. Ocular pharmacology and short-term ocular hypotensive effect in glaucomatous eyes. Arch Ophthalmol 100:1916–1919, 1982.
265. Bietti GB, Bucci MG, Pescosolido N: Topical oxprenolol in the treatment of various forms of glaucoma. Klin Monatsbl Augenheilkd 170:824–830, 1977.
266. Holt JPA, Waddington E: Short report: Oculocutaneous reaction to oxprenolol. BMJ 2:539–540, 1975.
267. Bonomi L, Perfetti S, Noya E, et al: Comparison of the effects of nine beta-adrenergic blocking agents on intraocular pressure in rabbits. Graefes Arch Clin Exp Ophthalmol 210:1–8, 1979.
268. Smith SE, Smith SA, Reynolds F, Whitmarsh VB: Ocular and cardiovascular effects of local and systemic pindolol. Br J Ophthalmol 63:63–66, 1979.
269. Man In T'Veld AJ, Schalekamp MADH: How intrinsic sympathomimetic activity modulates the haemodynamic responses to beta-adrenoceptor antagonists. A clue to the nature of their antihypertensive mechanism. Br J Clin Pharmacol 13:245S–257S, 1982.
270. Sakimoto G, Une H, Ohba N: Effects of topically applied bupranolol on the intraocular pressure: Effects on the untreated eye. Ophthalmologica 179:214–219, 1979.
271. Krieglstein GK, Sold-Darseff J, Leydhecker W: The intraocular pressure response of glaucomatous eyes to topically applied bupranolol. A pilot study. Graefes Arch Clin Exp Ophthalmol 202:81–86, 1977.
272. Demmler N: Langzeitbehandlung des weitwinkelglaukoms mit bupranolol. Klin Monatsbl Augenheilkd 177:523–526, 1980.
273. Miki H: Longterm bupranolol therapy in glaucoma eyes: a one to two year follow up study. Nippon Ganka Gakkai Zasshi 86:269–278, 1982.

274. Leydhecker W, Krieglstein GK: The intraocular pressure responses of low-dose bupranolol (Ophtorenin) and methazolamide (Neptazane) in glaucomatous eyes. A controlled clinical study. Graefes Arch Clin Exp Ophthalmol 210:135–140, 1979.
275. Phillips CI, Gore SM, Gunn PM: Atenolol versus adrenaline eye drops and an evaluation of these two combined. Br J Ophthalmol 62:296–301, 1978.
276. Ros FE, Dake CL, Offerhaus L, Greve EL: Atenolol 4% eye drops and glaucoma: A double-blind short-term clinical trial of a new beta-1-adrenergic blocking agent. Graefes Arch Clin Ophthalmol 205:61–70, 1977.
277. Wettrell K, Wilke K, Pandolfi M: Effect of beta-adrenergic agonists and antagonists on repeated tonometry and episcleral venous pressure. Exp Eye Res 24:613–619, 1977.
278. Macdonald MJ, Cullen PM, Phillips CI: Atenolol versus propranolol. A comparison of ocular hypotensive effect of an oral dose. Br J Ophthalmol 60:789–791, 1976.
279. Colasanti BK, Trotter RR: Responsiveness of the rabbit eye to adrenergic and cholinergic agonists after treatment with 6-hydroxydopamine or alpha-methyl-para-tyrosine: Part II—Intraocular pressure changes. Ann Ophthalmol 10:1209–1214, 1978.
280. Katz IM: Beta-Blockers and the eye: An overview. Ann Ophthalmol 10:847–850, 1978.
281. Bill A, Nilsson SF: Control of ocular blood flow. J Cardiovasc Pharmacol (Suppl 3):S96–S102, 1985.
282. Ros FE, Dake CL, Nagelkerke NJD, Greve EL: Metoprolol eye drops in the treatment of glaucoma: A double-blind single-dose trial of a beta-1-adrenergic blocking drug. Graefes Arch Clin Ophthalmol 206:247–254, 1978.
283. Nielsen PG, Ahrendt N, Buhl H, Byrn E: Metoprolol eyedrops 3%, a short-term comparison with pilocarpine and a five-month follow-up study. (Multicenter). Acta Ophthalmol 60:347–352, 1982.
284. Alm A, Wickstrom CP: Effects of systemic and topical administration of metoprolol on intraocular pressure in healthy subjects. Acta Ophthalmol 58:740–747, 1980.
285. Nielsen NV, Eriksen JS: Timolol and metoprolol—Glaucoma: A comparison of the ocular hypotensive effect, local and systemic tolerance. Acta Ophthalmol 59:336–346, 1981.
286. Nielsen NV, Eriksen JS: Timolol and metoprolol: A diurnal study of the ocular and systemic effects in glaucoma patients. Acta Ophthalmol 59:517–525, 1981.
287. Nielsen NV: A diurnal study of the ocular hypotensive effect of metoprolol mounted on ophthalmic rods compared to timolol eye drops in glaucoma patients. Acta Ophthalmol 59:495–502, 1981.
288. Alm A, Wickstrom CP, Tornquist P: Initial and long-term effects of metoprolol and timolol on the intraocular pressure. A comparison in healthy subjects. Acta Ophthalmol 59:510–516, 1981.
289. Alm A, Wickstrom CP, Eckstrom C, Ohman L: The effect of metoprolol on intra-ocular pressure in glaucoma. A pilot study. Acta Ophthalmol 57:236–242, 1979.
290. Novack GD, Leopold IH: The toxicity of topical ophthalmic beta-blockers. J Toxicol-Cut Ocular Toxicol 6:283–297, 1987.
291. Akingbehin T, Sunder Raj P: Ophthalmic topical beta blockers: Review of ocular and systemic adverse effects. J Toxicol-Cut Oculr Toxicol 9:131–147, 1990.
292. Fraunfelder FT, Meyer SM: Systemic side effects from ophthalmic timolol and their prevention. J Ocular Pharmacol 3:177–184, 1987.
293. Schwartz JS, Weinstock SM: Side effects of topical epinephrine therapy. Glaucoma 5:21–23, 1983.
294. Theodore J, Leibowitz HM: External ocular toxicity of dipivalyl epinephrine. Am J Ophthalmol 88:1013–1016, 1979.
295. Flach AJ, Kramer SG: Supersensitivity to topical epinephrine after long-term epinephrine therapy. Arch Ophthalmol 98:482–483, 1980.
296. Spaeth GL: Place of timolol in the treatment of glaucoma. Symposium on Glaucoma: Transactions of the New Orleans Academy of Ophthalmology. St. Louis, CV Mosby, 1981, pp 368–378.
297. Van Joost TH, Hup JM, Ros FE: Dermatitis as a side-effect of long-term topical treatment with certain beta-blocking agents. Br J Dermatol 101:171–176, 1979.
298. Lamping K, Gofman J, Duzman E, et al: Effect of changing beta-blocker treatment in six patients allergic to timolol. J Toxicol-Cut Ocular Toxicol 6:179–181, 1987.
299. van Buskirk EM: Corneal anesthesia after timolol maleate therapy. Am J Ophthalmol 88:739–743, 1979.
300. van Buskirk EM: Adverse reactions from timolol administration. Ophthalmology 87:447–450, 1980.
301. Fraunfelder FT, Meyer SM: Corneal complications of ocular medications. Cornea 5:55–59, 1986.
302. Strempel I: Instensitat und dauer der Tranefnfilmaufrisszeitanderungen durch handelsubliche betablocker und ihre kombination mit tranenfilmersatzmitteln. Ophthalmologica 195:61–68, 1987.
303. Nielsen NV, Eriksen JS: Timolol in maintenance treatment of ocular hypertension and glaucoma. Acta Ophthalmol 57:1070–1077, 1979.
304. Kuppens EVM, Stolwijk TR, de Keizer RJ, van Best JA: Basal tear turnover and topical timolol in glaucoma patients and healthy controls by fluorophotometry. Invest Ophthalmol Vis Sci 33:3442–3448, 1992.
305. Wright P: Untoward effects associated with practolol administration: Oculomucocutaneous syndrome. BMJ 1:595–598, 1975.
306. McMahon CD, Shaffer RN, Hoskins HD, Hetherington J: Adverse effects experience by patients taking timolol. Am J Ophthalmol 88:736–738, 1979.
307. Passo MS, Palmer EA, van Buskirk EM: Plasma timolol in glaucoma patients. Ophthalmology 91:1361–1363, 1984.
308. Zimmerman TJ, Kooner KS, Kandarakis AS, Ziegler LP: Improving the therapeutic index of topically applied ocular drugs. Arch Ophthalmol 102:551–553, 1984.
309. Bobik A, Jennings GL, Ashley P, Korner PI: Timolol pharmacokinetics and effects on heart rate and blood pressure after acute and chronic administration. Eur J Clin Pharmacol 16:243–249, 1979.
310. Moroi SE, Lichter PR: Ocular pharmacology. *In* Hardman JG, Limbird LE, Molinoff PB, et al (eds): Goodman and Gilman's The Pharmacological Basis of Therapeutics, 9th ed. New York, McGraw Hill, 1996, pp 1619–1645.
311. Leier CV, Baker ND, Weber PA: Cardiovascular effects of ophthalmic timolol. Ann Intern Med 104:197–199, 1986.
312. Wellstein A, Palm D, Pitschner HF, Belz GG: Receptor binding of propranolol is the missing link between plasma concentration kinetics and the effect-time course in man. Eur J Clin Pharmacol 29:131–147, 1985.
313. van Buskirk EM, Fraunfelder FT: Timolol and glaucoma. Arch Ophthalmol 99:696, 1981.
314. Atkins JM, Pugh BR, Timewell RM: Cardiovascular effects of topical beta-blockers during exercise. Am J Ophthalmol 99:173–175, 1985.
315. Hernandez HH, Cervantes R, Frati F, et al: Cardiovascular effects of topical glaucoma therapies in normal subjects. J Toxicol-Cut Ocular Toxicol 2:99–106, 1983.
316. Berlin I, Marlel P, Uzzan B, et al: A single dose of three different ophthalmic beta-blockers antagonizes the chronotropic effect of isoproterenol in healthy volunteers. Clin Pharmacol Ther 41:622–626, 1987.
317. Doyle WJ, Weber PA, Meeks RH: Effect of topical timolol maleate on exercise performance. Arch Ophthalmol 102:1517–1518, 1984.
318. Jones FL Jr, Ekberg NL: Exacerbation of asthma by timolol [Letter]. N Engl J Med 301:270, 1979.
319. Charan NB, Lakshminarayan S: Pulmonary effects of topical timolol. Arch Intern Med 140:843–844, 1980.
320. Schoene R, Abuan T, Ward RL, Beasley H: Effects of topical betaxolol, timolol and placebo on pulmonary function in asthmatic bronchitis. Am J Ophthalmol 97:86–92, 1984.
321. Scharrer A, Ober M: Kardiovaskulare und pulmonare Wirkungen bei lokaler beta-blockergabe. Klin Monatsbl Augenheilkd 179:362–363, 1981.
322. Diggory P, Heyworth P, Chau G, McKenzie S: Unsuspected bronchospasm in association with topical timolol—A common problem in elderly people: Can we easily identify those affected and do cardioselective agents lead to improvement? Age Ageing 23:17–21, 1994.
323. Diggory P, Cassels-Brown A, Vail A, et al: Avoiding unsuspected respiratory side-effects of topical timolol with cardioselective or sympathomimetic agents. Lancet 345:1604–1606, 1995.
324. Lynch MG, Whitson JT, Brown RH, et al: Topical β-blocker therapy and central nervous system side effects: A preliminary study comparing betaxolol and timolol. Arch Ophthalmol 106:908–911, 1988.
325. Feiler-Ofry V, Godel V, Lazar M: Nail pigmentation following timolol maleate therapy. Ophthalmologica 182:153–156, 1981.
326. Coppeto JR: Timolol-associated myasthenia gravis. Am J Ophthalmol 98:244–245, 1984.
327. Fraunfelder FT, Meyer SM, Menacker SJ: Alopecia possibly secondary to topical ophthalmic beta-blockers [Letter]. JAMA 263:1493–1494, 1990.
328. Benitah E, Chatelain C, Cohen F, Herman D: Fibrose retroperitoneale: Effect systemique d'un collyre beta-bloquant? La Presse Med 16:400–401, 1987.

329. Shaivitz SA: Timolol and myasthenia gravis [Letter]. JAMA 242:1611–1612, 1979.
330. Lustgarten JS, Podos SM: Topical timolol and the nursing mother. Arch Ophthalmol 101:1381–1382, 1983.
331. Burggraf GW, Munt PW: Topical timolol therapy and cardiopulmonary function. Can J Ophthalmol 15:159–160, 1980.
332. Velde TM, Kaiser FE: Ophthalmic timolol treatment causing altered hypoglycemic response in a diabetic patient. Arch Intern Med 143:1627, 1983.
333. Angelo-Nielsen K: Timolol topically and diabetes mellitus [Letter]. JAMA 244:2263, 1980.
334. Sharir M, Zimmerman TJ, Crandall AS, Mamalis N: A comparison of the ocular tolerability of a single dose of timolol and levobunolol in healthy normotensive volunteers. Ann Ophthalmol 25:133–137, 1993.
335. Wilhelmus KR, McCulloch RR, Gross RL: Dendritic keratopathy associated with beta-blocker eyedrops. Cornea 9:335–337, 1990.
336. Novack GD, Tang-Liu D, Glavinos EP, et al: Plasma levels following topical administration of levobunolol. Ophthalmologica 194:194–200, 1987.
337. Charap AD, Shin DH, Petursson G, et al: The effect of varying drop size on the efficacy and safety of a topical beta-blocker. Ann Ophthalmol 21:351–357, 1988.
338. Hugues FC, Le Jeunne C, Munera Y, Dufier JL: Comparison des effets des collyres au carteolol et au metipranolol sur les fonctions ventilatoire et cardiovasculair de l'asthmatique. J Fr Ophthalmol 10:485–490, 1987.
339. Bacon PJ, Brazier DJ, Smith R, Smith SE: Cardiovascular responses to metipranolol and timolol eyedrops in healthy volunteers. Br J Clin Pharmacol 27:1–5, 1989.
340. Bauer K, Brunner-Ferber F, Distlerath LM, et al: Assessment of systemic effects of different ophthalmic beta-blockers in healthy volunteers. Clin Pharmacol Ther 49:658–664, 1991.
341. Le Jeunne C, Bringer L, Mondjee-Tahura Z, et al: Effets cardiovasculaires des collyres au timolol, au carteolol, au metipranolol, au betaxolol chez le sujet age. Therapie 43:89–92, 1988.
342. de Groot AC, Conemans J: Contact allergy to metipranolol. Contact Dermatitis 18:107–108, 1988.
343. Akingbehin T, Villada JR, Walley T: Metipranolol-induced adverse reactions. I: The rechallenge study. Eye 6:277–279, 1992.
344. Akingbehin AO: Granulomatous uveitis and metipranolol [Letter]. Br J Ophthalmol 77:536–537, 1993.
345. O'Connor GR: Granulomatous uveitis and metipranolol [Letter]. Br J Ophthalmol 77:536–537, 1993.
346. Melles RB, Wong IG: Metipranolol-associated granulomatous iritis. Am J Ophthalmol 118:712–715, 1994.
347. Kessler C: Possible bilateral anterior uveitis secondary to metipranolol (OptiPranolol) therapy [Letter]. Arch Ophthalmol 112:1277, 1994.
348. Kessler C, Christ T: The incidence of uveitis in glaucoma patients using metipranolol. J Glaucoma 2:166–170, 1993.
349. Beck RW, Moke P, Blair RC, Nissenbaum R: Uveitis associated with topical beta-blockers. Arch Ophthalmol 114:1181–1182, 1996.
350. Brogliatti B, Raveggi F, Moscone F, et al: Draeger's esthesiometer: Its employment to evaluate local anesthetic effect of 3 β-blockers (Timolol, Betaxolol, Corteolol). New Trends Ophthalmol 2:359–363, 1986.
351. Segawa K, Nagai T, Tanaka N, Nishiyama K: Effects of three beta-blocker eye drops on the rabbit cornea: An electron microscope study. Clin Ther 8:263–268, 1986.
352. Brazier DJ, Smith SE: Ocular and cardiovascular response to topical carteolol 2% and timolol 0.5% in healthy volunteers. Br J Ophthalmol 72:101–103, 1988.
353. Kendall K, Mundorf T, Nardin G, et al: Tolerability of timolol and betaxolol in patients with chronic open-angle glaucoma. Clin Ther 9:651–655, 1987.
354. Vogel R, Clineschmidt CM, Kulaga SF, et al: Comparison of the ocular tolerability of two beta-adrenergic antagonists: Timolol and betaxolol. Glaucoma 10:71–75, 1988.
355. Hoh H: Hornhautsensibilitat nach einzeldosen von timolol, betaxolol oder placebo bei augengesunden—Randomisierte, prospektive doppblindstudie. Fortschr Ophthalmol 85:132–138, 1988.
356. Weissman SS, Asbell PA: Effect of topical timolol (0.5%) and betaxolol (0.5%) on corneal sensitivity. Br J Ophthalmol 74:409–412, 1990.
357. Vogel R, Clineschmidt CM, Hoeh H, et al: The effect of timolol, betaxolol, and placebo on corneal sensitivity in healthy volunteers. J Ocular Pharmacol 6:85–90, 1990.
358. Nelson WL, Kuritsky JN: Early postmarketing surveillance of betaxolol hydrochloride, September 1985–September 1986. Am J Ophthalmol 103:592, 1987.
359. Dunn TL, Gerber MJ, Shen AS, et al: The effect of topical ophthalmic instillation of timolol and betaxolol on lung function in asthmatic subjects. Am Rev Respir Dis 133:264–268, 1986.
360. van Buskirk EM: Comparison of ocular and systemic side effects of betaxolol and timolol. New Trends Ophthalmol 2:140–144, 1987.
361. Pasquale LR, Nordlund JR, Robin AL, et al: A comparison of the cardiovascular and pulmonary effects of brimonidine 0.2%, timolol 0.5%, and betaxolol suspension 0.25% [Abstract]. Invest Ophthalmol Vis Sci Suppl 34(4):1139–1139, 1993.
362. Brooks AMV, Gillies WE, West RH: Betaxolol eye drops as a safe medication to lower intraocular pressure. Aust N Z J Ophthalmol 15:125–129, 1987.
363. Bleckmann H, Dorow P: Behandlung mit betaxolol und placebo-augentropfen bei patienten mit glaukom und reaktiven atemwegserkrankungen. Klin Monatsbl Augenheilkd 191:199–202, 1987.
364. Bleckmann H, Dorow P: Lokal applizierte kardioselektive betablocker und histaminprovokation bei patienten mit obstruktiven atemwgerkrankungen. Forstchr Ophthalmol 84:346–349, 1987.
365. Vukich JA, Leef DL, Allen RC: Betaxolol in patients with coexistent chronic open angle glaucoma and pulmonary disease. Invest Ophthalmol Vis Sci 26:227, 1984.
366. Pecori-Giraldi J, Collini S, Planner-Terzaghi A, et al: Timolol, betaxolol und befunolol in der glaukombehandlung: Untersuchung uber die bronchopulmonalen effekte. Forstschr Ophthalmol 85:235–238, 1988.
367. van Buskirk EM, Weinreb RN, Berry DP, et al: Betaxolol in patients with glaucoma and asthma. Am J Ophthalmol 101:531–534, 1986.
368. Weinreb RN, van Buskirk EM, Cherniack R, Drake MM: Long-term betaxolol therapy in glaucoma patients with pulmonary disease. Am J Ophthalmol 106:162–167, 1988.
369. De Vries J, Van de Merwe SA, De Heer LJ: From timolol to betaxolol. Arch Ophthalmol 107:634, 1989.
370. Spiritus EM, Casciari R: Letter to the editor. Am J Ophthalmol 100:492–493, 1985.
371. Berger WE: Betaxolol in patients with glaucoma and asthma. Am J Ophthalmol 103:600, 1987.
372. Phan TM, Nguyen KP, Giacomini JC, Lee DA: Ophthalmic beta-blockers: Determination of plasma and aqueous humor levels by a radioreceptor assay following multiple doses. J Ocular Pharmacol 7:243–252, 1991.
373. Cohn JB: A comparative study of the central nervous system effects of betaxolol vs. timolol. Arch Ophthalmol 107:633–634, 1989.
374. Ball S: Congestive heart failure from betaxolol. Arch Ophthalmol 105:320, 1987.
375. Chamberlain TJ: Myocardial infarction after ophthalmic betaxolol. N Engl J Med 321:1342–1342, 1989.
376. Harris LS, Greenstein MD, Bloom AF: Respiratory difficulties with betaxolol. Am J Ophthalmol 102:274–275, 1986.
377. Zabel RW, MacDonald IM: Sinus arrest associated with betaxolol ophthalmic drops. Am J Ophthalmol 104:431–431, 1987.
378. Orlando RG: Clinical depression associated with betaxolol. Am J Ophthalmol 102:275, 1986.
379. Roholt PC: Betaxolol and restrictive airway disease. Arch Ophthalmol 105:1172, 1987.
380. Sonntag JR, Brindley GO, Shields MB: Effect of timolol therapy on outflow facility. Invest Ophthalmol Vis Sci 17:293–296, 1978.
381. Coulangeon LM, Sole M, Menerath JM, Sole P: Aqueous humor flow measured by fluorophotometry: A comparative study of the effect of various beta-blocker eyedrops in patients with ocular hypertension. Ophthalmologie 4:156–161, 1990.
382. Brubaker RF: Flow of aqueous humor in humans [The Friedenwald Lecture]. Invest Ophthalmol Vis Sci 32:3145–3166, 1991.
383. Yablonski ME, Novack GD, Burke PJ, et al: The effect of levobunolol on aqueous humor dynamics. Exp Eye Res 44:49–54, 1987.
384. Hayashi M, Yablonski ME, Novack GD, Cook DJ: True outflow facility determined by fluorophotometry in human subjects. Exp Eye Res 48:621–625, 1989.
385. Sole P, Coulangeon L-M, Menerath JM, Dalens H: Effect of ophthalmic solutions of timolol 0.5% and other beta-blocking agents on aqueous humor inflow. Chibret Int J Ophthalmol 7:9–12, 1990.
386. Araie M, Takase M: Effects of S-596 and carteolol, new beta-adrenergic blockers, and flurbiprofen on the human eye: A fluorophotometric study. Graefes Arch Clin Exp Ophthalmol 222:259–262, 1985.
387. Yablonski ME, Novack GD, Cook D, et al: Aqueous humor dynamics

in humans of a combination of drugs affecting inflow and outflow. Invest Ophthalmol Vis Sci 28(3):12, 1987.
388. Krieglstein GK: Carteolol and tonography. Eur Glaucoma Soc Abstr L19–L19, 1988.
389. Yablonski ME, Mindel JS: Methods for assessing the effects of pharmacological agents on aqueous humor dynamics. *In* Duane TD (ed): Biomedical Foundations of Ophthalmology. Philadelphia, Harper & Row, 1985, pp 1–9.
390. Cruickshank JM, Prichard BNC: Beta-Blockers in Clinical Practice. Edinburgh, Churchill Livingstone, 1988, pp 1–1003.
391. Bloom A, Grunwald JE: Effect of one week of levobunolol HCl 0.5% on the human retinal circulation. Curr Eye Res 16:191–197, 1997.
392. Grunwald JE: Effect of topical timolol on the human retinal circulation. Invest Ophthalmol Vis Sci 27:1713–1719, 1986.
393. Grunwald JE: Effect of timolol maleate on the retinal circulation of human eyes with ocular hypertension. Invest Ophthalmol Vis Sci 31:521–526, 1990.
394. Grunwald JE: Effect of two weeks of timolol maleate treatment on the normal retinal circulation. Invest Ophthalmol Vis Sci 32:39–45, 1991.
395. Grunwald JE, Delehanty J: Effect of topical carteolol on the normal human retinal circulation. Invest Ophthalmol Vis Sci 33:1853–1856, 1992.
396. Gupta A, Chen HC, Rassam SM, Kohner EM: Effect of betaxolol on the retinal circulation in eyes with ocular hypertension: A pilot study. Eye 8:668–671, 1994.
397. Yoshida A, Feke GT, Ogasawara H, et al: Effect of timolol on human retinal, choroidal and optic nerve head circulation. Ophthalmic Res 23:162–170, 1991.
398. Newsom JH, Fiore JL Jr, Hackett E: Treatment of infestation with Phthirus pubis: Comparative efficacies of synergized pyrethrins and gamma-benzene hexachloride. Sex Transm Dis 6:203–205, 1979.
399. Ernest JT, Goldstick TK: Timolol maleate and choroidal blood flow. *In* Krieglstein GK, Leyydhecker W (eds): Glaucoma Update II. New York, Springer-Verlag, 1983, pp 45–51.
400. Steigerwalt RD Jr, Belcaro G, Cesarone MR, et al: Doppler ultrasonography of the central retinal artery in patients with diabetes and vascular disease treated with topical timolol. Eye 495–501, 1995.
401. Steigerwalt RD Jr, Belcaro G, Cesarone MR, et al: Doppler ultrasonography of the central retinal artery in normals treated with topical timolol. Eye 7:403–406, 1993.
402. Baxter GM, Williamson TH, McKillop G, Dutton GN: Color Doppler ultrasound of orbital and optic nerve blood flow: Effects of posture and timolol 0.5%. Invest Ophthalmol Vis Sci 33:604–610.
403. Harris A, Spaeth GL, Sergott RC, et al: Retrobulbar arterial hemodynamic effects of betaxolol and timolol in normal-tension glaucoma. Am J Ophthalmol 120:168–175.
404. Rosendorff C: Beta-blocking agents with vasodilator activity. J Hypertens Suppl 11:S37–S40, 1993.
405. Hester RK, Chen Z, Becker EJ, et al: The direct vascular relaxing action of betaxolol, carteolol and timolol in porcine long posterior ciliary artery. Surv Ophthalmol 38(Suppl):S125–S134, 1994.
406. Thoft RA, Mobilia EF: Complications with therapeutic extended wear soft contact lenses. Int Ophthalmol Clin 21:197–208, 1997.
407. Weissman BA, Mondino BJ, Pettit TH, Hofbauer JD: Corneal ulcers associated with extended-wear soft contact lenses. Am J Ophthalmol 97:476–481, 1984.
408. Morrison JC, Robin AL: Adjunctive glaucoma therapy: A comparison of apraclonidine to dipivefrin when added to timolol maleate. Ophthalmology 96:3–7, 1989.
409. Merkle W: Timolol in combination with other glaucoma drugs. Klin Monatsbl Augenheilkd 178:50–54, 1981.
410. Kass MA: Efficacy of combining timolol with other antiglaucoma medications. Surv Ophthalmol 28(Suppl): 274–279, 1983.
411. Knupp JA, Shields MB, Mandell AI, et al: Combined timolol and epinephrine therapy for open angle glaucoma. Surv Ophthalmol 28:280–285, 1983.
412. Airaksinen PJ, Valkonen R, Stenborg T, et al: A double-masked study of timolol and pilocarpine combined. Am J Ophthalmol 104:587–590, 1987.
413. Berson FG, Epstein DL: Separate and combined effects of timolol maleate and acetazolamide in open-angle glaucoma. Am J Ophthalmol 92:788–791, 1981.
414. Keates EU: Evaluation of timolol maleate combination therapy in chronic open-angle glaucoma. Am J Ophthalmol 88:565–571, 1979.
415. Kass MA, Korey M, Gordon M, Becker B: Timolol and acetazolamide: A study of concurrent administration. Arch Ophthalmol 100:941–942, 1982.
416. Korey MS, Hodapp E, Kass MA, et al: Timolol and epinephrine: Long-term evaluation of concurrent administration. Arch Ophthalmol 100:742–746, 1982.
417. Thomas JV, Epstein DL: Study of the additive effect of timolol and epinephrine in lowering intraocular pressure. Br J Ophthalmol 65:596–602, 1981.
418. Tsoy EA, Meekins BB, Shields MB: Comparison of two treatment schedules for combined timolol and dipivefrin therapy. Am J Ophthalmol 102:320–324, 1986.
419. Ohrstrom A, Kattstrom O, Polland W, et al: Oral and topical adrenergic beta-receptor blockers in glaucoma treatment. Acta Ophthalmol 62:681–695, 1984.
420. Ohrstrom A: Dose response of oral timolol combined with adrenaline. Br J Ophthalmol 66:242–246, 1982.
421. Batchelor ED, O'Day DM, Shand DG, Wood AJ: Interaction of topical and oral timolol in glaucoma. Ophthalmology 86:60–65, 1979.
422. O'Connor MA, Mooney DJ: The additional pressure-lowering effect in patients with glaucoma of pilocarpine 2 per cent, adrenaline 1 per cent, or guanethidine 3 per cent with adrenaline 0.5% per cent and timolol 0.25 per cent: A double-blind cross-over study. Trans Ophthalmol Soc UK 103:588–592, 1983.
423. Calissendorff B, Maren N, Wettrell K, Ostberg A: Timolol versus pilocarpine separately or combined with acetazolamide-effects on intraocular pressure. Acta Ophthalmol 58:624–631, 1980.
424. Airaksinen PJ: The long-term hypotensive effect of timolol maleate compared with the effect of pilocarpine in simple and capsular glaucoma. Acta Ophthalmol 57:425–434, 1979.
425. Allen RC, Epstein DL: Additive effect of betaxolol and epinephrine in primary open angle glaucoma. Arch Ophthalmol 104:1178–1184, 1986.
426. Wang YL, Zhan GL, Toris CB, Yablonski ME: Effects of topical epinephrine on aqueous humor dynamics in feline eyes. Invest Ophthalmol Vis Sci Suppl 34:934, 1993.
427. David R, Ober M, Masi R, et al: Levobunolol and pilocarpine: Combination therapy for the treatment of elevated intraocular pressure. Can J Ophthalmol 22:208–211, 1987.
428. Allen RC, Robin AL, Long D, et al: A combination of levobunolol and dipivefrin for the treatment of glaucoma. Arch Ophthalmol 106:904–907, 1988.
429. Akira Omi C, De Almeida GV, Belfort-Mattos R: Double masked study of levobunolol and timolol maleate in chronic open angle glaucoma or ocular hypertension patients. Arq Bras Oftalmol 51:190–194, 1988.
430. Allen RC, Bruce LA: Clinical evaluation of betaxolol: Intraocular pressure and adjunctive therapy. New Trends Ophthalmol 2:109–113, 1987.
431. Bloom HR, Cech JM, Eston AB, et al: Letter to the Editor re: Additive effect of betaxolol and epinephrine in primary open angle glaucoma [Letter]. Arch Ophthalmol 105:1317–1318, 1987.
432. Clark JB, Brooks AM, Harper CA, et al: A comparison of the efficacy of betaxolol and timolol in ocular hypertension with or without adrenaline. Aust N Z J Ophthalmol 17:173–177, 1989.
433. Weinreb RN, Ritch R, Kushner FH: Effect of adding betaxolol to dipivefrin therapy. Am J Ophthalmol 101:196–198, 1986.
434. Allen RC, Cagle GD, Bruce LA: Controlled clinical evaluation of betaxolol (0.5%) ophthalmic solution intraocular pressure and adjunctive therapy. Program and Abstracts, Glaucoma Society Meeting, Turin. XXVth International Congress on Ophthalmology. 1:20, 1986.
435. Leopold IH: Dipivalyl epinephrine. *In* Srinivasan BD (ed): Ocular Therapeutics. New York, Masson, 1980, pp 159–162.
436. Mandell AI, Stentz F, Kitabchi AE: Dipivalyl epinephrine: A new prodrug in the treatment of glaucoma. Ophthalmology 85:268–275, 1978.
437. Wei CP, Anderson JA, Leopold I: Ocular absorption and metabolism of topically applied epinephrine and a dipivalyl ester of epinephrine. Invest Ophthalmol Vis Sci 17:315–321, 1978.
438. Kaback MB, Podos SM, Harbin TS Jr, et al: The effects of dipivalyl epinephrine on the eye. Am J Ophthalmol 81:768–772, 1976.
439. Anderson JA, Davis WL, Wei CP: Site of ocular hydrolysis of a prodrug, dipivefrin, and a comparison of its ocular metabolism with that of the parent compound, epinephrine. Invest Ophthalmol Vis Sci 19:817–823, 1980.
440. Albracht DC, LeBlanc RP, Cruz AM, et al: A double-masked comparison of betaxolol and dipivefrin for the treatment of increased intraocular pressure. Am J Ophthalmol 116:307–313, 1993.

441. Mills KB, Jacobs NA: A single-blind randomised trial comparing adrenaline 1.0% with dipivalyl epinephrine (propine) 0.1% in the treatment of open-angle glaucoma and ocular hypertension. Br J Ophthalmol 72:465–468, 1988.
442. Axelrod J: Methylation reactions in the formation and metabolism of catecholamines and other biogenic amines. Pharmacol Rev 18:95–113, 1966.
443. Becker B, Montgomery SW, Kass MA, Shin DH: Increased ocular and systemic responsiveness to epinephrine in primary open-angle glaucoma. Arch Ophthalmol 95:789–790, 1977.
444. Obstbaum SA, Kolker AE, Phelps CD: Low-dose epinephrine. Arch Ophthalmol 92:118–120, 1974.
445. Becker B: Additive effect of epinephrine and acetazolamide in control of intraocular pressure. Am J Ophthalmol 45:639, 1958.
446. Kolker AE, Becker B: Epinephrine maculopathy. Arch Ophthalmol 79:552–562, 1968.
447. Hoskins HD Jr, Kass M: Becker-Shaffer's Diagnosis and Therapy of the Glaucomas. St. Louis, CV Mosby, 1989, p 443.
448. Hoskins HD Jr, Kass M: Becker-Shaffer's Diagnosis and Therapy of the Glaucomas. St. Louis, CV Mosby, 1989, p 444.
449. Wand M, Grant WM: Thymoxamine hydrochloride: An alpha-adrenergic blocker. Surv Ophthalmol 25:75–84, 1980.
450. Diehl DLC, Robin AL, Wand M: Iris pigmentation reduces the miotic effect of thymoxamine. Am J Ophthalmol 111:351–355, 1991.
451. Mittag TW, Tormay A, Severin C, Podos SM: Alpha-adrenergic antagonists correlation of the effect on intraocular pressure and on alpha-2-adrenergic receptor binding specificity in the rabbit eye. Exp Eye Res 40:591–600, 1985.
452. Bonomi L, Marchini G, De Franco I, et al: Effects of topical dapiprazole on the intraocular pressure in humans: A controlled study. Glaucoma 10:8–10, 1988.
453. Bonomi L, Marchini G, Marraffa M, et al: Effects of the association of alpha and beta-blocking agents in glaucoma. J Ocular Pharmacol 8:279–283, 1992.
454. Massari AM, Sorella S: Dose-finding study of the pharmacodynamics and tolerability of a new eye-drops formulation containing dapiprazole and timolol (glamidolot). A double blind trial comparative to timolol in glaucoma patients. Rass Int Clin Ter 74:145–161, 1994.
455. Ponte F, Cillino S, Faranda F, et al: Intraocular dapiprazole for the reversal of mydriasis after extracapsular cataract extraction with intraocular lens implantation. Part II: Comparison with acetylcholine. J Cataract Refract Surg 17:785–789, 1991.
456. Wilcox CS, Heiser JF, Crowder AM, et al: Comparison of the effects on pupil size and accomodation of three regimens of topical dapiprazole. Br J Ophthalmol 79:544–548, 1995.
457. Johnson ME, Molinari JF: Efficacy of dapiprazole. Optom Vis Sci 70:818–821, 1993.
458. Bonomi L, Bellucci R, Pagliarusco A, Stefani L: Apraclonidine protection of the blood-aqueous barrier from traumatic break-down. J Ocul Pharmacol Ther 11:25–35, 1995.
459. Lefkowitz RJ, Hoffman BJ, Taylor P: Neurohumoral transmission: The autonomic and somatic motor nervous systems. *In* Gilman AG, Rall TW, Nies AS, Taylor P (eds): Goodman and Gilman's The Pharmacological Basis of Therapeutics, 8th ed. New York, Pergamon, 1990, pp 84–121.
460. Havener WH: Ocular Pharmacology, 5th ed. St. Louis, CV Mosby, 1983.
461. Fraunfelder FT, Meyer SM: Drug-Induced Ocular Side Effects and Drug Interactions. Philadelphia, Lea & Febiger, 1982, pp 381–384.
462. Meyer SM, Fraunfelder FT: 3. Phenylephrine hydrochloride. Ophthalmology 87:1177–1180, 1980.
463. Kopin IJ: Biosynthesis and metabolism of catecholamines. Anesthesiology 29:654–660, 1968.
464. Ellis PP: Autonomic nervous system agents. *In* Ocular Therapeutics and Pharmacology, 5th ed. St. Louis, CV Mosby, 1981, p 53.
465. Smith RB, Everett WG: Physiology and pharmacology of local anesthetic agents. Int Ophthalmol Clin 13:35–60, 1973.
466. Meyers EF: Cocaine toxicity during dacryocystorhinostomy. Arch Ophthalmol 98:842–843, 1980.
467. Bryant JA: Local and topical anesthetics in ophthalmology. Surv Ophthalmol 13:263–283, 1969.
468. Robin AL, Pollack IP: A comparison of neodymium:YAG and argon laser iridotomies. Ophthalmology 91:1011–1016, 1984.
469. Thomas JV, Simmons RJ, Belcher CD: Argon laser trabeculoplasty in the presurgical glaucoma patient. Ophthalmology 89:187–197, 1982.
470. Krupin T, Kolker AE, Kass MA, Becker B: Intraocular pressure the day of argon laser trabeculoplasty in primary open-angle glaucoma. Ophthalmology 91:361–365, 1984.
471. Hoskins HD Jr, Hetherington J Jr, Minckler DS, et al: Complications of laser trabeculoplasty. Ophthalmology 90:796–799, 1983.
472. Hodapp E, Kolker AE, Kass MA, et al: The effect of topical clonidine on intraocular pressure. Arch Ophthalmol 99:1208–1211, 1981.
473. Robin AL: The role of apraclonidine hydrochloride in laser therapy for glaucoma. Trans Am Ophthalmol Soc 87:729–761, 1989.
474. Holmwood PC, Chase RD, Krupin T, et al: Apraclonidine and argon laser trabeculoplasty. Am J Ophthalmol 114:19–22, 1992.
475. Barnebey HS, Robin AL, Zimmerman TJ, et al: The efficacy of brimonidine in decreasing elevations in intraocular pressure after laser trabeculoplasty. Ophthalmology 100:1083–1099, 1993.
476. Coleman AL, Robin AL, Pollack IP, et al: Cardiovascular and intraocular pressure effects and plasma concentrations of apraclonidine hydrochloride. Arch Ophthalmol 108:1264–1267, 1990.
477. Robin AL: Effect of topical apraclonidine on the frequency of intraocular pressure elevations after combined extracapsular cataract extraction and trabeculectomy. Ophthalmology 100:628–633, 1993.
478. Gharagozloo NZ, Relf SJ, Brubaker RF: Aqueous flow is reduced by the alpha-adrenergic agonist, apraclonidine hydrochloride (ALO 2145). Ophthalmology 95:1217–1220, 1988.
479. Koskela T, Brubaker RF: Apraclonidine and timolol: Combined effects in previously untreated normal subjects. Arch Ophthalmol 109:804–806, 1991.
480. Gharagozloo NZ, Brubaker RF: Effect of apraclonidine in long-term timolol users. Ophthalmology 98:1543–1546, 1991.
481. Toris CB, Gleason ML, Camras CB, Yablonski ME: Effects of brimonidine on aqueous humor dynamics in human eyes. Arch Ophthalmol 113:1514–1517, 1995.
482. Ruiz RS, Rhem MN, Prager TC: Effects of carbachol and acetylcholine on intraocular pressure after cataract extraction. Am J Ophthalmol 107:7–10, 1989.
483. Hollands RH, Drance SM, Schulzer M: The effect of acetylcholine on early postoperative intraocular pressure. Am J Ophthalmol 103:749–753, 1987.
484. Percival SPB: Glaucoma triple procedure of extracapsular cataract extraction, posterior chamber lens implantation, and trabeculectomy. Br J Ophthalmol 69:99–102, 1985.
485. Kooner KS, Cooksey JC, Perry P, Zimmerman TJ: Intraocular pressure following ECCE, phacoemulsification, and PC-IOL implantation. Ophthalmic Surg 19:643–646, 1988.
486. Wiles SB, MacKenzie D, Ide CH: Control of intraocular pressure with apraclonidine hydrochloride after cataract extraction. Am J Ophthalmol 111:184–188, 1991.
487. Araie M, Ishi K: Effects of apraclonidine on intraocular pressure and blood-aqueous barrier permeability after phacoemulsification and intraocular lens implantation. Am J Ophthalmol 116:67–71, 1993.
488. Gramer E, Busche S, Kampik A, Parsons D: Efficacy of apraclonidine ophthalmic solution (Iopidine) in presumed silicon oil-induced glaucoma and primary open-angle glaucoma. Graefes Arch Clin Exp Ophthalmol 233:13–20, 1995.
489. Pulido JS, Mallic KS, Sneed SR, Blodi CF: Apraclonidine hydrochloride in vitreoretinal surgery. Arch Ophthalmol 107:316–317, 1989.
490. Makabe R: Ophthalmological studies with dichlorophenyl-aminoimidazoline. Dtsch Med Wochenschr 91:1686–1688, 1966.
491. Hasslinger R: Catapres: A new drug lowering intraocular pressure. Klin Monatsbl Augenheilkd 154:95–105, 1969.
492. Harrison R, Kaufmann CS: Clonidine. Effects of a topically administered solution on intraocular pressure and blood pressure in open-angle glaucoma. Arch Ophthalmol 95:1368–1373, 1977.
493. Heilmann K: Clonidine in glaucoma therapy—Inferences for therapy and obvious problems. Buch Augenarzt 63:56–59, 1974.
494. Loewenstein A, Varssano D, Lazar M, Geyer O: Clonidine in the treatment of post-YAG capsulotomy ocular hypertension. New Trends Ophthalmol 7:179–180, 1993.
495. Chien DS, Homsy JJ, Gluchowski C, Tang-Liu DD: Corneal and conjunctival/scleral penetration of p-aminoclonidine, AGN 190342, and clonidine in rabbit eyes. Curr Eye Res 9:1051–1059, 1990.
496. Bill A, Heilmann K: Ocular effects of clonidine in cats and monkeys (Macaca irus). Exp Eye Res 21:481–488, 1975.
497. Heilmann K: [Studies on the effect of Catapresan on the intraocular pressure. 3]. Klin Monatsbl Augenheilkd 161:425–430, 1972.
498. Abrams DA, Robin AL, Crandall AS, et al: A limited comparison of

apraclonidine's dose response in subjects with normal or increased intraocular pressure. Am J Ophthalmol 108:230–237, 1989.
499. Abrams DA, Robin AL, Pollack IP, et al: The safety and efficacy of topical 1% ALO 2145 (p-Aminoclonidine hydrochloride) in normal volunteers. Arch Ophthalmol 105:1205–1207, 1987.
500. Vocci MJ, Robin AL, Wahl JC, et al: Apraclonidine hydrochloride: An evaluation of reformulation and drop size. Am J Ophthalmol 113:154–160, 1992.
501. Jampel HD, Robin AL, Quigley HA, Pollack IP: Apraclonidine: A one-week dose-response study. Arch Ophthalmol 106:1069–1073, 1988.
502. Chacko DM, Camras CB: The potential of α_2-adrenergic agonists in the medical treatment of glaucoma. Curr Opin Ophthalmol 5:76–84, 1994.
503. Robin AL: Questions concerning the role of apraclonidine in the management of glaucoma [Editorial]. Arch Ophthalmol 113:712–714, 1995.
504. Robin AL, Ritch R, Shin DH, et al: Short-term efficacy of apraclonidine hydrochloride added to maximum-tolerated medical therapy for glaucoma. Am J Ophthalmol 120:423–432, 1995.
505. Burke J, Kharlamb A, Shan T, et al: Adrenergic and imidazoline receptor-mediated responses to UK-14, 304- 18 (brimonidine) in rabbits and monkeys. A species difference. Ann N Y Acad Sci 763:78–95, 1995.
506. Liu JH, Dacus AC, Bartels SP: Adrenergic mechanism in circadian elevation of intraocular pressure in rabbits. Invest Ophthalmol Vis Sci 32:2178–2183, 1991.
507. David R, Spaeth GL, Clevenger CE, et al: Brimonidine in the prevention of intraocular pressure elevation following argon laser trabeculoplasty. Arch Ophthalmol 111:1387–1390, 1993.
508. The Brimonidine-ALT Study Group: Effect of brimonidine 0.5% on intraocular pressure spikes following 360° argon laser trabeculoplasty. Ophthalmic Surg Lasers 26:404–409, 1995.
509. Derick RJ, Walters TR, Robin AL, et al: Brimonidine tartrate: A one-month dose response study [Abstract]. Invest Ophthalmol Vis Sci Suppl 34(4):1138, 1993.
510. Serle JB, Podos SM, Abundo GP, et al: The effect of brimonidine tartrate in glaucoma patients on maximal medical therapy [Abstract]. Invest Ophthalmol Vis Sci Suppl 34(4):1137, 1993.
511. Schuman JS: Clinical experience with brimonidine 0.2% and timolol 0.5% in glaucoma and ocular hypertension. Surv Ophthalmol 41(Suppl 1):S27–S37, 1996.
512. Stewart WC, Ritch R, Shin DH, et al: The efficacy of aprachlonidine as an adjunct to timolol therapy. Apraclonidine Adjunctive Therapy Study Group. Arch Ophthalmol 113:287–292, 1995.
513. Nagasubramanian S, Hitchings RA, Demailly P, et al: Comparison of apraclonidine and timolol in chronic open-angle glaucoma: A three-month study. Ophthalmology 100:1318–1323, 1993.
514. Robin AL: Short-term effects of unilateral 1% apraclonidine therapy. Arch Ophthalmol 106:912–915, 1988.
515. Serdahl CL, Galustian J, Lewis RA: The effects of apraclonidine on conjunctival oxygen tension. Arch Ophthalmol 107:1777–1779, 1989.
516. Robin AL, Coleman AL: Apraclonidine hydrochloride: An evaluation of plasma concentrations, and a comparison of its intraocular pressure lowering and cardiovascular effects to timolol maleate. Trans Am Ophthalmol Soc 88:149–162, 1990.
517. Nordlund JR, Pasquale LR, Robin AL, et al: The cardiovascular, pulmonary, and ocular hypotensive effects of 0.2% brimonidine. Arch Ophthalmol 113:77–83, 1995.
518. Serle JB: A comparison of the safety and efficacy of twice daily brimonidine 0.2% versus betaxolol 0.25% in subjects with elevated intraocular pressure. The Brimonidine Study Group III. Surv Ophthalmol 41(Suppl 1):S39–S47, 1996.
519. Burke J, Schwartz M: Preclinical evaluation of brimonidine. Surv Ophthalmol 41(Suppl 1):S9–S18, 1996.
520. Maier C, Steinberg GK, Sun GH, et al: Neuroprotection by the alpha 2-adrenoreceptor agonist dexmedetomidine in a focal model of cerebral ischemia. Anesthesiology 79:306–312, 1993.
521. Osborne NN, Cazevielle C, Carvalho AL, et al: In vivo and in vitro experiments show that betaxolol is a retinal neuroprotective agent. Brain Res 751:113–123, 1997.

CHAPTER 27

Nonsteroidal Antiinflammatory Drugs

King W. To, Mark B. Abelson, and Arthur H. Neufeld

Corticosteroids have long been the standard in antiinflammatory therapy. However, this remarkable class of compounds has many significant systemic and ocular side effects. Prior to the development of corticosteroids, aspirin was used to treat intraocular inflammation.[1] Salicylic acid (orthohydroxybenzoic acid) or aspirin (acetylsalicylic acid) was introduced over a century ago as an antipyretic and for the treatment of rheumatic fever. Aspirin reduces inflammation primarily by inhibiting the cyclooxygenase enzyme that is involved in the production of prostaglandins,[2, 3] although additional antiinflammatory actions are probably involved. Prostaglandins (PGs) are 20-carbon, unsaturated fatty-acid derivatives with a cyclopentane ring; these biologically active lipids have a diverse spectrum of actions, including the control of the inflammatory response, pain, body temperature, intraocular pressure, blood coagulation, lipid and carbohydrate metabolism, and cardiovascular, respiratory, and renal physiology. The PGs are eicosanoids, which are a family of molecules derived from arachidonic acid. The mechanism of action of PGs is not well understood. Some PGs act antagonistically with one another, whereas individual PGs can have different effects on different tissues. In addition, responses to certain PGs can vary significantly in different animal models and human studies. The ocular effects of PGs that have been isolated from the eye are summarized in Table 27–1.

In the past 20 years, research has led to the development of useful aspirin-like, nonsteroidal antiinflammatory drugs

TABLE 27–1. **Ocular Effects of Prostaglandins**

Prostaglandin	Effect
D	Stimulates vasodilation and chemosis
E_1, E_2	Increase inflammation Increase intraocular pressure Increase capillary permeability Stimulate vasodilation Stimulate miosis
F_2	Reduces intraocular pressure Has minimal effect on inflammation Has minimal effect on miosis

(NSAIDs) in medicine. The NSAIDs are among the most commonly prescribed drugs. Their most useful application is in the management of inflammation in diseases such as osteoarthritis, rheumatoid arthritis, and ankylosing spondylitis. This chapter provides an overview of NSAIDs and their applications.

Chemical Properties

The NSAIDs, a heterogeneous group of compounds, all have some degree of antiinflammatory, antipyretic, and analgesic properties; however, their therapeutic properties differ significantly. Because PGs have such a diverse range of actions, NSAIDs, which inhibit the production of PGs, also possess a broad range of pharmacologic properties. Systemic NSAIDs at therapeutic doses can produce adverse changes in the gastrointestinal, respiratory, hepatic, endocrine, coagulation, and renal systems.[4] The NSAIDs can be divided into the following groups: salicylates, fenamates, and derivatives of indole, pyrazolone, propionic acid, phenylacetic acid, and oxicam (Table 27–2). Only the derivatives of indole, propionic acid, and phenylacetic acid are commercially available as topical ophthalmic agents. Indocid, a commercial form of ophthalmic indomethacin solution, currently is not yet available in the United States. Four FDA-approved NSAID topical ophthalmic agents are currently available (Table 27–3).

Mechanisms of Action

Arachidonic acid is the primary precursor of PGs, leukotrienes (LTs), and related compounds (Fig. 27–1). Arachidonic acid may be ingested or derived from dietary linoleic acid. Arachidonic acid is bound to phospholipids in the plasma membrane; its release by phospholipases is closely regulated by a wide variety of chemical, physical, and hormonal factors. The blockage of PG biosynthesis by NSAIDs is primarily due to the inhibitory effects of NSAIDs on cyclooxygenase, which is responsible for the conversion of arachidonic acid to endoperoxides (PG G_2, PG H_2) in ocular and nonocular tissues.[5] Endoperoxides are precursors of all other PGs. The inhibitory activity of NSAIDs on cyclooxygenase demonstrably correlates with its antiinflammatory activity.[3] Experimental studies have shown that certain PGs are potent mediators of ocular inflammation.[6,7] Topical application of arachidonic acid or certain PGs produces dilation of conjunctival vessels with chemosis, changes in intraocular pressure, and miosis.[8] PG levels are elevated in the aqueous humor following argon laser iridectomy,[9] cataract surgery,[10] and trauma.[11] By inhibiting cyclooxygenase, NSAIDs have been shown to reduce the de novo synthesis of PGs.[11–13] Unlike NSAIDs, corticosteroids affect both the cyclooxygenase and lipoxygenase pathways by preventing the release of arachidonic acid.[14, 15] However, NSAIDs do not inhibit lipoxygenase and may lead to an increase in the production of leukotrienes by increasing the amount of arachidonic acid

TABLE 27–2. **Classes of NSAIDs Available in the United States**

Generic Name	Trade Name
Salicylates	
Aspirin	[Multiple names and manufacturers]
Fenamates	
Mefenamate	Ponstel
Meclofenamate	Meclomen
Indole Derivatives	
Indomethacin	Indocin
Ketorolac	Toradol, Acular*
Sulindac	Clinoril
Tolmetin	Tolectin
Pyrazolone Derivatives	
Phenylbutazone	Butazolidin
Propionic Acid Derivatives	
Fenoprofen	Nalfon
Flurbiprofen	Ansaid, Ocufen*
Ibuprofen	Advil, CoAdvil, IBU-TAB Medipren, Motrin, Nuprin, Children's Motrin, Rufen
Ketoprofen	Orudis
Naproxen	Naprosyn
Suprofen	Profenal*
Phenylacetic Acid Derivatives	
Diclofenac	Voltaren, Voltaren Ophthalmic*
Oxicam Derivatives	
Piroxicam	Feldene

*Ophthalmic topical agents.

TABLE 27–3. **Topical Ophthalmic-Suspension NSAIDs Available in the United States**

Generic Name and Solution Concentration	Trade Name (Manufacturer)	Indication(s) for Use Approved by the FDA
Ketorolac 0.5%	Acular (Allergan)	1. Seasonal allergic conjunctivitis 2. Intraocular inflammation after cataract surgery
Flurbiprofen 0.03% Suprofen 1%	Ocufen (Allergan) Profenal (Alcon)	Minimizing intraoperative miosis during cataract surgery
Diclofenac 0.1%	Voltaren (CibaVision)	Intraocular inflammation following cataract surgery

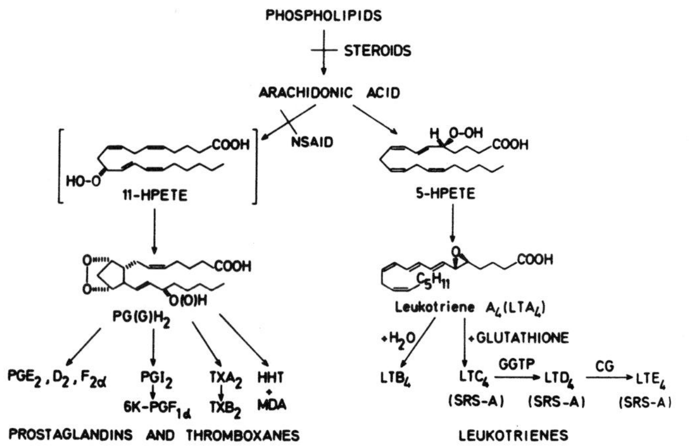

FIGURE 27–1. Structure of arachidonic acid cascade; synthesis of prostaglandins and related compounds.

available to be metabolized by lipoxygenase. The additional inhibition of leukotriene formation may be partially responsible for the greater antiinflammatory activity of corticosteroids. Other sources provide detailed discussion on the broad spectrum of actions of the PGs systemically[16] and in the eye.[17]

Pharmacokinetics

In general, orally ingested NSAIDs are rapidly absorbed and distributed throughout most body tissues. The NSAIDs are bound extensively to plasma proteins, and concentrations peak in blood 1 to 2 hours after administration. Biotransformation occurs primarily in the hepatic endoplasmic reticulum and mitochondria. The unchanged NSAID and its metabolic products are then eliminated in the urine. Therefore, patients with underlying liver or kidney dysfunction are at significant risk for the development of a wide range of toxic effects from normal doses of systemic NSAIDs.

Complications

Oral NSAID therapy is associated with a variety of complications. Only the most common and clinically significant adverse effects are addressed here. The most common undesirable effect is gastrointestinal irritation, which can lead to nausea, vomiting, cramps, and gastric or intestinal ulceration.[18, 19] Gastrointestinal ulceration can lead to significant blood loss and anemia. In addition to the local irritative effects of the NSAIDs on the gastrointestinal mucosa, inhibition of certain key gastric PGs (E_2, I_2) that normally protect against erosion may contribute to this side effect. The NSAIDs also increase the bleeding time by inhibiting platelet production of thromboxane A_2, a potent aggregating agent.[20] Although NSAIDs do not significantly affect renal function in healthy young patients, these aspirin-like drugs can produce acute renal failure in patients with chronic renal disease, congestive heart failure, cirrhosis with ascites, volume depletion secondary to diuretics, and hypotension secondary to hemorrhage. PGs protect the kidneys in disease states when renal perfusion is compromised by stimulating vasodilation and maintaining renal perfusion. NSAIDs block this PG-mediated compensatory response.[21] Therefore, it is not surprising that NSAIDs may produce renal compromise in the elderly,[22] which is important because the prevalence of rheumatic disease, in which the treatment of choice is NSAIDs, increases with age.

Topical NSAIDs generally appear to be significantly safer than oral NSAIDs. Application of these topical agents sometimes causes a stinging sensation. The benefits of greater comfort cannot be overemphasized, because comfort is clearly an important factor in a patient's adherence to a therapeutic regimen. Topical NSAIDs should be avoided in patients with a history of aspirin or NSAID sensitivity. Bronchospastic exacerbation was caused by topical ketorolac in a patient with asthma and nasal polyps.[23]

Some have suggested that the increased bleeding of ocular tissues (including hyphemas) in the setting of surgery and impairment of wound healing is associated with topical NSAID use.[24] In our clinical experience, the potential for increased bleeding and impairment of wound healing with topical NSAID use does not seem to be a problem. Whether topical NSAIDs may be used safely in the presence of fungal, bacterial, or viral infections remains unclear.

PREVENTION OF INTRAOPERATIVE MIOSIS

Miosis is a well-known complication of surgical trauma. In an effort to identify the agent responsible for stimulating miosis as part of the ocular response to trauma, researchers isolated a substance called irin more than 40 years ago.[25, 26] Irin, which was isolated from extracts of iris tissue, was found to produce miosis when introduced into the anterior chamber of animal eyes. PGs were later identified in these iris extracts. Although exactly how PGs mediate the miotic response and what other compounds in irin may be part of this reaction remain to be determined, topical application of cyclooxygenase blockers appears to help minimize the amount of intraoperative miosis. For many years, topical flurbiprofen has been used in preventing intraoperative miosis. Miosis during eye surgery, a common occurrence, can severely limit the surgeon's visualization and potentially increase the complication rate of the procedure. Surgical trauma that stimulates the production of PGs appears to play an integral role in the development of intraoperative miosis. PGs have been observed in the aqueous humor of traumatized eyes and appear to induce miosis independent of cholinergic mechanisms.[27] By inhibiting PG synthesis by blocking the cyclooxygenase pathway,[28] 0.03% flurbiprofen, when administered every 30 minutes beginning 2 hours preoperatively, has limited intraoperative miosis during anterior segment surgery in animal[29, 30] and human eyes.[31] Preoperative treatment is the key, because once the PGs are released, topical flurbiprofen does not block the PG's effect on the iris.

Some cataract surgeons have suggested that flurbiprofen may retard the reversal of the mydriasis by agents such as intracameral acetylcholine and carbachol, which potentially increase the chances of such complications as intraocular lens pupillary capture. Theoretically, flurbiprofen should have no effect on intracameral acetylcholine or carbachol; there is no known pharmacologic basis for any such interaction.[32] A possible explanation may be that some surgeons tend to rub the end of the cannula on the iris as the intraocular solution of acetylcholine or carbachol is injected to hasten the development of the miosis. In eyes without flurbiprofen, such as maneuver would likely stimulate the iris to produce PGs and induce miosis but not in eyes that have been previously treated with flurbiprofen.[32]

Topical flurbiprofen, however, does not appear to be as effective in minimizing miosis during vitreoretinal surgery.[33, 34] Whether this is because surgical manipulation is generally greater with vitreoretinal surgery than with anterior segment surgery and, therefore, more PGs are released, leading to miosis, remains to be determined. Another topical NSAID, suprofen, has been demonstrated to also be effective in reducing pupillary constriction during cataract surgery.[35] The relative efficacy of flurbiprofen and suprofen remains to be determined. Also, although topical diclofenac is only approved by the FDA for treatment of uveitis following cataract surgery, this drug can also minimize intraoperative miosis.[36]

The mechanisms involved in surgical miosis are complex. Although certain PGs have been associated with producing miosis, no single PG possesses a miotic effect in all species or is potent enough of a miotic to completely account for surgical miosis.[37, 38] The specific mechanism of action of cyclooxygenase blockers such as flurbiprofen may well have a variety of biologic effects that cannot be satisfactorily explained by inhibition of PG synthesis alone.

POSTSURGICAL INFLAMMATION AND DISCOMFORT

A number of topical NSAIDs have been tested as potential substitutes for topical corticosteroids for the treatment of postoperative inflammation. Because steroid use after cataract surgery may be associated with increased intraocular pressure and glaucoma, increased risk of infection, and inhibition of wound healing, a topical NSAID has been sought for the treatment of postsurgical inflammation. Because intraocular inflammation is associated with the breakdown of the blood-aqueous barrier, investigators have used the leakage of fluorescein into the anterior chamber after systemic administration to indirectly gauge the amount of inflammation.[39, 40] It has been suggested that a reduction in the leakage of fluorescein with NSAID treatment is an indication of a reduction in inflammation. The breakdown of the blood-aqueous barrier, assessed by fluorophotometry or slit-lamp examinations after cataract surgery, appears to be reduced by several topical NSAIDs, including ketorolac tromethamine, diclofenac sodium, and flurbiprofen.[41–45] Randomized, controlled studies to compare the antiinflammatory actions of 0.5% ketorolac tromethamine versus 0.1% dexamethasone[41] and 0.01%, 0.05%, or 0.1% diclofenac sodium versus 1% prednisolone sodium phosphate[43] demonstrated that topical NSAIDs were superior to the topical steroids in reducing breakdown of the blood-aqueous barrier as measured by fluorophotometry. These preliminary studies suggest that topical NSAIDs are a useful substitute for topical corticosteroids in the management of postoperative inflammation.

The only topical NSAIDs currently approved by the FDA for the treatment of inflammation following cataract surgery are diclofenac sodium 0.1% and ketorolac 0.5%.[46] The recommended dosage is one drop, four times a day, beginning 24 hours after cataract surgery.

Topical NSAIDs have recently found a new postsurgical role: The frequent occurrence of pain after refractive surgery, such as photorefractive keratectomy or radial keratotomy, has been reduced with the administration of topical ketorolac or diclofenac.[47–53] Topical diclofenac has also been shown to be a suitable replacement for topical steroids in managing postoperative inflammation following strabismus surgery.[54]

OCULAR INFLAMMATORY DISORDERS

Few areas in ophthalmology have received more attention than cystoid macular edema (CME). Although CME still remains poorly understood, most researchers would agree that inflammation is important to its pathogenesis. Preliminary studies involving topical or systemic NSAIDs have been encouraging.[55–59] These studies suggested that NSAIDs may be useful in the prophylaxis and treatment of CME following cataract surgery. In our clinical practice, we initially start our CME patients on intensive topical steroids (eight times a day) and topical NSAIDs (four to six times a day) for 2 weeks. If there is no response or if the CME worsens, topical NSAIDs are discontinued and the use of systemic NSAIDs is considered.

The NSAIDs have also been evaluated in the treatment of inflammatory diseases of the sclera. When taken orally, flurbiprofen may be effective in treating scleritis and episcleritis[60]; however, the topical form does not appear to be useful in the management of episcleritis.[61] Oral NSAIDs also may be useful as an adjunct in the management of chronic iridocyclitis in childhood.[62] When children with idiopathic iridocyclitis or iridocyclitis in association with juvenile rheumatoid arthritis were treated with oral NSAIDs, both inflammation in the anterior chamber and the need for topical and systemic steroids were reduced.[62]

Another potentially useful application of NSAIDs is in suppressing the inflammatory response associated with ocular infections. It is well known that topical steroid use can exacerbate viral, bacterial, and fungal infections of the eye. The effect of topical NSAIDs on corneal epithelial herpes simplex viral infections remains controversial; two experimental studies have found that topical NSAIDs did not worsen herpes simplex viral infections of the cornea,[63, 64] whereas an earlier study suggested that the exacerbation of ocular herpes simplex viral infections by topical flurbiprofen is similar to that of topical dexamethasone.[65] Preliminary studies have found that topical NSAIDs have no adverse effect on either bacterial[66] or fungal[67] ocular infections.

Traditional NSAIDs have also shown some promise in the management of allergic disorders of the eye. Topical flurbiprofen (0.03%) and suprofen (1%) may have a place in the treatment of allergic conjunctivitis[68] and vernal conjunctivitis,[69] respectively. Other topical NSAIDs, such as ketorolac and diclofenac, have also been effective in reducing symptoms associated with seasonal allergic conjunctivitis.[70, 71] However, topical ketorolac remains the only FDA-approved topical NSAID for seasonal allergic conjunctivitis. Oral aspirin has also been investigated and appears to be useful as both primary[72] and adjunctive[73] therapy with steroids in vernal conjunctivitis.

PREVENTION OF CATARACT FORMATION

Although corticosteroid use is associated with cataract formation, aspirin[74, 75] and other NSAIDs[76, 77] may protect against cataracts. The mechanism for this apparent protective effect remains nebulous; however, it may be related to aspirin's acetylation of the lens proteins, which protects these proteins from a variety of chemical insults.[78, 79] In addition, the lowering of blood glucose levels in diabetics and nondiabetics associated with NSAIDs may play a role in preventing cataracts.[77] Nearly half of all patients with cataracts have been estimated to have abnormal glucose tolerance.[80] Because diabetes is clearly associated with cataracts, perhaps the glucose-lowering effect of NSAIDs serves to favorably affect these patients with chronic elevation of glucose levels.[77] However, other observational studies[81–83] and a randomized study[84] did not find that aspirin lowered the incidence of cataracts. It seems that aspirin or aspirin-like agents do not prevent cataract formation or slow its progression, although a small benefit cannot be ruled out.[84]

REFERENCES

1. Gifford H: On the treatment of sympathetic ophthalmia by large doses of salicylate of sodium aspirin or other salicylic compounds. Ophthalmoscope 8:257, 1910.
2. Vane JR: Inhibition of prostaglandin synthesis as a mechanism of action for aspirin-like drugs. Nature 231:232, 1971.
3. Vane JR, Botting R: Inflammation and mechanism of action of anti-inflammatory drugs. FASEB J 1:89, 1987.
4. Rainsford KO: Inflammation Mechanisms and Actions of Traditional Drugs, Anti-Inflammatory and Anti-Rheumatic Drugs, vol I. Boca Raton, FL, CRC Press, 1985.
5. Bhattacherjee P: The role of arachidonate metabolites in ocular inflammation. Prog Clin Biol Res 312:211, 1989.
6. Eakins KE: Prostaglandin and non-prostaglandin-mediated breakdown of the blood-aqueous barrier: In the ocular and cerebrospinal fluid. Exp Eye Res 25:483, 1977.
7. Bhattacherjee P: Prostaglandin and inflammatory reactions in the eye. Methods Find Exp Clin Pharmacol 2:17, 1980.
8. Abelson MB, Butrus ST, Kliman GH, et al: Topical arachidonic acid: A model for screening anti-inflammatory agents. J Ocul Pharmacol 3:63, 1987.
9. Unger WG, Bass MS: Prostaglandin and nerve-mediated response of the rabbit eye to argon laser irradiation of the iris. Ophthalmologica 175:153, 1977.
10. Miyake K, Sugiyama S, Norimatsu L, et al: Prevention of cystoid macular edema after lens extraction by topical indomethacin (111): Radioimmunoassay measurement of prostaglandins in the aqueous during and after lens extraction procedures. Graefes Arch Klin Exp Ophthalmol 209:83, 1978.
11. Eakins KE: Prostaglandin and non-prostaglandin mediated break-down of the blood-aqueous barrier. Exp Eye Res 25:483, 1977.
12. Conquet P, Plazonnet B, LeDouarec J: Arachidonic acid-induced elevation of intraocular pressure and anti-inflammatory agents. Invest Ophthalmol 14:772, 1975.
13. Podos SM: Prostaglandin, nonsteroidal anti-inflammatory agents and eye disease. Trans Am Ophthalmol Soc 74:637, 1976.
14. Gryglewski RJ, Panczenko B, Korbut R, et al: Corticosteroids inhibit prostaglandin release from perfused lungs of sensitized guinea pig. Prostaglandins 10:343, 1975.
15. Hong SL, Levine L: Inhibition of arachidonic acid release from cells as the biochemical action of anti-inflammatory corticosteroids. Proc Natl Acad Sci U S A 73:1730, 1976.
16. Campbell WB, Halushka PV: Lipid-derived autocoids: Eicosanoids and platelet-activating factor. *In* Hardman JG, Limbird LE, Molinoff PB, et al (eds): Goodman and Gilman's The Pharmacological Basis of Therapeutics, 9th ed. New York, McGraw-Hill, 1996, pp 601–616.
17. Bito LZ: Ocular effects of prostaglandins and other eicosanoids. Surv Ophthalmol 41(Suppl 2):1–144, 1997.
18. Langman MJS: Peptic ulcer complications and the use of nonaspirin nonsteroidal anti-inflammatory drugs. Adverse Drug React Bull 120:448, 1986.
19. Paulus HE: Arthritis Advisory Committee Meeting. Risks of agranulocytosis aplastic anemia, flank pain and adverse gastrointestinal effects with the use of nonsteroidal anti-inflammatory drugs. Arthritis Rheum 30:593, 1987.
20. Hamberg M, Svensson J, Samuelsson B: Thromboxane: A new group of biologically active compounds derived from prostaglandin endoperoxides. Proc Natl Acad Sci U S A 72:2994, 1975.
21. Clive DM, Stoff JS: Renal syndromes associated with nonsteroidal anti-inflammatory drugs. N Engl J Med 310:563, 1984.
22. Gurwitz JH, Avorn J, Ross-Degnan D, et al: Nonsteroidal anti-inflammatory drug-associated azotemia in the very old. JAMA 264:471, 1990.
23. Sitenga GL, Ing EB, Van Dellen RG, et al: Asthma caused by topical application of ketorolac. Ophthalmology 103:890–892, 1996.
24. Miller D, Gruenberg P, Miller R, et al: Topical flurbiprofen or prednisolone: Effect on corneal wound healing in rabbits. Arch Ophthalmol 99:681, 1981.
25. Ambache N: Irin, a smooth-muscle contracting substance present in rabbit iris. J Physiol 129:65, 1955.
26. Ambache N: Properties of irin, a physiological constituent of the rabbit iris. J Physiol 135:114, 1957.
27. Cole DF, Unger WG: Prostaglandins as mediators for the responses of the eye due to trauma. Exp Eye Res 17:357, 1973.
28. Podos SM, Becker B: Comparison of ocular prostaglandin synthesis inhibitors. Invest Ophthalmol Vis Sci 15:841, 1976.
29. Anderson JA, Chen CC, Vita JB, et al: Disposition of topical flurbiprofen in normal and aphakic rabbit eyes. Arch Ophthalmol 100:642, 1982.
30. Duffin RM, Camras CB, Gardner SK, et al: Inhibitors of surgically-induced miosis. Ophthalmology 89:966, 1982.
31. Keates RH, McGowan KA: Clinical trial of flurbiprofen to maintain pupillary dilation during cataract surgery. Ann Ophthalmol 16:919, 1984.
32. Holmes JM, Jay WM: The effect of preoperative flurbiprofen on miosis produced by acetylcholine during cataract surgery. Am J Ophthalmol 111:735, 1991.
33. Vander JF, Greven CM, Maguire JI, et al: Flurbiprofen sodium to prevent intraoperative miosis during vitreoretinal surgery. Am J Ophthalmol 108:288, 1989.
34. Smiddy WE, Glaser BM, Michels RG, et al: Miosis during vitreoretinal surgery. Retina 10:42, 1990.
35. Stark WJ, Fagadau WR, Stewart RH, et al: Reduction of pupillary constriction during cataract surgery using suprofen. Arch Ophthalmol 104:364, 1986.
36. Roberts CW: A comparison of diclofenac sodium to flurbiprofen for maintaining intraoperative mydriasis. Invest Ophthalmol Vis Sci 35:1967, 1993.
37. Camras CB, Miranda OC: The putative role of prostaglandins in surgical miosis. *In* Bito LZ, Stjernschantz J (eds): The Ocular Effects of Prostaglandins and Other Eicosanoids. New York, Alan R. Liss, 1989, pp 197–210.
38. Miranda OC, Bito LZ: The putative and demonstrated miotic effects of prostaglandins in mammals. *In* Bito LZ, Stjernschantz J (eds): The Ocular Effects of Prostaglandins and Other Eicosanoids. New York, Alan R. Liss, 1989, pp 171–195.
39. Sanders DR, Kraff MC, Lieberman HL, et al: Breakdown and reestablishment of blood-aqueous barrier with implant surgery. Arch Ophthalmol 100:588, 1982.
40. Sanders DR, Kraff MC: Steroidal and nonsteroidal anti-inflammatory agents. Arch Ophthalmol 102:1453, 1984.
41. Flach AJ, Kraff MC, Sanders DR, et al: The quantitative effect of 0.5% ketorolac tromethamine solution and 0.1% dexamethasone sodium phosphate solution on postsurgical blood aqueous barrier. Arch Ophthalmol 106:480, 1988.
42. Araie M, Sawa M, Takase M: Topical flurbiprofen and diclofenac suppress blood-aqueous barrier breakdown in cataract surgery: A fluorophotometric study. Jpn J Ophthalmol 27:535, 1983.
43. Kraff MC, Sanders DR, McGuigan L, et al: Inhibition of the blood-aqueous barrier breakdown with diclofenac. Arch Ophthalmol 108:380, 1990.
44. Flach AJ, Graham J, Kruger LP, et al: Quantitative assessment of postsurgical breakdown of blood-aqueous barrier following administration of 0.5% ketorolac tromethamine solution: A double-masked, paired comparison with vehicle-placebo solution study. Arch Ophthalmol 106:344, 1988.
45. Flach AJ, Lavelle CJ, Olander KW, et al: The effect of ketorolac tromethamine solution 0.5% in reducing postoperative inflammation after cataract extraction and intraocular lens implantation. Ophthalmology 95:1279, 1988.

46. Vickers FF, McGuigan LJB, Ford C, et al: The effect of diclofenac sodium on the treatment of postoperative inflammation. Invest Ophthalmol Vis Sci 32(ARVO Suppl):793, 1991.
47. Eiferman RA, Hoffman RS, Sher NA: Topical diclofenac reduced pain following photorefractive keratectomy. Arch Ophthalmol 111:1022, 1993.
48. Sher NA, Frantz JM, Talley A, et al: Topical diclofenac in the treatment of ocular pain after excimer photorefractive keratectomy. Refract Corneal Surg 9:425–436, 1993.
49. Arshinoff EA: Use of topical nonsteroidal anti-inflammatory drugs in excimer laser photorefractive keratectomy. J Cataract Refract Surg 20:216–222, 1994.
50. Szerenyi K, Sorken K, Garbus JJ, et al: Decrease in normal human corneal sensitivity with topical diclofenac sodium. Am J Ophthalmol 118:312–315, 1994.
51. Epstein RL, Laurence EP: Relative effectiveness of topical ketorolac and topical diclofenac on discomfort after radial keratotomy. J Cataract Refract Surg 21:156–159, 1995.
52. Seitz B, Sorken K, LaBree LD, et al: Corneal sensitivity and burning sensation: Comparing topical ketorolac and diclofenac. Arch Ophthalmol 114:921–924, 1996.
53. Tomas-Barberan S, Törngren L, Lundberg K, et al: Effect of diclofenac on prostaglandin liberation in the rabbit after photorefractive keratectomy. J Refract Surg 13:154–157, 1997.
54. Wright M, Butt Z, McIllwaine G, et al: Comparison of the efficacy of diclofenac and betamethasone following strabismus surgery. Br J Ophthalmol 81:299–301, 1997.
55. Kraff MC, Sanders DR, Jampol LM, et al: Prophylaxis of pseudophakic cystoid macular edema with topical indomethacin. Ophthalmology 89:885, 1982.
56. Abelson MB, Smith LK, Ormerod LD: Prospective, randomized trial of oral piroxicam in the prophylaxis of postoperative cystoid macular edema. J Ocul Pharmacol 5:147, 1984.
57. Flach AJ, Dolan BJ, Irvine AR: Effectiveness of ketorolac tromethamine 0.5% ophthalmic solution for chronic aphakic and pseudophakic cystoid macular edema. Am J Ophthalmol 103:479, 1987.
58. Flach AJ, Stegman RC, Graham J, et al: Prophylaxis of aphakic cystoid macular edema without corticosteroids. Ophthalmology 92:807–810, 1990.
59. Solomon LD: Flurbiprofen-CME Study Group I. Efficacy of topical flurbiprofen and indomethacin in preventing pseudophakic cystoid macular edema. J Cataract Refract Surg 21:73–81, 1995.
60. Watson PG: Doyne Memorial Lecture. Trans Ophthalmol Soc UK 102:257, 1982.
61. Lyons CJ, Hakin KN, Watson PG: Topical flurbiprofen: An effective treatment for episcleritis? Eye 4:521, 1990.
62. Olson NY, Lindsley CB, Godfrey WA: Nonsteroidal anti-inflammatory drug therapy in chronic childhood iridocyclitis. Am J Dis Child 142:1289, 1988.
63. Fraser-Smith EB, Mathews TR: Effect of ketorolac on herpes simplex virus type one ocular infection in rabbits. J Ocul Pharmacol 4:321, 1988.
64. Colin J, Bodin C, Malet F, et al: La keratite herpetique experimentale du lapin. J Fr Ophtalmol 12:255, 1989.
65. Trousdale MD, Dunkel EC, Nesburn AB: Effect of flurbiprofen on herpes simplex keratitis in rabbits. Invest Ophthalmol Vis Sci 19:267, 1980.
66. Fraser-Smith EB, Mathews TR: Effect of ketorolac on Pseudomonas aeruginosa ocular infection in rabbits. J Ocul Pharmacol 4:101, 1988.
67. Fraser-Smith EB, Mathews TR: Effect of ketorolac on Candida albicans ocular infection in rabbits. Arch Ophthalmol 105:264, 1987.
68. Bishop K, Abelson M, Cheetharn J, et al: Evaluation of flurbiprofen in the treatment of antigen-induced allergic conjunctivitis. Invest Ophthalmol Vis Sci 31(ARVO Suppl):487, 1990.
69. Buckley DC, Caldwell DR, Reaves TA: Treatment of vernal conjunctivitis with suprofen, a topical nonsteroidal anti-inflammatory agent. Invest Ophthalmol Vis Sci 27(ARVO Suppl):29, 1986.
70. Tinkelman DG, Rupp G, Kaufman H, et al: Double-masked, paired-comparison clinical study of ketorolac tromethamine 0.5% ophthalmic solution compared with placebo eyedrops in the treatment of seasonal allergic conjunctivitis. Surv Ophthalmol 38:141–148, 1993.
71. Laibovitz RA, Koester J, Schaich L, et al: Safety and efficacy of diclofenac sodium 0.1% ophthalmic solution in acute seasonal allergic conjunctivitis. J Ocul Pharmacol 11:361–368, 1995.
72. Meyer E, Kraus E, Zonis S: Efficacy of antiprostaglandin therapy in vernal conjunctivitis. Br J Ophthalmol 71:497, 1987.
73. Abelson MB, Butrus SI, Weston JH: Aspirin therapy in vernal conjunctivitis. Am J Ophthalmol 95:502, 1983.
74. Cotlier E: Aspirin and senile cataract in rheumatoid arthritis. Lancet 1:338, 1981.
75. Cotlier E, Sharma YG, Niven T, et al: Distribution of salicylate in lens and intraocular fluids and its effects on cataract formation. Am J Med 74:83, 1983.
76. van Heyningen R, Harding JJ: Do aspirin-like analgesics protect against cataract? A case-control study. Lancet 1:1111, 1986.
77. Harding JJ, van Heyningen R: Drugs, including alcohol, that act as risk factors for cataract, and possible protection against cataract by aspirin-like analgesics and cyclopenthiazide. Br J Ophthalmol 72:809, 1988.
78. Crompton M, Rixon KC, Harding JJ: Aspirin prevents carbamylation of soluble lens proteins and prevents cyanate-induced phase separation opacities in vitro: A possible mechanism by which aspirin could prevent cataract. Exp Eye Res 40:297, 1985.
79. Rao GN, Lardis MP, Cotlier E: Acetylation of lens crystallins: A possible mechanism by which aspirin could prevent cataract formation. Biochem Biophys Res Commun 128:1125, 1985.
80. Dugmore WN, Tun K: Glucose tolerance tests in 200 patients with senile cataract. Br J Ophthalmol 64:689, 1980.
81. Siegel D, Sperduto RD, Ferris F: Aspirin and cataracts. Ophthalmology 89:47A, 1982.
82. Klein BK, Klein R, Moss S: Is aspirin use associated with lower rates of cataracts in diabetic individuals? Diabetes Care 10:495, 1987.
83. West SK, Munoz BE, Newland HS, et al: Lack of evidence for aspirin use and prevention of cataracts. Arch Ophthalmol 105:1229, 1987.
84. Seddon JM, Christen WG, Manson JE, et al: Low-dose aspirin and risks of cataract in a randomized trial of U.S. physicians. Arch Ophthalmol 109:252, 1991.

CHAPTER 28

Antihistamines and Mast Cell Stabilizers in Allergic Ocular Disease

Gregg J. Berdy and Mark B. Abelson

Ophthalmologists frequently see allergic diseases of the eye. They may be the most common clinical problems involving the external ocular adnexa. Approximately 18% of the U.S. population—about 40 million people—are affected with these disorders. Although allergic ocular diseases may affect the skin and subcutaneous tissues of the eyelids, it is the conjunctiva, the mucous membrane of the eye, that is more commonly and severely affected. In certain cases, the eye may be the only organ system involved. In most of these patients, however, the ocular tissues participate as part of a systemic allergic response to exogenous or intrinsic antigens.

Allergic diseases have been classified by Gell and Coombs[1] into four major categories of hypersensitivity reactions. Type I reactions include diseases in which antigen-specific immunoglobulin E (IgE) is responsible for the generation of the immune response. Type II responses occur as the result of antibody-dependent regulation of cell killing by subtypes of T lymphocytes. Diseases associated with antigen-antibody complex deposition within blood vessel walls and other tissues are classified as type III hypersensitivity responses. Lastly, type IV reactions are characterized by activity of T lymphocytes and their cytokines, resulting in a delayed response.

Ocular allergy encompasses a spectrum of diseases characterized by the type I hypersensitivity response. The most common ocular atopy is allergic conjunctivitis, the ocular counterpart of allergic rhinitis. Exposure to environmental allergens such as pollens, animal dander, and dust causes the symptoms and signs of ocular hay fever in sensitized persons. An acute attack is characterized by conjunctival injection, chemosis, tearing, eyelid swelling, burning, and ocular and periocular itching.

Mast Cell and Pathophysiology

Knowledge of the pathogenesis of ocular allergic disease is critical to understanding the role of therapeutic antiallergic compounds used in the treatment of these diseases. Allergic conjunctivitis is the prototype of this group of diseases and begins as an antigen–IgE antibody interaction on the surface of conjunctival mast cells.[2] Exposure of appropriately sensitized IgE-coated mast cells to airborne allergen is the initiating stimulus. The allergen binds to two separate IgE molecules, creating a dimer formation that initiates a chain of reactions in the mast cell plasma membrane.[3, 4]

It is thought that the bridging of mast cell IgE molecules (cross-linking) induces activation of membrane-associated enzymes, leading to an increase in the uptake of calcium.[5] Enzymes identified with intracellular calcium mobilization and initiation of the biochemical process of histamine release are membrane-associated proteolytic enzymes,[6] methyltransferases,[7] and adenylate cyclase.[8, 9] In addition, the cross-linking of membrane-bound IgE molecules induces the activation of phospholipase A_2 with subsequent release and metabolism of arachidonic acid.[10] This 20-carbon, unsaturated fatty acid serves as a precursor for newly synthesized substances, such as prostaglandins, leukotrienes,[11] and platelet-activating factor,[12, 13] that have been implicated as important mediators of clinical allergic disease.[14]

The intracellular biochemical events that follow cross-linking of IgE molecules have not been fully elucidated. However, methylation of membrane-bound phospholipids and phosphorylation of both membrane-bound and intracytoplasmic proteins are intricately involved in the release of intracytoplasmic granules. At the ultrastructural level, it has been demonstrated that human lung mast cells, once stimulated, show swelling of individual granules, with the subsequent fusion and formation of interconnected chains of altered granules. These intracellular cytoplasmic channels eventually fuse with the plasma membrane of the mast cell, thereby releasing their contents into the extracellular space.[15–17] These secretory granules contain several preformed mediators, including biogenic amines (histamine), neutral proteases (chymase, tryptase), proteoglycans (heparin), and acid hydrolases, that initiate and promulgate the allergic response.

Role of Histamine

The sentinel role of histamine in the acute allergic response has been well established. Histamine was first synthesized in 1907 and discovered to be an imidazolylethylamine.[18] In 1910, the biologic activity of this amine was discovered when it was detected as an uterine stimulant in extracts of ergot. Later that year, Dale and Laidlaw[19] observed bronchospastic and vasodilator activity in animals with the intravenous administration of histamine. In 1919, these authors observed that histamine applied locally produced redness, swelling, and edema. In addition, they noted that large doses of intravenous histamine produced a symptom complex that was identical to that of a systemic anaphylactic reaction.[20] Eight years later, investigators deduced that histamine was a humoral mediator involved in acute allergic reactions.[21]

In 1953, the presence of histamine was noted in mast cells taken from human skin.[22] This discovery spurred the interest of many researchers, leading to the elucidation of histamine's synthesis, secretion, metabolism, and biologic activity.[23, 24] It is the biologic activity of histamine that creates the signs and symptoms of the acute allergic reaction in ocular hay fever.

The physiologic and pharmacologic effects of histamine are mediated by specific receptor subtypes present on effector cell surfaces. In 1966, Ash and Schild[25] identified specific receptors that were blocked by the antihistamines known at that time and labeled them H_1 receptors. These authors discovered that only certain responses to histamine were blocked by the histamine antagonist mepyramine, and these responses were defined as being mediated by H_1 receptors. Six years later, Black et al.[26] identified a second histamine receptor subtype, H_2, by using specific antagonists that blocked only the H_2 receptors. They demonstrated that histamine-induced hypotension that was only partially relieved by mepyramine was totally blocked by the addition of the H_2-receptor antagonist burimamide.

Identification of the H_1 and H_2 receptors has permitted investigators to better understand histamine's role in human allergic disease. Owen and coworkers[27] concluded that the vasodilator response to histamine was mediated by both H_1 and H_2 receptors; however, the increase in vascular permeability was mediated solely by H_1 receptors. When injected intradermally, histamine causes a localized triple response. The initial component is the development of erythema immediately surrounding the injection site as the result of vasodilation mediated by both H_1 and H_2 receptors.[28, 29] A second component is the cutaneous flare that occurs as an indirect response to stimulation of histamine receptors on afferent nonmyelinated nerve endings. Antidromic nerve conduction initiates a reflex arc that culminates in the release of various neuropeptides, including substance P and calcitonin gene-related peptide, which directly affect arteriolar vasodilation.[30] The wheal results from exudation of plasma through gaps between vascular endothelium of postcapillary venules and is mediated by H_1 receptors.[31] Additionally, intradermal injection of histamine causes a sensory response that is manifested as the sensation of itching.

Allergic conjunctivitis can be characterized as ocular anaphylaxis occurring when a sensitized person is exposed to a specific aeroallergen. Abelson et al.[32] demonstrated the presence of mast cell–derived mediators in subconjunctival tissues and precorneal tear film in patients with ocular atopic diseases. This is not unexpected, because the human conjunctiva contains large numbers of mast cells subjacent to the epithelium.[33–35]

Previously, Abelson and coworkers[36] demonstrated the presence of histamine in the tear film of normal humans at concentrations of 5 to 10 ng/mL, whereas tear samples of patients with active vernal keratoconjunctivitis (VKC) contained significantly higher levels of histamine. These same investigators demonstrated that topical instillation of histamine produced the itching and redness associated with allergic conjunctivitis in a dose-dependent fashion.[37] Subsequently, identification of specific histamine receptors on the ocular surface has made it possible to selectively identify the pathologic effects of histamine. Stimulation of H_1 receptors with the highly selective H_1-receptor agonist 2-(2-aminoethyl) thiazoledihydrochloride elicited symptoms of ocular itching.[38] On the other hand, selective stimulation of H_2 receptors by dimethylaminopropylisothiourea, a highly selective H_2-receptor agonist, produced vasodilation of conjunctival vessels without itching.[39]

Therapeutic Options

Treatment of allergic ocular diseases, specifically allergic conjunctivitis, may be approached in the same manner as one would treat allergic rhinitis. Ideally, removing the offending allergen or modifying the patient's environment would be most effective. However, this is not always practical. Systemic medications such as oral antihistamines may be employed, but these agents do not reliably relieve ocular symptoms, and their soporific effects may mitigate their use. In most cases, treatment with topical medications in the form of eye drops has provided symptomatic relief without systemic side effects.

Topical corticosteroid preparations, such as fluorometholone and prednisolone 0.125%, are extremely effective in providing relief of itching, chemosis, and mucous discharge. These drugs should be used only in severe cases that do not respond to other, milder forms of therapy, because they have been associated with the development of glaucoma, cataract formation, and secondary bacterial, fungal, and viral infections.[40]

Mast cell stabilizer preparations have been purported to stabilize the mast cell plasma membrane, thereby preventing subsequent degranulation and release of inflammatory mediators. The ophthalmic literature has debated the therapeutic value of disodium cromoglycate in allergic conjunctivitis. Several studies have demonstrated a salutary effect,[41, 42] whereas others have shown no effect.[43, 44] A newer, second-generation preparation, lodoxamide 0.1%, has shown salutary effects in patients with VKC.[45, 46]

The drugs most commonly used to treat ocular hay fever are topical antihistamines. Their mechanism of action is competitive inhibition with histamine for the histamine receptors on effector cells. Currently, the only antihistamine preparations available are H_1-receptor antagonists. These agents reliably relieve the symptoms of itching found in allergic conjunctivitis; however, several preparations have little effect on chemosis and redness.[47] As such, these drugs are manufactured in combination with a vasoconstrictor agent that helps to relieve ocular injection. Recently, several H_1-selective receptor antagonists have been introduced that relieve both the itching and the redness associated with allergic conjunctivitis.[48, 49]

ANTIHISTAMINES

In 1927, Lewis[50] described the wheal-and-flare response seen in human skin and suggested that histamine could be released from intracellular stores by local injury. Armed with this information, investigators began the search to develop pharmacologic methods to blunt histamine's profound effects. In 1937, Bovet and Staub[51] fortuitously noted that a compound that they had been screening for adrenergic-blocking activity also possessed some antihistaminic activity. This compound, 2-isopropyl-5-methyl-phenoxyethyldiethylamine, when administered to guinea pigs protected them from lethal doses of histamine, antagonized histamine-induced smooth muscle contraction, and diminished the systemic symptoms of anaphylaxis. Unfortunately, this substance was too toxic for clinical use, but it led to the discovery of phenbenzamine (Antergan), a dimethylamine derivative that was the first antihistaminic compound to be used in humans.[52] In 1944, Bovet and coworkers[53] discovered another clinically effective compound, pyrilamine maleate (Neo-Antergan), which is still used today.

The first description of topical antihistamine use in the eye was published in 1946 by Bourquin.[54] He observed satisfactory results with the use of antazoline (Antistine) in patients with vernal catarrh, phlyctenular conjunctivitis, conjunctivitis associated with hay fever, and scleritis. Two years later, in the American literature, Hurwitz[55] reported favorable results with the same drug. Since the discovery that topical antihistamines could alleviate symptoms of allergic conjunctivitis, several authors have published results demonstrating that topical H_1 antihistamines were clinically effective.[56, 57]

MAST CELL STABILIZERS

Cromolyn sodium (DSCG), a derivative of khellin, a chromone found in *Ammi visnaga,* an eastern Mediterranean plant, was first synthesized in 1965. The drug is thought to act on the mast cell plasma membrane via control of transmembrane calcium flux. The effect of DSCG is to stabilize the membrane, thereby preventing degranulation and release of inflammatory mediators.[58, 59] Thus, DSCG must exert its effect prior to allergen binding or, at least, before the mast cell membrane is altered with subsequent mediator release.

Since its discovery, investigators have shown DSCG to have salutary effects in patients with allergic asthma and other IgE-mediated diseases.[60–67] In 1984, the U.S. Food and Drug Administration (FDA) granted approval of DSCG for ocular use in patients with VKC on the basis that the drug alleviated symptoms and signs of the disease and allowed a reduction in the frequency of steroid use in these patients.[68, 69] However, the ability of DSCG to suppress ocular allergic symptoms in environmental studies has yielded conflicting results.[70–74] To date, results of studies evaluating DSCG in allergic conjunctivitis have been encouraging, but the effectiveness of the drug in this condition remains controversial. However, both 4% DSCG and 0.1% lodoxamide have showed to be effective in controlling the signs and symptoms of VKC.[45, 68, 75]

Histamine H_1-Receptor Antagonists

CHEMISTRY

Histamine receptors were defined pharmacologically by the actions of their agonists and antagonists. Histamine H_1-receptor antagonists pharmacologically compete with histamine at the H_1-receptor site on effector cells and have been classified by their chemical structures into six groups: ethylenediamines, ethanolamines, alkylamines, phenothiazines, piperazines, and piperadines (Table 28–1). The H_1-receptor antagonist compounds can be described by the general structure shown in Figure 28–1. These compounds are composed of one or two aromatic (heterocyclic) rings connected via a nitrogen, carbon, or oxygen atom (X) to the ethylamine group. The nitrogen atom of the ethylamine group is tertiary—that is, it has two substituents. The H_1-receptor antagonists are structurally similar to histamine in that they both contain an ethylamine group. However, histamine consists of a single heterocyclic ring, in this case imidazole, which is connected directly to the ethylamine group. Unlike that of the H_1-receptor antagonists, the nitrogen atom of the ethylamine group is primary or unsubstituted.

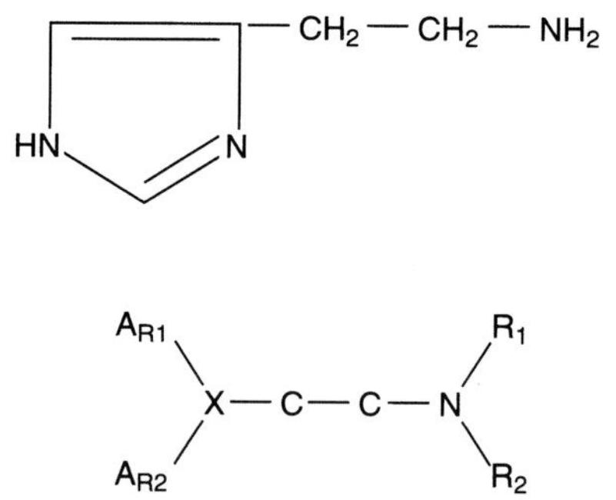

FIGURE 28–1. A comparison of the chemical structure of histamine *(top)* and of H_1-receptor antagonists *(bottom).*

STRUCTURE-ACTIVITY RELATIONSHIP

The H_1-receptor antagonists possess two chemical moieties that determine the pharmacokinetic properties of this group of drugs and thereby confer pharmacologic activity (Table 28–2). The H_1 antihistamines contain multiple aromatic rings, which make these compounds very lipophilic and contribute to receptor site binding via hydrophobic forces.[76] The second functional moiety is the positively charged side chain, which is usually an ammonium group. Both histamine and the H_1-receptor antagonists share an amino group that is believed to be important for H_1-receptor recognition.[77] Table 28–2 demonstrates the chemical structural similarities and differences between histamine and the H_1- and H_2-receptor antagonists.

MECHANISM OF ACTION

The H_1-receptor antihistamines act by occupying H_1 receptor on effector cells. Binding of antagonists to the receptor site does not initiate a response in the effector cell; rather, it prohibits histamine from binding. Therefore, histamine is unable to cause an effector cell response. The binding of the H_1-receptor antagonist is a reversible, competitive equilibrium reaction and is determined by the relative concentrations of histamine and H_1-receptor antagonist in the area of the receptor site. To ensure effective blockade of the H_1-receptor, the antihistamine concentration should be sufficiently high to compete with tissue histamine levels created by local mast cell degranulation.

PHARMACOKINETICS: ABSORPTION, DISTRIBUTION, BIOTRANSFORMATION, AND ELIMINATION

The majority of H_1-receptor antagonists are chemically stable and do not contain labile ester or amide moieties. The

TABLE 28–1. **The Six Major Groups of Classic H_1 Antihistamines**

Linkage Atom	General Class	Example	Other Members	General Comments
N	Ethylenediamines	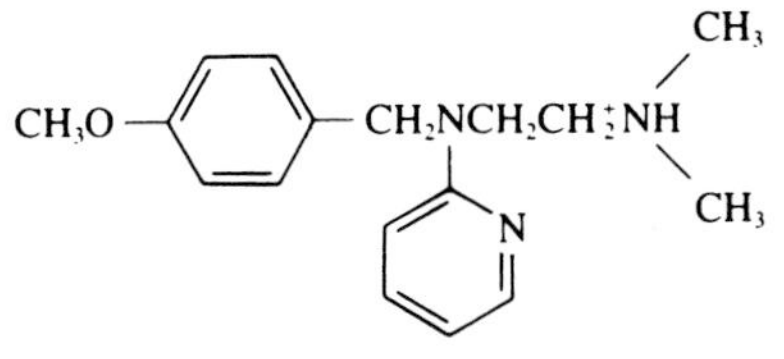 Pyrilamine	Antazoline Methapyrilene Tripelennamine	Relatively weak CNS effects, but drowsiness may occur in some patients; gastrointestinal side effects common
O	Ethanolamines (aminoalkyl ethers)	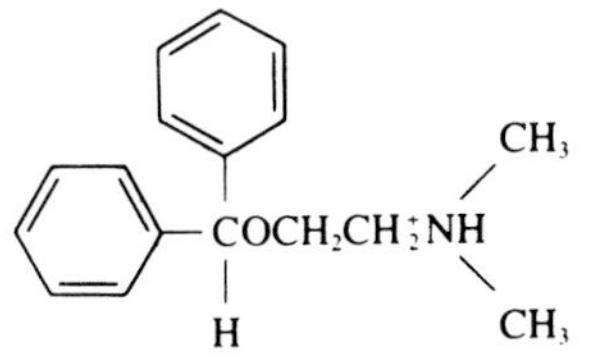 Diphenhydramine	Bromodiphenhydramine Carbinoxamine Clemastine Dimenhydrinate Diphenylpyraline Doxylamine Phenytoloxamine	Significant antimuscarinic activity; CNS depression common in about half of the patients using members of this group; relatively low incidence of gastrointestinal side effects
C	Alkylamines (propylamine derivatives)	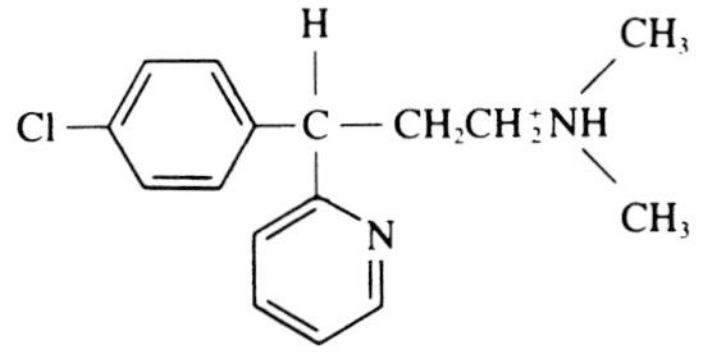 Chlorpheniramine	Brompheniramine Dexbrompheniramine Dexchlorpheniramine Dimethindene Pheniramine Pyrrobutamine Triprolidine	Cause less CNS depression than members of other groups; some CNS stimulation possible; best group of classic antihistamines for daytime use
N (in phenothiazine ring)	Phenothiazines	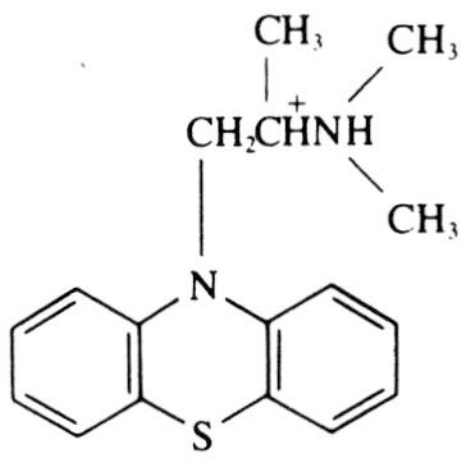 Promethazine	Methdilazine Trimeprazine	Sedative effects very prominent with this class; most have pronounced antimuscarinic activity; usually used primarily as antiemetics
N (in piperazine ring)	Piperazines	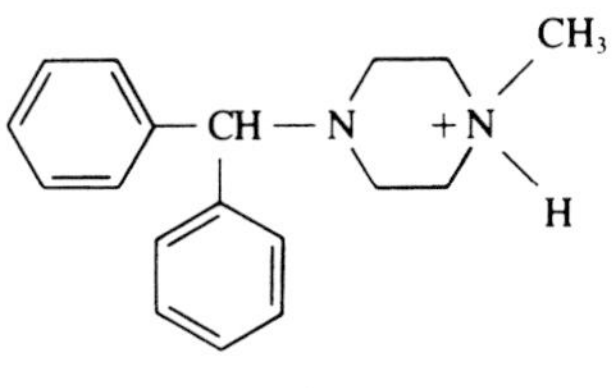 Cyclizine	Buclizine Chlorcyclizine Hydroxyzine Meclizine	Degree of sedation and antimuscarinic effects produced by this class is relatively mild; buclizine, cyclizine, and meclizine are used for treating motion sickness; hydroxyzine is used as sedative, tranquilizer, and antiemetic
N (in piperidine ring)	Piperidines	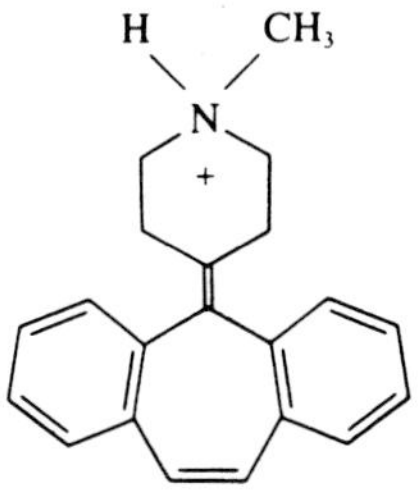 Cyproheptadine	Azatadine Phenindamine	Sedative potential is comparable to that of the ethylenediamine class; drowsiness is most common side effect

From Trzeciakowski JP, Mendelsohn N, Levi R: Antihistamines. *In* Middleton E, Reed CE, Ellis EF, et al (eds): Allergy Principles and Practice, 3rd ed. St. Louis, CV Mosby, 1988.

TABLE 28–2. **Chemical Differentiation Between Histamine and Its Respective Receptor Antagonists**

H_2 Antagonist	Histamine	H_1 Antagonist
Imidazole for analogous ring	Imidazole	Aryl rings
Hydrophilic	Hydrophilic	Lipophilic
Thiourea or guanidine	Ammonium	Ammonium (or similar group)
Preferably uncharged	Charged	Charged

From Ganellin CR: Chemistry and structure-activity relationship of H_2-receptor antagonists. *In* Rocha e Silva, M (ed): Handbook of experimental pharmacology, Vol 18, Part 2, Histamine II and Anti-Histaminics: Chemistry, Metabolism, Physiological, and Pharmacological Actions. New York, Springer-Verlag, 1978.

equilibrium constant of the base and its conjugate acid of the antihistamine compounds is greater than 8.0. Thus, at physiologic pH, all of the compounds would be at least 90% protonated and water-soluble. As a result of their basic properties, the H_1-receptor antihistamines may be administered orally. Following oral administration, the drugs are rapidly absorbed and render symptomatic relief beginning within 15 to 30 minutes. The duration of action usually is 3 to 6 hours. The H_1 receptor–blocking agents are widely distributed in body tissues and cross the blood-brain barrier. The compounds are metabolized in the liver and excreted in the urine within 24 hours of an oral dose.[78, 79]

Little information is available on the pharmacokinetics of topically applied ocular H_1 antihistamines. These drugs are administered to the ocular surface via application of water-soluble salts; maleate salts and phosphoric acid are most commonly used in ocular preparations. Currently, only three H_1 antihistamines are approved for use in the eye; these include pheniramine maleate, antazoline phosphate, and pyrilamine maleate. These preparations are well distributed in the preocular tear film and seem to have excellent penetration into the conjunctival epithelium and substantia propria. Systemic absorption occurs via drainage through the nasal lacrimal duct with subsequent absorption by the nasopharyngeal and oropharyngeal mucosal surfaces.

PHARMACOLOGIC PROPERTIES

The pharmacologic actions of the H_1-receptor antagonist subclasses are similar: They block the effects of histamine mediated by the H_1 receptors on effector cells. The effects of histamine on the vascular system are mediated by both H_1 and H_2 receptors.[80] Stimulation of H_1 receptors causes systemic vasodilation as well as localized cutaneous erythema due to capillary dilation.[29] However, when H_1 receptor–blocking agents are administered alone, the systemic hypotension caused by histamine-induced vasodilation is only partially blocked. When H_1- and H_2-receptor blockers are given concurrently prior to histamine challenge, the fall in blood pressure is negated. Cutaneous capillary permeability is increased after local injection of histamine, resulting in the formation of edema.[27] H_1-receptor antihistamines antagonize this action of histamine and inhibit the egress of plasma through capillary walls.

Histamine has a direct constrictor action on smooth muscle. In humans, histamine-induced bronchoconstriction of respiratory smooth muscle can be blocked with prophylactic administration of H_2-receptor antagonists.[81] In animal species, in vivo experiments have demonstrated histamine-induced contraction of gastrointestinal smooth muscle. The guinea pig ileum model had been used to provide early evidence for the effects of histamine and to document the presence of specific histamine-receptor subtypes. In addition, this animal model had been used to test various types of H_1-receptor antihistamines as these agents were developed.

In the eye, topical application of histamine induces ocular itching and conjunctival vasodilation. It has been demonstrated that the H_1 receptors mediate the symptoms of itching, whereas conjunctival vasodilation is mediated by both H_1 and H_2 receptors.[38, 39, 47] Pretreatment with topical H_1 antihistamines blocks the histamine-induced itching and decreases the amount of conjunctival hyperemia.

Many of the H_1 antihistamines possess pharmacologic properties unrelated to H_1-receptor blockade. These agents possess varying degrees of anticholinergic activity that is dose dependent and varies among the subclasses. The anticholinergic action has been used in treating several diseases, including motion sickness, vertigo resulting from vestibular disorders, and rigidity associated with Parkinson's disease.

Several H_1-receptor antagonist compounds have been demonstrated to possess local anesthetic action.[82] However, this effect occurs only with concentrations several orders of magnitude greater than the pharmacologic dosages employed to block the H_1 receptor. In eyes pretreated with antazoline phosphate, itching was blocked after topical histamine challenge, whereas corneal sensation was shown not to be decreased by anesthesiometry.[47]

ADVERSE EFFECTS

Systemic Administration

Therapeutic doses of oral H_1 antihistamines may be associated with mild systemic side effects; however, occasionally the untoward responses may necessitate drug withdrawal. The most common adverse effect observed with H_1-receptor antagonists is sedation, which varies between the drug subclasses and individual patient response.[83] Although sedation may not be problematic when medication is administered upon retiring for the night, this soporific effect may lead to potentially life-threatening accidents in patients who drive or operate heavy automated machinery. Other central nervous system (CNS) side effects include disturbed coordination, dizziness, fatigue, and difficulty in concentration, which result from a generalized depression of the CNS. Paradoxically, patients may also experience euphoria, nervousness, insomnia, and tremors.

Gastrointestinal adverse effects occur less frequently and include loss of appetite, nausea, vomiting, epigastric distress, and constipation or diarrhea. Occasionally, these symptoms are diminished by administering oral H_1 antihistamines with meals. Several less-frequent side effects of the H_1-receptor antagonists are attributable to their anticholinergic properties. Patients may note dryness of the mucous membranes of the oropharynx and the appearance of dry eye symptoms that may lead to contact lens intolerance or frank keratoconjunctivitis sicca. Other atropine-like effects include mydriasis that could precipitate an attack of acute angle-closure glaucoma in untreated, predisposed persons. Ciliary muscle paresis with an associated decrease in accommodation may account for visual difficulties experienced by some patients.

Systemic H_1 antihistamines should be used judiciously in young children; acute poisoning may result from an inability to metabolize the drugs rapidly and may produce dangerously high blood concentrations. The CNS effects of the H_1-receptor antagonists constitute the greatest danger to children, and the constellation of signs and symptoms are related to anticholinergic activity as evidenced by excitement, nervousness, irritability, incoordination, insomnia, and tremors.[84] Other signs associated with cholinergic blockage are fixed and dilated pupils, facial flushing, and elevated body temperature.

Safety in pregnancy for humans has not been established for systemic H_1 antihistamines.[85] However, the piperazine compounds may have teratogenic effects.

Topical Ocular Administration

Topical administration of H_1-receptor antagonists in the eye has been associated with a low incidence of systemic adverse effects. However, these agents are available only in combination with sympathomimetic decongestant agents that have been associated with systemic side effects. Ocular medications gain access to the systemic circulation via absorption through the nasal and oropharyngeal mucosae. Therefore, combination drugs should be used with caution in patients with poorly controlled hypertension, cardiovascular disease with arrhythmias, and poorly controlled diabetes mellitus. Additionally, patients using monoamine oxidase inhibitors for hypertensive disease may suffer a hypertensive crisis if administered a topical sympathomimetic decongestant agent.[86, 87]

Pupillary mydriasis may be induced by either component of an H_1-receptor antagonist/decongestant combination and may trigger an attack of acute angle-closure glaucoma. The combination drugs have not been evaluated for safety during pregnancy.

PREPARATIONS AND DOSAGES

Currently, both prescription and over-the-counter H_1-receptor antagonist antihistamine agents are available to treat disease. Three over-the-counter H_1-receptor antagonist antihistamines are available for topical ocular administration and are produced only as combination antihistamine/decongestant preparations. The H_1 antihistamines are 0.5% antazoline phosphate, 0.3% pheniramine maleate, and 0.1% pyrilamine maleate and are found in combination with either 0.025 to 0.05% naphazoline hydrochloride or 0.012% phenylephrine (Table 28–3). Each of the three H_1 antihistaminic agents is efficacious in reducing the chemosis and itching associated with allergic conjunctivitis. The decongestant agents are included for their vasoconstrictor properties and are efficacious in relieving conjunctival injection. The recommended dosage is one to two drops instilled in the eye up to four times daily as needed to control symptoms.

New H_1-selective receptor antagonist agents have been introduced that block both the itching and redness associated with allergic conjunctivitis. levocarbastine (Livostin) is a potent new topical ocular H_1-receptor antagonist that has been demonstrated to effectively control the symptoms of allergic conjunctivitis.[88] A topical preparation of 0.05% levocarbastine hydrochloride administered prior to conjunctival histamine challenge effectively prevented itching, conjunctival injection, and chemosis.[89] In conjunctival antigen challenge (CAC) studies, 0.05% levocarbastine hydrochloride has been shown to be more effective than placebo and 4% DSCG in inhibiting itching, hyperemia, eyelid swelling, chemosis, and tearing after allergen challenge.[48, 90]

TABLE 28–3. **Antihistamine-Decongestant Combinations**

Generic Name	Commercial Preparations	Recommended Dosage
Antazoline PO_4 (0.5%)	Albalon A	1–2 drops/eye q3–4hr or less to relieve symptoms
Naphazoline HCl (0.05%)	Vasocon A	
Pheniramine maleate (0.3%)	AK-Con A	1–2 drops/eye q3–4hr or less to relieve symptoms
Naphazoline HCl (0.025%)	Opcon A Naphcon A	
Pyrilamine maleate (0.1%)	Prefrin-A Prefrin-A	1–2 drops/eye q3–4hr or less to relieve symptoms
Phenylephrine (0.12%)		

From Pavan-Langston D, Dunkel EC: Handbook of Ocular Drug Therapy and Ocular Side Effects of Systemic Drugs. Boston, Little, Brown, 1991.

A second H_1-selective receptor antagonist agent, 0.1% olopatadine (Patanol), has been added to the armamentarium to treat allergic conjunctivitis. In CAC studies, 0.1% olopatadine has been shown to be more effective than placebo in inhibiting itching and redness after antigen challenge.[91] Additionally, the recommended dosing schedule of 0.1% olopatadine is twice daily, and it has been approved for use in children at least 3 years of age.

In addition to the antihistamine/decongestant preparations, several over-the-counter and prescription decongestant preparations and decongestant/astringent combinations are available (Table 28–4). These agents may be used in circumstances of mild ocular irritation or allergic conditions and are effective in reducing conjunctival injection and clearing mucus from the ocular surface.

NEW ADVANCES IN THERAPY

Recently, several new nonsedating H_1-receptor antagonists have been added to the array of agents used to treat allergic diseases. Astemizole (Hismanal)[92] and loratadine[93] have demonstrated efficacy in controlling ocular itching when given systemically to patients with seasonal allergic conjunctivitis. Ketotifen[94] and azelastine[95] have shown promise in the treatment of allergic rhinitis and asthma in multicenter studies and may prove to be helpful adjuncts in patients with allergic conjunctivitis.

Because of the success that H_1-receptor antagonists have had in controlling the symptoms of allergic rhinitis, we designed a study to determine the therapeutic value of a wide variety of H_1 antihistamines for ophthalmic use by performing ocular toxicity and efficacy tests in rabbits and humans.[96] Nontoxic compounds were tested in human subjects for comfort and efficacy in alleviating symptoms in the histamine model of allergic conjunctivitis and compared with 0.3% pheniramine. Dose-response curves for itching and conjunctival redness were generated to identify the ideal concentration for each antihistamine compound found to be

TABLE 28–4. **Ocular Decongestants, Decongestant-Astringents, and Decongestant-Antibacterials**

Generic Name	Commercial Preparations (drops)	Usual Recommended Dosage (7–14 Days)
Decongestants		
Naphazoline (0.12% [Rx]; 0.012% [OTC])	Albalon (OTC) Clear Eyes (OTC) Degest-2 (OTC) Opcon (OTC) Naphcon (OTC) Naphcon Forte (Rx) Vasoclear (OTC) Vasocon Regular (OTC)	1 drop/eye q3–4hr or less to relieve symptoms
Phenylephrine (0.12%)	AK-nephrine (OTC) Prefrin (OTC) Relief (OTC)	1 drop/eye q3–4hr or less to relieve symptoms
Tetrahydrozoline HCl (0.05%)	Collyrium (OTC) Murine PLUS (OTC) Visine (OTC)	1 drop/eye q3–4hr or less to relieve symptoms
Decongestant-Astringents		
Naphazoline (0.02%) Zinc SO_4 (0.25%)	Vasoclear A (OTC)	1–2 drops/eye up to 4 times daily
Phenylephrine HCl (0.12%) Zinc SO_4 (0.25%)	Visine AC (OTC)	1–2 drops/eye up to 4 times daily
Tetrahydrozoline HCl (0.05%) Zinc SO_4 (0.25%)	Zincfrin (Rx)	1–2 drops/eye up to 4 times daily
Decongestant-Antibacterials		
Phenylephrine HCl (0.12%) Sulfacetamide Na (15%)	Vasosulf (Rx)	1–2 drops/eye q4hr

Modified from Pavan-Langston D, Dunkel EC: Handbook of Ocular Drug Therapy and Ocular Side Effects of Systemic Drugs. Boston, Little, Brown, 1991.

efficacious. These compounds were then compared with 0.3% pheniramine.

Results of this study demonstrated that 0.1% chlorpheniramine (P = .03), 0.2% chlorpheniramine (P = .04), 0.3% chlorpheniramine (P = .04), 0.3% dexbrompheniramine (P = .01), 0.2% pyrilamine (P = .03), 0.4% pheniramine (P = .03), and 0.5% pheniramine (P = .003) were significantly more effective in preventing histamine-induced itching and were superior in preventing histamine-induced conjunctival injection when compared with 0.3% pheniramine maleate. The results suggest that these seven formulations were more efficacious in the symptomatic treatment of allergic conjunctivitis than compounds currently available and should be considered for possible use as ophthalmic antihistamines.

Histamine H_2-Receptor Antagonists

CHEMISTRY

The H_2-receptor antagonists were born of the idea to develop compounds that would block those responses induced by histamine that could not be blocked by the currently available H_1-receptor antagonists. The H_2-receptor antagonists were synthesized by a series of modifications of the histamine molecule and therefore have a structural relationship to histamine (Table 28–5). The first selective H_2-receptor antagonist, burimamide, was synthesized in 1969 by substituting bulkier, uncharged side chains to the imidazole ring.[26] Subsequently, two imidazole ring congeners—metiamide,[97] a thione-containing compound, and cimetidine,[98] a cyanimino compound—were developed. More recently, ranitidine, a furan derivative, has become available.[99] Each of these compounds contains a polar heterocyclic ring in its side chain.

STRUCTURE-ACTIVITY RELATIONSHIP

The H_2-receptor antagonists bear a closer structural relationship to histamine than do the H_1-receptor antagonists. Burimamide, metiamide, and cimetidine have an imidazole ring and are polar, hydrophilic compounds similar to histamine (see Table 28–2). It appears that the imidazole or another heterocyclic, side chain ring is critical for H_2-receptor site recognition and plays a role in determining drug activity.[76] The H_2-receptor antagonist compounds have similar equilibrium constants (pK_a values of approximately 14). These drugs are weak bases and highly water-soluble; thus, they exist in the uncharged form in aqueous solutions under physiologic conditions (pH of 7.4).[76]

MECHANISM OF ACTION

The H_2-receptor antagonists work in a manner similar to that of the H_1-receptor antihistamines. These agents bind reversibly and competitively to the histamine H_2 receptors on effector cells. When bound to the receptor site, the H_2-receptor antagonist agents do not elicit a tissue response and block the effect of histamine.

PHARMACOKINETICS: ABSORPTION, DISTRIBUTION, BIOTRANSFORMATION, AND ELIMINATION

Cimetidine, the prototype of the H_2-receptor antagonist drugs, is well absorbed after oral administration. After an oral dose, peak blood concentrations are reached in approximately 60 to 90 minutes with good tissue distribution throughout the body.[79] The one exception is the CNS; cimetidine penetrates the CNS poorly because the compound is poorly lipophilic. The drug has been found to cross the placental barrier and is excreted in breast milk.[79]

The majority of an oral dose of cimetidine is excreted in the urine, with a minor portion handled in the bile and by hepatic microsomal biotransformation. In patients with normal renal function, the plasma half-life ($t_{1/2}$) is approximately 2 hours. However, the $t_{1/2}$ increases in patients with impaired hepatic or renal function.[100]

PHARMACOLOGIC PROPERTIES

Cimetidine and the other H_2-receptor antagonist antihistamines are selective in their action and block the effects of histamine mediated through the H_2-receptor. The most noteworthy systemic effect is the ability of these agents to inhibit gastric secretion induced by histamine, gastrin, or pentagastrin in humans.[101–103] Cimetidine inhibits all phases of physiologic secretion of gastric acid. In humans, a single

TABLE 28–5. **Representative Histamine H_2-Antagonists Compared with Histamine**

Structure and Name	Ring Type	Relative Antagonist Potency	Reference
$CH_2CH_2NH_2$; HN, N (imidazole ring) Histamine	Imidazole	—	—
NH_2; CH_2CH_2NHC ⊕; NH_2; HN, N N^{α}-Guanylhistamine	Imidazole	.001	Durant et al. (1975)[108] Durant et al. (1977)[109] Ganellin (1978)[110]
$(CH_2)_4NHC$— NH CH_3; ‖ S; HN, N Burimamide	Imidazole	.1	Black et al. (1972)[101] Durant et al. (1977)[109] Ganellin (1978)[110]
$NHCH_3$; CH_3; $CH_2S(CH_2)_2NHC$; ‖ S; HN, N Metiamide	Imidazole	~1	Black et al. (1973)[103] Durant et al. (1977)[109] Forrest et al. (1975)[104] Ganellin (1978)[110]
$NHCH_3$; CH_3; $CH_2S(CH_2)_2NHC$; ‖ NCN; HN, N Cimetidine	Imidazole	1	Brimblecombe et al. (1975)[111] Durant et al. (1977)[109] Ganellin (1978)[110]
$NHCH_3$; $(CH_3)_2NCH_2$, O (furan ring), $CH_2S(CH_2)_2NHC$; ‖ HC—NO_2 Ranitidine	Furan	3-5	Brittain and Daly (1981)[112]
O; CH_2; N; O, CH_2, O; H_3C; $CH_2S(CH_2)_2NH$; N H; HN, N Oxmetidine	Imidazole	1-4	Blakemore et al. (1980)[113] Mills et al. (1982)[114]

From Trzeciakowski JP, Mendelsohn N, Levi R: Antihistamines. *In* Middleton E, Reed CE, Ellis EF, et al (eds): Allergy Principles and Practice, 3rd ed. St. Louis, CV Mosby, 1985.

300-mg dose decreases the fasting secretion of gastric acid and decreases the amount of acid induced by food or via vagal stimulation.[79]

When given intravenously in high doses, cimetidine may cause bradycardia and hypotension. However, when given to normal volunteer subjects, the cardiovascular changes were minor.[101] As previously mentioned, systemic administration of histamine caused vasodilation and severe hypotension that were completely blocked only by the concurrent use of both H_1- and H_2-receptor antihistamines.

In the eye, stimulation of H_2-receptors with a selective H_2 agonist produced diffuse conjunctival vasodilation.[39] Cimetidine has been the only H_2-receptor antagonist to be formulated into an ophthalmic preparation. Studies have shown that the addition of an H_2-receptor antagonist to a classic H_1 antihistamine reduced the amount of conjunctival vasodilation in response to histamine challenge.[57]

ADVERSE EFFECTS

Systemic Administration

The H_2-receptor antagonists are generally well tolerated when taken systematically. The side effects of cimetidine are minor, seldom posing a serious problem, and include headaches, fatigue, myalgias, constipation, and skin rashes. The CNS-depressive effects seen with the H_1 antihistamines are not seen with the H_2-receptor blockers, because these compounds are hydrophilic and penetrate the blood-brain barrier poorly. However, cimetidine has been associated with confusion, delirium, and convulsions, usually occurring in patients with concurrent liver or kidney disease.

Cimetidine possesses weak antiandrogenic effects and has been responsible for reports of gynecomastia in men and galactorrhea in women. These effects have occurred in patients treated for an extended length of time. Cimetidine has been demonstrated to release prolactin when given in large intravenous doses.[104, 105] There have been sporadic reports in the literature of bone marrow suppression associated with cimetidine therapy. Patients have experienced leukopenia, thrombocytopenia, and hemolytic anemia, which seems to be an idiosyncratic reaction.[106]

Cimetidine is metabolized partially by the hepatic microsomal enzyme system and therefore may impair the elimination of drugs that are catabolized in this manner. These drugs include oral anticoagulants,[107] theophylline,[108] benzodiazepines,[109] and propranolol.[110] Additionally, the pharmacokinetics of calcium channel blockers are altered by cimetidine.[111]

Topical Ocular Administration

Currently, no H_2-receptor antihistamines are approved for ocular use. However, it is conceivable that combination drops consisting of H_1 and H_2 antagonists have a place in the treatment of ocular allergic disorders. Studies have shown that combination drops have a synergistic effect in reducing conjunctival vasodilation and chemosis when compared with the individual agents alone.

PREPARATIONS AND DOSAGES

Studies evaluating cimetidine as a topical ocular preparation have found concentrations of 0.1%, 0.5%, and 1.0% to be well tolerated and efficacious in reducing ocular symptoms induced by histamine challenge.

NEW ADVANCES IN THERAPY

Since the discovery of cimetidine, two additional H_2-receptor antagonists have been developed, ranitidine and famotidine. Both of these agents are significantly more potent than cimetidine and may prove to be efficacious in the treatment of ocular allergic disorders.

Mast Cell Stabilizers

CHEMISTRY

The first mast cell–stabilizing compound was developed in the late 1960s from khellin, a chromone (benzopyrene) derived from *Ammi visnaga,* an eastern Mediterranean plant.[112] Successive modifications in structure yielded several *bis*-chromone compounds, one of which was DSCG. DSCG is the disodium salt of 1,3-*bis*(2-carboxychromon-5-yloxy)-2-hydroxypropane (Fig. 28–2). The compound is composed of two chromone rings joined by a flexible carbon chain, with each ring possessing a polar carboxyl group. The compound is an odorless, white, dehydrated crystalline powder that is moderately soluble in water but practically insoluble in alcohol.[113] The drug was first discovered to have antiasthma properties when Altounyan demonstrated on himself that cromolyn could afford protection against an asthmatic attack induced by bronchial provocation with pollen antigens.[60]

STRUCTURE-ACTIVITY RELATIONSHIP

Disodium cromoglycate forms complexes with divalent cations, including magnesium (Mg^{2+}), calcium (Ca^{2+}), strontium (Sr^{2+}), barium (Ba^{2+}), zinc (Zn^{2+}), and manganese (Mn^{2+}) when placed in organic solvents. These complexes are formed by an electrostatic interaction between the two carboxyl groups of DSCG and the divalent cations with a 1:1 stoichiometry.[114] Although cromolyn has been associated with reduced calcium flux across the mast cell membrane, chelation of calcium by cromolyn does not fully account for the drug's ability to inhibit mast cell degranulation. It has been demonstrated that DSCG interacts with a membrane-bound cromolyn receptor, which is a calcium-transporting protein necessary for the secretion of histamine. This interaction requires the presence of calcium ions in order to proceed.[115]

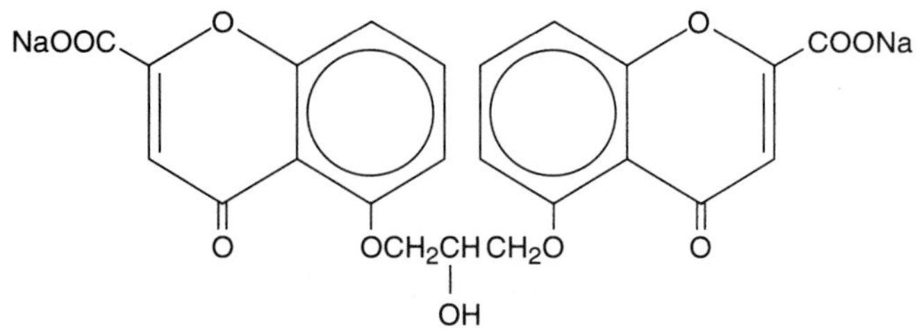

FIGURE 28–2. The chemical structure of disodium cromoglycate (cromolyn sodium) [1, 3-*bis*(2-carboxychromon-5-yloxy)-2-hydroxypropane].

MECHANISM OF ACTION

It had been thought that DSCG possessed membrane-stabilizing features in that the drug somehow modified the mast cell membrane to prevent histamine release in the presence of IgE antibody. When cromolyn was discovered, little was known of its mechanism of action. However, since the 1980s, evidence from research has shed light on the interaction between this drug and the mast cell. In 1980, Mazurek and coworkers identified a binding site on mast cells and basophils for DSCG.[115] The authors identified the cromolyn receptor as a membrane-binding protein that required the presence of calcium ions for the interaction to proceed. The evidence from the experiments suggests that the cromolyn-binding protein is a calcium-transporting protein that is necessary for the secretion of histamine after stimulation by an IgE antibody-antigen interaction.[116] It is theorized that the membrane-bound cromolyn-binding protein interacts with the Fc receptors for IgE in such a way that cross-linking of the Fc receptors does not occur upon antigen binding to the IgE molecule.[117]

Also in 1980, other researchers examined the association between DSCG and protein phosphorylation in the activation and regulation of histamine secretion in mast cells. Theoharides and associates demonstrated that cromolyn induced phosphorylation of a 78,000-Da mast cell protein.[118] These authors presented compelling data suggesting that DSCG and phosphorylation of the membrane-bound protein are intricately involved in the regulation of histamine secretion. The concentration range over which DSCG induced phosphorylation of proteins was similar to that for cromolyn-induced inhibition of histamine release stimulated by compound 48/80. Additionally, both activation of phosphorylation and inhibition of secretion by DSCG demonstrated tachyphylaxis—that is, a second exposure to cromolyn failed to induce phosphorylation in mast cells that were pretreated with the drug. Lastly, dephosphorylation after cromolyn-induced phosphorylation of the 78,000-Da protein had a time course identical to that of the loss of sensitivity of mast cells to the inhibition of histamine release caused by cromolyn.

The mechanism of protein phosphorylation has not been elucidated; however, it has been shown that cyclic guanosine monophosphate can phosphorylate the same 78,000-Da mast cell protein as cromolyn does. Thus, it has been theorized that cromolyn may act via a cyclic guanosine monophosphate–dependent protein kinase.[119] This is not surprising in that DSCG has been identified as an inhibitor of cyclic nucleotide phosphodiesterase.[120]

PHARMACOKINETICS: ABSORPTION, DISTRIBUTION, BIOTRANSFORMATION, AND ELIMINATION

DSCG is poorly absorbed from the gastrointestinal tract after oral administration. Therefore, it is available as an inhalant that can be administered via the nasal or respiratory tract. When given as an inhaled dose, approximately 8% is absorbed systematically through the bronchial tree.[121] The $t_{1/2}$ of the compound is approximately 80 minutes, with more than 98% being eliminated within 24 hours.[79] Cromolyn is not metabolized and is excreted unchanged in the urine and bile.

Little information is available on the pharmacokinetics of topically applied ocular disodium cromoglycate. Cromolyn is administered to the ocular surface via application of a water-soluble solution.

Currently, two mast cell-stabilizing drugs are approved for use in the eye: 4% DSCG (Crolom) and 0.1% lodoxamide tromethamine (Alomide). Both preparations are well distributed in the preocular tear film and seem to adequately penetrate the conjunctival epithelium and substantia propria. When administered to normal volunteer subjects, approximately 0.03% of DSCG was absorbed following an ocular dose.

PHARMACOLOGIC PROPERTIES

The pharmacologic actions of mast cell stabilizers result from the ability of the drug to bind to membrane-bound protein receptors on mast cells. This interaction inhibits histamine release when IgE-primed mast cells are challenged with antigen. Mast cell stabilizers do not interfere with the binding of IgE to the Fc receptors on mast cells or the interaction between mast cell–bound IgE and antigen. Mast cell stabilizers have no bronchodilator, antiinflammatory, or anticholinergic activity; rather, they suppress the mast cell secretory response to antigen. Thus, the drug is effective only when given prophylactically prior to an antigen–IgE antibody interaction.

Inhaled DSCG is recognized as an effective prophylactic drug for the treatment of asthma.[61–63] Cromolyn has also been demonstrated to have salutary effects in patients with food allergy,[64] systemic mastocytosis,[65] and seasonal allergic rhinitis.[66, 67] However, it should be noted that the effectiveness of the drug in these conditions remains controversial.

In the eye, 0.1% lodoxamide tromethamine[45, 46] and DSCG[68, 69] have shown effectiveness in relieving the signs and symptoms of VKC. The latter helped to reduce the frequency of steroid use in patients with VKC. When these two drugs were compared in a multicenter, double-masked, parallel-group clinical study, 0.1% lodoxamide was found to be statistically superior to 4% cromolyn in alleviating itching, tearing, foreign body sensation, and discomfort in patients with VKC.[45]

Likewise, clinical studies have demonstrated encouraging results with DSCG in acute allergic conjunctivitis. In general, investigators have reported satisfactory results with DSCG in acute allergic conjunctivitis. Greenbaum and associates[70] conducted the first environmental study evaluating 4% DSCG in a double-blind, placebo-controlled fashion and reported that eye symptom scores for patients receiving DSCG were significantly lower when compared with the previous year's ragweed season. In a double-masked, placebo-controlled, parallel-group prospective environmental study, Friday et al.[71] demonstrated that 4% DSCG was a safe and effective method of controlling the symptoms of ragweed conjunctivitis in patients with serum IgE levels less than 100 ng/mL. Patients with serum IgE levels greater than 100 ng/mL did not experience a significant improvement in symptoms. Leino and Tuovinen[72] evaluated DSCG in 33 patients with VKC, allergic conjunctivitis, or chronic conjunctivitis in a prospective uncontrolled study. The authors reported a beneficial effect associated with the use of DSCG; however, regression of the signs and symptoms varied widely.

Two well-designed, double-blind, placebo-controlled, comparative environmental studies reported that DSCG suppressed allergic eye symptoms in specific groups of patients identified by serum IgE antibody levels. However, the results were contradictory. Welsh et al.[73] showed that 4% DSCG caused a significant reduction in eye itching and irritation in subjects whose preseasonal IgE ragweed antibody level was less than 99 ng/mL; patients with IgE levels exceeding 100 ng/mL did not experience the same benefit. Kray et al.[74] stratified their subjects by radioallergosorbent (RAST) scores to IgE antibodies, including ragweed. These investigators noted a significant suppression of eye symptoms in subjects with class 3 or 4 RAST scores (higher antibody level). Subjects with classes 0, 1, and 2 RAST scores noted no significant difference between DSCG and placebo.

ADVERSE EFFECTS

Systemic Administration

Therapeutic doses of DSCG are well tolerated by patients. Most adverse reactions are mild and are associated with a direct irritant effect of the powder on the bronchial tree, including bronchospasm, wheezing, cough, sneezing, nasal congestion, and pharyngeal irritation.[79] Other adverse effects have been documented in case reports and consist of dermatitis, gastroenteritis, myositis, urethral burning, and pulmonary allergic granulomatosis.[122–125]

DSCG has no known effect on pregnancy in laboratory animals; however, safety for human use during pregnancy has not been established, and no controlled human studies have been performed.[79] It is not known whether the drug is excreted in human breast milk, and the safety and efficacy of cromolyn have not been established in children younger than 4 years.

Topical Ocular Administration

Topical administration of mast cell stabilizers in the eye has been associated with a low incidence of systemic adverse effects. Ocular side effects are common but usually mild and self-limited. Ocular administration of cromolyn has been associated with transient stinging and conjunctival injection. Other local adverse reactions include chemosis and ocular and periocular itching and irritation.

PREPARATIONS AND DOSAGES

Currently, the only mast cell–stabilizing drugs formulated for topical ocular use are 4% disodium cromoglycate (Opticrom) and 0.1% lodoxamide tromethamine. The former preparation, 4% disodium cromoglycate, contains 40 mg of DSCG in purified water with a preservative and is a clear, colorless, sterile solution with a pH of 4.0 to 7.0. The recommended dosage is one to two drops instilled in the eye four times daily. One drop of the solution contains approximately 1.6 mg of DSCG. The latter preparation, 0.1% lodoxamide tromethamine, contains 1.78 mg of lodoxamide tromethamine in purified water with EDTA, benzalkonium chloride, and other inactive ingredients. This preparation has been shown to be 2500 times more potent than DSCG[126] and has demonstrated satisfactory results in patients with atopic keratoconjunctivitis (AKC) and giant papillary conjunctivitis (GPC).[127] The recommended dosage is one drop applied four times daily, although patients have been able to use 0.1% lodoxamide tromethamine twice daily and still remain asymptomatic.

Because therapy with mast cell stabilizers is prophylactic, it is advisable to initiate treatment before the onset of allergic symptoms. It is not unexpected that symptomatic response to treatment may take up to 2 weeks with DSCG and up to 4 days with 0.1% lodoxamide tromethamine. Once therapy has commenced, it should be continuous and maintained even after symptomatic improvement.

NEW ADVANCES IN THERAPY

Currently, a new mast cell–stabilizing agent, a disodium salt of pyranoquinoline dicarboxylic acid (nedocromil), has demonstrated efficacy in patients with asthma.[128] Two percent nedocromil (Tilavist) was evaluated in allergic conjunctivitis and was found to be more effective than placebo in controlling itching and ocular irritation.[129, 130]

New Therapy for Ocular Allergy

Since the 1980s, researchers have explored different methods to block the allergic response in type I hypersensitivity reactions. It was discovered that Fc fragments from IgE antibody could competitively inhibit IgE binding to effector cells and block the Prausnitz-Küstner reaction when preinjected into skin.[131] HEPP (pentigetide), a synthetic pentapeptide derived from the Fc region of human IgE, was developed and consisted of an amino acid sequence of aspartyl-seryl-aspartyl-prolyl-arginine. In tests on atopic persons, HEPP blocked the Prausnitz-Küstner reaction[132]; however, its mechanism of action remains unknown. In a double-blind, randomized, parallel study, 0.5% pentigetide (Pentyde) ophthalmic solution was compared with 4% DSCG in patients with allergic conjunctivitis.[133] After a 2-week comparison, patients treated with 0.5% pentigetide experienced significant improvement in conjunctival hyperemia, chemosis, tearing, and itching. With further study, this drug may prove to be a useful adjunct in the treatment of allergic conjunctivitis.

As previously mentioned, other mediators of inflammation contribute to and help perpetuate the ocular allergic response. Several classes of pharmacologic agents have demonstrated efficacy in blocking the effects of these mediators of inflammation, and hence possess anti-allergic properties when used as ocular preparations. In CAC studies, topical nonsteroidal antiinflammatory drugs such as 0.5% ketorolac tromethamine (Acular), 0.03% flurbiprofen sodium (Ocufen), and 0.1% diclofenac sodium (Voltaren) and topical corticosteroid agents such as 0.5% loteprednol etabonate (Lotemax) and 1% rimexolone (Vexol) have demonstrated effectiveness in controlling the signs and symptoms of allergic conjunctivitis. Researchers are actively investigating compounds that blunt the response to or inhibit the action of these inflammatory mediators. In the future, we expect to have available topical medications such as anti–platelet activating factor and leukotriene inhibitors to add to our list of antiallergic drugs.

REFERENCES

1. Gell PGH, Coombs RRA: Clinical Aspects of Immunology, 2nd ed. Oxford, Blackwell Scientific, 1968, pp 575–596.
2. Allansmith MR, Abelson MB: Ocular allergies. *In* Smolin G, Thoft RA (eds): The Cornea. Boston, Little Brown, 1983, pp 231–243.
3. Ishizaka T, Ishizaka K: Biology of immunoglobulin E: Molecular basis of reaginic hypersensitivity. Prog Allergy 19:60, 1975.
4. Siraganian RP, Hook WA, Levine BB: Specific in vitro histamine release from basophils by bivalent haptens: Evidence for activation by simple bridging of membrane bound antibody. Immunochemistry 12:149, 1975.
5. Foreman FC, Hallett MB, Mangar J: The relationship between histamine secretion and ^{45}calcium uptake by mast cells. J Physiol (Lond) 271:193, 1977.
6. Austen KF, Brocklehurst WE: Anaphylaxis in chopped guinea pig lung. I. Effect of peptidase substrate and inhibitors. J Exp Med 133:521, 1960.
7. Hirata F, Axelrod J: Enzymatic synthesis and rapid translocation of phosphatidylcholine by two methyltransferases in erythrocyte membranes. Proc Natl Acad Sci U S A 75:2348, 1978.
8. Ishizaka T, Hirata F, Sterk AR, et al: Bridging of IgE receptors activates phospholipid methylation and adenylate cyclase in mast cell plasma membranes. Proc Natl Acad Sci U S A 78:6812, 1981.
9. Lewis RA, Holgate ST, Roberts LJ II, et al: Effects of indomethacin on cyclic nucleotide levels and histamine release from rat serosal mast cells. J Immunol 123:1633, 1979.
10. Flowers RJ, Blackwell GJ: The importance of phospholipase A^2 in prostaglandin biosynthesis. Biochem Pharmacol 25:285, 1976.
11. Warner JA, Peters SP, Lichtenstein LM, MacGlashan DW Jr: ^{3}H arachidonic acid incorporation and metabolism in purified human basophils. [Abstract] Fed Proc 45:735, 1986.
12. Hanahan DJ, Demopoulos CA, Liehr J, Pinckard RN: Identification of naturally occurring platelet activating factor as acetyl-glyceryl-ether-phosphorylcholine (AGEPC). J Biol Chem 255:5514, 1980.
13. Chilton FH, Ellis JM, Olson SC, Wykle RL: 1-O-alkyl-2 arachidonoyl-sn-glycero-3-phosphocholine: A common source of platelet activating factor and arachidonate in human polymorphonuclear leukocytes. J Biol Chem 259:12014, 1984.
14. Barnes PJ: New concepts in the pathogenesis of bronchial hyperresponsiveness and asthma. J Allergy Clin Immunol 83:1013, 1989.
15. Dvorak AM, Galli SJ, Schulman ES, et al: Basophil and mast cell degranulation: Ultrastructural analysis of mechanisms of mediator release. Fed Proc 42:2510, 1983.
16. Dvorak AM, Hammel I, Schulman ES, et al: Differences in behavior of cytoplasmic granules and lipid bodies during human lung mast cell degranulation. J Cell Biol 99:1678, 1984.
17. Dvorak AM, Schulman ES, Peters SP, et al: Immunoglobulin E–mediated degranulation of isolated human lung mast cells. Lab Invest 53:45, 1985.
18. Windaus A, Vogt W: Syntèse des imidazolylathylamins. Ber Dtsch Chem Ges 3:3691, 1907.
19. Dale HH, Laidlaw PP: The physiologic action of beta-imidazolethylamine. J Physiol (Lond) 41:318, 1910.
20. Dale HH, Laidlaw PP: Histamine shock. J Physiol (Lond) 52:355, 1919.
21. Best CH, Dale HH, Dudley HW, Thorpe WV: The nature of vasodilator constituents of certain tissue extracts. J Physiol (Lond) 62:397, 1927.
22. Riley JF, West GB: The presence of histamine in tissue mast cells. J Physiol (Lond) 120:528, 1953.
23. Schwartz LB, Austen KF: Structure and function of the chemical mediators of mast cells. Prog Allergy 34:271, 1984.
24. Snyder SH, Axelrod J: Tissue metabolism of histamine-^{14}C in vivo. Fed Proc 24:774, 1965.
25. Ash ASF, Schild HO: Receptors mediating some actions of histamine. Br J Pharmacol Chemother 27:427, 1966.
26. Black JW, Duncan WAM, Durant GJ, et al: Definition and antagonism of histamine H_2-receptors. Nature 236:385, 1972.
27. Owen DAA, Poy E, Woodward DF: Evaluation of the role of histamine H_1- and H_2-receptors in cutaneous inflammation in the guinea-pig produced by histamine and mast cell degranulation. Br J Pharmacol 69:615, 1980.
28. Robertson I, Greaves MW: Responses of human skin blood vessels to synthetic histamine analogues. Br J Clin Pharmacol 5:319, 1978.
29. Harvey RP, Schocket AL: The effect of H_1 and H_2 blockade on cutaneous histamine response in man. J Allergy Clin Immunol 65:136, 1980.
30. McCusker MT, Chung KF, Roberts NM, Barnes PJ: Effects of topical capsaicin on the cutaneous responses to inflammatory mediators and to antigen in man. J Allergy Clin Immunol 83:1118, 1989.
31. Smith JA, Mansfield LE, deShazo R, Nelson HS: An evaluation of the pharmacologic inhibition of the immediate and late cutaneous effects to allergen. J Allergy Clin Immunol 65:118, 1980.
32. Abelson MB, Baird RS, Allansmith MR: Tear histamine levels in vernal conjunctivitis and other ocular inflammations. Ophthalmology 87:812, 1980.
33. Levene RZ: Mast cells and amines in normal ocular tissues. Invest Ophthalmol 1:531, 1962.
34. Smelser GK, Silver S: The distribution of mast cells in the normal eye: A method of study. Exp Eye Res 2:134, 1963.
35. Allansmith MR, Greiner JV, Baird RS: Number of inflammatory cells in the normal conjunctiva. Am J Ophthalmol 86:250, 1978.
36. Abelson MB, Soter NA, Simon MA, et al: Histamine in human tears. Am J Ophthalmol 83:417, 1977.
37. Abelson MB, Allansmith MR: Histamine and the eye. *In* Silverstein AM, O'Connor GR (eds): Immunology and Immunopathology of the Eye. New York, Masson, 1979, pp 362–364.
38. Weston JH, Udell IJ, Abelson MB: H_1 receptors in the human ocular surface. Invest Ophthalmol Vis Sci 20(Suppl):32, 1981.
39. Abelson MB, Udell IJ: H_2-receptors in the human ocular surface. Arch Ophthalmol 99:302, 1981.
40. Friedlaender MH: Corticosteroid therapy of ocular inflammation. Int Ophthalmol Clin 23:175, 1983.
41. Greenbaum J, Cockcroft D, Hargreave FE, Dolovich J: Sodium cromoglycate in ragweed-allergic conjunctivitis. J Allergy Clin Immunol 59:437, 1977.
42. Friday GA, Biglan AW, Hiles DA, et al: Treatment of ragweed allergic conjunctivitis with cromolyn sodium 4% ophthalmic solution. Am J Ophthalmol 95:169, 1983.
43. Welsh PW, Yunginger JW, Tani DG, et al: Topical ocular administration of cromolyn sodium for treatment in seasonal ragweed conjunctivitis. J Allergy Clin Immunol 64:209, 1979.
44. Tani DG, Welsh PW, Bourne WM, et al: Cromolyn sodium treatment of seasonal ragweed conjunctivitis. Invest Ophthalmol Vis Sci 17(Suppl):227, 1978.
45. Caldwell DR, Verin P, Hartwich-Young R, et al: Efficacy and safety of lodoxamide 0.1% vs cromolyn sodium 4% in patients With vernal keratoconjunctivitis. Am J Ophthalmol 113:632, 1992.
46. Santos CI, Huang AJ, Abelson MB, et al: Efficacy of lodoxamide 0.1% ophthalmic solution in resolving corneal epitheliopathy associated with vernal keratoconjunctivitis. AM J Ophthalmol 117:488, 1994.
47. Abelson MB, Allansmith MR, Friedlaender MH: Effects of topically applied ocular decongestant and antihistamine. Am J Ophthalmol 90:254, 1980.
48. Abelson MB, George MA, Schaefer K, and Smith LM: Evaluation of the new ophthalmic antihistamine, 0.05% levocabastine, in the clinical allergen challenge model of allergic conjunctivitis. J Allergy Clin Immunol 94:458, 1994.
49. Sharif NA, Xu SX, Miller ST, et al: Characterization of the ocular antiallergic and antihistaminic effects of olopatadine (AL-4943A), a novel drug for treating ocular allergic diseases. J Pharm Exp Ther 278:1262, 1996.
50. Lewis T: The Blood Vessels of the Human Skin and Their Responses. London, Shaw, 1927.
51. Staub AM, Bovet D: Action de la thymoxyethyl-diethylamine (929F) et des ethers phenoliques sur le choc anaphylactique du cobaye. CR Soc Biol 125:818, 1937.
52. Halpern BN: Les antihistaminiques de syntèse: Essais de chimotherapie desétats alleriques. Arch Int Pharmacodyn Ther 68:339, 1942.
53. Bovet D, Horclois R, Walthort F: Proprietés antihistaminiques de la N-p-methoxybenzyl-N-dimethylaminoethyl amino-pyridine. CR Soc Biol 138:99, 1944.
54. Bourquin TB: A new synthetic antihistaminic substance (Antistine) and its use in ophthalmology. Schweiz Med Wochenschr 76:296, 1946.
55. Hurwitz P: Antistine in ocular allergy. Am J Ophthalmol 31:1409, 1948.
56. Miller J, Wolf EH: Antazoline phosphate and naphazoline hydrochloride, singly and in combination for the treatment of allergic conjunctivitis—A controlled, double-blind clinical trial. Ann Allergy 35:81, 1975.

57. Leon J, Charap A, Duzman E, Shen C: Efficacy of cimetidine/pyrilamine eyedrops, a dose response study with histamine challenge. Ophthalmology 93:120, 1986.
58. Mazurek N, Berger G, Pecht I: A binding site on mast cells and basophils for the anti-allergic drug cromolyn. Nature 286:722, 1980.
59. Theoharides TC, Sieghart W, Greengard P, Douglas WW: Antiallergic drug cromolyn may inhibit histamine secretion by regulating phosphorylation of a mast cell protein. Science 207:80, 1980.
60. Altounyan REC: Inhibition of experimental asthma by a new compound, disodium cromoglycate, "INTAL." Acta Allergol 22:487, 1967.
61. Bernstein IL, Siegel SC, Brandon ML, et al: A controlled study of cromolyn sodium sponsored by the Drug Committee of the American Academy of Allergy. J Allergy Clin Immunol 50:235, 1972.
62. Howarth PH, Durham SR, Lee TH, et al: Influence of albuterol, cromolyn sodium and ipratropium bromide on the airway and circulating mediator responses to allergen bronchial provocation in asthma. Am Rev Respir Dis 132:986, 1985.
63. Hughes D, Mindorff C, Levison H: The immediate effect of sodium cromoglycate on the airway. Ann Allergy 48:6, 1982.
64. Businco L, Cantani A, Benincori N, et al: Effectiveness of oral sodium cromoglycate (SCG) in preventing food allergy in children. Ann Allergy 51:47, 1983.
65. Dolovich J, Punthakee ND, MacMillan AB, Osbaldeston GJ: Systemic mastocytosis: Control of lifelong diarrhea by ingested disodium cromoglycate. Can Med Assoc J 111:684, 1974.
66. Sorri M, Jokinen K, Palva A: Disodium chromoglycate (sic) therapy in perennial rhinitis. Acta Otolaryngol 360(Suppl):30, 1979.
67. Pelikan Z: The effects of disodium cromoglycate and beclomethasone diproprionate on the late nasal mucosa response to allergen challenge. Ann Allergy 49:200, 1982.
68. Foster CS, Duncan J: Randomized clinical trial of topically administered cromolyn sodium for vernal keratoconjunctivitis. Am J Ophthalmol 90:175, 1980.
69. Easty DL, Rice NSC, Jones BR: Clinical trial of topical disodium cromoglycate in vernal kerato-conjunctivitis. Clin Allergy 2:99, 1972.
70. Greenbaum J, Cockcroft D, Hargreave FE, Dolovich J: Sodium cromoglycate in ragweed-allergic conjunctivitis. J Allergy Clin Immunol 59:437, 1977.
71. Friday GA, Biglan AW, Hiles DA, et al: Treatment of ragweed allergic conjunctivitis with cromolyn sodium 4% ophthalmic solution. Am J Ophthalmol 95:169, 1983.
72. Leino M, Tuovinen E: Clinical trial of the topical use of disodium cromoglycate in vernal, allergic and chronic conjunctivitis. Acta Ophthalmol 58:121, 1980.
73. Welsh PW, Yunginger JW, Tani DG, et al: Topical administration of cromolyn sodium for treatment in seasonal ragweed conjunctivitis. J Allergy Clin Immunol 64:209, 1979.
74. Kray KT, Squire EN, Tipton WR, et al: Cromolyn sodium in seasonal allergic conjunctivitis. J Allergy Clin Immunol 76:623, 1985.
75. Foster CS, Duncan J: Randomized clinical trial of topically administered cromolyn sodium for vernal keratoconjunctivitis. Am J Ophthalmol 90:175, 1980.
76. Ganellin CR: Chemistry and structure-activity relationships of H_2-receptor antagonists. *In* Rocha e Silva M (ed): Histamine II and Anti-Histaminics: Chemistry, Metabolism, and Physiological and Pharmacological Actions. Handbook of Experimental Pharmacology, vol 18, part 2. New York, Springer-Verlag, 1978, pp 251–294.
77. Ariens EJ, Simonis AM: Autonomic drugs and their receptors. Arch Int Pharmacodyn 127:479, 1960.
78. Rocha e Silva M: Kinetics of antagonist action. *In* Rocha e Silva M (ed): Histamine II and Anti-Histaminics: Chemistry, Metabolism, and Physiological and Pharmacological Actions. Handbook of Experimental Pharmacology, vol 18, part 2. New York, Springer-Verlag, 1978, pp 295–332.
79. Douglas W: Histamine and serotonin and their antagonists. *In* Goodman L, Gilman A, Rall T, Murad F (eds): The Pharmacologic Basis of Therapeutics, 7th ed. New York, Macmillan, 1985, pp 605–638.
80. Witiak DT, Lewis NJ: Absorption, distribution, metabolism and elimination of antihistamines. *In* Rocha e Silva M (ed): Histamine II and Anti-Histaminics: Chemistry, Metabolism, and Physiological and Pharmacological Actions. Handbook of Experimental Pharmacology, vol 18, part 2. New York, Springer-Verlag, 1978, pp 513–560.
81. Nathan RA, Segall N, Schocket AL: A comparison of the actions of H1 and H2 antihistamines on histamine-induced bronchoconstriction and cutaneous wheal response in asthmatic patients. J Allergy Clin Immunol 67:171, 1981.
82. Landau SW, Nelson NA, Gay LN: Antihistamine properties of local anesthetics and anesthetic properties of antihistaminic compounds. J Allergy 22:19, 1951.
83. Carruthers SG, Shoeman DW, Hignite CE, Azarnoff DL: Correlation between plasma diphenhydramine level and sedative and antihistamine effects. Clin Pharmacol Ther 23:375–382, 1978.
84. Crandall DC, Leopold IH: The influence of systemic drugs on tear constituents. Ophthalmology 86:115, 1979.
85. Loffler BH, Lemp MA: The effect of an antihistamine (chlorpheniramine maleate) on tear production in humans. Ann Ophthalmol 12:217, 1980.
86. Wyngaarten JB, Seevers MH: The toxic effect of antihistaminic drugs. JAMA 145:277, 1951.
87. Sadusk JF, Palmisano PA: Teratogenic effect of meclizine, cyclizine and chlorcyclizine. JAMA 194:987, 1965.
88. Pecoud A, Zuber P, Kolly M: Effect of a new selective H1 receptor antagonist (levocabastine) in a nasal and conjunctival provocation test. Int Arch Allergy Appl Immunol 82:541, 1987.
89. Abelson MB, Smith LM: Levocabastine evaluation in the histamine and compound 48/80 models of ocular allergy in humans. Ophthalmology 95:1494, 1988.
90. Abelson MB, George MA, Smith LM: Evaluation of 0.05% levocabastine versus 4% sodium cromolyn in the allergen challenge model. Ophthalmology 102:310, 1995.
91. Spitalny L, Abelson M: Olopatadine ophthalmic solution decreases itching and redness associated with allergic conjunctivitis. Invest Ophthalmol Vis Sci 37(Suppl):593, 1996.
92. Howarth PH, Emanuel MB, Holgate ST: Astemizole, a potent histamine H1-receptor antagonist: Effect in allergic rhinoconjunctivitis; on antigen and histamine induced skin wheal responses and relationship to serum levels. Br J Clin Pharmacol 18:1, 1984.
93. DelCarpio J, Kabbash L, Turenne Y, et al: Efficacy and safety of loratadine (10 mg once daily), terfenadine (60 mg twice daily), and placebo in the treatment of seasonal allergic rhinitis. J Allergy Clin Immunol 84:741, 1989.
94. Rackham A, Brown CA, Chandra RK, et al: A Canadian multicenter study with Zaditen (ketotifen) in the treatment of bronchial asthma in children aged 5 to 17 years. J Allergy Clin Immunol 84:286, 1989.
95. Meltzer EO, Storms WW, Pierson WE, et al: Efficacy of azelastine in perennial allergic rhinitis: Clinical and rhinomanometric evaluation. J Allergy Clin Immunol 82:447, 1988.
96. Berdy GJ, Smith LM, George MA, et al: Allergic conjunctivitis: A survey of new antihistamines. Ophthalmology 97(Suppl):136, 1990.
97. Black JW, Duncan WAM, Emmett JC, et al: Metiamide: An orally active histamine H_2-receptor antagonist. Agents Actions 3:133, 1973.
98. Colin-Jones DG, Langman MJS, Lawson DH, Vessey MP: Post-marketing surveillance of the safety of cimetidine: Mortality during second, third, and fourth years of follow up. Br Med J 291:1085, 1985.
99. Zeldis JB, Friedman LS, Isselbacher KJ: Ranitidine: A new H_2-receptor antagonist. N Engl J Med 309:1368, 1983.
100. Schentag JJ, Cerra FB, Calleri GM, et al: Age, disease and cimetidine disposition in healthy subjects and chronically ill patients. Clin Pharmacol Ther 29:737, 1981.
101. Bodemar G, Norlander B, Walan A: Cimetidine in the treatment of active peptic ulcer disease. *In* Burland WL, Simkins MA (eds): Cimetidine: Second International Symposium on Histamine H_2-Receptor Antagonists. Amsterdam, Excerpta Medica, 1977.
102. Brimblecombe RW, Duncan WAM: The relevance to man of preclinical data for cimetidine. *In* Burland WL, Simkins MA (eds): Cimetidine: Second International Symposium on Histamine H_2-receptor Antagonists. Amsterdam, Excerpta Medica, 1977.
103. Burland WL, Duncan WAM, Hessello T, et al: Pharmacological evaluation of cimetidine, a new histamine H_2-receptor antagonist, in healthy man. Br J Clin Pharmacol 2:481, 1975.
104. Lee PK, Lai LL, Lok ASF, et al: Haemodynamic responses to intravenous cimetidine in subjects with normal lung function and in subjects with chronic airway obstruction. Br J Clin Pharmacol 11:339, 1981.
105. Carlson HE, Ippoliti AF, Swerdloff RS: Endocrine effects of acute and chronic cimetidine administration. Dig Dis Sci 26:428, 1981.
106. MuGuigan JE: A consideration of the adverse effects of cimetidine. Gastroenterology 80:181, 1981.
107. Serlin MJ, Sibeon RG, Mossman S, et al: Cimetidine interaction with oral anticoagulants in man. Lancet 2:317, 1979.
108. Jackson JE, Powell JR, Wandell M, et al: Cimetidine decreases theophylline clearance. Am Rev Respir Dis 123:615, 1981.

109. Klotz U, Reiman I: Delayed clearance of diazepam due to cimetidine. N Engl J Med 302:1012, 1980.
110. Feely J, Wilkinson GR, Wood AJJ: Reduction of liver blood flow and propranolol metabolism by cimetidine. N Engl J Med 304:692, 1981.
111. Langman MJS: Gastrointestinal drugs. Side Eff Drugs Annu 10:323, 1986.
112. Cox JSG, Beach JE, Blair AMJN, et al: Disodium cromoglycate (Intal). Adv Drug Res 5:115, 1970.
113. Cox JSG: Disodium cromoglycate (FPL 67) (Intal): A specific inhibitor of reaginic antibody-antigen mechanisms. Nature 216:1328, 1967.
114. Mazurek N, Geller Bernstein C, Pecht I: Affinity of calcium ions to the antiallergic drug cromoglycate. FEBS Lett 111:194, 1980.
115. Mazurek N, Berger G, Pecht I: A binding site on mast cells and basophils for the antiallergic drug disodium cromoglycate. Nature 286:722, 1980.
116. Mazurek N, Bashkin P, Loyter A, Pecht I: Restoration of Ca^{2+} influx and degranulation capacity of variant RBL-2H3 cells upon implantation of isolated cromolyn binding protein. Proc Natl Acad Sci U S A 80:6014, 1983.
117. Mazurek N, Dulic V, Pecht I, et al: The role of Fc receptors in calcium channel opening in rat basophilic leukemic cells. Immunol Lett 12:31, 1986.
118. Theoharides TC, Sieghart W, Greengard P, Douglas WW: Antiallergic drug cromolyn may inhibit histamine secretion by regulating phosphorylation of a mast cell protein. Science 207:80, 1980.
119. Wells E, Mann J: Phosphorylation of a mast cell protein in response to treatment with antiallergic compounds: Implication for the mode of action of sodium cromoglycate. Biochem Pharmacol 32:837, 1983.
120. Bergstrand H, Lundquist B, Schurmann A: Rat mast cell high affinity cyclic nucleotide phosphodiesterases: Separation and inhibitory effects of two antiallergic agents. Mol Pharmacol 14:848, 1978.
121. Moss GF, Jones KM, Ritchie JT, et al: Plasma levels and urinary excretion of disodium cromoglycate after inhalation by human volunteers. Toxicol Appl Pharmacol 20:147, 1971.
122. Lobel H, Machtey J, Eldror MY: Pulmonary infiltrates with eosinophilia in an asthmatic patient treated with disodium cromoglycate. Lancet 2:1032, 1972.
123. Burgher LW, Kass I, Schenken JR: Pulmonary allergic granulomatosis: A possible drug reaction in a patient receiving cromolyn sodium. Chest 66:84, 1974.
124. Sheffer AL, Rocklin RE, Goetzl EJ: Immunologic components of hypersensitivity reactions to cromolyn sodium. N Engl J Med 293:1220, 1975.
125. Settipane GA, Klein DE, Boyd GK, et al: Adverse reactions to cromolyn. JAMA 241:811, 1979.
126. Johnson HG, VanHout CA, Wright JB: Inhibition of allergic reactions by cromoglycate and by a new anti-allergy drug U-42,585E. I: Activity in rats. Int Arch Allergy Appl Immunol 56:416, 1978.
127. Verstappen AA, Smith J, Rosenthal A: A double-masked efficacy and safety evaluation of lodoxamide 0.1% ophthalmic solution versus opticrom 2%: A multicenter study in patients with allergic eye disorders. Alcon Report No. 008:34350:1287, 1988.
128. Gonzalez JP, Brogden RN: Nedocromil sodium: A preliminary review of its pharmacodynamic and pharmacokinetic properties, and therapeutic efficacy in the treatment of reversible obstructive airways disease. Drugs 34:560, 1987.
129. Hirsh SR, Melamed J, Schwartz RH: Efficacy of nedocromil sodium 2% ophthalmic solution in the treatment of ragweed seasonal allergic conjunctivitis (SAC). J Allergy Clin Immunol 81:173, 1988.
130. Jarmoszuk I, Blumenthal M, Silvers W, et al: Nedocromil sodium 2% ophthalmic solution in the treatment of ragweed seasonal allergic conjunctivitis (SAC). J Allergy Clin Immunol 81:174, 1988.
131. Geha RS, Helm B, Gould H: Inhibition of the Prausnitz-Küstner reaction by an immunoglobulin E-chain fragment synthesized in *E. coli.* Nature 315:577, 1985.
132. Hamburger RN: Peptide inhibition of the Prausnitz-Küstner reaction. Science 189:389, 1975.
133. Kalpaxis JG, Thayer TO: Double-blind trial of pentigetide ophthalmic solution, 0.5%, compared with cromolyn sodium, 4%, ophthalmic solution for allergic conjunctivitis. Ann Allergy 66:393, 1991.

CHAPTER 29

Tear Film and Blink Dynamics

Marshall G. Doane

Dynamics of the Blinking Process

Blinking is usually performed as a nonconscious closing of the eyelids and serves to carry secreted tear fluid from the superior and inferior marginal menisci over the anterior surface of the eye, continuously reestablishing the tear film over the cornea. Also, the blinking action wipes debris and particulate matter from the surface of the cornea and sclera into the inferior marginal tear meniscus. As we shall see, once in the meniscus, such debris is effectively directed toward the medial canthal region by subsequent blinks and either drained with "used" tear fluid via the punctal openings or removed by a simple sweep of a finger. This constant drainage via the puncta is necessary to allow for the removal of used tear fluid, but it also removes instilled tear substitutes from the menisci, therefore limiting their effective residence time and requiring frequent reinstillation of such products.

Although the normal blink rate is often given as 12 to 15 per minute, this is, at best, an average of a greatly variable parameter, and it is strongly influenced by external events. A loud noise or bright flash of light, of course, immediately elicits a blink by reflex action, but more subtle events such as a visually intensive task (e.g., reading, watching a computer monitor) reduces the blink rate, thus increasing the length of interblink periods and minimizing how often vision is blocked by the closing of the eyelids. A person's tear film stability also can influence the blink rate; because discomfort is usually associated with the breakup and drying of the tear film on the cornea, this can stimulate blinking. Thus, many dry-eyed patients tend to have shortened blink intervals (i.e., high blink rates) as a result of the decreased tear film breakup time during interblink periods. A major goal of any tear substitute is to increase the stability of the tear film layer, usually by incorporating surfactants and viscosity agents, as described in the following section.

The details of the actual motion of the blinking eyelids occur too rapidly to see. With a high-speed motion picture or video camera, the recorded images can be replayed at a slower speed and the details of the motion accurately determined. Truly nonconscious blinks can only be recorded if the subject is *not* aware that such blinks are being measured or indeed that blinking is a subject of interest. Self-conscious blinks are invariably forced, and such blinks differ significantly in their dynamics and time course from the ordinary, nonconscious blinking that occurs thousands of times each day.

Studies using a high-speed camera and long telephoto lens placed behind a one-way mirror have recorded the normal, nonconscious blinks of an unknowing subject.[1] With a film-recording rate of up to 500 pictures per second, the resultant images were subsequently analyzed frame by frame for the details of motion of each lid, including their instantaneous velocities.

Motion of the Upper Lid

The upper lid is responsible for wiping the anterior surface of the globe and restoring a clean, "new" tear film with each blink. From its open, resting position, the upper lid rapidly accelerates downward until reaching the center of the cornea. It then decelerates, often slowing to a stop and reversing its motion before actually contacting the lower lid. Even when such contact does occur, it is seldom forceful except during strong, voluntary blinks. Figure 29–1 shows typical time and velocity profiles of the upper lid for four consecutive nonconscious blinks in four subjects. The point of zero velocity is the instant of reversal of motion between the closing and opening phase of the blink. Note that the opening phase consumes about twice the time of the closing phase and is particularly slow during the last few millimeters of lid opening. The reversal of lid motion is rapid, occurring in less than 2 msec; in voluntary blinking, the lid remains stationary for much longer, a consistent feature of such blinks. The maximum downward excursion of the upper lid is, of course, limited to the width of the palpebral fissure at the open, resting position of the lids. Many, if not most, blinks are less than complete, with the amount of lid excursion less than the maximum possible for a given individual. For the examples shown, the maximum excursion of the upper lid ranges from 5 to 13 mm and peak velocities from 80 to 300 mm/sec.

As indicated by the lid velocity profiles shown in Figure 29–1, blink velocities vary considerably among individuals and even between consecutive blinks in the same person. Nevertheless, by averaging the information for many nonconscious blinks, the data for a standard, nonforced blink have been obtained (Table 29–1).

TABLE 29–1. **Dynamics of Upper Eyelid Motion During a Blink***

Factor	Value
Duration of closing phase	82.1 ± 2.1 msec
Duration of opening phase	175.8 ± 11.0 msec
Total blink duration	257.9 ± 11.3 msec
Maximum closing velocity	18.7 ± 1.7 cm/sec
Maximum opening velocity	9.7 ± 0.7 cm/sec

*Each value given is an average of 40 blinks, ± standard error of the mean, in 10 different subjects.

From Doane MG: Interaction of eyelids and tears in corneal wetting and the dynamics of the normal human eyeblink. Am J Ophthalmol 89:507–516, 1980. Published with permission from the American Journal of Ophthalmology. Copyright by the Ophthalmic Publishing Company.

This blinking action of the upper lid efficiently spreads tear fluid from the marginal menisci over the entire anterior surface of the globe. This easily can be demonstrated by instilling a small drop of fluorescein solution from a micropipette into the tear meniscus along the inferior lid margin. A single blink uniformly distributes the fluorescein over the cornea. Thus, the instillation of a small quantity of a miscible tear substitute into the inferior tear meniscus can be reasonably expected to mix with the natural tear fluid in the meniscus and be spread over the entire anterior surface of the globe by the next few blinks of the lids.

Motion of the Lower Lid

The lower lid undergoes little vertical movement, its major motion being a horizontal translation directed toward the medial canthus during the closing of the upper lid. This motion reverses its direction in synchrony with the beginning of the opening phase of the upper lid. Total translation of the lower lid is proportional to the extent of movement of the upper lid, usually in the range of 2 to 5 mm. This horizontal motion is important in facilitating the turnover and drainage of the tear fluid via the punctal openings in the lid margin.

Tear Mixing, Turnover, and Drainage

Tear Volume and Mixing

As detailed earlier, the tear film is a quasilayered structure with numerous components secreted from many spatially separated sources. Although the main lacrimal gland secretes the major portion of the tear fluid volume, the contributions of the goblet cells in the conjunctiva (mucin glycoproteins) and the treelike meibomian glands in the lids (lipids) are no less important in maintaining a functional tear layer. Thus, in addition to the tear film resurfacing action of the blinking lids, the blink also serves the important function of combining and mixing these tear fluid components into a quasistable mixture. Included in this mixture would be any added tear substitute, suggesting the importance of the compatibility of the additive and the natural tear fluid.

The total tear volume on the anterior segment of the eye is usually between 6 and 7 μL,[2] and there is a certain amount of preferential compartmentalization for this fluid. When available fluid is deficient, the fornices "fill" first and can contain about 3 to 4 μL of fluid. Blinking carries fluid upward over the corneal surface, establishing the precorneal

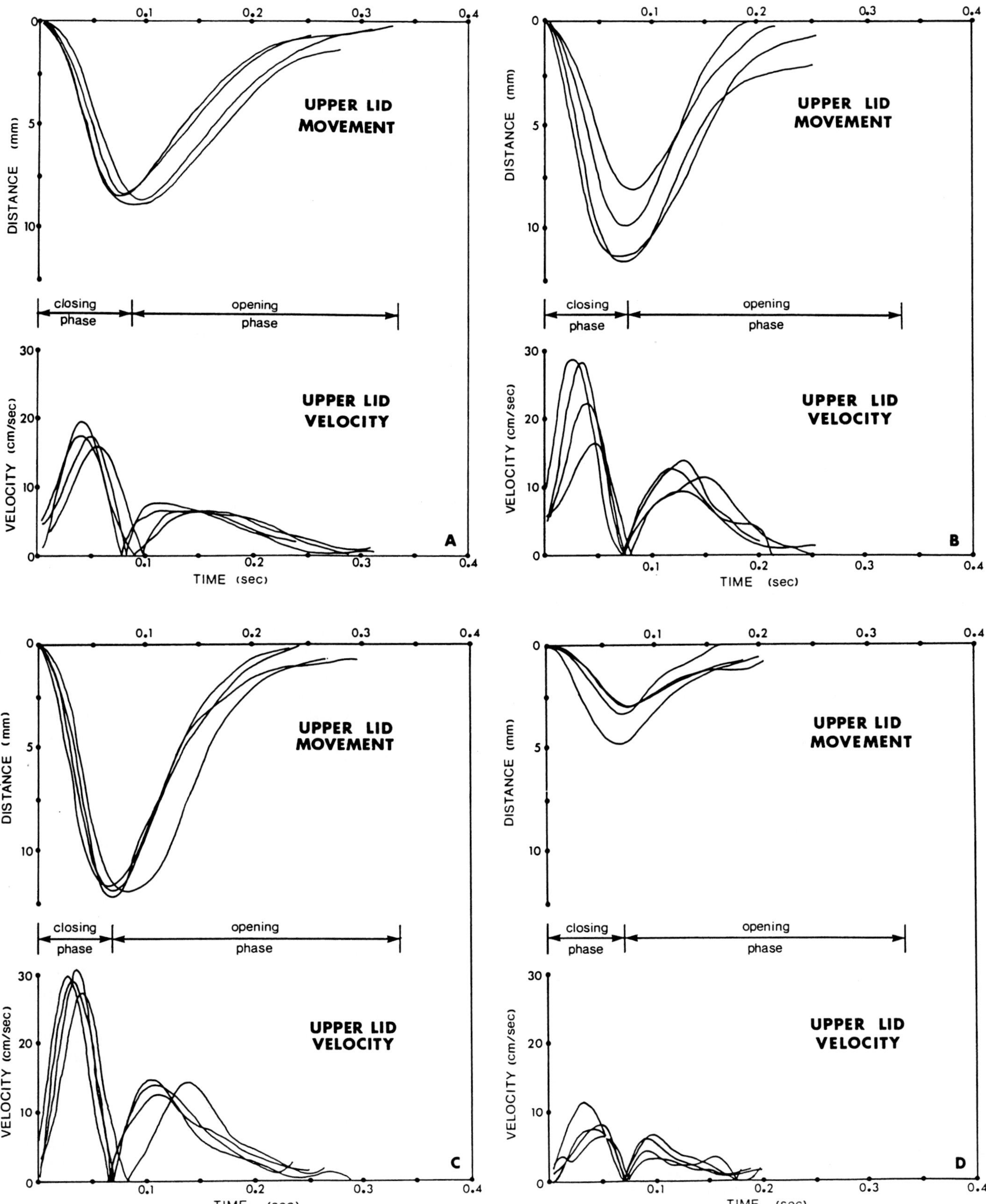

FIGURE 29–1. Plots of blink motion dynamics in four subjects. The upper curve of each pair represents the time course of the upper lid displacement during its closing and opening phases. The lower curve in each case is the time course of the instantaneous velocity of the upper lid, which is zero at the point where the lid reverses direction. Note the variation between individuals. The subject for plot *D* had a narrow palpebral fissure; consequently the lid excursions and velocities were less than normal. (From Doane MG: Interaction of eyelids and tears in corneal wetting and the dynamics of the normal human eyeblink. Am J Ophthalmol 89:507–516, 1980.)

tear film, requiring another 1 μL of fluid. The fornices cannot hold more fluid than their enclosed, defined space allows, nor can the tear film increase its fluid volume significantly. Once these "compartments" are filled, any *excess* fluid goes to fill the marginal tear menisci, which can hold 2 to 3 μL of tear fluid. Fluid much greater than this amount raises the level of the inferior meniscus above that of the punctal opening and, as described in following paragraphs, it is soon drained away via the canaliculi into the lacrimal sac. Thus, it is of little benefit to overfill the menisci with an instilled fluid, because any excess fluid that does not actually overflow onto the lids is quickly drained away by the blink-driven drainage system.

Within their sustainable volume range, the marginal menisci act as a variable reservoir. Often, the relative amount of tear volume in an eye can be semiquantitatively assessed by noting the height of the marginal tear menisci.[3] The height of the inferior tear meniscus often is reduced in patients with significant keratoconjunctivitis sicca, although individual variations in lid apposition, tightness, and thickness can also affect meniscus height.

Figure 29–2 is a schematic representation of this compartmentalization of the tear volume.

Mechanism of Tear Fluid Drainage

The single punctal opening in each of the lid margins is located at the apex of the lacrimal papillae, in the medial canthal region of the lids. Each punctal opening leads to a single tubular conduit, or canaliculus, which makes a right-angle bend about 2 mm from the edge of the lid and then parallels the lid margin for most of its length. The superior and inferior canaliculi usually join into a common pathway just before entering the lacrimal tear sac just posterior and superior to the center of its lateral wall. There is evidence for a one-way restriction, or valve, in this common canaliculus, allowing fluid to flow from the canaliculus into the lacrimal sac but restraining flow in the reverse direction. A duct, the nasolacrimal canal, descends from the inferior portion of the sac, opening into the nasal meatus.

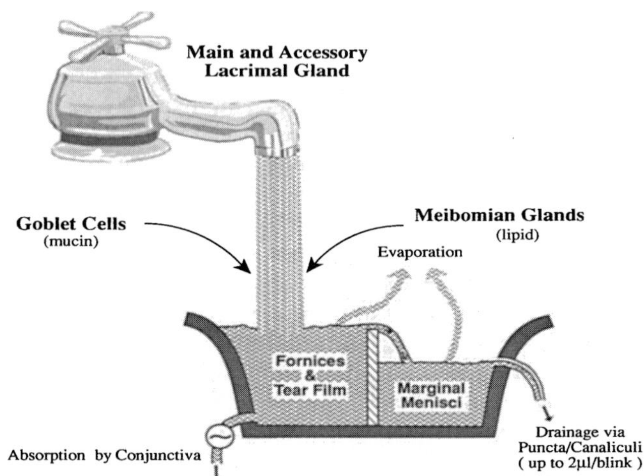

FIGURE 29–2. Schematic representation of tear fluid compartmentalization and outflow. Nearly all the effective tear volume is secreted by the main and accessory lacrimal glands, with an added contribution from the conjunctival goblet cells (mucin) and the meibomian glands in the lids (lipid). The tear fluid is first used to fill the volume between the globe and lids (superior and inferior fornices) and the tear film over the exposed globe. Any excess fluid then goes into the reservoir of the marginal menisci, from which drainage via the punctal openings occurs. Smaller amounts of fluid are lost by evaporation and absorption by the conjunctiva.

The passage of tear fluid through the punctal openings, into the canaliculi, and onward into the lacrimal sac is driven by the squeezing actions and muscular contractions associated with the blink action of the lids. This process involves a definitive, rapid sequence of events.[4] As the blinking action of the lids commences, the upper lid begins its downward sweep over the anterior portion of the globe, with the lower lid starting its movement medially, carrying with it the fluid in the marginal meniscus. The lacrimal papillae containing the punctal openings tend to extend and elevate themselves from the leading edge of the lids during the blink. Being located near the medial juncture of the lid structure, this region of the superior and inferior lid margins meet, often forcefully, by the time overall lid closure is only one-third to one-half complete. From this point to the completion of the lid motion associated with the blink, the punctal openings are largely occluded.

The primary effect of the second half of lid closure is to squeeze the elastic walls of the canaliculi, forcing any tear fluid within them onward into the lacrimal sac. Fluorescein experiments indicate minimal regurgitation of fluid out of the punctal openings, with the firm apposition of the lid margins minimizing this retrograde flow. Detailed high-speed, close-up photography shows that the region of the lid margins containing the punctal openings remains in tight contact until the lids are near the end of their opening phase. Then, the region of the lid margins containing the punctal openings suddenly pop apart when the force of the separating lids finally overcomes the suction force holding them together.[4] This suction is generated by the elastic walls of the canaliculi (and to some extent the lacrimal sac) trying to expand to contain their normal volume once the pressure of the closing lids is released.

Once the puncta are separated, a rapid, pulsatile flow of tear fluid is drawn into the puncta from the marginal menisci owing to the suction force generated within the canaliculi. When tear volume is normal, this flow typically lasts 1 or 2 seconds, *as long as the height of the fluid in the meniscus reservoir is sufficient to maintain contact with the punctal openings.* Any instillation of a tear substitute that temporarily increases the volume of fluid to a level above the punctal opening prolongs this exit flow, and the excess volume is quickly removed from the meniscus. Once the meniscus height falls below the slightly elevated position of the punctal openings, further drainage stops.[5] Because of differences in blink strength, degree of completion, and fluid volume in the marginal menisci, not all blinks result in equally efficient flow patterns. Because the puncta occlusion by the opposing lid margin occurs even with half blinks, with associated squeezing of the canaliculi, some tear fluid is often drawn into them even after incomplete blinks, although the amount of fluid drainage is reduced. Figure 29–3 is a schematic representation of this cycle.

From the time of initial instillation, any applied fluid is decreasing in its overall tear fluid concentration as time goes by. The time of contact between the ocular surface and the

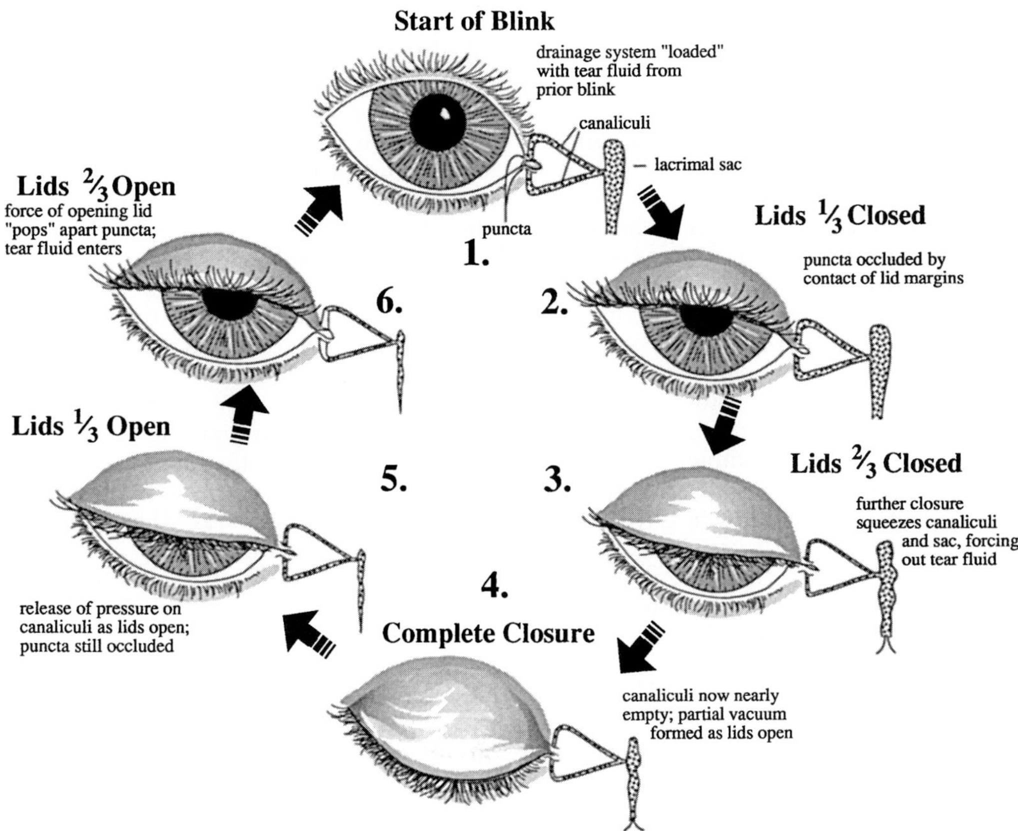

FIGURE 29–3. Mechanism of lacrimal drainage. Clockwise from the top: 1. At the start of the blink, the lacrimal drainage passages already contain tear fluid that has entered following the previous blink. 2. As the upper lid descends, the papillae containing the punctal openings elevate from the medial lid margin. By the time the upper lid has descended halfway, the papillae meet the opposing lid margin, occluding the puncta and resisting fluid regurgitation. 3. The remaining portion of the lid closure acts to squeeze the canaliculi and sac through the action of the orbicularis oculi, forcing out contained fluid that has not been absorbed by the mucosa of the sac and nasolacrimal duct. 4. At complete lid closure, the system is compressed and devoid of fluid. 5. During the start of the opening phase of the blink, the puncta are still occluded and valving action at the distal end of the canaliculi (and perhaps in the nasolacrimal duct) acts to prevent reentry of fluid or air. As lids open, compressive action ends and the elastic walls of the canaliculi attempt to expand to their normal shape. This elastic force causes a partial vacuum, or suction, to form within the canaliculi and sac. 6. The suction force holding the punctal region of the lid margins together is released when lid separation is sufficient, at about two thirds of the fully open position. The punctal openings are now accessible for fluid entry from the marginal tear menisci, and tear fluid is drawn into the canaliculi during the first few seconds following the blink. (From Doane MG: Blinking and the mechanics of the lacrimal drainage system. Ophthalmology 88:844, 1981.)

applied fluid is directly limited by the rate of drainage from the marginal menisci; in addition to drainage, the concentration of therapeutic agents that does remain is continuously diminished by newly secreted tear fluid. Thus, any means of increasing the retention time of instilled solutions at therapeutic levels is of crucial interest.

The stimulation of a faster blink rate (such as by the administration of a solution that stings or is otherwise uncomfortable) is undesirable, because this causes a more rapid drainage of tear fluid from the marginal menisci. An increase in the viscosity of a tear substitute *may* result in an effectively prolonged time of action. Recall that drainage from the inferior meniscus occurs from its highest, uppermost portion, which is drawn into the elevated punctal openings. If a viscous tear substitute is carefully instilled into the inferior cul-de-sac, it often acts as a longer-lasting depot of fluid that is not readily drained and is slowly mixed into the tear film by subsequent blinks. In fact, in monitoring the concentration of applied agents by interferometry, a few strong blinks often elicits a sudden increase in the amount of viscous agent in the tear film by forcing the "depot" out of the inferior cul-de-sac many minutes after initial instillation of the artificial tear solution. However, applied agents that are *too* viscous are detrimental to retention time, because they blur vision, elicit foreign body sensations that stimulate blinking, and are not well liked by users because of stickiness and the tendency to collect in the eyelashes.

Wetting and Drying of the Corneal Surface

Nature of the Wetting Process

We can define *wetting* as the spreading of a fluid over a solid surface, a complex process from a molecular, surface-chemical viewpoint. The degree of spreading depends on the relative forces of *cohesion* between the like molecules of the fluid and the forces of *adhesion* between the unlike molecules of the solid surface and those of the fluid. Thus, when a fluid rests on a solid surface, the relative strength of these two forces determines the degree of fluid spreading. The stronger the relative cohesive forces attracting the fluid molecules together, the less the fluid increases its surface area to spread out on the solid surface. Thus, in order to significantly spread and wet a surface, the fluid-solid adhesion forces must be greater than (or at least comparable to) the fluid-fluid cohesive forces.

However, wettability is more complex than this simple explanation; it also depends on the degree of polarity and type of charge of the molecular groups exposed on the surface of the solid. For instance, exposed polar groups tend to have an attraction for the polar molecules of water. Materials with nonpolar surfaces (Teflon, oils) have a low attraction for polar groups such as those in water and thus are inherently hydrophobic, or water-repelling. Surface-active agents, or *surfactants,* can greatly increase the wettability of a surface by acting as a bridge between polar and nonpolar molecules. Typically, such agents have molecules with some exposed moieties that are hydrophobic (such as alkyl groups) and others on the same molecule that are hydrophilic (such as carboxyl groups). Mucin glycoproteins are thought to act as a wetting agent in tear fluid. Virtually all artificial tear preparations contain one or more chemical surfactants that enhance their wetting of the cornea.

Surface tension is closely allied to wettability, because it is a measure of the relative strength of the intermolecular attraction of the surface molecules of a fluid. Obviously, in order for a fluid to flatten and spread, molecules from the interior of the fluid must move to the surface and spread the original molecules farther apart. The stronger the attraction, or cohesive force, between these molecules, the less that a given fluid easily expands its surface area and spreads over the solid surface. In the case of the tear film, surface tension at the fluid-air interface is lowered significantly by the presence of the superficial lipid layer floating on the surface, thus enhancing the spreading of the tear fluid in a thin film over the cornea. In addition, the surface of the cornea is covered by an adsorbed layer of mucin, perhaps 1 μm thick, which masks the normally hydrophobic corneal epithelium, allowing the tear fluid to spread easily over this surface.

Breakup of the Precorneal Tear Film

The surface of the cornea is rewet with a fresh layer of fluid, forming the precorneal tear film, by each blink of the eyelids. This periodic action is necessary owing to the deterioration of this thin fluid layer between blinks. Immediately after a new tear film is formed, it undergoes a progressive overall thinning owing to evaporation and, more importantly, begins to develop localized areas that thin even more rapidly than the tear layer as a whole. It is these localized regions, usually small in area, that result in the first "dry spots" observed after a blink. These spots appear as dark, nonfluorescent areas when fluorescein is in the tear fluid, because where there is no fluid, there is no fluorescein and hence no fluorescence. The time from the completion of a blink to the first appearance of these dark spots is the tear breakup time (BUT). Although BUTs vary from blink to blink and person to person, values shorter than about 10 seconds are often associated with dry eye symptoms, and BUT measurement is one of several diagnostic tools for this condition. Of course, persistently short blink intervals can somewhat moderate the effects of shortened BUTs.

Although evaporative effects progressively thin the tear film and promote eventual drying and breakup, theoretical calculations indicate that the times required to thin the tear layer to dryness should be much longer than those actually observed for measured BUTs.[6] Also, long before overall drying of the anterior surface of the eye occurs, the small, localized areas of drying discussed earlier are seen. Clearly, evaporation is not the sole (or even primary) cause of tear film breakup.

Several theories have been proposed to explain this, but the most likely and widely accepted mechanism was proposed by Holly[7] and Lemp[8]—that is, the development over short periods of time of local *nonwetting* areas on the corneal surface during each interblink period. Note that the corneal epithelial surface itself is hydrophobic, as can be demonstrated by carefully wiping the adsorbed mucin layer from the corneal surface with a cotton swab. The wiped surface, now consisting of mostly bare epithelial cells, does not wet by applied saline solutions. The wettability of the corneal surface is made possible by the presence of the relatively thick layer of adsorbed mucin. Highly hydrated mucin within the aqueous phase of the tear film itself also enhances the wetting process.

It is surmised that over time (i.e., within seconds after a blink), the mucin layer on the epithelium becomes contaminated by nonpolar components of the tear film, primarily lipid from the superficial layer. This oily layer is, of course, only about 5 or 6 μm above the surface of the mucin layer under the best of conditions. Microscopic flow patterns, either of thermal origin or due to the turbulence of the blink action, can bring this floating lipid into contact with the mucin on the corneal surface. Although a small amount of lipid contamination can be masked by the mucin molecules, sufficiently large areas eventually become contaminated whereby the mucin can no longer act as an effective surfactant. Then, nonwetting areas develop, with spontaneous thinning of the tear layer immediately above them, with eventual rupture of the tear film. When these localized nonwetting areas resist the formation of a new, clean mucin layer during blinking, persistent tear film breakup over the same area follows within a few seconds of each blink. A series of strong, forced blinks often reestablish tear film continuity over some of these areas by covering them with mucin.

There is no way to maintain an increase in the tear volume itself without either disabling the drainage mechanism (punctal plugs or surgery) or continuously instilling tear substitutes. Ideally, the application of a tear substitute should aid in wetting the corneal surface and prolong the BUT of the tear film for the entire time between instillations. Although the initial instillation of a drop of solution, of course, significantly increases tear volume and usually tear film thickness as well, this effect is largely transitory, and the tear volume quickly reverts to its prior value as the applied solution is drained away. Thus, it is unrealistic to expect retention of applied fluid volume per se to provide long-term benefit unless the solution is frequently applied to the eye. What is needed is a persistent agent in the applied solution that provides an increase in the tear film breakup times for long periods after the bulk of the applied solution is gone—that is, a component that binds to the eye tissues and does not leave with the fluid that is drained away. In theory, such an agent might be adsorbed to the surface of the epithelial cells of the cornea and conjunctiva or of the mucin layer that coats these surfaces and would act to improve the wetting action of the existing tear fluid, perhaps reducing the evaporation rate as well.

REFERENCES

1. Doane MG: Interaction of eyelids and tears in corneal wetting and the dynamics of the normal human eyeblink. Am J Ophthalmol 89:507–516, 1980.
2. Mishima S, Gasset A, Klyce SD, Baum JL: Determination of tear volume and tear flow. Invest Ophthalmol 5:264–275, 1966.
3. Scherz W, Doane MG, Dohlman CH: Tear volume in normal eyes and keratoconjunctivitis sicca. Graefes Arch Klin Exp Ophthalmol 192:141–150, 1974.
4. Doane MG: Blinking and the mechanics of the lacrimal drainage system. Ophthalmology 88:844–850, 1981.
5. Doane MG: Blinking and tear drainage. *In* Bosniak SB (ed): Advances in Plastic and Reconstructive Surgery, vol 3, The Lacrimal System. New York, Pergamon, 1984, pp 39–52.
6. Holly FJ: Tear film physiology and contact lens wear. I. Pertinent aspects of tear film physiology. Am J Optom Physiol Opt 58:324–330, 1981.
7. Holly FJ: Formation and rupture of the tear film. Exp Eye Res 15:515–525, 1973.
8. Lemp MA: Breakup of the tear film. Int Ophthalmol Clin 13:97–102, 1973.

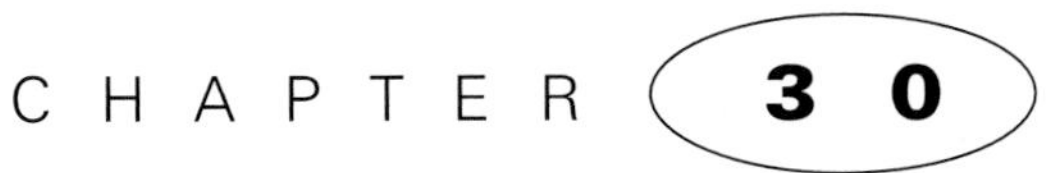

Tear Substitutes

J. Daniel Nelson and Mark B. Abelson

In the absence of any substantive cure for dry eye disorders, tear substitutes are the mainstay of therapy. No tear substitute, or individual component of such a formulation, has been approved for the treatment of dry eye based on a study demonstrating statistically significant clinical efficacy. For this reason, the components in tear substitutes are restricted within the confines of the U.S. Food and Drug Administration (FDA) monograph on over-the-counter products. This compendium lists all acceptable ingredients, both active and inactive, as well as acceptable concentration ranges allowed by the FDA in ophthalmic over-the-counter formulations. Ingredients that have been historically and traditionally used in ophthalmic products are included in this list based on the safety profile established through their numerous years of use. The various ingredients allowed by the FDA are classified as demulcents, emulsifiers, surfactants, viscosity agents, and preservatives.

The activity of a tear substitute, however, is difficult to detect. Proving that there is a significant difference between a complete tear formulation and one without its viscosity agent—the closest approximation to an active ingredient in a tear substitute—has proved nearly impossible. Lubrication of the ocular surface, which is the primary effect of available tear substitutes, is potentially achievable with any compatible formulation. However, the ability to design clinical trials sensitive enough to detect differences among topical lubricants is difficult with presently available measures of efficacy.

A tear substitute is generally used to supplement a tear film that is inferior in either quality or quantity in a patient with some dysfunction of the ocular surface or tear secretory system. As previously described, this system includes the main and accessory lacrimal glands, the meibomian glands, the glands of Zeis and Moll, and the goblet cells. Identification of the patient's specific dysfunction, whether it is an aqueous, lipid, or mucous layer deficiency, helps to determine optimal therapy. Whether dry eye is primary or secondary to lid conditions, such as blepharitis or ocular rosacea, must be determined in order to initiate the proper concomitant therapy, such as lid hygiene and oral tetracycline. Disorders of the ocular surface such as *ocular cicatricial* pemphigoid or Stevens-Johnson syndrome must be identified and treated as described in other chapters.

The primary objectives of the physician caring for patients with dry eye are to improve subjective comfort and to minimize ocular surface desiccation and cell death. Symptoms can often be reduced but rarely are eliminated. However, minimizing ocular surface desiccation and cell death prove much more difficult to accomplish with lubricants alone. Topical lubricants do improve comfort, but few, if any, well-designed clinical studies show that topical lubricants reduce ocular surface desiccation and cell death. Clinical studies also fail to show significant correlation among tests such as Schirmer's test, rose bengal staining, tear breakup time, and conjunctival impression cytology.[1, 2] Also, improvement in patient symptoms does not correlate with improvement in clinical test values.[1–3] Often, symptoms are reduced, but rose bengal staining persists in patients with moderate to severe dry eye placed on lubricants. Until we can mimic human tear composition, complete resolution of symptoms and of ocular surface and tear film abnormalities is unlikely.

Generally, tear substitutes are hypotonic or isotonic buffered solutions containing electrolytes, surfactants, and various types of viscosity agents that are added to increase the residency time on the ocular surface. The ideal artificial lubricant is preservative-free, contains potassium and bicarbonate at a slightly alkaline pH, and is slightly hypoosmotic (~290 mosm/L) with a polymeric system that increases retention time.[4–7] Historically, all formulations were preserved, multidose preparations. However, unit-dose, preservative-free systems are now common. The type and concentration of viscosity agent, preservative system, and electrolyte composition are the three primary variables in ophthalmic lubricant formulations.

Viscosity Agents

The stability of the tear film depends on the chemical-physical characteristics among the three layers. Classically, the mucin layer was thought to act as a surfactant by lowering the surface tension of the relatively hydrophobic ocular surface, rendering the corneal and conjunctival cells "wettable."[8] Recent evidence, however, suggests that the mucin layer is much thicker than previously thought, measuring 35 to 40 μm in thickness.[9] Its role may be similar to that of mucin in the stomach, where a mucin gel protects the surface epithelium from a harsh surrounding environment.[10] This may explain why water-containing lubricants are only partially effective in restoring the health of the ocular surface. Therefore, function of the mucin layer is more than that of a surfactant. The effect of most available lubricants is probably to hydrate available mucin and wash away irritating or toxic substances in the tear film. While some patients with dry eye have a deficiency in the aqueous layer, a primary or secondary disorder of one mucin layer may be present. The macromolecular complexes added to tear substitutes as viscosity agents lubricate and may fortify this mucous layer. The addition of a viscosity agent to increase residence time can play a role in active drug formulations by prolonging ocular surface contact, thereby increasing the drug's duration of action and comfort.

Polyvinyl alcohol, in concentrations ranging from 1.4 to 3%, is the most common viscosity agent added to tear substitutes. Polyethylene glycol, hydroxymethylcellulose, hydroxypropylcellulose, and carboxymethylcellulose are also present in tear substitutes in varying concentrations. Tables 30–1 and 30–2 list the marketed tear substitutes and combination tear substitute/vasoconstrictors, detailing the viscosity agent used and the concentration, if identified in *The Physicians Desk Reference*.[11]

Celluvisc (Allergan Pharmaceuticals, Irvine, CA), containing a 100,000 molecular weight carboxymethylcellulose (CMC) in a 1% solution, appears to have significantly enhanced viscosity and a greater residence time compared with currently available polymer-containing formulations. Gamma scintigraphy showed that an anionic charged CMC had a significantly slower rate of clearance from the eye than did a neutral hydroxymethylcellulose.[12] Furthermore, a clinical study of these same solutions showed significantly more improvement in the CMC-treated eyes with regard to patient symptoms, superficial punctate keratitis, and the degree of abnormal squamous metaplasia as demonstrated by impression cytology mapping.[13] These results are probably due to differences in residence time relating to increased viscosity.

The blurring of vision and esthetic disadvantages of caking and drying on eyelashes are drawbacks with highly viscous agents that patients with mild to moderate dry eye do not tolerate. A lower molecular weight (70,000) CMC in half the concentration of Celluvisc (Refresh Plus: 0.5% CMC, Allergan Pharmaceuticals) is an alternative formulation that may address some of these problems. Optimizing patient compliance, comfort, and convenience is important. The patient should thus be offered a range of tear substitute formulations with varying viscosities.

The effects of hydroxymethycellulose were evaluated in 20 patients with dry eye for both clinical and morphologic parameters identified by symptoms, slit-lamp examination, and electron microscopy of conjunctival biopsies.[14] The authors tested the hypothesis that hydroxymethylcellulose actually supplants a deficient mucous layer and reverses abnormal morphologic findings in patients with dry eye. Although morphologic aspects of the biopsies, specifically goblet cells, were unchanged before and after treatment, the study showed significant decreases in rose bengal staining after 15 days of treatment compared with baseline.

Hyaluronic acid is a viscosity agent that has been investigated for years as an "active" compound added to tear-substitute formulations for the treatment of dry eye. Using gamma scintigraphy, Snibson and associates reported that the ocular surface residence times of 0.2% hyaluronic acid were significantly longer than those of 0.3% hydroxymethylcellulose or 1.4% polyvinyl alcohol.[15] In 1982, Polack and McNiece reported subjective and objective improvement using a 0.1% solution in 20 patients with severe dry eye in whom other artificial tear preparations were ineffective.[16] In 1985, Stuart and Linn also evaluated 0.1% sodium hyaluronate in different ocular surface disorders and found significant relief in dry eye, epithelial corneal dystrophy, contact lens–induced irritation, and ocular pemphigoid.[17] In 1984, DeLuise and Peterson found improvement in 26 of 28 patients using the 0.1% solution.[18] In 1989, Sand and coworkers evaluated the effect of 0.1% and 0.2% sodium hyaluronate in 20 patients with severe dry eye in a double-masked crossover design against a placebo that contained all of the components except the sodium hyaluronate. The authors found significantly decreased rose bengal staining and increased tear breakup time after 0.2% treatment compared with placebo but no significant effect using the 0.1% solution.[19] In a multicenter, randomized, controlled clinical trial in patients with moderate to severe aqueous deficient dry eye, Nelson and Farris found that 0.1% sodium hyaluronate improved patient symptoms and reduced tear film osmolarity and ocular surface rose bengal staining. However, there were no statistically differences compared with the control preparation containing polyvinyl alcohol.[20] Sodium hyaluronate is not available in tear substitutes in the United States; however, it is included as a viscosity agent in formulations in some countries. Although many topical lubricants improve symptoms and objective findings, there is no evidence that any current viscous or polymer agent is better than another.

Other clinical trials have examined various topical agents to treat dry eye. Most clinical trials involving topical preparations document some improvement (but not resolution) of subjective symptoms and some objective findings.[1] However, these improvements are not any better than those produced by the vehicle or another nonpreserved artificial lubricant. This suggests that lubrication alone is insufficient to resolve the ocular surface disorder experienced by dry eye sufferers.

TABLE 30–1. **Currently Marketed Tear Substitutes***

Manufacturer and Drug System	Viscosity Agents	Preservative
Advanced Vision Research		
Theratears†	Carboxymethylcellulose 0.25%	None
Allergan Pharmaceuticals		
Celluvisc Lubricant Ophthalmic Solution†	Carboxymethylcellulose 1%	None
Refresh Tears	Carboxymethylcellulose 0.5%	Purite
Lacril Lubricant	Hydroxypropylmethylcellulose 0.5%	Chlorobutanol 0.5%
Liquifilm Forte	Polyvinyl alcohol 3%	Thimerosal 0.002%/EDTA
Liquifilm Tears	Polyvinyl alcohol 1.4%	Chlorobutanol 0.5%
Refresh Lubricant Ophthalmic Solution†	Polyvinyl alcohol 1.4% Povidone 0.6%	None
Refresh Plus† Ophthalmic Solution†	Carboxymethylcellulose 1% Povidone 0.6%	None
Tears Plus Lubricant Ophthalmic Solution	Polyvinyl alcohol 1.4% Povidone 0.6%	Chlorobutanol 0.5%
Cellufresh†	Carboxymethylcellulose 0.5%	None
Lacri-Lube NP	White petrolatum 57.3% Mineral oil 42.5%, lanolin	None
Lacri-Lube S.O.P.	White petrolatum 56.8% Mineral oil 42.5%, lanolin	Chlorobutanol 0.5%
Refresh PM	White petrolatum 56.8% Mineral oil 41.5%, lanolin	None
AKORN Pharmaceuticals		
AKWA Tears	Polyvinyl alcohol	BAC 0.001%/EDTA
AKWA Tears Ointment	White petrolatum; mineral oil	None
Tears Renewed	Dextran-70 Hydroxypropylmethylcellulose	BAC 0.001%/EDTA 0.05%
Alcon Laboratories		
Adsorbotear	Povidone 1.67% and water-soluble polymers, hydroxyethylcellulose	Thimerosal 0.004%/EDTA 0.1%
BION Tears†	Dextran, hydroxypropylmethylcellulose	None
Duratears Naturale Lubricant Eye Ointment	White petrolatum, mineral oil, anhydrous liquid lanolin	Unknown
Tears Naturale II	Dextran-70 0.1% Hydroxypropylmethylcellulose 0.3%	POLYQUAD (Polyquarternium-1 0.001%)
Tears Naturale Free†	Dextran, hydroxypropylmethylcellulose	None
Bausch and Lomb Pharmaceuticals		
Murocel	1% Methylcellulose	Methylparaben 0.023% Propylparaben 0.01%
CIBA Vision		
Aquasite†	Polyethylene glycol 400 0.2% Dextran-70 0.1% Polycarbophil	EDTA
Genteal Lubricating Eye Drops	Hydroxypropylmethylcellulose	Sodium perborate
Hypotears Lubricating Eye Drops	Polyvinyl alcohol 1% in polyethylene glycol 400 and dextrose	BAC/EDTA
Hypotears PF† Eye Drops	Polyvinyl alcohol 1% in polyethylene glycol 400 and dextrose	BAC/EDTA
Hypotears Ointment	White petrolatum, mineral oil	None
Ocumed		
Ocutears PF†	Polyvinyl alcohol	None
Ocutube	White petrolatum	Unknown
Ocu-Tears	Polyvinyl alcohol	Unknown
Pharmafair		
Lubrifair Ointment	White petrolatum, mineral oil, lanolin liquid	None
Lubrifair Solution†	Dextran-70, hydroxypropylmethylcellulose	None
Petrolatum Ointment-Sterile	White petrolatum	None
TearFair Ointment	White petrolatum, mineral oil, lanolin derivatives	None
Tearfair Solution†	Polyvinyl alcohol	None
Ross Laboratories		
Murine Eye Lubricant	1.4% Polyvinyl alcohol, 0.6% povidone	BAC/EDTA
Clear Eyes	Hydroxypropylmethylcellulose, glycerine	Sorbic acid/EDTA

*Concentrations of the listed components are identified when possible. Ethylenediaminetetraacetic acid (EDTA) is listed as a preservative in some product descriptions and as an inactive ingredient in others. If it is not specified that an ointment contains a preservative, it is listed as "unknown." (All information is available in Physician's Desk Reference for Ophthalmology, 26th ed. Oradell, NJ, Medical Economics, 1998.)

†Preservative-free, unit-dose vials.

TABLE 30–2. **Tear Substitute/Vasoconstrictor Combinations***

Manufacturer and Drug System	Active Compounds	Preservative
Allergan Pharmaceuticals		
Albalon	Naphazoline HCl 0.1% Liquifilm: Polyvinyl alcohol 1.4%	BAC 0.04%/EDTA
Pfizer, Inc.		
Visine Extra	Tetrahydrozoline HCl 0.05% Polyethylene glycol 400	BAC 0.013%/EDTA 0.1%
Ross Laboratories		
Clear Eyes	Naphazoline HCl 0.12% Glycerin 0.2%	BAC 0.01%/EDTA 0.1%
Murine Plus	1.4% Polyvinyl alcohol 0.6% Povidone 0.05% Tetrahydrozoline	BAC EDTA

*Concentrations of the listed components are identified when possible. Ethylenediaminetetraacetic acid (EDTA) is listed as a preservative in some product descriptions and as an inactive ingredient in others. (All information is available in Physician's Desk Reference for Ophthalmology, 26th ed. Oradell, NJ, Medical Economics, 1998.)

†Preservative-free, unit-dose vials.

Because one of the major causes of conjunctival redness and irritation may be mild dry eye, some available tear substitutes are combined with vasoconstrictors (see Table 30–2). However, in the more severe, aqueous-deficient dry eye, vasoconstrictors can be irritating.

Preservatives

The most important advancement in tear-substitute preparations was the introduction of preservative-free solutions in single-use vials. The absence of preservatives is more important than the particular viscous agent used in artificial lubricants. The epithelial toxic effects of frequent use of preservatives such as benzalkonium chloride (BAC) are well known.[21–25] BAC is the most frequently used preservative in both topical ophthalmic preparations and topical lubricants (see Tables 30–1 and 30–2). Yet, ophthalmic formulations used four times daily or less must be distinguished from those that are used, or have the potential to be used, more frequently. With normal dosing regimens, BAC is nontoxic to the corneal epithelium.[25] Thus, the use of BAC in prescribed ophthalmic formulations is not usually the main concern, except when multiple preserved topical medications are required, for example, in chronic glaucoma therapy. Problems can arise with over-the-counter products that contain BAC and can be abused by the patient or when patients with severe dry eye use these products more than six times daily. This frequency of BAC use can dramatically damage the corneal epithelium, causing a loss of cell-to-cell junctions and normal cell shape, a denuding of the microvilli, and cell necrosis leading to a sloughing of one to two layers of cells.[21, 23, 25, 26] Thus, the preservative-free formulations are an ideal solution for the patient with severe dry eye, the patient with ocular surface disease, or the patient on multiple, preserved topical medications for chronic ocular disease.

Edetate disodium is an additive that augments the preservative efficacy of BAC and other preservatives; however, it is not a true preservative by itself. In nonpreserved solutions, it may enhance and prolong the sterility in the unit-dose vial. Some preserved solutions have included edetate disodium in order to lower the concentration of preservative needed—a legitimate goal considering what is known about preservatives. Yet, the question of whether edetate disodium is also toxic in the concentrations used has arisen. One study compared two preservative-free solutions, Hypotears PF (Iolab Pharmaceuticals, Claremont, CA) containing edetate disodium and Refresh (Allergan Pharmaceuticals) without edetate sodium. With average and with exaggerated use, both formulations had identical safety profiles and were completely nontoxic to the rabbit corneal epithelium as shown by scanning electron microscopy.[25] Another study showed that preparations containing edetate sodium increased corneal epithelial permeability.[27, 28] Although edetate sodium may not be toxic to the normal rabbit corneal epithelium, patients with severe dry eye often find that preparations that contain edetate sodium cause increased irritation, even if they do not contain other preservatives.

Two drawbacks for the use of single unit-dose tear substitutes are the expense and the inconvenience of carrying many vials. Many patients therefore reuse their unit-dose vials by attempting to recap them or stand them upright until it is time for the next dose. A multidose, minimally filled vial that can be recapped and that contains a preservative-free solution that can remain sterile for at least 24 hours would be the ideal solution to this problem. Recently, a recappable vial containing Tears Natural Free (Alcon Laboratories, Fort Worth, TX) was introduced. Perhaps this will eliminate the worry of noncompliance and infection from improperly stored and capped unit-dose containers.

To avoid preservative toxicity and the disadvantages of unit-dose unpreserved vials, new preservatives, such as polyquad (polyquaternium-1), and other novel approaches have been used. A new artificial lubricant, Genteal (CIBA Vision, Duluth, GA), contains a novel preservative, sodium perborate, which is converted to water and oxygen on contact with the tear film. Whether these newer preservatives are less harmful to the ocular surface in patients with severe aqueous tear deficiency remains to be seen. The ideal packaging would contain a multidose, nonpreserved or a nontoxic, preserved preparation that maintains sterility with frequent use and is nontoxic to the ocular surface of patients with severe aqueous deficiency.

Currently, in preservative-free formulations, viscosities range widely (see Tables 30–1 and 30–2). Ointments are another alternative for long-acting protection of the ocular surface; however, blurring of vision limits their use to bedtime or in the most severe dry eye conditions. Most available ointments are formulated with an equal mixture of mineral oil and petrolatum. Some contain lanolin, a compound that may be irritating to the eye and delay corneal wound healing (see Table 30–1).[29] Wool-sensitive patients may show sensitivity to lanolin. Some ointments are preserved and others are not; however, not all ointment packaging clearly states this. In general, ointments containing parabens (acting as a preservative), lanolin, or both are less well tolerated in patients with more severe dry eye.

Electrolyte Composition

Electrolyte-containing solutions are beneficial in treating ocular surface damage due to dry eye.[4, 5, 28, 30, 31] Potassium seems to be one of the unique and beneficial constituents. Potassium is also important to maintain corneal thickness.[6] An electrolyte solution has been shown to increase conjunctival goblet cell density and corneal glycogen content, as well as to decrease elevated tear osmolarity and rose bengal staining after 2 weeks of treatment in rabbits with experimentally induced dry eye. Bicarbonate-containing solutions are superior to non–bicarbonate-containing solutions in promoting the recovery of the damaged corneal epithelial barrier function and in maintaining normal epithelial ultrastructure.[5] Topical lubricants that mimic the electrolyte composition of humans are now commercially available. TheraTears (Advance Vision Research, Woburn, MA) and BION Tears (Alcon Laboratories, Fort Worth, TX), which mimic the composition of human tears, also contain bicarbonate, which may be important in maintaining the mucin layer of the tear film.[5] Bicarbonate is known to be critical for forming and maintaining the protective mucin gel that lines the stomach.[10] Bicarbonate may play a similar role in forming the protective mucin gel on the ocular surface. When in contact with air, bicarbonate is converted to carbon dioxide, which can diffuse through the plastic unit-dose vials. To prevent this, special foil packaging is required for bicarbonate-containing solutions to maintain stability. In addition, patients are instructed to use the opened vials once and then discard them.

Osmolarity

Tears of patients with dry eye have a higher osmolarity (crystalloid osmolarity) than normal tears,[32–34] most likely owing to increased evaporation in patients with lipid layer deficiencies.[35] Hyperosmolarity may be toxic to the corneal epithelium, adding to the damage caused by the tear deficiency.[36] This knowledge has led to the development of hypoosmotic artificial tears such as Hypotears (CIBA Vision).

Colloidal osmolality, mainly dependent on macromolecule content, is another factor that varies in artificial tear formulations. Colloidal osmolarity, or oncotic pressure, is important for the control of water transport in tissues. It is defined as osmotic pressure due to the presence of colloids in a solution. Osmolality differences affect the net water flow across membranes. This water flow is eliminated by applying hydrostatic pressure to the downside of the water flow. The magnitude of this osmotic pressure is determined by osmolality differences on the two sides of the membrane. Damaged epithelial cells swell because of either cell membrane breaks or a dysfunction in the pumping mechanism. If a fluid with a high colloidal osmolality is added to this damaged and swollen cell surface, the oncotic pressure exerted causes cell deturgescence and a return to normal cell physiology. Thus, an artificial tear formulation with a high colloidal osmolality may be of value. In 1985, Holly and Esquivel evaluated many different formulations and found that Hypotears had the highest colloidal osmolality of all of the formulations tested.[37]

Investigational Compounds

Cyclosporine has been investigated as an immunosuppressive agent for ophthalmic indications such as the treatment of corneal graft rejection,[38] various autoimmune disease such as rheumatoid arthritis and Sjögren's syndrome,[39] and other inflammatory conditions, such as conjunctival pemphigoid[40] and vernal conjunctivitis.[41] Although certainly not a tear substitute, topical cyclosporine in an ophthalmic oil suspension is being investigated in clinical trials for the treatment of severe dry eye. In dogs with keratoconjunctivitis sicca, cyclosporine was shown to increase tear production and resolve corneal scarring.[42, 43] In human trials, cyclosporin A has shown some promise.[43–46]

Another investigational substance used for the treatment of dry eye is tretinoin or *trans*-retinoic acid, a derivative of vitamin A. Vitamin A is required for epithelial differentiation; a deficiency causes poorly differentiated lacrimal gland epithelium[47] with a decrease in the number of mucous-secreting cells,[48] in additional to squamous metaplasia and keratinization of the ocular surface.[49] Corneal and conjunctival epithelia also need vitamin A to maintain normal differentiation.[50] Because the corneal epithelium is avascular, the tear film must provide its vitamin A, and a deficiency could lead to pathologic changes in the lacrimal gland and in the corneal epithelium. Animal studies have shown that replenishing vitamin A reverts the abnormal morphology.[47] Although tear solutions containing retinyl palmitate (another derivative of vitamin A) are available, they do not contain the active form of vitamin A, tretinoin, which is not soluble in aqueous solutions.

REFERENCES

1. Nelson JD, Gordon JF: Topical fibronectin in the treatment of keratoconjunctivitis sicca. Chiron Keratoconjunctivitis Sicca Study Group. Am J Ophthalmol 114(4):441–447, 1192.
2. Schein O, Munoz B, Tielsch J, et al: Estimating the prevalence of dry eye among elderly Americans. Invest Ophthalmol Vis Sci 37(Suppl):S646, 1996.
3. Nelson JD: Impression cytology. Cornea 7:71–81, 1988.
4. Gilbard J, Rossi S, Heyda KG: Ophthalmic solutions, the ocular surface, and a unique therapeutic artificial tear formulation. Am J Ophthalmol 107:348, 1989.
5. Ubels J, McCartney M, Lantz W, et al: Effects of preservative-free artificial tear solutions on corneal epithelial structure and function. Arch Ophthalmol 113(3):371–378, 1995.
6. Green K, MacKeen DL, Slagle T, Cheeks L: Tear potassium contributes to maintenance of corneal thickness. Ophthalmic Res 24(2):99–102, 1992.
7. Holly F, Lemp M: Surface chemistry of the tear film: Implications for dry eye syndromes, contact lenses, and ophthalmic polymers. Contact Lens Soc Am J 5:12–19, 1971.
8. Holly F, Lemp M: Wettability and wetting of corneal epithelium. Exp Eye Res 11:239–250, 1971.
9. Prydal JI, Artal P, Woon H, Campbell FW: Study of human precorneal tear film thickness and structure using laser interferometry. Invest Ophthalmol Vis Sci 33(6):2006–2011, 1992.
10. Slomiany BL, Slomiany A: Role of mucus in gastric mucosal protection. J Physiol Pharmacol 42(2):147–161, 1991.
11. Physician's Desk Reference for Ophthalmology, 25th ed. Oradell, NJ, Medical Economics, 1997.
12. Hawi A, Smith T, Digenis G: A quantitative comparison of artificial tear clearance rates in humans using gamma scintigraphy. Invest Ophthalmol Vis Sci 31(Suppl):517, 1990.
13. Grene B, Harrold M, Mordaunt J, et al: A clinical study comparing the efficacy of two ophthalmic lubricating solutions using impression cytology. Invest Ophthalmol Vis Sci 31(Suppl):539, 1990.
14. Versura P, Maltarello M, Stecher F, et al: Dry eye before and after therapy with hydroxypropylmethylcellulose. Ophthalmologica 198:1989, 1989.
15. Snibson GR, Greaves JL, Soper ND, et al: Precorneal residence times

of sodium hyaluronate solutions studied by quantitative gamma scintigraphy. Eye 4(Pt 4):594–602, 1990.
16. Polack F, McNiece M: The treatment of dry eyes with Na hyaluronate (Healon). Cornea 1:1333, 1982.
17. Stuart J, Linn J: Dilute sodium hyaluronate (Healon) in the treatment of ocular surface disorder. Ann Ophthalmol 17:190, 1985.
18. DeLuise V, Peterson W: The use of topical Healon tears in the management of refractory dry-eye syndrome. Ann Ophthalmol 16:823, 1984.
19. Sand B, Marner K, Norn M: Sodium hyaluronate in the treatment of keratoconjunctivitis sicca. Acta Ophthalmol 67:181, 1989.
20. Nelson JD, Farris RL: Sodium hyaluronate and polyvinyl alcohol artificial tear preparations: A comparison in patients with keratoconjunctivitis sicca. Arch Ophthalmol 106:484–487, 1988.
21. Gassett A, Ishii Y, Kaufman H, et al: Cytotoxicity of ophthalmic preservatives. Am J Ophthalmol 78:98, 1974.
22. Wilson F: Adverse external effects of topical ophthalmic medications. Surv Ophthalmol 24:57–88, 1979.
23. Burstein N: Corneal cytotoxicity of topically applied drugs, vehicles and preservatives. Surv Ophthalmol 25:15, 1980.
24. Brubaker R, McLaren J: Uses of the fluorophotometer in glaucoma research. Ophthalmology 92:884–890, 1985.
25. Smith L, George M, Berdy G, Abelson M: Comparative effects of preservative free tear substitutes on the rabbit cornea: A scanning electron microscopic evaluation. Invest Ophthalmol Vis Sci 32 (Suppl):733, 1991.
26. Burstein N: The effects of topical drugs and preservatives on the tears and corneal epithelium in dry eye. Trans Ophthalmol Soc UK 104:402, 1985.
27. Lopez Bernal D, Ubels JL: Quantitative evaluation of the corneal epithelial barrier: Effect of artificial tears and preservatives. Curr Eye Res 10(7):645–656, 1991.
28. Bernal DL, Ubels JL: Artificial tear composition and promotion of recovery of the damaged corneal epithelium. Cornea 12(2):115–120, 1993.
29. Herrema J, Friedenwald J: Retardation of wound healing in the corneal epithelium by lanolin. Am J Ophthalmol 33:1421, 1950.
30. Nelson J, Drake M, Brewer J, Tuley M: Evaluation of physiologic tear substitute in patients with keratoconjunctivitis sicca. Adv Exp Med Biol 350:453–457, 1994.
31. Gilbard JP, Rossi SR: An electrolyte-based solution that increases corneal glycogen and conjunctival goblet-cell density in a rabbit model for keratoconjunctivitis sicca. Ophthalmology 99(4):600–604, 1992.
32. Gilbard J, Farris R: Tear osmolarity and ocular surface disease in keratoconjunctivitis sicca. Arch Ophthalmol 96:677, 1978.
33. Gilbard JP: Tear film osmolarity and keratoconjunctivitis sicca. CLAO J 11(3):243–250, 1985.
34. Gilbard J: Tear film osmolarity and keratoconjunctivitis sicca. Lubbock, TX, Dry Eye Institute, 1986.
35. Rolando M, Refojo M, Kenyon K: Increased tear film evaporation in eyes with keratoconjunctivitis sicca. Arch Ophthalmol 101:557, 1983.
36. Gilbard J, Carter J, Sang D, et al: Morphologic effect of hyperosmolarity on rabbit corneal epithelium. Ophthalmology 91:1205, 1984.
37. Holly F, Esquivel E: Colloid osmotic pressure of artificial tears. J Ocul Pharmacol 1:327, 1985.
38. Goichot-Bonnat L, De Beauregard C, Saragoussi J, et al: Usage de la cyclosporine A collyre dans la prevention du rejet de greffe de cornée chéz l'homme. J Fr Ophthalmol 10:207, 1987.
39. Drosos A, Skopouli F, Galanapoulou V, et al: Cyclosporin A therapy in patients with primary Sjögren's syndrome: Results at one year. Scand J Rheumatol 61(Suppl):246, 1986.
40. Sundmacher R, Peter H: Cyclosporin A after keratoplasty for rheumatoid corneal performation and for treatment of conjunctival pemphigoid. Spektrum Augenheilkd (Austria) 1:1987, 1987.
41. BenEzra D, Pe'er J, Brodsky M, et al: Cyclosporine eyedrops for the treatment of severe vernal keratoconjunctivitis. Am J Ophthalmol 101:278, 1986.
42. Kaswan R, Salisbury M, Ward D: Spontaneous canine keratoconjunctivitis sicca. A useful model for human keratoconjunctivitis sicca: Treatment with cyclosporine eye drops. Arch Ophthalmol 107:1210, 1989.
43. Kaswan R, Salisbury M: A new perspective on canine keratoconjunctivitis sicca. Treatment of ophthalmic cyclosporine. Vet Clin North Am Small Anim Pract 20:583, 1990.
44. Gunduz K, Ozdemir O: Topical cyclosporin treatment of keratoconjunctivitis sicca in secondary Sjögren's syndrome. Acta Ophthalmol Copenh 72(4):438–442, 1994.
45. Liu SH, Zhou DH, Gottsch JD, Hess AD: Treatment of experimental autoimmune dacryoadenitis with cyclosporin A. Clin Immunol Immunopathol 67(1):78–83, 1993.
46. Laibovitz RA, Sòlch S, Andriano K, et al: Pilot trial of cyclosporine 1% ophthalmic ointment in the treatment of keratoconjunctivitis sicca. Cornea 12(4):315–323, 1993.
47. Hayashi K, Reddy C, Hanninen L, et al: Pathologic changes in the exorbital lacrimal gland of the vitamin A–deficient rat. Invest Ophthalmol Vis Sci 31:1990, 1990.
48. Sullivan W, McCulley J, Dohlman C: Return of goblet cells after vitamin A therapy in xerosis of the conjunctiva. Am J Ophthalmol 75:720, 1973.
49. Tseng S, Hatchell D, Tierney N, et al: Expression of specific keratin markers by rabbit corneal, conjunctival, and esophageal epithelia during vitamin A deficiency. J Cell Biol 99:2279, 1984.
50. Kaswan RL, Salisbury M-A, Ward DA: Spontaneous canine keratoconjunctivitis sicca, a useful model for human keratoconjunctivitis sicca: Treatment with cyclosporine eye drops. Arch Ophthalmol 107:1210–1216, 1989.

CHAPTER 31

Viscoelastics

Jack V. Greiner and David Miller

The use of viscoelastics in ophthalmology has continued to increase, and viscoelastics are indispensable in certain surgical procedures. Viscoelastic solutions are characterized by a spectrum of viscosities that are related to their ability to resist mechanical deformation. They have been developed over the years as an extremely useful adjunct in various types of ophthalmic procedures, including cataract extraction, intraocular lens (IOL) implantation and exchange, keratoplasty, and vitreoretinal procedures. The adoption and further development of viscoelastics for use in the ophthalmologic field followed a number of interesting observations in our laboratory and others. In 1958, Balazs (Balazs EA, personal communication, 1959) began developing hyaluronic acid (HA) as a vitreous substitute. Initially isolated from the vitreous humor in 1934 by Meyer and Palmer,[1] HA is a mucopolysaccharide of repeating sodium glucuronate and *N*-acetyl-D-glucosamine units. It occurs naturally in many connective tissues of the body, the highest concentration being in the vitreous cortex. Balazs[2] later developed a method of purifying HA from umbilical cord and rooster combs. Ultimately, the Balazs material was improved on by Pharmacia Laboratories, Inc., of Uppsala, Sweden, and marketed as Healon. This viscoelastic substance became popular in ophthalmic surgery beyond its initial use as a vitreous substitute. In 1976, after the implantation of an IOL in an 82-year-old man by one of us (DM), it was noticed that the corneal endothelium remained edematous for about 1 month. Based on earlier studies by Kaufman and colleagues (Kaufman H, personal communication, 1976), it was reasoned that the IOL had touched a large portion of the corneal endothelium during surgery, resulting in the implant's pulling cells from the back of the cornea. Recalling the HA vitreous substitute developed by Balazs (Balazs EA, personal communication, 1959), we wondered whether such a thick jelly-like material could protectively coat the cornea during surgical procedures as well as retroplace the vitreous body and iris. After conferring with Balazs and receiving a number of syringes of sodium hyaluronate from him, we explored the use of this substance during implant surgery. In a large series of rabbits, lenses were implanted in one eye using Healon; these were compared with control eyes, in which implantation was achieved using air and balanced salt solution. Postoperatively, the Healon-treated eyes showed clearer corneas and fewer complications. There was no evidence of immunologically induced inflammation.

Human studies of the efficacy of Healon in intraocular procedures were carried out by Robert Stegmann and colleagues[3] of Pretoria, South Africa, who performed a slit-lamp examination on their patients on alternate days postoperatively. The results of the study confirmed the protective effect of HA on endothelial cells. As the material was used more extensively, we also found that it maintained the normal anatomic relationship within the eye during glaucoma surgery, corneal transplantation, and repair of ocular trauma.

Further confirmation of the usefulness of Healon was provided by Polack and his associates at Gainesville, Florida (Polack F, personal communication, 1979). Their histologic and clinical evidence demonstrated that Healon protected the cornea from the trauma of implant and instrument contact[4] and produced better results in corneal transplantation. Pape and Balazs[5] were also able to confirm its usefulness in glaucoma and cataract surgery.[5] They also reported that Healon could produce a transient rise in intraocular pressure (IOP) postoperatively and suggested that it be irrigated out at the end of surgery. This work was confirmed by Jaffe (Jaffe N, personal communication, 1980) and Alpar (Alpar JJ, personal communication, 1980). Holmberg and Philipson[6] further demonstrated the usefulness of Healon in extracapsular cataract extraction, and Lazenby and Broocker[7, 8] documented its usefulness in anterior chamber lens implantation. Stenkula and Tornquist[9] demonstrated Healon's effectiveness in vitrectomy and in repair of difficult retinal detachments. As Balazs looked over the many surgical applications of Healon (Healnoid), he coined the word *viscosurgery* to describe the use of a viscoelastic fluid during surgical manipulation of the eye.

Physical and Chemical Properties of Viscoelastic Materials

The ideal substance for use in viscosurgery would be a solution of high viscosity that was also noninflammatory, nonpyogenic, nontoxic, and nonantigenic. This jelly-like substance should also be endowed with a property called *pseudoplasticity*, which describes its ability to be passed through a small channel, for example, a fine cannula, a 30-gauge needle, or the pores of the trabecular meshwork. Further, elastic qualities would enable it to rebound after mechanical stress or compression. A number of viscoelastic polymers meeting these criteria have been derived from both natural and synthetic sources and are currently available to the ophthalmic surgeon. The most commonly used substances are listed in Table 31–1.

As mentioned previously, Healon was the first viscoelastic sodium hyaluronate solution to be marketed for ophthalmic use. Sodium hyaluronate's combined viscous, elastic, and pseudoplastic properties make it well suited for anterior

TABLE 31–1. **Comparative Properties of Viscoelastic Materials**

Material and Company	Cohesion	Composition	Molecular Mass (Daltons)	Viscosity (cSt)	pH	Osmolarity (mOsm/kg)	Storage Conditions (°C)	Shelf Life (Yr)
Amo Vitrax, *Allergan*	Low	3% NaHA	0.5 million	30,000	7.0–7.5	310	Room temp	1.5
Amvisc, *Chiron Vision*	High	1.2% NaHA	≥2.0 million	40,000	5.5–7.0	320	2–8	2
Amvisc Plus, *Chiron Vision*	Medium	1.6% NaHA	≈1.5 million	55,000	5.5–7.0	340	2–8	1
Cellugel,* *Alcon*	Data unavailable	2% HPMC	200,000	20,000	7.2	305	Room temp	1
Duovisc,† *Alcon*								
Provisc, *Alcon*	High	1% NaHA	2.4 million	39,000	7.2	310	2–8	3
Viscoat, *Alcon*	Low	3% NaHA and 4% CDS	NaHA: 0.5 million CDS: 22,000	≈40,000	7.2	325	2–8	2
Healon, *Pharmacia and Upjohn*	High	1% NaHA	3.8 million	35,000–40,000	7.0–7.5	302	2–8	3
Healon GV, *Pharmacia and Upjohn*	High	1.4% NaHA	5.0 million	200,000	7.0–7.5	302	2–8	3
Occucoat, *Storz Ophthalmics*	None	2% HPMC	>80,000	4,000	7.2	285	Room temp	1

Abbreviations: NaHA, sodium hyaluronate; HPMC, hydroxypropyl methylcellulose; CDS, chondroitin sulfate.
*Pending FDA approval.
†Duovisc = Provisc and Viscoat.

segment surgical applications. Healon is a 1% solution derived from a natural source (rooster combs) and is available as a sterile solution in sealed 0.5- to 1-mL glass syringes (10 mg/mL). Healon is also available with a blue tint in order to facilitate intraocular visualization of the polymer.[10] Provisc is comparable to Healon in terms of sodium hyaluronate concentration, viscosity, and cohesive properties.

Amvisc is similar to Healon in that it is a sodium hyaluronate solution purified from rooster combs. Unlike Healon, however, it is formulated to a consistent viscosity with a concentration varying between 1 and 1.4% hyaluronate, whereas Healon is prepared to a specific concentration (1%) with a variable viscosity. Amvisc Plus has a higher concentration of sodium hyaluronate (1.6%) and is 30% more viscous than Amvisc. Healon GV is also available, with a 1.4% sodium hyaluronate concentration and a viscosity considerably higher than that of other ophthalmic viscoelastic preparations.

Amo Vitrax contains 3% sodium hyaluronate, the highest concentration currently available. Viscoat combines 3% sodium hyaluronate with 4% chondroitin sulfate. Although the structure of chondroitin sulfate is similar to that of HA, the sulfate group of chondroitin sulfate results in a double negative charge per repeating disaccharide subunit compared with the single negative charge per subunit in HA. Chondroitin sulfate is not a pseudoplastic fluid; instead, it maintains a constant viscosity at various shear rates.

The choice of viscoelastic material should include consideration of the type of surgical procedure and the cohesive characteristics of the viscoelastic (see Table 31–1). Noncohesive (or dispersive) viscoelastics have a tendency to adhere to ocular surfaces, thereby providing a protective coating for the tissues and remaining in position without excessive leakage during irrigation. Thus, viscoelastics with low cohesive properties would be advantageous during iris plane and anterior chamber phacoemulsification, particularly where endothelial protection is critical, for example, cases of Fuchs' endothelial dystrophy. The disadvantages of these dispersive viscoelastic properties is the time and effort required for removal of the viscoelastics. In contrast, cohesive viscoelastics adhere more to themselves than to the ocular surfaces; as such they are easily aspirated from the eye. The more cohesive viscoelastics are desirable when anterior chamber maintenance, tissue manipulation, and easy removal are the principal goals. With high positive vitreous pressure, cohesive viscoelastics have the ability to create and maintain a deep anterior chamber. Cohesive viscoelastics would be effective during capsulorrhexis and IOL implantation, and particularly while unfolding a very fine foldable lens.

DuoVisc is a viscoelastic "system," containing Viscoat and Provisc in separate syringes, allowing the surgeon to customize the choice of viscoelastic materials to suit particular steps in a surgical procedure. Thus, Viscoat's tissue protection properties would be preferable in the initial stages of an anterior segment procedure such as extracapsular cataract extraction by phacoemulsification, whereas Provisc's cohesive properties would be advantageous for later phases of the procedure, such as expansion of the capsular opening, maintaining space, and IOL implantation.

Hydroxypropyl methylcellulose (2% solution) also has been used successfully as a viscoelastic material for anterior segment surgery. This linear polymer of glucose has a greater hydrophilic character than its parent molecule, cellulose, owing to the presence of hydroxypropyl and methyl groups. Occucoat and Cellugel are commercially available products of the same concentration but differ considerably in their viscosity (see Table 31–1). Both, however, are less viscous than Healon.

Indications for Use

Viscoelastics have been classified as devices (not drugs) by the U.S. Food and Drug Administration. As such, they can aptly be considered as surgical "tools" with which the intraocular environment can be manipulated. Viscoelastics are indispensable in certain procedures in which the maintenance of anatomic spaces and atraumatic tissue manipulation are required. Furthermore, their physical properties endow them with lubricating, wetting, and protective qualities.

The most common surgical application of viscoelastics in ophthalmology is cataract extraction. During such procedures, viscoelastic materials have been found to be indispensable in maintaining the anatomic space of the anterior chamber during surgical manipulation. Comparative studies have demonstrated that viscoelastics (see Table 31–1) are all effective in maintaining the intraocular space and manipulating intraocular tissues. All are also valuable in controlling posterior pressure.

When phacoemulsification is used for cataract extraction, injecting viscoelastics into the cleavage plane between the lens nucleus and cortex greatly facilitates phacoemulsification of the nucleus.[11] Such "viscodissection" may be especially useful in the case of cataracts with a soft nucleus in which there is difficulty negotiating the phacoemulsification tip beneath the nucleus, during which zonular tears or posterior lens capsular rupture could occur.[12] The technique of nuclear viscoexpression has been advocated after capsulorrhexis during extracapsular cataract extraction.[13–17]

Sodium hyaluronate has also been successfully used for the removal of severely subluxated lenses.[18] The injection of sodium hyaluronate beneath the lens results in lens elevation and prevention of total luxation, thus simplifying lensectomy. Viscoelastic dissection has also been used for relocation of off-axis IOL implants.[19]

Perhaps the greatest asset of viscoelastics in anterior chamber surgery is their ability to protect the corneal endothelium from mechanical trauma, particularly in IOL insertion and contact with neighboring tissues and surgical instruments. Glasser and colleagues[20] compared Healon, Amvisc, and Viscoat and found that all three viscoelastics provided complete corneal endothelium protection during contact with an IOL in vitro. However, a more recent study by Glasser and coworkers[21] cites the apparent superior ability of Viscoat to prevent endothelial cell loss in vivo during phacoemulsification with IOL implantation when compared with Healon. The authors attribute the difference in performance of these viscoelastics to the presence of chondroitin sulfate in Viscoat, which renders it more adherent to the corneal endothelium. This adherent layer would thus afford greater protection for the endothelial cells during surgery. The endothelium may also be spared physical trauma by coating the IOL with a viscoelastic polymer before implantation.

It has been reported that the use of hydroxypropyl methylcellulose resulted in patients' developing a nonreactive semidilated pupil when compared with eyes receiving sodium hyaluronate (Healonid).[22] However, a later study reported no statistical difference in pupil size or reactivity after the use of OcuCoat or Healonid in the course of cataract surgery.[23]

A number of reports have cited increased IOP postoperatively following the use of viscoelastics.[24] This transient rise in IOP characteristically occurs 6 to 24 hours after surgery and usually resolves spontaneously within 72 hours postoperatively.[25] Berson and associates[26] have suggested that such viscosurgery-associated IOP elevations may be due to mechanical obstruction of aqueous outflow by the viscoagent. It is recommended that the viscoagent be removed from the eye by thoroughly irrigating and aspirating with a balanced salt solution and that IOP be monitored postoperatively. In some instances, it may be necessary to treat the elevated IOP with antiglaucoma medications.

The protective effect of viscoelastics on corneal endothelial cells is the primary reason for their use in corneal surgery. However, we have used viscoagents on the corneal surface during anterior segment procedures and wound closure to prevent trauma to and desiccation of the corneal epithelium. In addition to these benefits of topical viscoagents during corneal surgery, Reed and colleagues[27] present evidence that such use results in significant improvement in corneal epithelial integrity 1 week after keratoplasty compared with corneas that were hydrated with a balanced salt solution.

Detachment of Descemet's membrane is a complication of intraocular surgery that may occur with the injection of sodium hyaluronate[28–30] as well as during insertion of IOLs or surgical instruments through the corneoscleral or corneal wound. Such trauma-induced detachment (stripping) of Descemet's membrane from the corneal stroma has been successfully repaired using sodium hyaluronate[31, 32] to move Descemet's membrane to its normal anatomic position as well as tamponade to avoid further detachment. Treatment of Descemet's membrane detachment is important in preventing localized corneal decompensation and consequent edema.

Glaucoma filtration procedures are further opportunities to employ viscoelastic materials. In these situations, viscoelastics have been shown to prevent the collapse of the anterior chamber as well as hyphema during the procedure in addition to stabilizing early postoperative pressure.[33–35] Alpar[36] reported that Healon use in glaucoma filtering procedures results in more permanent bleb formation and maintenance, more open clefts, less scarring, less peripheral anterior synechia formation, and significantly lower long-term IOP.

Sodium hyaluronate has been used in the treatment of incarceration of vitreous in patients with corneal decompensation.[37, 38] Before neodymium:yttrium-aluminum-garnet treatment for vitreolysis, the anterior chamber was filled with Healon, and postoperative corneal complications were reduced.

It has been suggested that viscoagents be used to control intraocular hemorrhage. In the case of blood in the anterior chamber, however, the use of viscoagents should be approached with caution, since the viscoelastic material may trap the clotted blood, causing it to be retained longer in the intraocular environment. In the case of suprachoroid hemorrhages, instillation of 10% sodium hyaluronate into the vitreous cavity has been used for postoperative management.[39, 40] Sodium hyaluronate offers certain advantages over intraocular air and balanced salt solution, which is similarly used. For example, the use of sodium hyaluronate allows good visualization of instruments in the eye and avoids image minification and distortion from the air-fluid interface. Although balanced salt solution can be used, sodium hyaluronate viscoelastic is less likely to egress through rents in the posterior lens capsule or between zonular fibers and consequently provides a more effective and durable expansion of intraocular volume.[39] Moreover, a viscoelastic may prolong the maintenance of the IOP after filtering surgery.[41]

Sustaining the IOP would help facilitate drainage of a suprachoroid hemorrhage and avoid choroid effusion and hemorrhage incurred by ocular hypotonia. Using a generous amount of Healon and flattening the retinochoroid elevations of a suprachoroid hemorrhage promotes expression of blood from the suprachoroid spaces.[42]

Viscoelastics have additional applications in vitreo-retinal surgery, including the repair of retinal detachments. For example, suprachoroid implantation of viscoelastic substances can result in the temporary induction of a choroid elevation for closing retinal tears.[43–47] Sodium hyaluronate has even been used for the repair of giant retinal tears. The technique allows unrolling of retinal flaps and apposing them to the underlying pigment epithelium.[48, 49]

The procoagulant effects of HA after diabetic vitrectomy have been reported,[50] and sodium hyaluronate has been used to perform delamination at the vitreoretinal juncture in diabetic eye disease. Such viscodelamination has been performed to separate attached vitreous cortex from fibrovascular epiretinal membranes.[51] Viscodelamination was especially of value in eyes with combined traction and rhegmatogenous retinal detachment; however, the viscodelamination technique has a significant risk of retinal breaks, which are especially likely to occur with attempts to elevate excessively adherent fibrovascular epiretinal membranes.[51] Methods of elevation of epiretinal membranes from the retina using sodium hyaluronate (Healon) have been described.[9]

Sodium hyaluronate has also been used in lacrimal surgery. When injected into the lacrimal sac, it is useful in identifying the extent of the sac lumen.[52, 53] Sodium hyaluronate has been reported to facilitate passage of lacrimal probes for repair of lacerated canaliculi.[54] The lacrimal sac is filled with hyaluronate via the intact lacrimal canaliculus and a pigtail probe or probes for bicanaliculonasal intubation performed. Hyaluronate is thought to coat and distend the lumen of the lacrimal passages, allowing the probe tip to find its way to the injured canaliculus.[54] Sodium hyaluronate injection into the lacrimal sac has been reported to facilitate locating cut medial canaliculi[55] with the viscoelastic presentation at a medial cut opening.[53]

Sodium hyaluronate has been used in strabismus surgery, with adjustable sutures to minimize tissue drag among conjunctiva, Tenon's capsule, and muscle and to facilitate suture adjustment.[56] Healon has been reported to reduce postoperative muscle adhesions[57] and to increase the period of suture adjustability in operated muscles.[58]

Nonsurgical applications of sodium hyaluronate include its use as a dry eye treatment; there have been several reports[59–66] of subjective and objective improvement in dry eye symptoms and patient comfort, particularly in those individuals with severe keratoconjunctivitis sicca.[67] Similarly, such patients have been reported to experience marked relief of symptoms after topical application of a chondroitin sulfate solution.[66]

Conclusions

Viscoelastic polymers are a valuable surgical adjunct owing to their ability to maintain anatomic space, manipulate intraocular tissues, and prevent mechanical trauma to critical fragile cells such as the corneal endothelium. The reported elevation of IOP after viscosurgery can be reduced by anterior chamber irrigation at the end of the procedure. Taken collectively, the comparative data suggest no major differences among commercially available viscosurgical agents in regard to optical clarity, ease of administration, tissue protection, postoperative IOP, and space maintenance.[68–70] When cost effectiveness is a major concern, consideration should be given to methylcellulose preparations. In summary, although a number of viscoelastic solutions are available to the ophthalmic surgeon, no single formulation appears significantly more efficacious than the other polymers.

REFERENCES

1. Meyer K, Palmer JW: The polysaccharide of the vitreous humor. J Biol Chem 107:629, 1934.
2. Balazs EA: Ultrapure hyaluronic acid and the use thereof. U.S. Patent No. 4, 141, 973, 1979.
3. Balazs EA, Miller D, Stegmann R: Viscosurgery and the use of Na-hyaluronate in intraocular lens implantation. Paper presented at the International Congress and First Film Festival on Intraocular Implantation, Cannes, France, 1979.
4. Graue EL, Polack FM, Balazs EA: The protective effect of Na-hyaluronate to corneal endothelium. Exp Eye Res 31:119, 1980.
5. Pape LG, Balazs EA: The use of sodium hyaluronate (Healon) in human anterior segment surgery. Ophthalmology 87:699, 1980.
6. Holmberg AS, Philipson BT: Sodium hyaluronate in cataract surgery. II: Report on the use of Healon in extracapsular cataract surgery using phacoemulsification. Ophthalmology 91:53, 1984.
7. Lazenby GW, Broocker G: The use of sodium hyaluronate (Healon) in intracapsular cataract extraction with insertion of anterior chamber intraocular lenses. Ophthalmic Surg 12:646, 1981.
8. Lazenby GW: Anterior chamber lens implantation combined with the use of Healon. *In* Miller D, Stegmann R (eds): Healon (Sodium Hyaluronate): A Guide to Its Use in Ophthalmic Surgery. New York, Wiley, 1983, p 69.
9. Stenkula S, Tornquist R: Use of Healon in vitrectomy and difficult retinal detachments. *In* Miller D, Stegmann R (eds): Healon (Sodium Hyaluronate): A Guide to Its Use in Ophthalmic Surgery. New York, Wiley, 1983, p 207.
10. Drews RC, Gabrawy L: Blue Healon. J Cataract Refract Surg 15:100, 1989.
11. Blaydes JE, Fritz KJ, Fogle JA: New techniques of viscosurgery with phacoemulsification. Am Intraocul Implant Soc J 11:395, 1985.
12. DeLuise VP: Viscodissection as an adjunct to phacoemulsification. Ophthalmic Surg 19:682, 1988.
13. Thim K, Krag S, Corydon L: Hydroexpression and viscoexpression of the nucleus through a continuous circular capsulorrhexis. J Cataract Refract Surg 19:209, 1993.
14. Burton RL, Pickering S: Extracapsular cataract surgery using capsulorrhexis with viscoexpression via a limbal section. J Cataract Refract Surg 21:297, 1995.
15. Bellucci R, Morselli S, Pucci V, Bonomi L: Nucleus viscoexpression compared with the other techniques of nucleus removal in extracapsular cataract extraction with capsulorrhexis. Ophthalmic Surg 25:432, 1994.
16. Schirmer K: Nuclear expression using viscoelastic versus small incision surgery. Ophthalmic Surg 26:169, 1995.
17. Korynta J: Viscoexpression of the lens nucleus in extracapsular cataract extraction. Cesk Oftalmol 52:179, 1996.
18. Toczolowski JR: The use of sodium hyaluronate (Hyalcon) for the removal of severely subluxated lenses. Ophthalmic Surg 18:214, 1987.
19. Mandelcorn M: Viscoelastic dissection for relocation of off-axis intraocular lens implant: A new technique. Can J Ophthalmol 30:34, 1995.
20. Glasser DB, Matsuda M, Edelhauser HF: A comparison of the efficacy and toxicity of and intraocular pressure response to viscous solutions in the anterior chamber. Arch Ophthalmol 104:1819, 1986.
21. Glasser DB, Katz HR, Boyd JE, et al: Protective effects of viscous solutions in phacoemulsification and traumatic lens implantation. Arch Ophthalmol 107:1047, 1989.
22. Tan AKK, Humphrey RC: The fixed dilated pupil after cataract surgery—is it related to intraocular use of hydromellose? Br J Ophthalmol 77:639, 1993.
23. Easen J, Seward HC: Pupil size and reactivity following hydroxypropyl methylcellulose and sodium hyaluronate. Br J Ophthalmol 79:541, 1995.

24. Kusman B, Jaffe NS, Clayman HM, Jaffe MS: Sodium hyaluronate (Healon) and intraocular pressure. *In* Miller D, Stegmann R (eds): Healon (Sodium Hyaluronate): A Guide to Its Use in Ophthalmic Surgery. New York, Wiley, 1983, p 195.
25. Larson RS, Lindstrom RL, Skelnik DL: Viscoelastic agents. CLAO J 15:151, 1989.
26. Berson FG, Patterson MM, Epstein DL: Obstruction of aqueous outflow by sodium hyaluronate in enucleated human eyes. Am J Ophthalmol 95:668, 1983.
27. Reed DB, Mannis MJ, Hills JF, Johnson CA: Corneal epithelial healing after penetrating keratoplasty using topical Healon versus balanced salt solution. Ophthalmic Surg 18:525, 1987.
28. Graether JM: Detachment of Descemet's membrane by injection of sodium hyaluronate (Healon). J Ocul Ther Surg 3:178, 1984.
29. Hoover DL, Giangiacomo J, Benson RL: Descemet's membrane detachment by sodium hyaluronate. Arch Ophthalmol 103:805, 1985.
30. Ostberg A, Törnquist G: Management of detachment of Descemet's membrane caused by injection of hyaluronic acid. Ophthalmic Surg 20:885, 1989.
31. McAuliffe KM: Sodium hyaluronate in the treatment of Descemet's membrane detachment. J Ocul Ther Surg 1:58, 1982.
32. Donzis PB, Karcioglu ZA, Insler MS: Sodium hyaluronate (Healon) in the surgical repair of Descemet's membrane detachment. Ophthalmic Surg 17:735, 1986.
33. Raitta C, Setälä K: Trabeculectomy with the use of sodium hyaluronate. One-year follow-up. Acta Ophthalmol 65:709, 1987.
34. Raitta C, Setälä K: Trabeculectomy with the use of sodium hyaluronate: A prospective study. Acta Ophthalmol 64:407, 1986.
35. Merriam JC, Wahlig JB, Konrad H, Zaider M: Extracapsular cataract extraction and posterior-lip sclerectomy with viscoelastic. Ophthalmic Surg 25:438, 1994.
36. Alpar JJ: Sodium hyaluronate (Healon) in glaucoma filtering procedures. Ophthalmic Surg 17:724, 1986.
37. Alpar JJ: The role of 1 percent sodium hyaluronate in treating vitreous incarceration with the neodymium: YAG laser in patients with corneal decompensation. J Cataract Refract Surg 12:502, 1986.
38. Alpar JJ: The role of 1 percent sodium hyaluronate in anterior capsulotomy with the neodymium: YAG laser in patients with diseased cornea. J Cataract Refract Surg 12:658, 1986.
39. Baldwin LB, Smith TJ, Hollins JL, Pearson PA: The use of viscoelastic substances in the drainage of postoperative suprachoroidal hemorrhage. Ophthalmic Surg 20:504, 1989.
40. Shin DH, Frenkel RE: The use of viscoelastic substances in the drainage of postoperative suprachoroidal hemorrhage. Ophthalmic Surg 20:895, 1989.
41. Gressel MG, Parrish RK, Heuer DK: Delayed nonexpulsive suprachoroidal hemorrhage. Arch Ophthalmol 102:1757, 1984.
42. Frenkel REP, Shin DH: Prevention and management of delayed suprachoroidal hemorrhage after filtration surgery. Arch Ophthalmol 104:1459, 1986.
43. Pruett RC, Schepens CL, Swan DA: Hyaluronic acid vitreous substitute: A six-year clinical evaluation. Arch Ophthalmol 97:2325, 1979.
44. Stenkula S, Ivert L, Gislason I, et al: The use of sodium-hyaluronate (Healon) in the treatment of retinal detachment. Ophthalmic Surg 12:435, 1981.
45. Poole TA, Sudarsky RD: Suprachoroidal implantation for the treatment of retinal detachment. Ophthalmology 93:1408, 1986.
46. Mittl RN, Tiwari R: Suprachoroidal injection of sodium hyaluronate as an "internal" buckling procedure. Ophthalmic Res 19:255, 1987.
47. Lavin MJ, Leaver PK: Sodium hyaluronate and giant retinal tears. Arch Ophthalmol 108:480, 1990.
48. Meredith TA: Giant retinal tears. Arch Ophthalmol 108:777, 1990.
49. Brown GC, Benson WE: Use of sodium hyaluronate for the repair of giant retinal tears. Arch Ophthalmol 107:1246, 1989.
50. Packer AJ, McCuen BW II, Hutton WL, Ramsay RC: Procoagulant effects of intraocular sodium hyaluronate (Healon) after phakic diabetic vitrectomy. A prospective randomized study. Ophthalmology 96:1491, 1989.
51. McLeod D, James CR: Viscodelamination at the vitreoretinal juncture in severe diabetic eye disease. Br J Ophthalmol 72:413, 1988.
52. Hurwitz JJ, Nik N: Lacrimal sac identification for dacryocystorhinostomy: The role of sodium hyaluronate. Can J Ophthamol 19:112, 1984.
53. Lerner HA, Boynton JR: Sodium hyaluronate (Healon) as an adjunct to lacrimal surgery. Am J Ophthalmol 99:365, 1985.
54. Vila-Coro AA, Vila-Coro AA: Hyaluronate facilitates passage of lacrimal probes for repair of lacerated canaliculi. Arch Ophthalmol 106:579, 1988.
55. Seiff SR, Ahn JC: Locating cut medial canaliculi by direct injection of sodium hyaluronate into the lacrimal sac. Ophthalmic Surg 20:176, 1989.
56. Clorfeine GS, Parker WT: Use of Healon in eye muscle surgery with adjustable sutures. Ann Ophthalmol 19:215, 1987.
57. Searl SS, Metz HS, Lindahl KJ: The use of sodium hyaluronate as a biologic sleeve in strabismus surgery. Ann Ophthalmol 19:259, 1987.
58. Manjoney D, Mathias S, Morris W, et al: Effect of Healon on adjustable suture strabismus surgery. Invest Ophthalmol Vis Sci (ARVO Suppl) 26:80, 1985.
59. Polack FM, McNiece MT: The treatment of dry eyes with Na hyaluronate (Healon). Cornea 1:133, 1982.
60. DeLuise VP: Viscodissection as an adjunct to phacoemulsification. Ophthalmic Surg 19:682, 1988.
61. Stuart JC, Linn JG: Dilute sodium hyaluronate (Healon) in the treatment of ocular surface disorders. Ann Ophthalmol 17:190, 1985.
62. Nelson JD, Farris RL: Sodium hyaluronate and polyvinyl alcohol artificial tear preparations. A comparison in patients with keratoconjunctivitis sicca. Arch Ophthalmol 106:484, 1988.
63. Laflamme MY, Swieca R: A comparative study of two preservative-free tear substitutes in the management of severe dry eye. Can J Ophthalmol 23:174, 1988.
64. Bohm E, Rama P, Tallandini L, et al: Low molecular weight sodium hyaluronate in the treatment of tear film changes and of dry eye. Ophthalmologie 2:353, 1988.
65. Orsoni JG, Chiari M, Guazzi A, et al: Efficacy of hyaluronic acid eyedrops in the treatment of dry eye. Cytologic study using an optical microscope and computerized microscope. Ophthalmologie 2:355, 1988.
66. Limberg MB, McCaa C, Kissling GE, et al: Topical application of hyaluronic acid and chondroitin sulfate in the treatment of dry eyes. Am J Ophthalmol 103:194, 1987.
67. Sand BB, Marner K, Norn MS: Sodium hyaluronate in the treatment of keratoconjunctivitis sicca. A double masked clinical trial. Acta Ophthalmol 67:181, 1989.
68. Genstler DE, Keates RH: Amvisc in extracapsular cataract extraction. Am Intra-ocular Implant Soc J 9:317, 1983.
69. Glasser DB, Matsuda M, Edelhauser HF: A comparison of the efficacy and toxicity of and intraocular pressure response to viscous solutions in the anterior chamber. Arch Ophthalmol 104:1819, 1986.
70. McKnight SJ. Giangiacomo J, Adelstein E: Inflammatory response to viscoelastic materials. Ophthalmic Surg 18:804, 1987.

CHAPTER 32

Osmotic Agents

James Lee

Osmotic phenomena occurring within the eye are the source of prominent signs and symptoms in many disease states. The origins of cataracts, aqueous humor formation, and some vitreous and retinal detachments are modified by the balance of osmotic forces within the membranes of the eye. Although the study of osmotic phenomena began in earnest toward the end of the 19th century,[1] it was greatly accelerated by the work of Friedenwald[18, 21, 22] and of Cogan.[2–14]

A review of the basic physiology of osmosis and its present applications in evaluation and treatment of the eye follows, including an overview of agents in each system.

Osmosis: Terms and Basic Physiology

If a membrane is permeable to water only, and if it separates two solutions with differing proportions of water, a net movement of water occurs through the membrane. *Osmosis* is the term used for the transfer of water. Kinetic movement of the water molecules provides the source of energy for the transfer. If a greater proportion of water molecules is on one side of the membrane, a larger number of water molecules come in contact with it; consequently, more molecules pass through the membrane from this side. The net flow of water can be prevented by the application of an opposing force, *osmotic pressure*. This pressure is directly proportional to the concentration of nondiffusible molecules on the other side and is not related to the molecular weight of the molecules. *Osmolarity* expresses osmoles per liter of water, and *osmolality* expresses osmoles per kilogram.

Diffusion is the constant movement of molecules among each other, which results in a solute or solvent moving to a region of lower concentration. It is a fundamental principle in the study of osmosis. If any part of the membrane interacts with the diffusing substance, such as a carrier protein in a cell wall aiding the passage of a given substance, diffusion is facilitated. A cell wall, which is a highly complex semipermeable membrane, has both outer and inner lipid layers and a middle aqueous layer. A lipid-soluble substance passes through the lipid-soluble layers with greater ease than a water-soluble substance, whereas the latter transgresses only the middle layer with comparative ease. The process of dialysis results when protein is on one side of the semipermeable membrane. Water moves toward the protein, and salt flows away from the protein. The final distribution of salt and protein is described by the Gibbs-Donnan equilibrium in which (1) the product of cations and anions is the same on both sides of the membrane and (2) the number of cations on the protein side equals the sum of anions and proteins on the same side. Ultrafiltration results when a hydrostatic force, such as blood pressure, acts on the solutions that contain protein.

Important Osmotic Phenomena in the Eye

CORNEA

Water movement within the epithelium is slowed by the presence of lipid membranes. Only lipid-soluble substances pass easily through the cell membranes. Epithelial cell junctions, the *zonulae occludens,* act as an additional barrier. In contrast, water moves rapidly within the stroma because of the abundance of collagen fibrils, which are separated by proteoglycans and water. Although endothelial cells have junctional complexes, they are much more leaky; the result is relative freedom of water movement.[2–10, 13–18] Thus, only lipid-soluble substances cross the epithelial and endothelial membranes, and water-soluble substances pass with equal freedom through the stromal layer. Substances soluble in both lipid and aqueous penetrate the cornea more easily.

AQUEOUS HUMOR

Within the ciliary epithelium, osmotic processes lead to the active secretion of Na^+ and HCO_3^-. The tight junctions of nonpigmented ciliary epithelium impede aqueous formation from plasma.[19, 20] Carbonic anhydrase catalyzes the reaction of $CO_2{}^+$ H_2O to H_2CO_3. Carbonic anhydrase inhibitors interfere with the rate of transfer of bicarbonate and sodium from plasma to aqueous humor, and the flow of aqueous is reduced.[21, 22]

The blood-aqueous barrier is a significant impediment to many osmotic processes, particularly those of higher molecular weight.[19, 20, 23–28] During inflammatory episodes, it becomes comparitively leaky.[24]

LENS

An active Na^+ ion-water pump, which is located within the epithelial cell membranes, is responsible for the relative low water content of the lens. During many disease processes, osmotic phenomena disrupt the balance of water. In diabetic cataract, excess glucose in the lens saturates hexokinase. As a result, glucose accumulates, some of which is converted to fructose and sorbitol. As sorbitol increases in concentration, water is drawn in to form vacuoles, and the initiation of cataract formation proceeds. The cataract formed in galactosemia results from an excessive amount of galactose, which is formed by the hydrolysis of lactose. As galactose builds up, galactitol forms, the presence of which is the basis for osmotic movement of water into the lens.[29–36]

VITREOUS

Movement of water from the vitreous follows several routes. The major portal for systemic circulation to the vitreous is the capillary system of the ciliary processes. The effect is chiefly on the anterior vitreous. For the posterior vitreous, the choroidal and retinal circulations present another portal. Solutes may pass from the systemic circulation into the vitreous. Polar molecules generally enter the vitreous through the ciliary processes, and lipid-soluble substances enter via the retina.[37–39]

Apposition of the retina to the choroid is largely due to the result of a pressure gradient of approximately 13 mm Hg between the two membranes. If the gradient is disturbed, which may occur during the infusion of a critically large quantity of intravitreal antibiotics, an osmotic detachment of the retina may result.[40]

TEARS

Cellular integrity of air-exposed cells of both the cornea and the conjunctiva is maintained by the presence of a complex barrier of isotonic fluid, the tear film. The outer layer is composed of lipid, which prevents excessive evaporation. Lipid is resurfaced over the aqueous layer during normal blinking. Approximately 10% of the normal tear volume is forced into the nasolacrimal passages during each blink. Baseline lacrimal secretion replaces the quantity of aqueous component that is lost through both evaporation and blinking. In keratoconjunctivitis sicca, tear replacement from the lacrimal gland is decreased, often with striking morphologic changes in both the conjunctival and the corneal epithelium. Disruptive osmotic forces within the epithelial cells are the principal cause of these changes.

Osmotic Agents

Both systemic and topically applied osmotic agents have been used in a variety of eye conditions. Only the currently available agents are presented.

SYSTEMIC

Treatment of ocular hypertension and preparation of the eye for intraocular surgery are the two prominent therapeutic indications for systemic delivery of osmotic agents.

Glycerin (Osmoglyn, Alcon)

Available as a 50% oral preparation in a flavored vehicle, glycerin produces rapid reduction in intraocular tension without the hazard of intravenous administration. It is rapidly metabolized to glucose and is excreted by the kidneys. Care must be taken when treating diabetics. Nausea and dehydration are frequent side effects.[41–43] Dosage is 1 to 1.5 g/kg body weight.

Isosorbide (Ismotic, Alcon)

Isosorbide is available in a 45% oral preparation in a vanilla-mint–flavored vehicle. Its physiologic properties are similar to those of glycerin.[44] It is essentially not metabolized and is excreted by the kidney. Dosage is 1.5 g/kg body weight.

Urea (Ureaphil)

Administered intravenously in a 30% solution, urea has hypotensive effects similar to those of other systemic osmotic agents. After urea achieves its maximal effect, its delayed entry into the vitreous may result in a concentration of urea higher than in the plasma. The result is a curious reverse osmotic effect, with water entering the vitreous from plasma.

Local thrombophlebitis is more common with urea, and extravasation into the surrounding tissues may lead to widespread tissue necrosis. Headaches are common. Dehydration can lead to confusion, stupor, and coma in the elderly. Stretching of the sagittal vein rarely leads to rupture of the bridging veins, with resulting subdural hematoma.[45]

Mannitol (Osmitrol)

Given intravenously, mannitol has osmotic effects similar to those of other agents.[46–48] It may be more effective during inflammation. It is not metabolized. Dosage is 1.5 to 2 g/kg body weight over 30 to 45 minutes.

LOCAL

Corneal Clearing

When visualization through the cornea becomes difficult because of stromal or epithelial edema, the following osmotic agents may provide rapid but only temporary improvement of both the examiner's visualization and the patient's vision.

Glycerin (Ophthalgan)

A single drop leads to rapid clearing (within 1 to 2 minutes). The effect may last several hours. Because glycerin is often painful, it is used only for diagnosis.[48]

Sodium Chloride (Adsorbonac Ophthalmic, 2% or 5% Solution; Ak-NaCl, 5% Solution and Ointment; Muro 128, 5% Solution and Ointment)

Administration leads to rapid osmotic movement of water from both epithelium and stroma. The effect lasts only a few minutes. When epithelium is partly or completely missing, the osmotic effect is much more rapid.

Glucose (Glucose-40 Ophthalmic, 40% Ointment)

The effect of glucose may last several hours. Administration may be repeated. Irritation may also occur.

Tear Substitutes

Some recent tear substitutes have closely approached the normal crystalline composition of tears. The goal is the

TABLE 32–1. **Artificial Tear Preparations**

Product	Manufacturer	Vehicle	Preservative
AKWA Tears	Akorn	Polyvinyl alcohol 1.4%	Benzalkonium chloride, edetate disodium
AquaSite	CIBA Vision	Polycarbophil, PEG-400 dextran-70	EDTA
Bion Tears	Alcon	Hydroxypropyl methylcellulose, dextran-70	Preservative-free
Boston Advance Reconditioning Drops	Polymer Technology	Patented hydrophilic polyelectrolyte	Polyaminopropyl biguanide edetate disodium
Celluvisc Lubricant	Allergan	Carboxymethylcellulose, polyvinyl alcohol	Preservative-free
Clear Eyes Ophthalmic Solution	Ross	Naphazoline hydrochloride	Edetate disodium, glycerin, benzalkonium chloride, chlorbutanol
Collyrium Fresh	Wyeth-Ayerst	Tetrahydrozoline hydrochloride, glycerin	Edetate disodium, benzalkonium chloride
Comfort Tears	Sola/Barnes-Hind	Hydroxyethycellulose benzalkonium chloride	Edetate disodium
Dry Eyes Lubricant	Bausch & Lomb	1.4% Polyvinyl alcohol	Chlorbutanol
GenTeal	CIBA Vision	0.3% Hydroxypropyl cellulose	Sodium perborate
HypoTears (hypotonic)	IOLAB	1% polyvinyl alcohol, PEG-400, dextran-70	Benzalkonium chloride
HypoTears PF	IOLAB	1% Polyvinyl alcohol, PEG-400, dextran-70	Preservative-free
Isopto Plain	Alcon	0.5% Hydroxypropyl methylcellulose	Benzalkonium chloride
Isopto Alkaline	Alcon	1% Hydroxypropyl methylcellulose	Benzalokonium chloride
Lacril	Allergan	Hydroxypropyl methylcellulose, gelatin A	Chlorobutanol, polysorbate-80
Lacrisert	MSD	Hydroxypropyl cellulose	Preservative-free
Liquifilm Forte	Allergan	1.4% Polyvinyl alcohol	EDTA, thimerosal
Liquifilm Tears	Allergan	1.4% Polyvinyl alcohol	Chlorbutanol
Murine	Ross	1.4% Polyvinyl alcohol, povidone	Benzalkonium chloride, edetate disodium
Muro 128	Bausch & Lomb	Sodium chloride 2% and 5%, propylene glycol, hydroxypropyl methylcellulose	Methylparaben, propylparaben
Murocel	Bausch & Lomb	1% Methylcellulose	Methyl-propylparabens
Neo-Tears		Hydroxyethyl cellulose	Thimerosal, EDTA
OcuCoat PF	Storz	Hydroxypropyl methylcellulose, dextran-70	Preservative-free
Refresh Plus	Allergan	0.5% Carboxymethylcellulose	Preservative-free
Refresh	Allergan	0.6% Polyvinyl alcohol, povidone	Preservative-free
Tears Naturale II	Alcon	Dextran-70, hydroxypropyl methylcellulose	Polyquaternium-1
Tears Naturale Free	Alcon	Dextran-70, hydroxypropyl methylcellulose	Preservative-free
Tears Plus	Allergan	Polyvinyl alcohol	Chlorbutanol
Tears Renewed	Akorn	Dextran-70, hydroxypropyl methylcellulose	Benzalkonium chloride, EDTA
Theratears	Advanced Vision Research	0.25% Carboxymethylcellulose, sodium chloride, potassium chloride, sodium bicarbonate, chloride, magnesium chloride, sodium phosphate	Preservative-free
Visine Extra	Pfizer	Tetrahydrozoline hydrochloride	Benzalkonium chloride, edetate disodium, polyethylene glycol
Visine L.R.	Pfizer	Oxymethazoline hydrochloride	Benzalkonium chloride, edetate disodium

EDTA, ethylenediaminetetraacetic acid.

maintenance of normal physiology of the tear film. Gilbard and associates have shown a 10% increase in the crystalloid osmolality of tears in dry-eye states.[49–51] This is not readily reversed with the application of topical isotonic solution.[49–51] Instead, hypotonic solutions are necessary to restore and maintain the normal osmolality of the tear film. The initial movement of water into the dehydrated cells results in a relative increase in osmolality of the tear substitute; continued evaporation of the solution from the surface of the eye also tends to increase osmolality.

Less viscous solutions disappear rapidly from the eye, and their effect is soon lost. Increasing viscosity with the addition of polymeric ingredients causes a longer interval of contact with the eye. A soft contact lens, with frequent instillation of saline or another tear substitute, also prolongs contact of the tear solution. Ointment greatly slows loss of water from the surface epithelium and is useful when frequent instillation is not possible. Finally, a moisture chamber prevents water loss through evaporation.

Beyond consideration of osmotic elements, other important considerations for tear replacements include pH, surface tension, mucomimetic action, interaction of the solution with mucus and lipid films, electrolyte composition, secondary effects of preservatives, lubricating properties, and finally actual comfort.[49–51] Table 32–1 lists many of the available tear substitutes.

Intraocular Irrigants

Contact of irrigating solutions with the corneal endothelium, lens, and vitreous may have important consequences for cellular survivability and function. Corneal endothelium is particularly vulnerable to disruptive osmotic forces.[52, 53] An irrigating solution must maintain both physiologic and anatomic integrity. Solutions that would preserve the corneal endothelial function should have buffering agents: glutathione to prevent oxidative damage, calcium and magnesium ions, and glucose. The lens epithelial cells require glucose, and during deprivation lens hexokinase shifts irreversibly to its insouble form. In diabetic patients, a posterior subcapsu-

TABLE 32–2. **Currently Available Intraocular Irrigating Solutions**

Product	Manufacturer	Composition
AMO Endosol	Alcon	Na^+, K^+, Ca^{2+}, Mg^{2+}, Cl^-, acetate, citrate
BSS (Balanced Salt Solution)	Alcon	NaCl, KCl, CaCl, MgCl, Na acetate, Na citrate
BSS Plus	Alcon	NaCl, KCl, CaCl, MgCl, Na phosphate, Na bicarbonate, dextrose, glutathione disulfide
IOCARE Balanced Saline Solution	IOLAB	NaCl, KCl, CaCl, MgCl, Na acetate, Na citrate

lar cataract is possible with prolonged irrigation.[54] The retina can withstand osmotic variations from 200 to 400 mOsm/L. Although isotonic by definition, NaCl 0.9% is toxic to intraocular tissues.

Table 32–2 presents currently available intraocular irrigating solutions.

REFERENCES

1. Duke-Elder S: System of Ophthalmology, vol 4. St. Louis, CV Mosby, 1969, pp 110–111.
2. Cogan DG: Studies on the clinical physiology of the cornea. Am J Ophthalmol 32:625, 1969.
3. Cogan DG, Hirsch E: The cornea: Permeability to weak electrolytes. Arch Ophthalmol 27:466, 1942.
4. Cogan DG, Kinsey VE: Transfer of water and sodium chloride by osmosis and diffusion through the excised cornea. Arch Ophthalmol 27:696, 1942.
5. Cogan DG, Kinsey VE: Hydration properties of the whole cornea. Arch Ophthalmol 28:449, 1942.
6. Cogan DG, Kinsey VE: Cornea: Physiologic aspects. Arch Ophthalmol 28:661, 1942.
7. Cogan DG: Clearing of edematous corneas by glycerin. Am J Ophthalmol 27:551, 1943.
8. Cogan DG, Hirsch E, Kinsey VE: Permeability characteristics of the excised cornea. Arch Ophthalmol 31:408, 1944.
9. Cogan DG, Kinsey VE: The cornea: Permeability to weak electrolytes. Arch Ophthalmol 32:276, 1955.
10. Kinsey VE: Transfer of ascorbic acid and related compounds across the blood-aqueous barrier. Am J Ophthalmol 31:1262, 1947.
11. Kinsey VE: Further study of the distribution of chloride between plasma and intraocular fluids of the eye. Invest Ophthalmol 6:395, 1967.
12. Kinsey VE, Reddy DVN: Chemistry and dynamics of aqueous humor. *In* Prince JH (ed): The Rabbit in Eye Research. Springfield, IL, Charles C Thomas, 1964.
13. Holt M, Cogan D: Permeability of the excised cornea to ions, as determined by measurements of impedance. Arch Ophthalmol 35:292, 1946.
14. Dohlman CH, Hedbys BO, Mishima S: The swelling pressure of the corneal stroma. Invest Ophthalmol 1:158, 1962.
15. Edelhauser HG, Hannekin AM, Pederson HJ, Van Horn DL: Osmotic tolerance of rabbit and human corneal endothelium. Arch Ophthalmol 99:1281, 1981.
16. Maurice DM, Giardini AA: Swelling of the cornea in vivo after the destruction of its limiting layers. Br J Ophthalmol 35:791, 1951.
17. Harris J: Transport of fluid from the cornea. *In* Duke-Elder S (ed): Transparency of the Cornea. Springfield, IL, Charles C. Thomas, 1960.
18. Friedenwald JS: The formation of the intraocular fluid. Am J Ophthalmol 32:9, 1949.
19. Bill A: A capillar permeability to and extravascular dynamics of myoglobin, albumen, and gamma globulin in the uvea. Acta Physiol Scand 73:204, 1968.
20. Bill A: A method to determine osmotically effective albumen and gamma globulin concentrations in tissue fluids, its application to the uvea and a note on the effects of capillary "leaks" on tissue fluid dynamics. Acta Physiol Scand 73:511, 1968.
21. Friedenwald JS, Becker B: Aqueous humor dynamics. Arch Ophthalmol 54:799, 1955.
22. Friedenwald JS, Hughes WF, Hermann H: Acid-base tolerance of the cornea. Arch Ophthalmol 31:279, 1944.
23. Maren TH: HCO_3^- formation in aqueous humor: Mechanism and relation to the treatment of glaucoma. Invest Ophthalmol 13:479, 1974.
24. Laties A, Armaly M, Rao R, et al: The blood-ocular barriers under stress. *In* Freeman HM, Hirose T, Schepens C (eds): Vitreous Surgery and Advances in Fundus Diagnosis and Treatment. New York, Appleton-Century-Crofts, 1977.
25. More E, Scheie HG, Adler FH: Chemical equilibrium between blood and aqueous humor; Further studies. Arch Ophthalmol 27:317, 1942.
26. Shakib M, Cunha-Vaz JG: Studies on the permeability of the blood-retinal barrier. IV, Junctional complexes of the retinal vessels and their role in the permeability of the blood-retinal barrier. Exp Eye Res 5:229, 1966.
27. Shiose Y: Electron microscopic studies on blood-retinal and blood-aqueous barriers. Jpn J Ophthalmol 14:73, 1970.
28. Vegge T: An epithelial blood-queous barrier to horseradish peroxidise in the ciliary processes of the vervet monkey *(Cercopithecus aethiops).* Z Zellforsch Mikrosk Anat 114:309, 1971.
29. Kinoshita JH, Merola IO, Dikmak E: Osmotic changes in experimental galactose cataracts. Exp Eye Res 1:405, 1962.
30. Kinoshita JH, Barber GW, Merola LO, Tung B: Changes in the levels of free amino acids and myo-inosotol in the galactose-exposed lens. Invest Ophthalmol 8:625, 1969.
31. Chylack LT, Kinoshita JH: The interaction of the lens and the vitreous. I: The high glucose cataract in a lens-vitreous preparation. Exp Eye Res 14:58, 1972.
32. Chylack LT, Schaefer FL: Mechanism of "hypoglycemic" cataract formation in the rat lens. II: Further studies on the role of hexokinase instability. Invest Ophthalmol 15:519, 1976.
33. Chylack LT: Mechanisms of senile cataract formation. Ophthalmology 96:888–892, 1984.
34. Haimann MH, Abrahams GW, Edelhauser HF, Hatchell DI: The effect of intraocular irrigating solution on lens clarity in normal and diabetic rabbits. Am J Ophthalmol 94:594, 1982.
35. Kawaba T, Cheng HM, Kinoshita JH: The accumulation of myoinositol and rubidium ions in galactose-exposed rat lens. Invest Ophthalmol Vis Sci 27:1522, 1986.
36. Coulter JB III, Eaton DK, Marr LK: Effects of diabetes and insulin treatment on sorbitol and water of rat lenses. Ophthalmic Res 18:357, 1986.
37. Maurice D: The exchange of sodium between the vitreous body and the blood and the aqueous humor. J Physiol (Lond) 137:110, 1957.
38. Duncan LS, Hostetter T, Ellis P: Vitreous osmolality changes following administration of hyperosmotic agents. Invest Ophthalmol 8:353, 1969.
39. Honda Y, Negri A, Kawano S: Mode of ion movements into vitreous-equilibration after vitrectomy. Arch Ophthalmol 101:105, 1983.
40. Marmor MJ: Retinal detachment from hyperosmotic intravitreal injection. Invest Ophthalmol Vis Sci 18:1237, 1979.
41. D'Alena P, Ferguson W: Adverse effects after glycerol orally and mannitol parenterally. Arch Ophthalmol 75:201, 1966.
42. McCurdy DK, Schneider B, Scheie HG: Oral glycerol: The mechanism of intraocular hypotension. Am J Ophthalmol 61:1244, 1966.
43. Wisznia KI, Lazare M, Leopold IH: Oral isosorbide and intraocular pressure. Am J Ophthalmol 70:630, 1970.
44. Galin MA, Davidson R: Hypotensive effect of urea in inflamed and noninflamed eye. Arch Ophthalmol 78:583, 1962.
45. Tarter RC, Linn JF: A clinical study of the use of intravenous urea in glaucoma. Am J Ophthalmol 52:323, 1960.
46. Spaeth GL, Spaeth EB, Spaeth PG, Lucier AC: Anaphylactic reaction to mannitol. Arch Ophthalmol 178:583, 1967.
47. Weaver A, Sica A: Mannitol-induced acute renal failure. Nephron 45:233, 1987.
48. Payrau P, Dohlman CH: Medical treatment of corneal edema. Int Ophthalmol Clin 8:601, 1968.
49. Gilbard JP, Faris LF: Tear osmolarity and ocular surface disease in keratoconjunctivitis sicca. Arch Ophthalmol 97:1642, 1979.
50. Gilbard JP, Rossi JP, Gray KL: A new rabbit model for keratoconjunctivitis sicca. Invest Ophthalmol Vis Sci 28:225, 1987.
51. Gilbard JP, Rossi SR, Heyda KG: Ophthalmic solutions, the ocular surface, and a unique therapeutic artificial tear formulation. Am J Ophthal 107(4):132, 1989.

52. Foulks GN, Thoft RA, Perry HD, Tolentino DI: Factors related to corneal epithelial complications after closed vitrectomy in diabetics. Arch Ophthalmol 97:1076, 1979.
53. Merrill DL, Fleming TC, Girard LJ: The effects of physiologic balanced salt solutions and normal saline on intraocular and extraocular tissues. Am J Ophthalmol 49:895, 1960.
54. Christiansen JM, Kollarits CR, Fukui H, Fishmen ML: Intraocular irrigating solutions and lens clarity. Am J Ophthalmol 82:594, 1976.
55. Bietti GB, Giraldi JP: Topical osmotherapy of corneal edema. Ann Ophthalmol 1:40, 1969.
56. Marici A, Aquavella JV: Hypertonic saline solution in corneal edema. Ann Ophthalmol 7:229, 1975.
57. Gilbard JP, Kenyon KR: Tear diluents in the treatment of keratoconjunctivitis sicca. Ophthalmology 92:236, 1985.
58. Holly FJ, Lamberts DW: Effect of nonisotonic solutions on tear osmolality. Invest Ophthalmol Vis Sci 20:236, 1985.

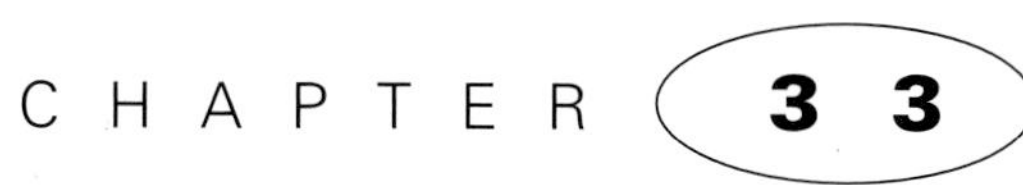

Carbonic Anhydrase Inhibitors

Abha R. Amin and Leon L. Remis

Carbonic anhydrase inhibitors (CAI) have reached a new level in the armamentarium of glaucoma therapies. Forty years after Becker first observed that acetazolamide lowered intraocular pressure (IOP), dorzolamide, a topical CAI, became the first drug in its class to be approved for clinical use.

Systemic CAIs are extremely useful antiglaucoma agents, although nearly half of all patients who take CAIs suffer a significant side effect, such as gastrointestinal disturbances or the "malaise symptom complex."[1] With the advent of laser trabeculoplasty and improved surgical outcomes, reliance on systemic agents has greatly diminished. Currently, topical CAIs are reinstating the importance of inhibition of the carbonic anhydrase (CA) enzyme in ciliary epithelium.

This chapter has undergone a shift in emphasis, from detailing the "older" systemic agents, toward revealing the present data on dorzolamide and its relationship to other glaucoma therapies.

Chemistry

CA is a 30,000-MW enzyme that incorporates three imidazole groups that bind Zn^{2+} and a fourth hydroxyl group.[2, 3] The active site is a Zn^{2+} moiety into which the inhibitors bind. This enzyme catalyzes the reversible reaction in which carbon dioxide (CO_2) is hydrated to form carbonic acid (H_2CO_3):

$$H_2O + CO_2 \leftrightarrows H_2CO_3$$

This acid then dissociates into bicarbonate ion and hydrogen ion:

$$H_2CO_3 \leftrightarrows H^+ + H^+CO_3^-$$

The aforementioned reaction can occur spontaneously but will occur several hundred to several thousand times faster in the presence of CA, depending on the tissue in which the reaction is taking place. At equilibrium, the concentration of CO_2 is 400 times greater than H_2CO_3.[4, 5]

At least four isoenzymes of CA are known to exist. Type I (CA-I) is found primarily in erythrocytes and in the corneal endothelium. Type II (CA-II) is the main isoenzyme in the eye and is found in the nonpigmented epithelium of the ciliary processes, the iris, and the retina.[2, 6] It is also found in the kidney, lungs, and gastrointestinal tract as well as in the glial cells in the brain, erythrocytes, gastric parietal cells, the lens, and Müller's cells of the retina. Type III (CA-III) is found in the skeletal muscle, and type IV (CA-IV) is found in the kidney.[7]

Physiology

Of the three main buffer systems within the body, the bicarbonate system is the most important because of its volume and capacity. The end-products of catabolism produce large amounts of CO_2, which is eliminated from the body by respiration and by the kidneys.[4, 5] CO_2 is transported by erythrocytes in the form of HCO_3^- to both the lungs and the kidneys. CA enhances the conversion of CO_2 and H_2O by a factor of several thousand, enabling the red blood cells (RBCs) to carry vast amounts of HCO_3^-. In the tubular cells of the kidneys, CA enhances the secretion of H^+ in exchange for Na^+, and bicarbonate is reabsorbed so that excess CO_2 can be transported via the blood stream to the lungs to be "blown off." Inhibition at this level can result in a metabolic acidosis that is due to the accumulation of H^+ in renal tubular cells. In the lungs, CO_2 is removed from the alveoli by respiration, thus ridding the body of excess acid.[4] Patients with limited lung capacity are unable to increase their respiratory rate to compensate for the acidosis produced by inhibition of CA and become even more severely acidotic (combined preexisting respiratory acidosis and metabolic acidosis) from the use of CAIs.

TABLE 33–1. **Pharmacokinetics of Carbonic Anhydrase Inhibitors**

	Plasma Binding (%)	Lipid Solubility	Plasma Half-life	Urinary Excretion (%)	Potency
Acetazolamide	95	+ +	2 hr	80	+ + +
Methazolamide	60	+ + +	15 hr	25	+ + +
Dichlorphenamide			2 hr	40	+
Ethoxzolamide	95	+ + + +	6 hr	40	+ + + +

Aqueous humor formation depends on the secretion of bicarbonate from the ciliary processes. Sodium is the sole cation tied to the bicarbonate anion and water follows, resulting in the formation of aqueous fluid.[8] "A key event is the catalytic formation of HCO_3^- from CO_2 and OH^-."[5] Inhibition of this step in the reaction results in reduced aqueous formation.

Although a similar process may be responsible for cerebrospinal fluid (CSF) production in the choroidal plexus of the brain, the role of CA in the stomach may be to buffer the excess of OH^- resulting from H^+ secretion.[3] In the kidney, HCO_3^- reabsorption is inhibited, resulting in metabolic acidosis, and may be related to the "malaise symptom complex," which consists of malaise, fatigue, weight loss, anorexia, loss of libido, and depression.[1] Acetazolamide is 20 times more active against CA-II than CA-I and is the least lipid-soluble of the CAIs.[9, 10] Other sulfonamides have greater lipid solubility and therefore greater ocular penetration.[5, 6] Inhibition of CA-II has therapeutic value by reducing fluid and electrolyte secretion in various tissues. Inhibition of the other forms has not yet been shown to be of therapeutic value.[2] CA-II is present in approximately 100-fold excess of its physiologic needs, and higher than 99% inhibition is required for a therapeutic effect owing to its rapid enzyme activity.[2, 4]

Carbonic Anhydrase Inhibitors

Acetazolamide, ethoxzolamide, methazolamide, and dichlorphenamide are all oral sulfonamides that have activity against CA. Dorzolamide and brinzolamide are topical sulfonamides that also inhibit CA. They produce their therapeutic effect by binding to the Zn^{2+} portion of the CA enzyme by the sulfamyl group $R—SO_2NH$.[2, 8] They are noncompetitive inhibitors that possess no bacteriostatic activity.[2, 3, 8] Acetazolamide, methazolamide, dorzolamide, and brinzolamide are discussed in this chapter.

SYSTEMIC ANHYDRASE INHIBITOR

Pharmacokinetics (Table 33–1)

CAIs will affect tissues that possess high amounts of CA, such as the renal cortex, liver, and erythrocytes and in decreasing amounts in the skeletal muscles, pulmonary alveoli, pancreas, gastric mucosa, choroidal plexus, and ciliary body. The highest concentration of CAIs is protein bound in the plasma. Because the oral CAIs are lipid soluble, they are able to penetrate the ciliary epithelial cells to the site of action.[2, 7]

Ninety-nine percent inhibition of CA in the nonpigmented ciliary epithelium reduces the rate of aqueous humor formation by up to 50%,[8] resulting in a reduction of IOP in more than 90% of patients. Acetazolamide and methazolamide are well absorbed after oral administration. Once in the general circulation, acetazolamide is 95% bound to plasma proteins compared with 60% binding of methazolamide.[7] Lower doses of methazolamide can produce the same level of effectiveness as acetazolamide owing to the higher amount of free (unbound) inhibitor and greater lipophilia.

The plasma half-life of acetazolamide is 4 hours. It is excreted unchanged by the kidney. Methazolamide has a plasma half-life of 15 hours.[2, 9] It is not primarily excreted by the kidney because only 25% of a single dose appears unchanged in the urine. Because it has greater lipid solubility than acetazolamide, methazolamide diffuses faster into ocular tissues.[9] In addition, its renal effects can be avoided at dosages of about 4 mg/mL, while preserving its ocular effects and preventing the acidosis that accompanies acetazolamide administration. The specific dosing, efficacy, and side effects of each drug are discussed separately.

Dosage and Administration (Table 33–2)

Acetazolamide

Acetazolamide is available in 125- and 250-mg tablets as well as 500-mg slow-release capsules. It is the only CAI

TABLE 33–2. **Dosage and Administration of Sulfonamide Carbonic Anhydrase Inhibitors**

	Route of Administration	How Supplied	Onset (Peak)	Duration of Action	Dosage (Frequency)	Brand Name
Acetazolamide tablet	Oral	Tablet	1 hr (2–4 hr)	6–8 hr	125 + 250 mg (2–4 × day)	Diamox Hydrazol
Azetazolamide capsule	Oral	Capsule	2 hr (4–6 hr)	18–24 hr	500 mg (1 or 2 × day)	Diamox Sequel
Acetazolamide	IM or IV	Vial	3 min (15 min)	4–5 hr	250–500 mg (q 4–6 hr)	Diamox
Dichlorphenamide	Oral	Tablet	45 min (2 hr)	6–12 hr	50 mg (1–3 × day)	Daranide Oratrol
Ethoxzolamide	Oral	Tablet	2 hr (5–6 hr)	8–12 hr	125 mg (2–4 × day)	Cardrase Ethamide
Methazolamide	Oral	Tablet	3 hr	8–12 hr	25 + 50 mg	Neptazane

available for parenteral use; it can be given intravenously or intramuscularly, although the latter can be painful owing to the alkaline pH of the solution.[10] Although dosages as low as 125 mg, two or three times daily, may be effective, plasma concentrations of 10 mg/mL are needed for maximum effect and can usually be achieved in patients taking 1 g/day.[11] Studies comparing the availability of the 250-mg tablets versus 500-mg capsules showed higher peak plasma concentrations in the 250-mg tablet than in the 500-mg capsule.[12] This result prompted the authors (Ledger-Scott and Hurst) to study patients taking 250-mg tablets twice daily, in whom they found equally satisfactory control of glaucoma as those taking 500-mg capsules twice daily. A satisfactory clinical effect may be obtained by utilizing the tablets two or three times a day or by supplementing a single 500-mg capsule with a 250-mg tablet 18 hours later.[13]

Methazolamide

Methazolamide is available in 25-mg and 50-mg tablets and is effective in doses as low as 25 mg twice daily.[9–14] Increasing the frequency to three times a day produced few additional side effects.[14] An increase in dosages from 25 mg three times a day to 50 mg three times a day to 100 mg three times a day resulted in increasingly lower pressures at the expense of increasingly troublesome side effects. Dosages in the range of 100 mg twice a day gave a substantial pressure lowering with tolerable side effects. Plasma levels in the 75 mg/day dose ranged between 3 and 4 mg/mL, and at the 150 mg/day dose between 6 and 8 mg/mL; at doses of 300 mg/day, the plasma level was 12 to 16 mg/mL.[15] The plasma levels of 8 to 10 mg/mL should produce a near-maximal therapeutic response and still be tolerated during long-term administration.

Toxicity

All the side effects known to occur in the sulfonamide family occur with the CAIs. Maculopapular skin rash, pruritus, urticaria, Stevens-Johnson syndrome, and toxic epidermolysis bullosa have all been described. Much worry and confusion exists on the part of clinicians regarding bone marrow depression. Hematopoietic toxicity can be dose-related or idiosyncratic and irreversible and is usually manifested by aplastic anemia or agranulocytosis.[16, 17] Two thirds of these hematologic effects occur within the first 6 months of therapy, and arguments are divided as to the need for routine blood testing. With the advent of topical CAIs, fewer patients are now taking systemic agents, making routine hematologic screening at 6 weeks and 6 months more practical.[17] Symptoms of anemia, fatigue, headache, leukopenia (frequent infections), and thrombocytopenia (easy bruising) should alert the clinician to the need for immediate hematologic work-up.

Paresthesias are probably the most commonly encountered side effects and are either circumoral or occur in the hands or feet. A flat or metalic taste to carbonated beverages is often present. The malaise symptom complex, as described by Epstein,[1] includes a feeling of being unwell, anorexia, weight loss, depression, and decreased libido and can be so troublesome that approximately 50% of patients taking either acetazolamide or methazolamide discontinue therapy. Supplemental sodium acetate alleviated symptoms in half of those affected.[18]

Gastrointestinal distress, such as cramping, burning, irritation, nausea, or diarrhea, may occur. Some of these symptoms may be due to CAI in the gastric and intestinal mucosae. Renal effects are directly related either to inhibition of CA, such as the alkalinization of urine resulting in metabolic acidosis, or to lowered citrate and magnesium excretion (by up to 80%) resulting in calcium phosphate stones.[19] In one study, none of the eight patients who had a previous history of idiopathic renal calculi developed an additional occurrence while taking acetazolamide, although 50% of patients who had calcium oxalate stones while on acetazolamide therapy developed additional calculi if treatment was continued.[20] Acute renal failure may result from tubular obstruction by acetazolamide crystalluria.

CAIs are contraindicated in patients with severely compromised lung capacity and in severe liver disease. Worsening of pulmonary insufficiency can result from the metabolic acidosis produced, because patients with pulmonary disease are unable to mount an additional respiratory drive needed to excrete excess CO_2. Blood pH and CO_2 combining power should be obtained before therapy in patients with mild pulmonary insufficiency.[21]

Induced myopia is the only known ocular side effect. Sexual dysfunction, such as decreased libido and organic impotence, has been associated with these drugs.[22] Teratogenesis occurs in a reproducible manner in bone development in adult mice that receive CAIs in utero.[23] An infant with a teratoma of the sacrococcygeal region was born to a mother taking acetazolamide during her first trimester.[24]

Interactions

Serious metabolic acidosis may also result from the combination of *salicylates* and CAIs. The coadministration of salicylates can result in both confusion and lethargy, by inhibiting both plasma binding and renal tubular secretion of acetazolamide. This increases the unbound fraction of acetazolamide from three to tenfold, greatly increasing plasma levels and the chances for any untoward reaction to occur.

TOPICAL CARBONIC ANHYDRASE INHIBITORS

Although oral CAIs work well to lower the IOP, none of the systemic agents discussed has activity as a topical medication. Therefore, a search commenced to find a topical CAI that would be as effective as the oral CAIs, yet not have all of the noxious side effects.

Aminozolamide, an analog of ethoxzolamide (a highly potent CAI), was placed in a "gel" vehicle to prolong corneal contact time and increase ocular penetration. The gel proved to have limited usefulness because it caused blurred vision and conjunctival injection. Sezolamide (MK-927) and dorzolamide (MK-507), both topically active CAIs, were found to be effective in lowering IOP. Dorzolamide hydrochloride was found to be the most potent and most selective for human CA isoenzyme II.[25, 26] Brinzolamide is the newest topical CAI currently available. It has similar efficacy to dorzolamide, yet with greater tolerability (personal communication).

Dosage and Administration

Dorzolamide

Dorzolamide is extraordinarily specific for CA-II. It has a 3000:1 affinity for isoenzyme II in relation to isoenzyme I, based on a ratio of dissociation constants of the inhibitor-enzyme complexes. Dorzolamide also has a strong affinity for CA-IV, which is found in the human eye but has not been observed in the ciliary processes. It is found, however, in the ciliary epithelium of the rabbit and mouse.[27]

Lippa and associates studied dorzolamide in patients with bilateral open-angle glaucoma with IOPs of 24 or greater, who were not on any concurrent ocular hypotensive medications. Dorzolamide demonstrated excellent IOP-lowering effect in both normal people and in patients with glaucoma or ocular hypertension.[26] Studies were performed using a two or three times daily regimen of 0.7%, 2%, and 3% dorzolamide. When given in low doses (0.7%), multiple drops were needed to achieve steady-state drug levels. Higher doses (3%) did not demonstrate a superior hypotensive effect over the 2% concentration of dorzolamide. Optimal dosing for 2% dorzolamide was determined to be three times daily.[28] The peak hypotensive effect was at 2 hours with a trough effect at 8 hours after administration of one drop.

Brinzolamide

Brinzolamide (Azopt) 1% suspension is a newly released topical carbonic anhydrase II inhibitor that was shown in two clinical trials to be equivalent to dorzolamide in reducing the IOP. It is absorbed systemically and is excreted unchanged in the urine. Although it accumulates within red blood cells, the levels do not have a pharmacologic effect on either the kidneys or the lungs. The major subjective difference between the two is that brinzolamide was associated with less stinging and burning upon instillation in clinical trials. Brinzolamide 1% is dosed one drop three times daily.

β-Blockers and Dorzolamide

Strahlman and associates conducted a study comparing the efficacy of 2% dorzolamide versus 0.5% betaxolol versus 0.5% timolol over 1 year. All three drugs had their peak ocular hypotensive effects 2 hours after the morning dose and their least effect 8 hours after the morning dose. The study concluded that dorzolamide given three times daily and betaxolol given twice daily had comparable ocular hypotensive efficacy. Timolol administered twice daily showed a greater hypotensive effect. The combined effect of twice daily 2% dorzolamide with either betaxolol or timolol produced a clinically significant drop in the IOP of 33% at peak and 27% at trough time.[30] Therefore, if a patient's IOP is insufficiently controlled on β-blockers, dorzolamide added twice daily will produce an additional IOP reduction.

Cosopt

Cosopt is a newly released combination drop of timolol and dorzolamide. Cosopt is administered twice daily, and results in a greater IOP lowering effect than either of its components taken alone; however, the reduction is not as much as when timolol twice daily and dorzolamide three times daily are administered concomitantly. The contraindications include bronchial asthma, severe obstructive lung disease, sinus bradycardia, heart block, and allergy to components of dorzolamide that includes sulfa. The advantages of this medication include simplification of the drug regimen, which may help to improve compliance.

Acetazolamide and Dorzolamide

Yamazaki and associates measured aqueous protein concentrations and IOPs after administration of a placebo, 1% dorzolamide, and 250 mg of acetazolamide in six normal patients. They found an equal amount of aqueous humor suppression of 20%, but dorzolamide showed a 1-hour delay in peak effect.[32]

Maus and associates measured aqueous flow rate by measuring fluorescein clearance. They found an almost twofold difference in aqueous suppression between 2% dorzolamide daily and 250 mg acetazolamide given three times daily. Acetazolamide reduced aqueous flow by 30% compared with 17% for dorzolamide. They concluded that topical dorzolamide is not as efficacious as orally administered acetazolamide.[31] When acetazolamide was added to dorzolamide, aqueous flow rate was further reduced by 16%. When dorzolamide was added to acetazolamide, no further reduction in aqueous flow rate was achieved. Therefore, when adding acetazolamide to better control IOP, discontinue the dorzolamide for two reasons: it is cost effective and it will simplify the patient's drug regimen. The combination of acetazolamide and dorzolamide provides no greater effect than acetazolamide alone.[33]

Pilocarpine and Dorzolamide

In a comparison study over 6 months, Strahlman and associates found that the addition of 2% dorzolamide twice daily to 0.5% timolol twice daily brought about an additional average IOP reduction of 13%. The addition of 2% pilocarpine four times daily to 0.5% timolol twice daily reduced the IOP by 10% on average. The difference in efficacy between adding dorzolamide and 2% pilocarpine was *not* statistically significant. However, pilocarpine was found to be less tolerable than dorzolamide because of side effects such as brow ache, headache, or decreased vision due to miosis.[34]

Toxicity

Strahlman and associates' study of 523 patients found that most patients tolerate dorzolamide well; however, a significant number of patients experience adverse side effects. The most common symptom was the bitter taste that patients experienced after taking the drug (27%), which was transient and did not decrease compliance. Patients also complained gastrointestinal disturbances (7%), headaches (5%), conjunctivitis (4%), burning (4%), eyelid inflammation (3%), itching eyes (3%), and eye pain (3%). The conjunctivitis and lid reactions were the main reasons why patients discontinued use of dorzolamide. These symptoms had a variable onset any time from 3 months to 1 year, and they appeared to be an allergy-type hypersensitivity reaction. It is interesting to note that the incidence of side effects typical of oral CAIs was very low for dorzolamide: fatigue (1%) and paresthesias (2%).[28]

Extensive testing was performed to determine what *systemic* effects dorzolamide may have. Wilkerson and colleagues performed blood and urine chemistries and electrocardiograms and measured CA levels in RBCs after 4 weeks of three times daily dorzolamide treatment.[25]

All were found to be unchanged from baseline. Interestingly, topically applied dorzolamide is systemically absorbed and excreted in the urine. During the dorzolamide clinical trials, two patients developed urolithiasis. This is the same rate of occurrence that occurs in the general population. Stone formation occurs with alkalinization of the urine as seen with oral CAIs. There is no change in urine pH in patients taking dorzolamide.[35]

The active metabolite, N-diethyl-dorzolamide, was observed to accumulate in RBCs during the 4-week trial. Accordingly, a decreased level (21%) of CA activity was measured. Although dorzolamide is absorbed systemically and inhibits CA in RBCs, it is felt that because 99% of the carbonic anhydrase is not inhibited, a physiologic effect is not seen. There was no evidence of metabolic acidosis or electrolyte disturbance.[36] It was noted, however, that the half-life of dorzolamide is 147 days, and there is a potential for accumulation with chronic use.[25] Other ocular and systemic adverse effects occurred infrequently including iritis, transient myopia, nausea, urolithiasis, dizziness, and skin rashes.[37]

Drug Warnings

Although the sulfonamide structure of dorzolamide differs from that of the oral CAIs, it is not known whether these structural differences will decrease the potential for sulfonamide-type adverse reactions. Although the risk may be small, the consequences may be severe.

Dorzolamide has not been tested in children or in patients with renal failure or liver disease. There have been no well-controlled studies on pregnant or nursing mothers either. Dorzolamide, like other CAIs, has teratogenic effects and may put the fetus at risk. The risks and benefits of treatment need to be weighed carefully in these cases. It is not known whether dorzolamide is excreted in human milk, thus either the medication or the nursing needs to be discontinued.[38]

Indications

Glaucoma

CAIs have been used systemically in the treatment of glaucoma since the mid-1950s. In most cases, topical antiglaucoma agents such as β-blockers and miotics had been previously utilized and had not produced the desired level of control. Dorzolamide, the new topical CAI, has become a commonly used drug to help further reduce the IOP. It is most often tried prior to the systemic CAIs.

Systemic CAIs are indicated when a lower IOP is desirable in a given patient who is already on topical CAIs. When prescribing oral CAIs, it is important to stop dorzolamide therapy. Most of the primary and secondary glaucomas respond well to the oral CAIs. Some clinicians advise against using an oral CAI in chronic angle-closure glaucoma because a normalization of IOP may lead to a false sense of control of the disease process while continued angle closure can occur.

The decision to institute systemic therapy with a CAI is often avoided or delayed owing to legitimate concern of inducing adverse side effects. These risks must be considered, but denying patients the substantial benefit obtainable from these agents is considered to be equally unwarranted. Many patients will derive a satisfactory reduction in pressure with few bothersome complaints. Medication in those who develop untoward effects can often be titrated to a proper dose, or the patient can be switched to a different dosage form of the drug with greater success. For an excellent discussion of good therapeutic techniques for a given patient, the reader is referred to review articles by Berson and Epstein[39] and Lichter.[40]

Pseudotumor Cerebri

Pseudotumor cerebri, or benign intracranial hypertension, is a condition in which increased intracranial pressure is found to be unassociated with a space-occupying intracranial lesion or other known cause of obstruction to the outflow of cerebrospinal fluid (CSF). This condition is often associated with obesity, a history of drug usage (often tetracycline or prednisone), or a number of other conditions or drugs. Clinical signs and symptoms often include headache and papilledema, which may result in visual field loss and eventual blindness. The CAIs can reduce CSF production in much the same way as aqueous production decreased. Increasing lipophilicity enhances the penetration of these drugs through the blood-brain barrier and reduces the renal effects as well.[2] Methazolamide is more lipophilic than acetazolamide and may be more suitable for this use because renal effects are avoided. In practice, many patients with this disease are in the younger age groups and tolerate the CAIs more readily than do the elderly.[10]

Cystoid Macular Edema

Macular edema can be reduced by taking 500 mg of acetazolamide daily. Both clinically detectable visual improvement and lessening of macular edema by angiography were noted in 10 of 12 patients studied with macular edema due to retinitis pigmentosa (even if the edema had been present for many years).[41] Other types of macular edema were also noted to improve, including pseudophakic macular edema and cystoid macular edema associated with choroidopathy.[42, 43] It has been shown that acetazolamide may reduce macular edema from chronic uveitis by angiography, but when acetazolamide therapy is stopped, the angiographic evidence of cystoid macular edema returns. Although some patients with aphakic and pseudophakic macular edema have improved on dosages between 125 and 1000 mg/day of acetazolamide, others have not benefited from this treatment. In particular, patients with diabetic retinopathy and vein occlusions have not shown improvement.[43, 44]

Although early results are encouraging, the tendency for spontaneous improvement, the variety of dosages used, and the differing indications for treatment make it difficult to draw any conclusions from these reports. Confirmation of these data by larger controlled prospective studies is needed before this form of treatment can be endorsed.

REFERENCES

1. Epstein DL, Grant WM: Carbonic anhydrase inhibitor side effects. Arch Ophthalmol 95:1378, 1977.
2. Lindskog S, Wistrand PJ: Inhibitors of carbonic anhydrase. *In* Sandler H, Smith HJ (eds): Design of Enzyme Inhibitors as Drugs. New York, Oxford University Press, 1987.
3. Maren TH: Carbonic anhydrase: Chemistry, physiology and inhibition. Physiol Rev 47:595, 1967.
4. Guyton AC: Textbook of Medical Physiology, 7th ed. Philadelphia, WB Saunders, 1986.
5. Maren TH: Carbonic anhydrase: General perspectives and advances in glaucoma research. Drug Dev Res 10:255, 1987.
6. Wistrand PJ, Schenholm M, Lonnerholm G: Carbonic anhydrase isoenzymes CA I and CA II in the human eye. Invest Ophthalmol Vis Sci 27:419, 1986.
7. Friedland BR, Maren TH: Carbonic anhydrase: Pharmacology of inhibitors and treatment of glaucoma. *In* Sears M (ed): Handbook of Experimental Pharmacology: Pharmacology of the Eye. Berlin, Springer-Verlag, 1984.
8. Maren TH: HCO_3^- formation in aqueous humor: Mechanism and relation to the treatment of glaucoma. Invest Ophthalmol 13:479, 1974.
9. Maren TH, Haywood JR, Chapman SK, et al: The pharmacology of methazolamide in relation to the treatment of glaucoma. Invest Ophthalmol Vis Sci 16:730, 1977.
10. Package insert.
11. Alm A, Berggren L, Hartvig P, et al: Monitoring acetazolamide treatment. Acta Ophthalmol 60:24, 1982.
12. Ledger-Scott M, Hurst J: Comparison of the bioavailability of two acetazolamide formulations. Pharm J 235:451, 1985.
13. Berson FG, Epstein DL, Grant WM, et al: Acetazolamide dosage forms in the treatment of glaucoma. Arch Ophthalmol 98:1051, 1980.
14. Stone RA, Zimmerman TJ, Shin DH: Low dose methazolamide and intraocular pressure. Am J Ophthalmol 83:674, 1977.
15. Dahlen K, Epstein DL, Grant WM, et al: A repeated dose-response of methazolamide in glaucoma. Arch Ophthalmol 96:2214, 1978.
16. Cohen AM, Prialnik M, Ben-Nissan DS, et al: Methazolamide-associated temporary leukopenia and thrombocytopenia. DICP 23:58, 1989.
17. Fraunfelder FT, Meyer SM, Bagby GC Jr, et al: Hematologic reactions to carbonic anhydrase inhibitors. Am J Ophthalmol 100:79, 1985.
18. Arrigg CA, Epstein DL, Giovanoni R, Grant WM: The influence of supplemental sodium acetate on carbonic anhydrase inhibitor-induced side effects. Arch Ophthalmol 99:1969, 1981.
19. Ahlstrand C, Tiselius HG: Urine composition and stone formation during treatment with acetazolamide. Scand J Urol Nephrol 21:225, 1987.
20. Wallace MR, MacDiarmid J, Reeder J: Exacerbation of nephrolithiasis by a carbonic anhydrase inhibitor. N Z Med J 79:687, 1974.
21. Block ER, Rostand RA: Carbonic anhydrase inhibition in glaucoma: Hazard or benefit for the chronic lunger? Surv Ophthalmol 23:169, 1978.
22. Wallace TR, Fraunfelder FT, Petursson GJ, et al: Decreased libido—a side effect of carbonic anhydrase inhibitor. Ann Ophthalmol 11:1563, 1979.
23. Deck SL: Assessment of adult skeletons to detect prenatal exposure to acetazolamide in mice. Teratology 28:45, 1983.
24. Worsham F Jr, Beckman EN, Mitchell EH: Sacrococcygeal teratoma in a neonate: Association with maternal use of acetazolamide. JAMA 240:251, 1978.
25. Lippa EA, Schuman JS, Higginbotham EJ, et al: MK507 vs. sezolamide: Comparative efficacy of two topically active carbonic anhydrase inhibitors. Ophthalmology 98:308, 1991.
26. Lippa EA, Carlson LE, Ehinger B, et al: Dose response and duration of action of dorsolamide, a topical carbonic anhydrase inhibitor. Arch Ophthalmol 110:495, 1992.
27. Sugru MF: The preclinical pharmacology of dorzolamide hydrochloride, a topical carbonic anyhydrase inhibitor. J Ocul Pharmacol 12(3):363, 1996.
28. Lippa EA, Carlson L, et al: Dose response and duration of action of dorzolamide: A topical carbonic anhydrase inhibitor. Arch Ophthalmol 110:495, 1992.
29. Azopt (brinzolamide ophthalmic suspension) 1%. Data available upon request from Alcon Labs., Inc., Fort Worth, TX 76134.
30. Strahlman E, Tipping R, et al: A double-masked, randomized 1-year study comparing dorzolamide (Trusopt), timolol, and betaxolol. Arch Ophthalmol 113:1009, 1995.
31. Cosopt (dorzolamide hydrochloride-timolol maleate ophthalmic solution) drug information. Data available upon request from Merck & Co., WPI-27, West Point, PA 19486.
32. Yamazaki Y, Miyamoto S, et al: Effect of MK-507 on aqueous humor dynamics in normal human eyes. Jpn J Ophthalmol 38:92, 1994.
33. Maus TL, Larsson L, et al: Comparison of dorzolamide and acetazolamide as suppressors of aqueous humor flow in humans. Arch Ophthalmol 115:45, 1997.
34. Strahlman ER, Vogel R, et al: The use of dorzolamide and pilocarpine as adjunctive therapy to timolol in patients with elevated intraocular pressure. Ophthalmology 103(8):1283, 1996.
35. Data available upon request from Merck & Co., WPI-27, West Point, PA 19486.
36. Palmberg P: A topical anhydrase inhibitor finally arrives. Arch Ophthalmol 113:985, 1995.
37. Trusopt (dorzolamide hydrochloride) drug information insert.
38. Whitcup SM, Csaky KG, Podgor MJ, et al: A randomized, masked, cross-over trial of acetazolamide for cystoid macular edema in patients with uveitis. Ophthalmology 103:1054, 1996.
39. Berson FG, Epstein DL: Carbonic anhydrase inhibitors: Management of side effects. Perspect Ophthalmol 4:91, 1980.
40. Lichter PR: Reducing side effects of carbonic anhydrase inhibitors. Am Acad Ophthalmol 161:266, 1980.
41. Fishman GA, Gilbert LD, Fiscella RG, et al: Acetazolamide for treatment of chronic macular edema in retinitis pigmentosa. Arch Ophthalmol 107:1445, 1989.
42. Steinmetz RL, Fitzke FW, Bird AC: Treatment of cystoid macular edema with acetazolamide in a patient with serpiginous choroidopathy. Retina 11(4):412, 1991.
43. Gelisken O, Gelisken F, Ozcetin H: Treatment of chronic macular edema with low dosage acetazolamide. Bull Soc Belge Ophtalmol 238:153, 1990.
44. Tripathi RC, Fekrat S, Tripathi BJ, et al: A direct correlation of the resolution of the pseudophakic cystoid macular edema with acetazolamide therapy. Ann Ophthalmol 23(4):127, 1991.

CHAPTER 34

Pharmacologic Treatment of Immune Disorders

C. Stephen Foster

In its broadest scope, the rubric *immune disorders* would include all disorders in which the immune system is abnormal. A treatise on the pharmacologic treatment of such immune disorders would necessarily include material devoted to the treatment of immunodeficiency diseases, including acquired immunodeficiency syndrome (AIDS) caused by the human immunodeficiency virus (HIV), as well as material on immunoregulatory disorders that result in autoimmunity or an overaggressive immune response. My charge for this chapter is to address the latter group of disorders. Because inflammation is the paradigm for the expression of autoimmune disease, a discussion of all therapies for inflammation might be appropriate here, but the pharmacology and use of the steroidal and nonsteroidal antiinflammatory drugs are dealt with in Chapters 25 and 27. This chapter therefore limits its discussion to the properties and uses of the immunosuppressive chemotherapeutic agents in the treatment of immune inflammatory or autoimmune diseases.

Although the use of immunosuppressive and biologic agents to inhibit immune reactions dates back at least half a century,[1] the mechanisms of action of most of the immunosuppressive agents are incompletely understood. Often we don't even know whether a particular agent is in fact suppressing immune responses or suppressing the inflammatory expression of these responses. By definition, immunosuppressive agents suppress the development of at least one type of immune reaction: They modify the specific immune sensitization of lymphoid cells.[2] Table 34–1 lists chemotherapeutic agents useful in the treatment of neoplastic disease, many of which are also commonly used to treat autoimmune inflammatory diseases. Usually only one, or at most two, agents from a given class of these chemotherapeutic agents has been used extensively enough as an immunosuppressive agent in the treatment of immune disorders to allow us to make wise choices about using such agents to treat autoimmune inflammatory disease. This is why only one or two agents are usually chosen to represent each class of chemotherapeutic agent in the following sections.

TABLE 34–1. **Agents Commonly Used to Treat Autoimmune Inflammatory Conditions**

Class	Type of Agent	Nonproprietary Names
Alkylating agents	Nitrogen mustards	Cyclophosphamide
		Chlorambucil
Antimetabolites	Folic acid analogs	Methotrexate
	Pyrimidine analogs	5-Fluorouracil
	Purine analogs	Azathioprine
Natural products	Antibiotics	Cyclosporine
		Dapsone
		Tacrolimus
		Mitomycin
	Antibodies	Antilymphocyte serum
		Anti–T-cell antibody
		Gamma globulin

One feature common to many of the immunosuppressive agents is their ability to interfere with synthesis of nucleic acid, protein, or both. This interference commonly is assumed to be the immunosuppressive mechanism, because lymphoid cells stimulated by antigen to proliferate and produce lymphokines are exquisitely sensitive to interference with nucleic acid or protein synthesis. Bach[2] and others have emphasized, however, that the effect of immunosuppressive agents cannot be explained solely by this simple notion. Considering the extraordinary complexity of the idiotypic-antiidiotypic immunoregulatory network of T-lymphocyte subsets, B-lymphocyte subsets, and antigen-presenting cells and macrophage subsets, it is remarkable that the first physicians to explore the possible use of immunosuppressive chemotherapeutic agents in the treatment of autoimmune inflammatory disorders discovered dosages that produced enough differential effect on subsets of helper and cytotoxic cells to cause immunosuppression.

Alkylating Agents

CHEMICAL PROPERTIES AND MECHANISM OF ACTION

Nitrogen mustards, ethylenimines and methylmelamines, alkylsulfonates, nitrosoureas, and triazenes all act in similar ways, through nucleophilic substitution reactions. Of these agents, only members of the nitrogen mustard family are commonly used as immunosuppressive chemotherapeutic agents in the treatment of autoimmune inflammatory disease; of the nitrogen mustards, only cyclophosphamide and chlorambucil have been used enough to warrant discussion here.

Cyclophosphamide (Cytoxan), the most potent of the therapeutic alkylating agents, is used extensively throughout the world to treat a variety of conditions (Fig. 34–1). All alkylating agents act through nucleophilic substitution reactions, and such reactions with DNA probably account for their predominant immunosuppressive activity (Fig. 34–2). Breaks occur in single-stranded DNA. When these breaks are repaired, phosphodiester bonds form and result in defective cell function. Cross-linking reactions occur between DNA

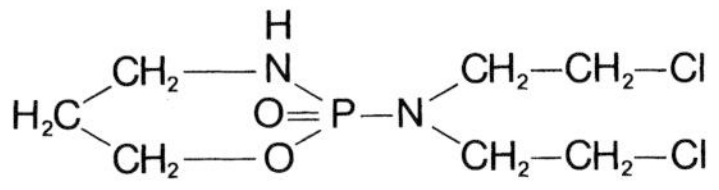

FIGURE 34–1. Chemical structure of cyclophosphamide.

strands, between DNA and RNA, and between these molecules and cell proteins, generally resulting in death of the affected cell.

Like most other immunosuppressive agents, cyclophosphamide is not immunosuppressive in its native state. After oral or intravenous administration, it is activated by the liver P-450 microsome system. Phosphoamidase, which is present in especially high concentrations in liver microsomes, catalyzes the conversion of the drug into its active principles, aldophosphamide and 4-hydroxycyclophosphamide. In clinical doses, alkylating drugs are very cytotoxic for lymphoid cells. The effect on B and T cells appears to be nearly equal, except that large doses enhance the effect on B cells. Cyclophosphamide has a potent effect on antibody responses when given with, or even up to 4 days after, antigen encounter. It suppresses secondary antibody responses in previously primed animals and patients. Cyclophosphamide effectively inhibits delayed hypersensitivity reactions and is as effective as azathioprine in liver, cardiac, bone marrow, skin, and pulmonary allograft rejection reactions. It is the only immunosuppressive agent that can induce immune tolerance to particulate antigen. The pharmacokinetics and kinetics of the development of such tolerance are complex. The drug

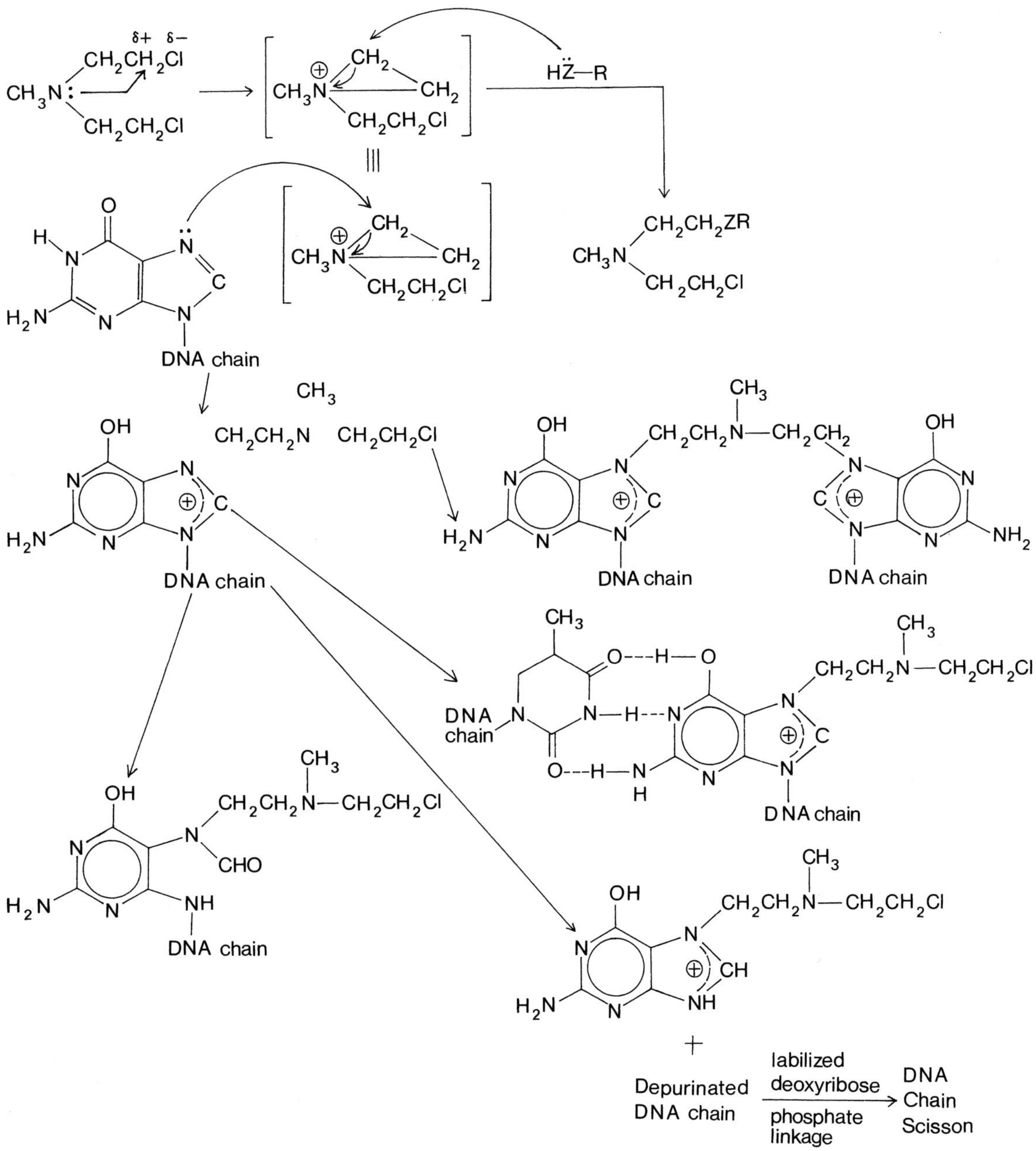

FIGURE 34–2. Diagrammatic representation of the mechanism of action of alkylating agents.

must be given 24 to 48 hours *after* antigen priming. Tolerance is probably mediated, at least predominantly, by regulatory T lymphocytes that develop after antigen priming. On the other hand, at least in the murine experimental model, low-dose cyclophosphamide therapy can eliminate regulatory T lymphocytes that actively mediate tolerance, resulting in release from tolerance and in expression of immunoreactivity in the form of a delayed hypersensitivity reaction to the relevant antigen. The dose and timing of administration of cyclophosphamide apparently are critical to its effect on lymphocyte subsets. This, of course, makes judgments about clinical use of the drug in new applications difficult. Cyclophosphamide inhibits monocyte precursor development but has little effect on fully developed macrophages. It is spectacularly effective in preventing the development of autoimmune disease in the NZB/NZW F1 mouse model of systemic lupus erythematosus. Cyclophosphamide is readily absorbed after oral administration. The standard initial daily dose is 1 to 2 mg/kg. The serum half-life is 7 hours, and allopurinol prolongs that half-life.

Chlorambucil (Leukeran) (Fig. 34–3) is also readily absorbed after oral administration. The standard initial daily dose is 0.1 to 0.2 mg/kg. The half-life in plasma is approximately 1 hour, and the drug is almost completely metabolized. It is the slowest-acting nitrogen mustard in clinical use, and its cytotoxic effects on bone marrow, lymphoid organs, and epithelial tissues are similar to those of the other nitrogen mustards.

NONOPHTHALMIC USES AND POTENTIAL SIDE EFFECTS

Cyclophosphamide is used extensively to treat Wegener's granulomatosis, polyarteritis nodosa, and other forms of systemic vasculitis. It is still sometimes used to treat human allograft recipients and often to treat bullous pemphigoid. It is sometimes used when severe rheumatoid arthritis is refractory to more conventional therapy, and it is a common drug of choice for nephrotic syndrome in children. It is also still sometimes employed in the "polydrug" approach to malignancies, including multiple myeloma; chronic lymphocytic leukemia; lung, breast, cervical, and ovarian carcinoma; neuroblastoma; retinoblastoma; and some other neoplasms of childhood.

Potential complications of cyclophosphamide therapy include severe bone marrow depression with resultant anemia, leukopenia, thrombocytopenia, and secondary infection; anorexia, nausea, vomiting, hemorrhagic colitis, and oral mucosal ulceration; jaundice; hemorrhagic cystitis; gonadal suppression; alopecia; and interstitial pulmonary fibrosis. Sterile hemorrhagic cystitis occurs in 5 to 10% of patients; this has been attributed to chemical irritation of the lining of the bladder produced by reactive metabolites of cyclophosphamide, particularly acrolein. This potentially devastating complication, which can lead to bladder carcinoma, can usually be avoided with correct administration (i.e., restricting consumption of cyclophosphamide to the early hours of the day and forcing fluid intake during the remainder of the day). Acetylcysteine or mesna (sodium 2-mercaptoethanesulfonate) can prevent or reverse cyclophosphamide-induced hemorrhagic cystitis. If a patient taking cyclophosphamide develops dysuria or microscopic hematuria, the physician should confirm that the patient is taking the drug correctly and is adequately hydrated and should perform emergency cystoscopy to confirm that the source of the blood is the lining of the bladder rather than the kidney. If, for example, a patient being treated for Wegener's granulomatosis develops microscopic hematuria, cessation of cyclophosphamide would be inappropriate if the red blood cells are coming from Wegener's inflammatory activity in the kidney rather than from cyclophosphamide-induced cystitis.

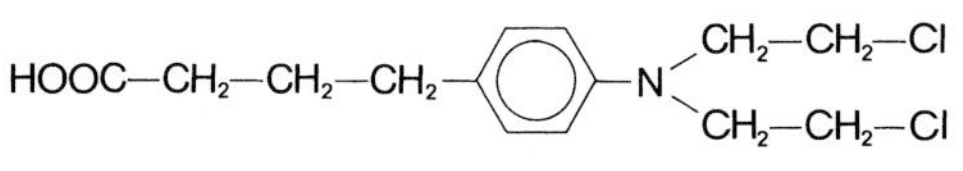

$$HOOC{-}CH_2{-}CH_2{-}CH_2{-}C_6H_4{-}N(CH_2{-}CH_2{-}Cl)_2$$

FIGURE 34–3. Structural formula of chlorambucil.

Chlorambucil is still the treatment of choice for chronic lymphocytic leukemia and primary (Waldenström's) macroglobulinemia. It is also sometimes used to treat Hodgkin's disease and other lymphomas as well as vasculitis associated with rheumatoid arthritis and autoimmune hemolytic anemia with cold agglutinins.

Potential complications of chlorambucil therapy include bone marrow suppression, gastrointestinal discomfort, azoospermia, amenorrhea, pulmonary fibrosis, seizures, dermatitis, and hepatotoxicity. A marked increase in the incidence of leukemia, lymphoma, and other neoplasms has been reported among patients receiving long-term adjuvant chemotherapy for breast cancer and patients being treated for polycythemia vera.

OPHTHALMIC INDICATIONS

Any patient who requires systemic immunosuppressive chemotherapeutic agents for a destructive ocular disease must be managed by an experienced chemotherapist who is, by virtue of formal training and experience, an expert in the use of immunosuppressive drugs and in the recognition and treatment of drug-induced side effects and potentially serious complications. My experience suggests that, in general, the chemotherapy experts with whom ophthalmologists can most consistently and effectively collaborate are oncologists or hematologists. The chemotherapist is completely responsible for the chemotherapeutic aspects of the patient's care. He or she personally sees the patient regularly; monitoring blood counts and blood chemistry without seeing the patient is inappropriate management. The ophthalmologist apprises the chemotherapist regularly of the status of the ophthalmic inflammatory condition. If the problem is not sufficiently controlled, it is the chemotherapist who decides, for instance, whether or not it is safe and appropriate to increase the patient's immunosuppressive medications, to add a second medication with or without stopping the initial one, or to supplement medications with systemic steroids. Foster and associates' published guidelines suggest initial doses of various agents and one routine for careful hematologic monitoring, avoiding depressing the white count below 3500 cells/mm^3 and the neutrophil count below 1500 cells/mm^3.[3] I also suggest avoiding thrombocytopenia below 75,000 platelets/mm^3. I suggest urinalysis every 2 weeks during the initial treatment period, and then once a month when the patient is on a steady maintenance drug program.

Cyclophosphamide is the treatment of choice for any

patient with ocular manifestations of Wegener's granulomatosis or polyarteritis nodosa. It is also unquestionably the most effective treatment for patients with highly destructive forms of inflammation in association with rheumatoid arthritis. Few other drugs have allowed us to intervene successfully in the progression of rheumatoid arthritis–associated necrotizing scleritis with associated peripheral ulcerative keratitis. Interestingly, Watson and Hazleman[4] find that the necrotizing scleritis and peripheral ulcerative keratitis in some patients with relapsing polychondritis may be more refractory to therapy than that associated with Wegener's granulomatosis, polyarteritis nodosa, or rheumatoid arthritis. Although dapsone is commonly effective in the extraocular manifestations of this disease, I have rarely found it effective in abrogating ocular inflammation in this disorder. Cyclophosphamide, with or without oral steroid and nonsteroidal antiinflammatory drug therapy, is often required to treat necrotizing scleritis associated with relapsing polychondritis.

Either cyclophosphamide or chlorambucil is an appropriate choice for effective treatment of posterior uveitis or retinal vasculitis manifestations of Behçet's syndrome. Chlorambucil may be the more effective of the two, but cyclophosphamide, particularly when given as intravenous pulse therapy, is highly effective. Baer and Foster[5] and others[6] find both drugs to be superior to cyclosporine (cyclosporin A, CsA) in the care of patients with posterior segment manifestations of Behçet's disease.

Cicatricial pemphigoid affecting the conjunctiva usually responds to cyclophosphamide therapy. If the patient with cicatricial pemphigoid has very active disease that is progressive, cyclophosphamide is the drug of first choice. Therapy typically lasts at least 1 year. The relapse rate after discontinuation of cyclophosphamide is approximately 20%.[7]

The use of cyclophosphamide or chlorambucil in the treatment of patients with other ocular inflammatory diseases is slightly more problematic. There is little question that each can be effective in the care of youngsters with juvenile rheumatoid arthritis (JRA)-associated iridocyclitis that does not respond to steroids and other conventional treatments, and that in this role these drugs can be sight-saving. This is a complex area, however, given the age of the patients and the potential risks for delayed malignancy or sterility associated with the treatment. The relative risks and benefits must be explored individually with patient and parents alike. I hope that longitudinal comparative trials in this patient group will help clarify the issue of relative risks and benefits of systemic immunosuppressive chemotherapeutic treatment *early* in the course of chronic iritis associated with JRA.

Other forms of uveitis that do not respond to conventional treatment or are associated with intolerable steroid-induced side effects may also respond to cyclophosphamide or chlorambucil therapy. The guidelines for such an approach vary from clinic to clinic around the world, but ample precedents exist for this alternative in patients with slowly blinding uveitis.[8–12] Whether the patient has pars planitis or uveitis associated with Reiter's syndrome, with ankylosing spondylitis, with inflammatory bowel disease, or even with "idiopathic" uveitis, I employ a stepladder approach to the treatment of that patient's ocular inflammation. I always use steroids first, and use them aggressively, via all potential routes of administration (topical, periocular injection, systemic) and in the largest doses tolerated. It is typical to obtain informed consent and dispense printed handouts that describe the potential risks of topical, periocular, and systemic steroids. If in spite of this approach, the patient's disease is chronic or relapses each time steroids are tapered or discontinued, I add oral nonsteroidal antiinflammatory drugs to the treatment plan (with the patient's consent). If this combination does not achieve the goal of total quiescence of all inflammation *off* all steroids, or if treatment-induced side effects appear that are unacceptable to patient or doctor, the patient is offered the alternative of a systemic immunosuppressive chemotherapeutic drug. The choice of that drug depends on the individual patient, the particular disease, the patient's age, and the patient's sex. Some of the entities I have treated successfully with systemic immunosuppressive chemotherapeutic agents, including cyclophosphamide and chlorambucil, are as follows: sympathetic ophthalmia; Vogt-Koyanagi-Harada syndrome; birdshot choroidopathy; multifocal choroiditis with panuveitis; retinal vasculitis associated with systemic lupus erythematosus; multifocal choroiditis associated with progressive systemic sclerosis; retinal vasculitis associated with sarcoidosis; pars planitis associated with multiple sclerosis; severe uveitis associated with ankylosing spondylitis, with Reiter's syndrome, or with inflammatory bowel disease; idiopathic uveitis; and bilateral Mooren's ulcer.[13]

Purine Analogs

CHEMICAL PROPERTIES AND MECHANISM OF ACTION

Thiopurines, such as mercaptopurine and azathioprine (Imuran) (Fig. 34–4), interfere with purine metabolism and, so, with synthesis of DNA, RNA, and protein. Purine analogs interfere with the synthesis of purine bases. They inhibit purine nucleotide interconversion reactions and the formation and function of coenzymes (such as coenzyme A), thereby inhibiting RNA and DNA synthesis. These agents or their metabolites are incorporated into DNA and RNA, but that probably is not the locus of their suppressive effect. These drugs must be converted to active principles, predominantly in the liver. One such metabolically active product is thioinosinic acid.

At clinical nontoxic doses of 2 to 3 mg/kg/day, azathioprine has little effect on humoral immunity. Immunoglobulin levels and specific antibody responses are relatively unaffected. In experimental systems, large doses of thiopurine given within 48 hours of antigen priming can suppress the antibody response and can induce temporary tolerance to the antigen when given in conjunction with large doses of the antigen.

Thiopurines appear to exert a *relatively* selective effect on T lymphocytes: They prolong renal, skin, lung, and cardiac allografts; suppress mixed lymphocyte reaction in vitro; depress recirculating T lymphocytes that are in the process of

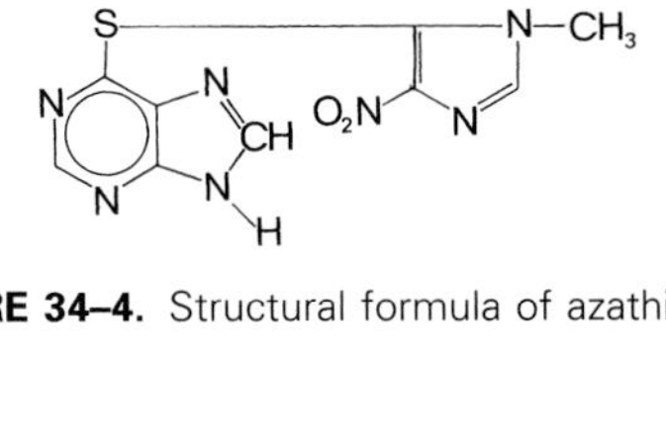

FIGURE 34–4. Structural formula of azathioprine.

homing; suppress development of monocyte precursor cells; inhibit participation of K cells (which arise from monocyte precursors) in antibody-dependent cytotoxicity reactions; and inhibit delayed type hypersensitivity reactions. On the other hand, they do not affect the onset or progression of the lupus-like autoimmune disease in NZB/NZW F1 mice, and their immunosuppression of renal transplant patients, for example, is partial because such patients consistently show lymphocyte responsiveness in vitro (proliferation, lymphokine production, cytotoxicity, cytotoxic antibody) to donor antigen.

NONOPHTHALMIC USES AND POTENTIAL SIDE EFFECTS

Purine analogs, most notably azathioprine, are used extensively in human heart, kidney, and lung allograft recipients. They have also been used to treat blistering dermatoses (pemphigus vulgaris and bullous pemphigoid), rheumatoid arthritis, and regional ileitis (Crohn's disease).

I have suggested an initial dose of 2 to 3 mg/kg/day; dose adjustments are based on clinical response and drug tolerance. Allopurinol inhibits xanthine oxidase and so inhibits the conversion of azathioprine to its inactive metabolites; the dose must be reduced accordingly.

Potential drug-induced complications of azathioprine therapy include hepatotoxicity, severe bone marrow depression with resultant anemia, leukopenia, thrombocytopenia, secondary infection, anorexia, nausea, vomiting, gastrointestinal distress, diarrhea, rash, fever, and arthralgia.

OPHTHALMIC INDICATIONS

Azathioprine can be effective in patients with ocular inflammatory manifestations of Behçet's syndrome.[14] In my experience, however, it is not the most effective drug for this purpose. Still, it can be effective and should be included in every doctor's therapeutic armamentarium for this potentially devastating, frequently blinding disease. Andrasch and coworkers[9] rigorously studied azathioprine in the treatment of uveitis of various causes. It was judged effective in 12 patients and ineffective in 10, either because of drug-induced side effects or because of inadequate response to treatment. Moore[15] stopped the inflammation associated with sympathetic ophthalmia, and Hemady and associates[16] have noted azathioprine's effectiveness in patients with JRA-associated uveitis that does not respond to conventional steroid therapy. It also can be effective in the treatment of cicatricial pemphigoid[17] and in the care of relapsing polychondritis-associated scleritis.[18] I have also used it as a steroid-sparing drug for patients with multifocal choroiditis with panuveitis, sympathetic ophthalmia, Vogt-Koyanagi-Harada syndrome, sarcoidosis, pars planitis, and Reiter's syndrome–associated iridocyclitis.

Folic Acid Analogs

CHEMICAL PROPERTIES AND MECHANISM OF ACTION

Methotrexate (Fig. 34–5), a folic acid analog also known as amethopterin, binds to folic reductase, thus blocking the conversion of dihydrofolic acid to tetrahydrofolic acid. This interferes with thymidine synthesis and, so, with DNA synthesis and cell division. Methotrexate has little effect on resting cells but pronounced effects on rapidly proliferating cells. It affects both B and T lymphocytes and can inhibit humoral and cellular responses when administered during antigenic encounter. The drug is excreted unchanged in the urine. Folinic acid can reverse the metabolic block produced by methotrexate, thus rescuing viable cells.

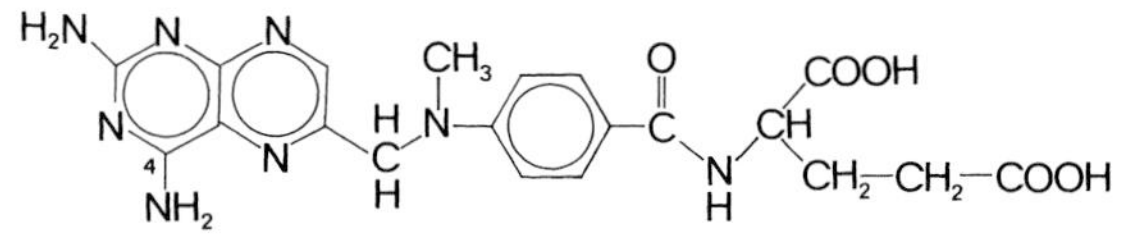

FIGURE 34–5. Structural formula of methotrexate.

Methotrexate is absorbed after oral administration, but the drug can also be given by intramuscular or intravenous routes. It is excreted unchanged in the urine within 48 hours. Renal compromise delays excretion and causes undesirable side effects. Consumption of sulfa drugs, salicylates, phenytoin, chloramphenicol, or tetracycline also increases the risk of methotrexate-induced complications through displacement of methotrexate from plasma proteins. The drug does not require metabolic conversion to active principles. The concurrent use of drugs that affect the kidney, such as nonsteroidal antiinflammatory agents, can delay drug excretion and lead to severe myelosuppression. Leucovorin "rescue" may help reverse some methotrexate-induced toxic effects.

5-Fluorouracil (5-FU) (Fig. 34–6) mimics uracil after intracellular conversion to nucleotide and subsequent incorporation into both DNA and RNA. The drug is especially toxic to rapidly dividing cells.

NONOPHTHALMIC USES AND POTENTIAL SIDE EFFECTS

Methotrexate is used to treat certain types of cancer, acute lymphoblastic leukemia, psoriasis, rheumatoid arthritis refractory to conventional therapy, JRA, and, in selected cases, sarcoidosis. Potential complications include severe bone marrow depression with resultant anemia, leukopenia, and thrombocytopenia; cirrhosis and hepatic atrophy; ulcerative stomatitis, nausea, vomiting, and diarrhea; interstitial pneumonitis; malaise, fatigue, and secondary infection; rash; cystitis; nephritis; headache, blurred vision, and drowsiness; and sterility. The hepatic fibrosis and cirrhosis associated with methotrexate therapy are related to dose and treatment duration, as well as to alcohol consumption. The risk of this potentially devastating complication can be minimized by administering it only once a week, insisting on total abstinence from alcohol, avoiding other drugs that may enhance the effects of methotrexate, and monitoring the liver care-

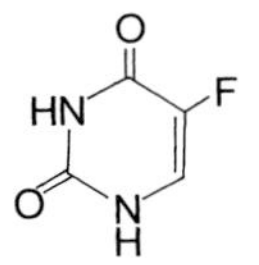

FIGURE 34–6. Structural formula of 5-fluorouracil.

fully and regularly. 5-FU is used intravenously to treat metastatic breast, liver, pancreatic, colon, ovarian, prostatic, and bladder cancer. Topical 5-FU is used to treat basal cell carcinomas.

OPHTHALMIC INDICATIONS

Idiopathic cyclitis,[12] sympathetic ophthalmia,[19] ocular manifestations of rheumatoid arthritis,[20] and the uveitis of JRA are particularly well suited for once-a-week therapy with oral methotrexate. Other varieties of uveitis, including that associated with Reiter's syndrome, ankylosing spondylitis, inflammatory bowel disease, or psoriasis, may also respond to methotrexate. This drug may be sufficient to control scleritis associated with the collagen diseases such as Reiter's syndrome and rheumatoid arthritis; I have found it effective in selected persons with progressive cicatricial pemphigoid. The suggested regimen is 2.5 to 7.5 mg once a week, with gradual escalation of the dose, as indicated by the clinical response, to a maximum of 15 mg/week.

Regrettably, despite abundant published evidence to the contrary, most ophthalmologists consider methotrexate "dangerous." They undoubtedly remember the complications associated with high-dose or daily methotrexate therapy in the care of patients with a malignancy or with psoriasis. Liver toxicity and bone marrow suppression were indeed prevalent in such patients. Although the potential risk for such problems in patients treated with a weekly low dose of methotrexate is not zero, the likelihood of such a problem is clearly low, provided the patient is managed and monitored correctly.[21–26] Proper monitoring is important; this obviously requires the involvement of an additional specialist and regular laboratory testing in these patients, but the alternative of slow degeneration in visual function is considerably more costly in both human and economic terms.

At the time of this writing, the sole ophthalmic application of 5-FU is subconjunctival injection after glaucoma filtering surgery in an effort to prevent subconjunctival fibrosis and bleb failure.[27] The primary toxic effect of subconjunctival 5-FU consists of superficial punctate keratopathy and persistent corneal epithelial defect.

Antibiotics

CHEMICAL PROPERTIES AND MECHANISM OF ACTION

CsA (Sandimmune, Neoral) (Fig. 34–7) is a fungal metabolite originally isolated from cultures of *Tolypocladium inflatum* Gams and *Cylindrocarpon lucidum* Booth by Sandoz Laboratories as part of a screening program of fungal products with antifungal activity. This undecacyclic peptide is also produced by *Cylindrocarpon lucidum.* Borel[28] found that it had potent immunosuppressive properties. Subsequent work in experimental models showed the drug to be truly immunosuppressive and capable of suppressing allograft reactions to heterotopic heart allografts in rats. CsA also prolonged the viability of renal allografts in dogs, heart allografts in pigs, and kidney allografts in rabbits.

Tacrolimus (FK-506, Prograf) is another fungus-derived immunosuppressant, isolated from *Streptomyces tsukubaensis.* It is structurally similar to rapamycin (Fig. 34–8) and is about 100 times more potent than CsA in preventing allograft rejection in animals.

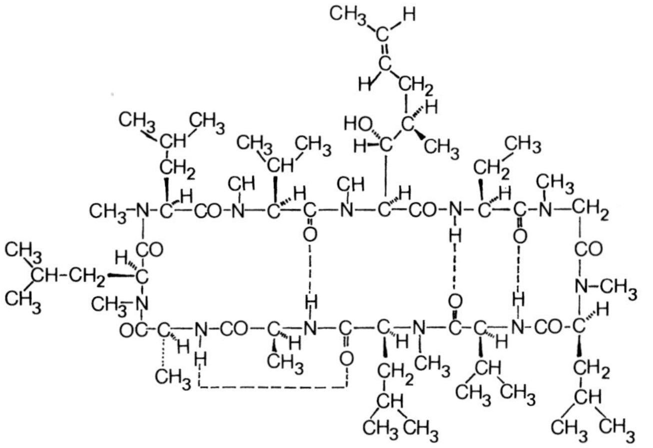

FIGURE 34–7. Structural formula of cyclosporine.

The mechanism of action of CsA's and tacrolimus' immunosuppressive properties is incompletely understood, but the best available evidence suggests that these drugs interfere with receptors on the surface membranes of certain T lymphocytes (particularly helper T cells) that recognize DR antigens on other cells, most notably antigen-presenting cells like macrophages. A 17-kDa protein, cyclophilin, which is a cytosolic protein, binds CsA and concentrates it intracellularly. Tacrolimus is similarly bound by another family of immunophilins, FKBP or FK-506–binding protein. These binding proteins are peptidyl-prolyl *cis-trans* isomerases; at least 26 have been identified to date. DR antigens participate in the production of interleukin-2 (IL-2) by helper T lymphocytes by rendering the IL-2–producing T cells sensitive to IL-1. CsA and tacrolimus interfere with helper T-cell response to IL-1 and blocks IL-2 production or IL-2 release from helper T cells. It appears that a complex composed of calcineurin A, CsA, or tacrolimus, and the relevant immunophilin, inhibits calmodulin binding, with resultant inhibition of a phosphatase activity and consequent inhibition of transport of cytoplasmic NFA-T and NFK6 into the nucleus; the result is inhibition of IL-2 mRNA transcription. CsA and tacrolimus also may inhibit IL-1 release from antigen-presenting cells such as macrophages. Both inhibit expression of IL-3, IL-4, IL-5, and interferon-γ.

CsA and tacrolimus have a fairly selective suppressive effect on T lymphocytes, which occurs early in the phase of T cell–subset interactions. The drugs profoundly decrease

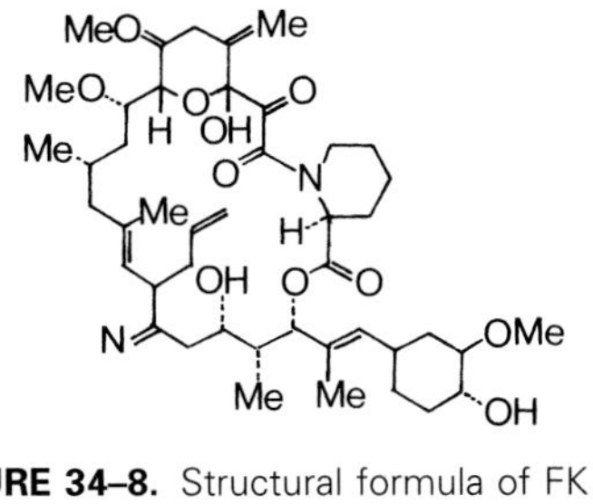

FIGURE 34–8. Structural formula of FK 506.

antibody production to T cell–dependent antigens, inhibit cytotoxic activity generated in mixed leukocyte reaction, and prolong the life of skin, kidney, and heart allografts in experimental animals and humans. They also may prevent or mitigate graft-versus-host disease and may prolong the life of other organ transplants, such as pancreas and cornea.

NONOPHTHALMIC USES AND POTENTIAL SIDE EFFECTS

CsA is used extensively for prevention of human allograft rejection and is being investigated for the treatment of a variety of other diseases, including psoriasis. Tacrolimus is in investigational studies for organ transplantation in humans, and has been approved by the Food and Drug Administration for prevention of human liver allograph rejection. Potential side effects associated with systemic use of CsA include an apparent increase in the incidence of B-cell lymphomas, interstitial pneumonitis, and opportunistic infections, particularly from herpes simplex virus and *Candida* and *Pneumocystis* organisms, as well as renal tubular necrosis with compromise of kidney function.

OPHTHALMIC INDICATIONS

CsA may be particularly useful in the treatment of various forms of posterior uveitis, especially when both retina and choroid are involved in the inflammatory process. Thus, sympathetic ophthalmia, Vogt-Koyanagi-Harada syndrome, multifocal uveitis with panuveitis, and posterior uveitis associated with Behçet's syndrome may lend themselves to effective treatment with CsA. I have been disappointed, however, with the effectiveness of CsA compared with cytotoxic immunosuppressive drugs in treating posterior uveitis associated with Behçet's syndrome when the dose of cyclosporine is in the acceptable range (5 to 7 mg/kg/day) from the standpoint of risk for kidney damage. Early enthusiastic reports of the effectiveness of CsA in the therapy of Behçet's syndrome were based on dosing schedules of 10 mg/kg/day.[22] Unfortunately, it was subsequently discovered that all patients who consumed this dose of CsA long enough to achieve the desired therapeutic effect in Behçet's disease developed renal damage from the drug. In my experience, the lower, less toxic dose of 5 to 7 mg/kg/day, is distinctly inferior to azathioprine, chlorambucil, and cyclophosphamide in the care of patients with ocular Behcet's disease. Others report similar disappointment.[23] In contrast, it is highly effective in the care of patients with birdshot retinochoroidopathy, even at low doses.[29] CsA may have a role in the care of patients with severe eczema, perhaps especially those with significant atopic keratoconjunctivitis. Topical CsA was investigated for the treatment of corneal graft rejection and keratoconjunctivitis sicca. The results were disappointing, but additional studies are in progress. Two other antibiotics with immunosuppressive properties that have ophthalmic indications are dapsone and mitomycin C.

DAPSONE

Dapsone (4,4′-diaminodiphenylsulfone, Fig. 34–9) is a sulfone used for the antibiotic treatment of leprosy. In addition to its antibacterial activity, it is a myeloperoxidase inhibitor and stabilizes lysosomal membranes. Its antiinflammatory and immunosuppressive effects are most dramatic in dermatitis herpetiformis and cicatricial pemphigoid. It is in the latter disease that ophthalmologists find it most useful. I found that, provided the cicatrizing conjunctivitis of cicatricial pemphigoid is not highly inflamed or rapidly progressive, dapsone halts progression of fibrosis in 70% of cases.[17] And although dapsone may help patients with relapsing polychondritis, Hoang-Xuan and coworkers found that treating the scleritis of this disease with dapsone was disappointing.[18]

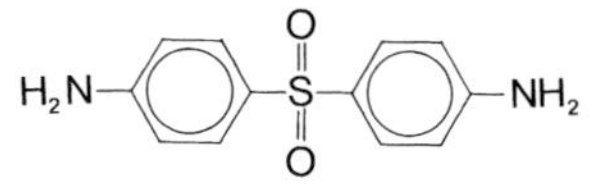

$$H_2N-C_6H_4-S(=O)_2-C_6H_4-NH_2$$

FIGURE 34–9. Structural formula of dapsone.

Dapsone may produce profound hemolysis in patients deficient in glucose-6-phosphate dehydrogenase, so any patient considered for dapsone therapy must first be evaluated for glucose-6-phosphate dehydrogenase level. I begin therapy with 25 mg twice daily; monitor the hemogram, reticulocyte count, and methemoglobin level biweekly; and increase to as much as 150 mg/day if needed and if tolerated. Additional toxic effects of dapsone include nausea, vomiting, hepatitis, peripheral neuropathy, blurred vision, psychosis, and a nephrotic-like syndrome.

MITOMYCIN C

Isolated from *Streptococcus calspitosus* in 1958, mitomycin (Fig. 34–10) reacts with DNA in ways similar to alkylating agents. It cross-links DNA and inhibits its synthesis. It is a highly effective antimitotic agent. It is used intravenously to treat carcinoma of the stomach and colon and sometimes as adjunctive therapy for cancer of the pancreas, breast, bladder, or lung. The major systemic side effect is myelosuppression.

The ocular indications for mitomycin C are recurrent pterygium and glaucoma filtering surgery. Kunitoma and Mori[30] and later Choon and Fong[31] reported favorably on the efficacy of mitomycin C eye drops in preventing pterygium recurrence after resection of pterygium that had recurred many times. Sing and colleagues confirmed these observations.[32] They also studied giving smaller doses of the drug than had been previously employed in an effort to avoid toxicity, and they compared the efficacy of topical mitomycin C with that of conjunctival transplantation for treatment of recurrent pterygium.[33] It is clear that topical mitomycin C is effective in this role. It is clearly simpler and cheaper than either conjunctival transplantation or β-irradiation. The smallest effective dose and shortest duration of therapy are not yet clear, however. I currently use a single application of 0.02% at the end of surgery.

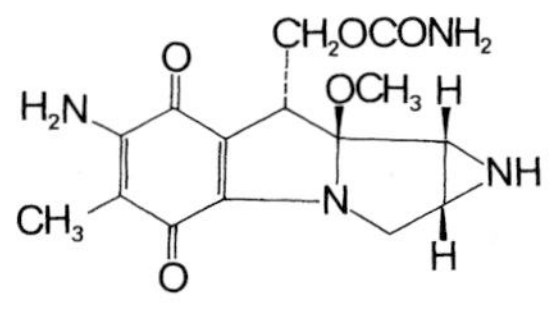

H_2N, CH_3, O, O, CH_2OCONH_2, OCH_3, H, N, NH, H

FIGURE 34–10. Structural formula of mitomycin C.

The efficacy of mitomycin C as an adjunctive component to glaucoma filtering surgery is now well established, although, as in pterygium surgery, in glaucoma surgery the "best" concentration of the drug and "best" technique and duration of application of the drug are not yet defined. I apply it to the scleral bed of the guarded trabeculectomy site, 0.4 mg/mL in saturated cellulose sponges, with conjunctiva draped over the sponges for 4 minutes, and then vigorously irrigate the area with 45 mL of balanced salt solution after removal of the sponges.

Potential complications of topical mitomycin C ocular therapy appear to be limited to instances of abuse and negligence, to drug dosage error, and to use of the drug in patients with ocular surface disorders, such as sicca syndrome and ocular rosacea. I am aware of four cases of scleral or corneal ulceration after such abuse: Applications were continued for 3 to 6 weeks after surgery rather than the prescribed 1 week.

Biologic Agents: Antibodies

CHEMICAL PROPERTIES AND MECHANISM OF ACTION

Heterologous antisera to leukocytes relevant to immune reactions have been used experimentally for immunosuppression since 1956 and clinically in humans since the late 1970s. The most extensively studied and widely used agent is antiserum prepared against human lymphocytes. Various antilymphocyte serum (ALS) preparations have been used; the most potent usually are obtained after immunization of horses with human thymus or thoracic duct cells. The greatest immunosuppressive activity usually appears in the immunoglobulin G (IgG) fraction of the immunized horse 2 to 4 weeks after immunization begins.

The effects of such antiserums after intravenous administration include leukopenia (highly immunosuppressive preparations of ALS sharply reduce the number of T lymphocytes); depletion of thymus-dependent areas in spleen and other lymphoid tissue; inhibition of delayed hypersensitivity reactions; prolonged viability of skin, renal, cardiac, liver, and lung allografts; and suppression of primary and secondary antibody responses if the antisera are given before antigen priming. Toxic effects of ALS include anaphylaxis and possible tumorigenesis.

Monoclonal antibodies directed against T lymphocytes (anti-OKT3 antibodies) have primarily the same effect as ALS, but their effect is more limited, being aimed only at T lymphocytes rather than all lymphocytes. Treatment with intravenous OKT3 antibodies (Orthoclone) can reverse renal allograft rejection reactions. Complications of anti-OKT antibody therapy include increased risk of malignancy, fever, malaise, severe nausea, and vomiting.

Pooled human immunoglobulin (Gamimune) is used not only for passive immunization to modify hepatitis A, prevent or modify measles, and provide replacement therapy for patients with agammaglobulinemia, but also, in its immunomodulatory role, to treat idiopathic thrombocytopenic purpura. It must be administered intravenously or intramuscularly and must be given repeatedly to achieve an immunomodulatory effect. Adverse reactions include malaise, nausea, vomiting, fever, chills, headache, arthralgia, and abdominal pain.

NONOPHTHALMIC USES AND POTENTIAL SIDE EFFECTS

ALS has been used in humans predominantly for organ transplantation, in conjunction with corticosteroid and cytotoxic drug therapy (usually azathioprine). As mentioned earlier, anti-OKT antibodies have been used exclusively in humans for attempted reversal of kidney transplant allograft rejection.

Human immunoglobulin has been used principally as replacement therapy for patients who are hypogammaglobulinemic or agammaglobulinemic and in treating hepatitis A infections, herpes zoster infections, and measles infections. Human immunoglobulin has also been used as an immunomodulatory agent for idiopathic thrombocytopenic purpura and in the experimental treatment of systemic lupus erythematosus and severe atopic dermatitis. Its toxic effects include malaise, fever, chills, headache, nausea, vomiting, shortness of breath, and back or hip pain. Patients with prior allergic responses to immunoglobulin may experience true anaphylactic reactions.

OPHTHALMIC INDICATIONS

To my knowledge, anti-OKT3 antibody therapy has been used only once for an ophthalmic indication. I treated a woman with bilateral keratoconus whose body was rejecting her fourth human leukocyte antigen–matched corneal graft, in the right eye, in spite of aggressive topical, regional injection, oral and intravenous pulse steroids, and topical and systemic CsA therapy with 7 days' intravenous OKT3 monoclonal antibody therapy. Her graft was saved, but this expensive in-hospital effort was an exercise in heroics that I suspect will find little use in ophthalmology. Intravenous gamma globulin therapy has been used extensively in the care of patients with severe eczema, and I have used this treatment modality in several patients whose severe atopic keratoconjunctivitis did not respond adequately to strict environmental controls and systemic antihistamine therapy. The drug must be given each week, and I prefer the intravenous route.

REFERENCES

1. Hektoen L, Corper JH: Effect of mustard gas on antibody formation. J Infect Dis 28:279, 1921.
2. Bach JF: The Mode of Action of Immunosuppressive Agents. Amsterdam, Elsevier/North Holland, 1975.
3. Foster CS, Wilson LA, Ekins MB: Immunosuppressive therapy for progressive ocular cicatricial pemphigoid. Ophthalmology 89:340, 1982.
4. Watson PG, Hazleman BL: The Sclera and Systemic Disorders. Philadelphia, WB Saunders, 1976, pp 90–154.
5. Baer JC, Foster CS: Ocular Behçet's disease in the United States: Clinical presentation and visual outcome in 29 patients. *In* Usui M, Ohno S, Aoki K (eds): Proceedings of the 5th International Symposium on the Immunology and Immunopathology of the Eye. Tokyo, March 13–15, 1990. Int Cong Ser 918. New York, Excerpta Medica, pp 383–386.
6. Fain O, Du B, Wechsler I, et al: Intravenous cyclophosphamide therapy in Behçet's disease. *In* O'Duffy JS, Kokinen E (eds): Behçet's Disease: Basic and Clinical Aspects. New York, Marcel Dekker, 1989, p 569.
7. Neumann R, Tauber J, Foster CS: Remission and recurrence after withdrawal of therapy for ocular cicatricial pemphigoid. Ophthalmology 98:858, 1991.
8. Godfrey WA, Epstein WV, O'Connor GR, et al: The use of chlorambucil in intractable idiopathic uveitis. Am J Ophthalmol 78:415, 1974.

9. Andrasch RH, Pirofsky B, Burns RP: Immunosuppressive therapy for severe chronic uveitis. Arch Ophthalmol 96:247, 1978.
10. Brubaker R, Font RL, Shephard EM: Granulomatous sclerouveitis. Regression of ocular lesions with cyclophosphamide and prednisone. Arch Ophthalmol 86:517, 1971.
11. Buckley CE III, Gills JP: Cyclophosphamide therapy of peripheral uveitis. Arch Intern Med 124:29, 1969.
12. Lazar M, Weiner MJ, Leopold IH: Treatment of uveitis with methotrexate. Am J Ophthalmol 67:383, 1969.
13. Foster CS: Immunosuppressive therapy for external ocular inflammatory disease. Ophthalmology 87:140, 1980.
14. Yazici H, Pazarli H, Barnes C, et al: A controlled trial of azathioprine in Behcet's syndrome. N Engl J Med 332:281, 1990.
15. Moore D: Sympathetic ophthalmia treated with azathioprine. Br J Pathol 52:688, 1968.
16. Hemady R, Baer JC, Foster CS: Immunosuppressive drugs in the management of progressive, corticosteroid-resistant uveitis associated with juvenile rheumatoid arthritis. Int Ophthalmol Clin 32(1):241, 1992.
17. Foster CS: Cicatricial pemphigoid. Trans Am Ophthalmol Soc 84:527, 1986.
18. Hoang-Xuan T, Foster CS, Rice BA: Scleritis in relapsing polychondritis. Ophthalmology 97:892, 1990.
19. Wong VG, Hersh EM, McMaster PRB: Treatment of a presumed case of sympathetic ophthalmia with methotrexate. Arch Ophthalmol 76:66, 1966.
20. Foster CS, Forstot SL, Wilson LA: Mortality rate in rheumatoid arthritis patients developing necrotizing scleritis or peripheral ulcerative keratitis: Effects of systemic immunosuppression. Ophthalmology 91:1253, 1984.
21. Graham LD, Myones BL, Rivas-Chacon RF: Methotrexate associated with long-term methotrexate therapy in juvenile rheumatoid arthritis. Pediatr Pharmacol Ther 120:468, 1992.
22. Giannini EH, Brewer EJ, Kuzmina N, et al: Methotrexate in resistant juvenile rheumatoid arthritis. N Engl J Med 326(16):1043, 1992.
23. Tagwell P, Bennett K, Bell M, et al: Methotrexate in rheumatoid arthritis. Ann Intern Med 110:581, 1989.
24. Lehman TJA: Aggressive therapy for childhood rheumatic diseases. Arthritis Rheum 36(1)71, 1993.
25. Wallace CA, Sherry DD: Preliminary report of higher dose methotrexate treatment in juvenile rheumatoid arthritis. J Rheumatol 19(10):1064, 1992.
26. Rose CD, Singsen BH, Eichenfield AH: Safety and efficacy of methotrexate therapy for juvenile rheumatoid arthritis. J Pediatr 117(4):655, 1990.
27. Fluorocil Filtering Study Group: Fluorocil filtering surgery study: One-year follow-up. Am J Ophthalmol 108:625, 1989.
28. Borel JF: Comparative study of in vitro and in vivo drug effects on cell-mediated cytotoxicity. Immunology 31:631, 1976.
29. Vitale AT, Rodriguez A, Foster CS: Low-dose cyclosporin therapy in the treatment of birdshot retinochoroidopathy. Ophthalmology 101(5):822, 1994.
30. Kunitoma N, Mori S: Studies on pterygium, IV. Treatment of pterygium by mitomycin C instillation. Acta Soc Ophthalmol Jpn 67:601, 1953.
31. Choon LK, Fong CY: The pterygium and mitomycin C therapy. Med J Malaysia 31:69, 1976.
32. Singh G, Wilson MR, Foster CS: Mitomycin eye drops as treatment for pterygium. Ophthalmology 95:813, 1988.
33. Singh G, Wilson MR, Foster CS: Long-term follow-up study of mitomycin eye drops as adjunct treatment for pterygium and its comparison with conjunctival autograft transplantation. Cornea 9:331, 1990.

CHAPTER 35

Antimetabolites for Trabeculectomy: 5-Fluorouracil and Mitomycin

Patricia A. Davis-Lemessy and Richard K. Parrish II

Antineoplastic antimetabolites are a group of specifically designed antitumor agents. They have two modes of function. The first is substitution for a component in a necessary cellular chemical compound. This yields a cell product that fails to function and subsequently blocks cell division. The second mode of function is inhibition of a key enzyme function, thus interfering with normal cellular metabolism.

Four groups of drugs are considered antineoplastic antimetabolites: folic acid antagonists, purine antagonists, pyrimidine antagonists, and alkylating agents. Methotrexate belongs to the folic acid antagonist group. Azathioprine, thioguanine, and mercaptopurine are members of the purine antagonist group. Floxuridine, cytosine arabinoside, and 5-fluorouracil (5-FU) comprise the pyrimidine antagonist group. Mitomycin C is a unique alkylating agent. This chapter focuses on 5-FU and mitomycin C because of their popularity for use in glaucoma filtering surgery.

The mechanism of action for each group of antimetabolite differs. Folic acid antagonists prevent the reduction of folic acid to tetrahydrofolic acid by inhibiting production of a native enzyme. Purine and pyrimidine antagonists interfere with nucleic acid biosynthesis. The alkylating agents are metabolized to active species that cross-link DNA and produce membrane-damaging free radicals.[1] In these ways, antimetabolites interrupt protein synthesis and thus prevent cells, including cancer cells, from reproducing and surviving. Antimetabolites destroy healthy as well as diseased cells. Their limited toxicity is attributed to the different rates at which different types of cells grow. Unfortunately, this group of drugs has a narrow therapeutic range of application.

5-Fluorouracil

In 1957, the synthesis of the simplest 5-fluoropyrimidines derivatives, 5-FU and 5-fluoroörotic acid was accomplished.[2] These compounds were designed to function as nucleic acid antagonists, namely for uracil and orotic acid, respectively, based on the observation that uracil is more rapidly used as a precursor of the nucleic acid pyrimidines in rat hepatoma.[3] Indeed, the compounds have displayed activity against bacteria in vitro, and in transplanted tumors in animals and are selectively localized in sarcoma 190 and randomly incorporated into RNA in mouse tissue and human tumor.[4] 5-FO is decarboxylated to 5-FU inside the cell, and then 5-FU is converted into nucleotides of all three levels of phosphorylation, as is true for orotic acid and uracil, respectively.

SYSTEMIC USE AND SIDE EFFECTS

Systemic 5-FU, alone or with other antimetabolites, is administered widely for treatment of carcinomas of the breast and gastrointestinal tract, especially adenocarcinoma of the colon. 5-FU is administered by intravenous infusion in dosages based on the patient's body weight. Side effects from the systemic use of 5-FU are numerous. The more common toxic side effects are on organ systems that normally have a rapid turnover of cells, such as the gastrointestinal tract, bone marrow, and integument, with major effects on the epithelial cells of the gastrointestinal tract and oral mucosa. Hair loss, leukopenia, thrombopenia, stomatitis, diarrhea, and anorexia are manifestations of 5-FU toxicity on susceptible healthy tissues. In addition, neurotoxicity as a result of systemic 5-FU use has been noted in about 1 to 2% of patients.[5–7] This neurotoxicity is believed to be a result of fluoroacetate intoxication.[5]

Oculomotor anomalies, primarily vergence disturbances, have been associated with 5-FU–related neurotoxicity.[8] Patients experience vertigo and blurred vision—symptoms that can easily be interpreted as ocular side effects. One report of excessive lacrimation from systemic 5-FU treatment included blurring of vision as a symptom.[9] Dacryostenosis, or fibrosis of the tear duct and adjacent tissue, has been attributed to 5-FU use.[10] Cicatricial ectropion, conjunctival irritation,[11] and punctal-canalicular stenosis[12] are causes of the observed excessive lacrimation in some patients on 5-FU therapy. Increased 5-FU concentration in the tears of patients with excessive lacrimation has been noted.[13] A recent review of oculotoxicities of systemically administered drug lists 5-FU as one such drug.[14] The possible role of intraocular structures and the issue of melanin binding for drug accumulation that leads to oculotoxicities has been discussed, but no definite conclusions have been reached.

TOPICAL USE AND SIDE EFFECTS

Topical use of 5-FU for carcinomas of the skin includes successful treatment of superficial premalignant keratoses, multiple basal cell carcinomas, late radiation dermatitis, squamous cell carcinomas, and leukoplakia of the mouth and lower female genitourinary tract.[15–19] Early topical 5-FU ointments contained 20% drug, a concentration that resulted in inflammation of the skin and conjunctival irritation.[17] Studies on optimal concentrations revealed that a 5% ointment is most effective but that 2.5% and 1% ointments are ineffective.[18] No reports have been made systemic side effects from topical 5-FU use. Moreover, only 6% of the topically applied 5-FU was absorbed systemically according to one study.[18] Ocular side effects, such as bilateral cicatricial ectropion,[19] were reported after topical application of 5-FU for treatment of facial keratoses.

OCULAR USE AND SIDE EFFECTS

Reports of ocular toxicities associated with systemic and topical uses of 5-FU have not dissuaded attempts to limit intraocular cellular proliferation with drugs such as 5-FU. After reviewing several antimetabolites,[20] fluorouracil was chosen for preliminary investigation as therapy for massive periretinal proliferation.[21] Then, 5-FU was successfully used as pharmacologic therapy for proliferative vitreoretinopathy (PVR).[22–24] No adverse systemic reaction was noted after intravitreal injection. Repeated injections reduced 5-FU toxicity threshold, and minor but irreversible corneal toxicities are associated with ocular use of 5-FU.

In the late 1980s, 5-FU emerged as an important drug for management of glaucoma filtration surgery in eyes that had poor prognoses.[25–32] Failure of filtering surgery is a major complication in the treatment of glaucoma. It usually results from postoperative trauma or excessive scarring that leads to closure of the filtering bleb. In animal models of glaucoma filtering surgery, proliferating fibroblasts close the wound in 14 days.[26] Postoperative subconjunctival injections of 5-FU inhibit the proliferation of fibroblasts and prevent scarring.[27–32] The toxicities observed were transient corneal filaments and mild corneal subepithelial opacification.[23, 31–32]

CHEMICAL PROPERTIES

The chemical properties of 5-FU are well documented.[33] 5-FU has a molecular weight of 130.08 (Fig. 35–1). A fluorine atom replaces the fifth carbon hydrogen in the uracil molecule. The solid form is an off-white crystalline material that is odorless. Reported physical properties of 5-FU include infrared spectrum, nuclear magnetic resonance spectrum, and ultraviolet spectrum. Other methods used to characterized 5-FU are differential scanning calorimetry and solubility in different solvents.

Hydrophilic 5-FU has poor solubility in common hydrophobic organic solvents but is sparingly soluble in water, methanol, and ethanol. 5-FU is stable in nonbasic solutions at pH below 9.00. Above pH 9.00, 5-FU hydrolyzes to urea, fluoride, and an aldehyde. Urea can further hydrolyze to ammonia and carbon dioxide. Of the physical properties mentioned previously, the ultraviolet spectral peak at 266

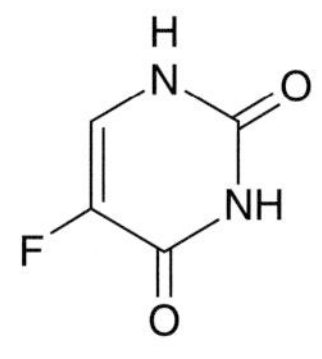

FIGURE 35–1. Structural formula of 5-fluorouracil.

nm is the most prevalent method used to assay for 5-FU in both in vitro and in vivo studies.[34, 35]

MECHANISM OF ACTION

Clues to the mechanism of action of 5-FU were available from early studies of the radiolabeled drug.[4] Figure 35–2 is a schematic of the mechanisms of 5-FU that have been verified during the past three decades.[3, 4, 36–44] 5-FU has two modes of action. The first mode entails enzyme inhibition. Before the activity of the drug is exerted, 5-FU is converted into 5′-fluoro-2′-deoxyuridine monophosphate (FdUMP) by 5′-fluoro-2′-deoxyuridine (FUdR). FdUMP is a potent inhibitor of the enzyme, thymidylate synthetase, which catalyzes the methylation of deoxyuridine monophosphate to thymine 5′-monophosphate. The FdUMP–thymidylate synthetase complex, $N^{5,10}$-methylene tetrahydrofolate, has been isolated[39–40] (see central portion of Fig. 35–2). Because thymine is one of the nucleotide bases found in DNA, the lack of thymine leads to imbalanced DNA growth, and finally cell death. Early rescue or reversal of the effect of 5-FU with thymine is possible.

The second mode of action is incorporation of 5-FU into RNA in place of uracil to make FU-RNA (see right portion of Fig. 35–2) after 5-FU is converted to the fluorouridine monophosphates, diphosphates, and triphosphates. FU-RNA synthesis occurs more readily in the nucleus than in the cytoplasm of the cell.[38] Accumulation of FU-sRNA retards ribosomal RNA synthesis[41] and makes the ribosomes more sensitive to enzymatic degradation. FU-rRNA prevents normal ribosomal maturation. Finally, FU-tRNA blocks the transfer of amino acids in protein synthesis.[42] Many of these proteins are necessary cellular enzymes.

PHARMACOKINETICS, ABSORPTION, FATE, AND EXCRETION

Pharmacokinetics studies of 5-FU have shown that it has a strong first-pass effect and exhibits nonlinear pharmacokinetics. Because 5-FU must be given to the point of toxicity for effectiveness against solid tumors, a narrow therapeutic index exists. The route of choice for administration is intravenous injection. The only formulation used is solution. Oral,[45–48] intramuscular,[49] and intraperitoneal[49] administration are associated with erratic drug absorption. For example, bolus intravenous administration yields plasma concentrations with half-lives ranging from 10 to 60 minutes,[34, 45–54] with peak levels appearing 7.5 to 30 minutes after injection and after 2 to 24 hours. Other administration routes have variable absorption rates and half-lives ranging from 30 minutes to 4 hours.

Systemically administered 5-FU is preferentially compartmentalized in tumors and intestinal mucosa.[4, 55] Rapid penetration of 5-FU into the brain,[7, 56] spinal fluid,[49] and eyes[57–60] occurs by simple diffusion. Metabolic degradation of 5-FU takes place in most normal tissue except the spleen and primarily in the liver.[49, 61, 62] The first step is conversion of 5-FU to dihydrofluorouracil. Then, conversion to α-fluoro-β-ureidopropionic acid (FUPA) and α-fluoro-β-guanidopropionic acid (FGPA) follows, as shown in Figure 35–3.[62] These conversions, excluding FGPA, are analogous to the degradation of uracil. Both FUPA and FGPA are further cleaved to urea, CO_2, and α-fluoro-β-analine (FBAL). Degradation products are nontoxic and are found in the liver, kidney, and intestines. 5-FU metabolism to FUdR (see Fig. 35–2) and catabolism to FDHU are responsible for its strong first-pass effect.

The degradation products of 5-FU account for up to 95% of urine radioactivity, according to one study.[55] Expired CO_2 is another major route of elimination of 5-FU. Minor routes may include tears because high tear concentration of 5-FU was found in patients displaying ocular toxicities to systemic 5-FU use.[13]

Mitomycin C

Mitomycin C was first isolated from the broth of *Streptomyces caespitosus* in 1958. A naturally occurring antibiotic antimetabolite, mitomycin C was initially found, in the late 1960s, to have clinical activity in a range of solid tumors in humans. Mitomycin C is an alkylating agent that is metabolized to active species that cross-link DNA and inhibit RNA and protein synthesis.[63–65] Mitomycin C is relatively phase specific for late G1 and early S phases of the cell cycle. It

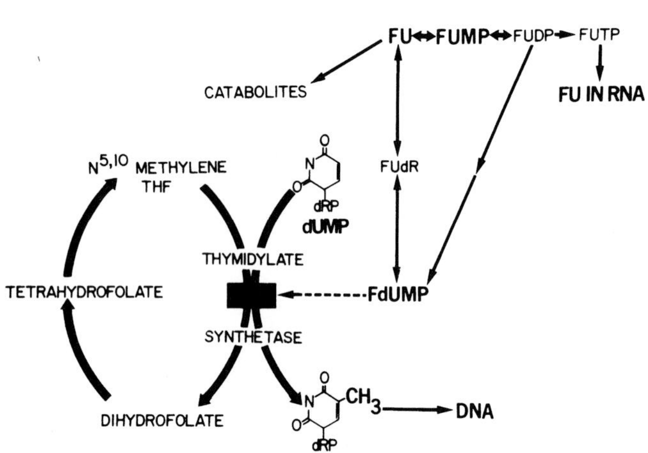

FIGURE 35–2. Mechanism of 5-fluorouracil (5-FU) action on the cell. At center, 5-FU is converted into FUdR, then to FdUMP, which blocks the action of thymidylate synthetase. This enzyme converts dUMP into dTMP—a necessary DNA nucleotide. Enzyme inhibition occurs by complexation of dUMP and thymidylate synthetase to form $N^{5,10}$ methylene tetrahydrofolate (*left* of figure). At right, 5-FU is converted to FUMP, FUDP, and FUTP, then becomes incorporated into RNA. FU, 5-fluorouracil; FUMP, fluorouridine monophosphate; FUDP, fluoroaridine diphosphate; FUTP, fluorouridine triphosphate; FUdR, 5′-fluoro-2′-deoxyuridine; FdUMP, 2′-deoxyuridine monophosphate; dTMP, thymine 5′-monophosphate; THF, tetrahydrofolate.

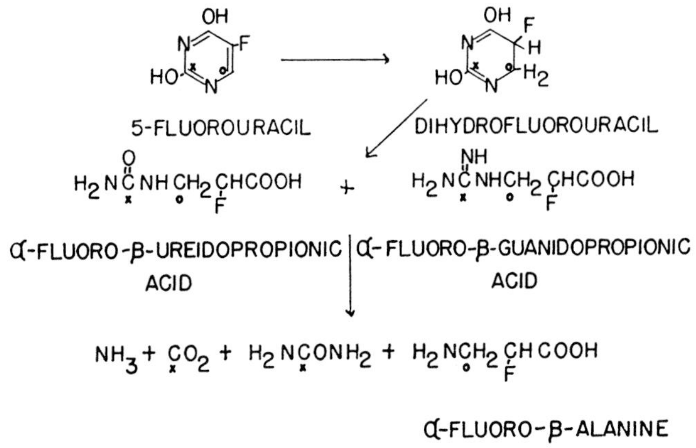

FIGURE 35–3. Metabolic degradation of 5-fluorouracil (5-FU). Conversion of 5-FU to dihydrofluorouracil (FDHU) is followed by conversion of FDHU to α-fluoro-β-ureidopropionic acid (FUPA) and α-fluoro-β-guanidopropionic acid (FGPA). Both FUPA and FGPA are further cleaved to urea, CO_2, and α-fluoro-β-analine (FBAL).

was found to be effective in breast, stomach, colorectal, head, neck, and pancreatic carcinomas.[65] Delayed, cumulative bone marrow depression is the severe toxicity observed with mitomycin C usage. Therefore, it is used for patients who have not responded to other treatments.[64–66]

SYSTEMIC USE AND SIDE EFFECTS

Mitomycin C is an antibiotic antineoplastic with activity against gram-positive bacteria. Cytotoxicity relates to cross-linking of DNA and inhibition of DNA synthesis. Mitomycin C also inhibits RNA and protein synthesis.[1] It has activity against carcinomas of the stomach, pancreas, colon, rectum, breast, lung, head, and neck as well as chronic myelogenous leukemia.[66] Intravenous use of mitomycin C is mutagenic, and myelosuppression has been reported. Myelosuppression resulted in leukopenia and thrombocytopenia.[65] Dose-related renal failure has been reported. Mitomycin C is teratogenic and carcinogenic in rodents.

OCULAR USE AND SIDE EFFECTS

Drops of a dilute solution of mitomycin C have been used in patients after pterygium surgery[67–69] to prevent recurrence. Drops of dilute solution of mitomycin C in concentrations ranging from 0.2 to 0.4 mg/mL were placed on the cornea daily for 1 to 3 weeks after pterygium surgery.[67–69] Pterygium excision with low concentration of mitomycin C resulted in less conjuctival scarring. Complications reported after topical use of mitomycin C in pterygium surgery include scleral ulceration and calcification, iridocyclitis, and secondary glaucoma.[69–71] Although mitomycin C is mutagenic and myelosuppressive with intravenous use, ocular surface neoplasia at the site of application has not been reported, nor has myelosuppression been associated with this drug's use as an adjunct to ocular surgery.[69]

CHEMICAL PROPERTIES

Mitomycin C forms blue-violet crystals that do not melt at temperatures below 360°C. The molecular weight is 334. It has a quinone group and mitosine ring as part of its chemical structure (Fig. 35–4). It has absorption maximums at 216, 360, and 560 nm in the ultraviolet-visible spectrum. Mitomycin C is highly soluble in methanol, acetone, butyl acetone, and cyclohexane and slightly soluble in benzene, carbon tetrachloride, and ether.[66] As with 5-FU, other methods used to characterized mitomycin C include differential scanning calorimetry and solubility in different solvents.

MECHANISM OF ACTION

Mitomycin C is metabolized to active agents that cross-link DNA and produce membrane-damaging free radicals. Before either of these metabolizing processes occurs, mitomycin C is enzymatically reduced by nicotinamide-adenine dinucleotide hydrogen phosphate (NADPH, Fig. 35–5). The mechanism involves an enzyme-mediated reduction to a mitomycin C radical or hydroquinone. Subsequently, mitomycin C becomes susceptible to nucleophilic attack by DNA bases. Several mitomycin C metabolites are created by nucleophilic attack of water or inorganic phosphorus.[64, 72]

Some controversy remains regarding the contributions of oxygen free radicals to the drug's toxicity and antitumor activity. Mitomycin C has been shown to generate superoxide, hydrogen peroxide, and hydroxyl free radical in isolated metabolic systems in vitro.[64, 72] These findings suggest that mitomycin C may produce toxic oxygen free radical in vivo. Damage to the unsaturated lipids of membranes is a consequence of significant oxygen free radical formation in vivo. Uncommon human pulmonary toxicity of mitomycin C has been noted; however, the etiology remains unclear.

The resistance of certain tumor cells to alkylating agents such as mitomycin C appears to correlate with enhanced DNA repair involving cross-link removal. Resistance develops after exposure to the drug. Human colon cancer cells that developed resistance to mitomycin C were not resistant to a number of other anticancer agents, such as deoxorubicin.[1]

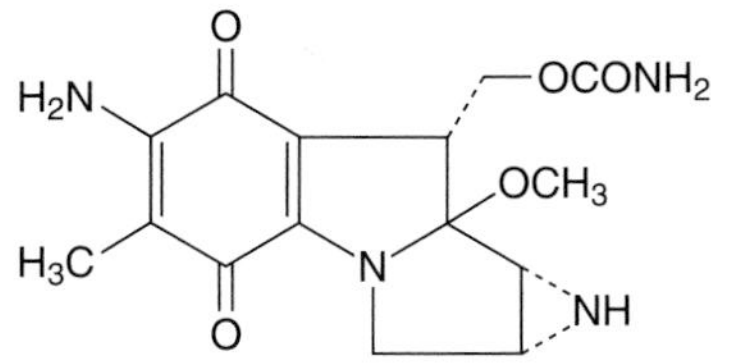

FIGURE 35–4. Chemical structure of mitomycin C.

MITOMYCIN C

NADPH ENZYME

H^+ O_2

$-CH_3OH$

$+ HO_2^{\bullet}$

$OH^{\bullet}$

DNA DEGRADATION

$-OCNH_2$

DNA CROSSLINKING

FIGURE 35–5. Mechanism of mitomycin C action on the cell. At top center, mitomycin C is enzymatically reduced using NADPH into a chemical species that undergoes further reaction. As shown on the right portion of the figure, the chemical species loses a methanol group (CH_3OH) and simultaneously reacts with DNA. Next, the new species loses an amide group ($OOCNH_2$) to effectuate DNA crosslinking. On the left portion of the figure, MMC reacts with hydrogen proton and oxygen to generate toxic oxygen free radicals, superoxide, and hydroxy radicals.

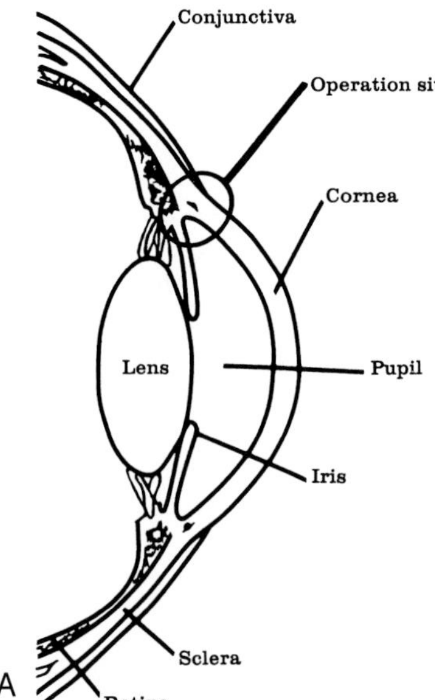

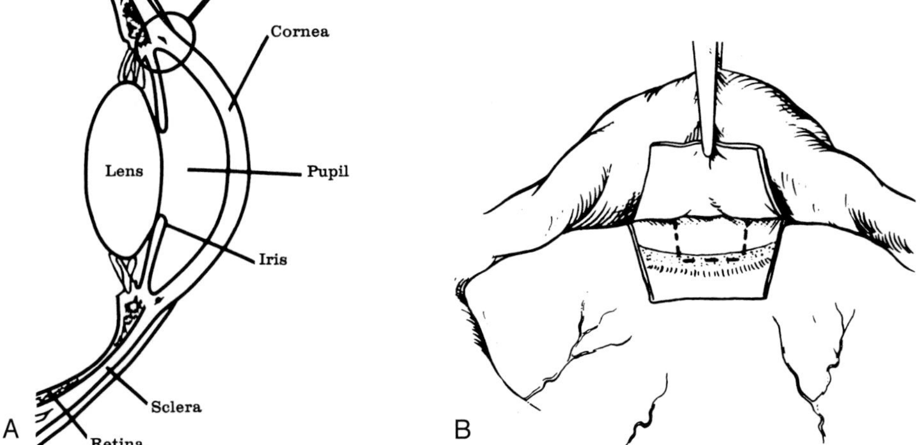

FIGURE 35–6. Surgical site for trabeculectomy *(A)* and nature of incision *(B)*. The incision shown on the right is made at the circled area labeled operation site.

PHARMACOKINETICS, ABSORPTION, FATE, AND EXCRETION

Mitomycin C is rapidly cleared from plasma by first-order elimination process. Plasma half-lives range from 30 to 70 minutes. The principle pathway is nonrenal and is most likely hepatic. No mitomycin C metabolites have been detected in plasma. Moreover, the absence of mitomycin C metabolites in plasma also suggests that the parent compound mediates cytotoxic activities. Mitomycin C metabolism is still not well understood, and future studies are needed to correlate plasma pharmacokinetics to response and toxicity.[1]

Ophthalmic Indications for 5-Fluorouracil and Mitomycin C

Proliferative vitreoretinopathy accounts for most of the surgical failures in the treatment of rhegmatogenous retinal detachment.[23] 5-FU has been successfully used in animals and humans to control massive periretinal cell proliferation.[23, 24] Dosages of up to 1.25[24] to 2.5 mg[23] were found to be safe for intraocular administration in humans.

Filtering surgery is performed to reduce intraocular pressure. This is accomplished by the creation of a small fistula through the sclera by means of which fluid flows from the eye. A bleb is produced that allows fluid outflow through either a transconjunctival route, a perivascular route, or a direct new recanalization.[73] Figure 35–6 gives an indication of the operation site and the bleb.[74]

When exaggerated wound healing by means of proliferating fibroblasts closes the bleb, filtering is prevented, and intraocular pressure rises. The successful use of 5-FU for PVR led to its investigation as an antiproliferative agent for use in glaucoma filtering surgery. Success with the owl monkey[27] was followed by human clinical trials.[28–30] The corticosteroids[75] class of drugs has also been used, with some success, in managing difficult trabeculectomies by maintaining a functional filtering bleb.

5-FLUOROURACIL

The ocular pharmacology of 5-FU parallels its systemic pharmacology. Animal studies indicate fibroblastic antiproliferative vitreous and aqueous levels of 5-FU after intravitreal[76] and subconjunctival[59, 60] injections as well as after topical administration.[57, 58] Moreover, significant plasma levels were attained after intravitreal injections.[76] High aqueous and tear levels were measured 1 hour after subconjunctival injection.[60] Corneal levels were greatest near the subconjunctival injection site, and transcorneal passage is the major route of ocular penetration after subconjunctival administration. A reservoir of the drug remains in the subconjunctival site and slowly releases into the tear film layer, from which it is absorbed through the cornea.[60] Another study determined peak serum levels of 5-FU 30 minutes after subconjunctival administration and documented the rapid distribution to the vitreous and aqueous chambers of the eye.[59] Topical ocular 5-FU application achieves sufficient therapeutic levels in one-half hour; however, the corneal levels are high, and corneal epithelial complications ensue.[57, 58] Ophthalmic excretion of 5-FU is through tears and the retrobulbar vascular network into serum.[59]

The optimal route of ocular 5-FU administration has been clarified. A report on 5-FU treatment of PVR acknowledged that the subconjunctival route of drug injection was preferred to the intravitreal route because gas bubbles developed after repeated intravitreal injections.[23] Although topical applications of 5-FU achieved aqueous and vitreous concentrations that inhibit fibroblast proliferation, corneal toxicities[31, 32] led investigators to select subconjunctival injections for 5-FU delivery to the area of the filtering bleb. Subconjunctivally administered 5-FU penetrates the sclera, cornea, and choroid and enters the eye.[59, 60] Risks of subconjunctivally administered 5-FU include hemorrhage, scarring, ocular penetration, and infection. Each repeated injection escalates the risks. However, subconjunctival injection remains the most predictable administration route until alternative methods such as site-implantable or injectable controlled release devices are developed.

In theory, a controlled-release device implanted at the time of surgery has many advantages. The maximal drug concentration, localized at the site of interest, could minimize the corneal toxicities associated with ocular 5-FU use. Repeated subconjunctival injections could be avoided and risk of ocular perforation eliminated. The controlled release of 5-FU for systemic chemotherapy is being investigated. Polymers have been used as nonactive matrices for drugs, including 5-FU. However, the concept of chemotherapeutic polymers—polymers containing drugs as parts of the backbone, pendant groups, or terminal groups on polymeric chains—is a recent biomedical application of polymers. Ouchi and colleagues[77] reported on the covalent attachment of 5-FU to poly(malic acid) and poly(α-malic acid–co-lactic acid) through amide, ester, and carbamoyl bonds.

In parallel to the development of polymeric drugs, current research has focused on the development of biodegradable ocular implants designed to release 5-FU slowly. Development of the ideal polymer and the most effective physical form, such as microencapsulated spheres[78, 79] or bioerodible[80–82] and nonerodible[82–84] monolithic matrices, is being investigated. At least one 5-FU liposomal ocular delivery system has been developed.[79] Lee and colleagues[81] published results on a bioerodible polyanhydride copolymer matrix for 5-FU release after glaucoma filtering surgery. The polyanhydride copolymer was composed of bis(p-carboxyphenoxy) hexane and sebacic acid. Concurrently, polyvinyl alcohol[83] and ethylene acetate copolymer[84] have been investigated as nonerodible ocular sustained-release systems. Charles and associates[85] obtained 200-hour release of mitomycin from polyanhdride P(CPP-SA) 25:75.

MITOMYCIN C

Unlike 5-FU, mitomycin C was used as early as 1962 as an adjunct to modify wound healing and fibrous tissue proliferation after pterygium surgery.[67–71] Limited research on the use of mitomycin C for PVR treatment has been performed. Two benefits of mitomycin use over 5-FU in glaucoma filtering surgery have been reported. The first is that only one application of mitomycin C is needed during surgery to inhibit fibroblast growth effectively and improve the surgical outcome. As initially described, a small sponge is soaked in 0.3 mL of the 0.2 mg/mL mitomycin C solution.[86] The cellulose sponge is placed under the flap (see Fig. 35–6) of the eye for 30 seconds to 5 minutes. Finally, the area is irrigated with balanced salt solution.[86–88]

With the intraoperative approach, the patient is much less inconvenienced than with multiple follow-up subconjunctival injections for the first 2 weeks after surgery. The second perceived benefit of mitomycin C is that the concentration needed to effect a good surgical outcome is much less than the concentration of 5-FU that is injected. One study followed the concentration of mitomycin C after a single subconjunctival injection in a rabbit.[89] Rapid disappearance of mitomycin C from the injected and adjacent tissues as well as the anterior chamber was noted, suggesting that its ocular half-life is similar to the serum half-life. The reported half-life in the conjunctiva, sclera, and aqueous humor ranged from 11 to 45 minutes. Similarly, reported 5-FU half-lives in the conjunctiva and sclera after a single subconjunctival injection were 23 and 26 minutes, respectively.

Other Ophthalmic Drugs for Trabeculectomy

Antineoplastics and corticosteroids have shown promise as pharmacologic agents for the alteration of wound healing after glaucoma filtering surgery in eyes with poor surgical prognoses. Triamcinolone, a corticosteroid that retards fibroblast proliferation by preventing cellular mobility, has historically been used as an antiinflammatory agent.[90] Triamcinolone exerts a bimodal effect. At low doses, it promotes fibroblast proliferation, but it inhibits proliferation at high doses.[20] The structures of triamcinolone and other drugs to be discussed in this section are shown in Figure 35–7. Daunomycin is an anthracycline glycoside antibiotic that belongs to the antineoplastic class of drugs. It inhibits DNA synthesis, DNA-dependent RNA synthesis, and polymerase activity.[90] Daunomycin is used with other antineoplastics for remission induction in leukemia patients. Cytosine arabinoside, like 5-FU, is a synthetic pyrimidine nucleoside that is converted intracellularly to the nucleotide cytarabine triphosphate. This complex inhibits DNA polymerase by competing with deoxycytidine triphosphate. As is the case with daunomycin, cytosine arabinoside is a component in chemotherapeutic regimens for leukemia remission induction.[90]

These drugs were investigated in terms of their abilities to inhibit fibroblast and epithelial cell proliferation in vitro, ocular therapeutic index, and in vivo posttrabeculectomy intraocular pressure management (Tables 35–1 through 35–3). The large differences in the reported ID_{50} levels could be explained by the use of different cells that were cultured. Therapeutic indices vary greatly from drug to drug, a likely result of different mechanisms of action; however, the large differences among groups for the same drug remain unexplained.

An indication of the ocular dosages and formulations that have been published for anti–fibroblast proliferation agents appears in Table 35–3. The formulations for effective inhibition of cell proliferation are in the microgram to milligram range. An excellent review of the pharmacologic management of trabeculectomy discusses the mechanisms of wound healing and the role that each antiproliferative agent plays in inhibiting the process.[111]

Subconjunctivally administered 5-FU can produce transiently decreased visual acuity and ocular discomfort as a result of corneal and conjunctival toxicity.[110] Mitomycin C use has been associated with the development of thin aeschemic blebs and epithelial surface breakdown with increased risk of infection.[112] The exact risk-to-benefit ratio of each treatment for controlling intraocular pressure remains to be determined.

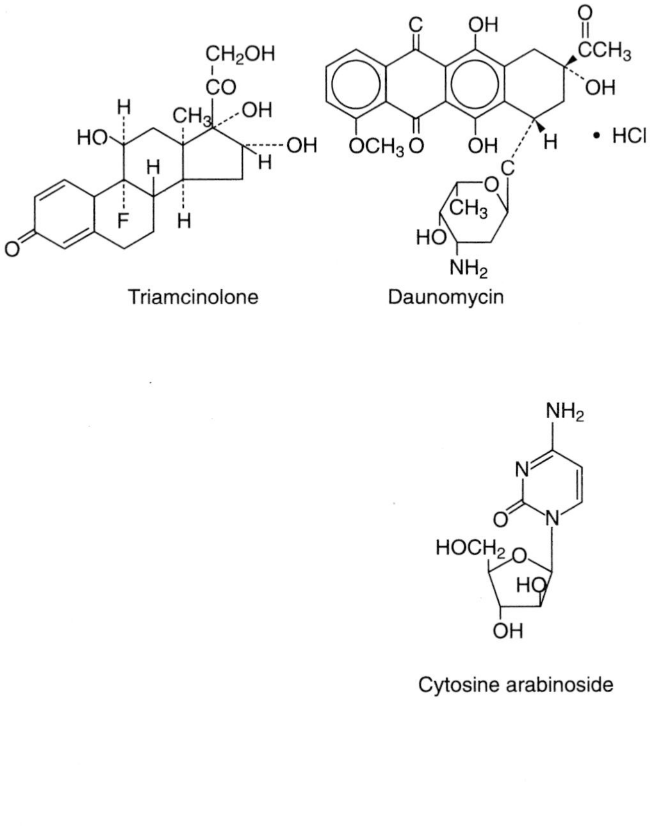

FIGURE 35–7. Chemical structures of the drugs used in posttrabeculectomy intraocular pressure management. Triamcinolone is a corticosteroid. Daunomycin and cytosine arabinoside are antineoplastics used in chemotherapy.

TABLE 35–1. **Toxicity Profiles of Mitomycin C and Daunomycin**

Drug	Cell Type	Source	ID_{50}* (mg/L)	Dose Applied (mg/mL)	Reference
Mitomycin C					
	Fibroblast	Cultured human tenon capsule			91
	Fibroblast	Cultured rabbit subconjunctiva	2×10^{-3}		92
	Corneal epithelium	Rabbit cornea organ preparation	6×10^{2}		63
	Fibroblast	Human subconjunctiva	1×10^{-1}		93
	Fibroblast	Rabbit tenon capsule posterior lip		0.5	94
	Fibroblast	Rabbit tenon capsule sclerotomy		0.2	95
	Fibroblast	Human tenon capsule-trabeculectomy		0.2	96
	Fibroblast	Cynomologus monkey tenon capsule		0.3–0.5	97
	Fibroblast	Human tenon capsule-trabeculectomy		0.5	65
	Fibroblast	Cultured human tenon capsule			98
	Fibroblast	Rabbit subconjunctiva posterior lip sclerectomy		0.4	99
	Corneal endothelium	Human donor buttons		0.2–0.5	100
	Ciliary body endothelium	Cynomologus monkey-whole		0.5	101
Daunomycin					
	Fibroblast	Rabbit dermis			102
	Epithelial cells	Rabbit lens	1×10^{-4}		103

*ID_{50} is the median effective dose required for 50% proliferation inhibition compared with control.

TABLE 35–2. **Toxicity Profiles of Triamcinolone, Cytosine Arabinoside, and 5-Fluorouracil***

Drug	Cell Type	Source	ID_{50}† (mg/L)	Reference
Triamcinolone (bimodal)				
	Fibroblast	Rabbit dermis	1.5×10^{3}	20
	Fibroblast	Rabbit conjunctiva	1.5×10^{3}	20
Arabinoside C				
	Fibroblast	Human conjunctiva	8×10^{-4}	104
	Epithelial	Rabbit lens	1×10^{2}	103
	Epithelial	Rabbit cornea	3×10^{1}	105
	Fibroblast	Rabbit conjunctiva	5×10^{1}	105
5-Fluorouracil				
	Fibroblast	Human subconjunctiva	2.5×10^{1}	104
	Fibroblast	Rabbit dermis	3×10^{-1}	20
	Fibroblast	Rabbit conjunctiva	2×10^{-1}	20
	Epithelial cells	Rabbit lens	3×10^{1}	103
	Epithelial cells	Rabbit cornea	6×10^{-1}	105
	Fibroblast	Rabbit conjunctiva	3×10^{-1}	105
	Fibroblasts	Cultured rabbit subconjunctiva	6×10^{-1}	92
	Fibroblasts	Cultured human tenon capsule		98
	Fibroblasts	Rabbit subconjunctival	4×10^{2}	99

*Little agreement can be found among researchers on ID_{50}, especially for 5-fluorouracil.
†ID_{50} is the median effective dose required for 50% proliferation inhibition compared with controls.

TABLE 35–3. **Ocular *in Vivo* Usage Profiles of the Drugs Used for Glaucoma Filtering Surgery***

Drug	Administration Route	Concentration (mg/mL	Single Dose (mg)	Reference
Mitomycin C	Subconjunctival: 5-minute soak (humans)	0.1, 0.2, 0.4	—	86
	Subconjunctival: 5 minute soak (humans)	0.2	—	87, 96, 106
	Subconjunctival: 2-minute soak (humans)	0.2	—	86, 107
	Subconjunctival: injection (rabbit)	0.2	—	108
Triamcinolone	Subconjunctival: injection 1 week before surgery (humans)	40	4	109
5-Fluorouracil	Subconjunctival: injection (humans)	10	3	28–30, 110
	Topical: (owl monkey)	2.4 mg/drop	7.2	58

*Subconjunctival injection is the most popular route of administration for 5-fluorouracil, whereas a 5-minute soak followed by irrigation is the method of choice for mitomycin C.

REFERENCES

1. Dorr RT: New findings in the pharmacokinetic, metabolic and drug-resistance aspects of mitomycin C. Semin Oncol 15(3–4):32, 1988.
2. Duschinsky R, Pleven E, Heidelberger C: The synthesis of 5-fluoropyrimidines. J Am Chem Soc 79:4559, 1957.
3. Heidelberger C: On the rational development of a new drug: The example of the fluorinated pyrimidines. Cancer Treat Rep 65:3, 1981.
4. Chaudhuri NK, Montag BJ, Heidelberger C: Studies of fluorinated pyrimidines. III: The metabolism of 5-fluorouracil-2-C^{14} and 5-fluorobrotic-2-C^{14} acid *in vivo*. Cancer Res 18:318, 1958.
5. Koenig H, Patel A: The acute cerebellar syndrome in 5-fluorouracil chemotherapy: A manifestation of fluoroacetate intoxication. Neurology 20:416, 1970.
6. Greenwald ES: Organic mental changes with fluorouracil therapy. JAMA 235:248, 1976.
7. Bourke RS, West CR, Chheda G, et al: Kinetics of entry and distribution of 5-fluorouracil in cerebrospinal fluid and brain following intravenous injection in a primate. Cancer Res 33:1735, 1973.
8. Bixenman WW, Nicholls JVV, Warwick OH: Oculomotor disturbances associated with 5-fluorouracil chemotherapy. Am J Ophthalmol 83:789, 1977.
9. Hamersley J, Luce JK, Florentz TR, et al: Excessive lacrimation from fluorouracil treatment. JAMA 225:747, 1973.
10. Haidak DJ, Hurwitz BS, Yeung KY: Tear duct fibrosis (dacryostenosis) due to 5-fluorouracil. Ann Intern Med 88:657, 1978.
11. Straus DJ, Mausoff FA, Ellerby RA, et al: Cicatricial ectropion secondary to 5-fluorouracil therapy. Med Pediatr Oncol 3:15, 1977.
12. Caravella LP, Burns JA, Zangrneister M: Punctal-canalicular stenosis related to systemic fluorouracil therapy. Arch Ophthalmol 99:284, 1981.
13. Christophidis N, Lucas I, Vajda FJE, et al: Lacrimation and 5-fluorouracil. Ann Intern Med 89:574, 1978.
14. Koneru PB, Lien EJ, Koda RT: Oculotoxicities of systemically administered drugs [Review]. J Ocul Pharmacol Ther 2:385, 1986.
15. Williams AC, Klein E: Experiences with local chemotherapy and immunotherapy in premalignant and malignant skin lesions. Cancer 25:450, 1970.
16. Kirwan P, Naftalin NJ: Topical 5-fluorouracil in the treatment of vaginal intraepithelial neoplasma. Br J Obstet Gynecol 92:287, 1985.
17. Dillaha CJ, Jansen UT, Honeycutt WM, et al: Further studies with topical 5-fluorouracil. Arch Dermatol 92:410, 1965.
18. Dillaha CJ, Jansen UT, Honeycutt WM, et al: Selective cytotoxic effect of topical 5-fluorouracil. Arch Dermatol 88:247, 1963.
19. Galentine P, Sloas H, Hargett N, et al: Bilateral cicatricial ectropion following topical administration of 5-fluorouracil. Ann Ophthalmol 13:575, 1981.
20. Blumenkranz MS, Claflin A, Hajek AS: Selection of therapeutic agents for intraocular proliferative disease: Cell culture evaluation. Arch Ophthalmol 102:598, 1984.
21. Blumenkranz MS, Avinoam O, Claflin AJ, et al: Fluorouracil for the treatment of massive periretinal proliferation. Am J Ophthalmol 94:458, 1982.
22. Stern WH, Lewis GP, Erickson PA, et al: Fluorouracil therapy for proliferative vitroretinopathy after vitrectomy. Am J Ophthalmol 96:33, 1983.
23. Blumenkranz MS, Hernandez E, Avinoam O, et al: 5-Fluorouracil: New applications in complicated retinal detachment for an established antimetabolilte. Ophthalmology 91:122, 1984.
24. Stern WH, Guerin CJ, Erickson PA, et al: Ocular toxicity of fluorouracil after vitrectomy. Am J Ophthalmol 96:43, 1983.
25. Heuer DK: Glaucoma update. Ophthalmology 95:282, 1988.
26. Desjardins DC, Parrish II RK, Folberg R, et al: Wound healing after filtering surgery in owl monkeys. Arch Ophthalmol 104:1835, 1986.
27. Gressel MG, Parrish II RK, Folberg R: 5-Fluorouracil and glaucoma filtering surgery. I: An animal model. Ophthalmology 91:378, 1984.
28. Heuer DK, Parrish II RK, Gressel MG, et al: 5-Fluorouracil and glaucoma filtering surgery. II: A pilot study. Ophthalmology 91:384, 1984.
29. Heuer DK, Parrish II RK, Gressel MG, et al: 5-Fluorouracil and glaucoma filtering surgery. III: Intermediate follow-up of a pilot study. Ophthalmology 93:1537, 1986.
30. Rockwood U, Parrish II RK, Heuer DK, et al: Glaucoma filtering surgery with 5-fluorouracil. Ophthalmology 94:1071, 1987.
31. Phelan MJ, Skuta GL: Reversible corneal keratinization following trabeculectomy and treatment with 5-fluorouracil. Ophthalmic Surg 21:296, 1990.
32. Shapiro MS, Thoft RA, Friend J, et al: 5-Fluorouracil toxicity to the ocular surface epithelium. Invest Ophthalmol Vis Sci 26:580, 1985.
33. Rudy BC, Senkowski BZ: Fluorouracil. *In* Florey K (ed): Analytical Profiles of Drug Substances, vol 2. New York, Academic Press, 1973.
34. Schaaf LJ, Ferry DG, Hung CT, et al: Analysis of 5′-deoxy-5-fluorouridine and 5-fluorouracil in human plasma and urine by high performance liquid chromatography. J Chromatogr 342:303, 1985.
35. Christophidis N, Mihaly G, Vajda F, et al: Comparison of liquid *and* gas-liquid chromatographic assays of 5-fluorouracil in plasma. Clin Chem 25:83, 1979.
36. Heidelberger C: Pyrimidine and pyrimidine nucleoside antimetabolites. *In* Holland JF, Frei III E (eds): Cancer Medicine, 2nd ed. Philadelphia, Lea & Febiger, 1982.
37. Heidelberger C: Fluorinated pyrimidines. Prog Nucleic Acid Res Mol Biol 4:1, 1965.
38. Mandel HG: Basic aspects of gynecologic cancer chemotherapy. *In* McGowan L (ed): Gynecologic Oncology. New York, Appleton-Century-Crofts, 1978.
39. Reyes P, Heidelberger C: Fluorinated pyrimidines. XXVI. Mammalian thymidylate synthetase: Its mechanism of action and inhibition by fluorinated nucleotides. Mol Pharmacol 1:14, 1965.
40. Danenberg PV, Langenbach RJ, Heidelberger C: Structures of reversible and irreversible complexes of thymidylate synthetase and fluorinated pyrimidine nucleotides. Biochemistry 13:926, 1974.
41. Wilkinson DS, Tlsty TD, Hanas RJ: The inhibition of ribosomal RNA synthesis and maturation in Novikoff hepatoma cells by 5-fluorouridine. Cancer Res 35:3014, 1975.
42. Mandel HG: The incorporation of 5-fluorouracil into RNA and its molecular consequences. Prog Mol Subcell Biol 1:82, 1969.
43. Wolberg WH: The effect of 5-fluorouracil on DNA-thymine synthesis in human tumors. Cancer Res 29:2137, 1969.
44. Mandel HG: The target cell determinants of the antitumor agent actions of 5-FU: Does PU incorporation into RNA play a role? Cancer Treat Rep 65:63, 1981.
45. Nadler SH: Oral administration of fluorouracil: A preliminary trial. Arch Surg 97:654, 1968.
46. Bruckner HW, Creasey WA: The administration of 5-fluorouracil by mouth. Cancer 33:14, 1974.
47. Clarkson B, O'Connor A, Winston L, et al: The physiologic disposition of 5-fluorouracil and 5-fluoro-2′-deoxyuridine in man. Clin Pharmacol Ther 5:581, 1964.
48. Cohen JL, Irwin LE, Marshall GJ, et al: Clinical pharmacology of oral and intravenous 5-fluorouracil (NSC-19893). Cancer Chemother Rep 58:723, 1974.
49. Mukherjee KL, Boohar J, Wentland D, et al: Studies on fluorinated pyrimidines, XVI: Metabolism of 5-fluorouracil-2-C^{14} and 5-fluoro-2′-deoxyuridine-2-C^{14} in cancer patients. Cancer Res 23:49, 1963.
50. Cohen JL, Brennan PB: GLC assay for 5-fluorouracil in biological fluids. J Pharm Sci 62:572, 1973.
51. Finn C, Sadee W: Determination of 5-fluorouracil (NSC-19893) plasma levels in rats and man by isotope dilution-mass fragmentography. Cancer Chemother Rep 59:279, 1975.
52. MacMillan WE, Wolberg WH, Welling PG: Pharmacokinetics of fluorouracil in humans. Cancer Res 38:3479, 1978.
53. De Leenheer AP, Cosyns-Duyck MCL: Flame-ionization GLC assay for fluorouracil in plasma of cancer patients. J Pharm Sci 68:1174, 1979.
54. Cano JP, Aubert C, Rigault JP, et al: Advantages and limitations of pharmacokinetic studies in the rationalization of anticancer therapy: Methotrexate and 5-FU. Cancer Treat Rep 65:33, 1981.
55. Mukherjee KL, Curreri AR, Javid M, et al: Studies on fluorinated pyrimidines. XVII: Tissue distribution of 5-fluorouracil-2-C^{14} and 5-fluoro-2′-deoxyuridine in cancer patients. Cancer Res 23:67, 1963.
56. Levin VA, Chadwick M: Distribution of 5-fluorouracil-2-^{14}C and its metabolites in a murine glioma. JNCI 49:1577, 1972.
57. Fantes FE, Heuer DK, Parrish II RK, et al: Topical fluorouracil: Pharmacokinetics in normal rabbit eyes. Arch Ophthalmol 103:953, 1985.
58. Heuer DK, Gressel MG, Parrish II RK, et al: Topical fluorouracil. II: Postoperative administration in an animal model of glaucoma filtering surgery. Arch Ophthalmol 104:132, 1986.
59. Rootman J, Tisdall J, Gudauskas G, et al: Intraocular penetration of subconjunctivally administered ^{14}C-fluorouracil in rabbits. Arch Ophthalmol 97:2375, 1979.

60. Fantes FE, Parrish II RK, Heuer GK, et al: Subconjunctival 5-fluorouracil mechanisms of ocular penetration. Ophthalmic Surg 18:375, 1987.
61. Chaudhuri NK, Mukherjee KL, Heidelberger C: Studies on fluorinated pyrimidines, VII: The degradative pathway. Biochem Pharmacol 1:328, 1958.
62. Mukherjee KL, Heidelberger C: Studies on fluorinated pyrimidines. IX: The degradation of 5-fluorouracil-6-C^{14}. J Biol Chem 235:433, 1960.
63. Ando H, Tadayoshi I, Kawai Y: Inhibition of corneal epithelial wound healing: A comparative study of mitomycin C and 5-fluorouracil. Ophthalmology 99(12):1809, 1992.
64. Dorr RT: New findings in the pharmacokinetic metabolic and drug-resistance aspects of mitomycin C. Seminars in Oncology 15:32, 1988.
65. Falck FY, Skuta GL, Klein TB: Mitomycin versus 5-fluorouracil antimetabolite therapy for glaucoma filtration surgery. Semin Ophthalmol 7(2):97, 1992.
66. Budavari S (ed): The Merck Index. Rahway, NJ, Merck and Company, 1989.
67. Kunitomo N, Mori S: Studies on the pterygium. Report IV: A treatment of the pterygium by mitomycin C instillation. Acta Soc Ophthalmol Jpn 67:601, 1963.
68. Hayasaka S, Noda S, Yamamoto Y, et al: Postoperative instillation of low-dose mitomycin C in the treatment of primary pterygium. Am J Ophthalmol 106:715, 1988.
69. Singh G, Wilson WR, Foster CS: Long-term follow-up of mitomycin eye drops as adjunctive treatment for ptyergia and its comparison with conjunctival autograft transplantation. Cornea 9:331, 1990.
70. Yamanouchi U, Mishima K: Eye lesions due to mitomycin C after pterygium operation. Folia Ophthalmol Jpn 18:854, 1967.
71. Rubinfield RS, Pfister RR, Stein RM, et al: Serious complications of topical mitomycin C after ptyergium surgery. Ophthalmology 99:1647, 1992.
72. Glaubiger D, Ramu A: Antitumor antibiotics. *In* Chabner BA (ed): Pharmacologic Principles of Cancer Treatment. Philadelphia, WB Saunders, 1982, p 407.
73. Teng CC, Chi HH, Katzin HM: Histology and mechanism of filtering operations. Am J Ophthalmol 47:16, 1959.
74. Van Buskirk EM: Clinical Atlas of Glaucoma. Philadelphia, WB Saunders, 1986.
75. Ball SF: Corticosteroids, including subeonjunctival triamcinolone, in glaucoma filtration surgery. Ophthalmol Clinics North Am 1:143, 1988.
76. Jarus G, Blumenkranz M, Hernandez E, et al: Clearance of intravitreal fluorouracil; Normal and aphakic vitrectomized eyes. Ophthalmology 92:91, 1985.
77. Ouchi T, Fujino A, Tanaka K, et al: Synthesis and antitumor activity of conjugates of poly (α-malic acid) and 5-fluorouracils bound via ester, amide or carbamoyl bonds. J Controlled Rel 12:143, 1990.
78. Wong VO: Biodegradable ocular implants. US Patent 4.853.224, 1989.
79. Simmons ST, Sherwood MB, Nichols DA, et al: Pharmacokinetics of a 5-fluorouracil liposomal delivery system. Br J Ophthalmol 72:688, 1988.
80. Lee DA, Flores RA, Anderson PJ, et al: Glaucoma filtration surgery in rabbits using bioerodible polymers and 5-fluorouracil. Ophthalmology 94:1523, 1987.
81. Lee DA, Leong KW, Panek WC, et al: The use of bioerodible polymers and 5-fluorouracil in glucoma filtration surgery. Invest Ophthalmol Vis Sci 29:1692, 1988.
82. Li NH, Richards M, Brandt K, et al: Poly(phosphate esters) as drug carriers. Polym Preprint 30:454, 1989.
83. Smith TJ, Maurin MB, Milosovich SM, et al: Polyvinyl alcohol membrane permeability characteristics of 5-fluorouracil. J Ocul Pharmacol Ther 4:147, 1988.
84. Wyszynski RE, Vahey JB, Manning L, et al: Sustained release of 5-fluorouracil from ethylene acetate copolymer. J Ocul Pharmacol Ther 5:141, 1989.
85. Charles JB, Ganthier R, Wilson MR, et al: Use of bioerodible polymers impregnated with mitomycin in glaucoma filtration surgery in rabbits. Ophthalmology 98:503, 1991.
86. Chen CW: Enhanced intraocular pressure controlling effectiveness of trabeculectomy by local application of mitomycin C. Trans Asia-Pacif Acad Ophthalmol 9:172, 1983.
87. Palmer SS: Mitomycin as adjunct chemotherapy with trabeculectomy. Ophthalmology 98:317, 1991.
88. Gardner S: Mitomycin C: Protocol for handling during trabeculectomy. Ocul Ther Management 3(1):13, 1992.
89. Kawase K, Matsushita H, Yamamoto T, et al: Mitomycin concentration in rabbit and human ocular tissues after topical administration. Ophthalmology 99(2):203, 1992.
90. McEvoy GK (ed): AHFS Drug Information. Bethesda, American Society of Hospital Pharmacists, 1990.
91. Lee CC, Chen CW, Chao MC: A study of inhibitory effect of mitomycin-C on fibroblasts in cell culture. Trans Ophthalmol Soc Rep China 25:752, 1986.
92. Yamamoto T, Varani J, Soong HK, et al: Effects of 5-fluorouracil and mitomycin on cultured rabbit subconjunctival fibroblasts. Ophthalmology 97:1204, 1990.
93. Lee DA, Lee TC, Cortes AE, et al: Effects of mithramycin, mitomycin, daunorubicin, and bleomycin on human subconjunctival fibroblast attachment and proliferation. Invest Ophthalmol Vis Sci 31:2136, 1990.
94. Bergstrom TJ, Wilkinson WS, Skuta GL, et al: The effects of subconjunctival mitomycin-C on glaucoma filtration surgery in rabbits. Arch Ophthalmol 109:1725, 1991.
95. Wilson MR, Lee DA, Baker RS, et al: The effects of topical mitomycin on glaucoma filtration surgery in rabbits. J Ocul Pharmacol Ther 7(1):1, 1991.
96. Kitazawa Y, Kawase K, Matsushita H, et al: Trabeculectomy with mitomycin. A comparative study with fluorouracil. Arch Ophthalmol 109:1693, 1991.
97. Pasquale LR, Thibault D, Dorman-Pease ME, et al: Effect of topical mitomycin on glaucoma filtration surgery in monkeys. Ophthalomolgy 99:14, 1992.
98. Khaw PT, Sherwood MB, MacKay SLD, et al: Five-minute treatments with fluorouracil, fluoruridine, and mitomycin have long-term effects on human tenon's capsule fibroblasts. Arch Ophthalmol 110:1150, 1992.
99. Khaw PT, Doyle JW, Sherwood MB, et al: Prolonged localized tissue effects from 5-minute exposures to fluorouracil and mitomycin C. Arch Ophthalmol 111:263, 1993.
100. McDermott ML, Wang J, Shin DH: Mitomycin and the human corneal endothelium. Arch Ophthalmol 112:533, 1994.
101. Kee C, Pelzeh CD, Kaufman PL: Mitomycin C suppresses aqueous humor flow in cynomolgus monkeys. Arch Ophthalmol 113:239, 1995.
102. Verdoorn C, Renardel de Lavalette VW, Dalma-Weizhausz, et al: Cellular migration, proliferation and contraction, An *in vitro* approach to a clinical problem—proliferative vitreoretinopathy. Arch Ophthalmol 104:1216, 1986.
103. McDonnell PJ, Krause W, Glaser BM: In vitro inhibition of lens epithelial cell proliferation and migration. Ophthalmic Surg 19:25, 1988.
104. Lee DA, Shapourifar-Tehrani S, Kitada S: The effect of 5-fluorouracil and cytarabine on human fibroblasts from Tenon's capsule. Invest Ophthalmol Vis Sci 31:1848, 1990.
105. Mallick KS, Hajek AS, Parrish RK II: Fluorouracil (5-FU) and cytarabine (ara-C) inhibition of corneal epithelial cell and conjunctival fibroblast proliferation. Arch Ophthalmol 103:1398, 1985.
106. Mermoud A, Salmon JF, Murray ADN: Trabeculectomy with mitomycin C for refractory glaucoma in blacks. Am J Ophthalmol 116:72, 1993.
107. Mégeuand GS, Salmon JF, Scholtz RP, et al: The effect of reducing the exposure time of mitomycin C in glaucoma filtering surgery. Ophthalmology 102:84, 1995.
108. Wang T-H, Hung PT, Ho T-C: THC:YAG laser sclerostomy with preoperative mitomycin-C subconjunctival injection in rabbits. J Glaucoma 2:260, 1993.
109. Giangiacomo J, Dueker DK, Adelstein EH: The effect of preoperative subconjunctival triamcinolone administration on glaucoma filtration. I: Trabeculectomy following subconjunctival triamcinolone. Arch Ophthalmol 104:838, 1986.
110. The Fluorouracil Filtering Surgery Study Group: Five-year follow-up of the Fluorouracil Filtering Surgery Study. Am J Ophthalmol 121:349, 1996.
111. Rader JE, Parrish RK: Update on adjunctive antimetabolites in glaucoma surgery. *In* Caprioli J (ed): Contemporary Issues in Glaucoma. Ophthalmol Clin North Am 4:861, 1991.
112. Yaldo MK, Stamper RL: Long-term effects of mitomycin on filtering blebs: Lack of fibrovascular proliferative response following severe inflammation. Arch Ophthalmol 111:824, 1993.

CHAPTER 36

Agents That Affect Corneal Wound Healing: Modulation of Structure and Function

James D. Zieske and Ilene K. Gipson

Corneal wound healing occurs in three basic phases (Fig. 36–1). The first phase involves epithelial cell migration and wound closure. During this phase the epithelium migrates as an intact sheet to cover the wound. The cells slide and flatten, with the leading edge tapering down to a single cell layer (see Fig. 36–1*A*). Except for very large wounds, this sliding phase is sufficient to cover the wound area.

In the second phase of corneal wound healing, the cell number is reestablished and the epithelial sheet regains its normal number of cell layers (see Fig. 36–1*B*). The primary events in this phase are cell proliferation and differentiation. Evidence suggests that epithelial stem cells localized in the limbus play a role in this phase of healing by undergoing proliferation to allow repopulation of the central corneal epithelium.[1, 2] In addition, transient amplifying cells in the peripheral cornea may remain hyperproliferative as long as 4 weeks after wounding.[3]

The third phase of corneal wound healing involves extracellular matrix synthesis and reassembly of adhesion structures (see Fig. 36–1*C* and *D*). Corneal epithelium is normally attached to its underlying stroma by an anchoring structure complex consisting of hemidesmosomes, basement membrane, and anchoring fibrils. After wounding, hemidesmosome components are rearranged,[4] resulting in the loss of functional hemidesmosomes, and, depending on the wound type, the basement membrane and anchoring fibril network may also be lost. During the cell migration of phase 1, a provisional adhesion structure—focal contacts—is formed.[5] During phase 3, resynthesis and reassembly of the hemidesmosomes, basement membrane, anchoring fibril components, and stromal matrix occur.[6] Fibroblasts are activated to produce matrix components, and fibroblasts and polymorphonuclear neutrophils may infiltrate the wound area. The first two phases of corneal wound healing generally proceed rapidly; the final phase may require months or even years.

Many agents affect corneal wound healing. In an effort to understand the physiologic processes involved as well as to find effective therapeutic modalities, a plethora of agents, experimental wound models, and animal species have been studied. Commonly used models involve removal of only the epithelium by scraping,[7] iodine vapors,[8] or *n*-heptanol application.[9] Others involve removal of both the epithelium and the stroma by mechanical or laser treatment.[10] Still others are simple incision wounds or wounds that chemically[11] or thermally[12] destroy large areas of cornea. The wounds may be allowed to heal in organ culture or in vivo. The most widely used species are rabbits, rats, and monkeys. Wound sizes range from limbus to limbus to a central abrasion 3 mm or smaller. Thus when comparing results, one must consider whether the epithelium is migrating over intact basement membrane, bare stroma, or another matrix; whether the wound closure involves healing by corneal, limbal, or conjunctival epithelium; whether (in primates) Bowman's layer is penetrated; and whether the endothelium is involved.

Phase 1: Epithelial Cell Migration and Wound Closure

Studies pertaining to the first phase of wound healing have been conducted for over 50 years.[13, 14] Subsequent studies of the reepithelialization phase of corneal wound healing are of three main types. The first group consists of efforts to document that certain compounds (e.g., drugs, analgesics, and preservatives) do not adversely affect wound repair. Table 36–1 lists some compounds shown to have little or no effect. The second group of studies consists of attempts to accelerate wound healing pharmacologically. Many of these studies have examined the effects of growth factors. More recently, a third type of study has addressed the physiologic alterations in gene expression during the healing process. A partial list of these gene products is given in Table 36–2.

EXTRACELLULAR MATRIX COMPONENTS

As seen in Table 36–2, many of the proteins whose expressions are altered during the migration phase of wound repair are either extracellular matric component (ECMs) (collagen I, III, IV, V; fibronectin; hyaluronan; and laminin 5)[15–18] or receptors for these components (APLP2, CD44, and integrin $\alpha_6\beta_4$).[15, 19–22] These studies suggest that there may be a therapeutic benefit to the addition of ECM components to the wound area. The rationale is that the addition of ECM components may provide a substrate for the epithelium to adhere to and migrate rapidly across. The most widely used and most controversial ECM component studied is fibronectin (FN). Nishida and collegues[23] were the first to report that FN stimulates corneal epithelial wound healing. They found that FN stimulated the rate of epithelial migration in an in vitro organ culture system in which the epithelium migrates down the side of a hand-cut corneal block. Their finding that FN stimulated migration by 29 to 44% encour-

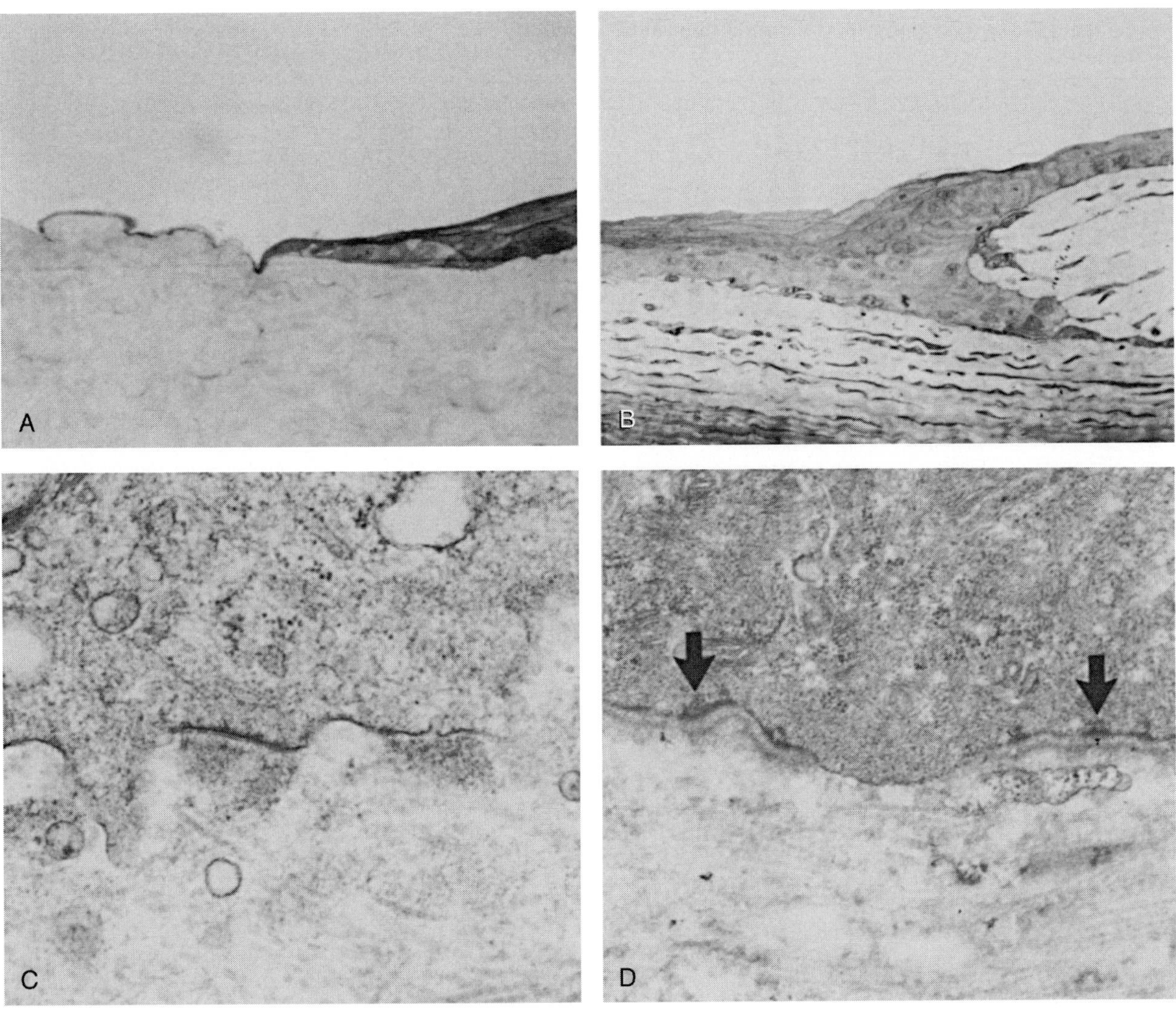

FIGURE 36–1. Light and electron micrographs demonstrating three phases of corneal epithelial wound healing. *A*, Light micrograph of the migratory phase. In corneal epithelium migrating to cover a keratectomy wound, the leading edge tapers to a single cell layer. ×300. *B*, Light micrograph demonstrating reestablishment of the cell layer phase. At the periphery of a keratectomy wound shown in the micrograph, reestablishment of cell numbers has occurred. ×300. *C* and *D*, Healing phase in which reestablishment of adhesion structures occurs is demonstrated in the electron micrographs of the basal cell–stroma interface of rabbit corneas healing at 66 hours (*C*) and 7 days (*D*). Note the small segment of newly assembled basement membrane and associated hemidesmosome in *C*. ×31,200. After 1 week (*D*) the segments of resynthesized basement membrane have increased in length and hemidesmosomes (*arrows*) are more numerous. ×31,200.

aged the use of FN, alone and in combination with various other compounds, to stimulate wound healing in a variety of models. However, other laboratories could not replicate the effect. Soong and associates,[24] using a serum-free rat corneal organ culture model, found no effect of FN on the rate of migration over an intact basement membrane. Using a similar model, Phan and coworkers[25] found that FN had no effect on healing rates in rabbit or guinea pig corneas after scrape or superficial keratectomy wounds. Newton and associates[26] noted no enhancement of epithelial migration after topical application of FN to rabbit corneas either after abrasion wounds or in a persistent epithelial defect model. Also, two double-blind clinical trials have reported no beneficial effects of fibronectin.[27, 28] These negative studies do not, however, rule out the possibility that FN enhances or facilitates epithelial adhesion. Indeed, FN has been demonstrated to enhance the formation of stress fibers and focal contacts in cultured fibroblasts.[29] Also, FN has been demonstrated to be synthesized by the wounded tissue itself.[18] Thus the presence of endogenous FN may diminish the effect of the addition of exogenous FN. Lastly, it should be noted that the wounded corneal tissues synthesize cellular FN, whereas the clinical studies have examined the effects of plasma FN.[27, 28]

Laminin, another component of the ECM, has also been examined for its effect on migration rates, but Gipson and colleagues[30] found no stimulation in rat or rabbit wound-healing models. However, recent reports suggest that an isoform, laminin 5, is upregulated during epithelial migration.[31] In addition, integrin $\alpha_6\beta_4$, which binds laminin 5, is also upregulated.[22] Investigations are currently under way assessing the therapeutic effects of the addition of laminin 5 in various wound models.[32] A third ECM component, sodium hyaluronate, has been reported to stimulate epithelial

TABLE 36–1. **Agents That Do Not Affect Corneal Epithelial Wound Healing**

Agent	Animal	Model
Acetylcysteine	Rabbit	Iodine vapor[97]
Acyclovir	Rabbit	Central abrasion[98]
Calmodulin inhibitors	Rabbit	Central abrasion[36]
Chloramphenicol	Rabbit	Central abrasion[99]
Colchicine	Rat	Central abrasion[37]
Collagen shields	Cat	Central abrasion[100]
EGF	Human	Penetrating keratoplasty[69]
EGF + colchicine	Rat	Central abrasion[61]
Fibronectin	Rabbit	Central abrasion or persistent defect[26]
Fibronectin	Rat	Central abrasion[24, 101]
Gentamicin	Rabbit	Total scrape[102]
Ketorolac	Rabbit	Central abrasion[103]
NaCl, 2%	Rabbit	Central abrasion[99]
Ophthalmic ointments	Rabbit	Central abrasion[104]
Pilocarpine	Rabbit	Heptanol[105]
Soybean agglutinin or lotus lectin	Rat	Central abrasion[38]
Tetracaine, 1%	Human	Photorefractive keratectomy[106]
Substance P	Rabbit	Heptanol[107]
Ketorolac tromethamine, 0.5%	Human	Corneal abrasion[108]
Morphine sulfate	Rabbit	Corneal abrasion[109]
Diclofenac	Rabbit	Photorefractive keratectomy[110]
Antimicrobials	Rabbit	Corneal block[111]

Abbreviations: EGF, epidermal growth factor.

migration. Both hyaluronan and its binding protein, CD44, are upregulated during corneal wound healing.[15]

OTHER PROTEINS ALTERED IN PHASE 1

In addition to the proteins listed in Table 36–2, a large number of other proteins and genes have been described as being altered during the initial phase of wound repair. Indeed, Ross and colleagues[33] identified 76 wound response complementary DNAs (cDNAs) through subtractive hybridization and partial sequencing of messenger RNA (mRNA) isolated from wounded and unwounded corneas. Many of these proteins are involved in energy production and cytoskeleton reassembly. These studies suggest several important mechanisms involved in phase 1 of wound healing: (1) alteration in adhesion complexes from hemidesmosomes to focal contact-like structures, (2) rearrangement of cell-cell attachments and cytoskeleton, and (3) upregulation of energy production. Although an increasing amount of information is known regarding the mechanisms involved in the epithelial migration phase of wound healing, there has been little success in finding agents to stimulate those processes and accelerate wound closure. One possible reason for this may be that the wound closure portion of wound healing is already nearly optimized in vivo. One compound that has been reported to stimulate cell migration during the first phase of corneal epithelial wound healing is vitamin A. Hatchell and associates[34] found that vitamin A, in the form of tretinoin (all-*trans*-retinoic acid), could stimulate migration rates by up to 30%. Ubels and coworkers[35] demonstrated that tretinoin stimulated corneal epithelial wound healing in rabbits by 18% and in monkeys by 22%. The mechanism involved is unclear; however, vitamin A remains

TABLE 36–2. **Partial List of Proteins Whose Expression or Localization Is Altered During Corneal Wound Repair**

Proteins	References
APLP2	Yu et al, 1995[20]
CD44	Asari et al, 1996[15]
Collagen I	Power et al, 1995[16]
Collagen III	Power et al, 1995[16]
Collagen IV	Power et al, 1995;[16] Saika et al, 1995[17]
Collagen V	Power et al, 1995[16]
Fibronectin	Nickeleit et al, 1996[18]
Fodrin	Amino et al, 1995[112]
Fos	Okada et al, 1996[113]
Glucose transporter 1	Takahashi et al, 1996[114]
Hyaluronan	Asari et al, 1996[15]
Integrin $\alpha_6\beta_4$	Latvala et al, 1996;[21] Stepp et al, 1996;[22] Gipson et al, 1993[95]
Jun	Okada et al, 1996[113]
Laminin 5	Fini et al, 1996[31]
Matrix metalloproteinases	Fini et al, 1996[31]
Protein kinase C	Lin and Bazan, 1995[115]
SPARC	Latvala et al, 1996[116]
Vinculin	Zieske et al, 1989[5]

Abbreviations: SPARC, secreted protein, acidic, rich in cysteine/osteonectin/BM-40.

one of the few compounds to stimulate migration rates without also stimulating cell proliferation.

INHIBITORS

An examination of compounds that inhibit epithelial migration (Table 36–3)[36–44] has demonstrated several events necessary for the first phase of corneal wound healing. Epithelial migration requires the synthesis of proteins and glycoproteins[42, 45, 46] (Fig. 36–2) and the formation of actin bundles.

TABLE 36–3. **Inhibitors of Corneal Epithelial Migration**

Agent	Animal	Model
β-Adrenergic antagonist	Rabbit	Iodine vapor[39]
Calmodulin inhibitors	Rat	Central abrasion[36]
	Rabbit	In vitro hemidesmosome[40]
Capsaicin	Rabbit	*n*-Heptanol[41]
Cytochalasins B and D	Rat	Central abrasion[37]
Glycoprotein synthesis inhibitors	Rat	Central abrasion[42]
Lectins (concanavalin A, wheat germ agglutinin)	Rat	Central abrasion[38]
PMN and PMN lysate	Rat	Central abrasion[43]
Protein synthesis inhibitors	Rat	Central abrasion[44]
Protease inhibitors	Rat	Central abrasion[44]
Wortmannin	Rabbit	Epithelial cell culture[55]
Protein kinase C inhibitors	Rat	Central abrasion[54]
Eosinophil major basic protein	Rat	Central abrasion[117]
TGF-β	Rabbit and cow	Central abrasion[67, 68]

Abbreviations: PMN, polymorphonuclear leukocytes; TGF-β, transforming growth factor-β.

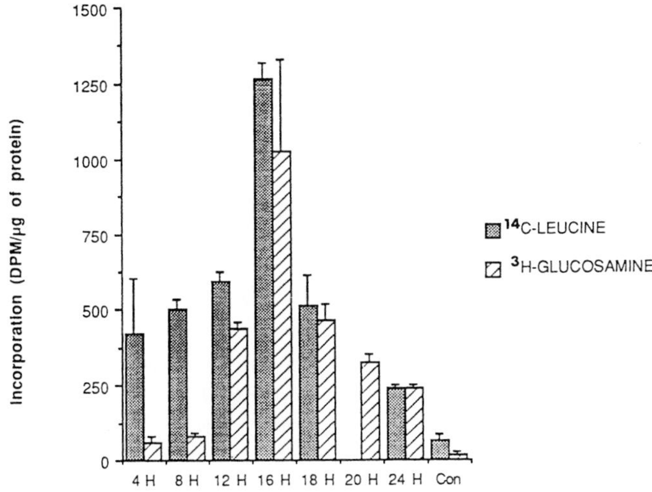

FIGURE 36–2. Incorporation of ^{3}H-glucosamine or ^{14}C-leucine into material precipitated by trichloroacetic acid (TCA). A wound 3 mm in diameter was created in situ by removing epithelium from rat corneas with a small scalpel. Corneas were removed and cultured 4 to 24 hours in a defined medium.[37] Unwounded corneas served as controls. Radiolabeled precursors were present for the final 3 hours of culture at a concentration of 2 μCi/mL. Migrating and control epithelium were harvested and washed in 7.5% TCA, and then radioactivity and protein concentrations were determined.[46] $N > 4$ for all time points. Wound closure occurs at 22 hours in this model.

Actin bundle formation during migration has been observed in both basal and suprabasal cells.[47] Colchicine has no effect on migration, indicating the lack of involvement of microtubules[37] and thus that cell proliferation is not required for epithelial sliding to cover the wound.

High levels of proteases apparently block migration in wound healing by digesting either matrix or cell surface molecules.[48, 49] Potential sources of proteases in wounds include inflammatory cells,[43] tears,[50, 51] and the corneal tissues themselves.[31, 52, 53] However, the finding that protease inhibitors slow migration suggests that low levels of proteases may be necessary for migration, perhaps by digesting temporary adhesion junctions or their associated matrix (Fig. 36–3).[44] The effects of lectins, vitamin A, and tunicamycin also suggest that the synthesis of cell surface molecules is necessary for healing.[34, 38, 41, 42] Perhaps tunicamycin blocks the synthesis of a cell surface glycoconjugate, whereas vitamin A would stimulate its synthesis, and the binding of lectins to the glycoconjugate could block its effectiveness. In addition, β-blockers inhibit migration, suggesting that cyclic AMP (cAMP) plays a role in migration.[39]

Protein kinase C inhibitors also slow epithelial healing rates.[54] Combined with the finding that calmodulin inhibitors slow migration, these data suggest that fluxes in Ca^{2+} levels are involved in migration.[36, 40] Interestingly, wortmannin, an inhibitor of phosphatidylinositol 3-kinase (PI-3 kinase) slows corneal epithelial migration.[55] Since PI-3 kinase is a common member of the signaling cascade of most growth factors, this finding suggests that activation of growth factor receptors is involved in wound repair. Indeed, inhibition of epidermal growth factor (EGF) receptor slows migration by over 50%.[56]

Phase 2: Reestablishment of Cell Number

GROWTH FACTORS

In the second phase of corneal wound healing, epithelial cells undergo cell proliferation to return the epithelium to its normal stratification. In wounds involving damage to the stromal matrix, fibroblasts become activated to begin the process of producing new matrix components. Research on this phase of corneal wound healing has centered around the use of various growth factors as possible therapeutic agents. The rationale is that they will stimulate cell proliferation, allowing rapid reestablishment of a normal stratified epithelium and the increased production of collagen by activated keratocytes leading to increased wound strength. EGF has been widely examined for its usefulness in corneal wound healing. Frati and associates[57] and Savage and Cohen[58] first demonstrated that EGF promotes corneal epithelial proliferation. Subsequently, several groups have quantitated the effect in various models. Petroutsos and colleagues[59] demonstrated a 23% increase in the healing rate over an intact basement membrane. Watanabe and coworkers[60] found up to a 60% increase in the epithelial migration rate in the corneal block model, and Soong and colleagues[61] reported a 20% increase in the rate induced by EGF in an in vitro model with epithelium migrating over denuded basement membrane. Epithelial proliferation has been shown to be stimulated by several other growth factors including transforming growth factor-α,[62] acidic and basic fibroblast growth factor,[63] keratinocyte growth factor,[64] hepatocyte growth factor,[65] and endothelin.[66] The extent of accel-

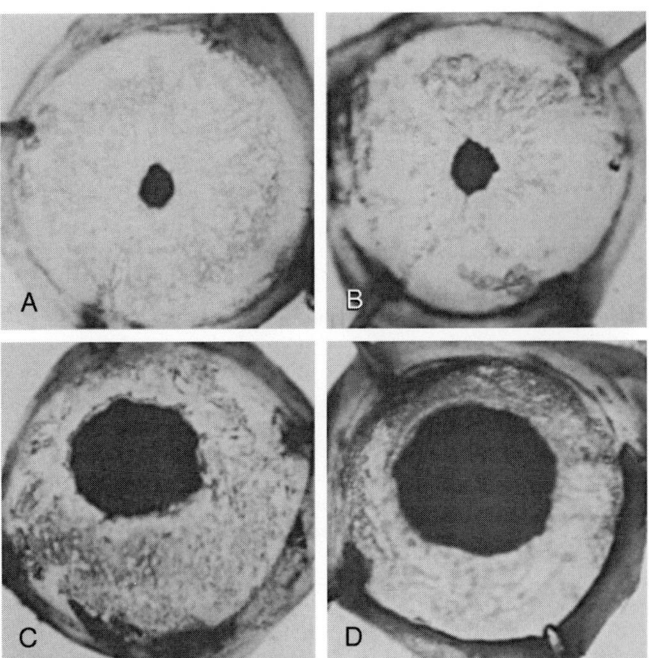

FIGURE 36–3. Effect of serine protease inhibitor phenylmethylsulfonyl fluoride (PMSF) on corneal epithelial migration. Three-mm epithelial débridement wounds were allowed to heal 18 hours in organ culture in the presence of (*A*) no additives, (*B*) 0.1 mM PMSF, (*C*) 0.5 mM PMSF, or (*D*) 1 mM PMSF. Corneas were stained with Richardson's stain to demarcate the remaining wound area. Epithelial migration was significantly slowed ($P \leq .01$) at concentrations of 0.5 and 1.0 mM PMSF.

eration of wound healing in almost all studies is within the range of 20 to 30%, suggesting that this percentage is the maximal effect of cell proliferation on wound closure. Transforming growth factor-β (TGF-β), to date, is unique among growth factors in that it inhibits epithelial healing rates.[67, 68] The therapeutic benefit of the addition of growth factors has been somewhat disappointing. For example, Kandarakis and colleagues[69] found no statistically significant effect of EGF in a clinical study examining healing after penetrating keratoplasty. Also, Singh and Foster[70] found in a double-masked study using alkali burns in rabbits that EGF stimulated healing by only 3% zero to 2 days after injury. However, at 3 to 5 days after wounding, EGF-treated corneas showed epithelial wound closure whereas the untreated controls did not. Furthermore, the wounds reopened when EGF treatment was stopped. One problem that is not generally addressed in the clinical studies is the expression and localization of the growth factor receptors in wounded corneas. Table 36–4 lists growth factor receptors present in the corneal epithelium. These receptors show distinct localization; for example, EGF receptor and TGF-β receptors I and II are primarily in the basal cell layer. Thus, endogenous growth factors may not reach their receptors after wound closure. Also, it is possible that receptors may be up- or downregulated after wounding; thus, attention should be given to determining the proper time to apply the growth factor.

INHIBITORS

One question raised by the stimulation of wound healing by growth factors is whether this effect is solely the result of the enhancement of the rate of proliferation or whether the factors may function through another mechanism. Studies using the inhibitors colchicine[37] and 5-fluorouracil[71] indicate that the stimulatory effect of growth factors is primarily through the enhancement of cell proliferation. Several groups have demonstrated that colchicine has no effect on healing rates, indicating that cell proliferation does not affect the first phase of corneal wound healing. Also, Soong and colleagues[24] found that although EGF stimulated healing by 20%, colchicine blocked this effect. 5-Fluorouracil, which also blocks mitosis, has been demonstrated to have no effect on the migration rate, but the epithelium did not regain normal stratification.[71] One potential problem in the interpretation of these results, however, is that the tear concentrations of some growth factors increase after wounding.[72] In addition, the corneal tissues may also upregulate the synthesis of growth factors; thus, the growth factor receptors may be activated to nearly maximal levels by endogenous growth factors, allowing only a minimal enhancement by exogenous addition of growth factors.

TABLE 36–4. **Growth Factor Receptors Expressed in Corneal Epithelium**

Receptor	References
Endothelin receptor	Tao et al, 1995[66]
Epidermal growth factor receptor	Wilson et al, 1992;[118] Zieske et al, 1993;[119] Hongo et al, 1992[120]
Hepatocyte growth factor receptor	Wilson et al, 1993;[121] Li et al, 1996[122]
Keratinocyte growth factor receptor	Wilson et al, 1993;[121] Sotozono et al, 1994[123]
Transforming growth factor receptor types I, II, and III	Joyce and Zieske, 1997;[124] Obato et al, 1995[125]

Phase 3: Extracellular Matrix Synthesis and Reassembly of Adhesion Structures

MATRIX METALLOPROTEINASES AND GROWTH FACTORS

In the third phase of wound healing the temporary adhesion junctions between epithelium and ECM are lost, and the normal permanent adhesion junctions are resynthesized or reassembled. This phase involves the restoration of hemidesmosomes, anchoring fibrils, the basement membrane, and the stromal matrix.[6] Potential therapeutic agents would include compounds that stimulate the synthesis of ECM components or block their degradation. ECM components that have been identified as being synthesized following wounding include FN,[73] laminin,[6] tenascin,[74] hyaluronan, and collagen types I, III, IV, V, VI, and VII.[6, 75, 76]

Phase 1 and phase 2, in general, occur uneventfully in most wounds; however, improper healing in phase 3 can lead to vision-threatening problems such as recurrent erosion and corneal ulceration. The key players in stromal remodeling after wounding are a family of matrix-degrading enzymes termed *matrix metalloproteinases* (MMPs). These enzymes function at neutral pH and can digest all the matrix macromolecules.[77] There are three main groups of MMPs: collagenases, which degrade native collagens; gelatinases, which degrade denatured collagen as well as collagen types IV, V, and VII; and stromelysins, which can degrade basement membrane collagens and proteoglycans. These enzymes are involved in the normal remodeling of corneal wounds[78, 79]; however, their overproduction (observed primarily in chemical and thermal injuries) may lead to stromal ulceration. This ulceration is generally preceded by epithelial erosion and breakdown of the basement membrane.[31, 53] The activity of the MMPs is regulated at several levels, including transcription and activation of enzyme activity, and by a naturally occurring group of inhibitors, tissue inhibitors of metalloproteinases (TIMPs). Three TIMPs have been cloned.[77] These TIMPs have an important role in modulating the actions of MMPs. Diseases in which tissue destruction is involved often correlate with imbalances of MMPs over TIMPs. Indeed, it has been observed in corneal ulceration that MMPs are upregulated, whereas TIMPs are downregulated.[80] Also, keratoconus corneas exhibit an imbalance of MMPs and TIMPs.[81]

Although several growth factors have been examined for their role in phase 3 of wound healing, TGF-β has received by far the most attention in the past several years. This is largely due to TGF-β's multifunctional role as an effector of cell proliferation as well as ECM synthesis and degradation. In general, TGF-β stimulates matrix deposition and inhibits degradation. TGF-β induces cell proliferation of keratocytes, inhibits proliferation of epithelial cells, enhances collagen and fibronectin synthesis, inhibits MMP expression, and appears to enhance TIMP expression.[82–86] In addition, TGF-β appears to stimulate the transformation of keratocytes to myofibroblasts, which are involved in wound remodeling and contraction.[83] Thus it has been postulated that TGF-β overproduction may result in excessive matrix deposition and scarring. To test this hypothesis, Jester and coworkers[86] added neutralizing antibodies to rabbit wounds and found that FN deposition and corneal fibrosis were significantly reduced.

CORTICOSTEROIDS

Another group of compounds that may affect the third phase of corneal wound healing is corticosteroids. These compounds, used clinically to suppress inflammation, have been shown to prevent neovascularization.[87] They have a slight or no effect on the first phase of wound healing involving migration of corneal epithelium, but they apparently do slow healing when the wound area must be covered by conjunctival cells.[88] Whether corticosteroids influence the third phase of wound healing by altering ECM synthesis or reassembly of adhesion structures is unclear. O'Brien and Geroski[89] found that methylprednisolone acetate inhibits macromolecular synthesis, but they did not examine the synthesis of ECM components. Also, Srinivasan and coworkers[90] found that prednisolone altered proteins synthesized by migrating epithelium, but they also did not assay for ECM components specifically.

The use of corticosteroids has received renewed interest since they have been used to slow regression after photorefractive surgery.[91] There appears to be no consensus, however, as to their therapeutic use in preventing corneal haze after these procedures.[91–94]

INHIBITORS

Several inhibitors have been tested for their effect on the resynthesis and reassembly of hemidesmosomes using the in vitro model devised by Gipson and associates.[95] Protein and glycoprotein synthesis inhibitors, calmodulin inhibitors, and EDTA all blocked the formation of hemidesmosomes, demonstrating that hemidesmosome formation requires protein and glycoprotein synthesis and the presence of Ca^{2+}.[40] The requirement of Ca^{2+} correlates well with the discovery that the $\alpha_6\beta_4$ form of integrin is present in hemidesmosomes[4]; Ca^{2+} has been shown to be necessary for ECM ligand binding to integrins.

Protease inhibitors, specifically aprotinin, have been suggested as potential therapeutic agents that would affect the third phase of corneal wound healing. The rationale is that aprotinin would block the digestion of ECM components necessary for cell attachment by plasmin in the tear fluid.[48] Aprotinin has been shown to aid healing in patients suffering from recurrent erosion and also in a rabbit model after alkali burns.[49] In both cases healing was stimulated, presumably by blocking the degradation of ECM components.

Finally, natural and synthetic inhibitors of MMPs have been examined for their ability to prevent ulceration after chemical or thermal burns. Paterson and coworkers[96] found that both TIMP1 and a synthetic MMP inhibitor reduced corneal ulceration following alkali burns in rabbits. Also, Fini and associates[31] reported that a synthetic inhibitor of MMPs slowed the degradation of the basement membrane and reduced ulceration in a rat thermal burn model. Lastly, in a combination therapy, Schultz and colleagues[62] observed that EGF, FN, a synthetic collagenase inhibitor, and aprotinin significantly blocked ulceration and enhanced epithelial regeneration.

Summary

Corneal epithelial wound healing requires normal, unimpeded migration of the epithelium to cover the wound, cell proliferation to reestablish the cell number, and reattachment of the epithelium to its ECM. Stromal healing requires the activation of keratocytes, the synthesis of matrix components, and unimpaired remodeling of the tissue, which requires a proper balance of MMPs and TIMPs. The first phase of healing, epithelial migration, normally occurs rapidly in response to all wounds and is relatively independent of the wound type. Epithelial migration is usually sufficient to cover most corneal wounds. The only agent that appears to speed this phase of healing in most wound models is vitamin A. The mechanism of this enhancement is unknown. A major clinical problem in which epithelial healing is blocked at this stage is persistent epithelial defect. This abnormality is uniformly correlated with the presence of inflammatory cells. Whether the inflammatory cells physically block migration or function by releasing proteases that digest ECM ligands necessary for migration is unclear.

In the second phase of healing, cell proliferation occurs to provide cells for reestablishing normal epithelial morphology. Growth factors may be beneficial in this phase, particularly when very large wounds are involved. The beneficial effect of growth factors may be very minor on small corneal wounds with an intact basement membrane.

Except for persistent epithelial defect, major clinical problems are seldom seen in the first two phases of epithelial healing. Epithelium normally migrates rapidly over most naturally occurring substrates, and cell proliferation proceeds unimpaired. In the third phase of epithelial wound healing, the major clinical abnormality is recurrent erosion. This disease is thought to involve improper reattachment of the epithelium to its underlying ECM. It is not known whether the impaired attachment results from a failure of the cells to produce the proper attachment proteins, for example, hemidesmosome components, anchoring fibril networks; whether the defect is in the existing or newly synthesized basement membrane and its association with the stroma; or whether ECM ligands necessary for attachment are being degraded by proteolytic enzymes. Therapies currently being explored include the use of FN to promote attachment; growth factors to increase cell density and the production of ECM; and protease inhibitors, which may block the degradation of attachment proteins.

Stromal healing requires the synthesis of new ECM components and their proper realignment to minimize light scattering. Current therapies focus on the use of steroids and of nonsteroidal antiinflammatory agents that inhibit inflammatory cells that may degrade ECM, and the use of growth factors, which activate keratocytes to produce ECM components to increase tensile strength. In addition, investigations are centering on the regulation of the balance of MMPs and TIMPs, and on the transformation of keratocytes to myofibroblasts.

In conclusion, the ultimate goal of studying corneal wound

healing remains the discovery of agents that will promote well-attached, healthy epithelium along with scar-free healing of the stroma. Research in the past 5 years has indicated that the expression of a large number of gene products is altered during the healing process. These studies indicate that, in most cases, proper wound healing requires a balanced response, making intervention with a single therapeutic agent difficult. However, the increase in knowledge regarding the basic mechanisms of corneal wound healing gives hope that beneficial therapies will continue to be developed.

REFERENCES

1. Schermer A, Galvin S, Sun T-T: Differentiation-related expression of a major 64 K corneal keratin in vivo and in culture suggests limbal location of corneal epithelial stem cells. J Cell Biol 103:49, 1986.
2. Cotsarelis G, Cheng S-Z, Dong G, et al: Existence of slow-cycling limbal epithelial basal cells that can be preferentially stimulated to proliferate: Implications on epithelial stem cells. Cell 57:201, 1989.
3. Chung E-H, DeGregorio PG, Wasson M, et al: Epithelial regeneration after limbus-to-limbus debridement: Expression of alpha-enolase in stem and transient amplifying cells. Invest Ophthalmol Vis Sci 36:1336, 1995.
4. Stepp MA, Spurr-Michaud S, Tisdale A, et al: $\alpha_6\beta_4$ Integrin heterodimer is a component of hemidesmosomes. Proc Natl Acad Sci USA 87:8970, 1990.
5. Zieske JD, Bukusoglu G, Gipson IK: Enhancement of vinculin synthesis by migrating stratified squamous epithelium. J Cell Biol 109:571, 1989.
6. Gipson IK, Spurr-Michaud S, Tisdale A, et al: Reassembly of the anchoring structures of the corneal epithelium during wound repair in the rabbit. Invest Ophthalmol Vis Sci 30:425, 1989.
7. Hanna C: Proliferation and migration of epithelial cells during corneal wound repair in the rabbit and the rat. Am J Ophthalmol 6:55, 1966.
8. Moses RA, Parkinson G, Schuchardt R: A standard wound of the corneal epithelium in the rabbit. Invest Ophthalmol Vis Sci 18:103, 1979.
9. Cintron C, Hassinger L, Kublin CL, et al: A simple method for the removal of rabbit corneal epithelium utilizing *n*-heptanol. Ophthalmic Res 11:90, 1979.
10. Lesperance FA, Taylor DM, Del-Pero RA, et al: Human Excimer laser corneal surgery: Preliminary report. Trans Am Ophthalmol Soc 86:208, 1989.
11. Pfister RR, Friend J, Dohlman CH: The anterior segments of rabbits after alkali burns: Metabolic and histologic alterations. Arch Ophthalmol 86:189, 1971.
12. Kenyon KR: Inflammatory mechanisms in corneal ulceration. Trans Am Ophthalmol Soc 83:610, 1985.
13. Friedenwald JS, Buschke W: Influence of some experimental variables on the epithelial movements in the healing of corneal wounds. Comp Physiol 23:95, 1944.
14. Smelser G, Ozanics V: Effect of chemotherapeutic agents on cell division and healing of corneal burns and abrasions in the rat. Am J Ophthalmol 27:1063, 1944.
15. Asari A, Morita M, Sekiguchi T, et al: Hyaluronan, CD44 and fibronectin in rabbit corneal epithelial wound healing. Jpn J Ophthalmol 40:18, 1996.
16. Power WJ, Kaufman AH, Merayo-Lloves J, et al: Expression of collagens I, III, IV and V mRNA in Excimer wounded rat cornea: Analysis by semi-quantitative PCR. Curr Eye Res 14:879, 1995.
17. Saika S, Kobata S, Hashizume N, et al: Type IV collagen in the basement membrane of the corneal epithelium after alkali burns in guinea pigs. Ophthal Res 27:129, 1995.
18. Nickeleit V, Kaufman AH, Zagachin L, et al: Healing corneas express embryonic fibronectin isoforms in the epithelium, subepithelial stroma, and endothelium. Am J Pathol 149:549, 1996.
19. Gipson IK, Spurr-Michaud S, Tisdale A, et al: Redistribution of the hemidesmosome components alpha 6 beta 4 integrin and bullous pemphigoid antigens during epithelial wound healing. Exp Cell Res 207:86, 1993.
20. Yu FX, Gipson IK, Guo Y: Differential gene expression in healing rat corneal epithelium. Invest Ophthalmol Vis Sci 36:1997, 1995.
21. Latvala T, Paallysaho T, Tervo K, et al: Distribution of alpha 6 and beta 4 integrins following epithelial abrasion in the rabbit cornea. Acta Ophthalmol Scand 74:21, 1996.
22. Stepp MA, Zhu L, Cranfill R: Changes in beta 4 integrin expression and localization in vivo in response to corneal epithelial injury. Invest Ophthalmol Vis Sci 37:1593, 1996.
23. Nishida T, Nakagawa S, Awata T, et al: Fibronectin promotes epithelial migration of cultured rabbit cornea in situ. J Cell Biol 97:1653, 1983.
24. Soong HK, Hassan T, Varani J, et al: Fibronectin does not enhance epidermal growth factor–mediated acceleration of corneal epithelial wound closure. Arch Ophthalmol 107:1052, 1989.
25. Phan TM, Foster CS, Zagachin LM, et al: Role of fibronectin in the healing of superficial keratectomies in vitro. Invest Ophthalmol Vis Sci 30:386, 1989.
26. Newton C, Hatchell DL, Klintworth GK, et al: Topical fibronectin and corneal epithelial wound healing in the rabbit. Arch Ophthalmol 106:1277, 1988.
27. McCulley JP, Horowitz B, Husseini ZM, et al: Topical fibronectin therapy of persistent corneal epithelial defects. Fibronectin Study Group. Trans Am Ophthalmol Soc 91:367, 1993.
28. Gordon JF, Johnson P, Musch DC: Topical fibronectin ophthalmic solution in the treatment of persistent defects of the corneal epithelium. Am J Ophthalmol 119:281, 1995.
29. Hynes RO: Fibronectins. *In* Rich A (ed): New York, Springer-Verlag, 1990.
30. Gipson IK, Azar DT, Zieske JD, et al: Effect of synthetic peptides of cell binding domain of fibronectin and laminin on corneal epithelial wound healing in vitro. Invest Ophthalmol Vis Sci 29(Suppl):54, 1988.
31. Fini ME, Parks WC, Rinehart WB, et al: Role of matrix metalloproteinases in failure to re-epithelialize after corneal injury. Am J Pathol 149:1287, 1996.
32. Tamura RN, Oda D, Quaranta V, et al: Coating of titanium alloy with soluble laminin-5 promotes cell attachment and hemidesmosome assembly in gingival epithelial cells: Potential application to dental implants. J Periodontal Res 32:287, 1997.
33. Ross LL, Danehower SC, Proia AD, et al: Coordinated activation of corneal wound response genes in vivo as observed by in situ hybridization. Exp Eye Res 61:435, 1995.
34. Hatchell DL, Ubels JL, Stekiel T, et al: Corneal epithelial wound healing in normal and diabetic rabbits treated with tretinoin. Arch Ophthalmol 103:98, 1985.
35. Ubels JL, Edelhauser HF, Foley KM, et al: The efficacy of retinoic acid ointment for treatment of xerophthalmia and corneal epithelial wounds. Curr Eye Res 10:1049, 1985.
36. Soong HK, Cintron C: Disparate effects of calmodulin inhibitors on corneal epithelial migration in rabbit and rat. Ophthalmic Res 17:27, 1985.
37. Gipson IK, Westcott MJ, Brooksby NG: Effects of cytochalasins B and D and colchicine on migration of the corneal epithelium. Invest Ophthalmol Vis Sci 22:633, 1982.
38. Gipson IK, Anderson RA: Effect of lectins on migration of the corneal epithelium. Invest Ophthalmol Vis Sci 19:341, 1980.
39. Liu GS, Trope GE, Basu PK: Beta adrenoceptors and regenerating corneal epithelium. J Ocul Pharmacol 6:101, 1990.
40. Trinkaus-Randall V, Gipson IK: Role of calcium and calmodulin in hemidesmosome formation in vitro. J Cell Biol 98:1565, 1984.
41. Gallar J, Pozo MA, Rebollo I, et al: Effects of capsaicin on corneal wound healing. Invest Ophthalmol Vis Sci 31:1968, 1990.
42. Gipson IK, Kiorpes TC, Brennan SJ: Epithelial sheet movement: Effects of tunicamycin on migration and glycoprotein synthesis. Dev Biol 101:212, 1984.
43. Wagoner MD, Kenyon KR, Gipson IK, et al: Polymorphonuclear neutrophils delay corneal epithelial wound healing in vitro. Invest Ophthalmol Vis Sci 25:1217, 1984.
44. Zieske JD, Bukusoglu G: Effect of protease inhibitors on corneal epithelial migration. Invest Ophthalmol Vis Sci 32:2073, 1991.
45. Gipson IK, Kiorpes TC: Epithelial sheet movement: Protein and glycoprotein synthesis. Dev Biol 92:259, 1982.
46. Zieske JD, Gipson IK: Protein synthesis during corneal epithelial wound healing. Invest Ophthalmol Vis Sci 27:1, 1986.
47. Gipson IK, Anderson RA: Actin filaments in normal and migrating corneal epithelial cells. Invest Ophthalmol Vis Sci 16:161, 1977.
48. Salonen E-M, Tervo T, Torma E, et al: Plasmin in tear fluid of patients with corneal ulcers: Basis for new therapy. Acta Ophthalmol 65:3, 1987.

49. Cejkova J, Lojda Z, Salonen E-M, et al: Histochemical study of alkali-burned rabbit anterior eye segment in which severe lesions were prevented by aprotinin treatment. Histochemistry 92:441, 1989.
50. Tervo T, Honkanen N, van Setten G: A rapid fluorometric assay for tear fluid plasmin activity. Cornea 13:148, 1994.
51. Cejkova J, Lojda Z, Dropcova S, et al: The histochemical pattern of mechanically or chemically injured rabbit cornea after aprotinin treatment: Relationships with the plasmin concentration of the tear fluid. Histochem J 25:438, 1993.
52. Berman M, Kenyon K, Hayashi K, et al: The pathogenesis of epithelial defects and stromal ulceration. *In* Cavanagh HD (ed): The Cornea: Transactions of the World Congress on the Cornea, vol III. New York, Raven, 1988, pp 35–43.
53. Matsubara M, Zieske JD, Fini ME: Mechanism of basement membrane dissolution preceding corneal ulceration. Invest Ophthalmol Vis Sci 32:3221, 1991.
54. Hirakata A, Gupta AG, Proia AD: Effect of protein kinase C inhibitors and activators on corneal re-epithelialization in the rat. Invest Ophthalmol Vis Sci 34:216, 1993.
55. Zhang Y, Akhtar RA: Epidermal growth factor stimulation of phosphatidylinositol 3-kinase during wound closure in rabbit corneal epithelial cells. Invest Ophthalmol Vis Sci 38:1139, 1997.
56. Zieske JD, Takahashi H, Kaminski AE: Epidermal growth factor receptor is activated during corneal epithelial migration. Invest Ophthalmol Vis Sci 37(Suppl):S460, 1996.
57. Frati L, Daniele S, Delogu A, et al: Selective binding of the epidermal growth factor and its specific effects on the epithelial cells of the cornea. Exp Eye Res 14:135, 1972.
58. Savage CR, Cohen S: Proliferation of corneal epithelium induced by epidermal growth factor. Exp Eye Res 15:361, 1973.
59. Petroutsos G, Courty J, Guimaraes R, et al: Comparison of the effects of EGF, pFGF and EDGF on corneal epithelium wound healing. Curr Eye Res 3:593, 1984.
60. Watanabe K, Nakagawa S, Nishida T: Stimulatory effects of fibronectin and EGF on migration of corneal epithelial cells. Invest Ophthalmol Vis Sci 28:205, 1987.
61. Soong HK, McClenic B, Varani J, et al: EGF does not enhance corneal epithelial cell motility. Invest Ophthalmol Vis Sci 30:1808, 1989.
62. Schultz G, Chegini N, Grant M, et al: Effects of growth factors on corneal wound healing. Acta Ophthalmol (Copenh) 70:60, 1992.
63. Dabin I, Courtois Y: Acidic fibroblast growth factor over expression in corneal epithelial wound healing. Growth Factors 5:129, 1991.
64. Sotozono C, Inatomi T, Nakamura M, et al: Keratinocyte growth factor accelerates corneal epithelial wound healing in vivo. Invest Ophthalmol Vis Sci 36:1524, 1995.
65. Wilson SE, He Y-G, Weng J, et al: Effect of epidermal growth factor, hepatocyte growth factor, and keratinocyte growth factor on proliferation, motility, and differentiation of human corneal epithelial cells. Exp Eye Res 59:665, 1994.
66. Tao W, Liou GI, Wu X, et al: ETB and epidermal growth factor receptor stimulation of wound closure in bovine corneal epithelial cells. Invest Ophthalmol Vis Sci 36:2614, 1995.
67. Nishida K, Ohashi Y, Nezu E, et al: Transforming growth factor-beta (TGF-beta) inhibits epithelial wound healing of organ-cultured rabbit cornea. Acta Ophthalmol Jpn 97:899, 1993.
68. Foreman DM, Pancholi S, Jarvis-Evans J, et al: A simple organ culture model for assessing the effects of growth factors on corneal reepithelialization. Exp Eye Res 62:555, 1996.
69. Kandarakis AS, Page C, Kaufman HE: The effect of epidermal growth factor on epithelial healing after penetrating keratoplasty in human eyes. Am J Ophthalmol 98:411, 1984.
70. Singh G, Foster CS: Epidermal growth factor in alkali-burned corneal epithelial wound healing. Am J Ophthalmol 103:802, 1987.
71. Capone A, Lance SE, Friend J, et al: In vivo effects of 5-FU on ocular surface epithelium following corneal wounding. Invest Ophthalmol Vis Sci 38:1661, 1987.
72. Vesaluoma M, Teppo AM, Gronhagen-Riska C, et al: Release of TGF-beta 1 and VEGF in tears following photorefractive keratectomy. Curr Eye Res 16:19, 1997.
73. Zieske JD, Higashijima SC, Spurr-Michaud SJ, et al: Biosynthetic responses of the rabbit cornea to a keratectomy wound. Invest Ophthalmol Vis Sci 28:1668, 1987.
74. Tervo K, Tervo T, van Setten GB, et al: Demonstration of tenascin-like immunoreactivity in rabbit corneal wounds. Acta Ophthalmol 65:347, 1989.
75. Smith RS, Smith LA, Rich L, et al: Effects of growth factors on corneal wound healing. Invest Ophthalmol Vis Sci 20:222, 1981.
76. Malley DS, Steinert RF, Puliafito CA, et al: Immunofluorescence study of corneal wound healing after Excimer laser anterior keratectomy in the monkey eye. Arch Ophthalmol 108:1316, 1990.
77. Reynolds JJ: Collagenases and tissue inhibitors of metalloproteinases: A functional balance in tissue degradation. Oral Dis 2:70, 1996.
78. Fini ME, Girard MT: The pattern of metalloproteinase expression by corneal fibroblasts is altered with passage in cell culture. J Cell Sci 32:3221, 1990.
79. Girard MT, Matsubara M, Kublin C, et al: Stromal fibroblasts synthesize collagenase and stromelysin during long-term remodeling repair tissue. J Cell Sci 104:1001, 1993.
80. Riley GP, Harrall RL, Watson P, et al: Collagenase (MMP-1) and TIMP-1 in destructive corneal disease associated with rheumatoid arthritis. Eye 9:703, 1995.
81. Kenney MC, Chwa M, Opbroek AJ, et al: Increased gelatinolytic activity in keratoconus keratocyte cultures: A correlation to an altered matrix metalloproteinases-2/tissue inhibitor of metalloproteinase ratio. Cornea 13:114, 1994.
82. Ohji M, SundarRaj N, Thoft RA: Transforming growth factor-beta stimulates collagen and fibronectin synthesis by human corneal stromal fibroblasts in vitro. Curr Eye Res 12:703, 1993.
83. Jester JV, Barry-Lane PA, Cavanagh HD, et al: Induction of alpha–smooth muscle actin expression and myofibroblast transformation in cultured corneal keratocytes. Cornea 15:505, 1996.
84. Fini ME, Girard MT, Matsubara M, et al: Unique regulation of the matrix metalloproteinase, gelatinase B. Invest Ophthalmol Vis Sci 36:622, 1995.
85. Girard MT, Matsubara M, Fini ME: Transforming growth factor-beta and interleukin-1 modulate metalloproteinase expression by corneal stromal cells. Invest Ophthalmol Vis Sci 31:2441, 1991.
86. Jester JV, Barry-Lane P, Petroll WM, et al: Inhibition of corneal fibrosis by topical application of blocking antibodies to TGF beta in the rabbit. Cornea 16:177, 1997.
87. Assouline M, Hutchinson C, Morton K, et al: In vivo binding of topically applied bFGF on rabbit corneal epithelial wound. Growth Factors 1:251, 1989.
88. Phillips K, Arffa R, Cintron C, et al: Effects of prednisolone and medroxyprogesterone on corneal wound healing, ulceration, and neovascularization. Arch Opthalmol 101:640, 1983.
89. O'Brien WJ, Geroski DH: The effects of methylprednisolone acetate on macromolecular synthesis and glycose oxidation in epithelial cells of the ocular surface. Invest Ophthalmol Vis Sci 23:501, 1982.
90. Srinivasan BD, Kulkarni PS, Bhat SP: Differential protein synthesis in steroid-treated ocular surface epithelium. Invest Ophthalmol Vis Sci 27:1005, 1986.
91. Arshinoff SA, Mills MD, Haber S: Pharmacotherapy of photorefractive keratectomy. J Cataract Refract Surg 22:1037, 1996.
92. O'Brart DP, Lohmann CP, Klonos G, et al: The effects of topical corticosteroids and plasmin inhibitors on refractive outcome, haze, and visual performance after photorefractive keratectomy: A prospective, randomized, observer-masked study. Ophthalmology 101:1565, 1994.
93. McCarey BE, Napalkov JA, Pippen PA, et al: Corneal wound healing strength with topical antiinflammatory drugs. Cornea 14:290, 1995.
94. Fagerholm P, Hamberg-Nystrom H, Tengroth B, et al: Effect of postoperative steroids on the refractive outcome of photorefractive keratectomy for myopia with the Summit Excimer laser. J Cataract Refract Surg 20 (Suppl.):212, 1994.
95. Gipson IK, Grill SM, Spurr SJ, et al: Hemidesmosome formation in vitro. J Cell Biol 97:849, 1983.
96. Paterson CA, Wells JG, Koklitis PA, et al: Recombinant tissue inhibitor of metalloproteinases type 1 suppresses alkali-burn-induced corneal ulceration in rabbits. Invest Ophthalmol Vis Sci 35:677, 1994.
97. Petroutsos G, Guimaraes R, Giraud JP, et al: Effect of acetylcysteine (Mucomyst) on epithelial wound healing. Ophthalmic Res 14:241, 1982.
98. Lass JH, Pavan-Langston D, Park NH: Acyclovir and corneal wound healing. Am J Ophthalmol 88:102, 1979.
99. Ali Z, Insler MS: A comparison of therapeutic bandage lenses, tarsorrhaphy, and antibiotic and hypertonic saline on corneal epithelial wound healing. Ann Ophthalmol 18:22, 1986.
100. Shaker GJ, Veda S, LoCascio JA: Effect of a collagen shield on cat corneal epithelial wound healing. Invest Ophthalmol Vis Sci 30:1565, 1989.

101. Wasson PJ, Fujikawa LS, Zagachin LM, et al: Role of fibronectin and fibrinogen in healing of corneal epithelial scrape wounds. Invest Ophthalmol Vis Sci 30:377, 1989.
102. Alfonso E, Kenyon KR, D'Amico DJ, et al: Effects of gentamicin on healing of transdifferentiating conjunctival epithelium in rabbit eyes. Am J Ophthalmol 105:198, 1988.
103. Waterbury L, Kunysz EA, Beuerman R: Effects of steroidal and nonsteroidal anti-inflammatory agents on corneal wound healing. J Ocul Pharmacol 3:43, 1987.
104. Hanna C, Fraunfelder FT, Cable M, et al: The effect of ophthalmic ointments on corneal wound healing. Am J Ophthalmol 76:193, 1973.
105. Robin JB, Kash RL, Azen SP, et al: Lack of effect of pilocarpine on corneal epithelial wound healing. Curr Eye Res 3:403, 1984.
106. Verma S, Corbett MC, Marshall J: A prospective, randomized, double-masked trial to evaluate the role of topical anesthetics in controlling pain after photorefractive keratectomy. Ophthalmology 102:1918, 1995.
107. Kingsley RE, Marfurt CF: Topical substance P and corneal epithelial wound closure in the rabbit. Invest Ophthalmol Vis Sci 38:388, 1997.
108. Donnenfeld ED, Selkin BA, Perry HD, et al: Controlled evaluation of a bandage contact lens and a topical nonsteroidal anti-inflammatory drug in treating traumatic corneal abrasions. Ophthalmology 102:979, 1995.
109. Peyman GA, Rahimy MH, Fernandes ML: Effects of morphine on corneal sensitivity and epithelial wound healing: Implications for topical ophthalmic analgesia. Br J Ophthalmol 78:138, 1994.
110. Loya N, Bassage S, Vyas S, et al: Topical diclofenac following Excimer laser: Effect on corneal sensitivity and wound healing in rabbits. J Refract Corneal Surg 10:423, 1994.
111. Nakamura M, Nishida T, Mishima H, et al: Effects of antimicrobials on corneal epithelial migration. Curr Eye Res 12:733, 1993.
112. Amino K, Takahashi M, Honda Y, et al: Redistribution of fodrin in an in vitro wound healing model of the corneal epithelium. Exp Eye Res 61:501, 1995.
113. Okada Y, Saika S, Hashizume N, et al: Expression of *fos* family and *jun* family proto-oncogenes during corneal epithelial wound healing. Curr Eye Res 15:824, 1996.
114. Takahashi H, Kaminski AE, Zieske JD: Glucose transporter 1 expression is enhanced during corneal epithelial wound repair. Exp Eye Res 63:649, 1996.
115. Lin N, Bazan HE: Protein kinase C substrates in corneal epithelium during wound healing: The phosphorylation of growth associated protein-43 (GAP-43). Exp Eye Res 61:451, 1995.
116. Latvala T, Puolakkainen P, Vesaluoma M, et al: Distribution of SPARC protein (osteonectin) in normal and wounded feline cornea. Exp Eye Res 65:579, 1996.
117. Trocmé SD, Gleich GJ, Kephart GM, et al: Eosinophil granule major basic protein inhibition of corneal epithelial wound healing. Invest Ophthalmol Vis Sci 35:3051, 1994.
118. Wilson SE, He Y-G, Lloyd SA: EGF, EGF receptor, basic FGF, TGF beta-1, and IL-1 alpha mRNA in human corneal epithelial cells and stromal fibroblasts. Invest Ophthalmol Vis Sci 33:1756, 1992.
119. Zieske JD, Wasson M: Regional variation in distribution of EGF receptor in developing and adult corneal epithelium. J Cell Sci 106:145, 1993.
120. Hongo M, Itoi M, Yamaguchi N, et al: Distribution of epidermal growth factor (EGF) receptors in rabbit corneal epithelial cells, keratocytes and endothelial cells, and the changes induced by transforming growth factor-beta1. Exp Eye Res 54:9, 1992.
121. Wilson SE, Walker JW, Chwnag EL, et al: Hepatocyte growth factor, keratinocyte growth factor, their receptors, fibroblast growth factor receptor-2, and the cells of the cornea. Invest Ophthalmol Vis Sci 34:2544, 1993.
122. Li Q, Weng J, Mohan RR, et al: Hepatocyte growth factor and hepatocyte growth factor in the lacrimal gland, tears, and cornea. Invest Ophthalmol Vis Sci 37:727, 1996.
123. Sotozono C, Kinoshita S, Kita M, et al: Paracrine role of keratinocyte growth factor in rabbit corneal epithelial cell growth. Exp Eye Res 59:385, 1994.
124. Joyce NC, Zieske JD: Transforming growth factor-beta receptor expression in human cornea. Invest Ophthalmol Vis Sci 38:1922, 1997.
125. Obata H, Kaburaki T, Kato M, et al: Expression of TGF-beta type I and type II receptors in rat eyes. Curr Eye Res 15:335, 1995.

CHAPTER 37

Angiogenic Factors and Inhibitors

Michael J. Tolentino, Anthony P. Adamis, and Joan W. Miller

New blood vessel formation can occur either through angiogenesis or vasculogenesis.[1] Vasculogenesis is the formation of new vessels from the differentiation of angioblasts that subsequently form primitive blood vessels. Formation of new blood vessels from preexisting microvasculature is called *angiogenesis*. Angiogenesis can occur both physiologically and pathologically. Physiologic angiogenesis occurs mainly in females, during menstruation, ovulation, and the development of the placenta. Pathologic angiogenesis, on the other hand, can occur in both sexes.

In the fully developed adult, ocular angiogenesis in most cases is pathologic and is a major component of several blinding conditions. These conditions include age-related macular degeneration (ARMD), diabetic retinopathy, neovascular glaucoma, corneal neovascularization, retinopathy of prematurity, and intraocular tumors and represent some of the most common causes of blindness in the United States. Understanding the cascade of events that result in angiogenesis can hopefully elucidate ways to inhibit this blinding process.

In this chapter we summarize the steps involved in new vessel formation, research techniques to study angiogenesis, angiogenic factors involved in ocular neovascularization, and newly discovered angiogenesis inhibitors.

Neovascularization

There are two types of angiogenesis, sprouting and nonsprouting (intussusception).[2] The cascade of events that leads to sprouting angiogenesis begins with a dissolution of vessel basement membrane and interstitial matrix. Angiogenesis occurs in response to angiogenic factors that stimulate the migration and proliferation of vascular endothelial cells. Canalization is followed by the formation of branches and loops of confluent sprouts that eventually support blood flow. New vessels can then begin the process of maturation and differentiation by the recruitment of pericytes and the deposition of basement membrane signaling the end of the neovascular cascade (Fig. 37–1).

Nonsprouting angiogenesis involves proliferation of endothelial cells that form a lumen within a preexisting vessel. Interstitial tissue columns in the lumen of preexisting vessels grow, stabilize, and partition the vessel lumen, resulting in new blood vessel formation. Nonsprouting angiogenesis has been described more in the embryonic lung and in tumor models; however, sprouting and nonsprouting angiogenesis can occur concurrently.[2]

Intervention at each step of angiogenesis can be used to inhibit or stimulate new vessel formation. A balance between endogenous stimulators and inhibitors leads to the maintenance of mature vessels, and the control of physiologic neovascularization. An imbalance results in pathologic neovascularization. In ocular neovascularization, overexpression of a stimulator of angiogenesis has been postulated since the late 1940s.[3] It was apparent then that hypoxia and ischemia result in a release of a "factor X" that results in the formation of new blood vessel growth.[4, 5] It is the identification of this factor X and the hope of inhibiting its effect that has spurred interest in angiogenesis research in ophthalmology.

Angiogenesis Research Methodology

The process of new blood vessel growth can be studied by several in vitro and in vivo bioassays. Bioassays are required to define the angiogenic properties of stimulators and inhibitors of angiogenesis. In vitro endothelial cell chemotaxis, proliferation, and lumen formation can be used to define angiogenic or angiostatic activity. In vivo, there are many bioassays of angiogenesis. The chick chorioallantoic membrane (CAM) assay is one of the first in vivo assays used. Many angiogenic assays of ocular neovascularization have been developed. The corneal neovascularization micropocket model is probably the most widely used. Others include the chemical injury– or cautery-induced corneal neovascularization model; the oxygen-cycling–induced model of retinopathy of prematurity; and retinal vein occlusion and laser-induced subretinal neovascularization models. A murine transgenic model of retinal vascular endothelial growth factor (VEGF) upregulation has been developed. Although these models do not fully mimic true ocular disease, they can be used to test the in vivo effects of angiogenic factors and inhibitors in the different vessel beds of the eye.

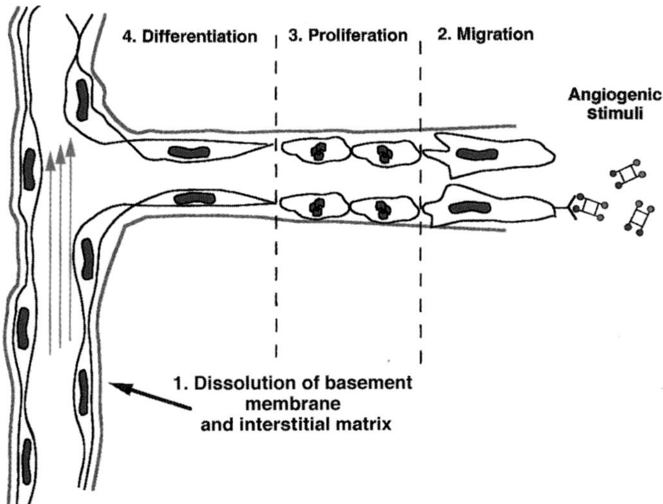

FIGURE 37–1. The cascade of angiogenesis begins with an angiogenic stimulus that leads to the dissolution of basement membrane and extracellular matrix. This allows the endothelial cell to migrate and proliferate. After proliferation, the endothelial cell can differentiate and recruit smooth muscle cells and pericytes, thus signaling the end of neovascularization.

IN VITRO

Capillary Endothelial Cell Culture

Capillary endothelial cell cultures were an important step to study the angiogenic activity of various factors.[6] This technique allows the angiogenic process to be dissected into several steps. With endothelial cell cultures, angiogenesis does not have to be measured as an all-or-nothing event; it can be divided into three steps: proliferation, motility, and capillary tube formation.

Endothelial cell proliferation can be measured by cell counts, thymidine uptake, and other markers of cellular proliferation and can be used to determine the endothelial cell mitogenic activity of various compounds. In the presence of a known angiogenic compound, cellular proliferation can be used to screen for angiostatic compounds. Endothelial cell migration can also be measured using the Boyden chamber assay.[7] This measures the chemotactic activity of various factors.

Capillary tube formation can be measured in several ways. In most cases it requires the growth of endothelial cells into a three-dimensional collagen matrix to form tubelike structures and lumens.[8] A fragment of human placental blood vessel embedded in a fibrin gel can give rise to a complex network of microvessels during a period of 7 to 21 days in culture.[9] Similar tube-formation models have been used to assay angiogenic factors and to screen for angiogenic inhibitors.[10–12] Fibrinolytic activity of cell types may also be predictive of the successful formation of capillary-like structures.[13] The mechanism underlying capillary formation in these in vitro assays is dependent on the matrix the cells are grown on. Plating human umbilical vein endothelial cells on Matrigel, results in a posttranslational-dependent capillary-like formation, whereas plating them on fibrin involves gene transcription and translation.[14] These findings may be helpful in further dissecting the angiogenic process.

IN VIVO

Chick Chorioallantoic Membrane Assay

The CAM assay most commonly involves removing a fertilized chicken egg from its shell and growing it in a Petri

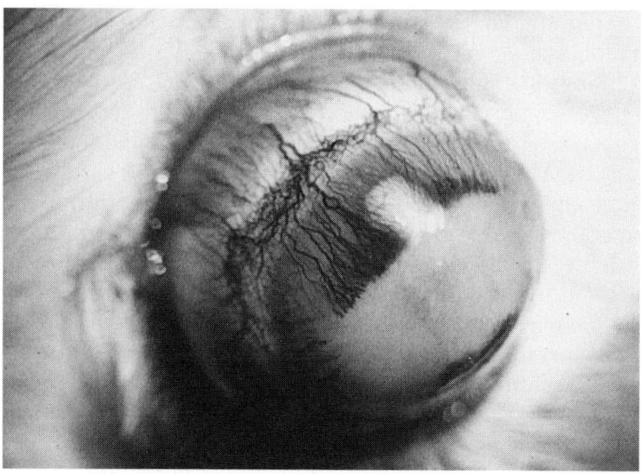

FIGURE 37–2. Corneal neovascularization induced in a mouse cornea by a Hydron pellet impregnated with basic fibroblast growth factor.

dish.[15] Potential angiogenic substances can be placed on the CAM to assay their ability to induce angiogenesis. To quantify angiogenesis, a collagen gel impregnated with an angiogenic factor is situated between nylon mesh and placed on the CAM surface. By counting the squares containing new vessels, one can quantify angiogenesis.[16, 17] This assay has been used to identify angiogenic factors and to test angiogenic inhibitors.[18]

Corneal Neovascularization

One of the most widely used angiogenesis assays involves the implantation of an angiogenic stimulant into a corneal micropocket, which induces vessel growth from the limbus toward the stimulant (Fig. 37–2). Various models have been described in mice, rats, and rabbits using endotoxin, basic fibroblast growth factor (bFGF), VEGF, and other angiogenic compounds contained within sustained-release polymers.[19–23] The rabbit models offer the advantage of size, but the mouse models offer the capability for genetic manipulation. A corneal micropocket model in a knockout or transgenic mice can be a useful assay to determine if a targeted endogenous factor can inhibit or accentuate neovascularization. For these assays to be effective, the bottom of the pocket has to be within a critical distance from the limbus.[20] Chemical cautery, epithelial scraping, and xenograft corneal transplants have been used to develop injury-induced models of corneal neovascularization.[24, 25]

Branch Retinal Vein Occlusion Model

Retinal vein occlusion models in rabbits, pigs, cats, and monkeys have been developed using diathermy and photocoagulation. Various degrees of retinal and iris neovascularization have developed in these models.[26, 27]

In a pig model, photodynamic, laser–induced, branch vein occlusion develops preretinal and optic nerve head neovascularization.[26, 28] A miniature pig model of laser-induced branch retinal vein occlusion develops only preretinal neovascularization.[29]

In monkeys, branch vein occlusions produce intraretinal without preretinal neovascularization.[30] When two temporal retinal veins were occluded, iris neovascularization and disc neovascularization developed in four of six monkeys. Occluding three retinal veins and performing vitrectomy-lensectomy resulted in 100% of monkeys developing iris neovascularization, and 2 of 12 monkeys developed neovascular glaucoma.[31] The use of dye yellow laser produced iris neovascularization in 70 to 95% of monkeys without the need for vitrectomy-lensectomy (Fig. 37–3).[32]

A grading system using standardized fluorescein iris angiograms and masked readers allows semiquantitative analysis in this monkey model. The development of this grading system has allowed the use of the model in the evaluation of angiogenic inhibitors.[27, 33, 34]

A laser-induced venous thrombosis rat model of preretinal neovascularization has been described.[28] With an argon blue-green laser, 70% of the eyes developed retinal neovascularization and traction retinal detachment. Retinal neovascularization included optic disc neovascularization and neovascularization elsewhere.

Retinopathy of Prematurity Model

Retinopathy of prematurity animal models expose the developing retinal vasculature to different cycles of relative hyperoxia and hypoxia. The hyperoxia produces vasoconstriction of the immature retinal vessels, whereas hypoxia produces vasoproliferation characteristic of retinopathy of prematurity.

Several species have been used, including rat, cat, mouse, and dog.[35–40] The models use alteration from high to low oxygen levels in newborn animals to produce preretinal neo-

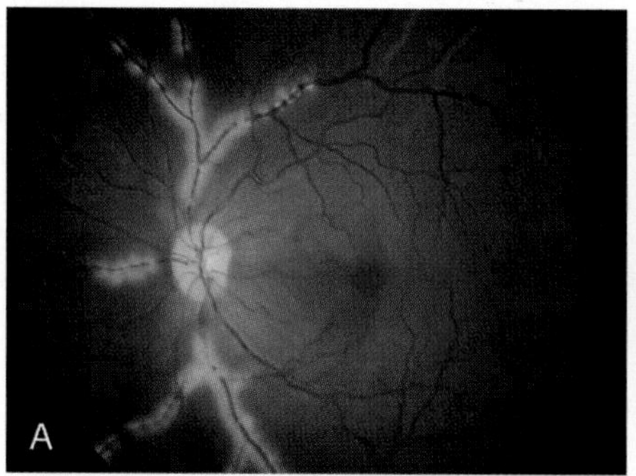

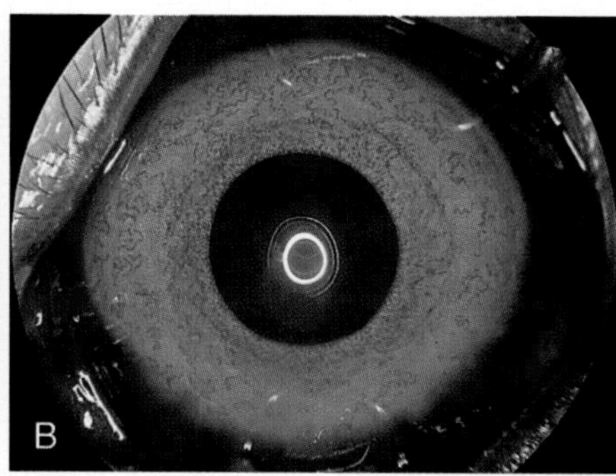

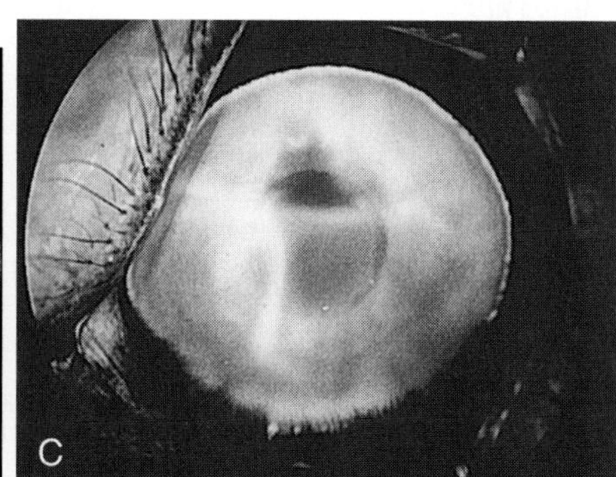

FIGURE 37–3. Iris neovascularization and laser-induced branch retinal vein occlusions. *A,* Laser-photocoagulated retinal veins in a monkey retina. *B,* Subsequent iris neovascularization. *C,* Leakage of fluorescein into the anterior chamber, demonstrating florid iris neovascularization.

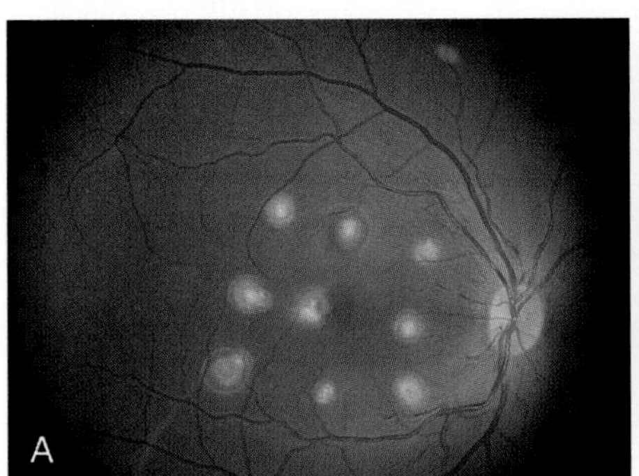

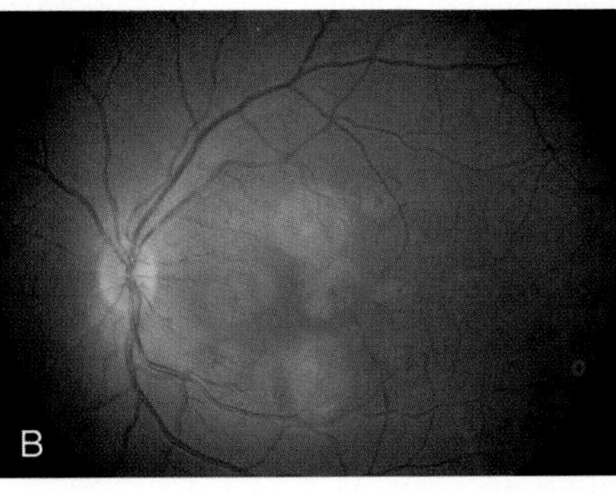

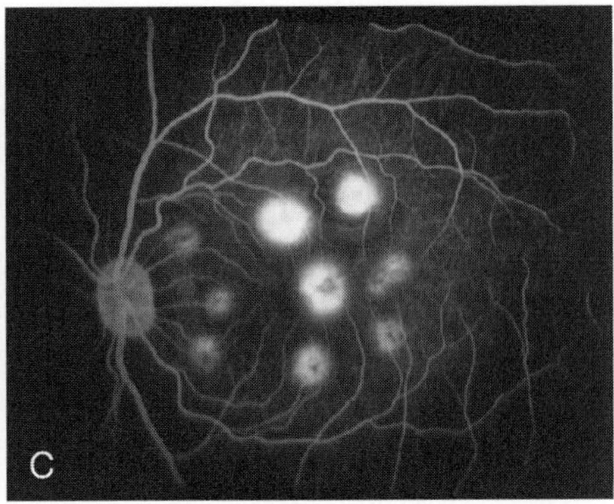

FIGURE 37–4. Laser-induced choroidal neovascularization. *A,* Day 1 after laser treatment. *B,* Four weeks after laser treatment, demonstrating subretinal neovascularization. *C,* Angiographically demonstrated choroidal neovascularization 4 weeks after laser treatment.

vascularization. In a rat model, alternating the oxygen levels from 40 to 80% for several days followed by room air produced histologically confirmed preretinal neovascularization in two-thirds of the animals.[36] In a newborn mouse model, 100% of the animals developed histologically determined preretinal neovascularization when placed in 75% oxygen for 5 days followed by room air.[39]

Laser-Induced Choroidal Neovascularization

A monkey model of choroidal neovascularization was first developed using laser-induced retinal vein occlusion and disruption of Bruch's membrane. The model was inconsistent, and 30% of the monkeys developed retinal neovascularization, with 33% developing vitreous hemorrhage.[41] Argon laser burns to the macular area without retinal vein occlusion produced a higher percentage of monkeys with choroidal neovascularization (Fig. 37–4).[42]

Unlike ARMD, this model is injury induced, but the development of choroidal neovascularization bears many similarities to that of ARMD. The model produces a membrane that leaks fluorescein into the subretinal space.[43] VEGF and -Vβ3 integrin, which have been implicated in choroidal neovascularization, are also expressed in this model.[44, 45]

Transgenic Vascular Endothelial Growth Factor–Dependent Mouse Model

A transgenic mouse overexpressing VEGF in the retina has been created. To produce a VEGF-induced transgenic model of retinal and subretinal neovascularization, a bovine rhodopsin promoter was linked to VEGF complementary DNA. This transgenic mouse produced upregulation of VEGF in the photoreceptors and very limited systemic expression of the transgene. Three transgenic founders were described, and one resulted in intraretinal neovascularization that grew into the subretinal space.[46] Although this pattern of retinal neovascularization is not seen in disease, this model can be a useful means of studying VEGF overexpression and its inhibitors in the eye.

Diabetes Models

Many models of diabetes have been developed using mice, rats, monkeys, and dogs.[47–49] Both bred rats and streptozocin-treated rats have produced consistent models of diabetes.[48] Galactose-fed dogs can produce retinopathy similar to that seen in diabetes.[50] The Koletsky spontaneous hypertensive, non–insulin-dependent rat was observed to have microangiopathic retinopathy with progressive retinal capillary dropout, and elevated vascular tortuosity with fluorescein leakage.[51] The Koletsky rat and galactose-fed dogs are the only two models of diabetes that develop proliferative retinopathy.

Angiogenic Factors

The discovery of specific factors that are operative in angiogenesis has facilitated the accelerated pace of angiogenesis research. Many angiogenic factors have been discovered to date (Table 37–1).

FIBROBLAST GROWTH FACTORS 1 TO 9

Fibroblast growth factors (FGFs) are a family of nine structurally related heparin-binding peptides the first of which was purified from bovine pituitary gland.[52, 53] They are synthesized by fibroblasts, macrophages, endothelial cells, and several neuronal cells.[54] They are acidic FGF(FGF-1), basic FGF (FGF-2; bFGF), int-2 (FGF-3), hst-1/kaposi-FGF

TABLE 37–1. **Angiogenesis Stimulators**

Fibroblast growth factor (FGF)
Vascular endothelial growth factor (VEGF)
Insulin-like growth factor (IGF)
Integrins
αVβ3
αVβ5
Platelet-derived growth factor (PDGF)
Transforming growth factor-α (TGF-α)
Transforming growth factor-β (TGF-β)
Tumor necrosis factor-α (TNF-α)
Matrix metalloproteinases (MMPs)
Placental-derived growth factor (PLGF)
Angiogenin
Angiotropin
Hepatocyte growth factor–scatter factor (HGF-SF)
Chemokines
Interleukin-8 (IL-8)
Low molecular weight factors

(FGF-4), FGF-5, hst-2 (FGF-6), keratinocyte growth factor (FGF-7), androgen-induced growth factor (FGF-8), and glia-activating growth factor (FGF-9).[55] There are four high-affinity tyrosine kinase FGF receptors (FGFr 1 to 4).[55] FGF-1 and FGF-2 are the most studied and well known angiogenic FGFs.

FGF-1[56] and FGF-2[57] are the archetypal members of this family of growth factors. Acidic FGF and bFGF, which share 53% sequence homology[58] and are differentiated by their isoelectric point, are mitogenic to endothelial cells. Acidic FGF has a low isoelectric point and bFGF has a high isoelectric point.

The distribution of the two factors differs in vivo. Although bFGF is found in all tissues, acidic FGF is found only in the neural tissue, including the retina.[59] In addition, bFGF is found in basement membranes bound to heparan sulfate proteoglycans.[60] Heparin protects bFGF from degradation[61] and has a threefold higher affinity for heparin than other growth factors as measured by heparin-Sepharose columns.[53]

There is evidence supporting the role of bFGF in ocular neovascularization. A potent angiogenic factor in vivo, bFGF was found to be responsible for the mitogenic activity[59] present in mammalian retinal extracts.[62] Ocular tissue, in particular retinal pigment epithelium cells[63, 64] and retinal vascular endothelial cells, can synthesize bFGF.[65] Levels of bFGF found in the vitreous specimens of diabetic retinopathy were high enough to produce angiogenesis in vitro. Levels of bFGF were increased in patients with active diabetic retinopathy.[66] In vivo, exogenous intravitreal bFGF increases the uptake of ^{3}H-thymidine in venule and capillary endothelial cells, implying a proliferative effect on retinal vasculature.[67] In addition, bFGF has been shown to upregulate another potent angiogenic factor, VEGF, in vitro, another avenue in which bFGF could stimulate ocular neovascularization.[68] VEGF-189 has also been shown to mediate its angiogenic activity by the release of bFGF in vitro. This could mean that VEGF and bFGF, both potent mitogens, may be involved in a positive-feedback loop that results in a stronger angiogenic response.[69]

Although bFGF may play a role in ocular neovascularization, its properties make it unlikely to be the only angiogenic factor involved. First, bFGF is not a secreted protein. The release of bFGF may occur during cell injury and death.[70] It can be released from the extracellular matrix by heparin displacement or heparinase degradation.[71] The 27-kDa heat shock protein can release bFGF from endothelial cells as well.[72]

The role of bFGF in ischemia-related ocular neovascularization is unclear. Although bFGF receptors are upregulated by hypoxia in vitro, bFGF production actually decreases with hypoxia in retinal cells in vitro.[73, 74] Furthermore, in human diabetic retinas, bFGF immunostaining was localized only with nonproliferating mature retinal vessels with thickened basement membranes but not with proliferating new vessels.[75]

FGF-4 also has been shown to be angiogenic. Its angiogenic activity in vitro is mediated by VEGF upregulation,[76] but its role in vivo is unclear.

VASCULAR ENDOTHELIAL GROWTH FACTOR

VEGF refers to a family of alternatively spliced peptides (121, 165, 189, 201).[77] VEGF is produced by macrophages, T cells, smooth muscle cells, astrocytes, Müller's cells, and retinal pigment epithelial cells.[78–82] VEGF has at least two tyrosine kinase receptors, flt-1 and flk-1/KDR, that mediate its activity[83, 84] and are found almost exclusively on vascular endothelial cells in vivo.[85–87]

VEGF was first described as a vascular permeability factor isolated from tumor-induced ascitic fluid.[88] Its permeability-enhancing property may be related to its fenestration-inducing ability in blood vessels.[89] It was later cloned and found to be angiogenic.[90, 91]

This angiogenic, endothelial-specific mitogen possesses many properties that implicate it in ocular neovascularization. VEGF is a soluble molecule[92] made and secreted by neural retinal cells[82] and glial cells in culture.[93, 94] In vitro, hypoxia upregulates VEGF in retinal and[74, 95] retinal glial cells[94] and is the major endothelial cell mitogen made by hypoxic retinal cells in vitro.[74]

In vivo, VEGF messenger RNA (mRNA) and protein levels were temporally and spatially correlated with the degree of iris neovascularization in a monkey branch retinal vein occlusion model[27] and in the mouse model of retinopathy of prematurity.[96] Specific inhibition of VEGF by a neutralizing antibody in the monkey model demonstrated a complete inhibition of iris neovascularization.[34] Retinal neovascularization was suppressed using a VEGF receptor chimeric protein in the mouse model.[97] Intravitreal injections of bioactive VEGF at regular intervals into a normal monkey eye produced stereotypical iris neovascularization and neovascular glaucoma.[98] In the retina, these injections cause hemorrhages, edema, microaneurysms, venous beading, capillary occlusion, and intraretinal vascular proliferation.[99]

The role of VEGF in nonproliferative and proliferative diabetic retinopathy is becoming better characterized. In patients with proliferative diabetic retinopathy, vitreous levels of VEGF protein[100–102] and mRNA are upregulated.[103] In patients who have nonproliferative diabetic retinopathy, VEGF protein has been localized to the glial cells of the retina and optic nerve.[93, 104] In a diabetic rat, VEGF mRNA expression and protein synthesis are increased in retinas with nonproliferative retinopathy.[105, 106]

Although the role of VEGF in early diabetic retinopathy is unclear, multiple potential stimuli for VEGF upregulation are present. Advanced glycation end products upregulate VEGF production in vitro and in vivo.[107] Reactive oxygen intermediates, a species of molecules associated with diabetic retinopathy, are known to upregulate VEGF.[108] Insulin-like growth factor (IGF) and hyperglycemia can also stimulate VEGF upregulation.[109] VEGF upregulation in a branch retinal vein occlusion monkey model can be reversed with systemic hyperoxia, implicating hypoxia as a critical stimulator of VEGF in vivo.[110] Furthermore, in the mouse model of retinopathy of prematurity, systemic hyperoxia also decrease retinal VEGF levels.[111] Panretinal photocoagulation, the present treatment for diabetic retinal neovascularization, is an example of how decreasing relative hypoxia in the retina can ameliorate retinal neovascularization.

VEGF is also critical in wound and inflammation-induced corneal neovascularization. Antibodies to VEGF in a sustained-release Hydron pellet were capable of inhibiting wound- and inflammation-induced corneal neovascularization.[25] This implicates VEGF in inflammatory-mediated neovascularization.

Indirect evidence demonstrates the involvement of VEGF in choroidal neovascularization. In laser-induced choroidal neovascularization models, VEGF expression was demonstrated.[44, 112, 113] Surgically removed choroidal neovascular membranes and autopsy specimens of patients with ARMD demonstrated immunopositive expression of VEGF.[114–117] Choroidal fibroblasts upregulate VEGF when challenged with transforming growth factor-β (TGF-β), interleukin-1 (IL-1), and phorbol esters,[118] more data supporting a role for VEGF in choroidal neovascularization.

Strong evidence supports VEGF's role in ischemia-related ocular neovascularization. Its role in choroidal neovascularization and inflammation-induced neovascularization is still under investigation.

INSULIN-LIKE GROWTH FACTOR-I

The insulin-like growth factors (IGF-I and IGF-II), single-chain peptides that share 70% homology with insulin,[119] were first identified as peptides that mediate the effects of growth hormone on the incorporation of sulfate by cartilage in vitro.[120] In the blood, multiple IGF-binding proteins modulate IGF's half-life and activity.[121] The major source of production is the liver, although many cell types produce IGF.

IGF-I is angiogenic in vitro and in vivo. It stimulates bovine aortic endothelial cell and retinal capillary endothelial cell proliferation and migration.[122] Cultured retinal pericytes and microvascular endothelial cells express IGF receptors and when challenged with IGF-I, demonstrate increased DNA synthesis.[123]

In the rabbit corneal micropocket model, Elvax pellets impregnated with IGF-I stimulated corneal neovascularization. Intravitreal injection of IGF-I, in pharmacologic amounts, produces vascular tortuosity, hemorrhage, optic disc hyperemia, and fluorescein angiographic leakage suggestive of neovascularization.[124] IGF-I also upregulates VEGF in vitro and in vivo, a possible mechanism for its angiogenic activity.[109]

IGF has been implicated in diabetic retinopathy. Hypophysectomy leads to the remission or reduction of the severity of diabetic retinopathy,[125, 126] and this is evidence that growth hormone–like factors may play a role in diabetic retinopathy. In diabetes, elevated IGF-I serum levels are correlated with proliferative diabetic retinopathy.[127] Vitreous levels of IGF-I, IGF-II, IGF-binding protein-3 and IGF-binding protein-2 are also increased in patients with proliferative diabetic retinopathy.[119] These correlations support this growth factor's role in diabetic-related ocular neovascularization.

INTEGRINS

Integrins are a family of cell adhesion proteins consisting of 15α and 8β subunits that combine and are expressed as heterodimers. These heterodimers bind to short-peptide-sequence extracellular matrix ligands. An example of a short peptide that is recognized by several integrins is the Arg-Gly-Asp (RGD) tripeptide.[128]

Both αVβ3 and αVβ5 have been implicated in angiogenesis. αVβ3 is upregulated on proliferating blood vessels induced by bFGF in the corneal micropocket assay and the CAM.[129, 130] Inhibition of αVβ3 inhibits angiogenesis, demonstrating the necessity of this integrin in the cascade of FGF-induced corneal neovascularization.[130] The mechanism by which antagonism of αVβ3 inhibits angiogenesis is by promoting programmed cell death (apoptosis) in newly sprouting blood vessels. This was observed in the bFGF-induced CAM and in tumors.[131]

In ocular neovascularization, αVβ3 is upregulated in a laser-induced choroidal neovascularization model.[45] Antagonism of this integrin may be a useful target in inhibiting choroidal neovascularization.

PLATELET-DERIVED GROWTH FACTOR

Platelet-derived growth factor (PDGF), is a dimeric molecule of disulfide-bonded A or B polypeptide chains, or both (PDGF-AA/AB/BB). Two PDGF receptors exist, α and β, which dimerize after ligand exposure. The α-receptor binds both A and B chains, whereas the β-receptor preferentially binds the B chain.[132] PDGF-BB has a greater angiogenic response on the CAM assay than PDGF-AA. In vitro, PDGF-BB is more potent than PDGF-AA in stimulating rat brain capillary endothelial cells chemotaxis.[133] Hypoxic macrophages upregulate PDGF, which is mitogenic for endothelial cells.[134] Macrophages may act in a paracrine way to stimulate angiogenesis in hypoxia-induced ocular neovascularization. PDGF can also act indirectly to stimulate angiogenesis by inducing connective tissue in the vicinity of endothelial cells to upregulate angiogenic factors.[135]

TRANSFORMING GROWTH FACTOR-α

Transforming growth factors (TGFs), polypeptides produced by tumors and transformed cells, can confer phenotypic properties associated with transformation on normal cells in culture; thus their name.[136] Transforming growth factor-α (TGF-α), a 50–amino acid polypeptide related to epidermal growth factor, binds to the EGF receptor.[137]

TGF-α is an angiogenic stimulator in vitro and in vivo. It binds endothelial cells and stimulates DNA synthesis in these cells. TGF-α also induced capillary-like tube formation into collagen gel in an in vitro model.[138] In vivo, TGF-α promotes angiogenesis.[137]

TRANSFORMING GROWTH FACTOR-β

Transforming growth factor-β (TGF-β) is a 25,000-kD polypeptide that is not biochemically related to TGF-α. There are three isoforms of TGF-β: β1, β2, and β3.[139] Of all the isoforms, TGF-β1 is the most abundant. TGF-β1 can be found in both latent and activated form. Activated TGF-β is a potent inhibitor of endothelial cell DNA synthesis and growth in vitro.[140] Conversely, in vivo it has angiogenic-promoting activity[141] and can promote tube formation in cultures.[142] One explanation for this dual role is that activated TGF-β1 is a potent angiogenesis inhibitor but can indirectly stimulate angiogenesis by upregulating VEGF. TGF-β1 has been shown to upregulate VEGF in endothelial and fibroblast cell cultures.[143]

It is apparent that the activity of TGF-β is regulated at the level of activation. Activators of TGF-β in vivo include plasminogen activator and type IV collagenase, a matrix metalloproteinase (MMP). Besides its angiogenic inhibitory and stimulatory properties, TGF-β can recruit inflammatory cells, which may contribute to its angiogenic activity in vivo.[144]

Another possible role of TGF-β may be as an endogenous angiogenic inhibitor. Pericytes inhibit the growth of endothelial cells in coculture systems. An active form of TGF-β was found to be responsible for this inhibition.[144] The loss of pericytes in the early stages of diabetic retinopathy can prime the endothelial cell to be more responsive to proliferative stimuli by eliminating the TGF-β–mediated steady-state inhibition of endothelial cell proliferation.

Maturation of newly formed vessels can signal the cessation of angiogenesis. Activated TGF-β1 has been shown to mature migrated and divided cells.[119, 141] This maturation signal may be involved in TGF-β's angiogenic inhibitory activity.

TGF-β is also a central factor in wound repair. It induces angiogenesis, fibrosis, and collagen formation.[145] In ocular neovascularization, TGF-β's role is probably dependent on its surrounding environment, which can either activate the factor or keep it latent.

TUMOR NECROSIS FACTOR-α

Tumor necrosis factor-α (TNF-α), a macrophage-monocyte–derived polypeptide, induces angiogenesis and modulates the expression of various genes in vascular endothelial cells. TNF-α, also named cachectin, is an inflammatory cytokine that is a central regulator of local inflammation. It is responsible for the activation of endothelial cells by inducing expression of many genes involved in thrombosis, cytoadhesion, and inflammation. TNF-α also affects many sites in the proteolytic cascade responsible for endothelial cell basement membrane breakdown and remodeling, one of the initial steps of angiogenesis.[146]

TNF-α promotes or inhibits angiogenesis. It induces new vessel growth in the rabbit cornea[147] and in the CAM assay.[148] It can stimulate endothelial cell chemotaxis in vitro.[148] TNF-α's ability to stimulate angiogenesis both in vitro and in vivo may result from upregulation of IL-8, VEGF, and bFGF.[149] Another mechanism could result from upregulation of MMP, which is an initiating step in the angiogenic cascade.[150]

TNF-α also inhibits angiogenesis. It inhibits FGF-induced endothelial cell proliferation,[147] monolayer integrity,[151] and tube formation in vitro.[152] The inhibitory activity of the endothelial cell is from the transcriptional downregulation of the VEGF KDR/flk-1 and flt-1 endothelial cell–specific receptors.[153] On the other hand, its inhibitory and stimulatory effect on endothelial cells is dependent on its concentration. Low levels of TNF-α are angiogenic, whereas high concentrations are angiostatic.[154] These properties allow TNF-α to influence the balance between angiogenic stimulation and inhibition.

Its role in ocular neovascularization is not determined, but there is evidence that TNF-α is upregulated in the vitreous of diabetic persons with neovascular eye disease.[155]

MATRIX METALLOPROTEINASES

MMPs are members of the multigene family of metal-dependent enzymes. They are zinc-binding, calcium-dependent neutral endopeptidases that degrade the extracellular matrix.[156] These enzymes are the collagenases (MMP-1, MMP-8, and MMP-13), the gelatinases (MMP-2 and MMP-9), and the stromelysins (MMP-3, MMP-10, MMP-11, and MMP-12).

There is strong evidence that the MMPs play a critical role in angiogenesis. It has been shown that a collagenase (MMP-1) capable of degrading type I collagen is required for angiogenesis in vitro.[157] Considering that type I collagen constitutes the major protein found in the perivascular extracellular matrix, type 1 collagen degradation would be an important step in the initiation of angiogenesis.

Further evidence for MMP's role in angiogenic initiation is bFGF's ability to upregulate MMP-1 and gelatinase in endothelial cells[152] and VEGF's ability to selectively upregulate MMP-1 in human umbilical vein endothelial cells.[158] MMP-2 alone can also enhance capillary tube formation in a Matrigel model of capillary tube formation.[159] Inhibition of MMPs resulting in inhibition of capillary tube formation in vitro provides further evidence of the critical role of MMPs. When an MMP inhibitor, BB-94 (batimastat), and tissue inhibitor of metalloproteinase-1 (TIMP-1) were used, both collagen degradation and in vitro capillary tube formation were significantly inhibited.[160]

PLACENTAL-DERIVED GROWTH FACTOR

The placental-derived growth factor (PLGF) is a dimeric glycoprotein showing a high degree of sequence similarity to VEGF. There are two alternatively spliced forms, PLGF-1 and PLGF-2, differing by the insertion of a highly basic carboxyl end 21–amino acid stretch. PLGF-1 is angiogenic on both the rabbit cornea and the chick CAM assays. In vitro, PLGF-1 induced cell growth and migration in bovine coronary postcapillary venules and in endothelial cells from human umbilical veins.[161] Its role in ocular angiogenesis is not known, but two isoforms of PLGF have been shown to be ligands for flt-1 but not KDR the two known tyrosine kinase receptors for VEGF. This suggests that PLGF plays a role as a redundancy mechanism in situations of limited VEGF.[162]

ANGIOGENIN

Angiogenin is a 14.4-kDa human secreted plasma protein with 65% homology to RNase A, a transfer RNA–specific RNase[163] that is a normal constituent of human plasma. Angiogenin is produced in various cells including vascular endothelial cells from saphenous and umbilical veins, aortic smooth muscle cells, fibroblasts, and tumor cells.[164] It was originally isolated from conditioned medium of human adenocarcinoma. Although not angiogenic in vitro, it is angiogenic in the rabbit cornea and CAM assay.[165] Its angiogenic activity appears to be dependent on two histidine residues, His-13 and His-114.[166] Two peptide antagonists of human angiogenin that inhibit its neovascular activity have been developed.[167] In ocular neovascularization, angiogenin levels are not significantly more elevated in eyes with proliferative diabetic retinopathy than in eyes with proliferative vitreoretinopathy,[168] but the levels are more elevated than in eyes without blood retinal barrier disruption. This factor may play a role as an indirect stimulator of angiogenesis.

ANGIOTROPIN

Angiotropin is a porcine peripheral monocyte-derived differentiation factor for microvascular endothelial cells. It is a copper-containing polyribonucleopeptide. Angiogtropin is not mitogenic for capillary endothelial cells but causes migration of endothelial cells and the formation of capillary-like structures in gelatinized plates. It is postulated that angiotropin is involved in monocyte-induced angiogenesis.[169] In an ear lobe model in rabbits, angiotropin induced angiogenesis. This ear lobe angiogenesis is not inhibited by local dexamethasone and resembles changes found in the undamaged skin margin of a primary healing wound during the inflammatory-proliferative phase.[170]

HEPATOCYTE GROWTH FACTOR–SCATTER FACTOR

Scatter factors (SFs), 90-kD heterodimeric proteins, are trypsin- and heat-sensitive cytokines secreted by vascular smooth muscle and fibroblastic cells. SF, a fibroblast-secreted epithelial motility factor, and hepatocyte growth factor (HGF), a hepatocyte mitogen, were found to be identical molecules.[171] Although this factor (HGF-SF) can stimulate motility in epithelial and endothelial cells, it is also chemotaxic and chemokinetic to vascular endothelium and can induce in vitro capillary-like structures on a basement membrane surface.[172] HGF-SF acts through a tyrosine kinase receptor encoded by the *MET* protooncogene and has been shown to be a potent stimulator of angiogenesis in vivo.[173, 174] Both bFGF and IL-1 upregulate HGF-SF in vitro.[175] HGF-SF mediates its angigogenic activity in vivo through platelet-activating factor.[176] HGF-SF is a multifunctional angiogenic factor whose role in ocular neovascularization is still under investigation.

CHEMOKINES

There are two classes of chemokines, a multigene family of low molecular weight proteins that share four highly conserved cysteine residues. The α class is characterized by a motif that has two cysteine residues separated by another amino acid at the amino terminus. The α-gene family includes several factors known to be angiogenesis stimulators and inhibitors of angiogenesis such as platelet factor 4, Gro-B, and interferon-inducible protein 10. The β-gene family, which is characterized by two adjacent cysteine residues at the amino terminus, has not been implicated in angiogenesis.

The presence or absence in its protein structure of the Glu-Leu-Arg sequence (the ELR motif) appears to determine the angiogenic stimulatory or inhibitory activity of chemokines. Chemokines platelet factor 4, interferon-γ–inducible protein 10, and monokine induced by interferon-γ are angiogenic inhibitors and do not have the ELR motif. Chemokines with the ELR motif such as IL-8 and epithelial neutrophil-activated protein (ENA-78) are angiogenic in vitro and in vivo.[177] In addition, when the ELR motif is substituted in IL-8, the mutated molecule is an inhibitor of angiogenesis.[177]

INTERLEUKIN-8

IL-8 is a chemokine angiogenic factor that is chemotactic for lymphocytes and neutrophils. It is potently angiogenic when implanted in the rat cornea and induces proliferation and chemotaxis of human umbilical vein endothelial cells. It seems to have a function in macrophage-associated, angiogenesis-dependent disorders such as rheumatoid arthritis, tumor growth, and wound repair.[178] IL-8 is upregulated by TNF-α and appears to mediate some of the angiogenic activity of TNF-α.[149] Its role in ocular neovascularization is still under investigation.

The existence of a multigene family that can act as both angiogenic inhibitors and angiogenic stimulators is consistent with the paradigm that angiogenesis is regulated by a balance of stimulators and inhibitors. The ELR motif appears to be important in the ligand-receptor interaction with neutrophils. Chemokines with this motif demonstrate biologic activation of neutrophils. This balance of angiostatic and angiogenic chemokines could play a role in the regulation of neovascularization.

LOW MOLECULAR WEIGHT ANGIOGENIC FACTORS

Several low molecular weight nonpolypeptide compounds such as 1-butyrylglycerol, prostaglandins E_1 and E_2, hyaluronic acid degradation products, nicotinamide, adenosine, and other factors isolated from tumors and tissues have shown angiogenic properties. They have yet to be fully characterized.[179]

Cofactors of Angiogenesis

FIBRONECTIN

Fibronectin is a component of the extracellular matrix of developing microvessels whose role in angiogenesis is poorly understood. It promotes the tube elongation of capillary structures but has no effect on microvascular DNA synthesis.[180] It is thought that fibronectin promotes angiogenesis and microvessel elongation as a result of an adhesion-dependent migratory recruitment of endothelial cells that does not require increased cell proliferation.[181]

ANGIOPOIETIN AND TIE

Angiopoietin 1 is a 70-kD glycoprotein that is the ligand for the endothelial cell–specific Tie2 tyrosine kinase receptor. It is a factor involved in angiogenesis but is neither an endothelial mitogen nor an inducer of tube formation. It is theorized that this factor may play a role in the assembly of nonendothelial cell components.[182] Mice deficient in angiopoietin 1 have shown a failure to recruit smooth muscle and pericyte precursors.[183]

Tie2 is a tyrosine kinase receptor expressed almost exclusively in endothelial cells and early hematopoietic cells. It is required for the normal development of vascular structures during embryogenesis. Both angiogenic and quiescent vasculature in adult tissue express activated Tie2 receptor, indicating a possible role of Tie2 in vascular maintenance.[184] Embryonic lethality results from disruption of the function of Tie2 in transgenic mice, indicating an important role for the Tie2—Tie2 ligand pathway during the development of the embryonic vasculature. A role for this ligand-receptor is seen in tumor angiogenesis as well.[185]

A unifying theory regarding angiopoietin 1 and Tie2's role in blood vessel formation is that angiopoietin, through Tie2, signals the production of PDGF-BB or PDGF-AA, which in turn recruit mesenchymal cells. Once mesenchymal cells contact endothelium, contact inhibition mediated by TGF-β occurs, and differentiation into pericytes and smooth muscle of the mesenchymal cell signals the maturation of the growing blood vessel.[182]

Angiopoietin 2, a molecule homologous to angiopoietin 1, is a naturally occurring antagonist for angiopoietin 1 and the Tie2 receptor. Transgenic overexpression of angiopoietin 2 disrupts blood vessel formation in the mouse embryo. Angiopoietin 2 is expressed only at sites of vascular remodeling.[186] The angiopoietin and Tie receptor role in ocular neovascularization is still under investigation.

Angiogenesis Inhibitors

In 1972, Dr. Judah Folkman proposed the potential therapeutic benefit of inhibiting new blood vessel growth in tumors.[187] At that time, there were no known angiogenesis inhibitors. The first inhibitor discovered was found in cartilage, although the actual factor was not fully purified.[188] Subsequently, protamine was reported to be an angiogenesis inhibitor.[189] Angiostatic steroids were the next inhibitors of angiogenesis discovered,[190] followed by the angioinhibins, a family of fungus-derived compounds that are relatives of fumagillin, an antiamebic drug. AGM-1470, renamed TNP-470, a synthetic analog of fumagillin, was found to inhibit both tumor and corneal neovascularization.[191, 192]

Interferon-α was initially described as an inhibitor of capillary endothelial cell migration in vitro.[193] It was later found to be a clinically useful angiogenic inhibitor in pulmonary hemangiomatosis.[194]

There has been explosion in the number of angiogenic inhibitors (Table 37–2). There is a multigene family of low molecular weight proteins with conserved N-terminal cysteine residues called *chemokines*. The specific inhibition of clinically relevant angiogenic factors has uncovered several potent inhibitors of angiogenesis. Several angiogenic inhibitors have been discovered to be endogenous proteins. These proteins are fragments of larger endogenous proteins. Angiogenic inhibitors have also been identified from antibiotics, sedatives, chemotherapeutic agents, and MMP inhibitors.

Efforts to identify angiogenic inhibitors from avascular tissue has been under way for many years. Avascular tissues being studied include cartilage, cornea, and vitreous. In addition, several dietary-derived inhibitors have been discovered. The screening of tumors for the secretion of angiogenic inhibitors has proved to be a promising strategy. Following is a summary of the known major inhibitors of angiogenesis.

TABLE 37–2. **Angiogenesis Inhibitors**

Angiogenesis Inhibitors
Angiostatic steroids
Angioinhibins
TNP-470 (AGM-1470)
Dietary-derived inhibitors
Thalidomide
Chemokines
Platelet factor 4 (PF-4)
Interferon-Inducible protein 10 (IP-10)
Interleukin-12 (IL-12)
Gro-β
Matrix metalloproteinases (MMPs)
Tissue inhibitors of matrix metalloproteinases (TIMPs)
VEGF inhibitors
VEGF upregulation inhibitors
Endogenous inhibitors
16-kDa N-terminal fragment of prolactin
Thrombospondin (TSP)
Angiostatin
Endostatin
Ion channel blockers
Chemotherapeutic agents
Antibiotics

ANGIOSTATIC STEROIDS

The first steroid inhibitor of angiogenesis was found when cortisone and heparin were applied together on a CAM assay. Interestingly, angiogenic inhibition was independent of heparin's anticoagulant activity and cortisone's glucocorticoid or mineralocorticoid activity.[190] Using the CAM as an assay for an antiangiogenic index, several steroid compounds were tested in the presence of heparin for relative angiostatic potency. In decreasing order of potency, tetrahydrocortisol followed by 17α-hydroxyprogesterone, hydrocortisone, 11α-epihydrocortisol, cortexolone, corticosterone, desoxycorticosterone, testosterone, and estrone were found to be angiostatic. Progesterone, pregnenolone, and cholesterol had no antiangiogenic effect.[195] Tetrahydrocortisol, a metabolite of cortisol with no glucocorticoid or mineralocorticoid properties, is the most potent angiostatic steroid. Other steroids such as cortexolone and 17α-hydroxyprogesterone also lack gluco- and mineralocorticoid activity but are antiangiogenic. Identification of the relative antiangiogenic activity of these steroids has allowed a rational approach in identifying likely angiostatic steroids.

A proposed mechanism by which angiostatic steroids and heparin effect their angiogenic inhibition may involve these compounds' ability to induce basement membrane breakdown, capillary retraction, and endothelial cell rounding.[196] The use of L-proline analogs, which inhibit collagen synthesis in combination with angiostatic steroids, demonstrated an increase in angiogenic activity.[197] In the chick CAM system, heparin plus cortisone caused a marked depression in the rate of collagenous protein biosynthesis during the inhibition of angiogenesis.[198] These observations support the role of extracellular matrix alteration as a potential mechanism for the inhibitory activity of angiostatic steroids.

Angiostatic steroids in combination with β-cyclodextrin tetradecasulfate, a heparin-like molecule with little or no anticoagulant activity, inhibit capillary endothelial cell migration in vitro.[199] In an endotoxin-induced corneal neovascularization model, this combination inhibited corneal neovascularization.[200] Two other compounds, both angiogenic inhibitors by themselves, aurintricarboxylic acid, a nonsulfated aromatic compound, and suramin, have both been shown to potentiate the angiogenic inhibitory effect of angiostatic steroids.[201, 202]

An angiostatic steroid that does not require heparin or a cyclodextrin for its antiangiogenic activity is 2-methoxyestradiol, an endogenous estrogen metabolite that inhibits endothelial cell proliferation, migration, and angiogenesis in vitro.[203] In vivo it was shown in the CAM assay to inhibit angiogenesis.[204] 2-Methoxyestradiol is a potent inhibitor of tubulin assembly.[204] Another tubulin assembly inhibitor, taxol, is an angiogenic inhibitor, but 2-methoxyestradiol is more potent. Vincristine and colchicine, both tubulin assembly inhibitors, demonstrate no antiangiogenic activity.[205]

Several angiostatic steroids have been tested in ocular neovascularization models. Intravitreal injection of triamcinolone acetonide inhibited neovascularization in a pig model of preretinal and optic nerve head neovascularization[206] and in a nonhuman primate model of subretinal neovascularization.[207] In a rabbit model of corneal neovascularization, topical application of novel angiostatic steroid AL-3789 inhibited neovascularization.[208]

ANGIOINHIBINS

TNP-470

TNP-470, formerly known as AGM-1470, is a synthetic analog of fumagillin, a naturally secreted antibiotic of *Aspergillus fumigatus fresenius.* This fungus was first isolated from a contaminated capillary endothelial cell culture that demonstrated capillary endothelial cell growth inhibition. Fumagillin was isolated and purified and found to inhibit endothelial cell proliferation in vitro and tumor-induced angiogenesis in vivo. TNP-470 is a potent inhibitor of angiogenesis.[191] Compared with its parent, fumagillin, TNP-470 is less toxic and more potent.[209]

The mechanism of action of TNP-470 may be related to its binding protein, which is found to be a metalloproteinase, methionine aminopeptidase, whose function has not yet been elucidated.[210, 211] It is possible that methionine aminopeptidase may play a role in the antiangiogenic effects of TNP-470. As a binding protein, it may prove to be a useful target in the development of future angiogenic inhibitors.

Although the exact mechanism of action of TNP-470's angiogenic inhibitory activity is not known, many studies have shown its ability to inhibit various tumors[212–219] as well as collagen-induced arthritis through its angiogenic activity.[220, 221] TNP-470 may also play a future role in the prevention of Tenon's fibroblast encapsulation, a common cause of bleb failure in glaucoma surgery. TNP-470 inhibits Tenon's fibroblast proliferation and may prove promising during filtering surgery.[222]

TNP-470 has undergone a dose-escalation phase 1 clinical trial in patients with human immunodeficiency virus–associated Kaposi's sarcoma. Concentrations of TNP-470 that show in vitro activity were achievable in vivo. Clearance of the drug was rapid.[223] Although no side effects were seen in humans, TNP-470 stimulates B-cell proliferation in mice.[224] The clinical relevance of this finding is not known.

Other Angioinhibins

Other fungus-derived compounds have been developed. One angioinhibin is FR-111142, which is produced by the fungus *Scolecobasidium arenarium.* It inhibits endothelial cell proliferation in vitro and angiogenesis in the growing chick CAM model in vivo and suppresses solid tumor growth in mice.[225]

DIETARY-DERIVED INHIBITORS OF ANGIOGENESIS.

Genistein is a synthetic isoflavonoid compound found in the fractionated urine of humans consuming a plant-based diet. It is an inhibitor of endothelial cell proliferation and in vitro angiogenesis.[226] More potent structurally related flavonoids have been isolated: 3-hydroxyflavone, 3′4′-dihydroxyflavone, 2′3′-dihydroxyflavone, fisetin, apigenin, and luteolin. These compounds inhibit both tumor cell proliferation and in vitro angiogenesis.[227] *Viscum album coloratum, a* Korean mistletoe, has been shown to inhibit angiogenesis by inducing TNF-α.[228]

THALIDOMIDE

The teratogen thalidomide has been resurrected as an inhibitor of angiogenesis, a property unrecognized due to its rat-based preclinical trials. Because thalidomide requires metabolism by the liver, in vivo assays such as the CAM assay do not demonstrate angiogenic inhibition. Orally administered thalidomide has, however, been shown to be an inhibitor of angiogenesis in the bFGF-induced rabbit cornea micropocket model[229] and mouse cornea micropocket assay. In the mouse model, intraperitoneal thalidomide but not orally administered thalidomide inhibits corneal neovascularization. Metabolites and analogs of thalidomide have been tested, and the $S(-)$ enantiomer of thalidomide shows the strongest antiangiogenic activity in both VEGF-induced and bFGF-induced corneal neovascularization.[230]

CHEMOKINES

Although the nonadjacent cysteine residues are highly conserved, in platelet factor 4 they do not appear to be important for their effect on endothelial cell inhibition. What appears to be important is the absence of the sequence Glu-Leu-Arg (the ELR motif). Chemokines platelet factor 4, interferon-γ–inducible protein 10, and monokine induced by interferon-γ are angiogenic inhibitors and do not have the ELR motif. Chemokines with the ELR motif such as IL-8 and epithelial neutrophil–activated protein (ENA-78) are angiogenic in vitro and in vivo.[177] In addition, when the ELR motif was substituted in IL-8, the mutated molecule was found to be an inhibitor of angiogenesis.[177] These data support the premise that the ELR motif is important in the angiogenic or anti-angiogenic activity of chemokines.

Platelet Factor 4

Platelet factor 4 is an α-class chemokine that was originally purified from the α-granules of platelets.[231] Platelet factor 4 was then found to inhibit endothelial cell migration and proliferation in vitro,[232] as well as in vivo angiogenesis in the CAM assay[233] and in a mouse tumor model.[234] In an animal model of intracerebral gliomas, treatment with a retroviral and adenoviral vector expressing secretable platelet factor 4 inhibited tumor-associated angiogenesis and prolonged animal survival.[235] Although it is a selective inhibitor of endothelial cells, it is not a potent inhibitor of angiogenesis. Proteolytic cleavage downstream of the N-terminal cysteine residues results in a 30- to 50-fold increase in endothelial cell inhibitory activity. The mechanism of its antiangiogenic effect is still not known, but it is thought that platelet factor 4 can block basic fibroblast growth factor's mitogenic effect on endothelial cells.[236] Its inhibitory activity is apparently independent of its heparin-binding capabilities. An analog of human platelet factor 4 lacking affinity for heparin demonstrated angiogenic inhibitory activity similar to that of native platelet factor 4.[237]

Interferon-Inducible Protein 10

Interferon-inducible protein 10 is an α-chemokine that is known to inhibit bone marrow colony formation, has antitumor activity in vivo, is chemoattractant for human monocytes and T cells, and promotes T-cell adhesion to endothelial cells. It is a potent angiogenic inhibitor that inhibits bFGF-induced in vivo neovascularization and capillary tube formation in vitro.[238] It has been shown to inhibit IL-8 and bFGF-induced angiogenic activity both in vitro and in vivo.[239] Its angiogenic inhibitory activity may be correlated to the absence of the ELR motif.[177]

Interleukin-12

IL-12 is a strong inhibitor of neovascularization. In vitro, it inhibits endothelial cell proliferation, and in vivo, it inhibits new vessel growth in the CAM assay and corneal micropocket model. Interferon-γ–neutralizing antibodies prevent its inhibitory activity, suggesting that IL-12's inhibitory activity is mediated through interferon-γ. IL-12 has been shown to induce interferon-γ, which, in turn, may mediate IL-12's antiangiogenic activity.[240]

Gro-β

Gro-β is an α-chemokine with the CXC and without the ELR motif. It inhibits growth factor–stimulated capillary endothelial cell proliferation. Gro-β can inhibit angiogenesis in vivo, in the CAM assay, and in the mouse model bFGF-induced corneal neovascularization.[241] Its role in ocular angiogenesis is still unknown, but it again demonstrates the role of the ELR motif in angiostatic activity.

MATRIX METALLOPROTEINASE AND TISSUE INHIBITORS OF METALLOPROTEINASE

MMPs appear to be involved in stimulating angiogenesis by degrading the perivascular extracellular matrix, a requirement for sprouting angiogenesis. These MMPs have endogenous inhibitors called *tissue inhibitors of metalloproteinases* (TIMPs). Four inhibitors have been cloned and expressed (TIMP-1, TIMP-2, TIMP-3, and TIMP-4).[242–246] Each TIMP can inhibit all the MMPs.[247, 248]

Evidence for a role of inhibitors of metalloproteinase as inhibitors of angiogenesis originate from studies that characterized the angiogenic activity of MMPs. TIMP-1 was capable of inhibiting capillary tube formation in vitro.[8, 160] Further evidence for angiogenic inhibitory activity came from the ability of cartilage to inhibit angiogenesis. First, rabbit cartilage explants inhibited the corneal micropocket assay.[188] It was later found that cartilage inhibited endothelial cell proliferation.[249] A cartilage-derived TIMP was the first TIMP identified to be a potent inhibitor of in vivo angiogenesis.[18]

Agents that inhibit collagenase such as minocycline,[250] TIMP-2,[251] batimastat, and α_2-macroglobulin[18] inhibit capillary endothelial cell proliferation. TIMP-1 promotes endothelial cell proliferation in vitro,[252] but in a rat corneal pocket model, it was an inhibitor of angiogenesis.[253] TIMP-1's inability to inhibit endothelial cell proliferation makes TIMP-2 a more promising candidate for angiogenic inhibitor.

TIMP-3 has been implicated in the pathogenesis of Sorsby's fundus dystrophy, an autosomal dominant macular dystrophy with usual onset in the third to fourth decade.[254] It is characterized by atrophy of the retinal pigment epithelium, choriocapillaris, and retina. Subretinal neovascularization is a prominent and blinding feature of this disorder. Lipid deposits in the inner portion of Bruch's membrane are thought to play a role in the pathogenesis of the disorder.[255]

A point mutation in the TIMP-3 gene has been found in Sorsby's fundus dystrophy patients.[256] In a study of fixed human eyes, TIMP-3 immunolabeling was seen in Bruch's membrane and drusen, with the strongest labeling in eyes from elderly donors. This study showed that TIMP-3 is an extracellular matrix component of Bruch's membrane. Thus, a malfunctioning TIMP-3 may lead to the characteristic findings in Sorsby's fundus dystrophy. Staining of drusen raises the possibility that altered TIMP-3–mediated matrix remodeling may contribute to age-related degenerative changes in Bruch's membrane.[257] As an inhibitor of angiogenesis,[258] TIMP-3 may be a physiologic regulator of angiogenic homeostasis. When TIMP-3 is inactivated by a gene mutation, the balance of angiogenic inhibitors and stimulators is disrupted, resulting in pathologic neovascularization.

TIMP-3 mRNA is found in cultured human retinal pigment epithelium, choroidal microcapillary endothelium, and pericytes. Retinal pigment epithelial cells also express and secrete TIMP-3 protein. TIMP-3 immunostaining shows a strong signal in Bruch's membrane, particularly near the basement membranes of the retinal pigment epithelium and endothelial cells, presumably in their basement membranes. TIMP-3 expression in the retinal pigment epithelium and Bruch's membrane supports a role for TIMP-3 in Sorsby's fundus dystrophy and possibly other choroidal dystrophies such as macular degeneration.

MMPS may play an indirect role, acting as proteolytic activators of endogenous protein inhibitors of angiogenesis. A macrophage metalloelastase has been shown to play a role in the cleavage of plasminogen into the angiogenic inhibitor angiostatin in the Lewis lung carcinoma, the tumor that was used to isolate angiostatin.[259]

Growth Factor Inhibition

VASCULAR ENDOTHELIAL GROWTH FACTOR INHIBITORS

VEGF's apparent role in ocular neovascularization makes it a likely target for inhibition. Several strategies have been identified to inhibit VEGF in hopes of developing an effective angiogenesis inhibitor (Fig. 37–5). One strategy involves inhibiting VEGF by binding and neutralizing the molecule. The soluble flt-1 receptor, which is actually encoded in the natural short message of the flt-1 gene, can bind VEGF

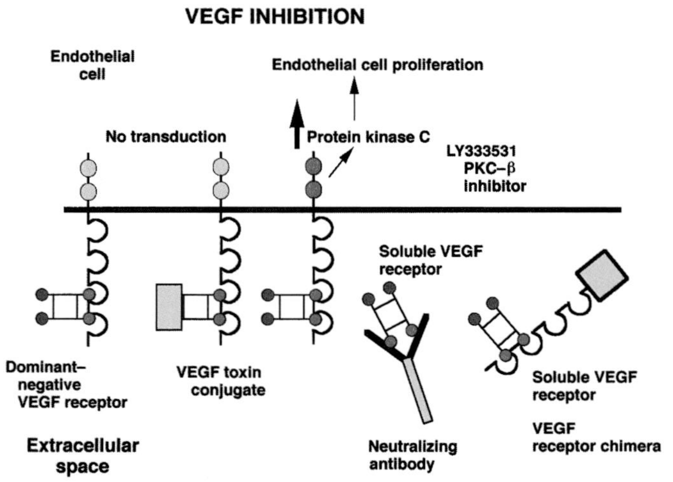

FIGURE 37–5. Inhibition of vascular endothelial growth factor (VEGF) as a means to inhibit angiogenesis. VEGF inhibition can be obtained by binding circulating VEGF with a neutralizing antibody, a soluble VEGF receptor, a dominant-negative VEGF receptor, or VEGF receptor chimera that does not transduce VEGF signal but competitively bind VEGF. Destruction of VEGF receptors can be accomplished with a VEGF-toxin conjugate. Blocking the cellular transduction cascade with a PKC protein kinase-β (PKC-β) inhibitor is another method to inhibit VEGF's mitogenic activity.

with high affinity and inhibits VEGF activity, presumably by binding free bioactive VEGF.[260] A dominant-negative VEGF receptor flk-1 has also been used to inhibit tumor angiogenesis by competitively binding to VEGF.[261, 262] Using the same strategy but a different delivery method, a gene for a VEGF receptor dominant-negative was used to transfect experimental brain tumors with success.[263]

Another strategy for inhibition of VEGF activity is to incapacitate the VEGF receptor. By chemically linking recombinant vascular endothelial growth factor (VEGF165) and a truncated diphtheria toxin molecule (DT385), both in vitro and in vivo angiogenesis was inhibited by this toxin-protein conjugate.[264]

Ocular neovascularization has been inhibited using both neutralizing antibodies and VEGF-inhibiting chimeric protein. Intravitreal injections of neutralizing antibodies inhibited iris neovascularization in a monkey model.[34] The intravitreal injection of a chimeric protein, a high-affinity VEGF receptor linked to the heavy chain of immunoglobulin G, decreased histologically evident retinal neovascularization in a mouse model of retinopathy of prematurity.[97] In models of both tumor and ocular neovascularization, inhibition of VEGF demonstrated potentiation of angiogenesis. This inhibition supports VEGF's role as a necessary factor in the development of both tumor and ocular neovascularization.

Inhibition of cellular transduction can be used to inhibit VEGF activity. Protein kinase C (PKC) activation (α and βII) increases after stimulation by VEGF. This upregulation is preceded by the activation of phospholipase C-γ, ^{3}H-inositol phosphate production, phosphatidylinositol 3-kinase, and ^{3}H-arachidonic acid–labeled diacylglycerol formation in bovine aortic endothelial cells. VEGF appears to mediate its mitogenic effects partly through the activation of the phospholipase C-γ and PKC pathway, involving predominately PKC-β isoform activation in endothelial cells.[265] VEGF can increase intraocular vascular permeability through the activation of PKC in vivo after the intravitreal injection of VEGF in rats.[266] This transduction pathway can be used to inhibit VEGF activity. Inhibition by intravitreal or oral administration of a PKC-β–isoform–selective inhibitor inhibits VEGF permeability activity.[266] In a pig model of intraocular neovascularization caused by branch retinal vein occlusion, a specific PKC-β inhibitor, Ly333531, effectively inhibited optic nerve and preretinal neovascularization.[267]

INHIBITION OF VASCULAR ENDOTHELIAL GROWTH FACTOR UPREGULATION

Inhibiting VEGF upregulation may be another useful strategy. VEGF upregulation is dependent on VEGF mRNA stability.[268] By selectively inhibiting VEGF mRNA translation, antisense oligodeoxynucleotides against VEGF can inhibit VEGF upregulation. Antisense oligodeoxynucleotides against VEGF inhibited retinal neovascularization in the mouse model of retinopathy of prematurity.[269] Ribozymes, cytosolic proteins that can selectively degrade specific mRNA, could be useful for decreasing mRNA stability. Decreasing tissue hypoxia is another method of inhibiting upregulation of VEGF.[29] Adenosine may be another possible target for inhibition. Hypoxia-induced accumulation of adenosine stimulates *VEGF* gene expression through stimulation of adenosine A2a receptor and subsequent activation of the cyclic AMP–dependent protein kinase.[270] Hypoxia-induced upregulation of VEGF receptor has also been shown to be adenosine mediated.[271] Other possible upregulators of VEGF that could be targeted include advanced glycation end products, IGF, and reactive oxygen intermediates (Fig. 37–6).

GROWTH HORMONE AND INSULIN-LIKE GROWTH FACTOR-I INHIBITION

Both growth hormone and IGF-I inhibition in the mouse model of retinopathy of prematurity demonstrated inhibition of retinal neovascularization independent of VEGF upregulation.[272] The inhibitor used in this study was MK678, a growth hormone secretion inhibitor. Future strategies to inhibit growth hormone or IGF-I may be useful as potential therapies for certain forms of pathologic neovascularization.

Endogenous Protein Inhibitors

CORNEAL ANGIOGENESIS INHIBITOR

A corneal angiogenesis inhibitor has been partially purified and has been shown to inhibit endothelial cell proliferation and migration as well as angiogenesis in the CAM assay.[273] Identification and characterization of this molecule is under active investigation.

16-kDa N-TERMINAL FRAGMENT OF PROLACTIN

A 16-kDa N-terminal fragment of prolactin is a potent inhibitor of angiogenesis.[274] Its ability to inhibit the activation of mitogen-activated protein kinases distal to autophosphorylation of the putative VEGF receptor, Flk-1, and phospholipase C-γ is the likely mechanism for its angiogenic inhibitory activity.[275] This inhibition is likely due to specific inhibition of

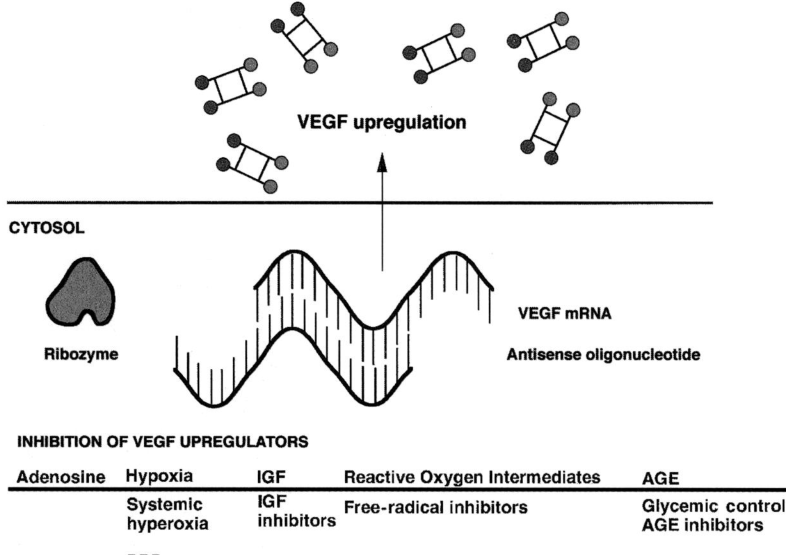

FIGURE 37–6. Inhibition of VEGF upregulation to inhibit angiogenesis. Inhibition of VEGF upregulators such as adenosine, hypoxia, insulin-like growth factor (IGF), reactive oxygen intermediates, and advanced glycation end products (AGE) can indirectly inhibit VEGF upregulation. Panretinal photocoagulation (PRP), the accepted treatment for diabetic retinopathy, decreases retinal hypoxia by destroying the retina and decreasing retinal hypoxia. Direct inhibition of VEGF upregulation can be accomplished by destroying or inactivating VEGF mRNA species with ribozymes specific for VEGF mRNA or antisense oligonucleotides that bind and inactivate VEGF mRNA.

raf-1, a signal transduction molecule.[276] Prolactin is normally released from the anterior pituitary and may play a role in the absence of direct arterial blood supply to the anterior pituitary.[277]

THROMBOSPONDIN

Thrombospondin-1 (TSP-1) is a large modular extracellular matrix-secreted glycoprotein that is a known potent inhibitor of neovascularization in vivo. In vitro it blocks the migration of endothelial cells and vascular smooth muscle cells but does not block the migration of fibroblasts, neutrophils, and keratinocytes. Inhibition of endogenous TSP-1 promotes the development of capillary tubes in vitro.[278, 279] TSP-1 was derived from platelets but has been shown to be produced by activated monocytes and macrophages as well.[280]

A possible mechanism for the antiangiogenic effects of TSP-1 could be its ability to bind angiogenic growth factors. Both HGF-SF[281] and bFGF bind TSP.[282] The angiogenic inhibitory activity of TSP has also been shown to involve MMP-9.[283]

TSP-2 has also been found to be an active inhibitor in vitro and in vivo, whereas TSP-5 is inactive. The angiogenic inhibitory activity of TSP-1 and TSP-2 and not TSP-5 suggests that the properdin-like type 1 module that is found in TSP-1 and TSP-2 but not in TSP-5 could contribute to this activity.[284]

P53, a tumor suppressor gene, seems to mediate its antitumor effect by an antiangiogenesis mechanism. Wild-type *p53* upregulates TSP-1, whereas mutated *p53* does not. *P53* and TSP may play a central role in the angiogenic switch of tumors.[285] Two other localized, but not identified, tumor suppressor genes upregulate TSP.[286, 287] This correlation between tumor suppressor genes and TSP implicates tumor suppressor genes in the angiogenic switch required in tumor growth and metastases.

ANGIOSTATIN

Angiostatin is a 38-kDa angiogenesis inhibitor isolated from a subclone of Lewis lung carcinoma that was known to inhibit its own metastases. Angiostatin was found to be an internal fragment of plasminogen. This fragment was found to inhibit endothelial cell proliferation and suppress tumor growth.[288] Different recombinant fragments of angiostatin have different inhibitory activities in vitro.[289] Other tumors have been shown to produce angiostatin.[290]

ENDOSTATIN

Endostatin is a 20-kDa angiogenesis inhibitor derived from the EOMA murine hemangioendothelioma cell line. It is the C-terminal fragment of collagen XVIII. Recombinant endostatin inhibits endothelial cell proliferation in vitro and angiogenesis in vivo. It also suppresses tumor growth.[291] It inhibits corneal neovascularization in the mouse bFGF-induced model. Otherwise this relatively new angiogenic inhibitor has not been evaluated in other models of ocular neovascularization.

ION CHANNEL BLOCKERS

The ion channel blocking agent amiloride has been shown to inhibit angiogenesis in an in vivo model, suggesting a vital role for Na^+-coupled transport processes in angiogenesis. Amiloride inhibits capillary morphogenesis completely and reversibly, and it appears to act by blocking endothelial cell proliferation but not migration.[292]

CHEMOTHERAPEUTIC AGENTS

Antineoplastic agents have been shown to inhibit angiogenesis. Alkyl-lysophospholipids are a group of anticancer compounds. One alkyl-lysophospholipid, et-18-OCH_3, inhibits induced angiogenesis at levels that do not affect the viability of endothelial cells.[293] The experimental antitumor agent titanocene dichloride also prevents angiogenesis in the CAM assay and tube formation in vitro. The antiangiogenic effect of titanocene are unrelated to metalloproteinase inhibition.[294] Pentosan polysulfate is a highly negatively charged polysaccharide that inhibits tubule formation in vitro and inhibits capillary formation in the CAM assay.[295] Other antineoplastic agents that have been shown to inhibit angiogenesis include mitoxantrone, bisantrene,[296] and flavone acetic acid.[297] Many others are undergoing investigation. None have yet been tested in ocular neovascularization.

ANTIBIOTICS

Many antibiotics have been tested for angiogenic activity. The anthracycline antibiotics daunorubicin, doxorubicin, and epirubicin inhibit in vitro and in vivo angiogenesis in noncytotoxic doses.[294] Eponemycin, a novel antibiotic, powerfully inhibits angiogenesis in the CAM assay. This powerful inhibition is dose dependent.[298] 15-Deoxyspergualin, an analog of spergualin;[299] minocycline, a semisynthetic tetracycline;[250] herbimycin;[299] and other antibiotics have been shown to inhibit angiogenesis in vivo and in vitro. Their mechanism has not yet been elucidated.

Summary

There are several resounding themes in angiogenesis research. The first is the balance between inhibitors and stimulators. This theme is played out in the chemokines, with which the mere presence of three amino acids can alter the angiogenic or angiostatic activity of a molecule. It is also seen in the discovery of angiogenic inhibitors in tumors. Tumors produce angiogenic stimulators and yet can also produce inhibitors of angiogenesis such as angiostatin and endostatin, which are actually cleavage fragments of endogenous proteins.

In ocular neovascularization, there is also a balance. Many ocular tissues such as the cornea, vitreous, and lens are avascular. With the overproduction of a growth factor such as VEGF and FGF, these tissues can develop new blood vessels. This implies that there is a yet-to-be-discovered inhibitor of angiogenesis in these avascular tissues, and only with the imbalance caused by excess stimulators can neovascularization occur.

The field of angiogenesis has exploded over the last decade with the discovery of many new stimulators and inhibitors of angiogenesis. Only a small number of these inhibitors have been tested in a clinical setting. In the future, many of the inhibitors described in this chapter will be used in clinical settings. One hopes that they can provide some hope in the treatment of several blinding conditions.

FUTURE DIRECTION

The future of angiogenesis research involves uncovering the cascade of events resulting in the inhibition or stimulation of angiogenesis. By understanding this cascade, one can develop new strategies to prevent the devastating effects of pathologic neovascularization. In ocular neovascularization, inhibition of angiogenesis is tantamount to preventing its blinding complications. In this chapter several promising inhibitors have been described that may in the future be developed into viable treatments. In addition, these inhibitors have identified strategies for developing new inhibitors of angiogenesis.

DISCOVERY OF NEW ANGIOGENIC INHIBITORS

The identification of the ELR motif in chemokines as a determinant of angiogenic activity will allow identification of likely angiogenic or angiostatic chemokines in the future. Chemokines yet to be discovered may be classified by the presence or absence of the ELR motif. New angiostatic chemokines will not have the ELR motif, whereas new angiogenic chemokines will. Design of new angiogenic inhibitors may be possible by substituting or eliminating the ELR motif in chemokines.

As mentioned, there is a physiologic balance between stimulators and inhibitors of angiogenesis in the normal eye. The cornea, vitreous, and lens harbor yet-unpurified inhibitors of angiogenesis that may lead to more physiologic strategies for the inhibition of ocular neovascularization. There is evidence that astrocytes produce angiogenic inhibitors that have not yet been identified.[300]

The isolation of both angiostatin and endostatin from tumors that inhibited their own metastases provides another strategy for identifying and isolating new angiogenic inhibitors. Several tumors have been screened for their ability to inhibit corneal neovascularization in a mouse model.[301] Protein purification strategies used in the purification of endostatin and angiostatin could be employed. Although these compounds have yet to be tested in ocularly relevant models other than corneal neovascularization, they may prove to be a promising treatment in the future.

Strategies that inhibit growth factors such as VEGF that are known to be involved in ocular neovascularization are probably the most promising. Inhibition of VEGF has been shown to inhibit ocular neovascularization in several animal models. The optimal technique for inhibiting VEGF is still not clear. But no matter which technique is utilized, the potential success of the strategy is great.

Although many angiogenesis inhibitors have been identified, their mechanisms of action are not fully understood. Understanding these mechanisms may lead to the design of more selective inhibitors of angiogenesis.

Besides inhibition, several fundamental questions are left unanswered. It is apparent that VEGF plays a role in hypoxia-mediated angiogenesis, but in ARMD, in which hypoxia is not clearly implicated, what is the order of events that results in the formation of choroidal neovascularization? Does TIMP-3 play a role in ARMD? How does the newly discovered gene for ARMD result in subretinal neovascularization? What factors play a role in ARMD? As the diabetic retinopathy and ischemia-related neovascularization puzzle has begun to be pieced together, there are many more questions than answers in the pathophysiology of ARMD. It is the promise of understanding the pathophysiology of disease along with the promise of possible treatment that spurs great interest in angiogenic research.

REFERENCES

1. Folkman J, Shing Y: Angiogenesis. J Biol Chem 267:10,931–10,934, 1992.
2. Risau W: Mechanisms of angiogenesis. Nature 386:671–674, 1997.
3. Michaelson I: The mode of development of retinal vessels, with some observations on its significance for certain retinal disease. Trans Ophthalmol Soc U K 68:137–180, 1948.
4. Ashton N: Retinal vascularization in health and disease. Am J Ophthalmol 44:7–24, 1957.

5. Wise G: Retinal neovascularization. Trans Am Ophthalmol Soc 54:729–826, 1956.
6. Folkman J, Haudenschild C: Angiogenesis by capillary endothelial cells in culture. Trans Ophthalmol Soc U K 100:346–353, 1980.
7. Boyden S: The chemotactic effect of mixtures of antibody and antigen on polymorphonuclear leukocytes. J Exp Med 115:453–466, 1962.
8. Montesano R, Orci L: Tumor-promoting phorbol esters induce angiogenesis in vitro. Cell 42:469–477, 1985.
9. Brown KJ, Maynes SF, Bezos A, et al: A novel in vitro assay for human angiogenesis. Lab Invest 75:539–555, 1996.
10. Montesano R, Vassalli JD, Baird A, et al: Basic fibroblast growth factor induces angiogenesis in vitro. Proc Natl Acad Sci U S A. 83:7297–7301, 1986.
11. Pepper MS, Ferrara N, Orci L, Montesano R: Leukemia inhibitory factor (LIF) inhibits angiogenesis in vitro. J Cell Sci 108:73–83, 1995.
12. Pepper MS, Montesano R, Vassalli JD, Orci L: Chondrocytes inhibit endothelial sprout formation in vitro: Evidence for involvement of a transforming growth factor-beta. J Cell Physiol 146:170–179, 1991.
13. Vailhe B, Ronot X, Lecomte M, et al: Description of an in vitro angiogenesis model designed to test antiangiogenic molecules. Cell Biol Toxicol 12:341–344, 1996.
14. Zimrin AB, Villeponteau B, Maciag T: Models of in vitro angiogenesis: Endothelial cell differentiation on fibrin but not Matrigel is transcriptionally dependent. Biochem Biophys Res Commun 213:630–638, 1995.
15. Auerbach R, Kubai L, Knighton D, Folkman J: A simple procedure for the long-term cultivation of chicken embryos. Dev Biol 41:391–394, 1974.
16. Nguyen M, Shing Y, Folkman J: Quantitation of angiogenesis and antiangiogenesis in the chick embryo chorioallantoic membrane. Microvasc Res 47:31–40, 1994.
17. Ribatti D, Vacca A, Roncali L, Dammacco F: The chick embryo chorioallantoic membrane as a model for in vivo research on angiogenesis. Int J Dev Biol 40:1189–1197, 1996.
18. Moses MA, Sudhalter J, Langer R: Identification of an inhibitor of neovascularization from cartilage. Science 248:1408–1410, 1990.
19. Kenyon BM, Voest EE, Chen CC, et al: A model of angiogenesis in the mouse cornea. Invest Ophthalmol Vis Sci 37:1625–1632, 1996.
20. Li WW, Grayson G, Folkman J, D'Amore PA: Sustained-release endotoxin: A model for inducing corneal neovascularization. Invest Ophthalmol Vis Sci 32:2906–2911, 1991.
21. Loughman MS, Chatzistefanou K, Gonzalez EM, et al: Experimental corneal neovascularisation using sucralfate and basic fibroblast growth factor. Aust N Z J Ophthalmol 24:289–295, 1996.
22. Fournier G, Lutty G, Watt S, et al: A corneal micropocket assay for angiogenesis in the rat eye. Invest Ophthalmol Vis Sci 21:351–354, 1981.
23. Muthukkaruppan V, Auerbach R: Angiogenesis in the mouse cornea. Science 205:1416–1418, 1979.
24. Benelli U, Ross JR, Nardi M, Klintworth GK: Corneal neovascularization induced by xenografts or chemical cautery. Inhibition by cyclosporin A. Invest Ophthalmol Vis Sci 38:274–282, 1997.
25. Amano S, Rohan R, Kuroki M, et al: Requirement of vascular endothelial growth factor in wound and inflammation related corneal neovascularization. Invest Ophthalmol Vis Sci 39:18–22, 1998.
26. Danis R, Yany Y, Massicotte S, Boldt H: Preretinal and optic nerve head neovascularization induced by photodynamic venous thrombosis in domestic pigs. Arch Ophthalmol 111:539–543, 1993.
27. Miller JW, Adamis AP, Shima DT, et al: Vascular endothelial growth factor/vascular permeability factor is temporally and spatially correlated with ocular angiogenesis in a primate model. Am J Pathol 145:574–584, 1994.
28. Saito Y, Park L, Skolik SA, et al: Experimental preretinal neovascularization by laser-induced venous thrombosis in rats. Curr Eye Res 16:26–33, 1997.
29. Pournaras C, Tsacopoulos M, Strommer K, et al: Experimental retinal branch vein occlusion in miniature pigs induced local tissue hypoxia and vasoproliferative microangiopathy. Ophthalmology 97:1321–1328, 1990.
30. Hamilton A, Marshall J, Kohner E, Bowbyes J: Retinal new vessel formation following experimental vein occlusion. Exp Eye Res 20:493–497, 1975.
31. Packer A, Gu X-Q, Servais G, Hayreh S: Primate model of neovascular glaucoma. Int Ophthalmol 9:121–127, 1986.
32. Miller J: Vascular endothelial growth factor and ocular neovascularization. Am J Pathol 151:13–23, 1997.
33. Miller JW, Stinson WG, Folkman J: Regression of experimental iris neovascularization with systemic alpha-interferon. Ophthalmology 100:9–14, 1993.
34. Adamis AP, Shima DT, Tolentino MJ, et al: Inhibition of vascular endothelial growth factor prevents retinal ischemia-associated iris neovascularization in a nonhuman primate. Arch Ophthalmol 114:66–71, 1996.
35. Reynaud X, Dorey CK: Extraretinal neovascularization induced by hypoxic episodes in the neonatal rat. Invest Ophthalmol Vis Sci 35:3169–3177, 1994.
36. Penn J, Tolman B, Lowery L: Variable oxygen exposure causes preretinal neovascularization in newborn rat. Invest Ophthalmol Vis Sci 34:576–585, 1993.
37. McLeod D, Crone S, Lutty G: Vasoproliferation in the neonatal model of oxygen-induced retinopathy. Invest Ophthalmol Vis Sci 37:1322–1333, 1996.
38. Chan-Ling T, Gock B, Stone J: The effect of oxygen on vasoformative cell division: Evidence that "physiological hypoxia" is the stimulus for normal retinal vasculogenesis. Invest Ophthalmol Vis Sci 36:1201–1214, 1995.
39. Smith L, Wesolowski E, McLellan A, et al: Oxygen-induced retinopathy in the mouse. Invest Ophthalmol Vis Sci 35:101–111, 1994.
40. Patz A: Clinical and experimental studies on retinal neovascularization. XXXIX Edward Jackson Memorial Lecture. Am J Ophthalmol 94:715–743, 1982.
41. Archer D, Gardiner T: Morphologic, fluorescein angiographic, and light microscopic features of experimental choroidal neovascularization. Am J Ophthalmol 91:297–311, 1981.
42. Ryan S: Subretinal neovascularization after argon laser photocoagulation. Graefes Arch Klin Ophthalmol 215:29–42, 1980.
43. Ryan S: Subretinal neovascularization: Natural history of an experimental model. Arch Ophthalmol 91:433–457, 1982.
44. Husain D, Ryan A, Cuthbertson R, et al: Vascular endothelial growth factor (VEGF) expression is correlated with choroidal neovascularization in a monkey model. Invest Ophthalmol Vis Sci 38:s501, 1997.
45. Corjay M, Husain D, Stoltenborg J, et al: Alpha V beta 3, alpha V beta 5, and ostopontin immunostaining in experimental choroidal neovascularization in the monkey. Invest Ophthalmol Vis Sci 38:s965, 1997.
46. Okamoto N, Tobe T, Hackett S, et al: Transgenic mice with increased expression of vascular endothelial growth factor in the retina: A model of intraretinal and subretinal neovascularization. Am J Pathol 151:281–291, 1997.
47. Danis RP, Yang Y: Microvascular retinopathy in the Zucker diabetic fatty rat. Invest Ophthalmol Vis Sci 34:2367–2371, 1993.
48. Kern TS, Engerman RL: A mouse model of diabetic retinopathy. Arch Ophthalmol 114:986–990, 1996.
49. Buchi ER, Kurosawa A, Tso MO: Retinopathy in diabetic hypertensive monkeys: A pathologic study. Graefes Arch Clin Exp Ophthalmol 234:388–398, 1996.
50. Kador PF, Takahashi Y, Wyman M, Ferris Fr: Diabeteslike proliferative retinal changes in galactose-fed dogs [see comments]. Arch Ophthalmol 113:352–354, 1995.
51. Huang S, Khosrof S, Koletsky R, et al: Characterization of retinal vascular abnormalities in lean and obese spontaneously hypertensive rats. Clin Exp Pharmacol Physiol 22 (Suppl 1):S129–S131, 1995.
52. Gospodarowicz D: Purification of fibroblast growth factor from bovine pituitary. J Biol Chem 250:2515–2520, 1975.
53. Klagsburn M: The fibroblast growth factor family: Structural and biological properties. Prog Growth Factor Res 1:207–235, 1989.
54. Sporn M, Roberts A: Peptide growth factors are multifunctional. Nature 332:217–219, 1988.
55. Klein S, Roghani M, Rifkin D: Fibroblast growth factors as angiogenesis factors: New insights into their mechanism of action. EXS (Basel) 79:159–192, 1997.
56. Jaye M, Howk R, Burgess W, et al: Human endothelial cell growth factor: Cloning, nucleotide sequence, and chromosome localization. Science 233:541–545, 1986.
57. Abraham J, Mergia A, Whang J, et al: Nucleotide sequence of a bovine clone encoding the angiogenic protein basic fibroblast growth factor. Science 233:545–548, 1986.
58. Esch F, Baird A, Ling N, et al: Primary structure of bovine pituitary basic fibroblast growth factor (FGF) and comparison with the amino-terminal sequence of bovine brain acidic FGF. Proc Natl Acad Sci U S A 82:6507–6511, 1985.

59. Baird A, Esch F, Gospadarowicz D, Guillemin R: Retina and eye-derived growth factor: Partial molecular characterisation and identity with acidic and basic fibroblast growth factors. Biochemistry 24:7855–7860, 1985.
60. Folkman J, Klagsbrun M, Sasse J, et al: A heparin-binding angiogenic protein—basic fibroblast growth factor—is stored within basement membrane. Am J Pathol 130:393–400, 1988.
61. Sommer A, Rifkin D: Interaction of heparin with human basic fibroblast growth factor: Protection of the angiogenic protein from proteolytic degradation by a glycosaminoglycan. J Cell Physiol 138:215–220, 1989.
62. Glaser B, D'amore P, Michels R, et al: Demonstration of vasoproliferative activity from mammalian retina. J Cell Biol 84:298–304, 1980.
63. Schweigerer L, Malerstein B, Neufeld G, Gospodarowicz D: Basic fibroblast growth factor is synthesized in cultured retinal pigment epithelial cells. Biochem Biophys Res Commun 143:934–940, 1987.
64. Sternfeld M, Robertson J, Shipley G, et al: Cultured human retinal pigment epithelial cells express basic fibroblast growth factor and its receptors. Curr Eye Res 8:1029–1037, 1989.
65. Schweigerer L, Neufeld G, Friedman J, et al: Capillary endothelial cells express basic fibroblast growth factor, a mitogen that promotes their own growth. Nature 325:257–259, 1987.
66. Sivalingam A, Kenney J, Brown GC, et al: Basic fibroblast growth factor levels in the vitreous of patients with proliferative diabetic retinopathy. Arch Ophthalmol 108:869–872, 1990.
67. De Juan E, Stefansson E, Ohira A: Basic fibroblast growth factor stimulates 3H-thymidine uptake in retinal venular and capillary endothelial cells in vivo. Invest Ophthalmol Vis Sci 31:1238–1244, 1990.
68. Stavri GT, Zachary IC, Baskerville PA, et al: Basic fibroblast growth factor upregulates the expression of vascular endothelial growth factor in vascular smooth muscle cells. Synergistic interaction with hypoxia. Circulation 92:11–14, 1995.
69. Jonca F, Ortega N, Gleizes PE, et al: Cell release of bioactive fibroblast growth factor 2 by exon 6–encoded sequence of vascular endothelial growth factor. J Biol Chem 272:24,203–24,209, 1997.
70. Muthukrishnan L, Warder E, McNeil P: Basic fibroblast growth factor is efficiently released from cytosolic storage site through plasma membrane disruptions of endothelial cells. J Cell Physiol 148:1–16, 1991.
71. Bashkin P, Doctrow S, Klagsbbrun M, et al: Basic fibroblast growth factor binds to subendothelial extracellular matrix and is released by heparinase and heparin-like molecules. Biochemistry 28:1737–1743, 1989.
72. Piotrowicz RS, Martin JL, Dillman WH, Levin EG: The 27-kDa heat shock protein facilitates basic fibroblast growth factor release from endothelial cells. J Biol Chem 272:7042–7047, 1997.
73. Khaliq A, Patel B, Jarvis-Evans J, et al: Oxygen modulates production of bFGF and TGF-beta by retinal cells in vitro. Exp Eye Res 60:415–424, 1995.
74. Shima DT, Adamis AP, Ferrara N, et al: Hypoxic induction of endothelial cell growth factors in retinal cells: Identification and characterization of vascular endothelial growth factor (VEGF) as the mitogen. Mol Med 1:182–193, 1995.
75. Hanneken A, de Juan E Jr, Lutty GA, et al: Altered distribution of basic fibroblast growth factor in diabetic retinopathy. Arch Ophthalmol 109:1005–1111, 1991.
76. Deroanne CF, Hajitou A, Calberg-Bacq CM, et al: Angiogenesis by fibroblast growth factor 4 is mediated through an autocrine up-regulation of vascular endothelial growth factor expression. Cancer Res 57:5590–5597, 1997.
77. Tischer E, Mitchell R, Hartman T, et al: The human gene for vascular endothelial growth factor. Multiple protein forms are encoded through alternative exon splicing. J Biol Chem 266:11,947–11,954, 1991.
78. Ijichi A, Sakuma S, Tofilon PJ: Hypoxia-induced vascular endothelial growth factor expression in normal rat astrocyte cultures. Glia 14:87–93, 1995.
79. Berse B, Brown L, VanDeWater L, et al: Vascular permeability factor (vascular endothelial growth factor) gene is expressed differentially in normal tissue, macrophages and tumors. Mol Biol Cell 3:211–220, 1992.
80. Freeman MR, Schneck FX, Gagnon ML, et al: Peripheral blood T lymphocytes and lymphocytes infiltrating human cancers express vascular endothelial growth factor: A potential role for T cells in angiogenesis. Cancer Res 55:4140–4145, 1995.
81. Iijima K, Yoshikawa N, Connolly DT, Nakamura H: Human mesangial cells and peripheral blood mononuclear cells produce vascular permeability factor. Kidney Int 44:959–966, 1993.
82. Adamis A, Shima D, Yeo K, et al: Synthesis and secretion of vascular permeability factor/vascular endothelial growth factor by human retinal pigment epithelial cells. Biochem Biophys Res Commun 193:631, 1993.
83. Ferrara N, Houck K, Jakeman L, Leung DW: Molecular and biological properties of the vascular endothelial growth factor family of proteins. Endocr Rev 13:18–32, 1992.
84. Quinn TP, Peters KG, De Vries C, et al: Fetal liver kinase 1 is a receptor for vascular endothelial growth factor and is selectively expressed in vascular endothelium. Proc Natl Acad Sci U S A 90:7533–7537, 1993.
85. Hewett PW, Murray JC: Coexpression of flt-1, flt-4 and KDR in freshly isolated and cultured human endothelial cells. Biochem Biophys Res Commun 221:697–702, 1996.
86. De Vries C, Escobedo JA, Ueno H, et al: The fms-like tyrosine kinase, a receptor for vascular endothelial growth factor. Science 255:989–891, 1992.
87. Terman B, Dougher-Vermazen M, Carrion M, et al: Identification of the KDR tyrosine kinase as a receptor for vascular endothelial growth factor. Biochem Biophys Res Commun 187:1579–1586, 1992.
88. Senger D, Galli S, Dvorak A, et al: Tumor cells secrete a vascular permeability factor that promotes accumulation of ascites fluid. Science 219:983–985, 1983.
89. Roberts WG, Palade GE: Increased microvascular permeability and endothelial fenestration induced by vascular endothelial growth factor. J Cell Sci 108:2369–2379, 1995.
90. Ferrara N, Henzel W: Pituitary follicular cells secrete a novel heparin-binding growth factor specific for vascular endothelial cells. Biochem Biophys Res Commun 161:851–858, 1989.
91. Keck P, Hauser S, Krivi G, et al: Vascular permeability factor, an endothelial cell mitogen related to PDGF. Science 246:1309–1312, 1989.
92. Leung DW, Cachianes G, Kuang WJ, et al: Vascular endothelial growth factor is a secreted angiogenic mitogen. Science 246:1306–1309, 1989.
93. Amin RH, Frank RN, Kennedy A, et al: Vascular endothelial growth factor is present in glial cells of the retina and optic nerve of human subjects with nonproliferative diabetic retinopathy. Invest Ophthalmol Vis Sci 38:36–47, 1997.
94. Hata Y, Nakagawa K, Ishibashi T, et al: Hypoxia-induced expression of vascular endothelial growth factor by retinal glial cells promotes in vitro angiogenesis. Virchows Arch 426:479–486, 1995.
95. Aiello LP, Northrup JM, Keyt BA, et al: Hypoxic regulation of vascular endothelial growth factor in retinal cells. Arch Ophthalmol 113:1538–1544, 1995.
96. Pierce E, Avery R, Foley E, et al: Vascular endothelial growth factor/vascular permeability factor expression in a mouse model of retinal neovascularization. Proc Natl Acad Sci U S A 92:905–909, 1995.
97. Aiello LP, Pierce EA, Foley ED, et al: Suppression of retinal neovascularization in vivo by inhibition of vascular endothelial growth factor (VEGF) using soluble VEGF-receptor chimeric proteins. Proc Natl Acad Sci U S A 92:10,457–10,461, 1995.
98. Tolentino M, Miller J, Gragoudas E, et al: Vascular endothelial growth factor is sufficient to produce iris neovascularization and neovascular glaucoma in a non-human primate. Arch Ophthalmol 114:964–970, 1995.
99. Tolentino MJ, Miller JW, Gragoudas ES, et al: Intravitreous injections of vascular endothelial growth factor produce retinal ischemia and microangiopathy in an adult primate. Ophthalmology 103:1820–1828, 1996.
100. Malecaze F, Clamens S, Simorre-Pinatel V, et al: Detection of vascular endothelial growth factor messenger RNA and vascular endothelial growth factor–like activity in proliferative diabetic retinopathy. Arch Ophthalmol 112:1476–1482, 1994.
101. Aiello LP, Avery RL, Arrigg PG, et al: Vascular endothelial growth factor in ocular fluid of patients with diabetic retinopathy and other retinal disorders. N Engl J Med 331:1480–1487, 1994.
102. Adamis AP, Miller JW, Bernal MT, et al: Increased vascular endothelial growth factor levels in the vitreous of eyes with proliferative diabetic retinopathy. Am J Ophthalmol 118:445–450, 1994.
103. Pe'er J, Shweiki D, Itin A, et al: Hypoxia-induced expression of vascular endothelial growth factor by retinal cells is a common factor in neovascularizing ocular diseases. Lab Invest 72:638–645, 1995.
104. Lutty G, Mcleod D, Merges C, et al: Localization of vascular endothelial growth factor in human retina and choroid. Arch Ophthalmol 114:971–977, 1996.

105. Murata T, Nakagawa K, Khalil A, et al: The relation between expression of vascular endothelial growth factor and breakdown of the blood-retinal barrier in diabetic rat retinas. Lab Invest 74:819–825, 1996.
106. Murata T, Ishibashi T, Khalil A, et al: Vascular endothelial growth factor plays a role in hyperpermeability of diabetic retinal vessels. Ophthalmic Res 27:48–52, 1995.
107. Lu M, Kuroki M, Amano S, et al: Advanced glycation endproducts increase retinal vascular endothelial growth factor expression. J Clin Invest 101:1219–1224, 1998.
108. Kuroki M, Voest EE, Amano S, et al: Reactive oxygen intermediates increase vascular endothelial growth factor expression in vitro and in vivo. J Clin Invest 98:1667–1675, 1996.
109. Punglia RS, Lu M, Hsu J, et al: Regulation of vascular endothelial growth factor expression by insulin-like growth factor I. Diabetes 46:1619–1626, 1997.
110. Pournaras CJ, Miller JW, Gragoudas ES, et al: Systemic hyperoxia decreases vascular endothelial growth factor gene expression in ischemic primate retina. Arch Ophthalmol 115:1553–1558, 1997.
111. Pierce E, Foley E, Smith L: Regulation of vascular endothelial growth factor by oxygen in a model of retinopathy of prematurity. Arch Ophthalmol 114:1219–1228, 1996.
112. Yi X, Ogata N, Komada M, et al: Vascular endothelial growth factor expression in choroidal neovascularization in rats. Graefes Arch Clin Exp Ophthalmol 235:313–319, 1997.
113. Ishibashi T, Hata Y, Yoshikawa H, et al: Expression of vascular endothelial growth factor in experimental choroidal neovascularization. Graefes Arch Clin Exp Ophthalmol 235:159–167, 1997.
114. Kvanta A, Algvere PV, Berglin L, Seregard S: Subfoveal fibrovascular membranes in age-related macular degeneration express vascular endothelial growth factor. Invest Ophthalmol Vis Sci 37:1929–1934, 1996.
115. Kliffen M, Sharma HS, Mooy CM, et al: Increased expression of angiogenic growth factors in age-related maculopathy. Br J Ophthalmol 81:154–162, 1997.
116. Amin RH, Frank RN, Kennedy A, et al: Vascular endothelial growth factor is present in glial cells of the retina and optic nerve of human subjects with nonproliferative diabetic retinopathy. Invest Ophthalmol Vis Sci 38:36–47, 1997.
117. Lopez PF, Sippy BD, Lambert HM, et al: Transdifferentiated retinal pigment epithelial cells are immunoreactive for vascular endothelial growth factor in surgically excised age-related macular degeneration–related choroidal neovascular membranes. Invest Ophthalmol Vis Sci 37:855–868, 1996.
118. Kvanta A: Expression and regulation of vascular endothelial growth factor in choroidal fibroblasts. Curr Eye Res 14:1015–1020, 1995.
119. Forrester JV, Shafiee A, Schroder S, et al: The role of growth factors in proliferative diabetic retinopathy. Eye 7:276–287, 1993.
120. Salmon W Jr, Daughaday W: A hormonally controlled serum factor which stimulates sulfate incorporation by cartilage in vitro. J Lab Clin Med 49:825–836, 1957.
121. LeRoith D, Roberts C Jr: Insulin-like growth factors. Ann N Y Acad Sci 692:1–9, 1993.
122. Grant M, Jerdan J, Merimee T: Insulin-like growth factor-1 modulates endothelial cell chemotaxis. J Clin Endocrinol Metab 65:370–371, 1987.
123. King G, Goodman A, Buzney S, et al: Receptors and growth promoting effects of insulin and insulinlike growth factors on cells from bovine retinal capillaries and aorta. J Clin Invest 75:1028–1036, 1985.
124. Grant M, Mames R, Fitzgerald C, et al: Insulin-like growth factor I as an angiogenic agent. In vivo and in vitro studies. Ann N Y Acad Sci 692:230–242, 1993.
125. Poulsen J: Recovery from retinopathy in a case of diabetes with Simmond's disease. Diabetes 2:7–12, 1953.
126. Luft R, Olivecrona H, Ikkos D, et al: Hypophysectomy in man: Further experiences in severe diabetes mellitus. BMJ 2:752, 1955.
127. Merimee TJ, Zapf J, Froesch ER: Insulin-like growth factor: Studies in diabetes with and without retinopathy. N Engl J Med 309:994–1007, 1983.
128. Hynes R: Integrins: Versatility, modulation and signaling in cell adhesion. Cell 69:11–25, 1992.
129. Brooks P, Clark R, Cheresh D: Requirement of vascular integrin AVB3 for angiogenesis. Science 264:569–571, 1994.
130. Friedlander M, Brooks P, Shaffer R, et al: Definition of two angiogenic pathways by distinct AV integrins. Science 270:1500–1502, 1995.
131. Brooks P, Montgomery A, Rosenfeld M, et al: Integrin alpha V beta 3 antagonist promotes tumor regression by inducing apoptosis of angiogenic blood vessels. Cell 749:1157–1164, 1994.
132. Hoppenreijs VP, Pels E, Vrensen GF, et al: Platelet-derived growth factor: Receptor expression in corneas and effects on corneal cells. Invest Ophthalmol Vis Sci 34:637–649, 1993.
133. Risau W, Drexler H, Mironov V, et al: Platelet-derived growth factor is angiogenic in vivo. Growth Factors 7:261–266, 1992.
134. Kuwabara K, Ogawa S, Matsumoto M, et al: Hypoxia-mediated induction of acidic/basic fibroblast growth factor and platelet-derived growth factor in mononuclear phagocytes stimulates growth of hypoxic endothelial cells. Proc Natl Acad Sci U S A 92:4606–4610, 1995.
135. Sato N, Beitz JG, Kato J, et al: Platelet-derived growth factor indirectly stimulates angiogenesis in vitro. Am J Pathol 142:1119–1130, 1993.
136. Todaro G, Fryling C, DeLarco J: Transforming growth factors produced by certain human tumor cells: Polypeptides that interact with epidermal growth factor receptor. Proc Natl Acad Sci U S A 7:5258, 1980.
137. Schreiber AB, Winkler ME, Derynck R: Transforming growth factor-alpha: A more potent angiogenic mediator than epidermal growth factor. Science 232:1250–1253, 1986.
138. Okamura K, Morimoto A, Hamanaka R, et al: A model system for tumor angiogenesis: Involvement of transforming growth factor-alpha in tube formation of human microvascular endothelial cells induced by esophageal cancer cells. Biochem Biophys Res Commun 186:1471–1479, 1992.
139. Roberts A, Sporn M: Physiological actions and clinical applications of transforming growth factor-β (TGF-β). Growth Factors 8:1–9, 1993.
140. Jennings J, Mohans S, Linkhart T, et al: Comparison of the biological actions of TGF-beta-1 and TGF-beta-2: Differential activity in endothelial cells. J Cell Physiol 137:167–172, 1988.
141. Yang E, Moses H: Transforming growth factor beta induced changes in cell migration, proliferation, and angiogenesis in the chick chorioallantoic membrane. J Cell Biol 111:731–741, 1990.
142. Merwin J, Newman W, Beall L, et al: Vascular cells respond differentially to transforming growth factors beta1 and beta2 in vitro. Am J Pathol 138:37–51, 1991.
143. Pertovaara L, Kaipainen A, Mustonene T, et al: Vascular endothelial growth factor is induced in response to transforming growth factor-beta in fibroblastic and endothelial cells. J Biol Chem 269:6271–6274, 1994.
144. Antonelli-Orlidge A, Saunders K, Smith S, D'Amore P: An activated form of transforming growth factor B is produced by cocultures of endothelial cells and pericytes. Proc Natl Acad Sci U S A 86:4544–4548, 1989.
145. Roberts A, Sporn M, Assoian R, et al: Transforming growth factor type B: Rapid induction of fibrosis and angiogenesis in vivo and stimulation of collagen formation in vitro. Proc Natl Acad Sci U S A 83:4167–4171, 1986.
146. Inagaki Y, Truter S, Tanaka S, et al: Overlapping pathway mediates the opposing actions of tumor necrosis factor-alpha and transforming growth factor-beta on alpha 2(I) collagen gene transcription. J Biol Chem 270:3353–3358, 1995.
147. Frater-Schroeder M, Risau W, Hallman R, Gautsch P: Tumor necrosis factor type alpha, potent inhibitor of endothelial cell growth in vitro, is angiogenic in vivo. Proc Natl Acad Sci U S A 84:5277–5281, 1987.
148. Leibovich S, Polverini P, Shepard H, et al: Macrophage-induced angiogenesis is mediated by tumor necrosis factor alpha. Nature 329:630–632, 1987.
149. Yoshida S, Ono M, Shono T, et al: Involvement of interleukin-8, vascular endothelial growth factor, and basic fibroblast growth factor in tumor necrosis factor alpha-dependent angiogenesis. Mol Cell Biol 17:4015–4023, 1997.
150. Hanemaaijer R, Koolwijk P, le Clercq L, et al: Regulation of matrix metalloproteinase expression in human vein and microvascular endothelial cells. Effects of tumour necrosis factor alpha, interleukin 1 and phorbol ester. Biochem J 296:803–809, 1993.
151. Burke-Gaffney A, Keenan A: Does TNF-alpha increase endothelial cell monolayer permeability? Agent Actions 38:83–85, 1993.
152. Sato N, Nariuchi H, Tsuruoka N, et al: Actions of TNF and IFN-gamma on angiogenesis in vitro. J Invest Dermatol 95:85s–89s, 1990.
153. Patterson C, Perrella MA, Endege WO, et al: Downregulation of vascular endothelial growth factor receptors by tumor necrosis factor-alpha in cultured human vascular endothelial cells. J Clin Invest 98:490–496, 1996.
154. Fajardo LF, Kwan HH, Kowalski J, et al: Dual role of tumor necrosis factor-alpha in angiogenesis. Am J Pathol 140:539–444, 1992.

155. Spranger J, Meyer-Schwickerath R, Klein M, et al: [TNF-alpha level in the vitreous body. Increase in neovascular eye diseases and proliferative diabetic retinopathy]. Med Klin 90:134–137, 1995.
156. Matrisian L: The matrix degrading metalloproteinases. Bioessays 14:455–463, 1992.
157. Fischer C, Gilbertson-Beadling S, Power E, et al: Interstitial collagenase is required for angiogenesis in vitro. Dev Biol 162:499–510, 1994.
158. Unemori EN, Ferrara N, Bauer EA, Amento EP: Vascular endothelial growth factor induces interstitial collagenase expression in human endothelial cells. J Cell Physiol 153:557–562, 1992.
159. Schnaper H, Grant D, Stetler-Stevenson W, et al: Type IV collagenase(s) and TIMPs modulate endothelial cell morphogenesis in vitro. J Cell Physiol 156:235–246, 1993.
160. Taraboletti G, Garofalo A, Belotti D, et al: Inhibition of angiogenesis and murine hemangioma growth by batimastat, a synthetic inhibitor of matrix metalloproteinases. J Natl Cancer Inst 87:293–298, 1995.
161. Ziche M, Maglione D, Ribatti D, et al: Placenta growth factor-1 is chemotactic, mitogenic, and angiogenic. Lab Invest 76:517–531, 1997.
162. Park J, Chen H, Winer J, et al: Placenta growth factor potentiation of vascular endothelial growth factor bioactivity, in vitro and in vivo, and high affinity binding to FLT-1 but not too Flk-1/KDR. J Biol Chem 269:25,646–25,654, 1994.
163. Saxena SK, Rybak SM, Davey RT Jr, et al: Angiogenin is a cytotoxic, tRNA-specific ribonuclease in the RNase A superfamily. J Biol Chem 267:21,982–21,9826, 1992.
164. Moenner M, Gusse M, Hatzi E, Badet J: The widespread expression of angiogenin in different human cells suggests a biological function not only related to angiogenesis. Eur J Biochem 226:483–490, 1994.
165. Fett J, Strydom D, Lobb R, et al: Isolation and characterization of angiogenin, an angiogenic protein from human carcinoma cells. Biochemistry 24:5480, 1986.
166. Shapiro R, Vallee BL: Site-directed mutagenesis of histidine-13 and histidine-114 of human angiogenin. Alanine derivatives inhibit angiogenin-induced angiogenesis. Biochemistry 28:7401–7408, 1989.
167. Gho YS, Chae CB: Anti-angiogenin activity of the peptides complementary to the receptor-binding site of angiogenin. J Biol Chem 272:24,294–24,299, 1997.
168. Ozaki H, Hayashi H, Oshima K: Angiogenin levels in the vitreous from patients with proliferative diabetic retinopathy. Ophthalmic Res 28:356–360, 1996.
169. Hockel M, Sasse J, Wissler JH: Purified monocyte-derived angiogenic substance (angiotropin) stimulates migration, phenotypic changes, and “tube formation” but not proliferation of capillary endothelial cells in vitro. J Cell Physiol 133:1–13, 1987.
170. Hockel M, Jung W, Vaupel P, et al: Purified monocyte-derived angiogenic substance (angiotropin) induces controlled angiogenesis associated with regulated tissue proliferation in rabbit skin. J Clin Invest 82:1075–1090, 1988.
171. Weidner KM, Arakaki N, Hartmann G, et al: Evidence for the identity of human scatter factor and human hepatocyte growth factor. Proc Natl Acad Sci U S A 88:7001–7005, 1991.
172. Rosen EM, Grant D, Kleinman H, et al: Scatter factor stimulates migration of vascular endothelium and capillary-like tube formation. EXS (Basel) 59:76–88, 1991.
173. Grant DS, Kleinman HK, Goldberg ID, et al: Scatter factor induces blood vessel formation in vivo. Proc Natl Acad Sci U S A 90:1937–1941, 1993.
174. Bussolino F, Di Renzo MF, Ziche M, et al: Hepatocyte growth factor is a potent angiogenic factor which stimulates endothelial cell motility and growth. J Cell Biol 119:629–641, 1992.
175. Roletto F, Galvani AP, Cristiani C, et al: Basic fibroblast growth factor stimulates hepatocyte growth factor/scatter factor secretion by human mesenchymal cells. J Cell Physiol 166:105–111, 1996.
176. Camussi G, Montrucchio G, Lupia E, et al: Angiogenesis induced in vivo by hepatocyte growth factor is mediated by platelet-activating factor synthesis from macrophages. J Immunol 158:1302–1309, 1997.
177. Strieter RM, Polverini PJ, Kunkel SL, et al: The functional role of the ELR motif in CXC chemokine-mediated angiogenesis. J Biol Chem 270:27,348–27,357, 1995.
178. Koch AE, Polverini PJ, Kunkel SL, et al: Interleukin-8 as a macrophage-derived mediator of angiogenesis [see comments]. Science 258:1798–1801, 1992.
179. Folkman J: Tumor angiogenesis. *In* Holland J, Frei E, et al (eds): Cancer Medicine, 3rd ed. Malvern, PA, Lea & Febiger, 1991.
180. Nicosia RF, Bonanno E, Smith M: Fibronectin promotes the elongation of microvessels during angiogenesis in vitro. J Cell Physiol 154:654–661, 1993.
181. Murata J, Saiki I, Makabe T, et al: Inhibition of tumor-induced angiogenesis by sulfated chitin derivatives. Cancer Res 51:22–26, 1991.
182. Folkman J, D'Amore P: Blood vessel formation: What is its molecular basis? Cell 87:1153–1155, 1996.
183. Suri C, Jones PF, Patan S, et al: Requisite role of angiopoietin-1, a ligand for the TIE2 receptor, during embryonic angiogenesis [see comments]. Cell 87:1171–1180, 1996.
184. Wong AL, Haroon ZA, Werner S, et al: Tie2 expression and phosphorylation in angiogenic and quiescent adult tissues. Circ Res 81:567–574, 1997.
185. Lin P, Polverini P, Dewhirst M, et al: Inhibition of tumor angiogenesis using a soluble receptor establishes a role for Tie2 in pathologic vascular growth. J Clin Invest 100:2072–2078, 1997.
186. Maisonpierre PC, Suri C, Jones PF, et al: Angiopoietin-2, a natural antagonist for Tie2 that disrupts in vivo angiogenesis [see comments]. Science 277:55–60, 1997.
187. Folkman J: Anti-angiogenesis: New concept for therapy of solid tumors. Ann Surg 175:409–416, 1972.
188. Brem H, Folkman J: Inhibition of tumor angiogenesis mediated by cartilage. J Exp Med 141:427–438, 1975.
189. Taylor S, Folkman J: Protamine is an inhibitor of angiogenesis. Nature 297:719–725, 1982.
190. Folkman J, Langer R, Linhardt R, et al: Angiogenesis inhibition and tumor regression caused by heparin or a heparin fragment in the presence of cortisone. Science 221:719–725, 1983.
191. Ingber D, Fujita T, Kishimoto S, et al: Synthetic analogues of fumagillin that inhibit angiogenesis and suppress tumour growth. Nature 348:555–557, 1990.
192. Gonzalez E, Adamis A, Folkman J: Systemic administration of an angiogenesis inhibitor (AGM-1470) inhibits bFGF induced corneal neovascularization. Invest Ophthalmol Vis Sci 33:424a, 1992.
193. Broutye-Boye D, Zetter B: Inhibition of cell motility by interferon. Science 108:516, 1980.
194. White C, Sondheimer H, Crouch E, et al: Treatment of pulmonary hemangiomatosis with recombinant interferon alpha 2a. N Engl J Med 320:1197, 1989.
195. Crum R, Szabo S, Folkman J: A new class of steroids inhibits angiogenesis in the presence of heparin or a heparin fragment. Science 230:1375–1378, 1985.
196. Ingber DE, Madri JA, Folkman J: A possible mechanism for inhibition of angiogenesis by angiostatic steroids: Induction of capillary basement membrane dissolution. Endocrinology 119:1768–1775, 1986.
197. Ingber D, Folkman J: Inhibition of angiogenesis through modulation of collagen metabolism. Lab Invest 59:44–51, 1988.
198. Maragoudakis ME, Sarmonika M, Panousacopoulou M: Antiangiogenic action of heparin plus cortisone is associated with decreased collagenous protein synthesis in the chick chorioallantoic membrane system. J Pharmacol Exp Ther 251:679–682, 1989.
199. Pereles T, Ingber D, Folkman J: Inhibition of capillary endothelial colony outgrowth: The role of complex formation between an angiostatic steroid and beta-cyclodextrin tetradecasulfate. J Cell Biol 109:311, 1989.
200. Li WW, Casey R, Gonzalez EM, Folkman J: Angiostatic steroids potentiated by sulfated cyclodextrins inhibit corneal neovascularization. Invest Ophthalmol Vis Sci 32:2898–2905, 1991.
201. Gagliardi A, Hadd H, Collins DC: Inhibition of angiogenesis by suramin. Cancer Res 52:5073–5075, 1992.
202. Gagliardi AR, Collins DC: Inhibition of angiogenesis by aurintricarboxylic acid. Anticancer Res 14:475–479, 1994.
203. Fotsis T, Zhang Y, Pepper MS, et al: The endogenous oestrogen metabolite 2-methoxyoestradiol inhibits angiogenesis and suppresses tumour growth. Nature 368:237–239, 1994.
204. D'Amato RJ, Lin CM, Flynn E, et al: 2-Methoxyestradiol, an endogenous mammalian metabolite, inhibits tubulin polymerization by interacting at the colchicine site. Proc Natl Acad Sci U S A 91:3964–3968, 1994.
205. Klauber N, Parangi S, Flynn E, et al: Inhibition of angiogenesis and breast cancer in mice by the microtubule inhibitors 2-methoxyestradiol and taxol. Cancer Res 57:81–86, 1997.
206. Danis RP, Bingaman DP, Yang Y, Ladd B: Inhibition of preretinal and optic nerve head neovascularization in pigs by intravitreal triamcinolone acetonide. Ophthalmology 103:2099–2104, 1996.
207. Ishibashi T, Miki K, Sorgente N, et al: Effects of intravitreal adminis-

tration of steroids on experimental subretinal neovascularization in the subhuman primate. Arch Ophthalmol 103:708–711, 1985.
208. Ben Ezra D, Griffin BW, Maftzir G, et al: Topical formulations of novel angiostatic steroids inhibit rabbit corneal neovascularization. Invest Ophthalmol Vis Sci 38:1954–1962, 1997.
209. Kusaka M, Sudo K, Fujita T, et al: Potent anti-angiogenic action of AGM-1470: Comparison to the fumagillin parent. Biochem Biophys Res Commun 174:1070–1076, 1991.
210. Sin N, Meng L, Wang MQ, et al: The anti-angiogenic agent fumagillin covalently binds and inhibits the methionine aminopeptidase, MetAP-2. Proc Natl Acad Sci U S A 94:6099–6103, 1997.
211. Griffith EC, Su Z, Turk BE, et al: Methionine aminopeptidase (type 2) is the common target for angiogenesis inhibitors AGM-1470 and ovalicin. Chem Biol 4:461–471, 1997.
212. Ahmed MH, Konno H, Nahar L, et al: The angiogenesis inhibitor TNP-470 (AGM-1470) improves long-term survival of rats with liver metastasis. J Surg Res 64:35–41, 1996.
213. Kanai T, Konno H, Tanaka T, et al: Effect of angiogenesis inhibitor TNP-470 on the progression of human gastric cancer xenotransplanted into nude mice. Int J Cancer 71:838–841, 1997.
214. Xia JL, Yang BH, Tang ZY, et al: Inhibitory effect of the angiogenesis inhibitor TNP-470 on tumor growth and metastasis in nude mice bearing human hepatocellular carcinoma. J Cancer Res Clin Oncol 123:383–387, 1997.
215. Futami H, Iseki H, Egawa S, et al: Inhibition of lymphatic metastasis in a syngeneic rat fibrosarcoma model by an angiogenesis inhibitor, AGM-1470. Invasion Metastasis 16:73–82, 1996.
216. Taki T, Ohnishi T, Arita N, et al: Anti-proliferative effects of TNP-470 on human malignant glioma in vivo: Potent inhibition of tumor angiogenesis. J Neurooncol 19:251–258, 1994.
217. Yamamoto T, Sudo K, Fujita T: Significant inhibition of endothelial cell growth in tumor vasculature by an angiogenesis inhibitor, TNP-470 (AGM-1470). Anticancer Res 14:1–3, 1994.
218. Morishita T, Mii Y, Miyauchi Y, et al: Efficacy of the angiogenesis inhibitor O-(chloroacetyl-carbamoyl)fumagillol (AGM-1470) on osteosarcoma growth and lung metastasis in rats. Jpn J Clin Oncol 25:25–31, 1995.
219. Yamaoka M, Yamamoto T, Masaki T, et al: Inhibition of tumor growth and metastasis of rodent tumors by the angiogenesis inhibitor O-(chloroacetyl-carbamoyl)fumagillol (TNP-470; AGM-1470). Cancer Res 53:4262–7, 1993.
220. Peacock DJ, Banquerigo ML, Brahn E: Angiogenesis inhibition suppresses collagen arthritis. J Exp Med 175:1135–1138, 1992.
221. Oliver SJ, Cheng TP, Banquerigo ML, Brahn E: Suppression of collagen-induced arthritis by an angiogenesis inhibitor, AGM-1470, in combination with cyclosporin: Reduction of vascular endothelial growth factor (VEGF). Cell Immunol 166:196–206, 1995.
222. Wong J, Wang N, Miller JW, Schuman JS: Modulation of human fibroblast activity by selected angiogenesis inhibitors. Exp Eye Res 58:439–451, 1994.
223. Figg WD, Pluda JM, Lush RM, et al: The pharmacokinetics of TNP-470, a new angiogenesis inhibitor. Pharmacotherapy 17:91–97, 1997.
224. Antoine N, Bours V, Heinen E, et al: Simulation of human B-lymphocyte proliferation by AGM–1470, a potent inhibitor of angiogenesis. J Natl Cancer Inst 87:136–139, 1995.
225. Otsuka T, Shibata T, Tsurumi Y, et al: A new angiogenesis inhibitor, FR-111142. J Antibiot (Tokyo) 45:348–354, 1992.
226. Fotsis T, Pepper M, Adlercreutz H, et al: Genistein, a dietary-derived inhibitor of in vitro angiogenesis. Proc Natl Acad Sci U S A 90:2690–2694, 1993.
227. Fotsis T, Pepper MS, Aktas E, et al: Flavonoids, dietary-derived inhibitors of cell proliferation and in vitro angiogenesis. Cancer Res 57:2916–2921, 1997.
228. Yoon TJ, Yoo YC, Choi OB, et al: Inhibitory effect of Korean mistletoe (*Viscum album coloratum*) extract on tumour angiogenesis and metastasis of haematogenous and non-haematogenous tumour cells in mice. Cancer Lett 97:83–91, 1995.
229. D'Amato RJ, Loughnan MS, Flynn E, Folkman J: Thalidomide is an inhibitor of angiogenesis. Proc Natl Acad Sci U S A 91:4082–4085, 1994.
230. Kenyon BM, Browne F, D'Amato RJ: Effects of thalidomide and related metabolites in a mouse corneal model of neovascularization. Exp Eye Res 64:971–978, 1997.
231. Zucker M, Katz I: Platelet factor 4: Production, structure, and physiologic and immunologic action. Proc Soc Exp Biol Med 198:693–702, 1991.
232. Teicher B, Sotomayor E, Huang Z: Anti-angiogenic agents potentiate cytotoxic cancer therapies against primary and metastatic disease. Cancer Res 52:6702–6704, 1992.
233. Maione TE, Gray GS, Petro J, et al: Inhibition of angiogenesis by recombinant human platelet factor-4 and related peptides. Science 247:77–79, 1990.
234. Kolber D, Knisely T, Maione T: Inhibition of development of murine melanoma lung metastases by systemic administration of recombinant platelet factor 4. J Natl Cancer Inst 87:304–309, 1995.
235. Tanaka T, Manome Y, Wen P, et al: Viral vector-mediated transduction of a modified platelet factor 4 cDNA inhibits angiogenesis and tumor growth. Nat Med 3:437–442, 1997.
236. Voest EE: Inhibitors of angiogenesis in a clinical perspective. Anticancer Drugs 7:723–727, 1996.
237. Maione TE, Gray GS, Hunt AJ, Sharpe RJ: Inhibition of tumor growth in mice by an analogue of platelet factor 4 that lacks affinity for heparin and retains potent angiostatic activity. Cancer Res 51:2077–2083, 1991.
238. Angiolillo AL, Sgadari C, Taub DD, et al: Human interferon-inducible protein 10 is a potent inhibitor of angiogenesis in vivo. J Exp Med 182:155–162, 1995.
239. Strieter RM, Kunkel SL, Arenberg DA, et al: Interferon gamma–inducible protein 10 (IP-10), a member of the C-X-C chemokine family, is an inhibitor of angiogenesis. Biochem Biophys Res Commun 210:51–57, 1995.
240. Voest EE, Kenyon BM, O'Reilly MS, et al: Inhibition of angiogenesis in vivo by interleukin 12. J Natl Cancer Inst 87:581–586, 1995.
241. Cao Y, Chen C, Weatherbee JA, et al: Gro-beta, a -C-X-C- chemokine, is an angiogenesis inhibitor that suppresses the growth of Lewis lung carcinoma in mice. J Exp Med 182:2069–2077, 1995.
242. De Clerck YA, Darville MI, Eeckhout Y, Rousseau GG: Characterization of the promoter of the gene encoding human tissue inhibitor of metalloproteinases-2 (TIMP-2). Gene 139:185–91, 1994.
243. Stetler-Stevenson WG, Krutzsch HC, Liotta LA: Tissue inhibitor of metalloproteinase (TIMP-2). A new member of the metalloproteinase inhibitor family. J Biol Chem 264:17,374–17,378, 1989.
244. Pavloff N, Staskus PW, Kishnani NS, Hawkes SP: A new inhibitor of metalloproteinases from chicken: ChIMP-3. A third member of the TIMP family. J Biol Chem 267:17,321–17,326, 1992.
245. Leco KJ, Apte SS, Taniguchi GT, et al: Murine tissue inhibitor of metalloproteinases-4 (Timp-4): cDNA isolation and expression in adult mouse tissues. FEBS Lett 401:213–217, 1997.
246. Liu YE, Wang M, Greene J, et al: Preparation and characterization of recombinant tissue inhibitor of metalloproteinase 4 (TIMP-4). J Biol Chem 272:20,479–20,483, 1997.
247. Ward R, Hembry R, Reynolds J: The purification of tissue inhibitor of metalloproteinase-2 from its 72kDa progelatinase complex. Demonstration of biochemical similarities. Biochem J 278:179–187, 1991.
248. Apte SS, Olsen BR, Murphy G: The gene structure of tissue inhibitor of metalloproteinases (TIMP)-3 and its inhibitory activities define the distinct TIMP gene family [published erratum appears in J Biol Chem 271(5):2874, 1996]. J Biol Chem 270:14,313–14,318, 1995.
249. Einstein R, Kuettner K, Neopolitan C, et al: The resistance of certain tissue to invasion. III: Cartilage extracts inhibit the growth of fibroblasts and endothelial cells in culture. Am J Pathol 81:337–347, 1975.
250. Tamargo R, Bok R, Brem H: Angiogenesis inhibition by minocycline. Cancer Res 51:672–675, 1991.
251. Murphy A, Unsworth E, Stetler-Steve: Tissue inhibitor of metalloproteinase-2 inhibits bFGF-induced human microvascular endothelial cell proliferation. J Cell Physiol 157:351–358, 1993.
252. Takigawa M, Nishida Y, Suzuki F, et al: Induction of angiogenesis in chick yolk-sac membrane by polyamines and its inhibition by tissue inhibitors of metalloproteinases (TIMP-1 and TIMP-2). Biochem Biophys Res Commun 171:1264–1271, 1990.
253. Johnson M, Kim H, Chester L, et al: Inhibition of angiogenesis by tissue inhibitor of metalloproteinase. J Cell Physiol 160:194–202, 1994.
254. Sorsby A, Mason M, Gardener N: A fundus dystrophy with unusual features. Br J Ophthalmol 33:67–97, 1949.
255. Capon M, Marshall J, Krafft J, et al: Sorsby's fundus dystrophy—A light and electron microscopy study. Ophthalmology 96:1769–1777, 1989.
256. Weber B, Vogt G, Pruett R, et al: Mutation in the tissue inhibitor of metalloproteinases-3 (TIMP-3) in patients with Sorsby's fundus dystrophy. Nature Genetics 8:353–356, 1994.
257. Fariss RN, Apte SS, Olsen BR, et al: Tissue inhibitor of metalloprotei-

nases-3 is a component of Bruch's membrane of the eye. Am J Pathol 150:323–328, 1997.

258. Anand-Apte B, Pepper MS, Voest E, et al: Inhibition of angiogenesis by tissue inhibitor of metalloproteinase-3 [see comments]. Invest Ophthalmol Vis Sci 38:817–823, 1997.
259. Dong Z, Kumar R, Yang X, Fidler I: Macrophage-derived metalloelastase is responsible for generation of angiostatin in Lewis lung carcinoma. Cell 88:801–810, 1997.
260. Kendall R, Thomas K: Inhibition of vascular endothelial growth factor activity by endogenously encoded soluble receptor. Proc Natl Acad Sci U S A 90:10,705–10,709, 1993.
261. Millauer B, Shawver LK, Plate KH, et al: Glioblastoma growth inhibited in vivo by a dominant-negative Flk-1 mutant. Nature 367:576–579, 1994.
262. Millauer B, Longhi MP, Plate KH, et al: Dominant-negative inhibition of Flk-1 suppresses the growth of many tumor types in vivo. Cancer Res 56:1615–1620, 1996.
263. Stratmann A, Machein MR, Plate KH: Anti-angiogenic gene therapy of malignant glioma. Acta Neurochir Suppl 68:105–110, 1997.
264. Ramakrishnan S, Olson TA, Bautch VL, Mohanraj D: Vascular endothelial growth factor–toxin conjugate specifically inhibits KDR/flk-1–positive endothelial cell proliferation in vitro and angiogenesis in vivo. Cancer Res 56:1324–1330, 1996.
265. Xia P, Aiello LP, Ishii H, et al: Characterization of vascular endothelial growth factor's effect on the activation of protein kinase C, its isoforms, and endothelial cell growth. J Clin Invest 98:2018–2026, 1996.
266. Aiello LP, Bursell SE, Clermont A, et al: Vascular endothelial growth factor–induced retinal permeability is mediated by protein kinase C in vivo and suppressed by an orally effective beta-isoform–selective inhibitor. Diabetes 46:1473–1480, 1997.
267. Danis R, Bingaman D, Jirousek M, Yang Y: Inhibition of intraocular neovascularization caused by retinal ischemia in pig PKCB inhibition with LY333531. Invest Ophthalmol Vis Sci 39:171–179, 1998.
268. Shima DT, Deutsch U, D'Amore PA: Hypoxic induction of vascular endothelial growth factor (VEGF) in human epithelial cells is mediated by increases in mRNA stability. FEBS Lett 370:203–208, 1995.
269. Robinson G, Pierce E, Rook S, et al: Oligodeoxynucleotides inhibit retinal neovascularization in a murine model of proliferative retinopathy. Proc Natl Acad Sci U S A 93:4851–4856, 1996.
270. Takagi H, King GL, Robinson GS, Ferrara N, Aiello LP: Adenosine mediates hypoxic induction of vascular endothelial growth factor in retinal pericytes and endothelial cells. Invest Ophthalmol Vis Sci 37:2165–2176, 1996.
271. Takagi H, King GL, Ferrara N, Aiello LP: Hypoxia regulates vascular endothelial growth factor receptor KDR/Flk gene expression through adenosine A2 receptors in retinal capillary endothelial cells. Invest Ophthalmol Vis Sci 37:1311–1321, 1996.
272. Smith L, Kopchick J, Chen W, et al: Essential role of growth hormone in ischemia-induced retinal neovascularization. Science 276:1706–1709, 1997.
273. Mun E, Doctrow S, Carter R, Ingber D: An angiogenesis inhibitor from the cornea. Invest Ophthalmol Sci 30:151, 1989.
274. Clapp C, Martial J, Guzman R, et al: The 16-kilodalton *N*-terminal fragment of human prolactin is a potent inhibitor of angiogenesis. Endocrinology 133:1292–1299, 1993.
275. D'Angelo G, Struman I, Martial J, Weiner RI: Activation of mitogen-activated protein kinases by vascular endothelial growth factor and basic fibroblast growth factor in capillary endothelial cells is inhibited by the antiangiogenic factor 16-kDa N-terminal fragment of prolactin. Proc Natl Acad Sci U S A 92:6374–6378, 1995.
276. Weiner R, D'Angelo G: Signaling for the antiangiogenic action of 16kD prolactin. Proc Am Assoc Cancer Res 37:667–668, 1996.
277. Ferrara N, Clapp C, Weiner R: The 16 kD fragment of prolactin inhibits basal or fibroblast growth factor stimulated growth of capillary endothelial cells. Endocrinology 129:896, 1991.
278. Tolsma SS, Stack MS, Bouck N: Lumen formation and other angiogenic activities of cultured capillary endothelial cells are inhibited by thrombospondin-1. Microvasc Res 54:13–26, 1997.
279. Iruela-Arispe ML, Bornstein P, Sage H: Thrombospondin exerts an antiangiogenic effect on cord formation by endothelial cells in vitro. Proc Natl Acad Sci U S A 88:5026–5030, 1991.
280. Di Pietro LA, Polverini PJ: Angiogenic macrophages produce the angiogenic inhibitor thrombospondin 1. Am J Pathol 143:678–684, 1993.
281. Lamszus K, Joseph A, Jin L, et al: Scatter factor binds to thrombospondin and other extracellular matrix components. Am J Pathol 149:805–89, 1996.
282. Taraboletti G, Belotti D, Borsotti P, et al: The 140-kilodalton antiangiogenic fragment of thrombospondin-1 binds to basic fibroblast growth factor. Cell Growth Differ 8:471–479, 1997.
283. Qian X, Wang TN, Rothman VL, et al: Thrombospondin-1 modulates angiogenesis in vitro by up-regulation of matrix metalloproteinase-9 in endothelial cells. Exp Cell Res 235:403–412, 1997.
284. Volpert OV, Tolsma SS, Pellerin S, et al: Inhibition of angiogenesis by thrombospondin-2. Biochem Biophys Res Commun 217:326–332, 1995.
285. Dameron KM, Volpert OV, Tainsky MA, Bouck N: Control of angiogenesis in fibroblasts by p53 regulation of thrombospondin-1. Science 265:1582–1584, 1994.
286. Good DJ, Polverini PJ, Rastinejad F, et al: A tumor suppressor–dependent inhibitor of angiogenesis is immunologically and functionally indistinguishable from a fragment of thrombospondin. Proc Natl Acad Sci U S A 87:6624–6628, 1990.
287. Hsu SC, Volpert OV, Steck PA, et al: Inhibition of angiogenesis in human glioblastomas by chromosome 10 induction of thrombospondin-1. Cancer Res 56:5684–5691, 1996.
288. O'Reilly M, Holmgren L, Shing Y, et al: Angiostatin: A novel angiogenesis inhibitor that mediates the suppression of metastases by a Lewis lung carcinoma. Cell 79:315–328, 1994.
289. Cao Y, Ji RW, Davidson D, et al: Kringle domains of human angiostatin. Characterization of the anti-proliferative activity on endothelial cells. J Biol Chem 271:29,461–29,467, 1996.
290. Gately S, Twardowski P, Stack M, et al: Human prostate carcinoma cells express enzymatic activity that converts human plasminogen to the angiogenesis inhibitor, angiostatin. Cancer Res 56:4887–4990, 1996.
291. O'Reilly MS, Boehm T, Shing Y, et al: Endostatin: An endogenous inhibitor of angiogenesis and tumor growth. Cell 88:277–285, 1997.
292. Alliegro MC, Alliegro MA, Cragoe EJ Jr, Glaser BM: Amiloride inhibition of angiogenesis in vitro. J Exp Zool 267:245–252, 1993.
293. Candal FJ, Bosse DC, Vogler WR, Ades EW: Inhibition of induced angiogenesis in a human microvascular endothelial cell line by ET-18-OCH3. Cancer Chemother Pharmacol 34:175–178, 1994.
294. Maragoudakis ME, Peristeris P, Missirlis E, et al: Inhibition of angiogenesis by anthracyclines and titanocene dichloride. Ann N Y Acad Sci 732:280–293, 1994.
295. Nguyen NM, Lehr JE, Pienta KJ: Pentosan inhibits angiogenesis in vitro and suppresses prostate tumor growth in vivo. Anticancer Res 13:2143–2147, 1993.
296. Polverini PJ, Novak RF: Inhibition of angiogenesis by the antineoplastic agents mitoxantrone and bisantrene. Biochem Biophys Res Commun 140:901–907, 1986.
297. Lindsay CK, Gomez DE, Thorgeirsson UP: Effect of flavone acetic acid on endothelial cell proliferation: Evidence for antiangiogenic properties. Anticancer Res 16:425–431, 1996.
298. Oikawa T, Hasegawa M, Shimamura M, et al: Eponemycin, a novel antibiotic, is a highly powerful angiogenesis inhibitor. Biochem Biophys Res Commun 181:1070–1076, 1991.
299. Oikawa T, Hasegawa M, Morita I, et al: Effect of 15-deoxyspergualin, a microbial angiogenesis inhibitor, on the biological activities of bovine vascular endothelial cells. Anticancer Drugs 3:293–299, 1992.
300. Behzadian MA, Wang XL, Jiang B, Caldwell RB: Angiostatic role of astrocytes: Suppression of vascular endothelial cell growth by TGF-beta and other inhibitory factor(s). Glia 15:480–490, 1995.
301. Chen C, Parangi S, Tolentino MJ, Folkman J: A strategy to discover circulating angiogenesis inhibitors generated by human tumors. Cancer Res 55:4230–4233, 1995.

CHAPTER 38

New Directions for the Medical Treatment of Glaucoma

Arthur H. Neufeld

Concepts of Neuroprotection Based on Studies of the Central Nervous System

Recent advances in the understanding of the underlying biology of neurodegenerative diseases of the central nervous system have offered new hope for developing pharmacologic treatment of these diseases. Pharmacologic neuroprotection can be broadly envisioned as using classic, low molecular weight, pharmacologic type molecules; high molecular weight biologics generated by biotechnology; or vector-targeted alterations in gene expression to prevent or to slow the loss of nerve cells in neurodegenerative diseases. A huge, ongoing research effort and numerous clinical trials are aimed at providing pharmacologic neuroprotection for patients suffering from stroke, spinal cord trauma, epilepsy, multiple sclerosis, acquired immunodeficiency syndrome (AIDS) dementia, amyotrophic lateral sclerosis, and Parkinson's, Huntington's, or Alzheimer's disease. Although this research has not yet actually brought new medical treatments to many patients, this work will undoubtedly prove fruitful and eventually lead to new treatment modalities. Because glaucoma has come to be described as an optic neuropathy, new treatments are being sought that are not based solely on lowering intraocular pressure. We can expect progress in the development of neuroprotective pharmacologic agents for the treatment of glaucomatous optic neuropathy.

Recent basic research has yielded several concepts describing neurodegeneration that have provided the framework for beginning to consider approaches to pharmacologic neuroprotection. We now know that in addition to nerves dying because of direct physical stresses, such as transection, crush, toxic chemicals, or anoxia, neuronal degeneration also occurs as an orderly process of programmed cell death, often called apoptosis.[1–4] Apoptosis is triggered by activation or inhibition of physiologic or pathologic stimuli and is accomplished by the expression of specific gene products and the activation of intracellular enzymes.

The concept of excitotoxicity has also provided new insights into stimuli that can cause neuronal degeneration.[5, 6] The amino acid glutamate is important physiologically as a neurotransmitter in the central nervous system. At increased levels, however, glutamate is toxic to nerve cells; this toxicity is mediated through physiologic glutaminergic receptors on the nerve. Inhibiting the excitotoxic activity of glutamate at its receptor, or the release of excessive neurotransmitter, is now a major target for pharmacologic intervention for stroke and spinal cord trauma.

Another concept that has come out of studies of neurodegeneration of the central nervous system describes primary and secondary events that cause death of nerve cells.[7, 8] For example, initial loss of neurons due to physical trauma or an ischemic event may be relatively local, caused by a necrotic mechanism, and can occur quickly within minutes or hours, causing a modest amount of damage and loss of function. However, this primary event may set up secondary events, involving inflammatory or toxic mediators, that cause more widespread degeneration of neurons by an apoptotic mechanism; such events can occur over days or weeks and can lead to more serious loss of function. These secondary events may be due to reperfusion, neurotoxic mediators, increased calcium levels, reactivated astrocytes, altered energy metabolism by the mitochondria, or a combination thereof. When a stroke occurs, there may be little that can be done for the initial loss of neurons, but many workers in the field believe that early pharmacologic intervention aimed at secondary events will reduce the subsequent damage and loss of function.

Extrapolations from these concepts indicate that neuronal degeneration is a complex series of events and, therefore, that there are many potential points of intervention. Many of the findings on neuronal degeneration in the central nervous system undoubtedly apply to the optic neuropathy associated with glaucoma and will be pursued as new treatments for the disease.

Potential Pharmacologic Approaches for Neuroprotection in Glaucoma

The changes in the visual field and loss of vision that are characteristic of glaucoma are due to degeneration of retinal ganglion cells and often are associated with elevated intraocular pressure. Clinically, axonal loss of the retinal ganglion cells is a thinning of the nerve fiber layer and an excavation of the optic disk. Previous research in humans with glaucoma and in monkeys with experimentally induced glaucoma suggested that the initial site of damage to the axons of the retinal ganglion cells occurs at the level of the lamina cribrosa in the optic nerve head.[9, 10] As nerve fibers are lost in this region, the remaining connective tissue, glia, and blood vessels are extensively remodeled to form the characteristic clinical appearance of the glaucomatous optic nerve head.

Glaucomatous optic neuropathy should not be thought of as a chronic degeneration of the optic nerve but as an acute death of individual axons of the optic nerve, which can progress throughout the tissue. Clearly, all of the axons of the optic nerve do not die at the same time, in the same year, or even in the same decade. Glaucomatous optic neuropathy is a slow disease process that progresses over years and often decades. Neuronal degeneration, as may occur by apoptosis, takes approximately 24 hours, start to finish. Obviously, then, all of the axons of the optic nerve and their associated retinal ganglion cells are not undergoing degeneration at the same time. Considering that the human optic nerve contains approximately 1 million axons, at any given time there are probably relatively few nerve cells that are degenerating in a glaucomatous eye. Thus, our conception of a glaucomatous optic nerve with mild disease must envision a tissue with some degenerating nerve fibers and many perfectly normal nerve fibers. With moderate disease, areas of the optic nerve in which axons previously degenerated are filled in by extracellular matrix and glial hyperplasia, but these optic nerves must still contain many healthy nerve fibers and some currently degenerating nerve fibers. Even in cases of severe disease in which the optic nerve head has been extensively excavated, there must still be normal, functioning retinal ganglion cells and their corresponding axons coursing through the remodeled tissue.

The concept of optic nerve degeneration as the progressive sum of acute degenerative processes of the individual axons suggests targets for neuroprotection that are related to primary or secondary events. Several recent advances in studying optic nerve degeneration and loss of retinal ganglion cells will help to establish the potential points of intervention for pharmacologic neuroprotection in glaucoma. These new findings include the demonstration of apoptosis of retinal ganglion cells and the identification of neurotoxic molecules in human glaucomatous tissue.

Using several animal models of optic nerve degeneration, researchers have demonstrated that retinal ganglion cells die by apoptosis.[11–13] The universality of this programmed cell death pathway, following both optic nerve transection and crush as well as acutely elevated high intraocular pressure and chronically elevated moderate intraocular pressure, strongly suggests the relevance of apoptotic mechanisms to glaucomatous optic neuropathy as the final common pathway by which retinal ganglion cells die. Interestingly, we know from models of cell death in spinal cord injury that apoptosis is the mechanism used in response to secondary stimuli. Inhibition of apoptosis, somewhere along the cascade of genes and enzymes that are implementing the program, is a reasonable goal for intervention.

During neuronal cell death by apoptosis, a variety of proteins and enzymes are activated or newly synthesized via gene expression.[1–4] There are proteins such as Bcl 2 and related molecules that tend to suppress apoptotic mechanisms and Bax and p53 that promote apoptosis. Much of the activity of these molecules centers around changes in mitochondrial permeability, thus affecting the energy state of the neuron.[14] Certain specific enzymes, such as those of the caspase family, are aimed at the enzymatic denaturation of key protein substrates within the neuron. Eventually, the nuclear DNA is fragmented by specific endonucleases. All of this activity occurs while the cell membrane remains intact. Thus, the cell does not lyse and release its internal contents but forms characteristic apoptotic blebs containing denatured material. The cellular material is phagocytosed by neighboring cells, and an inflammatory response is avoided.

The mechanism of apoptosis is important developmentally in the central nervous system.[15] During embryonic development, many more nerve cells are made than will survive postnatally. As neurons send out their axons and make synapses with other nerves in their target region, many axons do not make contact and presumably do not receive the appropriate neurotrophic factor. As shown in models of neurotrophic factor withdrawal, these nerves degenerate by apoptosis.[16] Exposure to neurotrophic factors for maintenance of nerves appears relevant to retinal ganglion cells. In animal models of transected or crushed optic nerves, intravitreal injection or enhanced retinal expression of neurotrophic factors such as brain-derived neurotrophic factor (BDNF) significantly decreases the rate of retinal ganglion cell loss.[17]

Currently, we do not have the means to intervene in the process of apoptosis in nerve cells. Experiments using transgenic animals and knockout animals demonstrate that overexpression or underexpression of certain gene products can interfere with the apoptotic mechanism in retinal ganglion cells.[18] Thus, a therapy based on vector-targeted gene transfer to retinal ganglion cells, most likely through intravitreal administration, may prove useful for glaucoma.[19] An alternative therapeutic approach would be to supply retinal ganglion cells with neurotrophic factors that may have lost access to the retinal ganglion cells and therefore triggered the cell's death cascade. A current hypothesis of several investigators is that the blockage of axoplasmic flow, at the level of the lamina cribrosa, prevents the transport of neurotrophic factors from the lateral geniculate nucleus to the retinal ganglion cell body and thus triggers apoptosis in a manner similar to that which occurs developmentally.[12] Therefore, an alternative approach to try to prevent activation of the apoptosis cascade would be to supply the missing neurotrophic factors to the stressed retinal ganglion cells. As pharmacologic neuroprotection, this therapeutic approach would need a long-term, local method to expose the retinal ganglion cells to the appropriate neurotrophic factor.

Glutamate probably plays an excitotoxic role in the death of retinal ganglion cells.[20] Within the retina, photoreceptors and bipolar cells contain high concentrations of glutamate, which they use as a neurotransmitter. Müller's cells are actively involved in maintaining extracellular glutamate levels by taking up the transmitter. The surface of many retinal neurons has glutaminergic receptors. There are four types of glutaminergic receptors: metabotropic receptors, α-amino-3-hydroxy-5-methylisoxazole-4-propionate (AMPA) receptors, kainate receptors, and *N*-methyl-D-aspartate (NMDA) receptors. Stimulation of the NMDA receptors leads to activation of a variety of intracellular calcium-dependent processes and is responsible for glutamate excitotoxicity and neuronal damage.

Recent evidence demonstrates the presence of elevated glutamate in the vitreous of patients with glaucoma and in the vitreous of experimental animals with elevated intraocular pressure and degeneration of retinal ganglion cells.[21] This work implies that excessive glutamate in the retina, due to increased release or decreased uptake, may be at least partially responsible for the death of retinal ganglion cells. If the initial events in glaucomatous optic neuropathy occur in the optic nerve, glutamate excitotoxicity in the retina may be a secondary event. Nevertheless, inhibition of this secondary event could have important consequences for saving additional retinal ganglion cells.

In several clinical trials aimed at central nervous system pathology, the use of specific antagonists of the glutamate receptors has failed because of intolerable side effects. As more specific glutamate antagonists are developed that are relatively free of side effects, a new glaucoma therapy based on blocking the excitotoxic activity of glutamate may emerge.

Another molecule of potential importance to optic nerve degeneration is nitric oxide.[22] Under physiologic conditions, nitric oxide (NO), synthesized by the enzyme nitric oxide synthase (NOS) from arginine, is an important mediator of neurotransmission and vasodilation. However, NO in excessive amounts can also kill cells and has been implicated in various neurodegenerative diseases as either a primary or secondary event.

Three isoforms of NOS have been localized in the central nervous system.[23] NOS-1, or neuronal NOS, is found constitutively in neurons and astrocytes and synthesizes NO as a transmitter. NOS-3, or endothelial NOS, is found constitutively in the vascular endothelia and stimulates vasodilation. NOS-2 is the inducible form of the enzyme and is not found constitutively in the central nervous system. NOS-2 can be induced in astrocytes in response to hypoxia, inflammatory mediators, and neuronal damage and can produce excessive NO that can damage the nearby nerve fibers. Nevertheless, both NOS-1 and NOS-2 apparently contribute to neuronal degeneration. Experimental models have demonstrated that NO synthesized by NOS-1 mediates early neuronal injury, and NOS-2 contributes to late neuronal injury. Because NO synthesized by NOS-3 causes vasodilation, this isoform offers some degree of neuroprotection from ischemic injury.

Recent evidence indicates the presence of the inducible isoform of NOS in the cells of the lamina cribrosa of patients with glaucoma.[24] In glaucomatous optic nerve heads, this enzyme may be causing nerve damage by local release of excessive NO. Pharmacologic inhibitors of the inducible form of NOS are being developed to treat diseases in which NO has been implicated and may one day help to accomplish neuroprotection in glaucoma.

Additional pharmacologic approaches based in neurodegenerative diseases of the central nervous system may affect glaucomatous neuropathy. Because elevated calcium has been implicated in neuronal cell death,[25] calcium channel blockers have been tried for the treatment of ischemic injury. Several reports in the glaucoma literature, on relatively small groups of patients, have claimed some success in slowing visual field loss, particularly in normal-pressure glaucoma. Adenosine agonists and drugs that increase adenosine appear to reduce neuronal damage in cerebrovascular disease.[26] Adenosine is a mediator of preconditioning, blocks neuronal damage experimentally in reperfusion injury, and causes vasodilation of retinal vessels. Conceivably, adenosine agonists could improve blood flow to a compromised optic nerve in glaucoma. To the extent that compromised vascular perfusion of the optic nerve head due to vasoconstrictors such as the endothelins may occur in glaucoma, antagonists at the receptors of these mediators may prove useful to restore optic nerve blood flow.[27] Neurotoxic free fatty acids such as platelet-activating factor may be produced from endogenous phospholipids in the glaucomatous optic nerve. In experimental models of retinal injury, platelet-activating factor antagonists reduce neuronal damage and may prove to be relevant to glaucoma.[28]

Developing a pharmacologic neuroprotective agent for the treatment of glaucoma presents significant obstacles that must be overcome in order to bring about a new drug therapy. Better animal or in vitro models for screening classes of compounds and candidate molecules need to be developed, and the experimental end-points used in these models have to be shown to be clinically relevant. Delivery of the pharmacologic agent must be addressed. For ophthalmic pharmaceuticals, delivery is usually topical to maximize the amount of drug reaching the target and to minimize the systemic side effects. A neuroprotective agent, such as one aimed at glutamate excitotoxicity or inhibition of nitric oxide synthase, will probably have to be administered systemically, i.e., orally. Considering that such a drug may have to be used chronically for the remainder of the patient's life, the side effect profile will have to be minimal. Possible delivery of a gene or neurotrophic factor to retinal ganglion cells will have to be accomplished locally and constantly in order to ensure continuous neuroprotection. This will be a formidable technical task.

Once a pharmacologic neuroprotective agent is in development for the treatment of glaucoma, clinical trials will have to focus on the measurement of a meaningful clinical end-point that can be measured at multiple participating clinical sites. The choice of this clinical end-point, such as visual fields, will have to be standardized at different sites and be robust enough to measure changes in any one patient in a reasonable time frame. Overcoming these obstacles will require a pharmaceutical company with sufficient resources in terms of researchers, time, and money as well as a long-range view of the significance of introducing a new glaucoma therapy based on pharmacologic neuroprotection.

REFERENCES

1. Johnson EM, Deckwerth TL, Deshmukh M: Neuronal death in developmental models: Possible implications in neuropathology. Brain Pathology 6:397–409, 1996.
2. Raff MC, et al: Programmed cell death and the control of cell survival: Lessons from the nervous system. Science 262:695–700, 1993.
3. Rubin LL, et al: The molecular mechanisms of neuronal apoptosis. Curr Opin Neurobiol 4:696–702, 1994.
4. Mattson MP, Furukawa K: Programmed cell life: Anti-apoptotic signaling and therapeutic strategies for neurodegenerative disorders. Restor Neurol Neurosci 9:191–205, 1996.
5. Choi DW: Glutamate neurotoxicity and diseases of the nervous system. Neuron 1:623–634, 1988.
6. Lipton SA, Rosenberg PA: Excitatory amino acids as a final common pathway for neurologic disorders. N Engl J Med 330:613–622, 1994.
7. Lipton SA: Similarity of neuronal cell injury and death in AIDS dementia and focal cerebral ischemia: Potential treatment with NMDA open-channel blockers and nitric oxide-related species. Brain Pathol 6:507–517, 1996.
8. Choi DW: Ischemia-induced neuronal apoptosis. Curr Opin Neurobiol 6:667–672, 1996.
9. Quigley HA, et al: Morphologic changes in the lamina cribrosa correlated with neural loss in open angle glaucoma. Am J Ophthalmol 95:673–691, 1983.
10. Quigley HA, Anderson DR: The dynamics and location of axonal blockade by acute intraocular pressure elevation in primate optic nerve. Invest Ophthalmol 15:606–616, 1976.
11. Garcia-Valenzuela E, et al: Programmed cell death of retinal ganglion cells during experimental glaucoma. Exp Eye Res 61:33–44, 1995.
12. Quigley HA, et al: Retinal ganglion cell death in experimental glaucoma and after axotomy occurs by apoptosis. Invest Ophthalmol Vis Sci 36:774–786, 1995.

13. Garcia-Valenzuela E, et al: Apoptosis in adult retinal ganglion cells after axotomy. J Neurobiol 25:431–438, 1994.
14. Kroemer G: Mitochondrial control of apoptosis. Immunol Today 18:44–51, 1997.
15. Johnson EM, Deckwerth TL: Molecular mechanisms of developmental neuronal death. Annu Rev Neurosci 16:31–46, 1993.
16. Silos-Santiago I, et al: Molecular genetics of neuronal survival. Curr Opin Neurobiol 5:42–49, 1995.
17. Mey J, Thanos S: Intravitreal injection of neurotrophic factors support the survival of axotomized retinal ganglion cells in adult rats in vivo. Brain Res 602:304–317, 1993.
18. Bonfanti L, et al: Protection of retinal ganglion cells from natural and axotomy-induced cell death in neonatal transgenic mice overexpressing bcl-2. J Neurosci 16:4186–4194, 1996.
19. Cayouette M, Gravel C: Adenovirus-mediated gene transfer to retinal ganglion cells. Invest Ophthalmol Vis Sci 37:2022–2028, 1996.
20. Olney JW: Glutamate-induced retinal degeneration in neonatal mice: Electron microscopy of the acutely evolving lesion. J Neuropathol Exp Neurol 28:455–474, 1969.
21. Dreyer EB, et al: Elevated glutamate levels in the vitreous body of humans and monkeys with glaucoma. Arch Ophthalmol 114:299–305, 1996.
22. Dawson TM, Dawson VL: Nitric oxide: Actions and pathological roles. Neuroscientist 1:9–20, 1994.
23. Samdani AF, Dawson TM, Dawson VL: Nitric oxide synthase in models of focal ischemia. Stroke 28:1283–1288, 1997.
24. Neufeld AH, Hernandez MR, Gonzalez M: Nitric oxide synthase in the human glaucomatous optic nerve head. Arch Ophthalmol 115:497–503, 1997.
25. McConkey DJ, Orrenius S: The role of calcium in the regulation of apoptosis. J Leukocyte Biol 59:775–783, 1996.
26. Guieu R, et al: Adenosine and the nervous system: Clinical implications. Clin Neuropharmacol 19:459–474, 1996.
27. Pang I-H, Yorio T: Ocular actions of endothelins. Proc Soc Exp Biol Med 215:21–34, 1997.
28. Bazan NG: Inflammation: A signal terminator. Nature 374:501–502, 1995.

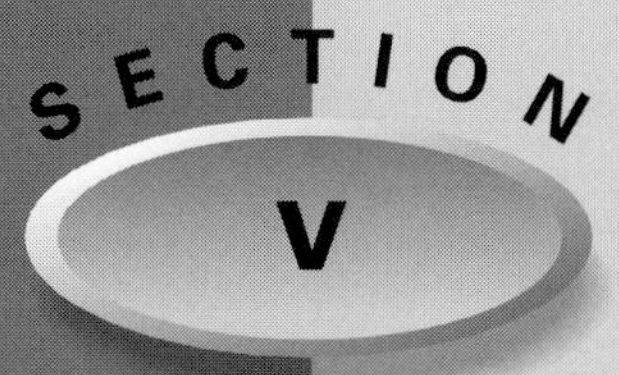

Toxicology

Edited by

TRAVIS A. MEREDITH

CHAPTER 39

Toxicology of Corticosteroids and Other Antiinflammatory Agents

Millicent L. Palmer and Robert A. Hyndiuk

The use of antiinflammatory agents is common in ophthalmic practice because inflammation, a nonspecific response to tissue injury,[1, 2] is frequently encountered. In this chapter, we review adverse effects caused by local (topical and periocular) administration of corticosteroids (CSs), the most commonly used antiinflammatory agents. We also review the adverse ocular and systemic effects of other agents used to treat ocular inflammations, including nonsteroidal antiinflammatory drugs (NSAIDs), antihistamines and decongestants, mast cell–stabilizing agents, and immunosuppressive drugs. This chapter focuses primarily on conditions of the anterior segment.

Emphasis is placed on dose-response relationships (Fig. 39–1), which have important implications for both therapeutic efficacy and drug toxicity.[3–5] Time-response relationships are also highlighted when appropriate. In a dose-response curve, as the dosage is increased, the increment in response becomes smaller until a maximum is reached. Each drug has a dose-response relationship, which may vary with disease states and is dependent on the therapeutic index of the drug as well as on host factors. Each drug also has a toxicity-response curve, which is located somewhere to the right of the therapeutic response curve. Different toxicity curves for different adverse effects may be generated for a single drug.

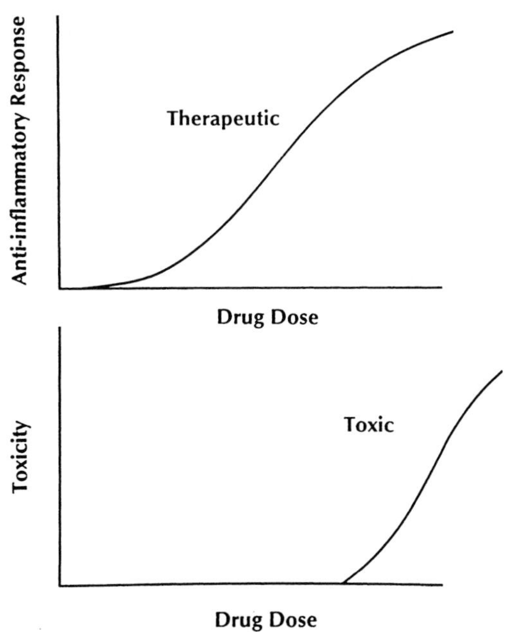

FIGURE 39–1. Hypothetical dose-response curve for therapeutic efficacy and drug toxicity. Each drug has a dose-response relationship, which may vary with the status of the disease and is dependent on the therapeutic index of the drug as well as host factors. As the drug dosage is increased, the increment in response becomes smaller until a maximum is reached. The toxic response curve is located somewhere to the right of the therapeutic response curve.

Systemic Side Effects Due to Local Corticosteroid Administration

Systemic complications due to the systemic use of CSs are discussed in detail elsewhere (see Chapter 101). Systemic side effects due to topical administration are unusual even with long-term therapy.[5] Measurable and physiologically significant systemic effects associated with frequent topical use of concentrated preparations of potent CSs have been reported. Burch and Migeon[6] described a 19 to 72% reduction of urinary excretion of 17-hydroxy CSs after bilateral administration of 0.01% dexamethasone every 2 hours for 4 days (daily systemic dose 0.75 mg); the cortisol production rate decreased by more than 50% during the experimental period. Prednisone, 10 mg, or its equivalent daily for 4 weeks may suppress normal growth in the pediatric population.[5] The administration of a single drop of 0.1% dexamethasone sodium phosphate four times daily in each eye yields a systemic dose of 0.25 mg.[5] Lowering of plasma cortisol levels after 6 weeks of such a regimen has been observed; the hypothalamic-pituitary axis functions normally as measured by metyrapone testing.[7] Prolonged orbital injections of CSs may also have systemic side effects, such as adrenal suppression.[8]

Corticosteroid-Induced Ocular Side Effects

SYSTEMIC ADMINISTRATION

Several adverse ocular side effects specifically related to systemic CS therapy are highlighted in Table 39–1 and summarized in detail elsewhere.[9] Pseudotumor cerebri and papilledema may occur after abrupt cessation or reduction of prolonged CS therapy, especially in children.[10] Similar case reports have been recorded in adults.[11] Treatment usually involves an increase in CS dosage followed by cautious tapering.[5] Long-term systemic CS therapy may induce exophthalmos in patients with no underlying thyroid disease;

TABLE 39–1. **Ocular Side Effects of Topical, Periocular, and Systemic Corticosteroids**

Local Ophthalmic Use (Topical or Periocular)	Systemic Administration	Common to Both
Irritation	Myopia	Cataract
Punctate keratitis	Visual hallucinations	Glaucoma
Optic atrophy	Diplopia	Mydriasis
Granulomas	Pseudotumor cerebri or papilledema	Ptosis
May aggravate Behçet's disease	Exophthalmos	Altered defense against infection
Corneal "melting" syndromes	Decreased tear lysozyme	Delayed wound healing
Scleromalacia perforans	Central serous chorioretinopathy	
Eales' disease		
Toxoplasmosis		
Paralysis of accommodation		
Alteration of corneal or scleral thickness		
Enhancement of lytic action of collagenase		
Anterior uveitis		
Scarring (subconjunctival injection)		
Fat atrophy (retrobulbar or subcutaneous injection)		
Skin atrophy (subcutaneous injection)		
Retinal or choroid embolic phenomena (injection)		

the exophthalmos resolves slowly but incompletely with the cessation of treatment.[12]

The decrease in tear lysozyme levels by CSs may have some role, although minor, in increasing the risk of bacterial infections of the conjunctiva and cornea.[13] Lysozyme is normally present in tears in high concentration and is bacteriolytic for gram-positive organisms.[13, 14]

LOCAL (TOPICAL AND PERIOCULAR) ADMINISTRATION

Lids, Conjunctiva, and Cornea

Allergic dermatoconjunctivitis is a cell-mediated (type IV hypersensitivity) contact allergy that involves the conjunctiva and periocular skin.[15] Although other topical ophthalmic drugs, for example, neomycin, gentamicin, and idoxuridine, are common sensitizers,[15] CSs have also been associated with contact allergic responses.[15–17] Ethylenediamine tetraacetate (disodium edetate, EDTA), a chelating agent and solution stabilizer, and benzalkonium chloride (BAK), a preservative, are commonly used in ophthalmic medications, including CS drop preparations, and may also play a role in inciting contact allergy.[15, 18] Patients usually complain of itching. The initial signs of allergic dermatoconjunctivitis are noted in the inferior or inferonasal aspect of the conjunctiva and medial aspect of the lower eyelid; this corresponds to the normal flow of tears, drugs, and ocular secretions. Eventually more generalized conjunctival, lid, and adjacent facial skin involvement may be observed.[15] Cutaneous manifestations of contact allergy are itching, erythema, papulation, vesiculation, oozing, crusting, scaling, thickening, and pigmentation.[15] Contact dermatitis may be confirmed by a patch test; however, this test is not without its limitations.[19] A careful history is often more helpful. The best treatment of contact allergies is discontinuation or avoidance of the inciting agent.

Many topical drugs, preservatives, and drug vehicles may be irritating to the corneal epithelium, as well as the conjunctiva, resulting in a nonspecific papillary, irritative, or toxic keratoconjunctivitis.[15] A coarse or punctate keratitis, occurring particularly inferiorly and inferonasally, is the most common manifestation. A similar form of keratopathy may also be seen in association with allergic contact dermatoconjunctivitis. Irritative or toxic keratoconjunctivitis is usually associated with a variable degree of drug-induced conjunctival hyperemia.[15] The preservative BAK, which is a quaternary ammonium cationic detergent, can be very irritating.[15, 18] Significant corneal epithelial cytotoxicity of this agent has been demonstrated by laboratory studies.[20, 21]

Transient irritation has also been attributed to the mechanical effects of aggregates of steroid particles in suspension.[15] This may be a particular problem in vernal and atopic keratoconjunctivitis or keratoconjunctivitis sicca.[22] Particles of CS in suspension become trapped among papillae and giant papillae and produce a mechanical epithelial keratitis.[23] Moreover, if there is inadequate tear production, the CS particles in suspension are unable to dissolve and persist as small, irritating foreign bodies.

Corneal penetration of CS suspensions is dependent on solubilization by the tears,[22, 24] which may lead to unpredictable bioavailability of CSs.[24, 25] This problem is enhanced in patients with dry eye syndromes. Moreover, CS suspensions must be shaken to disperse particles of the drug evenly. Poor patient compliance with instructions to shake suspension eye drops has been reported by Apt and coworkers;[26] this is likely to alter the amount of drug dispensed.[27] The use of soluble CS preparations averts this problem. As a rule, the use of topical CS suspensions should be avoided in allergic forms of keratoconjunctivitis, dry eye syndromes, and forms of inflammatory keratitis in which it is critical not to have significant variability in ocular bioavailability of the drug. This is a special problem in the "taper" of topical CSs, for example, in herpetic stromal keratitis or corneal graft rejection, when a severe inflammatory rebound may occur with inconsistent corneal concentrations.

Ocular Hypertension and Glaucoma

Ocular hypertension and glaucoma have been well documented after both topical and systemic CS administration (see Table 39–1).[28–44] In 1950, McLean[28] suggested that topical steroid therapy might increase intraocular pressure (IOP);[28] the first case of "cortisone glaucoma" was reported by Franois in 1954.[29]

The dose-response relationship is particularly important

in understanding this undesirable side effect.[40, 45, 46] Steroid-induced ocular hypertension can reach clinically significant levels in approximately 36% of normal subjects on a short-term steroid regimen.[45] A differential susceptibility among individuals expressed as a skewed distribution has been observed.[40] A more pronounced effect of increased IOP or disturbed aqueous fluid dynamics has been noted in individuals with suspected glaucoma,[35, 38, 47–51] in those with myopia,[52] in older patients,[53] in patients with glaucoma,[31, 35, 38, 47, 48, 50, 51, 54, 56] in relatives of glaucoma patients,[44, 50, 55–58] in patients with Krukenberg's spindle,[59] and in diabetic patients.[60]

The skewed distribution of frequency of elevated IOP may be interpreted on the basis of a mendelian genetic model. Armaly[33, 56] and Becker and coworkers[38, 54] proposed such a model consisting of subpopulations of low, intermediate, and high responders based on homozygous or heterozygous alleles. According to Becker's hypothesis, homozygous poor responders had IOP responses of less than 20 mm Hg; heterozygous intermediate responders had IOP responses between 20 and 31 mm Hg; and homozygous high responders had IOPs exceeding 31 mm Hg. Becker and Hahn[54] postulated that there is a high degree of correlation between the clinical state of glaucoma and the ocular hypertensive response to topical CSs; glaucoma is considered a recessive trait, whereas CS responsiveness is inherited dominantly. Armaly proposed a similar genetic model. He stressed the relative change in IOP rather than absolute range of pressure values and assumed that steroid responsiveness was transmitted in a dominant fashion.[56] The heritable nature of CS responsiveness has been questioned by studies demonstrating no greater similarity of IOP response in identical than in nonidentical twins.[61, 62] An alternative, multifactorial mode of inheritance has also been proposed.[40]

Factors affecting the dose-response relationship include the concentration of drug, the antiinflammatory potency, and the duration and frequency of use.[45] A positive correlation between ocular hypertensive effect and antiinflammatory potency of CSs has been observed by an in vitro assay reported by Cantrill and colleagues.[63] The authors noted a dissociation of antiinflammatory potency and IOP-elevating effects with medrysone and fluorometholone. A favorable modification of the toxic-therapeutic index may be achieved by a reduced frequency of administration, dilution of the more potent agents, or the use of CSs such as fluorometholone, which is rapidly degraded, or medrysone, which has poor ocular penetration.[39, 41, 45, 64–67]

A time-response relationship of CS-induced ocular hypertensive response has important implications. A clinically significant rise in IOP typically, but not always, requires greater than 1 to 2 weeks of topical therapy.[45] With systemic steroid administration, the ocular hypertensive response may require longer treatment.[43] A dose-dependent response after systemic CS therapy has also been observed.[36] A smaller concentration of drug reaches ocular sites by the systemic route and may explain the difference in the IOP response time between topical and systemic routes of administration.[45] The magnitude of the ocular hypertensive response after systemic administration has been noted to be similar to the response following topical therapy.[43]

The mechanism of the steroid ocular hypertensive response appears to involve an initial increase in aqueous inflow, as suggested by Linner,[68] with a secondary effect on the facility of outflow.[66] Several biochemical mechanisms have been proposed to explain the decrease in outflow facility based on CS effects on cells of the trabecular meshwork. These include inhibition of prostaglandin mediators[69] and alteration of glycosaminoglycan production or metabolism.[34, 66, 70–72]

The CS-induced ocular hypertensive response is usually reversible, especially with short-duration therapy (weeks);[45] however, irreversible steroid-induced glaucoma has been clearly documented, especially in patients with myopia.[34, 52, 73–76] Discontinuation of CSs may result in normalization of the IOP, but visual field abnormalities and optic nerve damage may be permanent.[34, 73, 74] Many patients respond to medical antiglaucomatous therapy. When medical treatment fails and the continued use of CSs is required to control ocular inflammatory disease, argon laser trabeculoplasty and glaucoma filtering procedures may be required.[74]

Rimexolone 1% (Vexol 1%) is a CS preparation that is indicated for the treatment of postoperative inflammation following ocular surgery, and for the treatment of anterior uveitis.[77–80] Rimexolone is chemically and pharmacologically related to other CSs such as prednisolone acetate but differs from prednisolone acetate by modifications to the cyclopentane ring and its side chain.[80]

Rimexolone is suspended in a vehicle stabilized by carbomer polymer. This not only limits phase separation of the drug but also results in an increased viscosity and a reduced drainage rate, leading to increased retention in the precorneal tear film after instillation. The latter is also thought to account for its limited systemic side effects.

Rimexolone is generally well tolerated. The ophthalmic preparation is near the physiologic pH and tonicity of tear film, and the drug has been micronized to a particle size of less than 5 μm. The small particle size facilitates its solubility in the tear film. The manufacturer recommends shaking before administration for a homogeneous suspension.

Although rimexolone's efficacy as an antiinflammatory agent is comparable to that of prednisolone acetate, rimexolone was found to be more similar to fluorometholone 0.1% in its lesser effect on IOP elevation.[30, 37, 38, 41, 77] A time-response relationship has also been demonstrated with rimexolone. Controlled clinical trials in steroid responders showed that treatment with rimexolone resulted in a longer average time to raise IOP and produced a lower mean end-point IOP than did treatment with other commonly prescribed steroids, such as prednisolone acetate 1% and dexamethasone phosphate 0.1%.[79]

Corticosteroid-Induced Cataract Formation

It is generally accepted that CSs are cataractogenic, commonly producing posterior subcapsular cataracts (PSCs). The association of PSCs with systemic CS use was first reported by Black and associates in 1960.[81] PSCs developed in patients receiving moderate or high doses of CSs for greater than 1 year's duration. Further work by Oglesby and coworkers,[82] Giles and colleagues,[83] and Crews[84] indicated that patients receiving doses of less than 10 mg/day of prednisone or its equivalent or patients receiving CS therapy for less than 1 year were unlikely to develop PSCs. However, cataracts have been observed after even short-term CS therapy,[85] and some authors now argue against the concept of a "safe" noncataractogenic dose.[86] Both systemic and topical administration of CS may induce PSC formation; those caused by systemic use are bilateral.[81–89] Although steroid-induced PSCs occurrence is dose and duration dependent, the precise relationship of lens changes to the total dose, the intensity of the dose, and the duration of therapy is not fully understood.[86] Some studies suggest that individual susceptibility and perhaps even genetic determinants may be important.[85, 86, 90] Children[85, 89] and diabetic patients[91, 92] appear to be more susceptible.

The pathophysiology of steroid-induced cataracts is similar to the mechanism of cataract formation proposed for galactose in that steroids increase the influx of cations,[93] resulting in an increase in the cellular water content, producing cellular intumescence and disparity of the refractive index from that of the surrounding medium.[74] Glucocorticoids also bind to specific amino acid groups of the lens cell fibers, leading to a conformational change and exposure of buried sulfhydryl groups.[74] These moieties (i.e., the sulfhydryl groups) form disulfide bonds and create protein aggregation and a change in the refractive index.[74]

Early PSC changes that are part of the "senile" cataract and early PSC changes caused by steroids are similar to but distinguishable from other secondary cataracts because initially, in the former, there is no involvement of the adjacent posterior cortex. Later, however, CS-induced lens changes are virtually indistinguishable from those of other secondary cataracts associated with intraocular inflammation, retinitis pigmentosa, or irradiation. Posterior subcapsular lens changes that are part of the "senile" cataract are also often associated with other aging lens changes, such as nuclear sclerosis or cortical opacities.[91] Greiner and Chylack[94] noted the same basic histopathologic features of senile PSCs and CS-induced PSCs, but the organization and localization of these abnormalities may be distinguishable features.

The majority of patients who develop steroid PSCs do not have clinically significant visual impairment; approximately 7% require cataract surgery.[91] Reversibility of steroid-induced PSCs has been described in children with nephrotic syndrome after the cessation of steroid therapy;[90] however, progression of lens changes may also occur despite the cessation of steroid therapy.[66]

There are insufficient data to determine which steroid preparations or what mode of delivery is more likely to predispose to PSC formation. Hyndiuk[95] showed that in the monkey the lens concentrates methylprednisolone more than other ocular tissues, but comparative studies evaluating other periocular steroid preparations have not been performed.

Delayed Wound Healing and Effects on Corneal Reepithelialization

The effect of CSs on corneal wound healing has been the focus of several investigations.[96–109] Corneal wound integrity has been evaluated by determining the tensile strength,[3, 99, 100, 102, 104, 105] histologic appearance,[96, 99, 101] and uptake of tritiated thymidine by keratocytes.[103] Although the results of these studies are somewhat inconsistent, a dose-response effect of CSs on corneal wound healing has been demonstrated.[104] Impaired corneal wound healing has been less pronounced when steroids were withheld until after the tenth postoperative day, after which topical CS treatment did not significantly interfere with the tensile strength of the healing wound.[3]

Topical and systemic cortisone derivatives have a depressant effect on many phases of the healing process. Alterations in fibroblast proliferation, vascularization, and deposition of extracellular matrix have been observed.[97] CSs primarily affect stromal rather than epithelial healing. Effects of CSs on corneal epithelial healing have been observed and may be related to the extent of epithelial injury. Topical CSs do not impair epithelialization after partial corneal denudation,[107, 108] but impairment is observed after complete denudation in a rabbit model.[107]

Investigative studies have demonstrated that the enzyme collagenase is produced in *Pseudomonas* and herpes simplex corneal ulcers; alkali burns; and ulcerations associated with collagen vascular diseases and Stevens-Johnson syndrome.[106] CSs may induce rapid destruction or corneal "melting" and even perforation in these conditions, possibly by enhancing collagenase activity.[5, 106]

There is disagreement regarding the use of topical steroids in the therapy of alkali corneal burns. This unique form of injury destroys keratocytes, leaving the collagen vulnerable to collagenolysis without the capacity for renewal.[5] Studies have indicated that topical CSs can be used in the first week after an alkali injury to suppress the inflammatory response without the risk of corneal melting.[110] After this time, topical CSs exacerbate corneal ulceration. The mechanism is thought to be due to impaired reparative processes.[110] Medroxyprogesterone inhibits collagenolytic activity and has been shown to substantially reduce the incidence of deep ulceration and perforation in alkali-burned rabbit corneas.[111]

The healing process is already faulty in patients with rheumatoid arthritis, keratoconjunctivitis sicca, rosacea keratitis, and neurotrophic keratitis.[22] The use of CSs in these patients may exacerbate healing problems, and careful clinical monitoring is advised.

Corticosteroids and Infectious Keratitis

Because CSs alter the host immunologic responses to infection, their use in the presence of an active infectious process is often contraindicated.[5, 108] In addition, chronic use of CSs may alter normal and pathogenic flora of the lids and conjunctiva.[15] The incidence of corneal thinning and perforation in severe infectious keratitis may be increased owing to the potential enhancement of collagenolytic enzymes or decreased collagen synthesis and wound healing.[5, 22] In certain cases, judicious use of CSs may be appropriate to limit the structural damage related to the inflammatory process. In general, the use of CSs should be avoided until the infectious process has been controlled by specific antimicrobial therapy. In the following sections, important issues regarding the use of CSs are briefly reviewed by the category of infectious agents: viral, bacterial, fungal, and parasitic.

VIRAL AGENTS

Herpes Simplex Virus

Topical CS therapy is contraindicated in the presence of active viral replication associated with herpes simples virus

(HSV) epithelial keratitis.[112] The deleterious effects of CSs in management of HSV infection have been clearly documented.[113–115] Local CSs, however, do not reactivate latent HSV keratitis or stimulate an episode of dendritic or stromal keratitis.[116] CS therapy plays a role in controlling the immunologically mediated inflammation of HSV stromal disease. The results of the Herpetic Eye Disease Study, a multicenter, randomized, double-masked clinical trial, revealed the efficacy of topical CSs in HSV stromal keratitis.[117] The initiation of CS therapy should be avoided if steroids were never used previously. Clinically, a careful risk-benefit analysis should be made on an individual basis.

In most cases of stromal involvement occurring in uncomplicated HSV infection, the stromal keratitis is mild and self-limited and does not call for immediate treatment with CSs. If the stromal edema is persistent and causes impairment of vision, however, topical CSs may be tried, using the lowest concentration of steroid to control the edema or vascular infiltration. The patient should be started on weak CS solution, two to three times each day, and the dose-response curve should climb from that point until the beginning of inflammatory suppression is seen. Dilute strengths of CSs such as prednisolone phosphate ⅛% or its equivalent once or twice daily are almost always effective if the patient has not been treated with CSs in the previous 3 to 4 months.

Starting at the top of the CS dose-response curve maximally compromises the host response, which may interrupt normal healing and lead to reinfection or thinning and perforation.[22] If an active recurrence develops during treatment with high-dose CSs, a fulminant stromal keratitis may ensue; this is a dose-related complication.[22]

During the treatment of active HSV stromal keratitis with CSs, an antiviral "umbrella" should be used concomitantly to prevent or limit recurrences of dendritic keratitis.[118, 119] Antiviral drops four to five times daily or ointment three times daily may be used. Antiviral coverage should be continued until the steroid dosage is less than the equivalent of one drop of prednisolone 1% daily. Use of prophylactic topical antibiotics is also important to minimize bacterial superinfection when a long-standing epithelial defect is present.[118]

A severe necrotizing inflammatory reaction with subsequent scarring and perforation may develop if topical CSs are abruptly stopped or tapered too rapidly (Fig. 39–2).[118] A temporary, usually aggressive increase in steroids is required to control this inflammation.

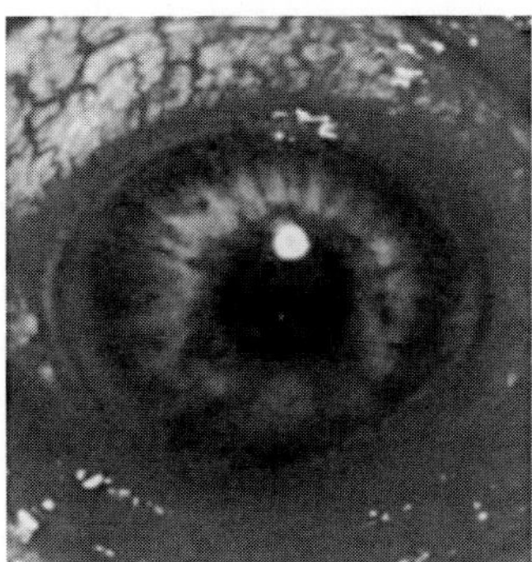

FIGURE 39–2. Rebound herpes simplex virus keratouveitis after abrupt tapering of topical corticosteroids. Note the intense ciliary injection. Short-term pulse corticosteroid therapy is required to control the inflammation.

Herpes Zoster

Topical CSs do not increase viral replication in cases of herpes zoster epithelial keratitis.[120, 121] Owing to the neurotrophic problem that may result, the cornea is susceptible to ulceration, and steroids should therefore be used with caution when they are indicated for significant stromal or uveal inflammation.

Adenovirus

The use of CSs for cases of epidemic keratoconjunctivitis is usually not necessary. In severe cases in which subepithelial infiltrates interfere significantly with vision or comfort, a trial of CS may be indicated if one is sure of the diagnosis. Caution should be exercised in the use of CSs in epidemic keratoconjunctivitis owing to the possibility of misdiagnosis of HSV or adult inclusion conjunctivitis, especially early in the course of disease.[112]

Cytomegalovirus

Cytomegalovirus (CMV) retinitis is a well-recognized opportunistic infection associated with acquired immunodeficiency disease, administration of immunosuppressive or cytotoxic agents, and systemic CS therapy in renal transplantation recipients and patients with neoplastic disease.[122] A culture-proven case of bilateral panuveitis due to CMV in a patient receiving immunosuppressive doses of CS has been described.[123]

BACTERIAL KERATITIS

The risks associated with CS therapy in the management of bacterial keratitis are a subject of controversy. Several reports favor adjunctive CS therapy in bacterial keratitis. Davis and coworkers[124] demonstrated that concurrent treatment with CSs did not inhibit the effect of antibiotics in *Pseudomonas* keratitis. Aronson and Moore[125] claimed that CS treatment promoted the resolution of inflammation associated with infectious keratitis in their series. A favorable visual outcome, however, was observed only in mild cases of paracentral keratitis. Leibowitz and Kupferman[126] concluded that the concurrent use of topical CSs with an effective bactericidal antibiotic regimen did not enhance the replication of *Staphylococcus aureus* or *Pseudomonas aeruginosa* if the CS was not instilled more frequently than the antibiotic.

CSs have been shown to enhance *P. aeruginosa* replication within the cornea if there is inadequate antimicrobial therapy.[127, 128] Animal studies have indicated that despite 5 days of treatment with an effective antibiotic, corneas infected with *Pseudomonas* were not sterilized.[129] Further recurrences of *Pseudomonas* keratitis have been reported in eyes treated with CSs.[130] CSs are contraindicated in eyes that have advanced corneal thinning with the potential for perforation, owing to possible enhancement of collagenolytic enzymes or inhibition of collagen synthesis.[22] A controlled prospective clinical study by Carmichael and coworkers[131] evaluated CS therapy with and without antibiotic therapy in bacterial ulcers and found no differences in visual outcome. Considering the risks, steroids should not be used if there is not a significant chance of preventing visual loss or of recovering lost vision; that is, control of inflammation alone should not be the deciding factor.

FUNGAL KERATITIS

The use of CSs in the early treatment of fungal keratitis is generally contraindicated owing to an enhancement of growth of both yeast and opportunistic fungi.[132] A clinical worsening of fungal keratitis has been demonstrated after treatment with CSs.[133–136] In contrast to the number of available antibiotics, there are relatively few antifungal agents. In general, these agents are poorly soluble and have limited ocular penetration; therefore, ocular bioavailability and the efficacy of antifungal agents are less than ideal, reaching only fungistatic, as opposed to fungicidal, corneal levels.[137] CSs may negate the effects of antifungal therapy and suppress host immune responses. Host immune responses may be particularly critical in controlling the inflammation of keratomycoses. The use of CSs to reduce stromal scarring, intraocular inflammation, and corneal neovascularization continues to be controversial.[138] Adjunctive CS therapy should be considered only in combination with an effective antifungal agent or agents in the later stages of a healing fungal keratitis.[138]

ACANTHAMOEBIC KERATITIS

Acanthamoeba keratitis is a chronic, potentially devastating infection that has received increasing recognition.[139] The role of CSs in the treatment of *Acanthamoeba* infection is unclear. The effect of CSs on the organism's morphogenesis (from cyst to trophozoite and vice versa) has not been fully elucidated. Osato and associates[140] reported that morphogenesis could be inhibited by dexamethasone in broth suspensions. The authors claim that by preventing free transformation of the two existing forms of *Acanthamoeba*, CSs may allow amebicidal agents to destroy the trophozoites, while the host response clears the amebic cysts. Clinical experience with *Acanthamoeba* keratitis, however, has demonstrated no uniform response to CS therapy.[141, 142] In a report by Rabinovitch and coworkers[143] on the evaluation of clinical signs and predictors of outcome, multivariate analysis indicated that the use of steroids was the sole parameter predicting medical failure. CSs may facilitate the establishment of disease and may also prolong the course and severity of the disease. Therefore, their use should probably be discouraged.

Mydriasis and Ptosis

Armaly[32] first reported the mydriasis associated with topical administration of CS preparations. Animal studies confirmed that mydriasis and ptosis observed with topical dexamethasone therapy is due to the vehicle and not to the steroid itself.[144] The vehicle, which contains a combination of preservatives, antioxidants, and surface-active agents, namely polysorbate 80, phenylethanol, and EDTA, is responsible for a direct myopathic effect.[144] The constituents of the vehicle apparently disturb the permeability of the cell membrane.[5, 144] The mydriasis may precipitate acute angle-closure glaucoma in susceptible individuals.

Anterior Uveitis

Topical administration of CSs may induce a nongranulomatous anterior uveitis.[145–147] Krupin and coworkers[145] first described this entity in two patients undergoing topical CS provocative testing with 0.1% dexamethasone sodium phosphate. Additional cases have also been reported.[146] The development of CS-induced uveitis may correlate with a high prevalence of positive results on fluorescent treponemal antibody absorption testing.[147] There is no direct proof, however, that this inflammatory response represents an activation of latent spirochetes in ocular tissue.

Periocular Corticosteroids

Severe, sight-threatening ocular inflammatory conditions, particularly inflammation involving ocular tissues of the posterior segment, may be more effectively managed with periocular steroid injections.[148–151] Specific sites for periocular steroid injections are advocated depending on the location of the ocular inflammation: (1) the subconjunctival route in the treatment of corneal disease, e.g., graft rejection; (2) anterior sub-Tenon's injection for iritis or iridocyclitis; (3) posterior sub-Tenon's injection for equatorial and midzone posterior uveitis; and (4) retrobulbar administration for inflammation of the macula, optic nerve, or disc.[66] The goal of periocular steroid injections is to maximize the delivery of steroid in close proximity to the site of the inflammatory process.

The type of steroid formulation plays an important role in determining the rate of drug release from the depot and therefore in the duration of steroid effects.[66] The site of injection and tissue distribution as well as drug metabolism and degradation[24, 74] are also important. Water-soluble compounds such as dexamethasone sodium phosphate (Decadron) or hydrocortisone sodium succinate (Solu-Cortef) tend to be short acting. Moderately soluble preparations include triamcinolone diacetate (Aristocort) and methylprednisolone acetate (Depo-Medrol). Triamcinolone acetonide (Kenalog) and triamcinolone hexacetonide (Aristospan) are poorly soluble agents. Betamethasone sodium phosphate and betamethasone acetate (Celestone Soluspan) are a mixture of soluble and moderately soluble compounds.[152]

A rare but dreaded complication of periocular injection of CSs is penetration of the globe and intraocular injection.[151, 153–157] This is associated with sudden visual loss and acute ocular pain. Significant damage to the retina, retinal degeneration, preretinal membrane formation, and cataract formation due to the preservatives and osmolarity of the vehicles have been described.[156] In an animal study by Hida and associates,[156] four of the six CS vehicles—betamethasone sodium phosphate and betamethasone acetate, methylprednisolone acetate; dexamethasone sodium phosphate, and dexamethasone acetate—showed obvious or potential retinal toxicity after intravitreal injection. The betamethasone sodium phosphate and betamethasone acetate preparation was the most toxic. This agent also had the lowest osmolarity. The methylprednisolone acetate vehicle demonstrated lenticular toxicity and caused retinal toxicity only after doubling of the standard dose. Double-strength solutions of dexamethasone sodium phosphate and dexamethasone acetate also produced retinal damage. No retinal or lens damage was observed with triamcinolone diacetate or triamcinolone acetonide. The toxic elements of the vehicles were thought to be their preservatives, such as BAK and myristyl γ-picolinium chloride, benzyl alcohol, parabens, and EDTA.[156] Other ocular complications may include transient increased IOP, hypotony, vitreous hemorrhage, retinal detachment, choroidal hemorrhage, ascending optic atrophy, endophthalmitis, and even phthisis bulbi.[157] Surgical removal of iatrogenic intraocular injection of depot CS by the pars plana approach has been reported by Zinn.[157] Intravascular injection of CSs resulting in embolic phenomena of the retinal or choroidal circulation as a complication of retrobulbar injections has also been reported.[158–160] Retrobulbar hemorrhage, proptosis of the globe, and extraocular muscle fibrosis are also potential complications from periocular injection.[74] A delayed hypersensitivity response to retrobulbar injections of methylprednisolone acetate has been described by Mathias and coworkers.[161] The patient developed hyperemia of the episclera and bulbar conjunctival vessels associated with chemosis. Confirmation was obtained by intradermal testing.

Elevated IOP may also occur with long-acting depot steroids.[74, 151, 152, 162] This may lead to prolonged elevation of the IOP. In some cases, surgical removal of the depot of steroid is required.[162]

Periocular steroids in patients with scleritis may cause staphyloma formation and globe perforation and should be avoided. They should also be avoided in ocular toxoplasmosis because they suppress the host immune defenses needed in eradicating the organism.[74]

Several complications of intralesional CS injection for juvenile capillary hemangioma of the ocular adnexa have been described. Treatment usually consists of a 50:50 mixture of triamcinolone acetonide (40 mg/mL) and betamethasone sodium phosphate/betamethasone acetate (Celestone Soluspan), (6 to 8 mg/mL).[163–167] Eyelid depigmentation,[163] eyelid necrosis,[164] central retinal artery occlusion,[167] subcutaneous fat atrophy,[166] and adrenal suppression[165] have been reported.

Permanent depigmentation of eyelid skin has been observed in an African American child after the injection of a chalazion with CS preserved with benzyl alcohol.[168] Such injections should be avoided in African American patients. The mechanism of this depigmentation may be CS inhibition of melanosome synthesis, impaired transfer of melanosome to the keratinocyte, or melanocyte ischemia.[168a] Benzyl alcohol is structurally related to substances that inhibit melanosome synthesis.[168] Subconjunctival injection may result in conjunctival scarring.[9] Fat atrophy has been noted to occur with both subcutaneous and retrobulbar injection of CSs.[9] Skin atrophy may be induced by periocular subcutaneous administration of CSs.[9]

Nonsteroidal Antiinflammatory Drugs

NSAIDs have analgesic, antiinflammatory, and antipyretic properties.[169–174] The antiinflammatory activity is related to the inhibition of the enzyme cyclooxygenase; this enzyme is responsible for the conversion of arachidonic acid to prostaglandins, which are potent inflammatory mediators.[169–172] A summary of the chemical classification of NSAIDs available in the United States and the usual dosages is presented in Table 39–2.[169, 174–184] These agents are widely used in the treatment of musculoskeletal disorders such as osteoarthritis, rheumatoid arthritis, ankylosing spondylitis, and acute gout.[169] Both systemic and topical NSAIDs also play a role in the management of ocular inflammatory conditions.

Oral NSAIDs have been useful in the management of patients with uveitis, particularly recurrent anterior uveitis.[171] Foster[171] has reported that diflunisal (Dolobid) was the safest and most effective; naproxen (Naprosyn) and indomethacin (Indocin-SR) were of intermediate efficacy; and piroxicam (Feldene), sulindac (Clinoril), and ibuprofen (Motrin) have been the least effective. Long-term maintenance therapy on oral NSAIDs may help to control inflammation caused by anterior uveitis without steroids and thereby reduce the steroid requirement.[171] In addition, oral NSAIDs may play a role in the management of cystoid macular edema (CME) associated with posterior uveitis and secondary retinal vasculitis; NSAID therapy has not been of benefit in the management of primary retinal vasculitis.[171]

These agents share several important systemic side effects.[169] The most common is the induction of gastric or intestinal ulceration. In some cases, anemia from gastrointestinal blood loss may occur. Gastrointestinal side effects are explained on the basis of two mechanisms. First, local irritation by orally administered agents allows back-diffusion of acid into the gastric mucosa, resulting in tissue damage. Parenteral administration may also induce similar gastrointestinal side effects. Inhibition of the biosynthesis of gastric prostaglandins that inhibit gastric acid secretion and induce gastric secretion of cytoprotective mucus in the intestine is the proposed mechanism.[169]

Additional untoward effects of these agents that are related to inhibition of the synthesis of endogenous prostaglandins include altered platelet function, impairment of renal function, and prolongation of gestation or spontaneous labor.[169] NSAIDs prevent the formation by platelets of thromboxane A_2, a potent platelet-aggregating agent. This results in an increased bleeding time.[169] These agents have a known effect on renal hemodynamics and fluid and electrolyte balance. In normal patients, little effect of NSAIDs is seen because the production of vasodilatory prostaglandins plays a minor role in the presence of normal sodium balance.[169, 185] NSAIDs, however, promote a decrease in renal blood flow and glomerular filtration in patients with congestive heart failure, chronic renal disease, hepatic cirrhosis with ascites, or hypovolemia of any cause.[169] Salt and water retention may also be induced secondary to the reduction of prostaglandin-induced inhibition of both reabsorption of chloride and function of antidiuretic hormone.[169] Edema may result in some patients. Hyperkalemia is also promoted by the use of NSAIDs.[169, 185] Another renal side effect is acute interstitial nephritis, with nephrotic-range proteinuria in 73% of cases.[185] Renal failure may be severe enough to require temporary dialysis in 32% of patients.[185] Propionic acid derivatives have been most often associated with acute interstitial nephritis (see Table 39–2).[185]

NSAIDs bind firmly to plasma proteins and therefore may displace certain other drugs from binding sites.[169] Thus, with concurrent use of drugs such as warfarin, sulfonylurea hypoglycemic agents, or methotrexate, an adjustment in the dosage of these drugs may be required.[169] This is particularly

TABLE 39–2. **Chemical Classification of Nonsteroidal Antiinflammatory Drugs in the United States**

Chemical Class	Generic Name	Trade Name	Usual Dosage
Salicylates	Acetylsalicylic acid; aspirin	—	300 mg–1 g q 4 hr
	Diflunisal	Dolobid	500 mg b.i.d.
	Salsalate	Disalcid	500–750 mg b.i.d.–q.i.d.
Naphthylalkanones	Nabumetone	Relafen	1000–2000 mg q.d.
Indoles	Indomethacin*	Indocin-SR	25–75 mg b.i.d.
	Etodolac	Lodine	75 mg b.i.d.
	Tolmetin sodium†	Tolectin	400 mg t.i.d.
Indenes	Sulindac	Clinoril	150–200 mg b.i.d.
Phenylacetic acids	Diclofenac sodium	Voltaren	50 mg t.i.d.–q.i.d.
	Diclofenac sodium 0.1%‡	Voltaren	1 drop q.i.d.
Propionic acids	Fenoprofen	Nalfon	300–600 mg t.i.d.–q.i.d.; max. 3200 mg/day
	Flurbiprofen sodium	Ansaid	300 mg b.i.d.–q.i.d.
	Flurbiprofen sodium 0.03%	Ocufen	1 drop q ½ hr × 4; 2 hr preoperatively
	Ibuprofen	Motrin, Advil, Rufen	1200–3200 mg/day divided t.i.d.–q.i.d.
	Ketoprofen	Orudis (Oruvail)	150–300 mg t.i.d. or q.i.d.
	Naproxen	Naprosyn	250–500 mg b.i.d.
	Naproxen sodium	Anaprox	
	Suprofen 1%	Profenal	2 drops at 3, 2, and 1 hr preoperatively
	Oxaprozin	Daypro	1200–1800 mg q.d.
Pyrrolopyrroles	Ketorolac tromethamine	Toradol (intramuscular)	Load 30–60 mg IM, 15 or 30 mg q.i.d.
		Toradol (oral)	20 mg load, 10 mg PO q 4–6 hr
	Ketorolac tromethamine 0.5%§	Acular	1 drop q.i.d.
Oxicam or enolic acids	Piroxicam	Feldene	10–20 mg q.d.
Pyrazolones	Phenylbutazone‖	Butazolidin	100–600 mg/day
Fenamates	Meclofenamate sodium	Meclomen	200–400 mg t.i.d.–q.i.d.
	Mefenamic acid	Ponstel	Load 500 mg; 250 mg q.i.d.

* Ophthalmic indomethacin suspension, Indocid 1%, is available in Canada and parts of Europe.[171]
† Structurally similar to indomethacin, but activity and toxicity are similar to those of propionic acid derivatives.[168]
‡ Useful in management of inflammation and pain after excimer photorefractive keratectomy.[181]
§ Clinical trials of topical ketorolac tromethamine 0.5% report benefit in inflammation after cataract surgery,[175–177] chronic aphakic cystoid macular edema,[178, 179] and inflammation and pain after excimer photorefractive keratectomy[182] and allergic keratoconjunctivitis.[183, 184]
‖ Serious toxic effects including agranulocytosis and aplastic anemia limit its long-term use.[168]

important in patients receiving the anticoagulant warfarin, in view of the effect of NSAIDs on platelet function.

Use of these aspirin-like agents is contraindicated in patients with hypersensitivity to NSAIDs and in those with the syndrome of nasal polyps, angioedema, and bronchospastic response to aspirin.[171] The use of NSAIDs in children should be restricted to those agents extensively tested in the pediatric population, namely aspirin, naproxen, and tolmetin.[169] Owing to the association of Reye's syndrome with aspirin treatment of children with febrile viral illness, NSAIDs should be strictly avoided in this clinical setting.[169]

NSAIDs have the potential to produce photosensitivity reactions and are a frequent cause of cutaneous reactions. Cutaneous reactions such as vesiculobullous eruptions, serum sickness, exfoliative erythroderma, erythema multiforme, and toxic epidermal necrolysis are well summarized in a report by Stern and Bigby.[186] Reactions to piroxicam were reported most frequently.[186]

OCULAR SIDE EFFECTS OF SYSTEMIC NSAIDs

Adverse ocular effects of NSAIDs have been reported; however, in many cases these are isolated reports or data obtained from retrospective studies in which a cause-and-effect relationship cannot be clearly established.[9] Generally, NSAIDs are photosensitizers and have the potential for inducing phototoxicity of the anterior and posterior segments of the eye.[9] Optic neuritis has been associated with this class of drugs and is presumed to occur as an idiosyncratic response that is reversible on cessation of therapy.[9] In the case of ibuprofen, a widely used NSAID, there have been enough occasional cases in which the drug has been rechallenged that changes in refractive error, diplopia, and diminished color vision seem to be well documented.[9, 187, 188] The occurrence of a reversible toxic amblyopia has also been described.[189–192] Patients taking this drug should be advised to stop if a sudden decrease in vision occurs.

Interpretation of reports of indomethacin-induced retinal and macular disease is complicated by almost equal numbers of contradictory studies.[9, 193, 194] Nevertheless, the potential for ocular toxicity exists. There are data to support the occurrence of superficial corneal crystalline deposits secondary to indomethacin that resolve with discontinuation of the drug.[193, 195] There have also been several reports of papilledema associated with pseudotumor cerebri.[9, 196]

Aspirin has been implicated in increasing the incidence of rebleeding in traumatic hyphema.[197] Therefore, this agent as well as the aspirin-like NSAIDs should be avoided in this condition.

OPHTHALMIC (TOPICAL) NSAIDs—INDICATIONS AND ADVERSE EFFECTS

The ophthalmic NSAIDs currently available include flurbiprofen sodium 0.03% (Ocufen), suprofen 1% (Profenal), diclofenac sodium 0.1% (Voltaren), and ketorolac tromethamine 0.5% (Acular).[172] Both flurbiprofen and suprofen are approved for the prevention of intraoperative miosis.[172, 172a, 197a, 198–200] Ketorolac tromethamine 0.5% is indicated for the treatment of ocular itch due to seasonal allergic conjunctivitis.[183, 184] Both diclofenac sodium 1% and ketorolac tromethamine 0.5% are indicated for the treatment of postoperative inflammation associated with cataract surgery.[198] In addition, diclofenac sodium 1% and ketorolac tromethamine 0.5% have also been effective in the reduction of pain and inflammation after excimer laser photorefractive keratectomy.[181, 182, 200a]

Caution is advised in using topical diclofenac sodium 1% and ketorolac tromethamine 0.5% after excimer laser photorefractive keratectomy without concomitant use of topical steroids. Subepithelial sterile corneal infiltrates have been reported in some patients when topical NSAIDs were used with a bandage contact lens after photorefractive keratectomy without concomitant topical steroids.[201] It is theorized that this may be due to suppression of the cyclooxygenase pathway via NSAIDs, leaving the lipooxygenase pathway active or unchecked, resulting in an increased polymorphonucleocyte response. Sterile subepithelial infiltrates are a well-recognized adverse effect of hydrogel contact lenses in the absence of surgery.[202, 203] The infiltrates, however, are usually marginal and not central or paracentral as noted with excimer photoreactive keratectomy.

Several double-masked, randomized studies of the effects of flurbiprofen on postoperative inflammation have been published.[204–207] Topical administration of flurbiprofen has also been shown to reduce the inflammation of experimental anterior uveitis.[208] These studies indicate that flurbiprofen does have some potential as an antiinflammatory agent, but additional well-controlled clinical trials are needed.

In general, flurbiprofen sodium 0.03% is well tolerated. The most frequent side effect is transient burning and stinging with instillation.[198] Flurbiprofen has been shown to inhibit corneoscleral wound healing[208, 209] and exacerbate epithelial HSV keratitis,[210] effects similar to those seen with topical CSs. A more recent report by Asbell and coworkers,[211] however, demonstrated that flurbiprofen sodium did not enhance HSV epithelial keratitis. The strain of HSV, however, was not specified in this report, and the timing of CS intervention after infection differed. In a review of topical antiinflammatory agents in an experimental model of microbial keratitis, a worsening of *Pseudomonas* keratitis with topical CSs was confirmed, and a greater worsening was observed with flurbiprofen sodium 0.03%.[212] Concomitant therapy with an effective antibiotic prevented the steroid- and flurbiprofen-induced worsening of *Pseudomonas* keratitis. Pneumococcal keratitis was not worsened by the use of either CSs or flurbiprofen in the presence of appropriate antimicrobial therapy.[212]

There have been reports that flurbiprofen sodium may promote bleeding of ocular tissues in the setting of ocular surgery, particularly in the case of concomitant systemic dipyridamole, an antiplatelet agent, or oral NSAIDs.[198, 213] The manufacturers of all of the currently available topical NSAIDs advise caution with the use of these agents in patients with bleeding disorders or individuals taking systemic medications that may prolong the bleeding time.[198, 214]

A double-masked study evaluating the effects of topical flurbiprofen sodium 0.03% on the IOP revealed that this agent did not alter the IOP in known CS responders. In this study, treatment with flurbiprofen did not prevent the steroid-induced increase in IOP or the decrease in outflow facility.[215]

Suprofen may cause minor irritation, itching, redness, allergic reaction, iritis, pain, chemosis, photophobia, and punctate keratopathy.[197a] The use of diclofenac may be associated with minor symptoms of irritation. Concurrent use of diclofenac and hydrogel contact lenses may cause burning and redness.[197a] Ketorolac tromethamine 0.5% ophthalmic solution may cause mild, transient burning and stinging on instillation.[183]

A case of asthma exacerbated by topical ketorolac has been reported. Caution must be exercised in prescribing topical NSAID eye drops for patients with a history of asthma, nasal polyps, and allergy to aspirin or NSAIDs.[216]

Antihistamines and Decongestants

Symptoms of itching, vasodilation (hyperemia), and chemosis of the acute inflammatory response are due primarily to histamine released from mast cell granules, platelets, and basophils.[217] Histamine receptors are distributed on leukocytes and on the ocular surface.[217] There are two types of histamine receptors on cells: the H_1 and the H_2 receptors.[217–219] Activation of H_1 receptors in the eye is associated with ocular allergy.[217, 218]

Antihistamines inhibit the effects of histamine by occupying histamine receptor sites. The five basic classes of H_1 antagonists include alkylamines, ethanolamines, ethylenediamines, phenothiazines, and piperazines.[9, 217, 220] The H_1 antihistamines used commonly in topical ophthalmic agents are ethylenediamines (antazoline phosphate and pyrilamine maleate) and an alkylamine (pheniramine maleate).[9, 198]

Levocarbastine hydrochloride (Livostin 0.05%), a potent H_1 antagonist, has demonstrated proven efficacy in reducing signs and symptoms of allergic conjunctivitis, with a duration of action of at least 4 hours. No severe adverse effects have been reported.[221] A tolerability profile similar to that of placebo was observed in several controlled studies.[222, 223–227]

Topical antihistamines, with a noted exception of levocarbastine hydrochloride, are commercially available as antihistamine-decongestant combinations. The most commonly used decongestants or vasoconstrictors are naphazoline hydrochloride, phenylephrine, and tetrahydrozoline.[198, 217]

Antihistamines may cause allergic responses and local irritation.[15] H_1 blockers also have local anesthetic properties; however, the concentrations required for this effect are much greater than those used therapeutically to antagonize the histamine response.[220]

Adverse systemic reactions to topical vasoconstrictors are uncommon, but headache,[228–230] dizziness,[229] nervousness,[231] hypotension,[232, 233] hypertension,[228, 229, 234–236] and cardiac dysrhythmias[229] have been reported. The most commonly reported ocular side effect is stinging on instillation. Blurred vision,[230, 237] mydriasis,[237–241] epithelial erosions,[242, 243] punctal stenosis,[244, 245] corneal pigment deposition,[246] iris pigment release,[239, 247] iritis,[248] change in IOP[228, 237, 239, 240, 249, 250] and acute angle closure have also been described.[230, 240, 241]

A case series report identified acute and chronic conjunctivitis due to over-the-counter ophthalmic decongestants.[251] Three clinical patterns in order of decreasing frequency were observed and include: (1) a pharmacologically induced rebound conjunctival hyperemia, (2) a toxic follicular conjunctivitis, and (3) an allergic, eczematoid blepharoconjunctivitis. The authors note that the longer the duration of eye drops use before presentation, the longer the recovery period required.

SYSTEMIC ANTIHISTAMINES

Many oral antihistamines may be used for adjunctive treatment of allergic symptoms, particularly itching.[217, 252–255] The agents used most commonly in the past include diphenhydramine, tripelennamine, chlorpheniramine maleate, and hydroxyzine hydrochloride.[217] Newer agents of the piperidine class include astemizole (Hismanal) and terfenadine (Seldane),[220, 253] loratadine (claritin), and fexofenadine (Allegra), an active acid metabolite of terfenadine.

Oral antihistamines have a drying effect on the eye that may worsen or induce keratoconjunctivitis sicca and cause contact lens intolerance.[217, 254] Chlorpheniramine maleate, a commonly prescribed oral antihistamine, which is also available over the counter, has been shown to decrease tear production significantly, as measured by standard Schirmer testing, in normal patients.[255]

The most common adverse effect of systemic administration of antihistamines is drowsiness.[217, 220, 256] This may be hazardous to those patients who must drive or operate machinery. These agents also enhance the action of narcotics and sedatives.[220] Astemizole, terfenadine, loratadine, and fexofenadine have fewer sedative and anticholinergic side effects.[175, 220] Gastrointestinal side effects of oral antihistamines such as nausea, emesis, anorexia, epigastric distress, and altered bowel habits may be reduced by ingestion of the medication with meals.[217] Less common central nervous system effects may include lassitude, dizziness, tinnitus, incoordination, blurred vision, diplopia, euphoria, nervousness, tremors, and insomnia.[217] The anticholinergic action of these drugs may induce mydriasis, triggering acute angle-closure glaucoma as well as a reduction in accommodation by effects on ciliary muscles.[9, 217] Rare side effects of visual hallucinations, temporary blindness, and an absence of pupillary light reflexes have been induced by overdosage.[217]

Serious adverse cardiovascular events, including death, cardiac arrest, torsades de pointes, and other ventricular arrhythmias have been reported with concomitant use of terfenadine with erythromycin and related macrolide antibiotics, ketoconazole, or itraconazole, and significant hepatic dysfunction. Use of terfenadine is therefore contraindicated in these situations.

Fexofenadine, a new antihistamine of the piperidine class of agents, has been approved. The previously described systemic cardiovascular event seen with terfenadine have not been reported with this newer agent.[257]

Loratadine, an antihistamine, has also been safely coadministered with erythromycin, cimetidine, and ketoconazole. There have been no significant effects on the QT interval and no reports of sedation or syncope with this agent.[198]

Ocular Mast Cell–Stabilizing Agents

Disodium cromoglycate (DSCG) 4%, cromolyn sodium (Opticrom), and lodoxamide tromethamine 0.1% (Alomide) are mast cell–stabilizing agents used in the treatment of vernal and atopic keratoconjunctivitis, giant papillary conjunctivitis, and allergic (hay fever) keratoconjunctivitis.[253, 258–265] Topical use of these agents is well tolerated in most instances.

Commonly reported side effects of disodium cromoglycate are transient burning and stinging on instillation.[198, 258, 260] Hyperemia and bulbar conjunctival chemosis have been reported in 35% of patients.[260] Less common adverse effects include watery and itchy eyes, sties, puffiness, and dryness around the eyes.[259] EDTA, a solution stabilizer in DSCG, has been implicated as the cause of conjunctival injection in some cases.[259]

Clinical trials have indicated that treatment-related ocular adverse effects of lodoxamide are mild, nonserious, and transient. Reported adverse effects include minor discomfort, itching, and pain.[263–265] Headache[265] and nausea[263] are nonocular side effects that have been reported in rare instances.

Both disodium cromoglycate and lodoxamide may decrease the steroid requirement, thus reducing the potential adverse effects from long-term corticosteroid therapy.[253, 258, 259, 261, 263–265] Acute exacerbations and severe forms of ocular allergy may require topical steroids, however. In these cases a pulse steroid regimen with aggressive but brief corticosteroid treatment with rapid tapering and maintenance therapy with these mast cell–stabilizing agents may have a therapeutic advantage while minimizing risks of steroid therapy. The therapeutic effect of mast cell–stabilizing agents is not as immediate as that of corticosteroids, taking usually several weeks of regular use for a desired therapeutic response. Patients should be advised of this when using these drugs, or compliance may be a problem.

Immunosuppressive Agents

In ophthalmic practice, immunosuppressive agents are used in the treatment of active bilateral, sight-threatening endogenous uveitis that has failed to respond to maximally tolerated systemic CSs. Immunosuppressive agents are often used in combination with low-dose steroid therapy. The potential life-threatening side effects of these agents warrant clear indications for instituting therapy. Such recommendations have been reviewed by the International Uveitis Study Group.[148] Behçet's disease and sympathetic ophthalmia are now considered absolute indications for cytotoxic therapy.[148, 266]

ALKYLATING AGENTS

Cyclophosphamide (Cytoxan) is a potent immunosuppressive agent that has been used in the treatment of Behçet's disease,[267–271] external ocular inflammatory disease due to Wegener's granulomatosis, Mooren's ulcer, cicatricial pemphigoid, and rheumatoid arthritis as well as advanced Graves' ophthalmopathy.[272, 273] The oral dosage is usually 1 to 2 mg/kg/day; this is titrated according to the patient's peripheral leukocyte count.[74] Bone marrow toxicity resulting in anemia, leukopenia, thrombocytopenia, and secondary infection is common.[74, 148, 171, 266] Careful monitoring of complete blood counts, platelets, and differential counts is crucial. A reduction in dosage is indicated if the total white blood cell count is less than 3000/mm^2 or the neutrophil count is less than 1500 to 2000/mm^2.[74, 148] An increased risk of opportunistic infection is more likely when blood counts are below these levels.[74] Hemorrhagic cystitis is a serious adverse effect.[74, 148, 171, 266] This may be an indication for cessation of therapy.

Patients who develop hemorrhagic cystitis are at increased risk of developing urinary bladder malignancies.[9, 148, 271] Patients should be instructed to drink at least 3 to 4 L/day to facilitate adequate urine output and reduce the risk of hemorrhagic cystitis.[74] Patients of child-bearing age should be cautioned about gonadal suppression. Men should bank their sperm in view of the risk of oligospermia, azoospermia, and testicular atrophy. Women should also be advised of potential ovarian failure.[74] Leukemia, lymphomas, and solid tumors have been reported to be more common in this population.[272] Other complications include renal and hepatic toxicity, alopecia, interstitial fibrosis, visual blurring, blepharoconjunctivitis, and keratoconjunctivitis sicca.[9, 74, 171, 273]

Chlorambucil exerts its effect primarily on B cells. This agent is used in the treatment of Behçet's disease, sympathetic ophthalmia, chronic cyclitis, and rheumatoid sclero-uveitis.[74, 148, 274] An initial dose of 2 mg/day is increased every 2 or 3 weeks until clinical improvement or toxicity develops.[74, 148] The usual therapeutic dose is 6 to 10 mg/day. Bone marrow toxicity is a major side effect. Irreversible bone marrow depression may occur with doses greater than 6.5 mg/kg.[74] Gonadal suppression and sterility may result. This agent also has carcinogenic, mutagenic, and teratogenic potential.[74] Notable ocular side effects include reversible pseudotumor cerebri with papilledema, diplopia, and keratoconjunctivitis sicca.[9, 275, 276]

ANTIMETABOLITES

Azathioprine (Imuran) has been used in the management of rheumatoid arthritis, pars planitis, sympathetic ophthalmia, Vogt-Koyanagi-Harada syndrome, and Behçet's disease.[74, 148, 274] It interferes with purine metabolism, which results in altered DNA, RNA, and protein synthesis. The usual dose is 150 mg/day for 1 month, which is tapered to 100 mg/day.[74] Complications of therapy include severe bone marrow suppression, hepatotoxicity, gastrointestinal symptoms (anorexia, nausea, vomiting, diarrhea), fever, and arthralgias.[9, 74, 148, 171, 266]

Methotrexate is a folic acid antagonist used in the treatment of Mooren's corneal ulcer,[269] sympathetic ophthalmia, and chronic cyclitis.[148, 268] It inhibits the enzyme folic acid reductase, thus blocking the conversion of dehydrofolic acid to tetrahydrofolic acid, which ultimately inhibits DNA synthesis and cell division.[74, 148] It affects both B- and T-lymphocyte functions.[74] The initial dose is 7.5 mg/wk in three divided doses over 36 hours.[74] Adverse side effects include acute and chronic pneumonitis.[277, 278] This complication, thought to be due to a hypersensitivity response or an idiosyncratic reaction, usually resolves with discontinuation of therapy and systemic steroids.[74] Hepatotoxicity is one of the more common complications. Careful monitoring of liver enzymes and periodic liver biopsies are important in monitoring these patients.[74, 148, 266] Alternative therapy should be considered in elderly patients and in patients with a history of alcoholism, diabetes mellitus, or obesity.[74] The pathophysiology of the hepatotoxicity has not been fully elucidated. Proposed mechanisms, however, include hepatocellular folate deficiency or toxicity due to the drug's metabolites.[74] It has been noted that frequent administration of lower doses is associated with greater hepatotoxicity than is weekly high-dose therapy.[279] Other complications include mucosal ulcerations, gastrointestinal symptoms, bone marrow depression, and teratogenicity.[74, 280] Reversible ocular irritation characterized by burning and itching from high-dose methotrexate therapy has been reported.[9] High levels of this agent found in the tears may explain the ocular irritation.[281] Approximately 25% of patients develop periorbital edema, blepharitis, conjunctival hyperemia, epiphora, and photophobia.[9, 275, 276] A toxic interaction between NSAIDs and methotrexate may result in severe bone marrow and renal toxicity.[282]

5-FLUOROURACIL

5-Fluorouracil (5-FU) is a fluorinated pyrimidine antimetabolite and a commonly used cytotoxic agent in the palliative treatment of solid tumors; it is also used topically for actinic keratoses and intradermally for skin cancer.[9] The subconjunctival administration of 5-FU is used in patients who are at high risk for bleb failure, as well as primary trabeculectomies in both adults and children.[283–287] 5-FU inhibits fibroblast proliferation stimulated by filtering surgery.[74]

The therapeutic dose is often close to the toxic level of drug, and 25 to 35% of patients on systemic therapy develop adverse ocular effects.[9] The most common ocular side effects are mild blepharitis and conjunctival irritation.[9, 275] Neurotoxicity with brain stem involvement may produce oculomotor disturbances.[9] With long-term systemic therapy, the drug has been found in tears, which may be responsible for the local irritation leading to cicatricial changes in the conjunctiva and lacrimal drainage system as well as cicatricial ectropion.[9, 275]

Topical application in the form of ointment used to treat skin lesions around the eye may cause ocular burning, irritation, and lacrimation as well as changes in lids and conjunctiva and cicatricial ectropion.[9] Subconjunctival administration may cause the development of prolonged corneal epithelial defects owing to the effect of 5-FU on corneal epithelial proliferation; other adverse effects are related to poor wound healing and include needle tract wound leaks and conjunctival dehiscence.[283–286] Subconjunctival hemorrhage at the site of injection has also been observed.[283] More serious late complications are corneal ulceration, perforation, and scarring in patients with underlying corneal disease.[288] Owing to the corneal epithelial toxicity of 5-FU, patients receiving this drug must have their corneal status closely monitored. The potential risk of perforation, infection, and fibrosis also exists as with all subconjunctival injections.

An increased incidence of late bleb infections and bleb-related endophthalmitis has been reported since 1984.[289] Wolner and associates[290] reported late infection rates of approximately 3% after filtering surgery with 5-FU superiorly and 9% inferiorly.

A preendophthalmitis bleb infection should be suspected in the presence of irritation, tearing or mucopurulent discharge, conjunctival hyperemia, or clouding of the bleb fluid with or without an obvious wound leak. The presence of aqueous or vitreous inflammatory cells suggests endophthalmitis. Signs of external bleb infection in the presence of hypopion is indicative of endophthalmitis.

CYCLOSPORINE

Cyclosporine (cyclosporin A [CsA]; Sandimmune) is a fungal metabolite whose immunosuppressive properties were first described by Borel at Sandoz, Ltd. in Basel, Switzerland.[74, 148, 288] Unlike other immunosuppressive agents, CsA specifically modulates T-lymphocyte proliferation and recruitment and lacks the bone marrow toxicity and hematopoietic complications.[148, 291] It is used to prevent kidney, liver, or heart allograft rejection. A masked, randomized clinical trial is in progress in the United States to evaluate the role of systemic CsA in the prevention of corneal graft rejection. CsA is also used to treat many resistant uveitic conditions and is considered the drug of choice in bilaterally active Behçet's disease.[74, 148, 288, 292] The agent is metabolized in the liver by the cytochrome P-450 microsomal enzyme system.[148] CsA tends to concentrate in lipid-containing tissues. Although higher doses were formerly used, the currently recommended dosage is 5 to 7 mg/kg/day given in a single dose or twice daily.[148] The dosage is adjusted based on the clinical response and renal function parameters. A relative contraindication to therapy is a history of renal disease associated with reduced creatinine clearance and uncontrolled hypertension.[74] Elderly patients with reduced renal reserve must undergo careful monitoring.

The most notable complication of CsA therapy is nephrotoxicity, manifested by decreased creatinine clearance, elevated serum creatinine levels, and a disproportionate increase in blood urea nitrogen with preserved urine output and sodium reabsorption.[293] It is important to note that the serum creatinine level underestimates the glomerular filtration rate and therefore should not be the sole marker of renal toxicity.[294] The renal toxicity occurs at the level of the arteriole, glomerulus, and proximal tubule.[74, 293] CsA-induced alteration in renal hemodynamics has been proposed.[251] Systemic hypertension is another significant side effect, occurring in 25% of patients; it tends to be more frequent in those with impaired renal function.[74] The exact mechanism remains unknown but appears to be dose-related. Hypertension is also more common in patients receiving CsA and steroids than in those receiving CsA alone.[295] Leukopenia is not seen with CsA; however, a normochromic normocytic anemia is observed in 25% of patients, and other causes of anemia should be ruled out.[74] An increase in the erythrocyte sedimentation rate has been noted in 40% of patients, but this does not correlate with the clinical course of the underlying disease and should not be used as an index of disease activity.[74] An increased incidence of lymphoma was once thought to be related to CsA use; however, in a large clinical series of 5000 transplant recipients, the incidence of lymphoma was no greater in patients receiving CsA than in those receiving other immunosuppressive agents.[291] Other side effects of CsA include hirsutism, gingival hyperplasia, central nervous system toxicity, and an increased incidence of viral infections.[74, 148, 291, 296] Several important drug interactions observed with the administration of CsA[74, 293, 293a, 297–303] are summarized in Table 39–3. Ocular side effects reportedly due to systemic use include decreased vision, eyelid or conjunctival erythema, nonspecific conjunctivitis, urticaria, visual hallucinations, and conjunctival and retinal hemorrhages related to drug-induced anemia.[9]

Topical CsA therapy has generated increasing interest in the treatment of corneal graft rejection[291, 304–306] and severe vernal keratoconjunctivitis.[307] CsA eye drops are generally well tolerated, although occasional eyelid irritation has been noted.[9] A report of skin maceration of the lateral canthus

TABLE 39–3. **Cyclosporine and Drug Interactions**

Drug	Mechanism
Drugs That Increase CsA Plasma Concentration or Toxicity	
Nonsteroidal antiinflammatory drugs	Altered renal blood flow[74, 293]
Aminoglycosides	Tubulotoxin[74, 293, 297]
Amphotericin B	Tubulotoxin[74, 293, 293a]
Co-trimoxazole/trimethoprim	Tubulotoxin[74, 293, 293a]
Ketoconazole	Inhibition of hepatic microsomal enzymes[297a]
Erythromycin	Inhibition of CsA metabolism or increased absorption[74, 299, 300]
Verapamil HCl Diltiazem HCl	Decreased CsA metabolism[74, 301]
Drugs That Decrease CsA Plasma Concentration or Toxicity	
Phenytoin (Dilantin) Phenobarbital	Increased activity of hepatic microsomal enzyme metabolism[298, 302]
Drug Toxicity Induced by CsA	
Digoxin (dysrhythmias, atrioventricular block)	Use with CsA results in reduced volume distribution and plasma clearance[74, 303]

Abbreviation: CsA, cyclosporine.

after 1 week of CsA therapy for severe vernal disease has been reported.[308] Hoffman and Wiederholt[307] noted that all patients developed a mild conjunctivitis and punctate keratitis after topical CsA therapy; however, topical steroids were used concomitantly.

THIOTEPA

Thiotepa (triethylenethiophosphoramide), an antimetabolic agent, is chemically and pharmacologically related to the nitrogen mustards. Thiotepa is used as a topical agent to inhibit pterygium recurrence and to prevent corneal neovascularization resulting from chemical injuries.[309–311] The mode of action is thought to be the release of ethylenimine radicals and their effect on actively dividing cells. Inhibition of neovascularization appears to be due to inhibition of capillary endothelial proliferation.[310]

Ocular irritation and allergic reactions are the most common side effects.[9, 311] Eyelid depigmentation is often the most bothersome adverse effect.[309, 311–314] This reaction occurs primarily in darkly pigmented patients and may be enhanced by excessive exposure to sunlight.[9] Prolonged, frequent administration of thiotepa has been associated with significant keratitis and conjunctivitis.[9] Lacrimal punctal occlusion has also been associated with topical use.[9]

MITOMYCIN C

Mitomycin C is an antibiotic antineoplastic agent isolated from *Streptomyces caespitosus*.[315] In ophthalmology, this agent is sometimes used after pterygium surgery to prevent recurrence.[9] In addition, mitomycin C is used as an adjunctive agent in primary and high-risk or complicated glaucoma filtering surgery.[316–318] It is used systemically to treat a variety of malignant diseases. Ocular side effects related to systemic use are generally reversible and self-limited.[9]

In a double-masked, prospective clinical trial by Singh

and coworkers,[315] topically applied mitomycin (1 mg/mL) caused conjunctival irritation, excessive lacrimation, and mild superficial punctate keratitis; these adverse effects were minimized with the lower (0.4 mg/mL) dosage; this lower dose was equally effective in preventing pterygium recurrence, and no systemic toxicity after topical administration was noted.

More serious complications of topical mitomycin C therapy after pterygium surgery were reported by Rubinfeld and coworkers.[319] In this case series of 10 patients, complications observed include severe secondary glaucoma, corneal perforation, corneal edema, scleral calcification, a sudden onset of mature cataract, iritis, intolerable pain, and photophobia. The authors advise extreme caution in the use of mitomycin and suggest that the lowest possible drug concentration be administered for the shortest time period, in an effort to avoid these serious, potentially sight-threatening complications.

Adverse effects of mitomycin C in glaucoma filtering surgery include sequelae of wound-healing inhibition and compromise of the conjunctival barrier, including bleb, wound leaks, and infection. A high rate, 8%, of late infection over 3 years after trabeculectomy inferiorly with mitomycin C and an overall late infection rate of 2.6% were described by Higginbotham and associates.[320]

Acknowledgment

Supported in part by an unrestricted grant from Research to Prevent Blindness, Inc., and Core Center Grant EYO1931.

REFERENCES

1. Leopold IH, Gaster RN: Ocular inflammation and anti-inflammatory drugs. *In* Kaufman HE, Barron BA, McDonald MB, Waltman SR (eds): The Cornea. New York, Churchill Livingstone, 1988, p 67.
2. Richardson KT: Pharmacology and pathophysiology of inflammation. Arch Ophthalmol 86:706, 1971.
3. Lorenzetti DWC: Therapeutic and toxic dose-response effect of corticosteroids. *In* Kaufman HE (ed): Symposium on Ocular Anti-inflammatory Therapy. Springfield, IL, Charles C Thomas, 1970, p 205.
4. Harter JG, Borgmann AR, Leaders FE: Steroid potency and the determination of potency, effectiveness and toxicity of anti-inflammatory drugs for use in the eye. *In* Kaufman HE (ed): Symposium on Ocular Anti-inflammatory Therapy. Springfield, IL, Charles C Thomas, 1970, p 234.
5. Havener WH: Anti-inflammatory agents. *In* Havener WH (ed): Ocular Pharmacology. St. Louis, CV Mosby, 1994, p 350.
6. Burch PG, Migeon CJ: Systemic absorption of topical steroids. Arch Ophthalmol 79:174, 1968.
7. Krupin T, Mandell AI, Podos SM, Becker B: Topical corticosteroid therapy and pituitary-adrenal function. Arch Ophthalmol 94:919, 1976.
8. O'Day DM, McKenna TJ, Eliott JH: Ocular corticosteroid therapy: Systemic hormonal effects. Trans Am Acad Ophthalmol Otolaryngol 79:71, 1975.
9. Fraunfelder FT, Meyer SM (eds): Drug-Induced Ocular Side Effects and Drug Interactions. Philadelphia, Lea & Febiger, 1989.
10. Walker AE, Adamkiewicz JT: Pseudotumor cerebri associated with prolonged corticosteroid therapy. JAMA 188:779, 1964.
11. Ivey KJ, Denbesten L: Pseudotumor cerebri associated with corticosteroid therapy in an adult. JAMA 208:1698, 1969.
12. Sloansky HH, Kolbert G, Gartner S: Exophthalmos induced by steroids. Arch Ophthalmol 77:579, 1967.
13. Nassif KF: Ocular surface defense mechanisms. *In* Tabbara KF, Hyndiuk RA (eds): Infections of the Eye. Boston, Little, Brown, 1986, p 37.
14. Ridley F: Lysozyme. An antibacterial present in great concentrations in tears and its relation to infection of the human eye. Proc R Soc Med 21:1495, 1978.
15. Wilson FM: Adverse external ocular effects of topical ophthalmic medications. Surv Ophthalmol 24:57, 1979.
16. Smolin G: Medrysone hypersensitivity. Report of a case. Arch Ophthalmol 85:478, 1969.
17. Alania UD, Alania SD: Allergic contact dermatitis to corticosteroid. Ann Allergy 30:181, 1972.
18. Fisher AF, Stillman MA: Allergic contact sensitivity to benzalkonium chloride: Cutaneous, ophthalmic and general medical implications. Arch Dermatol 106:169, 1972.
19. Sulzberger MB, Wise F: The contact or patch test: Its uses, advantages and limitations. Arch Dermatol Syph 23:519, 1931.
20. Gasset AR, Ishii Y, Kaufman HE, Miller T: Cytotoxicity of ophthalmic preservatives. Am J Ophthalmol 78:98, 1974.
21. Pfister RR, Burstein N: The effects of ophthalmic drugs, vehicles and preservatives on corneal epithelium: A scanning electron microscope study. Invest Ophthalmol Vis Sci 15:246, 1976.
22. Hyndiuk RA, Chin GN: Corticosteroid therapy in corneal disease. Int Ophthalmol Clin 13:103, 1973.
23. Jones BR: Vernal keratitis. Trans Ophthalmol Soc UK 81:215, 1961.
24. Olejnik O, Weisbecker CA: Ocular bioavailability of topical prednisolone preparations. Clin Ther 12:1, 1990.
25. Hull DS, Hine JE, Edelhauser HF, Hyndiuk RA: Permeability of the isolated rabbit cornea to corticosteroids. Invest Ophthalmol Vis Sci 13:457, 1974.
26. Apt L, Henrick A, Silverman LM: Patient compliance with the use of topical ophthalmic corticosteroid suspensions. Am J Ophthalmol 87:210, 1979.
27. Pernarowski M: Solutions, emulsions and suspensions. *In* Havener JE (ed): Remington's Pharmaceutical Sciences, 15th ed. Easton, PA, Mack, 1975, p 1436.
28. McLean JM: Clinical and experimental observation on the use of ACTH and cortisone in ocular inflammatory disease. Trans Am Ophthalmol Soc 48:259, 1950.
29. Franois J: Cortisone et tension oculaire. Ann Ocul 187:805, 1954.
30. Armaly MF: Effects of corticosteroids on intraocular pressure and fluid dynamics. I: Effect of dexamethasone in the normal eye. Arch Ophthalmol 70:482, 1963.
31. Armaly MF: Effect of corticosteroids on intraocular pressure and fluid dynamics. II: Effect of dexamethasone in the glaucomatous eye. Arch Ophthalmol 70:98, 1963.
32. Armaly MF: Effect of corticosteroids on intraocular pressure and fluid dynamics. III: Change in visual function and pupil size during topical dexamethasone application. Arch Ophthalmol 71:636, 1964.
33. Armaly MF: Statistical attributes of the steroid hypertensive response in the clinically normal eye. I: The demonstration of three levels of response. Invest Ophthalmol Vis Sci 4:187, 1965.
34. Spaeth GL, Rodriques MM, Weinreb S: Steroid induced glaucoma. A: Persistent elevation of intraocular pressure. B: Histopathological aspects. Trans Am Ophthalmol Soc 75:353, 1977.
35. Becker B, Mills DW: Corticosteroids and intraocular pressure. Arch Ophthalmol 70:500, 1963.
36. Bernstein HN, Mills DW, Becker B: Steroid-induced elevation of intraocular pressure. Arch Ophthalmol 70:15, 1963.
37. Goldmann H: Cortisone glaucoma. Arch Ophthalmol 68:621, 1962.
38. Becker B: Intraocular pressure response to topical corticosteroids. Invest Ophthalmol Vis Sci 4:198, 1965.
39. Fairbairn WD, Thorson JC: Fluorometholone. Anti-inflammatory and intraocular pressure effects. Arch Ophthalmol 86:138, 1971.
40. Schwartz B: The response of ocular pressure to corticosteroids. Int Ophthalmol Clin 6:929, 1966.
41. Mindel JC, Tavitian HO, Smith H, Walker EC: Comparative ocular pressure elevation by medrysone, fluorometholone and dexamethasone phosphate. Arch Ophthalmol 98:1577, 1980.
42. Palmberg PF, Mandell A, Wilensky JT, et al: The reproducibility of the intraocular pressure response to dexamethasone. Arch Ophthalmol 80:844, 1975.
43. Bernstein HN, Schwartz B: Effects of long-term systemic steroids on ocular pressure and tonographic values. Arch Ophthalmol 68:742, 1962.
44. Lee PF: The influences of systemic steroid therapy on the intraocular pressure. Am J Ophthalmol 46:328, 1958.
45. Armaly MF: Factors affecting the dose-response relationship in steroid-induced ocular hypertension. *In* Kaufman HE (ed): Symposium

on Ocular Anti-inflammatory Therapy. Springfield, IL, Charles C Thomas, 1970, p 88.
46. Hovland KR, Ellis PP: Ocular changes in renal transplant patients. Am J Ophthalmol 63:283, 1967.
47. Nicholas JP: Topical corticosteroids and aqueous humor dynamics. Arch Ophthalmol 72:189, 1964.
48. Spaeth GL: Effects of topical dexamethasone on intraocular pressure and the water drinking test. Arch Ophthalmol 76:772, 1966.
49. Levene R, Wigdor A, Edelstein A, Baum J: Topical corticosteroid in normal patients and glaucoma suspects. Arch Ophthalmol 77:593, 1967.
50. Spiers F: Topical steroids and intraocular pressure. I: Clinical investigation on the reactions of 93 outpatients to monocular steroid provocation and to subsequent water drinking test. Acta Ophthalmol 43:735, 1965.
51. Weekers R, Grieten J, Collignon-Brach J: Contribution à l'étude de l'hypertension oculaire provoquée par la dexamethasone dans le glaucoma à angle ouvert. Ophthalmologica 152:81, 1966.
52. Podos SM, Becker B, Morton WR: High myopia and primary open angle glaucoma. Am J Ophthalmol 62:1039, 1966.
53. Paterson GD, Owen R: Studies of the response to topical dexamethasone of glaucoma relatives. Trans Ophthalmol Soc UK 85:295, 1965.
54. Becker B, Hahn KA: Topical corticosteroids and heredity in primary open angle glaucoma. Am J Ophthalmol 57:543, 1974.
55. Ballin N, Becker B: Provocative testing for primary open angle glaucoma in "senior citizens." Invest Ophthalmol Vis Sci 61:121, 1967.
56. Armaly MF: Inheritance of dexamethasone hypertension and glaucoma. Arch Ophthalmol 77:747, 1967.
57. Becker B, Ballin N: Glaucoma and corticosteroid provocative testing. Arch Ophthalmol 74:621, 1965.
58. Becker B, Chevrette L: Topical corticosteroid testing in glaucoma siblings. Arch Ophthalmol 76:484, 1966.
59. Becker B, Podos SM: Krukenberg's spindle and primary open angle glaucoma. Arch Ophthalmol 76:635, 1966.
60. Becker B: Diabetes mellitus and primary open angle glaucoma. Am J Ophthalmol 71:1, 1971.
61. Schwartz JT, Reuling FH, Feinleib M, et al: Twin study on ocular pressure after topical dexamethasone. I: Frequency distribution of pressure response. Am J Ophthalmol 76:126, 1973.
62. Schwartz JT, Reuling FH, Feinleib M, et al: Twin study on ocular pressure following topically applied dexamethasone. II: Inheritance of variation in pressure response. Arch Ophthalmol 90:281, 1973.
63. Cantrill HL, Palmberg PF, Zink HA: Comparison of in vitro potency of corticosteroids with ability to raise intraocular pressure. Am J Ophthalmol 79:1012, 1975.
64. Podos SM, Kolker AE, Becker B: Topical corticosteroids: Dissociation of effects. *In* Kaufman HE (ed): Symposium on Ocular Anti-inflammatory Therapy. Springfield, IL, Charles C Thomas, 1970, p 106.
65. Armaly MF: Dexamethasone ocular hypertension in the clinically normal eye. II: The untreated eye, outflow facility and concentration. Arch Ophthalmol 75:776, 1966.
66. Polansky JR, Weinreb RN: Anti-inflammatory agents-steroids as anti-inflammatory agents. *In* Sears ML (ed): Pharmacology of the Eye. New York, Springer-Verlag, 1984, p 459.
67. Spaeth GL: Hydroxymethylprogesterone. Arch Ophthalmol 75:783, 1966.
68. Linner E: Adrenocorticosteroids and aqueous humor dynamics. Doc Ophthalmol 13:210, 1959.
69. Weinreb RN, Mitchell M, Polansky JB: Prostaglandin synthesis by human trabecular cells: Inhibitory effect of dexamethasone. Invest Ophthalmol Vis Sci 24(Suppl):136, 1983.
70. Francois J, Victoria-Troncoso V: Corticosteroid glaucoma. Ophthalmologica 174:195, 1977.
71. Knepper PA, Brun M, Weinstein HG, Black LT: Intraocular pressure and glycosaminoglycan distribution in the rabbit eye: Effect of age and dexamethasone. Exp Eye Res 27:567, 1978.
72. Polanksy JR, Gospodarowicz D, Weinreb RN, Alvarado JJ: Human trabecular meshwork cell culture and glycosaminoglycan synthesis. Invest Ophthalmol Vis Sci 17(Suppl):207, 1978.
73. Yoshiaki K, Horie T: The prognosis of corticosteroid-responsive individuals. Arch Ophthalmol 99:819, 1981.
74. Rubin B, Palestine AG: Complications of ophthalmic drugs and solutions. Int Ophthalmol Clin 29:159, 1989.
75. Briggs HH: Glaucoma associated with the use of topical corticosteroids. Arch Ophthalmol 70:312, 1963.
76. Goldmann H: Cortisone glaucoma. Arch Ophthalmol 68:621, 1962.
77. Foster CS, Alter G, De Barge LR, et al: Efficacy and safety of rimexolone 1% ophthalmic suspension vs. 1% prednisolone acetate in the treatment of uveitis. Am J Ophthalmol 122:171, 1996.
78. Lehmann R, Assil K, Stewart R, Fox K: Comparison of rimexolone 1% ophthalmic suspension to placebo in control of postcataract surgery inflammation. Invest Ophthalmol Vis Sci 36:S793, 1995.
79. Leibowitz HM, Bartlett J, Rich R, et al: IOP raising potential of rimexolone 1% in patients responding to corticosteroids. Arch Ophthalmol 114:933, 1996.
80. Alcon Laboratories: New Drug Application, 1994.
81. Black RL, Oglesby RB, von Sallman L, Bunim JJ: Posterior subcapsular cataracts induced by corticosteroids in patients with rheumatoid arthritis. JAMA 174:150, 1960.
82. Oglesby RB, Black RL, von Sallman T, Bunim JJ: Cataracts in rheumatoid arthritis patients treated with corticosteroids. Arch Ophthalmol 66:519, 1961.
83. Giles CL, Mason GL, Duff IF, McLean JA: The association of cataract formation and systemic corticosteroid therapy. JAMA 182:179, 1962.
84. Crews SJ: Posterior subcapsular lens opacities in patients on long-term corticosteroid therapy. Br J Med 5346:1644, 1963.
85. Loredo A, Rodriquez RS, Murillo L: Cataracts after short-term corticosteroid treatment. N Engl J Med 286:160, 1962.
86. Skalka H, Prchal JT: Effect of corticosteroids on cataract formation. Arch Ophthalmol 98:1773, 1980.
87. Urban RC, Cotlier E: Corticosteroid-induced cataracts. Surv Ophthalmol 31:102, 1986.
88. Sundmark E: The cataract-inducing effect of systemic corticosteroid therapy. Acta Ophthalmol 44:291, 1966.
89. Braver DA, Richards RD, Good TA: Posterior subcapsular cataracts in steroid-treated children. Arch Ophthalmol 77:161, 1967.
90. Forman AR, Loreto JA, Tina LU: Reversibility of corticosteroid-associated cataracts in children with nephrotic syndrome. Am J Ophthalmol 84:75, 1977.
91. Spaeth GL, von Sallmann L: Corticosteroids and cataracts. Int Ophthalmol Clin 6:915, 1966.
92. Yablonski ME, Burde RM, Kolker AE, Becker B: Cataracts induced by topical dexamethasone in diabetics. Arch Ophthalmol 96:474, 1978.
93. Harris JE, Gruber L: The electrolyte and water balance of the lens. Exp Eye Res 1:372, 1962.
94. Greiner JV, Chylack LT: Posterior subcapsular cataracts: Histopathologic study of steroid-associated cataracts. Arch Ophthalmol 97:135, 1979.
95. Hyndiuk RA: Radioactive depot-corticosteroid penetration into monkey ocular tissue. II: Subconjunctival administration. Arch Ophthalmol 82:259, 1969.
96. Ashton N, Cook C: Effect of cortisone on healing of corneal wounds. Br J Ophthalmol 35:708, 1951.
97. Aquavella JV, Gasset AR, Dohlman CH: Corticosteroids in corneal wound healing. Am J Ophthalmol 58:621, 1964.
98. Beams R, Linabery L, Grayson M: Effect of topical corticosteroids on corneal wound strength. Am J Ophthalmol 66:1131, 1968.
99. Newell FW, Dixon JM: Effect of subconjunctival cortisone upon the immediate union of experimental corneal grafts. Am J Ophthalmol 34:979, 1952.
100. Gasset AR, Dohlman CH: The tensile strength of corneal wounds. Arch Ophthalmol 79:595, 1968.
101. Palmerton ES: The effect of local cortisone on wound healing in rabbit corneas. Am J Ophthalmol 40:344, 1955.
102. Fink AI, Baras I: Effect of steroids on tensile strength of corneal wounds. Am J Ophthalmol 42:759, 1956.
103. Polack FM, Rosen PN: Topical steroids and tritiated thymidine uptake. Effect on corneal healing. Arch Ophthalmol 77:400, 1967.
104. Gasset AR, Lorenzetti DWC, Ellison EM, Kaufman HE: Quantitative corticosteroid effect on corneal wound healing. Arch Ophthalmol 81:589, 1969.
105. McDonald TO, Borgmann AR, Roberts MD, Fox LG: Corneal wound healing. I: Inhibition of stromal healing by three dexamethasone derivatives. Invest Ophthalmol Vis Sci 9:703, 1970.
106. Brown SI, Weller CA, Vadrich AM: Effect of corticosteroids on corneal collagenase of rabbits. Arch Ophthalmol 70:744, 1970.
107. Srinivasan BD, Kulkarni PS: The effect of steroidal and nonsteroidal anti-inflammatory agents on corneal re-epithelialization. Invest Ophthalmol Vis Sci 20:688, 1981.
108. Ho PC, Elliott JH: Kinetics of corneal epithelial regeneration. II:

Epidermal growth factor and topical corticosteroids. Invest Ophthalmol Vis Sci 4:630, 1973.
109. Leopold IH, Purnell JE, Cannon EJ, et al: Local and systemic cortisone in ocular disease. Am J Ophthalmol 34:361, 1951.
110. Donshik PC, Berman MB, Dohlman CH, et al: Effect of topical corticosteroids on ulceration in alkali-burned corneas. Arch Ophthalmol 96:2117, 1978.
111. Newsome DA, Gross J: Prevention by medroxyprogesterone of perforation in the alkali-burned rabbit cornea: Inhibition of collagenolytic activity. Invest Ophthalmol Vis Sci 16:21, 1977.
112. Kleinert RW, Palmer MP: Anti-inflammatory agents. *In* Tabbara KF, Hyndiuk RA (eds): Infections of the Eye. Boston, Little, Brown, 1996, p 301.
113. Hughes WF: Treatment of HSV keratitis: A review. Am J Ophthalmol 80:499, 1968.
114. Jones BR: Prospects in treating viral disease of the eye. Trans Ophthalmol Soc UK 87:537, 1967.
115. Laibson PR: Ocular inflammation, viruses and the two-edged sword of corticosteroid. Med Clin North Am 53:1145, 1969.
116. Kubrick S, Takahashi GH, Leibowitz HM, Laibson PR: Local corticosteroid therapy and reactivation of herpetic keratitis. Arch Ophthalmol 86:694, 1971.
117. Wilhelmus KR, Gee L, Hauck WW, et al: Herpetic eye disease study: A controlled trial of topical corticosteroids for herpes simplex stromal keratitis. Ophthalmology 101:1883, 1994.
118. Hyndiuk RA, Glasser DB: Herpes simplex keratitis. *In* Tabbara KF, Hyndiuk RA (eds): Infections of the Eye. Boston, Little, Brown, 1996, p 361.
119. Pavan-Langston D: Viral diseases: Herpetic infections. *In* Smolin G, Thoft RA (eds): The Cornea. Boston, Little, Brown, 1994, p 183.
120. Pavan-Langston D, McCulley J: Herpes zoster dendritic keratitis. Arch Ophthalmol 89:25, 1973.
121. Piebenga L, Laibson P: Dendritic lesions in herpes zoster ophthalmicus. Arch Ophthalmol 90:268, 1973.
122. Culbertson WW: Viral retinitis. *In* Tabbara KF, Hyndiuk RA (eds): Infections of the Eye. Boston, Little, Brown, 1996, p 499.
123. Berger BB, Weinberg RS, Tessler HH, et al: Bilateral CMV panuveitis after high-dose corticosteroid therapy. Am J Ophthalmol 88:1020, 1979.
124. Davis SD, Sarff LD, Hyndiuk RA: Corticosteroid in experimentally induced *Pseudomonas* keratitis: Failure of prednisolone to impair the efficacy of tobramycin and carbenicillin therapy. Arch Ophthalmol 96:126, 1978.
125. Aronson SB, Moore TE: Corticosteroid therapy in central stromal keratitis. Am J Ophthalmol 64:873, 1969.
126. Leibowitz HM, Kupferman A: Topically administered corticosteroids—effect on antibiotic-treated bacterial keratitis. Arch Ophthalmol 98:1287, 1980.
127. Stern GA, Okumoto M, Friedlander M, Smolin G: The effect of combined gentamicin-corticosteroid treatment on gentamicin-resistant *Pseudomonas* keratitis. Ann Ophthalmol 12:1011, 1980.
128. Badenoch PR, Hay GJ, McDonald PJ, Coster DJ: A rat model of bacterial keratitis: Effect of antibiotics and corticosteroid. Arch Ophthalmol 103:718, 1985.
129. Davis SD, Sarff LD, Hyndiuk RA: Antibiotic therapy of experimental *Pseudomonas* keratitis in guinea pigs. Arch Ophthalmol 95:1638, 1977.
130. Harbin T: Recurrence of a corneal *Pseudomonas* infection after topical steroid therapy. Am J Ophthalmol 58:670, 1974.
131. Carmichael TR, Gelfand Y, Welsh NH: Topical steroids in the treatment of central and paracentral corneal ulcers. Br J Ophthalmol 74:528, 1990.
132. Liesegang TJ: Bacterial and fungal keratitis. *In* Kaufman HE, Barron BA, McDonald MB, Waltman SR (eds): The Cornea. New York, Churchill Livingstone, 1988, p 217.
133. Kaufman HE: Use of corticosteroids in corneal disease and external diseases of the eye. Int Ophthalmol Clin 6:827, 1966.
134. Mitsue Y, Hanabusa J: Corneal infections after cortisone therapy. Br J Ophthalmol 39:244, 1955.
135. Ley AP: Experimental fungal infections of the cornea. Am J Ophthalmol 42:59, 1966.
136. Jones DB: Principles in the management of oculomycoses. Am J Ophthalmol 79:719, 1975.
137. O'Day DM, Ray WA, Robinson R, Head WS: Efficacy of antifungal agents in the cornea. II: Influence of corticosteroids. Invest Ophthalmol Vis Sci 2:331, 1984.
138. Koenig SB: Fungal keratitis. *In* Tabbara KF, Hyndiuk RA (eds): Infections of the Eye. Boston, Little, Brown, 1986, p 331.
139. Stehr-Green JK, Bailey TM, Visvesara GS: Epidemiology of *Acanthamoeba* keratitis in the U.S. Am J Ophthalmol 107:331, 1989.
140. Osato MS, Robinson NM, Wilhelmus K, Jones D: Morphogenesis of *Acanthamoeba castellan*. Titration of the steroid effect. Invest Ophthalmol Vis Sci 27(Suppl):37, 1986.
141. Auran JD, Starr MB, Jakobiec FA: *Acanthamoeba* keratitis. A review of the literature. Cornea 6:2, 1987.
142. Berger ST, Mondino BJ, Hoft RH, et al: Successful medical management of *Acanthamoeba* keratitis. Am J Ophthalmol 110:395, 1990.
143. Rabinovitch T, Weissman SS, Sheppard JD, Ostler HB: *Acanthamoeba* keratitis: Clinical signs and analyses of factors that affect outcome. Invest Ophthalmol Vis Sci 30(Suppl):38, 1989.
144. Newsome DA, Wong VG, Cameron TP, Anderson RR: "Steroid-induced" mydriasis and ptosis. Invest Ophthalmol Vis Sci 10:424, 1971.
145. Krupin T, LeBlanc RP, Becker B, et al: Uveitis in association with topically administered corticosteroid. Am J Ophthalmol 70:883, 1970.
146. Martins JC, Wilensky JT, Asseff CF, et al: Corticosteroid induced uveitis. Am J Ophthalmol 77:433, 1974.
147. Shin DH, Kass MA, Kolker AE, et al: Positive FTA-Abs tests in subjects with corticosteroid induced uveitis. Am J Ophthalmol 82:259, 1976.
148. Nussenblatt RN, Palestine AP: Uveitis: Fundamentals and Clinical Practice. Chicago, Year Book, 1989.
149. Aronson SB, Moore TE, Williams FC, Goodner EK: Corticosteroids in infectious ocular disease. *In* Kaufman HE (ed): Symposium on Ocular Anti-inflammatory Therapy. Springfield, IL, Charles C Thomas, 1970, p 15.
150. Smith R, Nozik RA: Uveitis. A Clinical Approach to Diagnosis and Management. Baltimore, Williams & Wilkins, 1982.
151. Schlaegel TF: Depot corticosteroid injection by the cul-de-sac route. *In* Kaufman HE (ed): Symposium on Ocular Anti-inflammatory Therapy. Springfield, IL, Charles C Thomas, 1970, p 117.
152. Herschler J: Increased intraocular pressure induced by repository corticosteroids. Am J Ophthalmol 82:90, 1976.
153. Giles CL: Bulbar perforation during periocular injection of corticosteroids. Am J Ophthalmol 77:438, 1974.
154. Schlaegel TF Jr, Wilson FM: Accidental intraocular injection of depot corticosteroids. Trans Am Acad Ophthalmol Otolaryngol 78:847, 1974.
155. Nozik RA: Periocular injection of steroids. Trans Am Acad Ophthalmol Otolaryngol 76:695, 1972.
156. Hida T, Chandler D, Arena JE, Machemer R: Experimental and clinical observation of the intraocular toxicity of commercial corticosteroid preparations. Am J Ophthalmol 101:190, 1986.
157. Zinn KM: Iatrogenic intraocular injection of depot corticosteroid and its surgical removal using the pars plana approach. Arch Ophthalmol 88:13, 1981.
158. Ellis PP: Occlusion of the central retinal artery after retrobulbar corticosteroid injection. Am J Ophthalmol 85:352, 1978.
159. McLean EB: Inadvertent injection of corticosteroid into the choroidal vasculature. Am J Ophthalmol 80:835, 1975.
160. Morgan CM, Schatz H, Vine AK, et al: Ocular complications associated with retrobulbar injections. Ophthalmology 95:650, 1988.
161. Mathias GGT, Maibach HI, Ostler HB, Conant MA: Delayed hypersensitivity to retrobulbar injections of methylprednisolone acetate. Am J Ophthalmol 86:816, 1978.
162. Mills DW, Siebert LF, Climenhoga DB: Depot triamcinolone induced glaucoma. Can J Ophthalmol 21:150, 1986.
163. Cogen MS, Elsas FJ: Eyelid depigmentation following injection for infantile ocular adnexal hemangioma. J Pediatr Ophthalmol Strabismus 26:35, 1989.
164. Sutula FC, Glover AT: Eyelid necrosis following intralesional corticosteroid injection for capillary hemangioma. Ophthalmic Surg 18:103, 1987.
165. Weiss AH: Adrenal suppression after corticosteroid injection of periocular hemangiomas. Am J Ophthalmol 107:518, 1989.
166. Droste PJ, Ellis FD, Sondhi N, Helveston EM: Linear subcutaneous fat atrophy after corticosteroid injection of periocular hemangiomas. Am J Ophthalmol 105:65, 1988.
167. Shorr N, Seiff SR: Central retinal artery occlusion associated with periocular corticosteroid injection for juvenile hemangioma. Ophthalmic Surg 17:229, 1986.
168. Cohen BZ, Tripathi RC: Eyelid depigmentation after intralesional injection of a fluorinated corticosteroid for chalazion. Am J Ophthalmol 88:269, 1979.

168a. Kligman AM, Williams IW: A new formula for depigmenting skin. Arch Dermatol 111:40, 1975.
169. Insel PA: Analgesic-antipyretics and anti-inflammatory agents; drugs employed in the treatment of rheumatoid arthritis and gout. *In* Gilman AG, Rall TW, Nies AS, Taylor P (eds): Goodman and Gilman's The Pharmacological Basis of Therapeutics, 8th ed. New York, Macmillan, 1990, p 638.
170. Masudu K: Anti-inflammatory agents. Nonsteroidal anti-inflammatory drugs. *In* Sears ML (ed): Pharmacology of the Eye. New York, Springer-Verlag, 1984, p 539.
171. Foster CS: Nonsteroidal anti-inflammatory drugs and immunosuppressives. *In* Lamberts DN, Potter DE (eds): Clinical Ophthalmic Pharmacology. Boston, Little, Brown, 1987, p 173.
172. Flach AJ: Cyclo-oxygenase inhibitors in ophthalmology. Surv Ophthalmol 36:259, 1992.
172a. Flach AJ: Non-steroidal anti-inflammatory agents. *In* Olin BR (ed): Drug Facts and Comparisons. St. Louis, Wolters Kluwer, 1991, p 488a.
172b. Kraff MC, Sanders DR, McGulgan L, Raanan MG: Inhibition of blood–aqueous humor barrier breakdown with diclofenac. A fluorophotometric study. Arch Ophthalmol 108:380, 1990.
172c. Sher NA, Barak M, Daya S, et al: Excimer laser photorefractive keratectomy in high myopia. Arch Ophthalmol 110:935, 1992.
173. Simon LS, Mills JA: Nonsteroidal anti-inflammatory drugs. Part I. N Engl J Med 302:1179, 1980.
174. Simon LS, Mills JA: Nonsteroidal anti-inflammatory drugs. Part II. N Engl J Med 302:1237, 1980.
175. Physicians' Desk Reference. Montvale, NJ, Medical Economics, 1997.
176. Flach AJ, Lavelle CJ, Olander KW, et al: The effect of ketorolac tromethamine solution 0.5% in reducing postoperative inflammation of the cataract extraction and intraocular lens implantation. Ophthalmology 95:1279, 1988.
177. Flach AJ, Graham J, Kruger LP, et al: Quantitative assessment of postsurgical breakdown of the blood-aqueous barrier following administration of 0.5% ketorolac tromethamine solution. Arch Ophthalmol 106:344, 1988.
178. Flach AJ, Kraff MC, Sanders DR, Tanenbaum L: Quantitative effect of 0.5% ketorolac tromethamine solution and 0.1% dexamethasone sodium phosphate solution on postsurgical blood-aqueous barrier. Arch Ophthalmol 106:480, 1988.
179. Flach AJ, Dol AN, Irvine AR: Effectiveness of ketorolac 0.5% solution for chronic aphakic and pseudophakic cystoid macular edema. Am J Ophthalmol 103:479, 1987.
180. Flach AJ, Stegman RC, Graham J, Kruger LP: Prophylaxis of aphakic cystoid macular edema without corticosteroids—a paired-comparison, placebo-controlled double-masked study. Ophthalmology 97:1253, 1990.
181. Sher NA, Frantz JM, Talley A, et al: Topical diclofenac in the treatment of ocular pain after excimer PRK. Refract Corneal Surg 9:425, 1993.
182. Arshinoff S, D'Addario D, Sadler C, et al: Use of topical NSAIDs in excimer PRK. J Cataract Refract Surg 20(Suppl):216, 1994.
183. Tinkleman DG, Rupp G, Kaufman H, et al: Double-masked, paired comparison clinical study of ketorolac tromethamine 0.5% ophthalmic solution. Surv Ophthalmol 38(Suppl):133, 1993.
184. Ballas Z, Blumenthal M, Tinkleman DG, et al: Clinical evaluation of ketorolac tromethamine 0.5% ophthalmic solution for the treatment of seasonal allergic conjunctivitis. Surv Ophthalmol 38(Suppl):141, 1993.
185. Pirson Y, van Ypersele de Strihou C: Renal side effects of nonsteroidal anti-inflammatory drugs: Clinical relevance. Am J Kidney Dis 8:338, 1986.
186. Stern RS, Bigby M: An expanded profile of cutaneous reactions to NSAIDs. Reports to a specialty-based system for spontaneous reporting of adverse reactions to drugs. JAMA 252:1433, 1984.
187. Asherov J, Schoenberg A, Weinberger A: Diplopia following ibuprofen administration. JAMA 248:649, 1982.
188. Registry of possible drug-induced ocular side effects. Ophthalmology 87:87, 1980.
189. Palmer CAL: Toxic amblyopia from ibuprofen. Br Med J 23:765, 1972.
190. Tullio CJ: Ibuprofen-induced visual disturbance. Am J Hosp Pharm 38:1362, 1981.
191. Callum LMT, Bowen DI: Ocular side effects of ibuprofen. Br J Ophthalmol 55:472, 1971.
192. Hamburger HA, Beckman H, Thompson R: Visual evoked potentials and ibuprofen (Motrin) toxicity. Ann Ophthalmol 16:328, 1984.
193. Burns CA: Indomethacin, reduced retinal sensitivity, and corneal deposits. Am J Ophthalmol 66:825, 1968.
194. Carr RE, Siegel IM: Retinal function in patients treated with indomethacin. Am J Ophthalmol 75:302, 1973.
195. Tillmann W, Keitel L: Indomethacin-induced corneal deposits. Klin Monatsbl Augenheilkd 170:756, 1977.
196. Katzman B: Pseudotumor cerebri: An observation on review. Ann Ophthalmol 13:887, 1981.
197. Crawford JS, Lewandowski RL, Chan W: The effect of aspirin on rebleeding in traumatic hyphema. Am J Ophthalmol 80:543, 1978.
198. Physicians' Desk Reference for Ophthalmology. Montvale, NJ, Medical Economics, 1997.
199. Keates RH, McGowan KA: Clinical trial of flurbiprofen to maintain pupillary dilation during cataract surgery. Ann Ophthalmol 16:919, 1984.
200. Flurbiprofen results in 1,000 cases described. Ocul Surg 5:11, 1987.
201. Sher NA, et al: The role of topical steroidal and NSAIDs in etiology of stromal infiltrates after excimer PRK. J Refract Corneal Surg 10:587, 1994.
202. Wilhelmus KR: Microbial keratitis associated with contact lens wear. *In* Dabezies OH Jr (ed): The CLAO Guide to Basic Science and Clinical Practice, 2nd ed, vol 2. Boston, Little, Brown, 1988, p 41.1.
203. Stein RM, Clinch TE, Cohen EJ, et al: Infected versus sterile corneal infiltrates in contact lens wearers. Am J Ophthalmol 10:632, 1988.
204. Hotchkiss ML, Robin AL, Pallock IP, Quigley HA: Nonsteroidal anti-inflammatory agents after argon laser trabeculoplasty. A trial with flurbiprofen and indomethacin. Ophthalmology 91:969, 1984.
205. Sabiston D, Tessler H, Sumers K, et al: Reduction of inflammation following cataract surgery by the NSAID, flurbiprofen. Ophthalmic Surg 18:873, 1987.
206. Weinreb RN, Robin AL, Baerveldt G, et al: Flurbiprofen pretreatment in argon laser trabeculoplasty for primary open angle glaucoma. Arch Ophthalmol 102:1629, 1984.
207. Hurwitz LM, Spaeth CL, Zakhour I, et al: Comparison of the effect of flurbiprofen, dexamethasone, and placebo on cyclocryotherapy induced inflammation. Ophthalmic Surg 15:394, 1984.
208. Leopold IH, Murray D: Noncorticosteroidal anti-inflammatory agents in ophthalmology. Ophthalmology 86:142, 1979.
209. Miller D, Gruenberg P, Miller R, Bergamini MVW: Topical flurbiprofen or prednisolone: Effect on corneal wound healing in rabbits. Arch Ophthalmol 99:681, 1981.
210. Trousdale MD, Dunkel EC, Nesburn AB: Effect of flurbiprofen on herpes simplex keratitis in rabbits. Invest Ophthalmol Vis Sci 19:267, 1980.
211. Asbell PA, Kenamar T, Torres MA: Effect of flurbiprofen on herpes simplex keratitis in rabbits. Invest Ophthalmol Vis Sci 31(Suppl):221, 1990.
212. Gritz DC, Lee TY, Kwitko S, McDonnell PJ: Topical anti-inflammatory agents in an animal model of microbial keratitis. Arch Ophthalmol 108:1001, 1990.
213. Feinstein NC, Rubin B: Toxicity of flurbiprofen sodium. Case report. Arch Ophthalmol 106:311, 1988.
214. Harker LA, Slichter SJ: The bleeding time as a screening test for evaluation of platelet function. N Engl J Med 287:155, 1972.
215. Gieser DK, Hodapp E, Goldenberg I, et al: Flurbiprofen and intraocular pressure. Ann Ophthalmol 13:831, 1981.
216. Sitenga GL, Ing EB, Van Dellen RG, et al: Asthma caused by topical ketorolac. Ophthalmology 103:890, 1996.
217. Abelson MB, Weston JH: Antihistamines. *In* Lamberts DN, Potter DE (eds): Clinical Ophthalmic Pharmacology. Boston, Little, Brown, 1987, p 417.
218. Weston JH, Udell IJ, Abelson MB: H_1 receptors in the human ocular surface. Invest Ophthalmol Vis Sci 20(Suppl):32, 1981.
219. Abelson MB, Udell IJ: H_2 receptors in the human ocular surface. Arch Ophthalmol 99:302, 1981.
220. Garrison JC: Histamine and 5-hydroxytryptamine (serotonin) and their antagonists. *In* Gilman AG, Rall TW, Nies AS, Taylor P (eds): Goodman and Gilman's The Pharmacological Basis of Therapeutics, 8th ed. New York, Macmillan, 1990, p 575.
221. Abelson MB, George MA, Schaefer K, et al: Evaluation of the new antihistamine, 0.05% levocabastine, in the clinical allergen challenge model of allergic conjunctivitis. J Allergy Clin Immunol 94:458, 1994.
222. Noble S, McTavish D: Levocabastine: An update of its pharmacology, clinical efficacy and tolerability in the treatment of allergic rhinitis and conjunctivitis. Drugs 50:1037, 1995.
223. Dechant KL, Goa KL: Levocabastine: A review of its pharmacological properties and therapeutic potential as a topical antihistamine in allergic rhinitis and conjunctivitis. Drugs 41:202, 1991.

224. Janssens M, Blockhuys S: Tolerability of levocabastine eye drops. Doc Ophthalmol 84(2):111, 1993.
225. Bonini St, Pierdomenico R, Bonini S: Levocabastine eye drops in vernal keratoconjunctivitis. [Abstract] Allergy 48(Suppl):40, 1993.
226. Howarth PH, Fell P, Selvam A: Levocabastine in allergic conjunctivitis. [Abstract] Clin Exp Allergy 24:184, 1994.
227. Goes F, Blockhuys S, Janssens M: Levocabastine eye drops in the treatment of vernal conjunctivitis. Doc Ophthalmol 87:271, 1994.
228. Caputo AR, Schnitzer RE: Systemic response to mydriatic eye drops in neonates: Mydriatics in neonates. J Pediatr Ophthalmol Strabismus 15:109, 1979.
229. Fraunfelder FT, Scafidi AF: Possible adverse effects from topical ocular 10% phenylephrine. Am J Ophthalmol 85:447, 1978.
230. Meyer SM, Fraunfelder FT: Phenylephrine hydrochloride. Ophthalmology 87:1177, 1980.
231. Mertins PS: Excessive self-medication with naphazoline hydrochloride (privine hydrochloride). JAMA 134:1175, 1947.
232. Mindlin RL: Accidental poisoning from tetrahydrozoline eyedrops. N Engl J Med 275:112, 1966.
233. Rogers GW: Safe use of eye drops. N Engl J Med 275:447, 1966.
234. Lansche RK: Systemic reactions to topical epinephrine and phenylephrine. Am J Ophthalmol 61:95, 1966.
235. Heath P: Neosynephrine hydrochloride: Some uses and effects in ophthalmology. Arch Ophthalmol 16:839, 1936.
236. Rosales T, Isenberg S, Leake R, Everett S: Systemic effects of mydriatics in low-weight infants. J Pediatr Ophthalmol Strabismus 18:42, 1981.
237. Hurwitz P, Thompson JM: Uses of naphazoline (Privine) in ophthalmology. Arch Ophthalmol 43:712, 1950.
238. Gordon DM: Ocular decongestants. Am J Ophthalmol 48:395, 1959.
239. Epstein DL, Boger WP III, Grant WM: Phenylephrine provocative testing in the pigmentary dispersion syndrome. Am J Ophthalmol 85:43, 1978.
240. Rumelt MB: Blindness from misuse of over-the-counter eye medications. Ann Ophthalmol 20:26, 1988.
241. Weiss DI, Shaffer RN: Mydriatic effects of one-eight percent phenylephrine: A potential cause of angle-closure glaucoma. Arch Ophthalmol 68:41, 1962.
242. Hanna C, Brainard J: Allergic dermatoconjunctivitis caused by phenylephrine. Am J Ophthalmol 95:703, 1983.
243. Komi T, Maeda I, Uno Y, Otsuka H: Inhibitory effect of sodium chondroitin sulfate on epithelial keratitis induced by naphazoline. Nippon Geka Gakkai Zasshi 68:154, 1964.
244. Lisch K: Conjunctival alterations by sympathomimetic drugs. Klin Monatsbl Augenheilkd 173:404, 1978.
245. Saraux H, Offret H, de Rancourt de Mimerand E: Pseudopemphigus oculaire induit par les collyres: à propos de 3 observations. Bull Soc Ophthalmol Fr 80:41, 1980.
246. Herman DC, Bartley GB: Corneal opacities secondary to topical naphazoline and antazoline (Albalon-A). Am J Ophthalmol 103:110, 1987.
247. Mathias CGT, Maibach HI, Irvine A, Adler W: Allergic contact dermatitis to echothiophate iodide and phenylephrine. Arch Ophthalmol 97:286, 1979.
248. Aronson SB, Yamamoto EA: Ocular hypersensitivity to epinephrine. Invest Ophthalmol 5:75, 1966.
249. Hill K: What's the angle on mydriasis? Arch Ophthalmol 79:804, 1968.
250. Lee PF: The influence of epinephrine and phenylephrine on intraocular pressure. Arch Ophthalmol 60:863, 1958.
251. Soparkar CN, Wilhelmus KR, Koch DD, et al: Acute and chronic conjunctivitis due to over-the-counter ophthalmic decongestants. Arch Ophthalmol 115:34, 1997.
252. Rhoades RB, Leifer KN, Cohan R, et al: Suppression of histamine-induced pruritus by three antihistamine drugs. J Allergy Clin Immunol 55:180, 1975.
253. Foster CS, Calonge M: Atopic keratoconjunctivitis. Ophthalmology 97:992, 1990.
254. Farber AS: Ocular side effects of antihistamine-decongestant combinations. Am J Ophthalmol 94:565, 1962.
255. Koffler BH, Lemp MA: The effect of an antihistamine (chlorpheniramine maleate) on tear production in humans. Ann Ophthalmol 12:217, 1980.
256. Carruthers SG, Shoeman DW, Hignite CE, Azarnoff DL: Correlation between plasma diphenhydramine levels and sedative and antihistamine effects. Clin Pharmacol Ther 23:375, 1978.
257. Fexofenadine data on file. Kansas City, MD, Hoechst Marion Roussel, 1997.
258. Ostler HB, Martin RG, Dawson CR: The use of disodium cromoglycate in the treatment of atopic ocular disease. *In* Leopold IH, Burns RP (eds): Symposium on Ocular Therapy. New York, Wiley, 1977, p 99.
259. Butrus SI, Weston JH, Abelson MB: Ocular mast cell stabilizing agents. *In* Lamberts DN, Potter DE (eds): Clinical Ophthalmic Pharmacology. Boston, Little, Brown, 1987, p 483.
260. Foster CS: The Cromolyn Sodium Collaborative Study Group: Evaluation of topical cromolyn sodium in the treatment of vernal keratoconjunctivitis. Ophthalmology 95:194, 1988.
261. Allansmith MR, Rose RN: Ocular allergy and mast cell stabilizers. Surv Ophthalmol 30:229, 1986.
262. Easty D, Rice NSC, Jones BR: Disodium cromoglycate (Intal) in the treatment of vernal keratoconjunctivitis. Trans Ophthalmol Soc UK 91:491, 1971.
263. Caldwell DR, Verin P, Hartwich-Young R, et al: Efficacy and safety of lodoxamide 0.1% versus cromolyn sodium 4% in patients with vernal keratoconjunctivitis. Am J Ophthalmol 113:632, 1992.
264. Fahy GT, Easty DL, Collum MT, et al: Randomized double-masked trial of lodoxamide and sodium cromoglycate in allergic eye disease. A multicenter study. Am J Ophthalmol 2:144, 1992.
265. Santos CL, Huong AJ, Abelson MB, et al: Efficacy of lodoxamide 0.1% in resolving corneal epitheliopathy associated with vernal keratoconjunctivitis. Am J Ophthalmol 117:488, 1994.
266. Gery I, Nussenblatt RB: Immunosuppressive drugs. *In* Sears ML (ed): Pharmacology of the Eye. New York, Springer-Verlag, 1984, p 587.
267. Oniki S, Kurakazu K, Kawata K: Immunosuppressive treatment of Behçet's disease with cyclophosphamide. Jpn J Ophthalmol 20:32, 1976.
268. Wong VG: Immunosuppressive therapy of ocular inflammatory diseases. Arch Ophthalmol 81:628, 1969.
269. Foster CS: Immunosuppressive therapy for external ocular inflammatory disease. Ophthalmology 87:140, 1980.
270. Bigos ST, Nisula BC, Daniels GH, et al: Cyclophosphamide in the management of advanced Graves' ophthalmopathy. A preliminary report. Ann Intern Med 90:921, 1979.
271. Nashel DJ: Mechanisms of action and clinical applications of cytotoxic drugs in rheumatic disorders. Med Clin North Am 69:817, 1985.
272. Ward JR: Role of disease modifying antirheumatic drugs versus cytotoxic drugs in the therapy of rheumatoid arthritis. Am J Med 85:39, 1988.
273. Kende G, Sirkin SR, Thomas PRM, et al: Blurring of vision, a previously undescribed complication of cyclophosphamide therapy. Cancer 44:69, 1979.
274. Andrasch RH, Pirofsky B, Burns RP: Immunosuppressive therapy for senile chronic uveitis. Arch Ophthalmol 96:247, 1978.
275. Vizel M, Oster MN: Ocular side effects of cancer chemotherapy. Cancer 49:1999, 1982.
276. Fraunfelder FT, Meyer SM: Ocular toxicity of anti-neoplastic agents. Ophthalmology 90:1, 1983.
277. Green L, Schattner A, Berkenstadt H: Severe reversible interstitial pneumonitis induced by low-dose methotrexate: Report of a case and review of the literature. J Rheumatol 15:110, 1988.
278. Ridley MG, Wolfe CS, Mattheus JA: Life-threatening acute pneumonitis during low-dose methotrexate treatment for rheumatoid arthritis: A case report and review of the literature. Ann Rheum Dis 47:784, 1988.
279. Kevat S, Ahern M, Hall P: Hepatotoxicity of methotrexate in rheumatic diseases. Med Toxicol 3:197, 1988.
280. Williams HJ, Willkens AF, Samuelson CO, et al: Comparison of low-dose oral pulse methotrexate and placebo in the treatment of rheumatoid arthritis. Arthritis Rheum 28:721, 1985.
281. Doroshow JH, Locker GY, Gaasterland DE, et al: Ocular irritation from high-dose methotrexate therapy: Pharmacokinetics of drug in the tear film. Cancer 48:2158, 1981.
282. Daly HM, Boyle J, Roberts CTC, Scott GL: Interaction between methotrexate and nonsteroidal anti-inflammatory agents. Lancet 1:557, 1986.
283. Fluorouracil Filtering Surgery Study Group: Fluorouracil filtering surgery study one-year follow-up. Am J Ophthalmol 108:625, 1989.
284. Gressel MG, Parrish RK, Folberg R: 5-Fluorouracil and glaucoma filtering surgery. I: An animal model. Ophthalmology 91:378, 1984.
285. Heuer DK, Parrish RK, Gressel MG, et al: 5-Fluorouracil and glaucoma filtering surgery. II: A pilot study. Ophthalmology 91:384, 1984.

286. Heuer DK, Parrish RK, Gressel MG, et al: 5-Fluorouracil and glaucoma filtering surgery. III: Intermediate follow-up of a pilot study. Ophthalmology 93:1537, 1986.
287. Skuta GL, Parrish RK: Wound healing in glaucoma filtering surgery. Surv Ophthalmol 32:149, 1987.
288. Knapp A, Heuer DK, Stern GA, Driebe WT: Serious complications of glaucoma filtering surgery with postoperative 5-fluorouracil. Am J Ophthalmol 103:183, 1987.
289. The Fluorouracil Filtering Surgery Group: Five-year follow-up with a fluorouracil filtering surgery study. Am J Ophthalmol 121:349, 1996.
290. Wolner B, Liebmann JM, Sassani JW, et al: Lead bleb-related endophthalmitis after trabeculectomy with adjunctive 5-fluorouracil. Ophthalmology 98:1053, 1991.
291. Nussenblatt RB, Palestine AG: Cyclosporine: Immunology, pharmacology and therapeutic uses. Surv Ophthalmol 31:159, 1986.
292. Nussenblatt RB, Palestine AG, Chan CC: Cyclosporin A therapy in the treatment of intraocular inflammatory disease resistant to systemic corticosteroids and cytotoxic agents. Am J Ophthalmol 96:275, 1983.
293. Kahan BD: Cyclosporine nephrotoxicity: Pathogenesis, prophylaxis, therapy and prognosis. Am J Kidney Dis 8:323, 1986.
293a. Hunnisett ABW, et al: Nephrotoxicity of trimethoprim-co-trimoxazole in renal allograft recipients treated with cyclosporine. Transplantation 36:204, 1983.
294. Tomlanovich S, Golbetz H, Pelrath M, et al: Limitations of creatinine in quantifying the severity of cyclosporine-induced chronic nephropathy. Am J Kidney Dis 8:332, 1986.
295. Loughran TP, Deeg HJ, Dahlberg S, et al: Incidence of hypertension after marrow transplantation among 112 patients randomized to either cyclosporine or methotrexate as graft vs. host disease prophylaxis. Br J Haematol 59:547, 1985.
296. Atkinson K, Biggs J, Darveniza P, et al: Cyclosporine-associated CNS toxicity after allogeneic bone marrow transplantation. N Engl J Med 310:527, 1984.
297. Morales JM, Andres A, Priete C, et al: Reversible acute renal toxicity synergistic effect between gentamicin and cyclosporine. Clin Nephrol 29:272, 1988.
297a. Morganstern GR, Powles R, Robinson B, et al: Cyclosporin interaction with ketoconazole and melphalan. Lancet 2:1342, 1982.
298. Handschumacher RE: Drugs used for immunosuppression. *In* Gilman AG, Rall TW, Nies AS, Taylor P (eds): Goodman and Gilman's The Pharmacological Basis of Therapeutics, 8th ed. New York, Macmillan, 1990, p 1264.
299. Kessler M, Louis J, Renoult E, et al: Interaction between cyclosporin and erythromycin in a kidney transplant patient. Eur J Clin Pharmacol 30:633, 1986.
300. Gupta SK, Barkan A, Johnson RWG, Rowland M: Erythromycin enhances the absorption of cyclosporin A. Br J Clin Pharmacol 25:401, 1988.
301. Robson RA, Fraenkel M, Barratt LJ, Birkett DJ: Cyclosporin-verapamil interaction. Br J Clin Pharmacol 25:402, 1988.
302. Freeman DJ, Laupacis A, Keown PA, et al: Evaluation of cyclosporin-phenytoin interaction with observation of cyclosporin metabolite. Br J Clin Pharmacol 18:887, 1984.
303. Dorian P, Strauss M, Cardella C, et al: Digoxin-cyclosporine interactions: Severe digoxin toxicity after cyclosporine treatment. Clin Invest Med 11:108, 1988.
304. Foets B, Missotten L, Vandervelren P, Goossens W: Prolonged survival of allogeneic corneal grafts in rabbits treated with topically applied cyclosporin A: Systemic absorption and local immunosuppressive effect. Br J Ophthalmol 69:600, 1985.
305. Hunter PA, Wilhelmus KR, Rice NSC, Jones BR: Cyclosporin A applied topically to the rabbit eye inhibits corneal graft rejection. Clin Exp Immunol 45:173, 1981.
306. Hunter PA, Garner A, Wilhelmus KR, et al: Corneal graft rejection: A new rabbit model and cyclosporin A. Br J Ophthalmol 66:292, 1982.
307. Hoffman F, Wiederholt M: Lokale Behandlung des hornhaut Transplantates beim Menscher mit Cyclosporin A. Klin Monatsbl Augenheilkd 187:92, 1985.
308. Ben Ezra D, Pe'er J, Brodsky M, Cohen E: Cyclosporine eye drops for the treatment of severe vernal keratoconjunctivitis. Am J Ophthalmol 95:502, 1983.
309. Asregadoo ER: Surgery, thio-tepa and corticosteroid in the treatment of pterygium. Am J Ophthalmol 74:960, 1972.
310. Meacham CT: Triethylene thiophosphoramide in the prevention of pterygium recurrence. Am J Ophthalmol 54:751, 1962.
311. Howitt D, Karp EJ: Side-effect of topical thiotepa. Am J Ophthalmol 68:473, 1969.
312. Berkow JW, Geils JB, Wise JB: Depigmentation of eyelids after topically administered thiotepa. Arch Ophthalmol 82:415, 1969.
313. Hornblass A, Adler RI, Vukcevich WM, Gombos GM: A delayed side effect of topical thiotepa. Ann Ophthalmol 6:1155, 1974.
314. Greenspan EM, Jaffrey I, Bruckner H: Thiotepa, cutaneous reactions and efficacy. JAMA 237:2288, 1977.
315. Singh G, Wilson MR, Foster CS: Mitomycin eye drops as treatment for pterygium. Ophthalmology 95:813, 1988.
316. Kitazawa Y, Kawase K, Matsushita H, Minobe M: Trabeculectomy with mitomycin. Arch Ophthalmol 109:1693, 1991.
317. Palmer SS: Mitomycin as an adjunct chemotherapy with trabeculectomy. Ophthalmology 98:317, 1991.
318. Skuta GL, Beeson CC, Higginbotham EJ, et al: Intraoperative mitomycin versus postoperative 5-fluorouracil in high-risk glaucoma filtering surgery. Ophthalmology 99:438, 1992.
319. Rubinfeld RS, Pfister RR, Stein RM, et al: Serious complications of topical mitomycin-C after pterygium surgery. Ophthalmology 99:1647, 1992.
320. Higginbotham EJ, Stevens RK, Musch D, et al: Bleb-related endophthalmitis after trabeculectomy with MMC. Ophthalmology 105:650–656, 1996.

CHAPTER 40

Toxicity of Ocular Antiinfectives

Mark S. Hughes and Ann Sullivan Baker†

Ocular toxicology is a rapidly growing field that encompasses local and systemic side effects of ocular medications as well as adverse ocular reactions from systemic medications. This chapter reviews the ocular toxicity of common topical, subconjunctival, and intraocular antibiotic, antifungal, and antiviral agents. The medications discussed are available in the United States; those available elsewhere are not covered.

Antibiotics

Appropriate use of antibiotics can significantly reduce the morbidity associated with a wide range of ocular infections and salvage useful vision in many cases of serious bacterial infection.[1] Successful antibiotic treatment is based on identification of the organism, sensitivity of the organism to the antibiotic, bioavailability of the antibiotic at the site of infection, and low antibiotic toxicity.[2]

Investigation of the effects of topical antibiotics on the healing of corneal epithelial wounds reveals that commercially available topical preparations do not significantly delay healing of experimental wounds.[3, 4] Toxicity of a topically applied antibiotic may be related to the antibiotic itself[5, 6] or to the preservatives and vehicle used in the formulation.[7, 8] Thimerosal, a mercurial preservative, has been reported to cause toxic effects (superficial punctate keratopathy) and hypersensitivity reactions, including keratoconjunctivitis and giant papillary conjunctivitis.[1, 9] Another commonly used preservative, benzalkonium chloride, is a quaternary ammonium compound that inhibits epithelial adhesion, causes loss of superficial epithelial cells, and retards healing of epithelial defects.[10] Of note, this epithelial toxicity may enhance the penetration of topical formulations. Benzalkonium chloride and chlorhexidine are toxic to the corneal endothelium and are contraindicated for intraocular use.[10]

The intraocular use of antibiotics has been evaluated extensively.[11–13] This method of delivery affords high ocular concentrations of antibiotics but is complicated by the risk of intraocular penetration and the potential for intraocular toxicity. Intracameral injections of antibiotics can destroy the endothelium, with resultant corneal opacification, or produce iritis with rubeosis and cataract formation.[14] Intravitreal injections must be distinguished from continuous infusion of antibiotic-containing solution. The tolerated dose of an antibiotic is much less when given in a continuous flow of long duration than in a single injection placed in the midvitreous.[15]

Safe use of intravitreal antibiotics requires an understanding of the intravitreous pharmacokinetics and the retinal toxicity of the formulations. Maurice and Mushme have shown that injected water-soluble drugs diffuse freely throughout the vitreous.[16] Elimination of these agents occurs anteriorly through the trabecular meshwork and Schlemm's canal or posteriorly via diffusion and active transport across the retina. The limiting factor in intravitreal antibiotic injections is retinal toxicity.

The narrow therapeutic index for drugs in the vitreous cavity mandates accurate dose administration to achieve therapeutic levels and avoid toxicity.[16] Jeglum and associates[18] compared the accuracy of preparation of a 400-μg dose by pharmacists and physicians. They found that pharmacists were more accurate (433 μg ± 5%) than physicians (484 μg ± 61%). They recommend that pharmacists prepare intravitreal injections. The method advocated was to draw up 1 mL of stock solution in a 1-mL syringe and inject it into a 30-mL empty sterile container, then draw up 9 mL of diluent in a 10-mL syringe and inject it into the same vial, mixing thoroughly, and withdraw 0.1 mL with a fresh 1-mL syringe. Conway and Campochiaro[19] advocated using a 27-gauge hubless insulin syringe to draw up 0.9 mL of diluent, then 0.1 mL of active agent, then an air bubble, and expel all except 0.1 mL.

The antibiotic section briefly covers the ocular toxicity of aminoglycoside, cephalosporins, penicillins, bacitracin, chloramphenicol, clindamycin, erythromycin, fluoroquinolones, polymyxin, sulfonamides, and vancomycin. Emphasis is placed on the ocular toxicity of aminoglycosides, cephalosporins, and vancomycin, because they are more commonly employed. For many antibiotics, the mechanism of toxicity is ill understood. Table 40–1 contains the topical and subconjunctival doses of commonly administered antibiotics; Table 40–2 lists the intravitreal doses.

AMINOGLYCOSIDES

The aminoglycosides are bactericidal antibiotics that irreversibly inhibit protein synthesis and ribosome function. Amikacin, gentamicin, neomycin, and tobramycin are in common use today. The narrow therapeutic index of the aminoglycosides has stimulated extensive investigation into the mechanism of aminoglycoside toxicity. The mechanism of toxicity is discussed with each individual aminoglycoside.

Amikacin. Amikacin is a semisynthetic aminoglycoside antibiotic that is a derivative of kanamycin sulfate. Because of its unique structure, it has a wider antibiotic spectrum than kanamycin, and only aminoglycoside acetyl transferase 6′ has been found capable of inactivating the drug. Hansen and Meyer[20] reported a case of gentamicin-resistant *Pseu-*

†Deceased.

TABLE 40–1. **Topical and Subconjunctival Antibiotic Doses**

Drug	Topical	Fortified Topical	Subconjunctival
Aminoglycoside			
Amikacin		50 mg/mL	250 mg
Gentamicin	3 mg/mL	14–20 mg/mL	20–40 mg
Neomycin	5–8 mg/mL	33 mg/mL	250–500 mg
Tobramycin	3 mg/mL	14–20 mg/mL	20–40 mg
Cephalosporins			
Cefamandole		50 mg/mL	100 mg
Cefazolin	50 mg/mL	100 mg/mL	100 mg
Cefuroxime	50 mg/mL	100 mg/mL	100 mg
Ceftazidime	50 mg/mL	100 mg/mL	100 mg
Cephalothin		65 mg/mL	100 mg
Penicillins			
Ampicillin		50 mg/mL	25–125 mg
Carbenicillin	4 mg/mL	50 mg/mL	100 mg
Methicillin		50 mg/mL	100 mg
Oxacillin		66 mg/mL	100 mg
Penicillin G		50,000–100,000 U/mL	1,000,000 U
Ticarcillin		6 mg/mL	
Other			
Bacitracin	500 U/g	10,000 U/mL	10,000 U
Chloramphenicol	5 mg/mL		100 mg
Clindamycin		20 mg/mL	150 mg
Erythromycin	5 mg/g (ung)		100 mg
Polymyxin B	10,000 U/mL		100,000 U
Sulfacetamide	100 mg/mL	300 mg/mL	
Vancomycin	14 mg/mL	25 mg/mL	25 mg/mL

domonas aeruginosa keratitis that was successfully treated hourly with amikacin drops (100 μg/mL) and intravenous amikacin. Nelsen and associates[21] evaluated intravitreal amikacin for treatment of *Pseudomonas* endophthalmitis in a rabbit model. Of note, they used a 0.5% topical solution and a 25-mg subconjunctival injection, which produced no evidence of ocular toxicity. The intravitreal doses evaluated ranged from 100 to 6000 μg. Doses higher than 1000 μg produced retinal degeneration, with diffuse disorganization of all layers and loss of retinal pigment integrity. Eyes treated with doses higher than 3000 μg developed cataracts.

Bennett and Peyman[22] initially evaluated amikacin in owl monkeys and found no evidence of retinal toxicity at doses less than 2 mg when evaluated by light microscopy and electrophysiology; they did note transient posterior subcapsular lens opacification. Conway[23] confirmed the nontoxicity of intravitreal amikacin in cynomolgus monkeys. Light microscopy revealed no evidence of toxicity with doses of 900 to 5000 μg. Conway concluded that amikacin is significantly less toxic to the primate retina than gentamicin, even taking into account its three- to fivefold lesser potency.

Talamo and colleagues[24] reported four cases of bilateral endophthalmitis treated with intravitreal amikacin and cephalosporin. Intravitreal doses ranged from 100 to 400 μg, and there was no evidence of ocular toxicity at these doses. Oum and coworkers[25, 26] evaluated the retinal toxicity of combined and repetitive vancomycin and aminoglycoside intravitreal injections. They documented retinal toxicity with repeated injections of 1 mg of vancomycin and 400 μg of amikacin, despite an interval of 48 hours between injections. Histologic findings included macrophages in the subretinal space, numerous lamellar lysosomal inclusions in the retinal pigment epithelium (RPE), focal areas of RPE hypertrophy or hyperplasia, and disorganization of photoreceptor outer segments. Stainer and coworkers[27] evaluated the toxicity of vitrectomy infusions containing amikacin and found 10 μg/mL to be nontoxic in a rabbit model. Concentrations of 20 and 50 μg/mL resulted in an extinguished electroretinogram (ERG). Amikacin is currently used in the treatment of endophthalmitis with intravitreal injection of 400 μg/0.1 mL. This concentration is generally tolerated well, although cases of macular infarction have been reported at these doses.[28]

TABLE 40–2. **Intravitreal Antibiotic Doses**

Drug	Intravitreal Dose
Aminoglycoside	
Amikacin	400 μg
Gentamicin	100 μg
Tobramycin	200 μg
Cephalosporins	
Cefamandole	1 mg
Cefazolin	2 mg
Cefuroxime	1 mg
Ceftazidime	2.25 mg
Penicillins	
Ampicillin	500 μg
Carbenicillin	2.0 mg
Methicillin	1–2 mg
Oxacillin	500 μg
Penicillin G	1000–4000 IU
Other	
Chloramphenicol	1–2 mg
Clindamycin	1 mg
Erythromycin	500 μg
Vancomycin	1 mg

Gentamicin. Gentamicin is a broad-spectrum aminoglycoside antibiotic. Topical formulations of gentamicin have been used extensively to treat conjunctivitis and keratitis.[29] The adverse side effects of topical gentamicin include bulbar injection, white discharge, punctate corneal staining, toxic conjunctivitis, and chemosis and erythema of the eyelids.[30] Subconjunctival injections[31–33] and transcorneal iontophoresis[34] have been documented as effective forms of delivery. Barza and coworkers[35] demonstrated the efficacy and safety of repetitive transscleral iontophoresis of gentamicin in monkeys. Fishman and associates[36] evaluated the intraocular penetration of gentamicin (50 mg/mL) into aphakic rabbit eyes following anodal iontophoresis. They documented therapeutic vitreous levels and no evidence of significant ocular toxicity. Different delivery systems have been evaluated for the ocular application of gentamicin; Barza and colleagues[37] studied the effects of liposome encapsulation as a method of slowing the release of subconjunctival gentamicin. Although the dose employed (5 mg) was small, there was no evidence of significant ocular toxicity. An injection of subconjunctival gentamicin can cause mydriasis and conjunctival paresthesia.[38] Apparently, gentamicin can compete with calcium for the receptor sites on the nerve terminals, thus blocking the release of acetylcholine.[39] Chapman and colleagues demonstrated subconjunctival gentamicin can cause an acute toxic reaction myopathy of the extraocular muscles.[40] In addition, Medin found that 3 mg/mL of gentamicin in an organ culture medium caused endothelial dysfunction with a resultant increased stromal weight of the corneal buttons.[41] Kanter and Brucker reported a case of macular infarction after cataract surgery with the placement of a postoperative gentamicin-soaked collagen shield.[42]

The intraocular use of gentamicin has been evaluated extensively.[11, 12, 43–45] Bennett and Peyman[22] evaluated the toxicity of intravitreal gentamicin in owl monkeys and found extensive retinal degeneration and extinguished ERG with doses of 2 mg, whereas animals given doses of 1 mg developed lens vacuoles but retained normal electrophysiologic function and histologic appearance. Peyman and associates[46, 47] evaluated the toxicity of injected intraocular gentamicin in rabbits. Intracameral doses of 250 to 8000 μg were evaluated; none was associated with histologic evidence of toxicity. Intravitreal injections of 250 to 10,000 μg were evaluated. Doses higher than 1000 μg caused significant retinal degeneration, and doses higher than 3000 μg caused cataracts. Band keratopathy was noted with intravitreal doses of 8000 to 10,000 μg. Electrophysiologic findings after intravitreal doses of 500 μg were normal. In contrast, Peyman and associates[48] found 4000 μg of intravitreal gentamicin to be toxic by histologic and electrophysiologic evaluation in rabbits undergoing lensectomy. Zachary and Forster[49] determined the nontoxic dose of intravitreal gentamicin in a rabbit model evaluated by clinical examination, electrophysiology, and light microscopy. They found an extinguished ERG with inner retinal edema and pigment epitheliopathy with intravitreal doses of 4 μg. If gentamicin is injected close to the retina, edema and RPE changes occur. Certainly, the surgical state of the eye,[50, 51] the animal model evaluated (smaller vitreous volume means higher concentration), and whether the retina is foveate (rabbit versus primate) alter interpretation of toxicity data.

Aminoglycosides are believed to exit the eye via the anterior route. Without an active transport system, these drugs are limited in the route of exit.[52] Cobo and Forster[53] documented enhanced turnover of gentamicin with intravitreal injection after lens or vitreous removal or in the presence of intraocular infection. Although Kane and colleagues[54] came to the same conclusions, they raised the issue of gentamicin binding to pigment as a possible explanation for some differences in toxicity.

A number of investigators have examined the toxicity of intraocular gentamicin at the electron microscopic level. Ling and coworkers[55] documented normal electron microscopic and electrophysiologic studies in cynomolgus monkeys (vitreous volume of 2 to 3 mL) treated with 400 μg of intravitreal gentamicin. In contrast, D'Amico and associates[56] documented retinal ultrastructural changes with intraocular gentamicin doses ranging from 100 to 4000 μg. Injections of 200 to 250 μg resulted in lamellar material in round storage lysosomes of the basal portion of the RPE cells, although the inner retina was normal. Injections of 400 to 500 μg resulted in lysosomal storage of complex lipid in the RPE cells, loss of polarity of the RPE cells, and photoreceptor outer segment disintegration. Intravitreal doses of 800 to 1000 μg produced more extensive changes: focal RPE necrosis, mitochondrial swelling, focal inner plexiform and inner nuclear necrosis, and photoreceptor degeneration. Injections of 1600 to 2000 μg resulted in frank retinal necrosis with loss of RPE, whereas injections of 2000 to 4000 μg led to retinal necrosis, atrophy, and gliosis.

A number of reports of macular infarction after intraocular aminoglycoside injection have appeared. McDonald and associates[57] presented five cases of severe retinal ischemia associated with gentamicin injection (doses ranged from 400 to 40,000 μg). Prominent findings included early superficial and intraretinal hemorrhage, opaque and edematous retina, cotton-wool spots, arteriolar narrowing, and venous beading. Fluorescein angiography revealed severe retinal vascular nonperfusion. Conway and Campochiaro[19] reported two cases of macular infarction after vitrectomy and intravitreal gentamicin (400 μg), cefazolin (1 mg), and dexamethasone (320 μg) for endophthalmitis. A primate model of the retinal toxic reaction to intravitreal gentamicin has been evaluated.[59] Marked capillary occlusion in the posterior pole with retinal edema and intravitreal hemorrhages was noted. Electron microscopy revealed primary inner retinal neuronal swelling with no evidence of vasculitis.

Intravitreal liposomes have been evaluated for a number of drugs. The rate of elimination of the drug is determined in part by the composition of the liposome and in part by the rate of clearance of the liposome itself.[1] Fishman and associates[60] have evaluated the efficacy of intravitreal liposome-encapsulated gentamicin in a rabbit model. There was no toxicity evaluation. The toxicity may be less with liposomes as the peak concentrations are lower, although exposure to the drug lasts longer.

Gentamicin is currently used as a topical agent for bacterial conjunctivitis or keratoconjunctivitis as well as an intravitreal agent for endophthalmitis.[61] Current recommendations for intravitreal injections are 100 μg/0.1 mL; even at this level cases of macular infarction have been reported.

Neomycin. Neomycin is a broad-spectrum aminoglycoside antibiotic. It is used almost exclusively as a topical agent. Local toxicity includes superficial punctate keratopathy, conjunctival injection, and periorbital skin rash or edema.[62]

Tobramycin. Tobramycin is a broad-spectrum aminoglycoside antibiotic. Although the drug was available in 1979, it was not until 1981 that a topical ophthalmic formulation became commercially available. Like gentamicin, topical tobramycin can cause bulbar injection, white discharge, superficial punctate keratopathy, toxic conjunctivitis, chemosis, and erythema of the conjunctiva.[30, 63] Purnell and McPherson[64, 65] evaluated 1 and 5% topical tobramycin solutions and 5% tobramycin subconjunctival injections and found little evidence of ocular toxicity. Topical solutions of tobramycin ranging from 0.3 to 400 mg/mL have been evaluated for efficacy in the treatment of *Pseudomonas* keratitis; however, no toxicologic studies were performed.[66] Iontophoresis of tobramycin also has been evaluated for the treatment of *Pseudomonas* keratitis[67] in a rabbit model. Iontophoresis was more effective than fortified (13.6 mg/mL) tobramycin, but no toxicologic studies were performed even though tobramycin concentrations as great as 40 mg/mL were used.

Intravitreal tobramycin has been evaluated by a number of investigators. Bennett and Peyman[22] evaluated the toxicity of intravitreal tobramycin in owl monkeys and found that doses of 2 mg resulted in an extinguished ERG and retinal degeneration, whereas doses of 1 mg produced posterior subcapsular cataracts but retained normal electrophysiologic function and histopathologic appearance. Bennett and Peyman[68] found that a dose of 750 μg was nontoxic by histopathologic and electrophysiologic evaluation in a rabbit model of *P. aeruginosa* endophthalmitis. They evaluated doses from 100 to 8000 μg; doses greater than 4000 μg resulted in extinguished ERGs. They recommend intravitreal injections of 500 μg. These findings were confirmed by Atkins and McPherson.[69, 70] Kawasaki and associates found that doses of 80 μg caused no change in the a-wave, b-wave, c-wave and oscillatory potentials. Whereas 200 to 500 μg slightly suppressed the b-wave and oscillatory potentials, but recovery occurred within 48 hours in the rabbit model.[71] Balian[72] reported a case of accidental intraocular tobramycin injection. Inadvertent intraocular injection of 20 mg of tobramycin resulted in optic atrophy and retinal degeneration. Vitrectomy infusions containing 10 μg/mL tobramycin were nontoxic in a rabbit model when evaluated by light microscopy and electrophysiologic testing,[27] whereas concentrations of 50 μg/mL resulted in an extinguished ERG. Judson[73] reported a case of tobramycin macular toxicity after subconjunctival injection after cataract surgery. The opaque retina and intraretinal hemorrhage in the posterior pole with vascular obliteration on fluorescein angiography are consistent with aminoglycoside macular toxicity. Judson speculates that the toxicity may result from seepage through the corneoscleral wound as opposed to occult perforation with intraocular injection. Interestingly, Yoshizumi[74] evaluated an aphakic rabbit model with extensive topical treatment and subconjunctival injections and was unable to achieve toxic intravitreal levels of gentamicin.

Mechanism of Toxicity

Extensive studies of the mechanism of aminoglycoside toxicity have been performed owing to the oto- and nephrotoxicity associated with systemic use of aminoglycoside. Previous investigators have demonstrated selective accumulation of aminoglycoside within the lysosomes of cultured fibroblasts.[75, 76] This may result from the protonation of aminoglycoside molecules, thus trapping the drug in the low-pH lysosomal environment. The accumulation of aminoglycoside produces disturbances in phospholipid catabolism, possibly through lowered activity of sphingomyelinase and phospholipases as demonstrated by Aubert-Tulkens and associates in cultured rat fibroblasts.[75]

Libert and colleagues[77] evaluated the cellular toxicity of subconjunctival gentamicin. Electron microscopy revealed an accumulated substance within the lysosomes that consisted of granular material with a pleomorphic lamellar structure, corresponding to the presence of complex lipids. Laurent and coworkers[78] demonstrated that systemic gentamicin induces a loss of activity of lysosomal sphingomyelinase and phospholipase A in rats. Furthermore, they found that amikacin binds more loosely to phospholipid bilayers, induces less inhibition of phospholipases in vitro, and is taken up less by tubular cells in vivo. Given amikacin's lesser nephro- and retinotoxicity, lysosomal alterations may be an early step in aminoglycoside-induced toxicity.

Intravitreal injection of aminoglycoside antibiotics is an established mode of therapy for bacterial endophthalmitis. D'Amico and coworkers[79] have evaluated the comparative toxicity of intravitreal aminoglycoside antibiotics in a rabbit model. The observations ranked gentamicin as the most toxic, then tobramycin, and amikacin as the least toxic: full-thickness retinal necrosis was induced with 800, 1600, and 3000 μg, respectively. Toxic lesions secondary to intravitreal aminoglycoside injection consist of focal areas of lysosomal storage, with outer retinal necrosis, whereas other areas of the retina appear normal with the exception of mild accumulation of complex lysosomal lipids. Owing to the focal areas of toxicity and the potential that pigmented eyes may raise the threshold for toxicity,[54] it is particularly difficult to determine the threshold toxic dose.

After intravitreal aminoglycoside injection, the area of toxicity is localized to the RPE-photoreceptor outer segment complex.[80, 81] The production of lamellar lysosomal inclusions in the RPE indicates the accumulation of complex lipids. The aminoglycoside concentrates within the lysosomes and may interfere with one or more lysosomal enzymes, causing accumulation of unmetabolized substrates.[80] A number of possible mechanisms have been proposed. Gentamicin-treated cells exhibit a greater decrease in the activity of sphingomyelinase than amikacin.[75, 76] Alternatively, the cytoplasmic enzyme phospholipase C correlates well with the nephrotoxicity. Finally, investigators have proposed a direct effect on the mitochondria, with disruption of oxidative phosphorylation with aminoglycoside toxicity. Fleisher and associates[83] reported that intraocular injections of tunicamycin produce photoreceptor-specific degeneration. The glycosylation of opsin can be blocked by tunicamycin in vitro in conditions where polypeptide synthesis is only slightly decreased. Thus, aminoglycoside toxicity may be mediated by disturbance in glycoprotein metabolism. Certainly, some combination of these mechanisms could be responsible for the pathogenesis of aminoglycoside toxicity.

Some have proposed that the toxicity of intravitreal antibiotics can also be effected by the surgical status of the eye.[53] Talamo and coworkers[84] showed that posterior capsulectomy and vitrectomy do not change the therapeutic index (toxic dose:therapeutic dose) for intravitreal aminoglycoside despite the dramatic reduction in vitreous half-life. Retinal damage may be related to the peak concentration of the drug to which the retina is exposed after intravitreal injection. No additional protection from aminoglycoside toxicity is noted after vitrectomy.

Macular infarction has been reported after intravitreal aminoglycoside injection.[19, 57] Conway and associates[59] evaluated the effect of intravitreal gentamicin in the primate retina. Intravitreal gentamicin doses of 1000 and 3000 μg were employed. The inner retinal layers exhibited considerable swelling of the nerve fiber and ganglion cell layers; however, the outer segments and RPE appeared normal by light microscopy. Electron microscopy of the 3000-μg intravitreal gentamicin specimens revealed intracellular edema with massive thickening of the ganglion cell axons. A prominent inflammatory response was noted on the internal limiting membrane. Despite these findings there was no evidence of retinal vasculitis. In areas of the retina that had shown nonperfusion of the capillary bed, granulocyte plugs were seen filling the vessels. The authors hypothesize that the inflammation of the inner layers of the retina associated with the toxic effects of gentamicin may induce granulocytic plugging with permanent closure of the capillary bed.[59, 85] Granulocytes obstruct the lumen by adhering to the endothelium; this occlusion, combined with oxygen-free radical formation and lysosomal enzyme activity, may cause ischemic injury.[86] The findings of Conway and coworkers provide strong evidence that gentamicin toxicity occurs in normal retinal tissue.[59] This effect is in keeping with the known neurotoxicity of gentamicin.[87] Tabatabay and associates[88] examined the immunohistochemical localization of gentamicin in the rabbit after a single intravitreal injection. Initially, gentamicin was localized to the ganglion cell layer, inner plexiform and nuclear layers, and the photoreceptors. By 24 hours, gentamicin was predominantly in the RPE and choriocapillaris. Haines and associates evaluated the morphologic changes after intravitreal injection of gentamicin in pig eyes. Three mg of gentamicin was injected intravitreally to observe the toxicity-related changes that occurred in the retina. Vacuolization of the nerve fiber layer and perivascular swelling was seen within 6 hours and subsequently descended deeper into the retina. Vascular endothelial cells, photoreceptors, and the RPE appeared to be spared from the toxic effect of gentamicin. By 48 and 72 hours after injection, numerous large and small retinal vessels showed congestion and leukocyte margination. These changes could not be prevented by changing the pH to the gentamicin to 7.2. Thus, the authors conclude that the gentamicin toxicity effect is not a pH-related phenomenon but that the primary targets for gentamicin are the neurons and the glia of the inner retina, and as a result, retinal infarction occurs secondarily owing to leukocyte plugging.[89] In addition, Haines and colleagues speculate that the predisposition for macular infarction is due to the dependent position of the macula during surgery as well as the higher density of ganglion cells in the perimacular area.[89]

A survey of retinal specialists from the Retina, Macula, and Vitreous Societies revealed 101 cases of macular infarction due to aminoglycoside administration.[28] Interestingly, 93 cases were associated with gentamicin, five with amikacin, and three with tobramycin. Of the 93 gentamicin cases, 21 used intravitreal doses of 100 to 200 μg, a dose considered to be nontoxic. Twenty-three cases of gentamicin toxicity resulted from prophylactic subconjunctival injections after cataract extraction. Although dilution errors cannot be ruled out, this reference clearly points out that the safe therapeutic window for ocular use of aminoglycoside is sufficiently narrow to be a significant clinical problem. The authors advocate reserving aminoglycoside for known or highly suspicious gram-negative infections.[28] They recommend: (1) abandoning routine use of subconjunctival aminoglycoside after ocular surgery (using cefazolin instead), and (2) avoiding intravitreal aminoglycoside in the prophylaxis of penetrating ocular trauma.[90] The authors[28] recommend vancomycin (or clindamycin) and ceftazidime or imipenem[91] for penetrating ocular trauma.

More recently, Campochiaro and Lim reported on the results of a survey of 13 patients who received 200 to 400 μg of amikacin sulfate or 100 to 200 μg of gentamicin sulfate for prophylaxis or treatment of endophthalmitis. Low-dose gentamicin or amikacin can cause macular infarction, even with doses prepared by hospital pharmacists using typewritten protocol. Of note, several cases exhibited very discrete macular involvement, causing the authors to speculate on the role of a localized increase in concentration in dependent areas of the retina.[28a] Table 40–2 lists the more commonly employed intravitreal doses of antibiotics. Generally, retinal specialists recommend vancomycin, 1 mg, and ceftazidime, 2.25 mg, for intravitreal injections. Although antibiotic choice may vary based on the patient's clinical circumstances.

CEPHALOSPORINS

Cephalosporins are β-lactam antibiotics that interfere with bacterial cell wall synthesis. The first-generation cephalosporins include cefazolin, cephalothin, cephapirin, cephradine, cephaloxin, and cefadroxil. The second-generation cephalosporins include cefamandole, cefuroxime, cefonicid, cefoxitin, ceforanide, and cefaclor. The third-generation cephalosporins include cefepime, cefoperazone, cefotaxime, ceftizoxime, moxalactam, ceftazidime, and ceftriaxone. Although many cephalosporins have been evaluated for use in ocular infections, cefazolin, ceftazidime, and cefuroxime are the most often used cephalosporins. The intravitreal use of cefazolin has been supplanted mainly by vancomycin.

Cefamandole. Cefamandole is a second-generation cephalosporin. Barza and associates[92] evaluated the intraocular levels after subconjunctival cefamandole in a rabbit model after *Staphylococcus aureus* endophthalmitis. Subconjunctival doses of 100 mg/0.5 mL saline (1156 mOsm) resulted in conjunctival chemosis, pronounced lid edema, conjunctival necrosis, and peripheral stromal edema with areas of corneal opacification. The same dose reconstituted in 0.5 mL distilled water (871 mOsm) was significantly less irritating and produced chemosis and mild conjunctival necrosis.

Cefazolin. Cefazolin, a first-generation cephalosporin, is tolerated well when given topically and subconjunctivally. Barza and associates[92, 93] evaluated the intraocular levels of cefazolin after subconjunctival injection in an experimental model of *S. aureus* endophthalmitis. Subconjunctival doses of 100 mg/0.5 mL saline (855 mOsm) were well tolerated, as were doses of 100 mg reconstituted in distilled water (599 mOsm).

Fischer and colleagues[94, 95] evaluated the toxicity, efficacy, and clearance of intravitreal cefazolin in a rabbit model of *S. aureus* endophthalmitis. The doses evaluated ranged from 0.25 to 45 mg. Of note, no generalized changes in the fundus were seen at any doses tested. There was a decrease in scotopic electrophysiologic testing with doses higher than 5 mg. Histologic examination by light microscopy revealed no evidence of pathologic change in any of the retinal layers. The authors concluded that doses up to 2.25 mg were safe for intravitreal injection. Ficker and coworkers[96] evaluated cefazolin levels after intravitreal injection of 2.25 mg in phakic, aphakic, and aphakic-vitrectomized rabbit eyes. The effect of ocular inflammation (induced by injection of heat-killed *Staphylococcus epidermidis*) was to prolong the half-life of cefazolin, presumably because the inflammation reduced elimination via the posterior route (interfering with active pump mechanism). Despite the change in half-life induced by surgical manipulation and the effect of inflammation, there was no evidence of clinical toxicity, although electrophysiologic and histopathologic studies were not performed. The use of intravitreal cefazolin has been largely supplanted by vancomycin.

Cefepime. Cefepime is a new third-generation cephalosporin. Jay and Schockley[97] evaluated the dose- and time-dependent retinal toxic effects following intravitreal injection of cefepime in a rabbit model. Doses ranged from 0.5 to 20 mg/0.1 mL; electrophysiologic testing at 1 and 2 weeks revealed evidence of toxicity with doses of 20 mg.

Cefoperazone. Cefoperazone is a broad-spectrum third-generation cephalosporin. Okumoto and associates[98] performed studies in vitro and in vivo on cefoperazone. Subconjunctival doses of 50 mg in an experimental *Pseudomonas* keratitis rabbit model revealed no evidence of ocular toxicity. O'Hara and colleagues[99] evaluated the retinal toxicity of intravitreal cefoperazone in a rabbit model. Doses ranged from 2 to 32 mg/0.1 mL and evaluation included serial indirect ophthalmoscopy, electrophysiology testing, and histopathologic examination. Concentrations up to 8 mg/0.1 mL were found to be nontoxic. Injections of 16 mg and 32 mg/0.1 mL extinguished electroretinograms at 1 week, although some of the 16 mg/0.1 mL group had recovered electrophysiologic function by 2 weeks. Histopathologic examination revealed diffuse vacuolization of the RPE and photoreceptor disruption and epiretinal inflammation with injections of 32 mg/0.1 mL. The degree of toxicity was roughly proportional to the concentration of cefoperazone. The authors suggested that hyperosmolarity could be a mechanism of retinal toxicity. Marmor[100] demonstrated that the weakest solutions that produced ophthalmoscopically visible changes in the retina were near 500 mOsm. However, the 32 mg/0.1 mL of cefoperazone produced a 371.2-mOsm solution, making osmotic pressure an unlikely mechanism of toxicity. Okayama and coworkers[101] demonstrated the nontoxic concentration of cefoperazone for vitrectomy infusion to be 0.2 mg/mL. At this concentration there was no effect on the a-wave, b-wave, or oscillatory potential in perfused rabbit eye preparation. After infusion of 0.33 mg/mL, rabbits demonstrated decreased amplitude and prolonged latency with mild change in a- and b-waves and significant changes in oscillatory potentials.

Ceftazidime. Ceftazidime is a third-generation cephalosporin that is resistant to β-lactamase and exhibits a broad range of activity against gram-negative and gram-positive organisms. Shockley and associates[102] evaluated the intraocular kinetics of subconjunctival ceftazidime in phakic and aphakic pigmented rabbit eyes. Subconjunctival injections of 100 mg in aphakic and phakic rabbits exhibited grade 1 irritation on the Draize scale at the site of injection. Findings of ophthalmoscopic examinations and scotopic ERG were normal. Jay and colleagues[103] evaluated dose- and time-dependent toxicity of intravitreal ceftazidime. Intravitreal doses ranging from 0.5 to 50 mg/0.1 mL were evaluated. Electrophysiologic testing at days 1 and 7 revealed a flat b-wave with doses of 20 to 50 mg. Concentrations of 2, 5, and 10 mg decreased the b-wave amplitude to zero at 24 hours after injection, but it returned to normal by 1 week after injection. The authors theorize that this transient ERG alteration may be due to osmolar load added to the vitreous cavity by the injected drug. Campochiaro and Green evaluated the toxicity of intravitreous ceftazidime in the squirrel monkey. Injection of 1 mg, 2.5 mg, and 10 mg of intravitreal ceftazidime was performed. At 10 mg of ceftazidime, there was a marked cystic change in the macula. There was disruption of the photoreceptors (primarily outer segments) in the fovea with cystic changes in all three monkeys as well as macular holes in two of the three. Electromicroscopic studies revealed mild swelling of the mitochondria and perinuclear halos around the photoreceptor nuclei in both control eyes and in eyes injected with 1 mg and 2.25 mg. An eye injected with 10 mg showed severe damage to the central photoreceptor inner segments consisting of disruption of the plasma membranes and accumulation of intracytoplasmic granular material. The inner segments also showed a mild change; there was loss of apical microvilli in the RPE. The authors conclude that high doses of intravitreal ceftazidime exhibited toxicity primarily in the photoreceptor cells; however, doses of 2.25 mg are safe in this intravitreal model.[104] In addition, Meredith studies of intravitreal ceftazidime reinforce the importance of the status of the vitreous gel (as well as the issue of inflammation) in the pharmacokinetics of intravitreal ceftazidime.[105]

Ceftriaxone. Ceftriaxone is a third-generation cephalosporin with a broad spectrum of activity against gram-negative and gram-positive pathogens. Jay and associates[106] evaluated the ocular pharmacokinetics of ceftriaxone following subconjunctival injections in rabbits. Subconjunctival doses of 100 mg produced grade-1 irritation on the Draize scale but normal ophthalmoscopic appearance and normal scotopic ERGs.

Shockley and colleagues[107] evaluated doses of intravitreal ceftriaxone from 0.5 to 50 mg in a rabbit model. Evaluations consisted of ophthalmoscopy, electrophysiology, and histopathologic examination. Injections of 0.5 to 5 mg revealed no evidence of toxicity by electrophysiology or histopathology. Concentrations of 7.5 to 20 mg produced a transient decrease in b-wave amplitude ratio at 24 hours, which recovered by 7 days. Concentrations of 50 mg produced a flat b-wave at 24 hours, which was still two standard deviations below normal 2 weeks after the injection. Of note, the injection of 50 mg caused histopathologic changes at 24 hours, including retinal edema and disruption of retinal layers with a fibrinous exudate in the anterior chamber. By 2 weeks, however, there was no evidence of histologic alterations in the eye injected with 50 mg. These studies were performed with light microscopy and not with electron microscopy. The authors postulate that the transient ERG alterations may be attributed to the osmolar load that the injected drug adds to the vitreous cavity.[100] The osmolarities of the ceftriaxone ranged from 4 to 886 mOsm. Jay and coworkers[108] investigated the pharmacokinetics of intravitreal ceftriaxone in monkeys. Single intravitreal doses of 2, 2.5, and 3 mg/0.1 mL were injected; specimens were evaluated by ophthalmoscopy, electrophysiologic study, and histopathologic examination. There was no evidence of toxicity with the doses evaluated.

Cephaloridine. Cephaloridine is a broad-spectrum cephalosporin that has been largely replaced by safer and less nephrotoxic cephalosporins.[109] Graham and associates[110] evaluated the ocular toxic effects of intravitreal cephaloridine (0.1 mg to 60 mg/0.1 mL) in rabbits. They found that 0.25 mg of intravitreal cephaloridine was nontoxic by electrophysiologic and histopathologic evaluation. Doses higher than 0.5 mg produced clumping of the outer segments of the photoreceptors and destruction of the RPE. Doses greater than 5 mg resulted in punctate hemorrhages in the vascularized retina and destruction of the photoreceptor outer segment. Doses higher than 10 mg exhibited serous exudate in the anterior chamber and vitreous cavity with inflammation around the retinal vessels and disruption of photoreceptor outer segments with RPE destruction.

Cephalothin. Cephalothin is a first-generation cephalosporin. Boyle and associates[111] evaluated intraocular penetration of cephalothin after subconjunctival injection in 22 patients. Doses of 50 mg were tolerated, although significant pain and chemosis were associated. Rutgard and colleagues[112] evaluated intravitreal cephalothin in an experimental rabbit staphylococcal endophthalmitis model. They evaluated doses of 0.125 to 8 mg; injections of 2 mg were to found to be nontoxic by light microscopy. Doses of 4 to 8 mg produced focal areas of disorganization of the retinal nuclear layers.

Moxalactam. Moxalactam, a third-generation cephalosporin, is out of favor because of bleeding associated with systemic use. Leeds and associates[113] evaluated it in the treatment of experimental staphylococcal endophthalmitis. Subconjunctival injections of 75 mg produced no sign of ocular toxicity. Topical solution of 10% given every 5 minutes for 2 hours created no gross ocular toxicity. Intravitreal injections of 0.05 to 16 mg were evaluated. At doses higher than 4 mg there was evidence of retinal disorganization. A concentration of 2 mg was nontoxic by histopathologic examination and electrophysiologic testing. Fett and colleagues[114] evaluated the retinal toxicity of moxalactam in a rabbit model by ophthalmoscopy, electrophysiologic testing, and light and electron microscopy. They evaluated concentrations from 0.125 to 10 mg. The ERGs were normal up to and including intravitreal doses of 1.25 mg; marked decreases in photopic amplitudes were observed at doses of 5 and 10 mg. Light and electron microscopy revealed no abnormalities up to 1.25 mg; at 2.5 mg focal swelling of the photoreceptors was present on electron microscopy. Intravitreal doses of 10 mg resulted in destruction of the entire retinal architecture by 1 week.

PENICILLINS

Penicillins are bactericidal agents that act by interfering with bacterial cell wall peptidoglycan synthesis. Penicillins possess a β-lactam ring attached to a thiazolidine ring and an acyl side chain. Potassium penicillin G, procaine penicillin G, benzathine penicillin G, and phenoxymethyl penicillin have essentially the same antibacterial effect and differ only in solubility and stability. The semisynthetic β-lactamase-resistant penicillins, which include methicillin, oxacillin, cloxacillin, dicloxacillin, and nafcillin, retain activity against penicillinase-producing staphylococci.[115] The semisynthetic extended-spectrum penicillins, which include ampicillin, amoxicillin, azlocillin, carbenicillin, mezlocillin, piperacillin, and ticarcillin, are active against certain gram-negative bacilli.

Carbenicillin. Carbenicillin is a semisynthetic extended-spectrum penicillin. Boyle and associates[116] evaluated the intraocular penetration of disodium carbenicillin after subconjunctival injection in humans. Doses ranged from 50 to 500 mg; adverse side effects were limited to marked burning pain and chemosis.

Schenk and colleagues evaluated the retinal toxicity of intravitreal carbenicillin in a rabbit model of *Pseudomonas* endophthalmitis.[117] The doses employed ranged from 0.5 to 20 mg. Intravitreal doses higher than 10 mg resulted in transient diffuse speckling of the posterior lens, which cleared in 4 to 5 weeks. A number of retinal detachments were noted with intravitreal doses of 15 and 20 mg. Histopathologic examination revealed disorganization of the nuclear layers and retinal attenuation with outer layer disorganization in other areas in doses of 15 to 20 mg. Intravitreal doses of 8 to 10 mg resulted in circumscribed areas of thinning in the nuclear layers and disappearance of the outer segments. There was no evidence of histopathologic abnormalities by light microscopy with doses less than 7 mg. Unfortunately, electron microscopy was not performed, and only one eye, injected with 5 mg, was examined electrophysiologically, which was normal.

Barza and coworkers examined the effects of inflammation due to *S. aureus* endophthalmitis and of probenecid on the kinetics of intravitreally injected carbenicillin in rabbits. At the dose employed (1 mg/0.1 mL) there was no ocular toxicity noted; however, the study documented the increased half-life with probenecid administration and inflammation. Organic ions such as penicillin and cephalosporins are thought to be eliminated via the retinal route by an active transport pump. The pump is believed to reside in the pigment epithelium or vascular endothelium of the retina. Owing to the large surface area of the retina, the β-lactam antibiotics have a short vitreous half-life and low aqueous:vitreous ratio.[43] Of note, probenecid also inhibits the elimination of prostaglandins from the eye. Thus, use of probenecid may increase the level of prostaglandins that are released in the course of ocular inflammation and may increase retinal damage.

Methicillin. Methicillin is a semisynthetic β-lactamase-resistant penicillin. Brick and coworkers[115] demonstrated mild chemosis and injection with subconjunctival injections of 100 mg of methicillin. Daily and associates[119] evaluated the toxicity, clearance, and therapeutic efficacy of intravitreal methicillin in a rabbit model of *S. aureus* endophthalmitis. Intravitreal injections ranged from 0.1 mg to 10 mg. Electrophysiologic and histopathologic (light microscopy) study revealed no evidence of toxicity at the doses employed. Grant[120] evaluated the effect of probenecid on intravitreal methicillin. The half-life of intravitreal methicillin increased from 3.5 to 4.25 hours with probenecid. Cazeau and colleagues[121] evaluated the toxicity of vitrectomy infusions containing methicillin doses of 10, 20, and 50 μg/mL. There was no clinical evidence of toxicity at these doses except, however, histopathologic examination revealed focal photoreceptor damage and focal pigment epithelial disturbance with infusion concentrations of 50 μg/mL. Removal of the vitreous gel may expose the retina to high concentrations of the drug, thus facilitating its toxic effect. This may explain why doses of antibiotics that are nontoxic by intravitreal injection differ from nontoxic doses of vitrectomy infusion solutions.[15]

Oxacillin. Oxacillin is a semisynthetic β-lactamase-resistant penicillin. Barza and associates evaluated subconjunctival oxacillin in the treatment of *S. aureus* endophthalmitis in a rabbit model.[93, 122] They found no evidence of ocular toxicity with subconjunctival injections of 100 mg. Cazeau and colleagues[121] evaluated the toxicity of vitrectomy infusions containing oxacillin doses of 10, 20, and 50 μg/mL. Observation of animals treated with infusions of 50 μg/mL revealed severe conjunctival injection, corneal edema, and vitreous haze. Electrophysiologic testing of eyes treated with 50 μg/mL revealed a flat ERG. Even doses of 20 μg/mL produced focal areas of photoreceptor damage and pigment epithelium disturbances. Only infusions of 10 μg/mL were found to be nontoxic by electrophysiologic and light microscopic evaluation.

Penicillin. von Sallmann and associates[123] studied the toxicity of intravitreal penicillin in an experimental rabbit model of *S. aureus* endophthalmitis. Several eyes that were injected intravitreally with 0.5 mg of highly purified penicillin revealed focal areas of retinal atrophy with outer segment disintegration and outer nuclear layer changes. The authors postulated that the retinal toxicity was caused by the proximity of the intravitreal injections to the retina.

Leopold[14] evaluated the efficacy of subconjunctival, intracameral, and intravitreal injection of penicillin in the *S. aureus* endophthalmitis model. Intracameral doses of 500 units of penicillin were tolerated without ocular toxicity. Intravitreal injections ranging from 5 to 2500 units were evaluated. Unfortunately, no histopathologic data are available from this study. Early penicillin was quite impure and intraocular injection often produced inflammatory reactions. Mann[124] demonstrated that intracameral doses of penicillin as large as 1500 units were generally tolerated, whereas 100 units of pure intravitreal penicillin produced no pathologic reaction. Sorsby and Ungar[125] evaluated crystalline penicillin intravitreal injections for the treatment of *S. aureus* endophthalmitis in a rabbit model. Intravitreal purified crystalline penicillin in concentrations higher than 5000 units is toxic to the retina. Retinal findings include retinal edema, localized RPE atrophy, pigment migration, vacuolization of the nerve fiber layer, and preretinal exudate.

Purified crystalline penicillin is virtually nontoxic to the external eye. In order to avoid toxicity with concentrated solutions of penicillin, it has been suggested that concentrated solutions be made up with distilled water as opposed to saline, otherwise the solution is hypertonic.

Schaeffer and Krohn[126] studied the effect of topically applied liposomes containing penicillin G. They found that transcorneal flux of penicillin was enhanced by charged liposomes without evidence of ocular toxicity. Electrostatic adsorption allows the liposomes to transfer their membrane-associated drug to the corneal epithelial cell membrane, thus facilitating drug transport across the cornea.

Piperacillin. Piperacillin is a semisynthetic extended-spectrum penicillin. Semple and associates[127] evaluated the toxicity of intravitreal piperacillin in a rabbit model. Doses ranged from 50 to 3000 μg. Only doses of 3000 μg revealed outer retinal degeneration and diminished electrophysiologic function.

Ticarcillin. Ticarcillin is a water-soluble, semisynthetic, extended-spectrum carboxy penicillin. Ticarcillin is available as a topical preparation (4 to 6 mg/mL) for the treatment of *P. aeruginosa* keratitis. This preparation is tolerated well.[128] It should, however, be administered in conjunction with a second antibiotic, generally an aminoglycoside, to provide a synergistic effect.[129] Heigle and Peyman[130] evaluated the intravitreal toxicity of ticarcillin in a rabbit model. Doses ranged from 50 to 3000 μg; there was no evidence of toxicity by electrophysiologic or histopathologic evaluation. Light microscopy revealed no focal areas of retinal damage, no retinal detachment, and no thinning of the retina due to photoreceptor outer segment loss.

OTHER ANTIBIOTICS

Bacitracin and Gramicidin. Bacitracin and gramicidin are bactericidal peptide antibiotics. Bacitracin affects cell wall peptidoglycan synthesis and wall permeability. Topical and subconjunctival administration of bacitracin results in therapeutic aqueous levels only in the presence of an epithelial defect or ocular inflammation.[1] Bacitracin solutions of 1000 μg/mL are not irritating clinically. Stronger formulations may be irritating and locally toxic.[131]

Chloramphenicol. Chloramphenicol is a bacteriostatic antibiotic that reversibly inhibits bacterial protein synthesis. Roberts[132] evaluated the topical use of chloramphenicol for external ocular infection. He found that the formulations of 1% ointment and 0.2 and 0.5% solutions were not toxic to the eye. Beasley and coworkers[133] found no evidence of ocular toxicity with 0.5% ophthalmic solutions with excellent intracameral penetration. Interestingly, Mitsiu and associates[134] found deposits of mucosubstances on the cornea after administration of topical 1% chloramphenicol. They postulated that the roughened proliferative corneal surface and the mucosubstances may accelerate *Pseudomonas* keratitis after application of chloramphenicol. A case of optic atrophy was reported after chloramphenicol irrigation of the lacrimal duct (with inadvertent orbital injection). Stainer[27] found that vitrectomy infusions containing 5 μg/mL of chloramphenicol in a rabbit model produced no evidence of toxicity by electrophysiologic or histopathologic study.

Clindamycin and Lincomycin. Clindamycin, a bacteriostatic chlorinated derivative of lincomycin, acts by reversibly inhibiting bacterial protein synthesis. Kleinberg and coworkers[135] evaluated the intraocular penetration of topically applied lincomycin hydrochloride in rabbits. A 1% topical solution was clinically nontoxic and, with removal of the corneal epithelium, produced 10-fold higher intracameral drug levels. Boyle and associates[136] evaluated subconjunctival lincomycin and found that 300 mg/0.25 mL produced significant chemosis and subconjunctival hemorrhage that was not the result of mechanical trauma. Devlin and colleagues[137] evaluated intraocular penetration of topical clindamycin in rabbits. Clindamycin hydrochloride, 0.2%, was nontoxic and resulted in two to six times higher levels than clindamycin phosphate, 0.2%. Tabbara and Salamoun[138] reported a case of accidental posterior chamber injection of 300 mg lincomycin. Clinically there was no evidence of toxicity, although immediately after injection of lincomycin, the posterior chamber was irrigated with 2.5 mL balanced salt solution. Paque and Peyman[139] evaluated the toxicity of intravitreal clindamycin phosphate in a rabbit model of *S. aureus* endophthalmitis. They found that doses higher than 5 mg produced severe retinal toxicity with focal areas of retinal destruction, disorganization, and disruption of the nuclear layers, thinning of all layers, and attenuation and disruption of the photoreceptor outer segments. Doses of 1.5 mg or less were apparently nontoxic by light microscopy. Stainer[27] evaluated the toxicity of clindamycin in vitreous infusions and found that concentrations of 10 μg/mL were nontoxic by electrophysiologic and histopathologic evaluation. Concentrations of 50 μg/mL resulted in extinguished ERG.

Erythromycin. Erythromycin is a bacteriostatic inhibitor of bacterial protein synthesis and can be bactericidal in high concentrations. Topical erythromycin in available as a 0.5% ophthalmic ointment and is not irritating. Naib and associates[140] evaluated the ocular effects of erythromycin. Topical solutions ranging from 1 to 20 mg/mL given four times a day for 3 days produced no toxicity, although subconjunctival doses of 20 mg caused conjunctival injection with corneal haze and lid edema. Doses of 2 mg or less are tolerated well. Intracameral erythromycin can be destructive; a 5-mg injection resulted in conjunctival injection, hazy cornea with denuded epithelium, iris injection with a pronounced anterior chamber exudate, and posterior synechiae. Intracameral doses of 0.5 and 1 mg produced a mild inflammatory response with conjunctival injection and small flakes in the aqueous. Meisels and Peyman[141] evaluated intravitreal erythromycin in the treatment of experimentally induced staphylococcal endophthalmitis. They found that doses of erythromycin gluceptate higher than 1 mg caused segmented and diffuse lenticular opacities and retinal disorganization and atrophy, whereas doses of 0.5 mg were tolerated without evidence of toxicity by light microscopy.

Fluoroquinolones. The fluoroquinolones are structurally related to nalidixic acid. These agents block enzymatic activity of bacterial DNA gyrase and alter the structure and functioning ability of bacterial DNA. Currently, ciprofloxacin, norfloxacin, and ofloxacin are available in the United States, although a number of fluoroquinolones are under study, including pefloxacin.[142] Topical 0.3% ciprofloxacin is tolerated well. Only mild untoward ocular events are noted, the most frequent one being a white crystalline precipitate, commonly located in the superficial portion of the corneal defect. This precipitate has been identified as ciprofloxacin. Hodden and colleagues demonstrated the efficacy of transcorneal iontophoresis of 1% ciprofloxacin for therapy of aminoglycoside-resistant *Pseudomonas* keratitis.[143] They found no evidence of toxicity with the 1% formulation.

Stamer and coworkers[144] evaluated the effect of ciprofloxacin on rabbit corneal endothelial viability. A concentration of 10 μg/mL of ciprofloxacin had no effect on endothelial cell counts or viability, whereas 100 μg/mL caused a 2% reduction in viable endothelial cells. Haller-Yeo and associates[145] evaluated intravitreal ciprofloxacin; they reported no toxicity in cat eyes with doses of 1, 10, 100, and 1000 μg when evaluated by light microscopy and electrophysiology. Steven and coworkers[146] evaluated the intraocular use of ciprofloxacin in phakic and aphakic rabbits. Corneal decompensation occurred in aphakic vitrectomized rabbits with intravitreal doses of 100 μg of ciprofloxacin, whereas retinal toxicity was noted on electron microscopy with doses higher than 250 μg. At 1000 μg, electron microscopy revealed loss of the outer rod segments, followed by atrophic changes of the inner rod segments as well as the outer and inner nuclear cell layers. Marchese and colleagues evaluated the toxicity and pharmacokinetics of ciprofloxacin. They studied the pigmented rabbit model and injected doses of 100 μg, 200 μg, 500 μg, and 1000 μg. An evaluation was performed by indirect ophthalmoscopy, electrophysiology study, and histology. Focal areas of retinitis were observed after injections of both 500 μg and 1000 μg but not with 250 μg of ciprofloxacin. In addition, electrophysiology revealed that the amplitude ratios were significantly reduced after the 1000-μg dose. At the 100- or 250-μg ciprofloxacin dose, histologic sections were comparable between control eyes, and ERG ratios were unchanged from the baseline level.[147]

Kawasaki and associates found that 200 μg of ofloxacin did not cause deterioration of the b-wave, c-wave, or the oscillatory potential over a 2-month period in the rabbit model.[71] Mochizuki and colleagues studied the effects of ofloxacin on the rabbit ERG in vivo.[149] They also determined that 200 μg of ofloxacin did not cause an alteration in the ERG in the rabbit model.[149]

Polymyxins. Polymyxin B and polymyxin E (colistin) are bactericidal peptide antibiotics that increase cell membrane permeability. Concentrations of polymyxin B of 2.5% (2.5 mg/mL) are not irritating; however, Williams and coworkers[150] documented that subconjunctival injections of 10 mg of polymyxin B produced severe chemosis, localized necrosis, and bloody discharge in rabbits, whereas 0.5 mg was tolerated well. Pryor and associates[151] found that 0.12% colistin solution was nontoxic. Subconjunctival injections of 10 mg of colistin produced no evidence of toxicity. Although polymyxin E is one fourth as potent as polymyxin B, polymyxin E is much less irritating.

Sulfonamides. The sulfonamides interfere with bacterial utilization of *p*-aminobenzoic acid (PABA). These drugs are bacteriostatic, and the various preparations have different chemical, pharmacologic, and antibacterial properties. Flach and associates[152] demonstrated that topical 25% sulfisoxazole diolamine ointment and exposure to ultraviolet light resulted in a phototoxic reaction. Boettner and coworkers[153] found that topical use of sulfadiazine ointment for 1 year caused formation of multiple small white concretions in cysts of the palpebral conjunctiva, identified by spectroscopy as sulfadiazine. Hook and colleagues[154] reported a case of transient myopia induced by sulfonamides. A-scan measurements and cycloplegic refraction demonstrated the primary mechanism of sulfonamide-induced myopia to be lens thickening from ciliary body edema.

Vancomycin. Vancomycin is a bactericidal antibiotic that inhibits bacterial cell wall synthesis through interference with glycopeptide polymerization. Pryor and associates[151] evaluated topical and subconjunctival administration of vancomycin in rabbits. They found no evidence of toxicity with subconjunctival doses of 12.5 or 25 mg, whereas a 5% aqueous solution given every 5 minutes for 30 minutes revealed minimal superficial punctate keratopathy. Fortified vancomycin in doses of 14 to 25 mg/mL has been reported to cause irritation, conjunctival injection, and superficial punctate keratopathy. Although subconjunctival vancomycin injections have been reported to cause conjunctival necrosis and sloughing,[155] Lindquist and coworkers demonstrated the safety and efficacy of vancomycin in corneal storage media.[156] They found no evidence of endothelial damage at doses of 150 μg/mL vancomycin in gentamicin-free Dex-Sol. Kattan and Pflugfelder[157] evaluated the corneal toxicity of vancomycin in corneal storage media and found no evidence of endothelial damage with concentrations of 5 mg/mL. Garcia-Ferrer and associates[155] evaluated the antimicrobial efficacy and lack of corneal endothelial toxicity of Dex-Sol corneal storage medium supplemented with vancomycin, 10 μg/mL. Choi and Lee[158] documented an 8.8% decrease in endothelial cell counts with transcorneal iontophoresis of vancomycin in rabbit eyes, compared with 5.4% decrease with balanced saline solution.

Intravitreal vancomycin has been evaluated extensively. Homer and associates evaluated the toxicity, clearance, and therapeutic effectiveness of intravitreal vancomycin in a rabbit model of staphylococcal endophthalmitis.[159] Concentrations of vancomycin ranged from 0.25 to 500 mg/0.1 mL. At doses higher than 5 mg/0.1 mL the vitreous exhibited a whitish reaction, although ERG abnormalities were associated with doses higher than 2 mg. Histologic study of doses of 2 to 5 mg revealed toxicity localized to the retina with photoreceptor outer segment degeneration. In contrast, Smith and coworkers[160] evaluated the toxicity, clearance, and efficacy of intravitreal vancomycin in an experimental rabbit model of methicillin-resistant *S. epidermidis* endophthalmitis. Doses of 1, 2, and 5 mg were evaluated by light microscopy. There were no discernible retinal abnormalities except one eye injected with 5 mg confirmed the absence of extensive toxicity. Smith and coworkers believe that the histologic change noted by Homer and coworkers[159] might be the result of tissue processing. Borhani and associates evaluated vancomycin in the vitrectomy infusion solution. They found that concentrations of 8 μg/mL, 16 μg/mL, and 32 μg/mL of vancomycin in infusion solution caused no abnormal ERG or histologic changes. However, electrophysiologic depression and abnormal histologic changes occurred with concentrations of 100 μg/mL of vancomycin in the infusion solution.[148]

Pflugfelder and colleagues[161] evaluated the retinal toxicity, clearance, and interaction of intravitreal vancomycin with gentamicin in phakic and aphakic vitrectomized rabbits. Clinically, with doses higher than 2 mg there was immediate clouding of the vitreous and within 24 hours opacification of the retina. By 2 weeks the retinal opacification had cleared, but the RPE showed pigment clumping and atrophy. Electrophysiologic testing revealed no evidence of toxicity up to 2 mg; however, there was marked reduction in the a- and b-wave amplitudes in the eye that received a 5-mg dose. Ultrastructural studies of doses greater than 2 mg revealed a number of pathologic changes, including: (1) hypertrophy of the RPE with abnormal clustering of pigment granules in the cytoplasm; (2) loss of photoreceptor outer segment-RPE interdigitation due to retraction of apical microvilli of RPE; (3) appearance of lucent vacuoles in the RPE basal cytoplasm beneath the plasmalemma infoldings; (4) gross disorganization of the photoreceptor outer segments with distention and displacement of the inner segments past the external limiting membrane; and (5) accumulation of cellular debris in the subretinal space. Pflugfelder and colleagues[161] found that lensectomy and vitrectomy increased the intraocular clearance of vancomycin but did not alter the threshold for retinal toxicity. Oum and associates[25, 26] studied the effect of combined and repeated injections of intravitreal vancomycin and aminoglycoside. They found increasing retinal toxic reaction with repeated injections. The exact biochemical mechanism of toxicity is unknown.[162]

Imipenem. Imipenem (*N*-formimidoyl thienamycin), a stable derivative of thienamycin, combined with cilastatin, an inhibitor of the renal dehydropeptidase that inactivates the drug, form an antibiotic preparation with an unusually broad spectrum of activity for a β-lactam antibiotic. Loewenstein and colleagues evaluated the intravitreal use of imipenem in the albino rabbit model. Imipenem did not affect the ERG and the VEP responses or the morphology of the retina up to a total injected dose of 0.9 mg (2 mg of Tienam). This is over 500-fold higher than the effective dose needed against a bacterial infection.[163]

Aztreonam. Aztreonam is a monocyclic antibiotic with excellent activity against members of the family Enterobacteriaceae, inhibiting 50% of islets of most species at concentrations lower than 2 μg/mL. Loewenstein and coworkers also evaluated the use of aztreonam in the albino rabbit model. They found that aztreonam was not toxic to the albino rabbit retina up to a total injected dose of 2.8 mg (5 mg of aztreonam). Severe functional and morphologic retinal damage was seen when 10 mg of aztreonam was injected. Of note, a similar degree of damage was seen when a dose of 5 mg of L-arginine, an active ingredient of aztreonam was injected into the vitreous.[163]

Antifungal Agents

Ocular fungal infections continue to challenge ophthalmologists.[164] The selection of appropriate antifungal chemotherapy is limited by the paucity of effective drugs.[165, 166] The only approved ophthalmic antifungal is 5% natamycin; however, amphotericin B, flucytosine, miconazole, and ketoconazole have a role in the management of ocular fungal infections.[167, 168] Table 40–3 outlines the nontoxic topical, subconjunctival, and intravitreal doses of commonly used antifungals.

TABLE 40–3. **Antifungal Doses**

Drugs	Topical (%)	Subconjunctival	Intravitreal (μg)
Amphotericin	0.15	500 μg	5–10
Fluconazole	1		100*
Flucytosine	1	2.5 mg	100*
Ketoconazole	1		540*
Miconazole	1	5–10 mg	25*
Natamycin	5		
Itraconozole			10*

*Experimental animal data.

POLYENES

The polyenes consist of a conjugated double-bond system of variable size linked to mycosamine, an amino acid sugar. Polyenes bind preferentially to ergosterol in the fungal plasma membrane, thus altering membrane permeability and disrupting the fungal cell.

Natamycin. Natamycin is a tetraene polyene and is the only antifungal available in the United States in a topical form. Topical natamycin is well tolerated. Superficial punctate keratopathy has been reported with prolonged use.[17, 169] Foster and coworkers[170] demonstrated that natamycin did not retard the healing of corneal epithelial defects. Ellison and Newmark[171] demonstrated conjunctival necrosis after subconjunctival injection of natamycin.

Intraocular use of natamycin is not well tolerated.[172] Anterior chamber injection of 250 μg of natamycin is tolerated in a rabbit model; however, with a dose of 500 μg corneal decompensation and iridocyclitis develop. Ellison and Newmark[173] reported the intravitreal effects of pimaricin: 25 μg was not toxic but was not therapeutic either; doses higher than 50 μg destroy the retina.

Amphotericin B. Amphotericin B is a heptaene polyene available in an intravenous formulation. Amphotericin B is stabilized with a bile salt (sodium deoxycholate) to form a colloidal dispersion.

Local application of amphotericin B has been evaluated extensively because of its systemic toxicity. Montana and Sery[174] found no evidence of toxicity in rabbits with an amphotericin B (5 mg/mL in 5% glucose) solution applied as drops three times a day or as a subconjunctival injection (0.3 mL = 1.5 mg). In contrast, Foster and associates[175] found that subconjunctival injections greater than 500 μg of amphotericin B in sterile distilled water were toxic to rabbits, which developed corneal epithelial defects, conjunctival injection, and iritis. Green and coworkers[176] evaluated subconjunctival amphotericin B in rabbits and found that 150 μg were well tolerated, although there was poor intraocular penetration. Jones and associates[177] found that topical amphotericin B in a sodium deoxycholate vehicle causes pain, brow ache, and superficial punctate keratopathy. This formulation consisted of 3 to 5 mg/mL (at 4 mg/mL pH of 5.5 and 55 mOsm), and they found that the vehicle alone was toxic to corneal epithelium.

Bell and Ritchey[178] found that a subconjunctival dose of 5.5 mg of amphotericin B resulted in severe pain, marked chemosis, and conjunctival necrosis; at doses of 7.5 mg a salmon-colored subconjunctival nodule developed, consisting of a diffuse proliferation of histiocytes against a background of fibrous proliferation with scattered lymphocytes and plasma cells. Wood and Williford[179] found that 0.15% topical amphotericin B was tolerated well and the ocular toxicity of 0.3% amphotericin was due to the toxicity of sodium deoxycholate. Confirming this, Foster and coworkers[170, 180] found that 1% topical amphotericin B with sodium deoxycholate greatly delays the healing of corneal epithelial defects and causes marked conjunctival injection in a rabbit model.

Other formulations of amphotericin B have been evaluated topically. Amphotericin B methyl ester, which is water soluble and has reduced toxicity, has been evaluated in a 1% formulation and has been found to be nontoxic and to penetrate better than amphotericin B.[181] Owing to leukoencephalopathy associated with systemic administration, further work on amphotericin B methyl ester has not been pursued.

The effects of intracameral amphotericin B have been evaluated. Foster and coworkers[175] found that 25 μg of intracameral amphotericin B resulted in transient iris and conjunctival congestion, lens opacities, and, at doses smaller than 35 μg, corneal edema, iris congestion, and lens opacities that lasted 4 days. At doses of 125 μg, intracameral amphotericin B produced irreversible opacification of the cornea.[180, 182]

Intravitreal injection of amphotericin B has been studied in detail. Foster and associates[175] reported a case of *Volutella* fungal infection after cataract extraction that was treated with three intravitreal injections of 35 to 40 μg over 1 month. The eye was sterilized, although blind with a corneal pannus, updrawn pupil, and total, funnel-shaped retinal detachment. Green and coworkers[176] reported successful sterilization of a postcataract fungal infection with 20 μg of intracameral amphotericin B combined with topical and subconjunctival amphotericin B, although the final acuity was extremely poor. Axelrod and associates[183] evaluated the toxicity of intravitreal amphotericin B in a rabbit model. They found that doses of 25 to 500 μg of intravitreal amphotericin B resulted in retinal detachment with a proteinaceous exudate and cloudy vitreous with monocytes in the vitreous cavity. They proposed that the amphotericin B alters cell membranes, with resultant transudation of subretinal fluid. Of note, they found that sodium deoxycholate is not toxic to the retina, and intravitreal doses of 5 to 10 μg of amphotericin B produced no abnormalities by electrophysiologic testing or light microscopy. In addition, 25 μg of amphotericin B injected close to the retina resulted in immediate focal retinal necrosis. Axelrod and Peyman[184] demonstrated that, in the setting of experimental fungal endophthalmitis, 5 μg of intravitreal amphotericin B was nontoxic (as determined by light microscopy) in rabbits. Souri and Green[185] documented that intravitreal doses of amphotericin B as small as 1 μg resulted in focal retinal necrosis in the rabbit when injected adjacent to the retina.

Stern and coworkers[186] reported a case of fungal endophthalmitis treated with 5 μg of intravitreal amphotericin B in which histopathologic examination revealed the infection was eradicated and there was no evidence of amphotericin B–induced toxicity.[186] Perrault and associates[188] reported a similar case treated with 5 μg of intravitreal amphotericin B and 190 mg of intravenous amphotericin B in which visual acuity was 20/25 and normal electrophysiologic function was observed 22 months after surgery. Stern and coworkers[189] reported a series of cases of postoperative *Candida parapsilosis* endophthalmitis in which one patient received a cumulative dose of 20 μg of intravitreal amphotericin B over 48 hours and another patient received 30 μg over 96 hours. There were no abnormalities of electrophysiologic tests in either patient. Finally, Brod and associates[190] reported successful treatment of endogenous *Candida* endophthalmitis after vitrectomy with intravitreal doses of 5 μg in six patients and 10 μg in two patients, all without clinical evidence of toxicity.

The effect of vitrectomy on the toxicity of intravitreal amphotericin has been investigated.[50] Vitrectomy may allow increased retinal toxicity or may accelerate the disappearance of amphotericin B. Huang and associates[191] found that the method of injection and proximity to the retina were most important. There was no evidence of toxicity by electrophysiologic testing or light microscopy at doses up to 5 μg of intravitreal amphotericin B after vitrectomy in rabbits. Doft and coworkers[192] found that vitrectomy and lensectomy accelerate the disappearance kinetics of amphotericin B, whereas the presence of *Candida* endophthalmitis has a negligible effect on them. Baldinger and associates[193] found that intravitreal doses of 5 to 10 μg produced minimal retinal toxicity in both vitrectomized and nonvitrectomized rabbits and identical pathologic findings (small areas of retinal necrosis) and normal electrophysiologic studies. Wingard and coworkers[194] investigated the intraocular distribution of intravitreally injected amphotericin B in rabbits. Using radiolabeled carbon-14 amphotericin B, they found that amphotericin B demonstrates faster physical disappearance from the aphakic-vitrectomized eye (half-life of 1.8 versus 8.2 to 8.9 days); this suggests that repeated intravitreal injections are safer for aphakic-vitrectomized eyes.

Pflugfelder and associates[195] reported 19 cases of exogenous fungal endophthalmitis. Patients who received anterior chamber amphotericin B administration showed no clinical evidence of corneal decompensation, even with repetitive anterior chamber doses of 10 μg. One patient had posttreatment visual acuity of 20/30 with a normal-looking fundus after a total of 25 μg (in divided doses) of intravitreal amphotericin B.

Different formulations and delivery systems for intravitreal amphotericin B have been evaluated. Amphotericin B methyl ester, although it has much less antifungal activity, is a water-soluble compound with a much wider range of therapeutic doses. McGetrick and associates[196] found that amphotericin B methyl ester showed no evidence of retinal toxicity by light microscopy or electrophysiologic studies when intravitreal doses were 50 μg or less. Doses of 100 μg of amphotericin B methyl ester resulted in degeneration of the photoreceptor layer; this was caused by the drug and not by the ascorbic acid used to solubilize the antifungal agent. Raichand and coworkers[197] evaluated the toxicity of amphotericin B methyl ester in vitrectomy infusion fluid and found that the maximal nontoxic dose was 75 μg/mL; at 100 μg/mL. Electrophysiologic studies revealed a decreased response, although no toxic damage was appreciated by light microscopy. Amphotericin B methyl ester was found to cause leukoencephalopathy when used systemically and has not, therefore, been a candidate for intraocular use.

Extensive evaluations of intravitreal amphotericin B liposomes have been performed after it was reported that liposome encapsulated amphotericin B treatment of disseminated candidiasis resulted in greater survival rates with less drug toxicity.[198] Tremblay and coworkers[199] found that liposomal amphotericin B retains its full antifungal activity in vitro. Amphotericin B is found within the walls of the liposomes, and they speculate that liposomal cholesterol competes for amphotericin B with the drug captured by fungal ergosterol. It is not known whether the drug is cleared as a drug-liposome complex or after it is separated from the liposome.[200] Tremblay and associates[201] observed reduced toxicity of intravitreal liposomal amphotericin B in rabbits. The liposomes were composed of phosphatidylcholine, cholesterol, and tocopherol succinate. There was no evidence of retinal toxicity in doses of 20 μg intravitreal liposomal amphotericin B, but doses of 10 and 20 μg of amphotericin B produced evidence of retinal damage.

Barza and coworkers[202] evaluated the toxicity of intravitreally injected liposomal amphotericin in rhesus monkeys. The liposomes were composed of phosphatidylcholine, cholesterol, and tocopherol succinate. A mild vitreal infiltrate was associated with large doses (30 μg of amphotericin B and 120 μg of liposomal amphotericin B). One eye treated with large doses of liposomal amphotericin B had small inferior chorioretinal scars in the periphery. By phase-contrast microscopy, the internal limiting membrane was intact; there was no evidence of gliosis and no retinal disorganization; and the photoreceptor outer segments were normal. It was postulated that the competitive binding between liposomal cholesterol and host cell membranes resulted in the greatly decreased toxicity of liposomal amphotericin B. The authors did point out that in the study each monkey was given several injections, which might have influenced the ocular response. Szoka and associates[203] evaluated the effects of lipid composition and liposome size on toxicity of liposomal amphotericin B. They found that cytotoxicity and lethality of liposomes were a function of their lipid composition and diameter. The reduced toxicity and equivalent efficacy were explained by the reduction in the rate of transfer of the drug from the liposome into the cellular membrane and not by the major redistribution of the drug in the organs. Interestingly, Liu and associates[204] evaluated the efficacy of amphotericin B in large, negatively charged liposomes and found reduced efficacy. The liposomal preparation was different from that used by Szoka and coworkers[203]; however, the authors believed that the reduced efficacy could be caused by the lipophilic nature of amphotericin B, which reduced the interaction of intercalated drug with *Candida* organisms. It was also possible that the negatively charged head groups may have inhibited contact between the fungi and liposomes.

Flucytosine. Flucytosine, a secondary agent in the treatment of fungal infections,[205] is a fluorinated pyrimidine that is transported across the fungal cell membrane by a specific permease elaborated by certain fungi. Flucytosine is then deaminated to fluorouracil, a thymidine analog that further blocks fungal thymidine synthesis.

The topical solution of flucytosine has been used with success in experimental fungal keratitis. Foster and coworkers[170, 180] evaluated the effects of topical 1% flucytosine and found no evidence of delay in corneal epithelial wound healing. O'Day and associates[206] found that 1% flucytosine was tolerated well but ranked behind amphotericin (0.15 or 0.075%) and 5% natamycin in efficacy. Walsh and coworkers[207] found that 2.5 mg of subconjunctival flucytosine was not toxic to rabbits. Yoshizumi and Silverman[208] evaluated the toxicity of intravitreal flucytosine. They found that 1000-μg injections resulted in a decline in flicker fusion and in the density of outer segments and damage to the inner segments of photoreceptors.

IMIDAZOLES

The imidazoles are a group of synthetic antifungals that are fungistatic in low concentration and fungicidal in high concentrations. They possess a broad spectrum of antifungal activity. They inhibit ergosterol synthesis at low concentrations and interfere with the mitochondrial oxidative and peroxidase enzymes.

Ketoconazole. Ketoconazole is a weakly dibasic synthetic imidazole that inhibits ergosterol synthesis. Foster and coworkers[170, 180] evaluated the toxicity of 1% ketoconazole with Cremophore EL as the carrier. They found a slight delay in corneal epithelial wound healing. Grossman and Lee[209, 210] evaluated transscleral and transcorneal iontophoresis of ketoconazole in a rabbit model. Subconjunctival ketoconazole (50-μg) injections were compared with iontophoresis and produced no evidence of toxicity at the doses employed. Intravitreal ketoconazole in dimethyl sulfoxide (DMSO) was evaluated by Yoshizumi and Banihashemi.[211] The ocular toxicity of experimental intravitreal DMSO has been evaluated[212]; a single 0.1-mL injection of 100% DMSO results in transient focal retinal edema and a 50% decrease in the amplitude of the photopic, flicker fusion, scotopic, and combined photopic and scotopic response. Electrophysiologic response returned to normal after 1 month and retinal edema resolved within a week. Intravitreal injections of ketoconazole in DMSO at doses of 2240 μg resulted in retinal edema and necrosis with marked photoreceptor outer segment loss; electron microscopy of the RPE revealed degeneration of mitochondria and a decline in the number of melanin granules.[211] Doses of 720 μg of intravitreal ketoconazole produced toxic vacuolizations of the inner segments of the photoreceptors detected by electron microscopy. The study determined that doses up to 540 μg produced no ocular toxicity, giving a much wider therapeutic window than miconazole.

Miconazole. Miconazole nitrate is an imidazole antifungal agent with broad-spectrum antifungal activity and low toxicity. Foster and Stefanyszyn[213] found that miconazole nitrate in Cremophore EL (polyethoxylated castor oil) is tolerated well as a 10-mg subconjunctival injection. Foster[214] found that topical 1% miconazole is tolerated well, although superficial punctate keratopathy occasionally occurs.[215] The topical solution with Cremophore EL as the carrier does not significantly retard corneal epithelial wound closure.[180]

Intraocular miconazole has been evaluated by a number of investigators. Jaben and Forster[216] found that a 25-μg dose of intravitreal miconazole was nontoxic and efficacious in a rabbit model of *Aspergillus* endophthalmitis. Osato and coworkers[216a] evaluated the toxicity of intravitreal miconazole and found that results of electrophysiologic studies did not correlate with histopathologic findings. At doses higher than 100 μg, lens opacities developed; at doses higher than 250 μg, lesions were seen clinically in the fundus corresponding with the focal site of photoreceptor obliteration with areas of photoreceptor atrophy, whereas the RPE exhibited elongated apical microvilli with intravitreal pigment migration.

Tolentino and associates[217] evaluated the toxicity of intravitreal miconazole in rabbits and owl monkeys. They found that doses of 100 μg or greater were toxic to the retina, and the concentration of solvent (polyethoxylated castor oil-Cremophore EL) equivalent to 100 μg of miconazole was also toxic to the retina in rabbits. With doses higher than 250 μg, histopathologic examination revealed extensive vitreous infiltration with neutrophils. There was severe retinal edema, with loss of cell architecture and pyknotic nuclei. In recent injections the RPE revealed intracellular edema and loss of cells, whereas in older injections the RPE had areas of hypertrophy and atrophy with hypopigmentation. In owl monkeys, they found that doses of 80 μg of intravitreal miconazole resulted in inferior segmental thinning of all retinal layers and formation of cystic spaces; electron microscopy demonstrated intercellular cystic spaces in the inner plexiform layer, with mild axonal degeneration. The authors concluded that an intravitreal injection of 40 μg of miconazole was not toxic.

Kawasaki and associates found that 100 to 500 μg of intravitreal miconazole caused transient changes in the ERG, whereas no change was seen with 50 μg of intravitreal miconazole injection.[71] Pflugfelder and associates[195] reported 19 cases of exogenous fungal endophthalmitis. One case was treated with multiple intravitreal injections of 25 μg of miconazole; final visual acuity was 20/40. Yoshizumi and coworkers evaluated the toxicity of intravitreal miconazole in DMSO in rabbits.[219] Unfortunately, intravitreal miconazole has a narrow therapeutic window. They found that doses of 30 μg or less of intravitreal miconazole in DMSO can be tolerated without ocular toxicity in rabbits. Doses of 40 to 100 μg produced focal retinal edema with a decrease in electrophysiologic tests, and doses of 200 μg resulted in frank retinal necrosis.

Itraconazole. Itraconazole is a triazole derivative with broad-spectrum antifungal activity in vitro and in animal models. This antifungal drug is lipophilic and practically insoluble in water. Schulman and colleagues injected intravitreal itraconazole in doses ranging from 10 to 100 μg devolved in 100% DMSO into the eyes of New Zealand rabbits. Ocular toxicity studies performed 5 weeks after administration showed no substantial retinal or histologic changes in eyes injected with either 100% DMSO or 10 μg of itraconazole. Higher doses cause focal areas of retinal necrosis.[220]

Fluconazole. Fluconazole is a *bis*-triazole, potent antifungal with low toxicity and excellent water solubility; it is currently available in oral and intravenous forms. Brooks and associates[221] found that topical fluconazole, 100 μg/mL, appeared to be equivalent to, and potentially less toxic than, amphotericin B in an experimental *Candida* keratitis model. Schulman and coworkers[222] evaluated the toxicity of intravitreal fluconazole in the rabbit. They found no corneal, lenticular, or retinal changes by light microscopy and no evidence of depressed electrophysiologic testing at doses of 100 μg. Fluconazole has excellent ocular penetration when taken systemically; further work is required to evaluate the efficacy and toxicity of ocular fluconazole treatment.

Antivirals

Great strides have been made in the chemotherapy of ocular viral diseases since the introduction of idoxuridine in 1962. Currently, ophthalmic preparations of idoxuridine (IDU), vidarabine, and trifluridine (TFT) are available. Acyclovir is available for systemic use and as a dermatologic preparation; ganciclovir is available for systemic and intraocular use.[223] Table 40–4 outlines the nontoxic topical and intravitreal doses of commonly used antivirals.

Idoxuridine. IDU is a halogenated pyrimidine in which the 5-methyl group of thymidine is replaced by iodine. IDU is phosphorylated by viral thymidine kinase and results in

TABLE 40–4. **Antiviral Doses**

Drug	Topical (%)	Intravitreal (μg)
Idoxuridine	0.1	—
Trifluridine	1.0	200
Vidarabine (Ara-A)	3.0	80
Acyclovir	—	240*
Ganciclovir	—	200
Foscarnet	—	1200
Cidofovir	—	20

*Experimental animal data.

defective viral DNA. Altered viral messenger RNA is produced after IDU is incorporated into DNA; this results in defective enzymes needed for DNA production.[62] IDU is available in a 0.1% ophthalmic solution and 0.5% ophthalmic ointment for the treatment of herpes simplex keratitis.[223]

The adverse ocular effects of topical IDU are common and result from direct toxicity or allergic reactions. Local irritation, with conjunctival injection, follicular conjunctivitis, allergic blepharoconjunctivitis,[224] and perilimbal filaments have been reported.[131] Lass and associates[118] have reported IDU-induced conjunctival cicatrization. Corneal problems such as superficial punctate keratitis, delayed corneal wound healing, and corneal edema have been reported.[131] Punctal scarring and occlusion have also been reported, particularly after long-term therapy. The mechanism for the observed toxicity is believed to be the activation of IDU in normal cells, particularly rapidly dividing cells, resulting in disruption of normal DNA synthesis.

Payrau and Dohlman[225] found that 0.1% IDU administered every hour did not significantly retard the healing of the corneal epithelium in a rabbit model, although it was noted that intensive topical 0.1% IDU did greatly retard the healing of penetrating corneal wounds as measured by tensile strength. Interestingly, Gasset and Katzin[226] found that 0.1% IDU, given four times daily did not significantly affect corneal wound healing in the rabbit model. Although topical IDU is well tolerated, noninfected corneal epithelial cell culture in 0.1% IDU was noted to cause increased granularity and vacuolization of the cytoplasm with shrinkage of the epithelial sheets and disruption of the intercellular boundaries.[227] It may be that the toxicity of IDU is related to its degradation products. Maloney and Kaufman[228] found that IDU in concentrations of 1 mg/mL exhibited no toxicity in rabbit kidney cell culture, whereas the degradation products of IDU (iodouracil and deoxyuridine) in concentrations of 0.001 mg/mL did exhibit cytopathic changes. These same corneal findings were mirrored in a trial with normal human volunteers.

New delivery vehicles for IDU have been evaluated. Smolin and associates[229] evaluated an IDU-liposome preparation in a rabbit model of herpes simplex keratitis. The liposomal preparation (phosphatidic acid, phosphatidylcholine, α-tocopherol in a 1:5:1 ratio) was nontoxic and resulted in greater corneal penetration and faster epithelial healing.[230] IDU has not been used for intraocular treatment of viral disease, although data have shown that 1 μg of IDU in human corneal cell culture significantly depresses cell mitosis.[231]

Vidarabine. Adenine arabinoside (vidarabine, Ara-A) is a purine analog. Ara-A is phosphorylated by viral thymidine kinase, then triphosphorylated. The active form inhibits DNA polymerase and ribonucleotide reductases, thus blocking viral DNA synthesis. Ara-A is available in a 3% ophthalmic ointment and an intravenous suspension (200 mg/mL).[223]

Similar to IDU, the adverse effects of Ara-A are due to direct toxicity or to allergic reactions. Local ocular reactions include conjunctival injection, follicular conjunctivitis, and punctal scarring. With prolonged treatment, conjunctival cicatrization, corneal scarring, or permanent punctal occlusion can result.[1] Lass has reported that Ara-A has insignificant effects on corneal epithelial wound healing, although there is significant delay in stromal wound healing.[1] Kaufman and associates[232] have found that subconjunctival injections of Ara-A can be toxic; daily subconjunctival injection of 5% Ara-A results in significant conjunctival inflammation; 20% injections result in the formation of conjunctival granuloma.

Different methods of delivery of Ara-A have been evaluated. Hill and associates[233] found that iontophoresis (0.5 mAmp in 4 minutes) of Ara-AMP (vidarabine adenosine-5-phosphate) resulted in higher corneal and intracameral levels without evidence of toxicity. Pulido and associates[234] evaluated the toxicity of intravitreal injections and infusions of vicarabine in rabbits. Intravitreal injections of 80 μg/0.1 mL Ara-A revealed no abnormalities in electrophysiologic testing or light microscopy. However, after vitrectomy/lensectomy, disorganization of the external retina was visible by light microscopy in rabbits that received infusions of 100 μg/mL Ara-A.

Trifluridine. TFT is a halogenated pyrimidine with three fluorines in place of the 5-methyl group of thymidylate. It is a potent inhibitor of thymidine synthesis, which in turn inhibits DNA synthesis. It is preferentially incorporated into viral DNA, thus producing defective DNA. TFT is available as a 1% ophthalmic solution. The adverse ocular effects of topical TFT are due to direct toxicity or to allergic reaction. Local reactions include conjunctival injections, superficial punctate keratopathy, filamentary keratitis, and punctal occlusion with prolonged treatment.[131] Udell[235] has reported conjunctival cicatrization after topical TFT, whereas Maudgal and associates[236] have reported corneal epithelial dysplasia after TFT.

Carmine and associates[237] reported no evidence of toxicity of 1% TFT in normal rabbit eyes. However, with a standard corneal epithelial defect and 8 days of 8-times-daily 1% TFT, they noted pathologic changes in the regenerating epithelium, which resolved when the TFT was discontinued. They also noted that stromal wound healing was affected with decreased tensile strength; this was confirmed by Gassett and Katzin.[226] Wellings and associates[238] have demonstrated that TFT is more effective than IDU, associated with fewer failures and less toxicity, although the toxicity may reflect failure to control the herpetic keratitis rather than a toxic reaction to IDU. Hyndiuk and associates[239] documented a case of reversible crystalline epithelial keratitis with 1% TFT, which presented with superficial punctate keratopathy and gray epithelium with fine linear retractile crystalline intraepithelial deposits. Maudgal and associates[240] did report on conjunctival ischemia, corneal epithelial dysplasia, filamentary keratitis, and punctal stenosis with the use of 2% TFT (with 1% neomycin) in an experimental model of herpes simplex keratouveitis. The complications increased with prolonged use.

Peyman and associates[241] have investigated the toxicity of intravitreal TFT. Pang and associates[242] found that intravitreal injections of 200 μg/0.1 mL and vitrectomy infusion solutions of 60 μg/mL were not toxic to rabbits. With injections of 500 μg a mild decrease in ERG functions was noted; however, no damage was seen by light microscopy. With injection of 1000 μg (and infusions of 100 μg/mL) there was a moderate depression in B-wave amplitudes, and photoreceptor clumping and degeneration were noted by light microscopy. Liu and associates[243] evaluated liposomal delivery of intravitreal TFT. Injections of 42.9 μg revealed no evidence of toxicity by clinical examination, ERG, or light microscopy, and vitreal drug levels remained for 28 days in the range of ID^{50} for many strains of herpesvirus and human cytomegalovirus (CMV).

Acyclovir. Acyclovir, a purine analog similar to Ara-A, is activated by virus-induced thymidine kinase to the monophosphate form and then to the triphosphate form. It inhibits viral DNA polymerase. Acyclovir is available as a 5% dermatologic ointment, a 3% ophthalmic ointment (not available in the United States), and in oral and intravenous formulations. The adverse ocular effects of topical acyclovir (not approved for ophthalmic use) are mild: local irritation with mild superficial punctate keratitis and follicular conjunctivitis.[244] One report of punctal stenosis with the topical preparation was reported,[1] but it is not known whether stenosis was due to acyclovir or to herpes zoster keratouveitis.

Because of the low toxicity of acyclovir, it has been investigated for intraocular injection. Pulido and associates[245] investigated intravitreal injections and infusion solutions of acyclovir in rabbits. They found that injections of 240 μg/0.1 mL revealed no evidence of abnormalities on histopathologic examination or electrophysiologic testing. Infusion solutions containing 400 μg/mL revealed disorganization of the external layers of the retina after lensectomy or vitrectomy.

Peyman and associates[246] reported two cases of vitrectomy, scleral buckle, and intravitreal acyclovir infusion in patients with acute retinal necrosis. Both were treated with systemic steroids and acyclovir during their illness. One patient received an intravitreal infusion of 10 μg/mL, the other 40 μg/mL; pre- and posttreatment electrophysiologic studies revealed no toxicity from the intravitreal medications.

Ganciclovir. Ganciclovir is a synthetic nucleoside analog of 2′-deoxyguanosine, similar to acyclovir. Virus-specified thymidine kinase converts ganciclovir to the monophosphate form, which is then converted to the di- and triphosphate form, which competitively inhibits virus DNA polymerase, thus preventing viral replication. Ganciclovir is available for systemic use.

The rising incidence of AIDS and the widespread use of immunosuppressive drugs have caused an increase in CMV and herpesvirus retinitis. In particular, ganciclovir is effective in CMV retinitis; unfortunately, its systemic toxicity (bone marrow suppression) has limited its use. Much research has focused on intraocular injections and new delivery systems for intraocular ganciclovir.

Pulido and associates[245] first investigated intravitreal ganciclovir in rabbits and with single doses of 400 μg found no evidence of toxicity by light microscopy and electrophysiologic testing. Schulman[247] evaluated the clearance of ganciclovir in a rabbit model, demonstrating that 60 hours after injection the intravitreal ganciclovir level was greater than ID^{50} for several CMV strains. They also demonstrated that subconjunctival injections of 1.25 mg are tolerated without toxicity but produce very low intraocular levels. Henry and associates[248] reported a patient with bilateral CMV retinitis who received 28 injections (200 μg/0.1 mL) in both eyes over a 3-month period without evidence of ocular toxicity.

Ussery and associates[249] reported a series of 14 eyes in 11 patients with CMV retinitis who received 200 μg ganciclovir intravitreally without short-term evidence of intraocular toxicity; many also received intravenous ganciclovir. Cantrill and associates[250] reported a series of 10 patients who were treated with 200 μg of intravitreal ganciclovir; patients received between nine and 30 injections without evidence of ocular toxicity. Heinemann[251] reported results of seven patients treated with repeated intravitreal ganciclovir (200 to 300 μg) injections over a period of 14 to 56 weeks; there was no evidence of ocular toxicity.

Peyman and associates[252] have evaluated the intravitreal injection of liposome-encapsulated ganciclovir in rabbits. This work demonstrated that 84.1 μg of ganciclovir is nontoxic to the eye and sustains the ganciclovir concentration above the ID^{50} (up to 28 days) for a number of strains of the herpes simplex virus (HSV) family. No evidence of gross retinal toxicity was found by clinical or light microscopy; however, electron microscopy and electrophysiologic studies are required to adequately evaluate retinal toxicity. Yoshizumi and coworkers[253] evaluated the ocular toxicity of multiple intravitreal ganciclovir injections in a rabbit model. They found electroretinographic evidence of retinal toxicity with doses as small as 100 μg, and electromicrographic studies show evidence of toxic vacuolization in the photoreceptor inner segments at doses of 25 μg. With repeated doses of 100 to 200 μg, electron microscopy revealed vacuolization of the outer nuclear layer and photoreceptor inner segments.

The intravitreal concentration of ganciclovir is affected by inflammation. Most toxicity studies are done in normal rabbit eyes. Kuppermann and coworkers[254] evaluated an HSV-infected rabbit model treated with 250 μg of intravitreal ganciclovir and demonstrated that infected eyes showed a sevenfold greater concentration of ganciclovir at 72 hours than did the control group.

Cochereau-Massin and colleagues[255] evaluated the efficacy and tolerance of intravitreal ganciclovir in CMV retinitis in AIDS. They found no evidence of toxicity either with electrophysiologic studies or anatomopathologic studies with 400 μg of ganciclovir injected on a weekly basis. In addition, Moschos and associates evaluated the intravitreal ganciclovir in the rabbit model.[256] Different doses of ganciclovir ranging from 200 to 600 μg/0.1 mL were injected intravitreously. Ganciclovir doses of 300 to 600 μg/0.1 mL have a toxic effect on the retina as shown by electrophysiologic changes. The electroretinogram was either distinguished or greatly suppressed 1 month after injection. Of note, a ganciclovir injection of 200 μg/0.1 mL does result in the b-wave showing a 20% reduction of its normal amplitude 4 months after the injection of ganciclovir. Electromicroscopy of the retina revealed in the inner segment of the receptor cells the existence of dilatation and vesiculation of the endoplasmic reticulum in the surrounding nuclear cytoplasm and swelling of the mitochondria with fragmentation of the cristae in several of them, while in the outer segment of the photoreceptors degeneration and destruction of the lamellae accompanied by disintegration of the adjacent protoplasm in parts of certain rods and cones appeared.[256] Saran and McGuire[257] reported the case of an inadvertent high dose of ganciclovir by injection in which a 44-year-old patient with AIDS received 40 mg in 0.1 mL of ganciclovir. The result was an immediate loss of vision accompanied by the appearance of a necrotizing vasculitis. The authors speculate that the possible mechanisms include the alkaline nature of the solution with subsequent saponification of fatty acids in the cell membranes. In addition, osmotic damage induced by the highly concentrated solution may induce hyperosmotic retinal damage.[257]

The ganciclovir implant has been evaluated extensively since 1991. Sanborn and associates[258, 259] reported the results of a phase I clinical study of the effectiveness of a drug delivery system utilizing polyvinyl alcohol, ethylene vinyl alcohol, and ganciclovir. They report sustained delivery for longer than 90 days without clinical evidence of toxicity. The implant has the advantage of high intraocular drug levels and no systemic toxicity and minimizes the disadvantage of repeated intraocular injections (scleral induration, vitreous haze, iritis, vitreous hemorrhage, retinal detachment, and endophthalmitis).

The original ganciclovir implant (mark I) will release ganciclovir at a rate of 2 μg/hr. The device consists of a 6-mg pallet of ganciclovir in 10% polyvinyl alcohol coated with ethylene vinyl acetate then again in 10% polyvinyl alcohol.[260, 261] Martin and associates evaluated 26 patients with the ganciclovir implant for evidence of progression of CMV retinitis.[262] Progression occurred in 226 days with the implant compared with 15 days with no therapy, and there was no clinical evidence of toxicity. Charles and Steiner performed a clinical pathologic study in four eyes of three patients with the implant.[263] None of the four globes revealed toxic or inflammatory adverse effects on the intraocular structures attributable to the implant.[263]

Foscarnet. Phosphonoformate (PFA, foscarnet) is a highly water-soluble pyrophosphate analog that effectively inhibits in vitro replication of HSV-1 and HSV-2, varicella zoster, and CMV through noncompetitive binding to the exchange site of virus DNA polymerase, thus blocking viral DNA synthesis. Foscarnet has been used as an alternative to ganciclovir in the systemic treatment of CMV infections. A number of investigators have evaluated the effects of intravitreal foscarnet. She and coworkers found that single doses of intravitreal foscarnet in doses ranging from 200 to 1000 μg/0.1 mL are nontoxic to the retina in New Zealand albino rabbits.[264] Of note, their evaluation consisted of clinical examinations and light microscopy. Dia-Llopis and colleagues reported no evidence of toxicity with intravitreal injection of 1200 μg in an AIDS patient with CMV retinitis; again toxicity was evaluated by post mortem light microscopy.[265]

In order to evaluate the effect of repeated intravitreal injections of foscarnet, Turrini and coworkers evaluated the retinal toxicity of 2, 4, and 6 intravitreal injections of 3.6 mg of foscarnet in 16 pigmented rabbits using ophthalmoscopy, histology, and electrophysiology.[266] All rabbits revealed evidence of yellowish punctate retinopathy in the midperiphery and posterior pole after the first injection. After four or six injections, there was a significant decrease in the scotopic ERG, whereaas after six injections there was a significant decrease in the mesopic ERG. Of note, light microscopy revealed mild vacuolization and rarefaction in the photoreceptors and inner nuclear layers. After six intravitreal injections, focal areas of photoreceptor layer destruction was observed.[266]

Noninvasive intravitreal foscarnet has been evaluated by Yoshizumi and colleagues.[267] Ten pigmented New Zealand rabbits were subjected to 10 minutes of iontophoresis (1aA with 0.19 mm^2 probe tip surface area) of foscarnet (0.5 mL of 24 mg/mL) and evaluated by a light microscopy, electromicroscopy, and Ganzfeld electrophysiologic studies. No ocular damage was detected in this study.

Cidofovir. [(s)-1-(3-hydroxy-2-phosphonylmethoxytrophyl)cytosine] is an acyclic nucleoside phosphonate analog with broad-spectrum anti-DNA virus activity and a potent and selected inhibitor of CMV in vitro. Cidofovir requires only a short exposure time to produce a marked inhibition of CMV cytopathogenicity and viral DNA synthesis. In addition, cidofovir produces a long-lasting antiviral effect. Cidofovir is a polar and highly water-soluble compound, thus making it more suitable for liposomal delivery systems in intraocular use. Initial animal studies were favorable. Dolnak and coworkers[268] evaluated 20 eyes in 10 New Zealand white rabbits with injections of normal saline or doses of cidofovir of 10, 50, 100, 300, or 1000 μg. Toxicity was assessed by indirect ophthalmoscopy, electroretinography, and light and electron microscopy. Both a- and b-wave ERG findings in ophthalmoscopy in all groups were normal. Light in electromicroscopy revealed no toxicity at doses of 100 μg or less. At doses of 300 and 1000 μg, there were scattered areas of vacuoles in the RPE and degeneration of the photoreceptor layer.

Davis and associates performed a retrospective review of three university outpatient ophthalmology clinics to describe intraocular inflammation with intravenous cidofovir for CMV retinitis.[269] They reported that 11 of 43 patients (26%) had significant iritis. Patients with iritis were more likely to be diabetic, previously treated for CMV retinitis, or receiving protease inhibitors. Hypotony was reported in six eyes of four patients who received intravenous cidofovir in this study.[270]

Kirsch and colleagues[270] evaluated intravitreal cidofovir as the treatment of CMV retinitis in patients with AIDS in a phase I/II study. In one group, 10 eyes in nine patients on intravenous ganciclovir were treated with 14 intravitreal injections of 20 μg of cidofovir, and no toxicity was noted clinically. In a second group, eight eyes were treated in seven patients on no systemic treatment with doses of 20, 40, and 100 μg. Both eyes at 100 μg developed vitritis and hypotony. All patients (after the two who received 100 μg) were treated with probenecid at the time of their intravitreal injections. Despite this, one of three patients who received 40 μg developed vitritis and hypotony. The postulated mechanism for vitritis and hypotony is that direct damage to the nonpigmented epithelium or the inner vasculature results in diminution of aqueous production similar to the acute tubular necrosis observed in the proximal renal tubules with systemic cidofovir.[271]

Besen and colleagues[272] evaluated the liposomal cidofovir.

Seven New Zealand white rabbits were evaluated with liposomal preparations of 100, 500, and 1000 μg of cidofovir. Clinical evaluations revealed no toxicity. The ERG findings for all concentrations showed normal b-wave amplitudes, implicit times, and waveforms. Light microscopy at all concentrations revealed no toxicity, whereas electron microscopy for the highest concentration revealed no evidence of toxicity.[272]

REFERENCES

1. Lamberts DW, Potter DE: Clinical Ophthalmic Pharmacology. Boston, Little, Brown, 1987.
2. Sears ML: Pharmacology of the Eye. Berlin, Springer-Verlag, 1984.
3. Marr WG, Wood R, Grieves M: Further studies on the effect of agents on regeneration of corneal epithelium. Am J Ophthalmol 37:544, 1954.
4. Marr WG, Wood R, Storck M: Effect of some agents on regeneration of corneal epithelium. Am J Ophthalmol 34:609, 1951.
5. Burnstein NL, Klyce SD: Electrophysiologic and morphologic effects of ophthalmic preparations on rabbit corneal epithelium. Invest Ophthalmol Vis Sci 16:899, 1977.
6. Stern GA, Schemmer GB, Farber RD, Gorovoy MS: Effect of topical antibiotic solutions on corneal epithelial wound healing. Arch Ophthalmol 101:644, 1983.
7. Petroutsos G, Guimaraes R, Giraud J, Pouliquen Y: Antibiotics and corneal epithelial wound healing. Arch Ophthalmol 101:1775, 1983.
8. Wilson FM: Adverse external ocular effects of topical ophthalmic medications. Surv Ophthalmol 24:57, 1979.
9. Pfister RR, Burstein NL: The effects of ophthalmic drug vehicles and preservatives on corneal epithelium: A scanning electron microscopy study. Invest Ophthalmol Vis Sci 15:246, 1976.
10. Lerman S, Tripathi RC: Ocular Toxicology. New York, Marcel Dekker, 1990.
11. Peyman GA, Vastine DW, Meisels H: Experimental and clinical use of intravitreal antibiotics to treat bacterial and fungal endophthalmitis. Doc Ophthalmol 39:183, 1975.
12. Peyman GA, Vastine DW, Crouch ER, Herbst RW Jr: Clinical use of intravitreal antibiotics to treat bacterial endophthalmitis. Trans Am Acad Ophthalmol Otolaryngol 78:OP862, 1974.
13. Waring GO III: Antibiotic administration in the treatment of bacterial endophthalmitis. Surv Ophthalmol 21:332, 1977.
14. Leopold IH: Antibiotics and antifungal agents. Invest Ophthalmol Vis Sci 3:504, 1964.
15. Morgan BS, Larson B, Peyman GA, West CS: Toxicity of antibiotic combinations for vitrectomy infusion fluid. Ophthalmic Surg 10:74, 1979.
16. Maurice DM, Mushme S: Pharmacology of the eye. *In* Sears ML (ed): Pharmacology of the Eye. Berlin, Springer-Verlag, 1984.
17. Newmark E, Ellison AC, Kaufman HE: Pimaricin therapy of cephalosporum and fusarium keratitis. Am J Ophthalmol 69:458, 1970.
18. Jeglum EL, Rosenberg SB, Benson WE: Preparation of intravitreal drug doses. Ophthalmic Surg 12:355, 1981.
19. Conway BP, Campochiaro PA: Macular infarction after endophthalmitis treated with vitrectomy and intravitreal gentamicin. Arch Ophthalmol 104:367, 1986.
20. Hansen KD, Meyer RF: Amikacin treatment of *Pseudomonas*-caused corneal ulcer. Arch Ophthalmol 98:1991, 1980.
21. Nelsen P, Peyman GA, Bennett TO: BB-K8: A new aminoglycoside for intravitreal injection in bacterial endophthalmitis. Am J Ophthalmol 78:82, 1974.
22. Bennett TO, Peyman GA: Toxicity of intravitreal aminoglycoside in primates. Can J Ophthalmol 9:475, 1974.
23. Conway BP: Amikacin is less toxic than gentamicin in the primate. Invest Ophthalmol Vis Sci 29(Suppl):404, 1988.
24. Talamo JH, D'Amico DJ, Kenyon KR: Intravitreal amikacin in the treatment of bacterial endophthalmitis. Arch Ophthalmol 104:1483, 1986.
25. Oum BS, D'Amico DJ, Wong KW: Intravitreal antibiotic therapy with vancomycin and aminoglycoside: An experimental study of combinations and repetition injections. Arch Ophthalmol 107:1055, 1989.
26. Oum B, Wong K, Kwak H, et al: Intravitreal antibiotic therapy with a combination of vancomycin and aminoglycoside: Examination of the influence of repetitive injections after vitreous and lens removal. Invest Ophthalmol Vis Sci 31(Suppl):510, 1990.
27. Stainer GA, Peyman GA, Meisels H, Fishman G: Toxicity of selected antibiotics in vitreous replacement fluid. Ann Ophthalmol 9:615, 1977.
28. Campochiaro PA, Conway BP: Aminoglycoside toxicity: A survey of retinal specialists. Arch Ophthalmol 109:946, 1991.

28a. Campochiaro PA, Lim JI: Aminoglycoside toxicity in the treatment of endophthalmitis. Arch Ophthalmol 112:48, 1994.

29. Bras JF, Coyle-Gilchrist MM: Gentamicin in conjunctivitis and keratitis. Br J Ophthalmol 52:560, 1968.
30. Laibson P, Michaud R, Smolin G, et al: A clinical comparison of tobramycin and gentamicin sulfate in the treatment of ocular infection. Am J Ophthalmol 92:836, 1984.
31. Barza M, Kane A, Baum J: Regional differences in ocular concentration of gentamicin after subconjunctival and retrobulbar injection in the rabbit. Am J Ophthalmol 83:407, 1977.
32. Barza M, Kane A, Baum J: Intraocular penetration of gentamicin after subconjunctival and retrobulbar injection. Am J Ophthalmol 85:541, 1978.
33. Baum JL, Barza M, Shushan D, Weinstein L: Concentration of gentamicin in experimental corneal ulcers. Arch Ophthalmol 92:315, 1974.
34. Chu DF, Lee DA: Regional ocular gentamicin levels following transcorneal iontophoresis. Invest Ophthalmol Vis Sci 29(Suppl):438, 1988.
35. Barza M, Peckman C, Baum J: Transscleral iontophoresis of gentamicin in monkeys. Invest Ophthalmol Vis Sci 28:1033, 1987.
36. Fishman PH, Jay WM, Rissing JP, et al: Iontophoresis of gentamicin into aphakic rabbit eyes. Invest Ophthalmol Vis Sci 25:343, 1984.
37. Barza M, Baum J, Szoka F: Pharmacokinetics of subconjunctival liposome-encapsulated gentamicin in normal rabbit eyes. Invest Ophthalmol Vis Sci 25:486, 1984.
38. Awan KJ: Mydriasis and conjunctival paresthesia from local gentamicin. Am J Ophthalmol 99:723, 1985.
39. Pittinger C, Adamson R: Antibiotic blockade of neuromuscular function. Annu Rev Pharmacol 12:169, 1972.
40. Chapman JM, Abdelatif OM, Cheeks L, Green K: Subconjunctival gentamicin induction of extraocular toxic muscle myopathy. Ophthalmic Res 24(4):189–196, 1992.
41. Medin W: A method for registration of toxic drug effects on corneal endothelium: Effect of gentamicin on rabbit corneal endothelium. Acta Ophthalmol (Copenh) 70(1):101–107, 1992.
42. Kanter E, Brucker A: Aminoglycoside macular infarction in association with gentamicin soaked collagen corneal shield. Arch Ophthalmol 113:1359–1360, 1995.
43. Barza M, Kane A, Baum J: Pharmacokinetics of intravitreal carbenicillin, cefazolin, and gentamicin in rhesus monkeys. Invest Ophthalmol Vis Sci 24:1602, 1983.
44. Barza M, Peckman C, Baum J: Transscleral iontophoresis of cefazolin, ticarcillin and gentamicin in the rabbit. Ophthalmology 93:133, 1986.
45. Baum J, Peyman GA, Barza M: Intravitreal administration of antibiotic in the treatment of bacterial endophthalmitis. III: Consensus. Surv Ophthalmol 26:204, 1982.
46. May DR, Ericson ES, Peyman GA, Axelrod AJ: Intraocular injection of gentamicin. Arch Ophthalmol 91:487, 1974.
47. Peyman GA, May DR, Ericson ES, Apple D: Intraocular injection of gentamicin. Arch Ophthalmol 92:42, 1974.
48. Peyman GA, Paque JT, Meisels H, Bennett TO: Postoperative endophthalmitis: A comparison of methods for treatment and prophylaxis with gentamicin. Ophthalmic Surg 6:45, 1975.
49. Zachary IG, Forster RK: Experimental intravitreal gentamicin. Am J Ophthalmol 82:604, 1976.
50. Cottingham AJ, Forster RK: Vitrectomy in endophthalmitis. Arch Ophthalmol 94:2078, 1976.
51. McGetrick JJ, Peyman GA: Vitrectomy in experimental endophthalmitis. Part II: Bacterial endophthalmitis. Ophthalmic Surg 10:87, 1979.
52. Ben-Nun J, Joyce DA, Cooper RL, et al: Pharmacokinetics of intravitreal injection. Invest Ophthalmol Vis Sci 30:1055, 1989.
53. Cobo LM, Forster RK: The clearance of intravitreal gentamicin. Am J Ophthalmol 92:59, 1981.
54. Kane A, Barza M, Baum J: Intravitreal injection of gentamicin in rabbits. Invest Ophthalmol Vis Sci 20:593, 1981.
55. Ling CH, Peyman GA, Raichand M: Electron microscopic study of toxicity of intravitreal injections of gentamicin in primates. Can J Ophthalmol 20:179, 1985.
56. D'Amico DJ, Libert J, Kenyon KR, et al: Retinal toxicity of intravitreal gentamicin: An electron microscopy study. Invest Ophthalmol Vis Sci 25:564, 1984.
57. McDonald HR, Schatz H, Allen AW, et al: Retinal toxicity secondary to intraocular gentamicin injection. Ophthalmology 93:871, 1986.

58. Schatz H, McDonald HR: Acute ischemic retinopathy due to gentamicin injection. JAMA 256:1725, 1986.
59. Conway BP, Tabatabay CA, Campochiaro PA, et al: Gentamicin toxicity in the primate retina. Arch Ophthalmol 107:107, 1989.
60. Fishman PH, Peyman GA, Lesar T: Intravitreal liposome-encapsulated gentamicin in a rabbit model. Invest Ophthalmol Vis Sci 27:1103, 1986.
61. Greenwald MJ, Wohl LG, Sell CH: Metastatic bacterial endophthalmitis: A contemporary reappraisal. Surv Ophthalmol 31:81, 1986.
62. Havener WH, Wachtel J: IDU therapy of herpetic keratitis. Am J Ophthalmol 55:234, 1963.
63. Leibowitz HM, Hyndiuk RA, Smolin GR, et al: Tobramycin in the external eye diseases: A double masked study vs. gentamicin. Curr Eye Res 1:259, 1981.
64. Purnell WE, McPherson SD: An evaluation of tobramycin in experimental corneal ulcers. Am J Ophthalmol 78:318, 1974.
65. Purnell WD, McPherson SD Jr: The effect of tobramycin on rabbit eyes. Am J Ophthalmol 77:578, 1984.
66. Davis SD, Sarff LD, Hyndiuk RA: Topical tobramycin therapy of experimental pseudomonas keratitis. Arch Ophthalmol 96:123, 1978.
67. Rootman DS, Hobden JA, Jantzen JA, et al: Iontophoresis of tobramycin for the treatment of experimental pseudomonas keratitis in the rabbit. Arch Ophthalmol 106:262, 1988.
68. Bennett TO, Peyman GA: Use of tobramycin in eradicating experimental bacterial endophthalmitis. Graefes Arch Klin Exp Ophthalmol 191:93, 1974.
69. Atkins WS, McPherson SD Jr: Intravitreal injection of tobramycin. Invest Ophthalmol Vis Sci 18(Suppl):8, 1976.
70. Atkins WS, McPherson SD: Intravitreal injection of ampicillin, cephaloridine, gentamicin and tobramycin. Surg Forum 26:542, 1975.
71. Kawasaki K, Mochizuki K, Torisaki M, et al: Antibiotic toxicity. Lens and Eye Toxicity Research 7:693–704, 1990.
72. Balian JV: Accidental intraocular tobramycin injection: A case report. Ophthalmic Surg 14:353, 1983.
73. Judson PH: Aminoglycoside macular toxicity after subconjunctival injection. Arch Ophthalmol 107:1282, 1989.
74. Yoshizumi MO: Gentamicin toxicity after cataract extraction or traumatic perforation in the eye. Presented at the Retina Society, Quebec City, September 13, 1991.
75. Aubert-Tulkens G, Van Hoof F, Tulkens P: Gentamicin induced phospholipidosis in cultured rat fibroblasts. Lab Invest 40:481, 1979.
76. Tulkens P, Trouet A: The uptake and intracellular accumulation of aminoglycoside antibiotics in lysosomes of cultured rat fibroblasts. Lab Invest 40:481, 1979.
77. Libert J, Ketelbart-Balasse PE, Van Hoof F, et al: Cellular toxicity of gentamicin. Am J Ophthalmol 87:405, 1979.
78. Laurent G, Carlier M-B, Rollman B, et al: Mechanism of aminoglycoside induced liposomal phospholipidosis: In vitro and in vivo studies with gentamicin and amikacin. Biochem Pharmacol 31:3861, 1982.
79. D'Amico DJ, Caspers-Velu L, Libert J, et al: Comparative toxicity of intravitreal aminoglycoside antibiotics. Am J Ophthalmol 100:264, 1985.
80. Tabatabay CA, D'Amico DJ, Hanninen LA, Kenyon KR: Experimental drusen formation induced by intravitreal aminoglycoside injection. Arch Ophthalmol 105:826, 1987.
81. Tabatabay CA, D'Amico DJ, Hanninen LA, et al: Residual bodies in the retinal pigment epithelium induced by intravitreal netilmicin. Invest Ophthalmol Vis Sci 28:1783, 1987.
82. Lullman-Rauch R: Experimentally induced lipidosis in rat retinal pigment epithelium. Graefes Arch Klin Ophthalmol 215:297, 1981.
83. Fleisher SJ, Rapp LM, Hollyfield JG: Photoreceptor-specific degeneration caused by tunicamycin. Nature 311:575, 1984.
84. Talamo JH, D'Amico DJ, Hanninen LA, et al: The influence of aphakia and vitrectomy on experimental retinal toxicity of aminoglycoside antibiotics. Am J Ophthalmol 100:840, 1985.
85. Mayrovitz HN, Tuma RF, Weidman MP: Leukocyte adherence in arterioles following extravascular tissue trauma. Microvasc Res 20:264, 1980.
86. Schmid-Schonbein GW: Capillary plugging by granulocytes and the no-reflow phenomenon in the microcirculation. Fed Proc 46:2397, 1987.
87. Hodges GR, Watanabe I: Chemical injury of the spinal cord of the rabbit after intracisternal injection of gentamicin. J Neuropathol Exp Neurol 39:452, 1980.
88. Tabatabay CA, Young LHY, D'Amico DJ, Kenyon KR: Immunocytochemical localization of gentamicin in the rabbit retina following intravitreal injection. Arch Ophthalmol 108:723, 1990.
89. Haines J, Vinores SA, Campochiaro PA: Evolution of morphologic changes after intravitreous injection of gentamicin. Curr Eye Res 12(6):521–529, 1993.
90. Peyman GA, Carrol CP, Raichand M: Prevention and management of traumatic endophthalmitis. Ophthalmology 87:320, 1980.
91. Derick RJ, Paylor R, Peyman GA: Toxicity of imipenem in vitreous replacement fluid. Ann Ophthalmol 19:338, 1987.
92. Barza M, Kane A, Baum JL: Intraocular levels of cefamandole compared with cefazolin after subconjunctival injection in rabbits. Invest Ophthalmol Vis Sci 18:250, 1979.
93. Barza M, Kane A, Baum J: Ocular penetration of subconjunctival oxacillin, methicillin, and cefazolin in rabbits with staphylococcal endophthalmitis. J Infect Dis 145:899, 1982.
94. Civiletto SE, Fisher JP: Toxicity, efficacy and clearance of intravitreal cefazolin. Invest Ophthalmol Vis Sci 18(Suppl):132, 1979.
95. Fisher JP, Civiletto SE, Forster RK: Toxicity, efficacy and clearance of intravitreal injected cefazolin. Arch Ophthalmol 100:650, 1982.
96. Ficker L, Merdith TA, Gardner S, Wilson I: Cefazolin levels after intravitreal injection. Invest Ophthalmol Vis Sci 31:502, 1990.
97. Jay WM, Shockley RK: Toxicity and pharmacokinetics of cefepime (BMY-28142) following intravitreal injection in pigmented rabbit eyes. J Ocul Pharmacol 4:345, 1988.
98. Okumoto M, Smolin G, Grabner G, et al: In vitro and in vivo studies on cefoperazone. Cornea 2:35, 1983.
99. O'Hara MA, Bude DD, Kincaid MC, et al: Retinal toxicity of intravitreal cefoperazone. J Ocul Pharmacol 2:177, 1986.
100. Marmor MF: Retinal detachment from hyperosmotic intravitreal injection. Invest Ophthalmol Vis Sci 18:1237, 1979.
101. Okayama Y, Kitano K, Shivao Y, et al: Nontoxic concentration of intravitreal antibiotics for vitrectomy: An evaluation by in vitro ERG of the rabbit. Invest Ophthalmol Vis Sci 31(Suppl):510, 1990.
102. Shockley RK, Fishman P, Aziz M, et al: Subconjunctival administration of ceftazidime in pigmented rabbit eyes. Arch Ophthalmol 104:266, 1986.
103. Jay WM, Wichman P, Aziz M, Shockley RK: Intravitreal ceftazidime in a rabbit model, dose and time dependent toxicity and pharmacokinetic analysis. J Ocul Pharmacol 3:257, 1987.
104. Campochiaro PA, Green WR: Toxicity of intravitreous ceftazidime in primate retina. Arch Ophthalmol 110(11):1625–1629, 1992.
105. Meredith TA: Antimicrobial pharacokinetics in endophthalmitis treatment: Studies of ceftazidime. Trans Am Ophthalmol Soc 91:653–699, 1993.
106. Jay WM, Shockley RK, Aziz AM, et al: Ocular pharmacokinetics of ceftriaxone following subconjunctival injection in rabbits. Arch Ophthalmol 102:430, 1984.
107. Shockley RK, Jay WM, Friberg TR, et al: Intravitreal ceftriazone in a rabbit model. Arch Ophthalmol 102:1236, 1984.
108. Jay WM, Aziz MZ, Rissing JP, Shockley RK: Pharmacokinetic analysis of intravitreal ceftriaxone in monkeys. Arch Ophthalmol 103:121, 1985.
109. Honda Y, Nagata M: A neurological side effect of cephaloridine: Enhancement of the electroretinogram. Ophthalmic Res 7:395, 1975.
110. Graham RO, Peyman GA, Fishman G: Intravitreal injection of cephaloradine in the treatment of endophthalmitis. Arch Ophthalmol 93:56, 1975.
111. Boyle GL, Abel R Jr, Lazechek GW, Leopold IH: Intraocular penetration of sodium cephalothin in man after subconjunctival injection. Am J Ophthalmol 74:868, 1972.
112. Rutgard JJ, Berkowitz RA, Peyman GA: Intravitreal cephalothin in experimental staphylococcal endophthalmitis. Ann Ophthalmol 10:293, 1978.
113. Leeds NH, Peyman GA, House B: Moxalactam (Moxam) in the treatment of experimental staphylococcal endophthalmitis. Ophthalmic Surg 13:653, 1982.
114. Fett DR, Silverman CA, Yoshizumi MO: Moxalactam retinal toxicity. Arch Ophthalmol 102:435, 1984.
115. Brick DC, West C, Ostler HB: Ocular toxicity of subconjunctival nafcillin. Invest Ophthalmol Vis Sci 18(Suppl):132, 1979.
116. Boyle GL, Gwon AE, Zinn KM, Leopold IH: Intraocular penetration of carbenicillin after subconjunctival injection in man. Am J Ophthalmol 73:754, 1972.
117. Schenk AG, Peyman GA, Paque JT: The intravitreal use of carbenicillin (Geopen) for treatment of *Pseudomonas* endophthalmitis. Acta Ophthalmol 52:707, 1974.

118. Lass JH, Thoft DA, Dohlman CH: Idoxuridine-induced conjunctival cicatrization. Arch Ophthalmol 101:747, 1983.
119. Daily MJ, Peyman GA, Fishman G: Intravitreal injection of methicillin for treatment of endophthalmitis. Am J Ophthalmol 76:343, 1973.
120. Grant S: Probenecid and intraocular methicillin. Ann Ophthalmol 13:209, 1981.
121. Cazeau T, Mason GI, Peyman GA: Effects of vitrectomy infusion solutions containing oxacillin, methicillin, or lincomycin. Ann Ophthalmol 11:1247, 1979.
122. Barza M, Kane A, Baum J: Oxacillin for bacterial endophthalmitis: subconjunctival, intravenous, both, or neither? Invest Ophthalmol Vis Sci 19:1348, 1980.
123. von Sallmann L, Meyer K, Di Grandi J: Experimental study on penicillin treatment of ectogenous infection of vitreous. Arch Ophthalmol 32:179, 1944.
124. Mann I: The intra-ocular use of penicillin. Br J Ophthalmol 30:134, 1946.
125. Sorsby A, Ungar J: Intravitreal injection of penicillin: Study on the levels of concentration reached and therapeutic efficacy. Br J Ophthalmol 32:857, 1948.
126. Schaeffer HE, Krohn DL: Liposomes in topical drug delivery. Invest Ophthalmol Vis Sci 21:220, 1982.
127. Semple HC, Liu JC, Peyman GA: Intravitreal injection of piperacillin. Ophthalmic Surg 20:588, 1989.
128. Waring GO III: Initial therapy of suspected microbial corneal ulcers. Surv Ophthalmol 24:105, 1979.
129. Baum J, Barza M: Topical vs. subconjunctival treatment of bacterial corneal ulcers. Ophthalmology 90:162, 1983.
130. Heigle TJ, Peyman GA: Retinal toxicity of intravitreal ticarcillin. Ophthalmic Surg 21:263, 1990.
131. Fraunfelder FT (ed): Drug-Induced Ocular Side Effects and Drug Interactions, 3rd ed. Philadelphia, Lea & Febiger, 1989.
132. Roberts W: Topical use of chloramphenicol in external ocular infections. Am J Ophthalmol 34:1081, 1951.
133. Beasley H, Boltralik JJ, Baldwin HA: Chloramphenicol in aqueous humor after topical application. Arch Ophthalmol 93:184, 1975.
134. Mitsiu Y, Takashima R, Fujimoto M, Kashyama T: Deposits of mucosubstances on the cornea by topical chloramphenicol: An electron microscopic study. Invest Ophthalmol Vis Sci 15:211, 1976.
135. Kleinberg J, Dea FJ, Anderson JA, Leopold IJ: Intraocular penetration of topically applied lincomycin hydrochloride in rabbits. Arch Ophthalmol 97:933, 1979.
136. Boyle GL, Lightig ML, Leopold IH: Lincomycin levels in human ocular fluids and serum following subconjunctival injection. Am J Ophthalmol 71:1303, 1971.
137. Devlin JL III, Mercer KB, Dea FJ, Leopold IH: Intraocular penetration of topical clindamycin in rabbits. Arch Ophthalmol 96:1650, 1978.
138. Tabbara KF, Salamoun SG: Accidental intraocular injection of lincomycin. Am J Ophthalmol 73:596, 1972.
139. Paque JT, Peyman GA: Intravitreal clindamycin phosphate in the treatment of vitreous infection. Ophthalmic Surg 5:34, 1974.
140. Naib K, Hallett JW, Leopold IH: Observations on the ocular effects of erythromycin. Am J Ophthalmol 39:395, 1955.
141. Meisels HI, Peyman GA: Intravitreal erythromycin in the treatment of induced staphylococcal endophthalmitis. Ann Ophthalmol 8:939, 1976.
142. Cochereau-Massir I, Bauchet J, Faurisson F, et al: Ocular kinetics of pefloxacin after intramuscular and intravitreal administration. Invest Ophthalmol Vis Sci 30:247, 1989.
143. Hodden JA, O'Callaghan RJ, Reidy JJ, et al: Transcorneal iontophoresis of ciprofloxacin for therapy of aminoglycoside resistant *Pseudomonas aeruginosa* keratitis. Invest Ophthalmol Vis Sci 31(Suppl 40):570, 1990.
144. Stamer WD, Jahnke J, McDermott ML, Snyder RW: Effect of ciprofloxacin on rabbit corneal endothelial viability. Invest Ophthalmol Vis Sci 32(Suppl):1063, 1991.
145. Haller-Yeo J, O'Brien TP, Green WR, et al: Ciprofloxacin: Oral penetration into the eye and retinal toxicity of intravitreal injection. Invest Ophthalmol Vis Sci 30:381, 1989.
146. Steven SX, Fouraker BD, Jensen HG: Intraocular safety of ciprofloxacin. Arch Ophthalmol 109:1737, 1991.
147. Marchese AL, Slana VS, Holmes EW, Jay WM: Toxicity on pharmacokinetics of ciprofloxacin. J Ocul Pharmacol 9:69–76, 1993.
148. Borhani H, Peyman GA, Wafapoor H: Use of vancomycin in vitrectomy infusion solution and the value and evaluation of retinal toxicity. Int Ophthalmol 17(2):85–88, 1993.
149. Mochizuki K, Torisaki M, Wakabayashi K: Effects of vancomycin and ofloxacin on rabbit ERG in vivo. Jpn J Ophthalmol 35(4):435–445, 1991.
150. Williams RK, Hench ME, Guerry D: Pyocyaneus ulcer. Am J Ophthalmol 37:538, 1954.
151. Pryor JG, Apt L, Leopold IH: Intraocular penetration of vancomycin. Arch Ophthalmol 67:608, 1962.
152. Flach AJ, Peterson JS, Toby Mathias CG: Photosensitivity to topically applied sulfisoxazole ointment. Arch Ophthalmol 100:1286, 1982.
153. Boettner EA, Fralick FB, Wolter JR: Conjunctival concretions of sulfadiazine. Arch Ophthalmol 92:446, 1974.
154. Hook SR, Holladay JT, Prager TC, Goosey JD: Transient myopia induced by sulfonamides. Am J Ophthalmol 101:495, 1986.
155. Garcia-Ferrer FJ, Pepose IS, Murray PR, et al: Antimicrobial efficacy and corneal endothelial toxicity of Dex-Sol corneal storage medium supplemented with vancomycin. Ophthalmology 98:863, 1991.
156. Lindquist TD, Roth BP, Fritsche TR: Safety and efficacy of corneal storage media. Invest Ophthalmol Vis Sci 32(Suppl):1063, 1991.
157. Kattan HM, Pflugfelder SC: Corneal endothelial toxicity of vancomycin in corneal preservation media. Invest Ophthalmol Vis Sci 32(Suppl):1063, 1991.
158. Choi TB, Lee DA: Transscleral and transcorneal iontophoresis of vancomycin in rabbit eyes. J Ocul Pharmacol 4:153, 1988.
159. Homer P, Peyman GA, Koziol J, Sanders D: Intravitreal injection of vancomycin in experimental staphylococcal endophthalmitis. Acta Ophthalmol 53:311, 1975.
160. Smith MA, Sorenson JA, Lowy FD, et al: Treatment of experimental methicillin-resistant *Staphylococcus epidermidis* endophthalmitis with intravitreal vancomycin. Ophthalmology 93:1328, 1986.
161. Pflugfelder SC, Hernandez E, Fleister SJ, et al: Intravitreal vancomycin: Retinal toxicity, clearance, interaction with gentamicin. Arch Ophthalmol 105:831, 1987.
162. Kattan HM, Pflugfelder SC, Hernandez E, Ravinowitz S: Retinal toxicity of combined intravitreal vancomycin and aminoglycoside in the rabbit's eyes. Invest Ophthalmol Vis Sci (Suppl)31:510, 1990.
163. Loewenstein A, Zemel E, Lazar M, Perlman I: Drug induced retinal toxicity in albino rabbits: The effects of imipenem and aztreonam. Invest Ophthalmol Vis Sci 34:3466–3476, 1993.
164. Ryan SJ (ed): Retina. St Louis, CV Mosby, 1989.
165. Jones DB: Therapy of postsurgical fungal endophthalmitis. Symposium on Postoperative Endophthalmitis 85:357–373, April 1978.
166. Noske W: Inaccuracy in preparation of intravitreal solutions. Arch Ophthalmol 104:1748, 1986.
167. Johns KJ, O'Day DM: Pharmacologic management of keratomycoses. Surv Ophthalmol 33:178, 1988.
168. Jones DB: New drugs for fungal bugs. Invest Ophthalmol Vis Sci 12:551, 1973.
169. O'Day DM, Head WS, Robinson RD, Clanton JA: Corneal penetration of topical amphotericin B and natamycin. Curr Eye Res 5:877, 1986.
170. Foster CS, Lass JH, Moran-Wallace K, Giovanoni R: Ocular toxicity of topical antifungal agents. Arch Ophthalmol 99:1081, 1981.
171. Ellison AC, Newmark E: Effects of subconjunctival pimaricin in experimental keratomycosis. Am J Ophthalmol 75:790, 1973.
172. Ellison AC: Intravitreal effects of pimaricin in experimental fungal endophthalmitis. Am J Ophthalmol 81:157, 1976.
173. Ellison AC, Newmark E: Intraocular effects of pimaricin. Ann Ophthalmol 8:897, 1976.
174. Montana JA, Sery TW: Effect of fungistatic agents on corneal infections with *Candida albicans*. Arch Ophthalmol 60:1, 1958.
175. Foster JBT, Almeda E, Littman ML, Wilson ME: Some intraocular and conjunctival effects of amphotericin B in man and in the rabbit. Arch Ophthalmol 60:555, 1958.
176. Green WR, Bennett JE, Goos RD: Ocular penetration of amphotericin B. Arch Ophthalmol 73:769, 1965.
177. Jones DB, Forster RK, Rebell G: *Fusarium solani* keratitis treated with natamycin (Pimaricin). Arch Ophthalmol 88:147, 1972.
178. Bell RW, Ritchey JP: Subconjunctival nodules after amphotericin B injection. Arch Ophthalmol 90:402, 1973.
179. Wood TO, Williford W: Treatment of keratomycosis with amphotericin B 0.15%. Am J Ophthalmol 81:847, 1976.
180. Foster CS, Lass JH, Moran K, Giovanoni R: Ocular toxicity of topical antifungal agents. Invest Ophthalmol Vis Sci 18(Suppl):132, 1979.
181. O'Day DM, Ray WA, Head WS, Robinson RD: Efficacy of antifungal agents in the cornea. IV. Amphotericin B methyl ester. Invest Ophthalmol Vis Sci 25:851, 1984.

182. Lavine JB, Binder PS, Wickhan MG: Antimicrobials and the corneal endothelium. Ann Ophthalmol 11:1517, 1979.
183. Axelrod AJ, Peyman GA, Apple DJ: Toxicity of intravitreal injection of amphotericin B. Am J Ophthalmol 76:578, 1973.
184. Axelrod AJ, Peyman GA: Intravitreal amphotericin B treatment of experimental fungal endophthalmitis. Am J Ophthalmol 76:584, 1973.
185. Souri EN, Green WR: Intravitreal amphotericin B toxicity. Am J Ophthalmol 78:77, 1974.
186. Stern GA, Fetkenhour CL, O'Grady RB: Intravitreal amphotericin B treatment of *Candida* endophthalmitis. Arch Ophthalmol 95:89, 1977.
187. Mosier MA, Lusk B, Pettit TH: Fungal endophthalmitis following intraocular lens implantation. Am J Ophthalmol 83:1, 1977.
188. Perrault LE Jr, Perrault LE, Bleiman B, Lyons J: Successful treatment of *Candida albicans* endophthalmitis with intravitreal amphotericin B. Arch Ophthalmol 99:1565, 1981.
189. Stern WH, Tamura E, Jacobs RA, et al: Epidemic postsurgical *Candida parapsilosis* endophthalmitis: Clinical findings and management of 15 consecutive cases. Ophthalmology 92:1701, 1985.
190. Brod RD, Flynn HW, Clarkson JG, et al: Endogenous *Candida* endophthalmitis. Ophthalmology 97:666, 1990.
191. Huang K, Peyman GA, McGetrick J: Vitrectomy in experimental endophthalmitis: Part 1. Fungal infection. Ophthalmic Surg 10:84, 1979.
192. Doft BH, Weiskopf J, Nilsson-Ehle I, Wingard LB: Amphotericin-B clearance in vitrectomized versus nonvitrectomized eyes. Ophthalmology 92:1601, 1985.
193. Baldinger J, Doft BH, Burns SA, Johnson B: Retinal toxicity of amphotericin B in vitrectomised versus non-vitrectomised eyes. Br J Ophthalmol 70:657, 1986.
194. Wingard LB, Zuravleff JJ, Doft BH, et al: Intraocular distribution of intravitreally administered amphotericin B in normal and vitrectomized eyes. Invest Ophthalmol Vis Sci 30:2184, 1989.
195. Pflugfelder SC, Flynn HW Jr, Zwickey TA, et al: Exogenous fungal endophthalmitis. Ophthalmology 95:19, 1988.
196. McGetrick JJ, Peyman GA, Nyberg MA: Amphotericin B methyl ester: Evaluation for intravitreous use in experimental fungal endophthalmitis. Ophthalmic Surg 10:25, 1979.
197. Raichand M, Peyman GA, West CS, et al: Toxicity and efficacy of vitrectomy fluids: Amphotericin B methyl ester in the treatment of experimental fungal endophthalmitis. Ophthalmic Surg 11:246, 1980.
198. Lopez-Bernstein G, Mehta R, Hopfer RL, et al: Treatment and prophylaxis of disseminated infection due to *Candida albicans* in mice with liposome-encapsulated amphotericin B. J Infect Dis 147:939, 1983.
199. Tremblay C, Barza M, Biore C, Szoka F: Efficacy of liposome-intercalated amphotericin B in the treatment of systemic candidiasis in mice. Antimicrob Agents Chemother 26:170, 1984.
200. Barza M, Stuart M, Szoka R Jr: Effect of size and lipid composition on the pharmacokinetics of intravitreal liposomes. Invest Ophthalmol Vis Sci 28:893, 1987.
201. Tremblay C, Barza M, Szoka F, et al: Reduced toxicity of liposome-associated amphotericin B injected intravitreally in rabbits. Invest Ophthalmol Vis Sci 26:711, 1985.
202. Barza M, Baum J, Tremblay C, et al: Ocular toxicity of intravitreally injected liposomal amphotericin B in rhesus monkeys. Am J Ophthalmol 100:259, 1985.
203. Szoka FC, Milholland D, Barza M: Effect of lipid composition and liposome size on toxicity and in vitro fungicidal activity of liposome-intercalated amphotericin B. Antimicrob Agents Chemother 31:421, 1987.
204. Liu K-R, Peyman GA, Khoobehi B: Efficacy of liposome-bound amphotericin B for the treatment of experimental fungal endophthalmitis in rabbits. Invest Ophthalmol Vis Sci 30:1527, 1989.
205. Montgomerie JZ, Edwards JE, Guze LB: Synergism of amphotericin B and fluorocytosine for *Candida* species. J Infect Dis 132:82, 1975.
206. O'Day DM, Robinson R, Head WS: Efficacy of antifungal agents in the cornea. I: A comparative study. Invest Ophthalmol Vis Sci 24:1098, 1983.
207. Walsh JA, Haft DA, Miller MH, et al: Ocular penetration of 5-fluorocytosine. Invest Ophthalmol Vis Sci 17:691, 1978.
208. Yoshizumi MO, Silverman C: Experimental intravitreal 5-fluorocytosine. Ann Ophthalmol 17:58, 1985.
209. Grossman R, Lee DA: Transscleral and transcorneal iontophoresis of ketoconazole in the rabbit eye. Invest Ophthalmol Vis Sci 30(Suppl):247, 1989.
210. Grossman R, Lee DA: Transscleral and transcorneal iontophoresis of ketoconazole in the rabbit eye. Ophthalmology 96:724, 1989.
211. Yoshizumi MO, Banihashemi AF: Experimental intravitreal ketoconazole in DMSO. Retina 8:210, 1988.
212. Silverman CA, Yoshizami MO: Ocular toxicity of experimental intravitreal DMSO. J Toxicol Cutan Ocul Toxicol 2:193, 1983.
213. Foster CS, Stefanyszyn M: Intraocular penetration of miconazole in rabbits. Arch Ophthalmol 97:1703, 1979.
214. Foster CS: Miconazole therapy for keratomycosis. Am J Ophthalmol 91:662, 1981.
215. Zaidman GW: Miconazole corneal toxicity. Cornea 10:90, 1991.
216. Jaben SL, Forster RK: Intraocular miconazole therapy in fungal endophthalmitis. Invest Ophthalmol Vis Sci 22(Suppl):109, 1981.
216a. Osato M, Broberg P, Mehta R, et al: Toxicity of intravitreal miconazole in the rabbit. Invest Ophthalmol Vis Sci 23(Suppl):250, 1982.
217. Tolentino FI, Foster CS, Lahav M, et al: Toxicity of intravitreous miconazole. Arch Ophthalmol 100:1504, 1982.
218. Yoshizumi MO, Vinci V, Fong KD: Toxicity of intravitreal miconazole in DMSO. J Toxicol Cutan Ocul Toxicol 6:19, 1987.
220. Schulman JA, Peyman GA, Didlein J, Fiscella R: Ocular toxicity of expermental intravitreal itraconozole. Int Ophthalmol 15:21–24, 1991.
221. Brooks JG, O'Brien T, Wilhelmus KR, et al: Comparative topical triazole therapy of experimental candida albicans keratitis. Invest Ophthalmol Vis Sci 31(Suppl):570, 1990.
222. Schulman JA, Peyman G, Fiscella R, et al: Toxicity of intravitreal injection of fluconazole in the rabbit. Can J Ophthalmol 22:304, 1987.
223. Walsh J, Gold A, Charles H (eds): PDR for Ophthalmology. Oradell, NJ, Medical Economics Co, 1991.
224. Pavan-Langston D: Clinical evaluation of adenine arabinoside and idoxuridine in the treatment of ocular herpes simplex. Am J Ophthalmol 80:495, 1975.
225. Payrau P, Dohlman CH: IDU in corneal wound healing. Am J Ophthalmol 57:999, 1964.
226. Gassett AR, Katzin D: Antiviral drugs and corneal wound healing. Invest Ophthalmol Vis Sci 14:628, 1975.
227. Krejci L, Krejcova H: Effects of IDU and corticosteroids on corneal epithelium. Can J Ophthalmol 9:221, 1974.
228. Maloney ED, Kaufman HE: Antagonism and toxicity of IDU by its degradation products. Invest Ophthalmol Vis Sci 2:55, 1963.
229. Smolin G, Okumoto M, Feiler S, Condon D: Idoxuridine-liposome therapy for herpes simplex keratitis. Am J Ophthalmol 91:220, 1981.
230. Dharma SK, Fishman PH, Peyman GA: A preliminary study of corneal penetration of 125 I-labelled idoxuridine liposomes. Acta Ophthalmol 64:298, 1986.
231. Dutt R, Dobrowski P, Centifanto Y, Caldwell D: Endothelial cell toxicity produced by commercially prepared solutions of anti-virals on cultured human corneal cells. Invest Ophthalmol Vis Sci 32:1066, 1991.
232. Kaufman HE, Ellison ED, Townsend WM: The chemotherapy of herpes iritis with adenine arabinoside and cytarabine. Arch Ophthalmol 84:783, 1970.
233. Hill JM, Park H-N, Gangarosa LP, et al: Iontophoresis of vidarabine monophosphate into rabbit eyes. Invest Ophthalmol Vis Sci 17:473, 1978.
234. Pulido JS, Palacio M, Peyman GA, et al: Toxicity of intravitreal antiviral drugs. Ophthalmic Surg 15:666, 1984.
235. Udell IJ: Trifluridine-associated conjunctival cicatrization. Am J Ophthalmol 99:363, 1985.
236. Maudgal PC, Van Damme B, Missoten L: Corneal epithelial dysplasia after trifluridine use. Arch Clin Exp 220:6, 1983.
237. Carmine AA, Brogden RN, Heel RC, et al: Trifluridine: A review of its antiviral activity and therapeutic use in the topical treatment of viral eye infections. Drugs 23:329, 1982.
238. Wellings PC, Awdry PN, Bors FH, et al: Clinical evaluation of trifluorothymidine in the treatment of herpes simplex corneal ulcers. Am J Ophthalmol 73:932, 1972.
239. Hyndiuk RA, Charlin RE, Alpren TVP, Schultz RO: Trifluridine in resistant human herpetic keratitis. Arch Ophthalmol 96:1839, 1978.
240. Maudgal PC, Vrijghem JC, Colemans M, Missoten L: Effect of topical acyclovir therapy on experimental herpes simplex keratouveitis. Arch Ophthalmol 103:1389, 1985.
241. Peyman GA, Schulman JA, Khoobehi B, et al: Toxicity and clearance of a combination of liposome-encapsulated ganciclovir and trifluridine. Retina 9:232, 1989.
242. Pang MP, Peyman GA, Nikoleit J, et al: Intravitreal trifluorothymidine and retinal toxicity. Retina 6:260, 1986.

243. Liu K-R, Peyman GA, Khoobehi B, et al: Intravitreal liposome-encapsulated trifluorothymidine in a rabbit model. Ophthalmology 94:1155, 1987.
244. Klauber A, Ottovay E: Acyclovir and idoxuridine treatment of herpes simplex keratitis: A double blind clinical study. Acta Ophthalmol 60:838, 1982.
245. Pulido JS, Peyman GA, Lesar T, Vernot J: Intravitreal toxicity of hydroxyacyclovir (BW-B759U): A new antiviral agent. Arch Ophthalmol 103:840, 1985.
246. Peyman GA, Goldberg MF, Uninsky E, et al: Vitrectomy and intravitreal antiviral drug therapy in acute retinal necrosis syndrome. Arch Ophthalmol 102:1618, 1984.
247. Schulman JA, Peyman GA, Horton MB, et al: Intraocular 9-([hydroxy-1-(hydroxymethyl) ethoxy] methyl) guanine levels after intravitreal and subconjunctival administration. Ophthalmic Surg 17:429, 1986.
248. Henry K, Cantrill H, Fletcher C, et al: Use of intravitreal ganciclovir for cytomegalovirus retinitis in a patient with AIDS. Am J Ophthalmol 103:17, 1987.
249. Ussery FM, Gibson SJ, Conklin RH, et al: Intravitreal ganciclovir in the treatment of AIDS–associated cytomegalovirus retinitis. Ophthalmology 95:640, 1988.
250. Cantrill HL, Henry K, Melroe H, et al: Treatment of cytomegalovirus retinitis with intravitreal ganciclovir: Long-term results. Ophthalmology 96:367, 1989.
251. Heinemann M-H: Long-term intravitreal ganciclovir therapy for cytomegalovirus retinopathy. Arch Ophthalmol 107:1767, 1989.
252. Peyman GA, Khoobehi B, Tawakol M, et al: Intravitreal injection of liposome-encapsulated ganciclovir in the rabbit model. Retina 7:227, 1987.
253. Yoshizumi MO, Lee D, Vinci V, Fajardo S: Ocular toxicity of multiple intravitreal DHPG injections. Graefes Arch Clin Exp Ophthalmol 228:350, 1990.
254. Kuppermann BD, Liggett PE, Trousdale MD: Intravitreal ganciclovir clearance in rabbits with experimentally induced herpes simplex virus retinitis. Invest Ophthalmol Vis Sci (ARVO Suppl)31:511, 1990.
255. Cochereau-Massin I, Lehoang P, Lautier-Frau M, et al: Efficacy and tolerance of intravitreal ganciclovir and cytomegalovirus retinitis in acquired immunodeficiency syndrome. Ophthalmology 98:1348–1355, 1991.
256. Moschos M, Vamvasakis M, Kontogeorgos G, et al: Intravitreal application of ganciclovir in rabbits: ERG and electron microscopic findings. Ophthalmologic A 210:215–222, 1996.
257. Saran BR, McGuire AM: Retinal toxicity of high dose intravitreal ganciclovir. Retina 14:248–255, 1994.
258. Sanborn GE, Anand R, Torti R, et al: Treatment of CMV retinitis with sustained release intravitreal ganciclovir. Invest Ophthalmol Vis Sci 32:765, 1991.
259. Sanborn GF, Amand R, Torti R: Treatment of cytomegaloretinitis with sustained intravitreal gancyclovir implantable device for sustained release of DHPG. Presented at the Retina Society Meeting, Quebec City, September 13, 1991.
260. Sanborn GF, Anand R, Torti RE, et al: Sustained release ganciclovir therapy for treatment of cytomegalovirus. Arch Ophthalmol 110:188–195, 1992.
261. Ashton P, Brown JD, Pearson PA, et al: Intravitreal ganciclovir pharmacokinetics in rabbits and man. J Ocul Pharmacol 8(4):343–357, 1992.
262. Martin DF, Parks DJ, Mellon SD, et al: Treatment of cytomegalovirus retinitis with an intraocular sustained release ganciclovir implant: Randomized control clinical trial. Ophthalmology 112:1531–1539, 1994.
263. Charles NC, Steiner GC: Ganciclovir intraocular implant: A clinical pathologic study. Ophthalmology 103:416–421, 1996.
264. She S, Peyman GA, Schulman JA: Toxicity of intravitreal injection of foscarnet in the rabbit eye. Int Ophthalmol 12:151–154, 1988.
265. Dia-Llopis M, Chipont E, Sanchez S, et al: Intravitreal foscarnet for cytomegalovirus retinitis in a patient with acquired immunodeficiency syndrome. Am J Ophthalmol 114:742–747, 1992.
266. Turrini B, Tognon MS, DeCaro E, Secoh AG: Intravitreal use of foscarnet: Retinal toxicity of repeated injections in the rabbit eye. Ophthalmic Res 26:110–115, 1994.
267. Yoshizumi MO, Lee DA, Sarraf DA, et al: Ocular toxicity of iontophoretic foscarnet in the rabbit. J Ocul Pharmacol Ther 11:183–189, 1995.
268. Dolnak DR, Munguia D, Wiley CA, et al: Lack of retinal toxicity of the anti-cytomegalovirus drug (s)-1-3 hydroxy-2-phosphonylmethoxytrophyl) cytosine. Invest Ophthalmol Vis Sci 33:1557–1563, 1992.
269. Davis JL, Taskintuna I, Freeman WR, et al: Iritis and hypotony after intravenous cidofovir for cytomegalovirus retinitis. Arch Ophthalmol 115:733, 1997.
270. Kirsch LS, Fernando-Arevalo J, Clereq E, et al: A phase I/II study of intravitreal cidofovir in the treatment of cytomegalovirus retinitis in a patient with acquired immunodeficiency syndrome. Am J Ophthalmol 119:466–476, 1997.
271. Bravo FJ, Stanberry LR, Kier AB, et al: Evaluation of HPMPC therapy for primary and recurrent genital herpes in mice and guinea pigs. Antiviral Res 21:59–72, 1993.
272. Besen G, Flores-Aguila M, Afil KK, et al: Long-term therapy for herpes retinitis in an animal model and high concentrated liposome encapsulated HPMPC. Arch Ophthalmol 113:661–668, 1995.

CHAPTER 41

Toxicology of Antiglaucoma Drugs

Kristine Erickson and Alison Schroeder

Medical intervention is the first choice of physicians in the treatment of primary open-angle glaucoma (POAG). The therapeutic basis for the use of pharmaceutical agents is their ability to lower intraocular pressure (IOP), delaying the loss of vision that eventually occurs after prolonged periods of elevated IOP. Although lowering the IOP with medical treatment is often effective, no medical treatment to date is curative. Patients often eventually fail to respond to medications owing either to disease progression or to an acquired subsensitivity to the treatment regimens. Ironically, some animal studies suggest that the loss of responsiveness may be due to the toxicity of chronic medical treatment to ocular tissues.[1–5] Further investigation is necessary to understand the mechanism underlying the loss of responsiveness to the therapeutic agents in order to facilitate a more effective treatment of POAG. Furthermore, rather than treating the symptom of glaucoma (elevated IOP), full-scale efforts need to be employed to understand the pathophysiology of POAG so that curative treatments can be employed.

Drugs that are used in the treatment of POAG exert their therapeutic effects by decreasing aqueous outflow resistance, reducing aqueous humor formation, or increasing uveal scleral flow. The four categories of drugs classically used that decrease IOP are cholinergic agonists and adrenergic agonists and antagonists and oral carbonic anhydrase inhibitors.

Cholinergic drugs used in the treatment of POAG include direct-acting agonists such as pilocarpine, aceclidine, and carbachol and indirect-acting cholinesterase inhibitors such as echothiophate iodide, demecarium bromide, isoflurophate, neostigmine, paraxon physostigmine, and tetraethyl pyrophosphate. These drugs contract the ciliary muscle, which leads to a reduction in the resistance to aqueous humor outflow by a mechanism that is not fully understood.[6] On the other hand, the adrenergic agonists, including epinephrine and norepinephrine, act directly on the outflow pathway to lower outflow resistance by a β-adrenergic receptor–mediated mechanism.[7–11]

β-Blockers, including timolol, L-bunolol, and betaxolol, exert their therapeutic effects by acting at the nonpigmented ciliary epithelium to reduce the inflow of aqueous humor. Carbonic anhydrase inhibitors such as acetazolamide dramatically decrease aqueous humor formation by acting on membrane-bound carbonic anhydrase in the ciliary processes (Table 41–1).

TABLE 41–1. **Mechanism of Intraocular Pressure Reduction Achieved by Classes of Drugs Commonly Used to Treat Primary Open-Angle Glaucoma**

Drug Class	Therapeutic Effect
Cholinergics—Direct Acting	Decreased outflow resistance
Pilocarpine	
Aceclidine	
Carbachol	
Cholinesterase Inhibitors	Decreased outflow resistance
Physostigmine	
Demecarium	
Edrophonium	
Echothiophate	
Isoflurophate	
Adrenergics	Decreased aqueous inflow
Epinephrine	
Dipivefrin	
Apraclonidine	
Brimonidine	
β-Adrenergic–Receptor Blockers	Decreased aqueous inflow
Timolol	
L-Bunolol	
Betaxolol	
Carteolol	
Metipranolol	
Carbonic Anhydrase Inhibitors	Decreased aqueous formation
Acetazolamide	
Methazolamide	
Dichlorophenamide	
Dorzolamide	

Several classes of drugs have recently been approved for the treatment of POAG. Included are two α-adrenergic agonists, apraclonidine[12] and brimonidine, that lower IOP by reducing aqueous humor formation; latanoprost, a prostaglandin $F_{2\alpha}$ analog, which lowers pressure presumably by increasing the outflow of aqueous humor through the unconventional uveal scleral route;[13, 14] dorzolamide, a topical carbonic anhydrase inhibitor; and a new form of timolol, timoptic-XE, which forms a gel on contact with the ocular surface, providing the necessity for once-daily dosing instead of the twice-daily dosing suggested for the conventional preparation.

This chapter describes the basic mechanism of action of specific drugs in each of these classes and summarizes the known nature and incidence of toxicity associated with the use of these compounds clinically and in experimental systems. For the most part, the literature covered includes reports published within the past 20 years. For a more comprehensive treatment of this subject, the reader is referred to the excellent summaries of Grant.[15] Further, the reader can refer to Tripathi and Tripathi[16] and Lütjen-Drecoll and associates[1–5] for reviews of the pathologic effects of some drugs.

Cholinergic Drugs

Much has been learned about the ophthalmic toxicology of cholinergic drugs from testing in animals and humans, from observations in accidental poisonings, and in connection with medical uses of both direct-acting agents and anticholinesterases in the treatment of glaucoma, accommodative strabismus, and myasthenia gravis. Most commonly known effects include miosis (constriction of the pupil), induction of pupillary cysts, enhancement of accommodation (i.e., adjustment of the lens of the eye to focus on near objects), formation of cataracts, and reduction of IOP. A variety of other effects are less well known or are less well established. Systemic poisoning, which has occasionally been caused by the use of anticholinesterase eye drops, is manifested by both muscarinic and nicotinic symptoms, which can include paralysis of the respiratory muscles mediated by stimulation of nicotinic receptors. Although the ocular and systemic side effects of anticholinesterases are generally more frequent, similar patterns are noted with direct-acting muscarinic agents such as pilocarpine. Therefore, direct-acting agonists and anticholinesterases are considered as a group (Table 41–2).

OCULAR SIDE EFFECTS

Cornea, Conjunctiva, and Lacrimal Apparatus

Clinical examination of the cornea and conjunctiva after application of anticholinesterase eye drops such as are used in the treatment of glaucoma or accommodative strabismus or after test exposures to anticholinesterase insecticides or nerve gases usually reveals only hyperemia of the conjunctiva from dilation of conjunctival blood vessels. The cornea usually shows no abnormality. Exceptionally, in rabbits, repeated exposures to 1% ethyl dimethyl thiophosphate (Hektion) is reported to have caused corneal ulceration and perforation,[17] and repeated exposure to fenitrothion (Sumithion) to have produced changes suggestive of conical cornea.[18] Also, there

TABLE 41–2. **Side Effects Associated With the Use of Cholinergic Drugs in the Treatment of Primary Open-Angle Glaucoma**

Ocular Side Effects
Conjunctival hyperemia and follicles
Miosis
Shallowing of the anterior chamber
Iritis
Pupillary cysts
Accommodation
Brow ache
Anterior and posterior subcapsular lens opacities
Retinal detachment
Acute alterations in the electrical properties of the retina
Systemic Side Effects
Diaphoresis
Salivation
Nausea
Tremor
Hypotension
Gastrointestinal disturbances
Bradycardia
Paralysis of respiratory muscles
Delayed peripheral neurotoxicity
Exacerbation of asthma

are scattered reports of cases of the development of pseudopemphigoid in the treated eye after several years of treatment with miotics, including echothiophate iodide and pilocarpine eye drops.[19–21] Long-term administration of pilocarpine has also been associated with conjunctival changes, including hyperemia and the appearance of follicles.[22] A diffuse corneal haze has also been noted during therapy with pilocarpine gel. However, the authors concluded that the apparent toxicity was probably secondary to chlorobutanol that was used as a preservative in the gel.[23] Similarly, band keratopathy has also been associated with long-term administration of pilocarpine drops containing the preservative phenyl mercuric nitrate.[24]

Although the function of the high levels of acetylcholine, choline acetylase, and cholinesterase in the corneal epithelium and endothelium of some species remains unknown, speculations have been offered that acetylcholine may contribute to ion movement across the epithelium and endothelium and to corneal sensation.[25, 26] However, it has been noted that corneal touch or pain stimuli are neither enhanced by physostigmine nor blocked by atropine.[27] Cultured corneal epithelium from rabbits and human beings has been reported to show cytotoxicity after the addition of extremely high dilutions of anticholinesterase eye drops. What significance, clinical or otherwise, this may have is unclear.[28]

Rarely, disturbances of the lacrimal apparatus have been reported after treatment with topical miotics. Also, a case of bilateral stenosis of the tear ducts has been reported after the use of echothiophate iodide eye drops twice a day for 13 years.[29] Excessive tearing from stimulation of the lacrimal glands has been noted in anticholinesterase poisoning.[30]

Iris

Cholinergic agents affect the iris in several ways, usually producing miosis but sometimes causing dilatation of the pupil. Certain concentrations of anticholinesterases and direct-acting agonists such as aceclidine in contact with the eye may cause the pupil to become extremely miotic but may affect accommodation only moderately.[31, 32]

In systemic poisoning by anticholinesterases, the pupils may become extremely small, but paradoxically in some cases of severe poisoning the pupils are found to be dilatated.[33, 34]

In some animals, a decrease in miosis is noted on repeated administration of anticholinesterase eye drops. In rabbits,[35, 36] cats,[36] monkeys,[37] and guinea pigs,[38] repeated application of anticholinesterase eye drops has resulted in a decrease in the amount of miosis induced and a decrease in miosis from carbachol and pilocarpine eye drops. However, in most cases, the maximal pupillary response to bright light was unaltered even after several weeks of anticholinesterase eye drop treatment.[37, 39]

Miosis in humans commonly brings with it a feeling that the surroundings are dim or that the illumination has been reduced.[40, 41] This is simply related to the decrease in pupillary area through which light can enter the eye.[40, 42] Dark adaptation has little effect on strong miosis from anticholinesterase agents.[40]

According to Romano and Jackson,[43] Wilkie and coworkers,[44] and Drance,[45] when miosis is maintained for weeks or months by daily anticholinesterase eye drops, there is a gradual shallowing of the anterior chamber. In rare instances, angle-closure glaucoma has resulted. The mean decrease in axial depth for a group of patients receiving echothiophate iodide was 0.2 and 0.44 mm at 1 week and 8 weeks, respectively. None of these patients developed glaucoma. When the administration of echothiophate iodide was discontinued, their axial depth gradually returned toward normal.[44]

Iritis from contact of the eye with anticholinesterases is an infrequent complication in humans. Iritis is usually associated with conjunctival hyperemia and consists of dilatation of the iris vessels with cells in the anterior chamber. It has usually been associated with the use of anticholinesterase eye drops but in one case has been described in both eyes from a spray of the insecticide bromophos.[46] In some cases, anticholinesterase-induced iritis responds well to anticholinergic treatment,[40] but in other cases response has been slow despite treatment with mydriatics, corticosteroids, and pralidoxime.[47]

The development of cysts of the pupillary border of the iris is a common complication of repeated application of anticholinesterases to the human eye. Efforts to reproduce the cysts in rabbits and guinea pigs have been unsuccessful.[48] Pupillary cysts were originally described after the use of physostigmine,[49] but they have been observed with most anticholinesterase eye drops. Characteristically, one to a dozen brown cysts, 0.1 to 1 mm in diameter, are seen along or behind the pupillary edge of the iris. In response to marked miosis such cysts may develop in 1 to 2 weeks.[50] If the miotic eye drops are discontinued, the cysts change to shrunken brown tags and slowly disappear within 2 to 40 weeks.[50] In adults, the cysts usually develop only in response to strong miosis, but in children they commonly develop in association with moderate miosis.[51–54] Rarely, the pupillary cysts interfere with vision, particularly in association with extreme miosis.[55, 56] The simultaneous use of phenylephrine eye drops can enlarge the pupil slightly and reduce the tendency to form cysts.[52–54, 57, 58] The ciliary processes have rarely been reported to have cysts in association with pupillary cysts from miotics.[59]

Histologically, Christensen and colleagues[60] found proliferations of iris pigment epithelium instead of cysts, but in another case Straub and Conrads[48] found that two posterior epithelial layers of the iris were separated in some places, forming fluid-filled cysts. The latter case fits better a suggested mechanism that miosis pinches the iris pigment epithelium against the lens, allowing retention of fluid between the layers, which produces cysts.[50, 55] Consistently, cysts are not produced by miotic eye drops in the absence of the lens.[55]

Depth perception may be unreliable after unequal contact of an anticholinesterase with a person's two eyes, producing unequal miosis and unequal amounts of light reaching the retinas of the two eyes.[41] Spatial movement of an object may be interpreted erroneously when seen more dimly by one eye than by the other.

Ciliary Body

The ciliary body, which consists of the ciliary muscle and ciliary processes, has two main functions that are affected by cholinergic agents. One is accommodation, that is, focusing of the eye, and the other is an action on the aqueous outflow system, which facilitates aqueous outflow and reduces IOP. Both are muscular functions. Also, there are responses of the nonmuscular portions of the ciliary body to cholinergic agents, which are described subsequently.

Anticholinesterase agents slow enzymatic destruction of tonically released acetylcholine, and direct-acting cholinergic agents stimulate ciliary muscle muscarinic receptors. Cholinergic stimulation produces ciliary muscle contraction, resulting in accommodation. In humans, the near point of accommodation may move in 10 cm and the amount of minus lens that can be overcome may be increased by more than 4 D at distance, yet when the effort to accommodate is relaxed, the focus of the eye and the visual acuity at distance may rapidly return to normal.[40, 41] The rate and completeness of recovery appear to be dose dependent. With submaximal dosage, one can easily demonstrate an abnormal slowness in relaxation of accommodation. With maximal dosage, some accommodative myopia may persist even when no effort at accommodation is being made. Aching discomfort in the eye or forehead is commonly noted when a person looks at a near object after the application of cholinergic agents because of the enhanced contraction of the ciliary muscle, and this discomfort fades away when the person shifts the gaze to the distance.

The fact that cholinergic agents can potentiate accommodation and induce a temporary functional myopia has led some investigators, especially in Japan, to wonder if chronic exposure to anticholinesterase eye drops or insecticides might induce a persistent or chronic form of myopia based on some structural change. No convincing evidence has been produced, although there have been some intriguing observations. In an extensive retrospective study, Tamura and Mitsui[61] reported on the correlation between the incidence of myopia in 40,000 school-aged children and the use of organophosphate insecticides in the Tokushima Prefecture between 1957 and 1973. In that study, peak incidences of myopia occurred that coincided with the peak use of organophosphorous insecticides. In another study, refractive errors occurred in 88% of 71 children (4 to 16 years old) from rural areas of the Saku district who visited Asama Hospital compared with a 2% incidence of myopia in an age-matched control group of patients in Tokyo University Hospital.[62] It is not at all clear that the exposure of the children of the Saku region to anticholinesterase insecticides was of sufficient magnitude and duration to cause significant sustained accommodation. Furthermore, myopia has not been demonstrated to be a side effect in children who have been chronically treated with anticholinesterase medication for esotropia.[63, 64] However, recent experimental models of myopia have suggested that cholinergic nerves may play a role in the development of myopia. Abnormal eye growth (axial myopia) is restricted to the childhood years and apparently can be stimulated by manipulation of the visual environment. One hypothesis is that axial myopia is caused by excessive accommodation. Data supporting this hypothesis come from experiments with subhuman primates as well as with tree shrews. Young[65] found that restriction of the visual space of rhesus monkeys led to the development of axial myopia, which was reversed in part by the administration of atropine. Similarly, axial myopia induced by suturing the lids closed in tree shrews[66] and in rhesus (but not *Macaca acctoides*) monkeys[67] was prevented by atropine.

Other experimental findings in laboratory animals tend to support the possibility that an anticholinesterase-induced myopia can occur in young animals and may be mediated by pathologic changes of the ciliary muscle. Beagle dogs treated daily with oral ethylthiometon (5 to 20 mg/dog/day) or fenitrothion (10 to 20 mg/dog/day) for 2 years developed myopia and corneal astigmatism.[68, 69] The myopia was presumed to be due to pathologic changes in the ciliary muscle rather than elongation of the globe, since widespread destruction of the ciliary muscle fibers was present, whereas the axial length of the treated globes was not significantly different from that in control eyes. Anticholinesterase-induced changes in the ciliary muscle also occur in the subhuman primate eye. Daily topical treatment with clinically relevant doses of echothiophate iodide (as used in the treatment of glaucoma) to the young adult cynomolgus monkey eye resulted in swelling of the mitochondria and thickening of the basement membrane of the ciliary muscle after 2 months.[1, 2] However, although muscle degeneration became progressively more severe after 6 months of treatment, no sign of myopia was ever evident in the treated eyes.

Unrelated to the induction of myopia but of interest in respect to persistent changes in the ciliary muscle after exposure to anticholinesterases, the administration of echothiophate eye drops in monkeys for 2 to 6 months results in a subsensitivity of the accommodative mechanism in response to parenteral pilocarpine, associated with alterations in muscarinic receptors that can persist for several months.[70, 71] Interestingly, the accommodative response appeared to recover in spite of widespread damage to the ciliary muscle.

Both direct-acting and indirect-acting cholinergic agents reduce the outflow resistance in normal and glaucomatous eyes via contraction of the ciliary muscle. The precise mechanism by which contraction of the ciliary muscle reduces resistance to the outflow of aqueous humor has not yet been defined. In human and other primate eyes, the "scleral spur" to which the ciliary muscle is attached is intimately related to aqueous outflow channels. Severing the attachment of the ciliary muscle to the scleral spur prevents the change in resistance to aqueous outflow that normally occurs in response to parasympathetic innervation or to the action of cholinergic or anticholinesterase agents.[6] In excised eyes, with the attachment to the scleral spur intact, mechanically manipulating the ciliary muscle by pulling on the zonules attached to the lens reversibly reduces resistance to aqueous outflow. This can be prevented by detaching the ciliary muscle, suggesting that this resistance is subject to physical modulation and that it is the potentiation of contraction of ciliary muscle that is important in the treatment of glaucoma by means of cholinergic agents.[72] With continuing treatment there may be a decrease in the effectiveness of cholinergic agents with time.[73] Lütjen-Drecoll and Kaufman[1, 2] have described microscopic structural alterations that may account for a decrease in the effectiveness of cholinergic agents in the treatment of glaucoma.

Lens

Anticholinesterase drugs that are used as eye drops in the treatment of glaucoma can cause changes in the transparency of the crystalline lens, leading to a decrease in vision in some patients.[15] The first systematic study was reported by Axelsson and Holmberg,[74] followed by a series of related reports by Axelsson,[38, 75–79] de Roetth,[80–82] Shaffer and Hetherington,[83, 84] Cinotti and Patti,[85] Thoft,[86] Abraham and Teller,[87] Drance,[45] Levene,[88] Morton and colleagues,[89] and Nordmann and Gerhard.[90, 91] Most have agreed that careful slit-lamp examination of the lens after several months of daily administration of anticholinesterase eye drops reveals anterior and posterior subcapsular vacuoles or small opacities in about half the patients studied. Axelsson[77] has provided good evidence that glaucoma itself does not produce cataracts. The length of treatment and observation and the incidence of lens changes vary from one reporter to another, but it is generally accepted that anticholinesterase drugs, including echothiophate iodide, demecarium bromide, diethyl *p*-nitrophenyl phosphate (Paraoxon), and isoflurophate, produce a much higher incidence of anterior and posterior subcapsular changes than do pilocarpine or carbachol eye drops or than occurs in untreated controls. Not all observers have been wholly in agreement.[85–87] It appears that eyes that have been treated with pilocarpine before shifting to anticholinesterase eye drops are somewhat protected from the effects of anticholinesterases on the lens.[83, 84, 88, 90, 91] The reason for this is unknown. Also unexplained is the fact that some adult glaucoma patients are highly resistant to the adverse effect of anticholinesterase eye drops on their lenses and despite the daily use of drops of maximal concentration for years maintain normal visual acuity and normal transparency of their lenses.[45, 80, 81, 83, 84]

Axelsson[77] and others[45, 89, 92] have described the lens changes produced by anticholinesterase eye drops as typically consisting of minute anterior subcapsular vacuoles in groups, very small anterior subcapsular woolly or mossy opacities in aggregates, often associated with nuclear sclerosis, and posterior subcapsular small vacuoles or opacities. The anterior changes are easily seen but usually do not interfere with vision, whereas the posterior changes are more difficult to see, and they often reduce visual acuity. In some patients, cataract extraction has been necessary.

Age influences the susceptibility to the induction of lens changes by anticholinesterase eye drops. Susceptibility is highest in elderly persons, whereas children receiving the drops for the treatment of accommodative strabismus rarely show lens changes.[54, 93–97]

Anticholinesterase drugs administered orally in the treatment of myasthenia gravis do not produce lens changes, but miosis does usually not develop in this type of treatment; therefore, the dose reaching the eyes must be much less than that from eye drops of ordinary strength.[98]

A series of experiments with cynomolgus and vervet monkeys has been particularly interesting. Kaufman and Bárány[70] and Kaufman and colleagues[99] showed that the daily administration of 0.25% echothiophate eye drops produced anterior and posterior subcapsular opacities in 2.5 to 14.0 weeks, the anterior opacities reaching a maximum at 3.0 to 4.0 months, and the posterior after 1.5 to 3.0 months. Kaufman and Bárány[70] and Kaufman and colleagues[99, 100] found that when the iris was removed beforehand, more opacities resulted, but if eye drops containing atropine in addition to echothiophate iodide were used, the development of anterior and posterior opacities was delayed and the number was reduced. Experiments have been reported by Albrecht and Bárány[101] and Kaufman and associates[102] in which accommodation was eliminated by disinserting the ciliary muscle from the scleral spur before the daily administration of echothiophate eye drops. Eyes so treated developed anterior and posterior opacities similar to those in eyes with normal accommodation.

Albrecht and Bárány[101] and Philipson and coworkers[103] observed that besides subcapsular opacities, there was swelling of the anterior cortex of the lens in monkeys in response to the daily administration of echothiophate eye drops. These results are reminiscent of the increase in permeability of cultured rabbit lenses described by Michon and Kinoshita.[104]

Aqueous Humor

Although anticholinesterases reduce the IOP in both normal and glaucomatous eyes, as previously described in discussing the ciliary muscle, a paradoxical transitory increase in IOP may occur in some patients due to a breakdown of the blood-aqueous barrier. This initial pressure increase can be extreme in rabbits. Application of physostigmine, prostigmine, or isoflurophate to rabbit eyes initially causes hyperemia of the iris, a rise in IOP, and an increase in capillary permeability, allowing the entry of proteins from the blood sufficient to produce a strong flare in the aqueous humor.[105, 106] This may be a prostaglandin-mediated reaction.

Rabbits can be made tolerant to anticholinesterases by repeated application, to which their eyes respond more like primate eyes, with a reduction in IOP and no inflammatory signs.[105, 106]

In humans, an acute iritic or iridocyclitic reaction to anticholinesterase eye drops reminiscent of the initial reaction seen regularly in rabbits does occasionally occur.[40, 47]

Retina and Optic Nerve

A review by Alpar[107] lists case reports in which retinal detachment occurred after the initiation of treatment of glaucoma with miotics, especially with anticholinesterase miotics. However, retinal detachment has also been noted after treatment with shorter-acting miotics such as pilocarpine.[108, 109] Although suggestive, a cause-effect relationship between the treatment with strong miotics and retinal detachment has not been established.

No mention is made of retinal detachment in reports describing the sequelae of poisoning with organophosphorous agents. Similarly, retinal detachment has not been noted in studies in experimental animals, including those involving long-term (e.g., up to 6 months) daily administration of anticholinesterase to monkey eyes.[70, 71] Therefore, it is likely that anticholinesterase-induced retinal detachment occurs only in eyes in which retinal abnormality preexists.

The results of a survey of 91 retinal surgeons and examination of data obtained from the National Registry of Drug-Induced Ocular Side Effects strongly suggest the possibility of miotic-induced retinal detachment in patients with preexisting retinal abnormality, including high myopia, lattice degeneration of the retina, and a previous history of retinal detachment.[110]

Several studies of humans as well as experimental animals suggest that exposure to anticholinesterases may lead to acute alterations in the electrical properties of the retina. Alpern and Jampel[111] reported that topical application of 1% physostigmine resulted in a decrease in the critical flicker frequency in human subjects, which on the basis of pharmacologic experiments was hypothesized to be due to a cholinergic mechanism. Gazzard and Thomas[112] analyzed the threshold luminance of the central visual fields of human subjects after exposure to sarin vapor. Results indicated that sarin vapor raises the visual threshold, influencing cone more than rod function. Other studies have demonstrated sarin-induced elevation of the absolute scotopic threshold in human subjects.[113, 114]

Retinal pigmentary degeneration has been reported in two patients after documented exposure to organophosphate insecticides.[115] Misra and colleagues[116] have also reported on the high incidence (22% of a sample population of 64) of macular degeneration among workers engaged in the spraying of organophosphate insecticides in India. The results of fluorescein angiography suggest that the macular lesions were due to a defect in the pigment epithelium. However, in that study, no information was provided with regard to whether or not the workers were also exposed to the antimalarial drug chloroquine that is known for its toxicity to the retinal pigment epithelium.

Toxic retinopathy has not been noted in the thousands of individuals who have received topical anticholinesterase treatment for glaucoma or esotropia. Although one could argue that retinal damage might not be differentiated from the disease process itself in glaucoma, this is certainly not the case in esotropia. Extensive reviews of the literature presented no evidence for retinal pathology in children treated for accommodative esotropia.[63, 64] Collectively, the weight of evidence suggests that the effect of sustained inhibition of cholinesterase per se is limited to acute alterations of the electrical properties of the retina with no long-term abnormality. However, several organophosphate compounds have other pharmacologic activity. For example, some organophosphates are capable of inhibiting esterases other than cholinesterase.[117] A spontaneous retinal degeneration is known to occur in the *rd* mouse owing to increased turnover of retinal cyclic guanosine monophosphate (cGMP) phosphodiesterase.[118] Phosphodiesterase inhibitors produce changes in the electroretinogram of the isolated perfused cat eye that are similar to electroretinogram abnormalities found in individuals with hereditary retinitis pigmentosa.[119] Collectively, these studies suggest the theoretical possibility that anticholinesterase-induced retinal degeneration could result if substantial inhibition of cGMP phosphodiesterase occurred in addition to cholinesterase inhibition.

SYSTEMIC TOXICITY

Acute poisoning with anticholinesterase agents produces the cholinergic crisis syndrome consisting of sweating, gastrointestinal disturbances, bradycardia, and paralysis of respiratory muscles.

Acute poisoning with direct-acting muscarinic agonists can also be life threatening and involves the cardiovascular system but not the diaphragm. The incidence of acute toxicity associated with the repeated application of pilocarpine eye drops, which consists of sweating, salivation, nausea, tremor, and decreased blood pressure, is reviewed by Grant.[15]

Delayed peripheral neurotoxicity from organophosphorous esters has been a well-known clinical entity for over 50 years, particularly from the contamination of food or drink by tri-*ortho*-cresyl phosphate. The anticholinesterases diisopropyl fluorophosphate and mipafox have caused delayed neurotoxicity involving axonal degeneration with secondary demyelination without clinically evident involvement of the eyes.[120, 121]

Caution should be exercised in the use of cholinergic agents in patients with asthma. The administration of pilocarpine in the subconjunctival sac has been associated with reports of bronchoconstriction in patients with asthma.[122, 123]

Adrenergic Agonists

Nonselective adrenergic agonists, such as epinephrine, stimulate both α- and β-adrenergic receptors. They exert their therapeutic effect on IOP by reducing aqueous outflow resistance. Although adrenergic agonists have been used in the treatment of POAG for over 100 years, the site of action of the outflow resistance–decreasing effect is unknown. The mechanism of action is through stimulation of the β-adrenergic receptors.[7–11] Adrenergic receptors are found on almost all ocular tissues, and adrenergic agonists are known to affect a number of ocular physiologic parameters, including smooth muscle tone in the iris and ciliary body, aqueous humor production, and intraorbital and extraorbital vascular tone. The incidence of cardiovascular stimulation after topical ocular treatment is a potential major side effect that limits the therapeutic use of epinephrine. The prodrug formulation dipivefrin has allowed smaller doses of epinephrine to be administered, limiting the risk of adverse systemic effects (Table 41–3).

TABLE 41–3. **Side Effects Associated With the Use of Adrenergic Drugs in the Treatment of Primary Open-Angle Glaucoma**

Ocular Side Effects	Systemic Side Effects
Epinephrine and Dipivefrin	
Ocular Side Effects	Systemic Side Effects
Allergic contact sensitivity of the cornea, conjunctiva, and lids	Hypertension
Adrenomelanin deposits	Heart palpitations
Pseudopemphigoid	Ventricular arrhythmia
Macular abnormalities	Cerebral hemorrhage
Apraclonidine and Brimonidine	
Ocular Side Effects	Systemic Side Effects
Hyperemia	Oral dryness
Burning and stinging	Headache
Blurred visual acuity	Fatigue and drowsiness
Foreign body sensation	Upper respiratory symptoms
Conjunctival follicles	Dizziness
Allergic reactions	Gastrointestinal symptoms
Pruritus	Asthenia
Corneal staining or erosion	Muscular pain
Photophobia	Abnormal taste
Eyelid erythema	Insomnia
Ocular ache or pain	Depression
Dryness	Hypertension
Tearing	Anxiety
Eyelid edema	Palpitations
Conjunctival edema	Nasal dryness
Blepharitis	Abdominal pain
Irritation	Diarrhea
Conjunctival blanching	Stomach discomfort
Abnormal vision	Emesis
Lid crusting	Bradycardia
Conjunctival hemorrhage	Vasovagal attack
Conjunctival discharge	Peripheral arrhythmia
Syncope	Somnolence
Upper lid elevation	Dream disturbance
Mydriasis	Irritability
Itching	Decreased libido
Hypotony	Paresthesia

OCULAR SIDE EFFECTS

Cornea and Conjunctiva

Frequently, patients develop allergic contact sensitivity to epinephrine characterized by itching and burning, epiphora, and hyperemia of the conjunctiva and lids.[15] Other conjunctival or scleral abnormalities include adrenomelanin deposits due to the accumulation of metabolic products of epinephrine. Whereas benign and symptomless, they resemble a malignant melanoma.[124] In the case of preexisting epithelial defects, a similar corneal discoloration, "black cornea," can occur.[15] The occurrence of dacryoliths has also been attributed to the build-up of epinephrine breakdown products after chronic topical treatment with 1% epinephrine.[125] Actual epithelial toxicity is rare. However, several reports of corneal and conjunctival epithelial toxicity, including pseudopemphigoid, have been summarized by Grant[15] and others.[20, 21]

Drug preservatives themselves can have toxicity. The corneal endothelium appears to be susceptible to commercial preparations of epinephrine. Intracameral epinephrine, containing bisulfate, has occasionally resulted in corneal endothelial swelling when administered during anterior chamber surgery. However, epinephrine without the bisulfate preservative does not produce significant swelling in an in vitro perfusion system. It is noted that the commercial preparation of epinephrine causes increased corneal thickness and loss of corneal endothelial cells.[126] There is evidence that some of the clinically observed toxicity may be mediated by the drug preservative benzalkonium chloride[127] or by the antioxidant bisulfite contained in the commercial preparation.[128] The long-term use of epinephrine drops containing preservative caused a slight decrease in the number of corneal endothelial cells. However, the number stayed within the normal range.[129] Dipivefrin-induced abnormalities have also been noted and include symblepharon,[130] conjunctival shrinkage,[130] and follicular conjunctivitis.[131, 132]

Aqueous Humor Outflow Pathway Tissues and the Ciliary Body

In in vitro studies, epinephrine in clinically relevant doses was toxic to trabecular cells.[133] In contrast, examination of the outflow pathway tissue of normal cynomolgus monkey eyes after 6 months of topical treatment with epinephrine revealed no apparent toxicity to the outflow pathway tissues.[4] However, the ciliary muscle appeared to be displaced anteriorly, narrowing the chamber angle. Also, changes in the ciliary processes consistent with hypersecretion were noted in some sections and hyposecretion in others.[3]

Experimentally, epinephrine dramatically reduces blood flow to the ciliary processes in the cynomolgus monkey[134] and the albino rat[135] but not to the ciliary muscle[134] as observed by a functional resin-casting method. Similar results were noted using radioactive microspheres in the albino rabbit eye, in which 2% epinephrine administered topically three times a day over a 5- to 6-week period resulted in decreased blood flow to the iris and ciliary processes but not to the posterior uvea or optic nerve head.[136]

Retina

As reviewed by Grant,[15] epinephrine-induced retinal toxicity was not recognized until the 1960s. A reduction in visual acuity can occur with the long-term administration of epinephrine. Generally, the reduction in visual acuity is reversible within several months.

Chronic topical treatment with epinephrine is associated with the development of various macular abnormalities. Acute macular neuroretinopathy has been reported to occur immediately after intravenous infusion of sympathomimetics, presumably caused by acute hypertension or to a direct retinal effect.[137] Retinal and choroidal blood flow as measured by laser Doppler methods is decreased by topically applied 2% epinephrine, which may be the mechanism underlying epinephrine-induced maculopathy.[138] However, when it was administered intravenously (1 to 10 mg/kg), an increase in blood flow was noted coincident with the elevation in systemic blood pressure. Further support for a causative role for epinephrine in macular edema comes experimentally from a study using pigmented rabbits. Topical administration of 1.5% epinephrine three times a day resulted in a breakdown of the blood-aqueous and blood-retinal barriers 2 to 3 months after the initiation of treatment, which could be blocked by coadministration of indomethacin, as measured by aqueous and vitreous fluorophotometry.[139] However, a study by the same authors in patients with glaucoma revealed that daily topical treatment with epinephrine resulted in a blood-aqueous barrier breakdown, blockable with indomethacin, but no change in blood-retinal barrier function.[140] The influence of epinephrine on prostaglandin synthesis is evident in the eye. Chronic treatment with epinephrine was associated with elevated prostaglandin E levels in both the aqueous and vitreous humors in rabbit eyes after 5 months of treatment.[141]

SYSTEMIC TOXICITY

Much has been written about the incidence of hypertension and heart palpitations after the administration of topical epinephrine. An extensive review is presented by Grant.[15] Additional caution is necessary when epinephrine is employed in combination with a local anesthetic, such as occurs in the course of otolaryngologic procedures. Additionally, if a patient is taking β-blockers, the possibility of serious complications resulting from additional epinephrine results.[142] What is sometimes observed is a hypertensive crisis that is immediately followed by cardiac slowing and possible cardiac arrest. Despite the potential for adverse cardiovascular effects, the use of intraocular epinephrine has become standard practice in cataract surgery, and no untoward effects on the cardiovascular system have been noted.[143–145]

Adrenergic β-Receptor–Blocking Drugs

The β-blockers timolol, betaxolol, and levobunolol are widely used in the treatment of primary open-angle glaucoma. Both timolol and levobunolol are nonselective β-blockers (e.g., they bind β_1- and β_2-receptors with nearly equal affinity). Betaxolol is somewhat selective for the β_1-receptor. More recently, carteolol has been introduced into the medical treatment of glaucoma. Carteolol is a nonselective β-blocker that also has some intrinsic sympathomimetic activity (ISA).

Much has been written about the tendency of β-blockers to cause cardiovascular and respiratory problems.[15, 146, 147] Theoretically, the selectivity of a β-blocker for β_1- or β_2-receptors would make it a better choice for use in patients with asthma and cardiovascular insufficiency, respectively. However, the drugs currently in use do not have a selectivity sufficient to prevent their binding of all β-receptors at therapeutic concentrations.

In addition to receptor selectivity, several other pharmacologic parameters determine the profile of side effects associated with a given β-blocker. β-Blockers with some ISA, such as carteolol, pindolol, acebutolol, and penbutolol, are less likely to cause cardiovascular insufficiency, bronchospasm, or adverse changes in serum lipids.[148] The degree of lipid solubility should influence how much drug needs to be given topically to reach therapeutic levels in the anterior chamber. Also, the degree of plasma protein binding influences how much free drug is available to the systemic circulation. β-Blockers also differ in their activity as membrane-stabilizing (and anesthetic) agents. All these factors influence the degree of local and systemic toxicity.

A recent area of investigation has involved the development of prodrugs of timolol and levobunolol that might allow greater corneal permeability; therefore, the required topical dose of drug could be reduced, minimizing possible systemic toxicity (Table 41–4).[149, 150] Timoptic-XE (a formulation of timolol that forms a gel on contact with the ocular surface) administered once a day was shown to be equally effective in lowering IOP as the equivalent concentration of topical timolol administered twice a day. The safety profile is similar to that of equivalent concentrations of timolol.[151]

TABLE 41–4. **Side Effects Associated With the Use of β-Blockers in the Treatment of Primary Open-Angle Glaucoma**

Ocular Side Effects
Reduction in tear production
Reduction in tear breakup time
Transient corneal irritation
Corneal anesthesia
Possible toxicity to corneal endothelium
Cataractogenesis
Changes in retinal blood flow
Cystoid macular edema
Choroidal detachment
Systemic Side Effects
Bronchial constriction
Cardiovascular effects (bradycardia, decreased cardiac contractility, prolongation of atrioventricular conduction)
Increased serum lipid levels
Alopecia
Arthropathy
Exacerbation of myasthenia gravis
Central nervous system effects (depression, sexual dysfunction, emotional lability)
Psoriasis

OCULAR SIDE EFFECTS

The most frequent ocular complaint with the administration of β-blockers is transient discomfort. Timoptic-XE has a higher incidence of transient blurred vision (30%) than timolol owing to the physical characteristics of the formulation.[151] A factor that may influence corneal irritation is the degree of membrane stabilization of the β-blocker; those producing less corneal desensitization causing less corneal irritation. However, other potentially more serious complications have been noted. The pattern of intraocular side effects may be mediated in part by the pigment-binding characteristics of the β-blockers.[152] Those drugs that bind more avidly to pigment may produce an enhanced toxicity due to the build-up of a substantial drug reservoir within the eye.

Lacrimal Apparatus

There have been reports of timolol-induced reduction in tear secretion, causing discomfort sufficient to stop treatment.[153] Systemic administration of β-blockers to rabbits, including metoprolol, betaxolol, butoxamine, timolol, propranolol, and oxprenolol, reduced tear production with all drugs tested. However, the reduction was less with the β_1-selective betaxolol, implicating a role of the β_2-receptor in tear production.[154] Further, with the exception of levobunolol,[155, 156] β-blockers, including timolol, metipranolol, befunolol, bupranolol, carteolol, pindolol, and betaxolol, also reduce tear break-up time.[155–157]

Conjunctiva

One case of conjunctival leukoplakia has been observed in a patient with glaucoma treated with topical metipranolol.[158]

There have also been rare reports of betaxolol-induced conjunctivitis.[159] Long-term therapy with timolol has not been associated with any conjunctival abnormality.[160] Timoptic-XE has been shown to be associated with conjunctivitis in 1 to 5% of patients.[151]

Cornea

There are conflicting reports on the occurrence of corneal anesthesia with chronic topical treatment of β-blockers. The propensity for causing corneal anesthesia appears to relate to the membrane-stabilizing properties of some of the β-blockers. In one study, decreased corneal sensitivity was not noted in patients treated with timolol, levobunolol, and betaxolol. Similarly, only a slight reduction in corneal sensitivity was noted in patients with glaucoma treated with timolol compared with pretreatment measurements.[161] However, there are apparently patients who are more responsive to the occurrence of corneal anesthesia than others.[162] Carteolol, a relatively newly introduced β-blocker with ISA, appears to lower IOP as effectively as timolol.[163–165] Carteolol does not appear to have anesthetic properties,[166] which may explain a lower incidence of ocular irritation.[165]

A number of studies have documented the toxicity of β-blockers to the ultrastructure of corneal epithelial cells after chronic topical administration.[167–169] Timolol seems to be more toxic than other topical β-blockers. In one study, a delay in reepithelization after corneal ulcer was noted with β-blocker administration. The results of this study showed that betaxolol was less toxic to rabbit cornea than timolol or levobunolol.[169] Similarly, a second study showed that reepithelization of rabbit cornea after abradement was slower with timolol than with betaxolol, and that at the twentieth day, plasma membrane defects were noted in the timolol group but not in the betaxolol group.[167]

β-Blockers reactivate latent herpes simplex virus type 1 corneal ulcers in rabbit and mouse eyes.[170, 171]

Changes in the morphology and physiology of the corneal endothelium have been noted after the administration of β-blockers. However, there have been conflicting reports on the toxicity of β-blocker administration to the corneal endothelium. In one study, the thickness of human corneas increased after 3 days of topical timolol administration.[172] In a second study, 8 months of topical treatment of the rat eye with 0.5% timolol, 1% befunolol, or 2% carteolol resulted in degeneration of the ultrastructure of the endothelium with both befunolol and timolol, whereas changes with carteolol were minimal.[173] There is some thought that topical drug-induced corneal toxicity might be due to the benzalkonium chloride present in the drug vehicle. Alanko and Airaksinen[174] and Nesher and coworkers[175] independently reported that no changes in corneal thickness or endothelial cell density were noted at either 2 weeks[174] or 60 weeks[175] in patients topically treated with timolol or vehicle compared with baseline values[176] or an external control group.[177] In contrast, Brubaker and colleagues[176] found a 6% decrease in endothelial cell density after 1 year of topical timolol treatment.

Lens

A possible cataractogenesis due to topical β-blocker treatment has been discussed. However, no evidence for transparency changes or energy metabolism were noted after chronic topical treatment of the rabbit eye with daily timolol, betaxolol, or befunolol for 2 months.[177] In contrast, postmortem examination of rabbit eyes chronically treated with timolol revealed a cocataractogenic potential for timolol and befunolol in animal models of ultraviolet[178, 179] and diabetic[178] cataract development. In humans, there have been isolated reports of timolol-induced cataractogenesis after long-term treatment with timolol.[15]

Ciliary Body

Toxicity of β-blockers to the ciliary body has not been noted clinically. However, several reports in experimental animal models have described morphologic changes to the ciliary body after β-blocker administration. Mitochondrial swelling was noted in the ciliary epithelium 30 minutes and 1 hour after topical application of timolol or befunolol to albino and pigmented rabbit eyes.[180, 181] Of considerable interest is the observation that 3 to 6 months of daily topical treatment with timolol resulted in changes in the ciliary processes in cynomolgus monkey eyes. These changes included narrowed stromal vessels, with few fenestrations, surrounded by a thickened fiber sheath; thickened pigmented epithelium basement membrane; few pigmented epithelium and nonpigmented epithelium infoldings; flattened nonpigmented epithelium with small mitochondria; and the presence of pigmented granules and large phagolysosomes in the nonpigmented epithelium.[3] In the same eyes, timolol also produced changes in the trabecular meshwork and ciliary muscle. The changes included focal degenerations of the trabecular meshwork endothelium, destruction of the central core of the lamellae, and a densification and collapse of the meshwork. The ciliary muscle was pulled inwardly, the intramuscular spaces were widened, and the shape of Schlemm's canal was altered.[4]

Retina and Optic Nerve Head

β-Adrenergic receptors are present in the human retinal pigmented epithelium in vitro. Stimulation of these receptors leads to cyclic adenosine monophosphate accumulation and alters the retinal pigmented epithelium–mediated electric current.[182] Intravitreal injection of 10μL of 1% befunolol into the vitreous chamber of rabbit eyes resulted in acute flattening of the retinal pigmented epithelium, atrophy of the microvilli, opening of basal infoldings, swollen mitochondria, decreases in the smooth endoplasmic recticulum, and marked vacuolization with recovery within 5 days of injection.[183] In a second study, twice-daily topical application of 1% befunolol to the rabbit eye for 3 to 6 months resulted in decreased microvilli, swollen mitochondria, accumulation of phagolysosomes and lipofuscin granules, and degeneration of the outer segments of the photoreceptors. These degenerative changes were reversible within 6 months of drug washout.[184] These morphologic alterations may relate to changes noted in retinal function with application of β-blockers. The β-adrenergic antagonists timolol, propranolol, and ICI 118551 caused a reversible reduction in the b-wave of the dark-adapted cat eye.[185] However, the significance of these findings to the human situation is unknown.

The ocular pulse pressure is affected differently by β-blockers. Two percent carteolol reduced the pulse pressure, whereas 0.5% timolol and 0.5% betaxolol had no effect on the pulse pressure, and levobunolol (0.5%) significantly increased the ocular pulse amplitude.[186]

The retinal circulation is affected by β-blocker administration. As measured by fluorescein angiography, timolol decreased the arteriovenous passage time and the dye bolus velocity in normal human subjects, implying that timolol increased retinal perfusion.[187] Similarly, topical timolol increased the blood flow rate in the retinas of normotensive and hypertensive human eyes as measured by bidirectional laser Doppler velocimetry and monochromatic fundus photography.[188–190] These changes in retinal blood flow are maintained for at least a 2-week period of chronic topical treatment.[191] These measured changes in retinal blood flow may relate to isolated reports of β-blocker–induced cystoid macular edema.[192]

Choroidal detachment due to β-blocker–induced hypotony has also been noted in eyes after postfiltration surgery with the administration of subsequent topical[193] or oral β-blockers.[194]

Systemic Toxicity

The ocular administration of β-blockers results in rapid systemic absorption of the drugs in sufficient quantities to affect the heart and the lungs.[195] Early clinical trials showed timolol to be without serious systemic side effects. However, as summarized by Nelson and colleagues,[196] many of these early studies did not include patients with underlying cardiovascular or respiratory problems. As of 1985, the U.S. Food and Drug Administration and the National Registry of Drug-Induced Ocular Side Effects have tabulated a total of 450 case reports of serious cardiovascular or respiratory complications, 32 of which resulted in death, after the administration of topical timolol. Of the 212 patients for which a medical history was provided, 92% had either cardiovascular or respiratory problems.[196] Therefore, a careful medical history is necessary before prescribing topical β-blockers for the treatment of glaucoma in order to eliminate the possibility of exacerbating an underlying condition.

In addition to the contraindications noted later, β-blockers should not be used in combination with calcium channel blockers, since sudden death has been reported after the systemic administration of a β-blocker and verapamil.[197, 198]

Bronchial Tract

β-Blockers cause bronchial constriction as a consequence of binding to β_2-receptors in the bronchi. β-blockers that are nonselective (such as timolol) may compromise ventilation in patients with obstructive lung disease, asthma, or bronchospasm. The National Registry of Drug-Induced Ocular Side Effects has received over 200 reports of topical timolol–induced respiratory problems. Sixteen fatal attacks of status asthmaticus have occurred after the application of topical timolol.[20]

β_1-Selective antagonists like betaxolol are expected to have less effect on respiratory function. For example, the expiratory volume was lowered and the airway resistance raised in patients with glaucoma after topical ocular treatment with the nonselective antagonist metipranolol but not with the β_1-selective antagonist pindolol.[199] Similarily, betaxolol, a β_1-selective blocker, lowers IOP to therapeutically acceptable levels but apparently has less effect on pulmonary function than timolol.[200, 201] In general, betaxolol is well tolerated in patients with underlying obstructive lung disease.[202–205] However, betaxolol has only a limited selectivity, and the therapeutic intraocular dose may actually be high enough to bind both β_1- and β_2-receptors.[206] Similarly, high concentrations may be achieved systemically so that binding of both β_1- and β_2-receptors occurs. Further, there is some indication that there are a substantial number of β_1-type receptors in the lung that may be coupled to airway constriction.[207] Finally, there have been scattered reports of respiratory problems after the use of topical betaxolol.[208–211] Collectively, these observations dictate that caution should be exercised even with the use of selective β_1-antagonists in patients with respiratory disease, a view that is shared by other authors who have reviewed the literature.[210, 212]

Cardiovascular System

Cardiovascular effects of β-blockers include decreases in the cardiac rate, contractility, and prolongation of atrioventricular conduction. Because of their cardiovascular effects, the use of β-blockers is contraindicated in patients with congestive heart failure, severe bradycardia, and high-grade atrioventricular block.[207] Topical timolol caused a reduction in the maximal heart rate and the time to exhaustion in healthy young subjects during a maximal exercise treadmill evaluation.[213] In another study, timolol decreased the resting and maximal exercise heart rate after the first dose and the maximal exercise heart rate with repeated dosing.[214] Topical timolol has been associated with serious cardiac decompensation when used in the treatment of glaucoma.[196] Although betaxolol is β_1 selective, it was thought to be an "oculoselective drug" owing to its high lipid solubility and its affinity for binding to plasma proteins.[215] However, instances of potentially dangerous cardiac decompensation associated with the use of topical betaxolol have been reported.[210, 216, 217] It appears that the β-blockers with ISA are associated with fewer cardiovascular problems. In one study, befunolol (which has ISA) was administered topically to patients with glaucoma for 1 week. No significant changes in the mean, maximal, and minimal blood pressure, heart rate, or PR intervals compared with baseline values were noted as measured by continuous electrocardiographic recording.[218]

Serum Lipids

β-Adrenergic antagonists adversely affect the serum lipid profile in patients who receive oral medical therapy for hypertension. Although one study did not document any changes after 1 year of timolol treatment,[219] a recent study designed to test the effect of topical ocular application of 0.5% timolol on serum lipids showed that after 76 days of timolol treatment, the high-density lipoprotein levels were lowered and plasma triglyceride levels were increased relative to baseline measurements.[220]

Alopecia

The National Registry of Drug-Induced Ocular Side Effects has reported 56 cases of hair loss after topical ocular administration of timolol, betaxolol, and levobunolol. Ninety percent of the instances involved females. Hair regrowth occurs after withdrawal of the β-blocker.[221]

Musculoskeletal System

Arthropathy has been reported to occur after the systemic administration of β-blockers. In one report, arthropathy occurred bilaterally to the knees of a 61-year-old woman after the initiation of topical timolol therapy for POAG.[222]

There have been reports of a worsening of myasthenia gravis with systemic β-blocker administration.[223–225] Isolated instances of exacerbation of myasthenia gravis have also been reported after topical timolol therapy.

Central Nervous System

Topical β-blockers have been associated with central nervous system side effects, including depression, sexual dysfunction, and emotional lability.[226–233] There is some evidence that the incidence and severity of these effects may be lower with the selective β_1-blocker betaxolol.[224, 234] However, at least one case report documents the occurrence of betaxolol-induced severe depression.[235]

Skin

Several reports have indicated the occurrence of psoriasis after the initiation of medical therapy with β-blockers.[236–239] In one report, psoriasis was associated with topical ocular timolol application.[240]

Adrenergic α-Receptor Blocking Drugs

Clonidine is a relatively selective α_2-adrenergic agonist that is used clinically as an antihypertensive agent. The hypotensive effect is mediated by the activation of α_2-receptors in the central nervous system.[241] Topically, clonidine reduces IOP[242–246] and aqueous humor flow.[247] It is thought to act by binding α_2-receptors in the ciliary body that inhibit adenylate cyclase.[248] Apraclonidine is a *p*-amino derivative of clonidine, which is incapable of penetrating the blood-brain barrier. Therefore, the use of topical apraclonidine should prevent the systemic hypotension that can occur with the use of topical clonidine. Apraclonidine is as effective as clonidine in lowering IOP[249, 250] and has seen use clinically in preventing the large elevations in IOP that occur after argon laser iridotomy,[251, 252] argon laser trabeculoplasty,[252, 253] and neodymium-yttrium-aluminum-garnet posterior capsulotomy.[252, 254] There are indications of possible usefulness in the treatment of POAG,[255, 256] particularly when a patient on maximally tolerated medical therapy is awaiting surgery. Long-term use of apraclonidine requires frequent monitoring due to the frequent occurrence of tachyphylaxis. Brimonidine, an α_2-adrenergic agonist that is 10-fold more selective than apraclonidine, also binds to imidazoline receptors. It functions similarly to apraclonidine, by reducing aqueous inflow and uvealscleral flow. Brimonidine (0.5%) was developed for post–argon laser iridotomy and (0.2%) for glaucoma treatment.[257] The advantage of brimonidine over apraclonidine is that there appears to be a lower incidence of allergic reaction and tachyphylaxis does not occur.

OCULAR SIDE EFFECTS

Possible ocular side effects of clonidine or apraclonidine may relate to their effects on hemodynamics. Clonidine constricts episcleral and fundal vessels in rabbits and minipigs. Additionally, in minipigs, a 2-second delay was seen in the filling of retinal vessels after intravenous injection, suggestive of vasoconstriction upstream from the retinal vessels.[258] In adult humans, the ocular perfusion pressure is decreased bilaterally after unilateral topical application of 0.125% clonidine. However, the decrease to the treated eye is greater, suggesting a local as well as a systemic effect on hemodynamics.[259] Additional ocular side effects of apraclonidine in 1% of patients include conjunctival blanching, upper lid elevation, mydriasis, burning, a foreign body sensation, hypotony, and blurred vision acuity.[260]

Treatment with brimonidine induced ocular hyperemia, burning and stinging, blurring, a foreign body sensation, conjunctival follicles, ocular puntis, and ocular allergic reaction in 10 to 30% of patients. Less common side effects include corneal erosion, photophobia, eyelid erythema, ocular pain, dryness, tearing, edema, blepharitis, and abnormal vision.[257]

The IOP-lowering effects of brimonidine are comparable to those of timolol, without contraindications in cardiopulmonary disease, and the allergic response is significantly less than that with apraclonidine (12.7% versus 23%).[261–266]

SYSTEMIC SIDE EFFECTS

Caution should be exercised in the use of clonidine to avoid systemic toxicity, especially in children. A recent report documented clonidine poisoning in a 2-year-old after the child ingested clonidine from a discarded patch used as an aid in smoking cessation.[267]

To date, it appears that apraclonidine obviates much of the systemic toxicity of clonidine. A number of studies have demonstrated minimal if any effects of apraclonidine on the resting heart rate or mean arterial blood pressure when applied locally to the eye.[220, 251–255, 268, 269]

Some of the systemic side effects that have occurred in less than 1% of patients include abdominal pain, diarrhea, stomach discomfort, emesis, dry mouth, bradycardia, vasovagal attack, palpitations, asthenia, peripheral arrhythmia, insomnia, somnolence, dizziness, dream disturbance, irritability, decreased libido, paresthesia, headache, and taste abnormalities.

Carbonic Anhydrase Inhibitors

Inhibition of carbonic anhydrase in the ciliary processes of the eye reduces aqueous humor secretion, presumably by slowing the formation of bicarbonate ions with a subsequent reduction in sodium and fluid transport. The result is a reduction in IOP.[270]

Acetazolamide (Diamox) has been used in the treatment of glaucoma. It has been administered orally on account of the inability of the compound or other carbonic anhydrase inhibitors such as methazolamide, ethoxzolamide, and dichlorphenamide to cross the cornea.[271] Even though systemically administered carbonic anhydrase inhibitors are effective in lowering IOP, the constellation of side effects associated with their use has limited the clinical usefulness of carbonic anhydrase inhibitors in the treatment of glaucoma (Table 41–5).

Recently, as summarized by Podos and Serle,[272] three derivatives of acetazolamide that are permeable to the cornea have been introduced. They are effective in reducing the IOP with systemic drug levels too low to produce systemic side effects.[273] Most literature concerns the effects of MK-927.[274–284] There is some evidence that MK-417, the enantiomer of MK-927, is slightly more effective in lowering the IOP with multiple-dose administration to patients with glaucoma.[283] Finally, early results with a third derivative, MK-507, suggest that it may be longer lasting than the other two derivatives.[284]

Dorzolamide has been developed as a long-awaited carbonic anhydrase inhibitor that can be administered topically rather than systemically. It inhibits carbonic anhydrase type II, reduces the IOP by 21.8% (b.i.d.) to 26.2% (t.i.d.), and is used alone or as an adjunctive therapy. Although it is administered topically, the potential for systemic absorption exists. Therefore, its use is contraindicated with oral carbonic anhydrase inhibitors.[270]

TABLE 41–5. **Side Effects Associated With the Use of Carbonic Anhydrase Inhibitors in the Treatment of Primary Open-Angle Glaucoma**

Oral

Ocular Side Effects
- Acute myopia
- Increased corneal thickness after cataract extraction

Systemic Side Effects
- Paresthesia
- Fatigue
- Weight loss
- Anorexia
- Impotence
- Depression
- Blood dyscrasias (thrombocytopenia, agranulocytosis, aplastic anemia)
- Respiratory difficulties
- Osteomalacia
- Rash
- Alopecia

Topical

Ocular Side Effects
- Burning and stinging
- Superficial punctate keratitis
- Blurred vision
- Tearing
- Dryness
- Photophobia
- Iridocyclitis
- Transient myopia
- Postmarketing hypersensitivity
- Allergic sensitivity

Systemic Side Effects
- Bitter taste
- Headache
- Nausea
- Fatigue
- Skin rash
- Urolithiasis
- Dizziness
- Paresthesia

OCULAR TOXICITY

The incidence of ocular toxicity with orally administered acetazolamide is rare. In rare cases, acute myopia is noted.[15] Typically, it occurs within 4 hours to 5 days of initiating therapy. Usually, there is a history of previously taking the medication, and the myopia occurs when treatment is resumed. It is doubtful that a contraction of the ciliary muscle mediates the myopia, since the myopia is not relieved by atropine. It is thought that an alteration of the hydration of the lens and the resulting change in refractive power could underlie the myopia. In almost all cases, the myopia is reversible within 2 days of discontinuing treatment.[15] In rare instances, the myopia has been more complicated. Further details can be found in reviews by Grant[15] and Berson.[285]

Although possible toxicity to the lens due to the reduced formation of aqueous humor was formerly a concern, no increased frequency of cataracts has been noted.[15] Similarly, although preexisting corneal abnormalities may predispose the cornea to acetazolamide-mediated thickening after cataract extraction, patients with normal corneas show no adverse effects of acetazolamide.[15] Finally, routine clinical testing reveals no abnormalities in retinal function. However, there have been reports of altered parameters as measured by the electroretinogram. Stanescu and Michels[286] reported increased b-wave amplitude and Yonemura[287] and Missotten and coworkers[288] have reported decreases in the dark component of the standing potential. Whether the relative lack of toxicity will be observed with topical administration should become evident within the next few years.

The most common ocular side effects of dorzolamide include ocular burning and stinging in 33% of patients, superficial punctate keratitis in 10 to 15%, an allergic reaction in 10%, and blurred vision, tearing, dryness and photophobia in 1 to 5%.[270]

SYSTEMIC SIDE EFFECTS

Oral administration of acetazolamide and dorzolamide results in side effects that range from minimal discomfort to life threatening. Detailed reviews of systemic toxicity have been published.[15, 279] A brief outline of systemic complications follows.

Paresthesias

Paresthesia consisting of a tingling in the extremities or the face occurs commonly with acetazolamide treatment. However, it is transient and is generally not severe enough to discontinue treatment. Paresthesias occur in less than 1% of patients after dorzolamide treatment.[270]

Malaise Syndrome

Of greater consequence is the malaise syndrome consisting of fatigue, weight loss, anorexia, impotence, and depression. It is this side effect that most often causes the patient to discontinue treatment.[289] The malaise syndrome is probably a consequence of acidosis, which can be relieved by treatment with sodium bicarbonate and titration of the drug dosage.[15, 289] Caution is necessary in patients with renal insufficiency or diseases affecting the urinary tract, as these patients are susceptible to excessive blood levels of acetazolamide with resulting severe acidosis.[290, 291] Cotreatment with salicylates is also contraindicated, since the combination of salicylates and acetazolamide can produce a serious acidosis.[15]

Blood Dyscrasias

The most serious side effect of acetazolamide is the rare but life-threatening occurrence of blood dyscrasias. Thrombocytopenia, agranulocytosis, and aplastic anemia have all been reported. There is controversy as to whether routine blood monitoring is useful in the early detection of blood dyscrasias. Although some authors have deemed such monitoring necessary,[20] others feel that it would be of no value, since the dyscrasias that occur are not dose related and are of an idiosyncratic nature.[292] Grant[15] points out that most of the blood dyscrasia results from an acute immunologic sensitivity reaction. The collective consensus among ophthalmologists appears to be that routine blood chemistry studies would not predict this complication.[15, 293]

Other Systemic Side Effects

Other complications resulting from oral acetazolamide use include respiratory difficulties in patients with chronic obstructive lung disease; osteomalacia with bone demineralization; skin rashes; and hair loss or excessive hair growth. Several studies have reported on the teratogenesis of acetazolamide in laboratory animals. The teratogenic potential in humans is unknown.

Most of the systemic side effects that occur with oral carbonic anhydrase inhibitors apparently do not occur with topical dorzolamide. However, treatment with dorzolamide resulted in a bitter taste in 25% of patients, and headache, nausea, fatigue, skin rashes, urolithiasis, and dizziness in less than 1%. Because dorzolamide and its metabolites are excreted predominantly by the kidneys, it is not recommended for use in patients with renal failure. In addition, dorzolamide is contraindicated in patients with an allergy to sulfa drugs.[270]

Prostaglandins

Prostaglandins were discovered in the eye in the course of a search for mediators of ocular inflammation. Prostaglandins D_2, E_2, and $F_{2\alpha}$ are synthesized by ocular tissues[294] and are actively transported out of the eye.[295] Aside from playing a role in intraocular inflammation, there is some evidence that prostaglandins play an endogenous role in normal physiologic processes.[295] Some prostaglandins may actually attenuate an inflammatory response.[296] Prostaglandin $F_{2\alpha}$ causes a dramatic reduction in IOP in monkey eyes,[297–303] and in normal[304, 305] and glaucomatous[306] human eyes, which is apparently mediated by increased nonconventional outflow.[298, 300–302, 296] Latanoprost, a prostaglandin $F_{2\alpha}$ analog that has been introduced for the treatment of glaucoma, is a prodrug and is metabolized by corneal esterases. Latanoprost reduces the IOP about 27% when administered once daily in the morning and, interestingly, about 35% when administered once daily in the evening. Prostaglandin E_2 also apparently reduces the IOP in human eyes.[307] However, the potential for an irritative response is apparently greater with prostaglandin E_1 and prostaglandin E_2 than with prostaglandin $F_{2\alpha}$.[303]

The major ocular side effects that result from prostaglandin use relate to their capacity to influence the blood-aqueous and blood-retinal barriers. Prostaglandin E_2 (0.02%) administration to human eyes is associated with a transient mild eye ache, photophobia, and conjunctival vasodilatation without clinical evidence of ciliary flush or anterior chamber cells and flare.[307] Intravenously administered prostaglandin E_1 resulted in retinal vasodilation in normal human adults.[308] In a single-dose study, administration of the trimethalamine salt of prostaglandin $F_{2\alpha}$ in doses ranging from 62.5 to 250 mg resulted in reddened skin of the lower lid, ocular irritation, conjunctival hyperemia, and headache without evidence of pupillary changes or anterior chamber cells or aqueous flare.[304]

In another study, chronic administration of the more lipid-soluble isopropylester of prostaglandin $F_{2\alpha}$ in doses of 1 mg once daily or 0.5 mg twice daily for 2 weeks resulted in a significant reduction in IOP in normal human eyes that was associated with a dose-dependent hyperemia, foreign body sensation, pain, and photophobia with no evidence of ocular inflammation.[305] No studies in animals or humans have noted a systemic side effect related to the topical application of prostaglandins.

The ocular side effects associated with latanoprost are a foreign body sensation, punctate epithelial keratopathy, stinging, conjunctival hyperemia, blurred vision, itching, burning, and iris pigmentation (Table 41–6). In preclinical studies, latanoprost was found to increase pigmentation in the iris of monkeys.[309] Additionally, in a 6-month study comparing latanoprost with timolol in open-angle glaucoma and ocular hypertensive patients, 10% of patients developed increased iris pigmentation. All these patients had hazel irises.[310] Latanoprost increases the amount of brown pigment in the iris by increasing the number of melanosomes within melanocytes, rather than melanocyte proliferation. The increase in brown pigment does not progress after discontinuation of treatment, but the resultant color change may be permanent.[309, 310]

TABLE 41–6. **Side Effects Associated With the Use of Latanoprost in the Treatment of Primary Open-Angle Glaucoma**

Ocular Side Effects
Foreign body sensation
Punctate epithelial keratopathy
Stinging
Conjunctival hyperemia
Blurred vision
Itching
Burning
Iris pigmentation
Systemic Side Effects
Respiratory tract infection or cold or flu
Muscle or joint or back pain
Chest pain or angina pectoris
Rash or allergic skin reaction

Acknowledgments

Professor W. Morton Grant generously shared with me his literature resources, time, and guidance, for which I am deeply appreciative.

The preparation of this manuscript was supported in part by grants from the National Eye Institute (EYO 7321), Research to Prevent Blindness, and the Massachusetts Lions Eye Research Fund.

REFERENCES

1. Lütjen-Drecoll E, Kaufman PL: Echothiophate-induced structural alterations in the anterior chamber angle of the cynomolgus monkey. Invest Ophthalmol Vis Sci 18:918, 1979.
2. Lütjen-Drecoll E, Kaufman PL: Biomechanics of echothiophate-induced anatomic changes in monkey aqueous outflow system. Graefes Arch Clin Exp Ophthalmol 224:564, 1986.
3. Lütjen-Drecoll E, Kaufman PL, Eichhorn M: Long-term timolol and epinephrine in monkeys. I: Functional morphology of the ciliary process. Trans Ophthalmol Soc UK 105:180, 1986.
4. Lütjen-Drecoll E, Kaufman PL: Long-term timolol and epinephrine in monkeys. II: Morphological alterations in trabecular meshwork and ciliary muscle. Trans Ophthalmol Soc UK 105:196, 1986.
5. Lütjen-Drecoll E, Rohen JW: Reactive changes in primate trabecular meshwork cells following surgical and pharmacological stimulation. Proc Int Soc Eye Res 1:4, 1980.
6. Kaufman PL, Wiedman T, Robinson JR: Cholinergics. *In* Sears ML (ed): Handbook of Experimental Pharmacology, vol 69. Berlin, Springer-Verlag, pp 150–191.
7. Kaufman PL, Robinson JC: Epinephrine, norepinephrine and timolol effects on outflow facility in the cynomolgus monkey. Invest Ophthalmol Vis Sci 30(ARVO Suppl):444, 1989.
8. Kaufman PL: The effects of drugs on the outflow of aqueous humor. *In* Drance SM (ed): Applied Pharmacology in the Medical Treatment of Glaucomas. New York, Grune & Stratton, 1984, pp 429–458.
9. Neufeld AH, Bartels SP: Receptor mechanisms for epinephrine and timolol. *In* Lütjen-Drecoll E (ed): Basic Aspects of Glaucoma Research. Stuttgart, FK Schattauer, 1982, pp 113–122.
10. Thomas JV, Epstein DL: Timolol and epinephrine in primary open angle glaucoma: Transient additive effect. Arch Ophthalmol 99:91, 1981.
11. Erickson-Lamy KA, Ostovar B, Hunnicutt EJ, et al: Epinephrine increases facility of outflow and trabecular meshwork cAMP content in the human eye in vitro. Invest Ophthalmol Vis Sci 31:184, 1990.
12. Gharagozloo NZ, Relf SJ, Brubaker RF: Aqueous flow is reduced by the alpha-adrenergic agonist apraclonidine hydrochloride (ALP 2145). Ophthalmology 95:1217, 1988.
13. Crawford K, Kaufman PL, Gabelt BT: Prostaglandins and aqueous humor dynamics. *In* Shields MB, Pollack IP (eds): Perspectives in Glaucoma: Transactions of First Scientific Meeting of the American Glaucoma Society. Thorofare, NJ, Slack, 1988, pp 259–267.
14. Kaufman PL, Crawford K, Gabelt BT: The effects of prostaglandins on aqueous humor dynamics. Ophthalmol Clin North Am 2:141, 1989.
15. Grant WM: Toxicology of the Eye, 3rd ed. Springfield, IL, Charles C Thomas, 1986.
16. Tripathi RC, Tripathi BJ: The eye. *In* Riddell RH (ed): Pathology of Drug-Induced and Toxic Diseases. New York, Churchill Livingstone, 1982, pp 377–456.
17. Slem G, Ayan Y, Baykal E: Experimental study on the effects of insecticides on the rabbit eye. Ann Ophthalmol 4:874, 1972.
18. Kawai M, Tojyo K, Miyazawa S, et al: The effects of organophosphorous compounds on the eyes of experimental animals. Boei Eisei 23:1, 1976.
19. Patten JT, Cavanagh HD, Allansmith MR: Induced ocular pseudopemphigoid. Am J Ophthalmol 82:272, 1976.
20. Fraunfelder FT, Meyer SM: Ocular toxicology update. Aust J Ophthalmol 12:391, 1984.
21. Pouliquen Y, Patey A, Foster CS, et al: Drug-induced cicatricial pemphigoid affecting the conjunctiva: Light and electron microscopic features. Ophthalmology 93:775, 1986.
22. Cvetkovic D, Parunovic A, Kontic D: Conjunctival changes in local long-term medical glaucomatous therapy. Fortschr Ophthalmol 83:407, 1986.
23. Johnson DH, Kenyon KR, Epstein DL, et al: Corneal changes during pilocarpine gel therapy. Am J Ophthalmol 101:13, 1986.
24. Brazier DJ, Hitchings RA: Atypical band keratopathy following long-term pilocarpine treatment. Br J Ophthalmol 73:294, 1989.
25. Petersen RA, Lee K, Donn A: Acetylcholinesterase in the rabbit cornea. Arch Ophthalmol 73:370, 1965.
26. Fitzgerald GG, Cooper JR: Acetylcholine as a possible sensory mediator in rabbit corneal epithelium. Biochem Pharmacol 20:2741, 1971.
27. van Alphen GWHM: Acetylcholine synthesis in corneal epithelium. Arch Ophthalmol 58:449, 1957.
28. Krejci L, Harrison R: Antiglaucoma drug effects on corneal epithelium: A comparative study in tissue culture. Ther Hung 18:766, 1970.
29. Wood JR, Anderson RL, Edwards JJ: Phospholine iodide toxicity and Jones' tubes. Ophthalmology 87:346, 1980.
30. Ecobichon DJ, Ozere RL, Reid E, et al: Acute fenitrothion poisoning. Can Med Assoc J 116:377, 1977.
31. Moylan-Jones RJ, Thomas DP: Cyclopentolate in treatment of sarin miosis. Br J Pharmacol 48:309, 1973.
32. Erickson-Lamy K, Schroeder A: Dissociation between the effect of aceclidine on outflow facility and accommodation. Exp Eye Res 50:143, 1990.
33. Leuzinger S, Pasi A, Dolder R: Synoptische Auswertung von Alkylphosphatvergiftungen. Schweiz Med Wochenschr 101:563, 1971.
34. Dixon EM: Dilatation of the pupils in parathion poisoning. JAMA 163:444, 1957.
35. Auricchio G, Diotallevi M: Ulteriori ricerche sull'influenza esercitata dal DFP sulla resistenza al deflusso in occhi di coniglio. Ann Ottalmol 85:567, 1959.
36. Bito LZ, Hyslop K, Hyndman J: Anti-parasympathomimetic effects of cholinesterase inhibitor treatment. J Pharmacol Exp Ther 157:159, 1967.
37. Bito LZ, Banks N: Effects of chronic cholinesterase inhibitor treatment. Arch Ophthalmol 82:681, 1969.
38. Axelsson U: Glaucoma miotic therapy and cataract. VI: Experimental studies on the guinea pig eye. Acta Ophthalmol 47:1057, 1969.
39. Harris LS, Shimmyo M, Mittag TW: Effects of echothiophate on cholinesterases in cat irides. Arch Ophthalmol 91:57, 1974.
40. Aldrige WH, Davson H, Dunphy EB, et al: The effects of di-isopropyl fluorophosphate vapor on the eye. Am J Ophthalmol 30:1405, 1947.
41. Upholt WM, Quinby GE, Batchelor GS, et al: Visual effects accompanying TEPP-induced miosis. Arch Ophthalmol 56:128, 1956.
42. Stewart WC, Madill HD, Dyer AM: Night vision in the miotic eye. Can Med Assoc J 99:1145, 1968.
43. Romano J, Jackson H: Clinical observations on the use of phospholine iodide in glaucoma. Br J Ophthalmol 48:480, 1964.
44. Wilkie J, Drance SM, Schulzer M: The effects of miotics on anterior chamber depth. Am J Ophthalmol 68:78, 1969.
45. Drance SM: The effects of phospholine iodide on the lens and anterior chamber depth. *In* Leopold IH (ed): Symposium on Ocular Therapy. St. Louis, CV Mosby, 1969, pp 25–31.
46. Deodati F, Bechac G, Philipott V, et al: Uveite bilaterale par insecticide organophosphore. Bull Soc Ophthalmol Fr 77:857, 1977.
47. Becker B, Pyle GC, Drews RC: The tonographic effects of echothiophate (phospholine iodide). Am J Ophthalmol 47:635, 1959.
48. Straub W, Conrads E: Beobachtungen über Mioticumcysten. Acta Ophthalmol 33:561, 1955.
49. Vogt A: Weitere Ergebnnisse der Spaltlampenmikroscopie des vorderen Bulbusabschnittes. Arch Ophthalmol 111:91, 1923.
50. Abraham SV: Intra-epithelial cysts of the iris. Am J Ophthalmol 37:327, 1954.
51. Hill K, Stromberg AE: Echothiophate iodide in the management of esotropia. Am J Ophthalmol 53:488, 1962.
52. Chin NB, Gold AA, Breinin GM: Iris cysts and miotics. Arch Ophthalmol 71:611, 1964.
53. Catros A, Cahn R, Guyader M: Effets secondaires des myotiques forts dans le traitement du strabisme accommodatif de l'enfant. Bull Soc Ophtalmol Fr 69:370, 1969.
54. Chamberlain W: Anticholinesterase miotics in the management of accommodative esotropia. J Pediatr Ophthalmol 12:151, 1975.
55. Swan KC: Iris pigment nodules complicating miotic therapy. Am J Ophthalmol 37:886, 1954.
56. Funder W: Pigmentzysten nach Mintacolgebrauch. Klin Monatsbl Augenheilkd 126:218, 1955.
57. Abraham SV: The use of an echothiophate-phenylephrine formulation (echophenyline-B3) in the treatment of convergent strabismus with special reference to cysts. J Pediatr Ophthalmol 4:29, 1967.

58. Haddad HM, Rivera H: Echophenyline-B3 and phospholine iodide 0.3% in the management of esotropia. J Pediatr Ophthalmol 4:24, 1967.
59. Kraft H: Auftreten von zystischen Veranderungen an den Ziliarörperforätzen bei langer dauerndem Gebrauch von cholinesterasehemmenden Medikamenten. Klin Monatsbl Augenheilkd 140:584, 1962.
60. Christensen L, Swan KC, Huggins HD: Histopathology of iris pigment changes induced by miotics. Arch Ophthalmol 55:666, 1956.
61. Tamura O, Mitsui Y: Organophosphorous pesticides as a cause of myopia in school children. Jpn J Ophthalmol 19:250, 1975; Jpn J Clin Ophthalmol 29:583, 1975.
62. Ishikawa S: Eye injury by organic phosphorous insecticides (preliminary report). Jpn J Ophthalmol 15:60, 1971.
63. Apt L: Toxicity of strong miotics in children. *In* Leopold IH (ed): Symposium on Ocular Therapy. St. Louis, CV Mosby, 1972, pp 30–35.
64. Apt L, Gaffney WL: Toxicity of topical eye medication used in childhood strabismus. *In* Leopold IH, Burns RP (eds): Symposium on Ocular Therapy. New York, Wiley, 1976, pp 1–9.
65. Young FA: The effect of atropine on the development of myopia in monkeys. Am J Optom 42:439, 1965.
66. McKanna JA, Casagrande VA: Atropine affects lid suture myopia development: Experimental studies of chronic atropinization in tree shrews. Doc Ophthalmol [Proc Ser] 28:187, 1981.
67. Raviola E, Wiesel TN: An animal model for myopia. N Engl J Med 312:1609, 1985.
68. Tokoro T, Suzuki K, Nakano H, et al: Chronic organic phosphorus pesticide intoxication of beagle dogs. Acta Soc Ophthalmol Jpn 77:1237, 1973.
69. Ishikawa S, Miyata M: Development of myopia following chronic organophosphate pesticide intoxication: An epidemiological and experimental study. *In* Merigan WH, Weiss B (eds): Neurotoxicology of the Visual System. New York, Raven, 1980, pp 233–254.
70. Kaufman PL, Bárány EH: Subsensitivity to pilocarpine in primate ciliary muscle following topical anticholinesterase. Invest Ophthalmol 14:302, 1975.
71. Erickson-Lamy KA, Polansky JR, Kaufman PL, et al: Cholinergic drugs alter ciliary muscle response and receptor content. Invest Ophthalmol Vis Sci 28:375, 1987.
72. Grant WM: Experimental aqueous perfusion in enucleated human eyes. Arch Ophthalmol 69:783, 1963.
73. Grant WM: Additional experiences with tetraethyl pyrophosphate in treatment of glaucoma. Arch Ophthalmol 44:362, 1950.
74. Axelsson U, Holmberg A: The frequency of cataract after miotic therapy. Acta Ophthalmol 44:421, 1966.
75. Axelsson U: Glaucoma miotic therapy and cataract. I: The frequency of anterior subcapsular vacuoles in glaucoma eyes treated with echothiophate (phospholine iodide) pilocarpine or pilocarpine-eserine and in nonglaucomatous untreated eyes with common senile cataract. Acta Ophthalmol 46:83, 1968.
76. Axelsson U: Glaucoma miotic therapy and cataract. II: The frequency of anterior subcapsular vacuoles in glaucoma eyes treated with paraoxon (Mintacol). Acta Ophthalmol 46:99, 1968.
77. Axelsson U: Glaucoma miotic therapy and cataract. III. Visual loss due to lens changes in glaucoma eyes treated with paraoxon (Mintacol) echothiophate (phospholine iodide) or pilocarpine. Acta Ophthalmol 46:831, 1968.
78. Axelsson U: Glaucoma miotic therapy and cataract studies on echothiophate (phospholine iodide) and Paraoxon (Mintacol) with regard to cataractogenic effect. Acta Ophthalmol 102(Suppl):1, 1969.
79. Axelsson U: Cataracts following the use of long-acting cholinesterase inhibitors in glaucoma patients. Proc Eur Soc Drug Toxicol 12:199, 1971.
80. deRoetth A Jr: Lenticular opacities in glaucoma patients receiving echothiophate iodide therapy. JAMA 195:665, 1966.
81. deRoetth A Jr: Lens opacities in glaucoma patients on phospholine iodide therapy. Am J Ophthalmol 62:619, 1966.
82. deRoetth A Jr: Lens opacities in glaucoma patients on phospholine iodide therapy. Trans Ophthalmol Soc UK 86:89, 1966.
83. Shaffer RN, Hetherington J Jr: Anticholinesterase drugs and cataracts. Trans Am Ophthalmol Soc 64:204, 1966.
84. Shaffer RN, Hetherington J Jr: Anticholinesterase drugs and cataracts. Trans Am Ophthalmol Soc 62:613, 1966.
85. Cinotti AA, Patti JC: Lens abnormalities in an aging population of nonglaucomatous patients. Am J Ophthalmol 65:25, 1968.
86. Thoft RA: Incidence of lens changes in patients treated with echothiophate iodide. Arch Ophthalmol 80:317, 1968.
87. Abraham SV, Teller JJ: Influence of various miotics on cataract formation. Br J Ophthalmol 53:833, 1969.
88. Levene RZ: Echothiophate iodide and lens changes. *In* Leopold IH (ed): Symposium on Ocular Therapy. St. Louis, CV Mosby, 1969, pp 45–52.
89. Morton WR, Drance SM, Fairclough M: Effects of echothiophate iodide on the lens. Am J Ophthalmol 68:1003, 1969.
90. Nordmann J, Gerhard JPA: Propos de la cataracte par miotiques. Bull Soc Ophthalmol Fr 69:649, 1969.
91. Nordmann J, Gerhard JP: La phospholine et le cristallin. Bull Soc Ophtalmol Fr 70:745, 1970.
92. Tarkkanen A, Karjalainen K: Cataract formation during miotic treatment for chronic open-angle glaucoma. Acta Ophthalmol 44:932, 1966.
93. Harrison R: Bilateral lens opacities associated with use of diisopropyl fluorophosphate. Am J Ophthalmol 50:153, 1960.
94. Baldone JA, Clark WB: Absence of lenticular changes from cholinesterase inhibitors in 205 eyes of children. J Pediatr Ophthalmol 6:81, 1969.
95. Axelsson U, Nyman KG: Side effects from use of long-acting cholinesterase inhibitors in young persons. Acta Ophthalmol 48:396, 1970.
96. Pietsch RI, Bobo CB, Finklea JF, Valotton WW: Lens opacities and organophosphate cholinesterase-inhibiting agents. Am J Ophthalmol 73:236, 1972.
97. Wolter JR, Lee MS: Free floating pigment cyst of the anterior chamber ten years after miotic therapy. J Pediatr Ophthalmol 15:33, 1978.
98. Lieberman TW, Leopold IH, Osserman KE, et al: Lens findings in patients with myasthenia gravis on long-term treatment with oral anticholinesterases. Mt Sinai J Med 38:324, 1971.
99. Kaufman PL, Axelsson U, Bárány EH: Induction of subcapsular cataracts in cynomolgus monkeys by echothiophate. Arch Ophthalmol 95:499, 1977.
100. Kaufman PL, Axelsson U, Bárány EH: Atropine inhibition of echothiophate cataractogenesis in monkeys. Arch Ophthalmol 95:1262, 1977.
101. Albrecht M, Bárány E: Early lens changes in *Macaca fascicularis* monkeys under topical treatment with echothiophate or carbachol studies by slit-image photography. Invest Ophthalmol 18:179, 1979.
102. Kaufman PL, Erickson KA, Neider MW: Echothiophate iodide cataracts in monkeys. Occurrence despite loss of accommodation induced by retrodisplacement of ciliary muscle. Arch Ophthalmol 101:125, 1979.
103. Philipson B, Kaufman P, Fayerholm P, et al: Echothiophate cataracts in monkeys. Electron microscopy and microradiography. Arch Ophthalmol 97:340, 1979.
104. Michon J Jr, Kinoshita JH: Experimental miotic cataract. I: Effects of miotics on lens structure cation content and hydration. Arch Ophthalmol 79:79, 1968.
105. Bárány E: The action of atropine homatropine eserine and prostigmine on the osmotic pressure of the aqueous humor. Acta Physiol Scand 13:95, 1947.
106. von Sallmann L, Dillon B: The effect of di-isopropyl fluorophosphate on the capillaries of the anterior segment of the eye in rabbits. Am J Ophthalmol 30:1244, 1947.
107. Alpar JJ: Miotics and retinal detachment: A survey and case report. Ann Ophthalmol 11:395, 1979.
108. Puustärvi T: Retinal detachment during glaucoma therapy. Ophthalmologica 190:40, 1985.
109. Schuman JS, Hersh P, Kylstra J: Vitreous hemorrhage associated with pilocarpine. Am J Ophthalmol 106:333, 1989.
110. Beasley H, Fraunfelder FT: Retinal detachments and topical ocular miotics. Ophthalmology 86:95, 1979.
111. Alpern M, Jampel RS: The effects of autonomic drugs on human flicker discrimination. Am J Ophthalmol 47:464, 1959.
112. Gazzard MF, Thomas DP: A comparative study of central visual field changes induced by sarin vapour and physostigmine eye drops. Exp Eye Res 20:15, 1975.
113. Rubin LS, Goldberg MN: Effect of sarin on dark adaptation in man: Threshold changes. J Appl Physiol 11:439, 1957.
114. Rubin LS, Krop S, Goldberg MN: Effect of sarin on dark adaptation in man: Mechanism of action. J Appl Physiol 11:445, 1957.
115. Ohto K: Long term follow up study of chronic organophosphate pesticide intoxication (Saku disease) with special reference to retinal pigmentary degeneration. Acta Soc Ophthalmol Jpn 78:237, 1974.
116. Misra UK, Nag D, Misra NK, Krishna Murti CR: Macular degeneration associated with chronic pesticide exposure. Lancet 1:288, 1982.
117. Su M-Q, Kinoshita FK, Frawley JP, DuBois KP: Comparative inhibi-

tion of aliesterases and cholinesterase in rats fed eighteen organophosphorus insecticides. Toxicol Appl Pharmacol 20:241, 1971.
118. Farber DB, Park S, Yamashita C: Cyclic GMP-phosphodiesterase of *rd* retina: Biosynthesis and content. Exp Eye Res 46:363, 1988.
119. Sandberg MA, Pawlyk BS, Crane WG, et al: Effects of IBMX on the ERG of the isolated perfused cat eye. Vision Res 27:1421, 1987.
120. Duffy FH, Burchfiel JL: Long-term effects of the organophosphate sarin on EEG's in monkeys and humans. Neurotoxicology 1:667, 1980.
121. Koelle GB: Anticholinesterase agents. *In* Goodman LS, Gilman A (eds): The Pharmacologic Basis of Therapeutics. New York, Macmillan, 1975, pp 445–466.
122. Bruchhausen D, Haschem J, Dardenne MU: Veränderungen des Bronchialwiderstandes bei Asthmatikern nach Applikation von Pilocarpin in den Konjunktivalsack. Deutsch Med Wochenschr 94:1651, 1969.
123. Bruchhausen D, Haschem J, Baack G, et al: Medikamentöse Provokation von Bronchospasmen bei Asthmatikern. Verh Dtsch Ges Inn Med 77:1321, 1971.
124. Soong HK, McKenney MJ, Wolter JR: Adrenochrome staining of senile plaque resembling malignant melanoma. Am J Ophthalmol 101:380, 1986.
125. Bradbury JA, Rennie IG, Parsons MA: Adrenaline dacryolith: Detection by ultrasound examination of the nasolacrimal duct. Br J Ophthalmol 72:935, 1988.
126. Edelhauser HF, Hyndiuk RA, Zeeb A, Schultz RO: Corneal edema and the intraocular use of epinephrine. Am J Ophthalmol 93:327, 1982.
127. Samples JR, Binder PS, Nayak S: The effect of epinephrine and benzalkonium chloride on cultured corneal endothelial and trabecular meshwork cells. Exp Eye Res 49:1, 1989.
128. Slack JW, Edelhauser HF, Helenek MJ: A bisulfite-free intraocular epinephrine solution. Am J Ophthalmol 110:77, 1990.
129. Waltman SR, Yarian D, Hart W Jr, et al: Corneal endothelial changes with long term topical epinephrine therapy. Arch Ophthalmol 95:1357, 1977.
130. Blanchard DL: Adrenergic-associated symblepharon. Glaucoma 9:18, 1987.
131. Liesegang TJ: Bulbar conjunctival follicles associated with dipivefrin therapy. Ophthalmology 92:228, 1985.
132. Coleiro JA, Sigurdsson H, Lockyer JA: Follicular conjunctivitis on dipivefrin therapy for glaucoma. Eye 2:440, 1988.
133. Tripathi BJ, Tripathi RC: Effect of epinephrine in vitro on the morphology, phagocytosis and mitotic activity of human trabecular endothelium. Exp Eye Res 39:731, 1984.
134. Funk R, Rohen JW: SEM studies of the functional morphology of the ciliary process vasculature in the cynomolgus monkey: Reactions after application of epinephrine. Exp Eye Res 47:653, 1988.
135. Seki R: Scanning electron microscopic observations on vascular casts of ciliary processes in normal and topical epinephrine-treated rats. Jpn J Ophthalmol 32:288, 1988.
136. Green K, Hatchett TL: Regional ocular blood flow after chronic topical glaucoma drug treatment. Acta Ophthalmol 65:503, 1987.
137. O'Brien DM, Farmer SG, Kalina RE, et al: Acute macular neuroretinopathy following intravenous sympathomimetics. Retina 9:281, 1989.
138. Chiou GCY, Girgis Z, Chiou FY: Effects of epinephrine on retinal and choroidal blood flow through different routes of drug administration. Ophthalmic Res 20:293, 1988.
139. Miyake K, Kayazawa F, Manabe R, et al: Indomethacin and the epinephrine-induced breakdown of the blood-ocular barrier in rabbits. Invest Ophthalmol Vis Sci 28:482, 1987.
140. Miyake K, Miyake Y, Kuratomi R: Long-term effects of topically applied epinephrine on the blood-ocular barrier in humans. Arch Ophthalmol 105:1360, 1987.
141. Miyake K, Shirasawa E, Hikita M, et al: Synthesis of prostaglandin E in rabbit eyes with topically applied epinephrine. Invest Ophthalmol Vis Sci 29:332, 1988.
142. Brummett RE: Warning to otolaryngologists using local anesthetics containing epinephrine: Potential serious reaction occurring in patients treated with beta adrenergic receptor blockers. Arch Otolaryngol 110:561, 1984.
143. Fiore PM, Cinotti AA: Systemic effects of intraocular epinephrine during cataract surgery. Ann Ophthalmol 20:23, 1988.
144. Yamaguchi H, Matsumoto Y: Stability of blood pressure and heart rate during intraocular epinephrine irrigation. Ann Ophthalmol 20:58, 1988.
145. Dupeyron G, Eledjan JJ, Poupard P, et al: Perfusion d'adrenaline intra-camerulaire dans la chirugie extra-capsulaire du cristallin interet et limites de la methode. Bull Soc Ophtalmol Fr 85:631, 1985.
146. Novack GD, Leopold IH: The toxicity of topical ophthalmic beta blockers. J Toxicol Cutan Ocul Toxicol 6:283, 1987.
147. Novack GD: Ophthalmic beta-blockers since timolol. Surv Ophthalmol 31:307, 1987.
148. James IM: Pharmacologic effects of beta-blocking agents used in the management of glaucoma. [Summary] Surv Ophthalmol 33:453, 1989.
149. Chang SC, Bundgaard H, Buur A, et al: Improved corneal penetration of timolol by prodrugs as a means to reduce systemic drug load. Invest Ophthalmol Vis Sci 28:487, 1987.
150. Potter DE, Shumate DJ, Bundgaard H, et al: Ocular and cardiac β-antagonism by timolol prodrugs timolol and levobunolol. Curr Eye Res 7:755, 1988.
151. Timoptic-XE (Timolol Maleate Ophthalmic Gel Forming Solution, 0.25% and 0.5%). Product insert. West Point, PA, Merck & Co, 1993.
152. Aula P, Kaila T, Huupponen R, et al: Timolol binding to bovine ocular melanin in vitro. J Ocul Pharmacol 4:29, 1988.
153. Bucci MG, Gualano A, Capra P, et al: Treatment of the tear hyposecretion after topical beta-blockers. Ann Ottalmol 114:1216, 1988.
154. Petounis AD, Akritopoulos P: Influence of topical and systemic β-blockers on tear production. Int Ophthalmol 13:75, 1989.
155. Strempel I: Influence of β-blockers on the tear film stability. Ophthalmologica 195:61, 1987.
156. Strempel I: The influence of topical β-blockers on the breakup time. Ophthalmologica 189:110, 1984.
157. Strempel I: Different β-blockers and their short-time effects on "breakup time." Ophthalmologica 192:11, 1986.
158. Derous D, de Keizer RJW, de Wolff-Rouendaal D, et al: Conjunctival keratinisation: An abnormal reaction to an ocular beta-blocker. Acta Ophthalmol 67:333, 1989.
159. Nelson WL, Kuritsky JN: Early post marketing surveillance of betaxolol hydrochloride. Sept 1985–Sept 1986. Am J Ophthalmol 4:592, 1987.
160. Quaranta CA, Russo L, Brunori PR, et al: Osservazioni ultrastrutturali sugli ipotetici danni congiuntivali da farmaci beta-bloccanti. Boll Ocul 67(Suppl):345, 1988.
161. Spinelli D, Vigasio F, Montanari P: Short-term and long-term timolol maleate effects on corneal sensitivity. Doc Ophthalmol 56:385, 1984.
162. Weissman SS, Asbell PA: Effects of topical timolol (0.5%) and betaxolol (0.5%) on corneal sensitivity. Br J Ophthalmol 74:409, 1990.
163. Avitabile T, Saraniti G, Spampinato D: Carteololo e glaucoma: Aspetti farmacologici e prospettive cliniche. Boll Ocul 67 (Suppl):271, 1988.
164. Brazier DJ, Smith SE: Ocular and cardiovascular response to topical carteolol 2% and timolol 0.5% in healthy volunteers. Br J Ophthalmol 72:101, 1988.
165. Scoville B, Mueller B, White BG, et al: A double-masked comparison of carteolol and timolol in ocular hypertension. Am J Ophthalmol 105:150, 1988.
166. Höh H: Local anesthetic effect and subjective tolerance of carteolol 2% and metipranolol 0.6% in subjects with healthy eyes. Klin Monatsbl Augenheilk 194:241, 1989.
167. Liu GS, Trope GE, Basu PK: A comparison of topical betoptic and timoptic on corneal re-epithelialization in rabbits. J Toxicol Cutan Ocul Toxicol 6:335, 1987.
168. Liu GS, Basu PK, Trope GE: Ultrastructural changes of the rabbit corneal epithelium and endothelium after timoptic treatment. Graefes Arch Clin Exp Ophthalmol 225:325, 1987.
169. Trope GE, Liu GS, Basu PK: Toxic effects of topically administered betagan betoptic and timoptic on regenerating corneal epithelium. J Ocul Pharmacol 4:359, 1988.
170. Haruta Y, Rootman DS, Hill JM: Recurrent HSV-1 corneal epithelial lesions induced by timolol iontophoresis in latently infected rabbits. Invest Ophthalmol Vis Sci 29:387, 1987.
171. Hill JM, Shimomura Y, Dudley JB, et al: Timolol induces HSV-1 ocular shedding in the latently infected rabbit. Invest Ophthalmol Vis Sci 28:585, 1987.
172. Nielsen CB, Nielsen PJ: Effect of α- and β-receptor active drugs on corneal thickness. Acta Ophthalmol 63:351, 1985.
173. Matsuda M, Ishii Y, Awata T, et al: The effect of long-term topical administration of commercial beta-blockers on the rat corneal endothelium. Int Ophthalmol 13:67, 1989.
174. Alanko HI, Airaksinen PJ: Effects of topical timolol on corneal endothelial cell morphology in vivo. Am J Ophthalmol 96:615, 1983.
175. Nesher R, Kass MA, Gans LA: Corneal endothelial changes in ocular

hypertensive individuals after long-term unilateral treatment with timolol. Am J Ophthalmol 110:309, 1990.
176. Brubaker RF, Nagataki S, Bourne WM: Effect of chronically administered timolol on aqueous humor flow in patients with glaucoma. Ophthalmology 89:280, 1982.
177. Eckerskorn U, Wegener A, Hockwin O, et al: Effect of topical β-blockers on the rabbit lens. Fortschr Ophthalmol 85:139, 1988.
178. Wegener A, Eckerskorn U, Hockwin O, et al: Investigations into the possible cocataractogenic potential of β-blockers in rat cataract models. Fortschr Ophthalmol 85:695, 1988.
179. Wegener A, Maierhofer O, Heints M, et al: Testing a possible cocataractogenic potential of befunolol (Glauconex) with animal cataract models. J Ocul Pharmacol 5:45, 1989.
180. Hiramatsu K, Yamashita H: Morphological changes in the ciliary epithelium after subconjunctival administration of befunolol (β-adrenergic blocker). Acta Soc Ophthalmol Jpn 86:1051, 1982.
181. Hiramatsu K, Yamashita H, Uyama M: Morphological changes in the ciliary epithelium after instillation of 1% befunolol (β-adrenergic blocker). Acta Soc Ophthalmol Jpn 88:251, 1984.
182. Frambach DA, Fain GL, Farber DB, et al: Beta adrenergic receptors on cultured human retinal pigment epithelium. Invest Ophthalmol Vis Sci 31:1767, 1990.
183. Makiura M, Uyama M: Morphological changes in the retinal pigment epithelium by intravitreal administration of β-blocker. Acta Soc Ophthalmol Jpn 86:1091, 1982.
184. Makiura M, Yamashita H, Uyama M: Morphological changes in the retinal pigment epithelium by a long term topical application of β-blocker. Acta Soc Ophthalmol Jpn 88:360, 1984.
185. Niemeyer G, Gerber U, Uji Y: Effects of β-adrenergic antagonists on rod-mediated retinal function in the perfused cat eye. Klin Monatsbl Augenheilkd 192:391, 1988.
186. Bucci MG, Pescosolido N, Mariotti SP, et al: Comportamento dell'ampiezza del polso oculare dopo instillazione di β-bloccanti. Boll Ocul 69:285, 1990.
187. Wolf S, Schulte K, Berg B, et al: Einfluss von β-blockern auf die retinale Ämodynamik. Klin Monatsbl Augenheilkd 195:229, 1989.
188. Grunwald JE: Effect of topical timolol on the human retinal circulation. Invest Ophthalmol Vis Sci 27:1713, 1986.
189. Grunwald JE: Topical timolol and the human retinal circulation. [Summary] Surv Ophthalmol 33(Suppl):415, 1989.
190. Grunwald JE: Effect of timolol maleate on the retinal circulation of human eyes with ocular hypertension. Invest Ophthalmol Vis Sci 31:521, 1990.
191. Grunwald JE: Effect of two weeks of timolol maleate treatment on the normal retinal circulation. Invest Ophthalmol Vis Sci 32:39, 1991.
192. Hesse RJ, Swan JL II: Aphakic cystoid macular edema secondary to betaxolol therapy. Ophthalmic Surg 19:562, 1988.
193. Vela MA, Campbell DG: Hypotony and ciliochoroidal detachment following pharmacologic aqueous suppressant therapy in previously filtered patients. Ophthalmology 92:50, 1985.
194. Perell H, Campbell DG, Vela A, et al: Choroidal detachment induced by a systemic β-blocker. Ophthalmology 95:410, 1988.
195. Kaila T, Salminen L, Huupponen R: Systemic absorption of topically applied ocular timolol. J Ocul Pharmacol 1:79, 1985.
196. Nelson WL, Fraunfelder FT, Sills JM, et al: Adverse respiratory and cardiovascular events attributed to timolol ophthalmic solution 1978–1985. Am J Ophthalmol 102:606, 1986.
197. Brown JH, McGeown MG: Chronic renal failure associated with topical application of paraphenylenediamine. Br Med J 294:155, 1987.
198. Collignon P: Cardiovascular and pulmonary effects of β-blocking agents: Implications for their use in ophthalmology. [Summary] Surv Ophthalmol 33(Suppl):455, 1989.
199. Bleckmann H, Dorow P: The effect of various β-blocker agents on intraocular pressure and ventilation. Fortschr Ophthalmol 83:567, 1986.
200. Bleckmann H, Dorow P: Cardioselective β-blockers locally applied and histamine provocation in patients suffering from obstructive airways disease. Fortschr Ophthalmol 84:346, 1986.
201. D'Andrea A, Ando F, De Natale R, et al: Studio della funzionalita respiratoria in soggetti glaucomatosi sottopositi a terapia con β-bloccanti. Boll Ocul 68:423, 1989.
202. Brooks AMV, Gillies WE, West RH: Betaxolol eye drops as a safe medication to lower intraocular pressure. Aust N Z J Ophthalmol 15:125, 1987.
203. Brooks AMV, Burdon JGW, Gillies WE: The significance of reactions to betaxolol reported by patients. Aust N Z J Ophthalmol 15:353, 1989.
204. Ofner S, Smith TJ: Betaxolol in chronic obstructive pulmonary disease. J Ocul Pharmacol 3:171, 1987.
205. Weinreb RN, Van Buskirk EM, Cherniack R, et al: Long-term betaxolol therapy in glaucoma patients with pulmonary disease. Am J Ophthalmol 106:162, 1988.
206. Gaul GR, Jo Will N, Brubaker RF: Comparison of a noncardioselective β-adrenoceptor blocker and a cardioselective blocker in reducing aqueous flow in humans. Arch Ophthalmol 107:1308, 1989.
207. Collignon P: Cardiovascular and pulmonary effects of β-blocking agents: Implications for their use in ophthalmology. [Summary] Surv Ophthalmol 33(Suppl):455, 1989.
208. Nelson WL, Kuritsky JN: Early postmarketing surveillance of betaxolol hydrochloride Sept 1985–Sept 1986. Am J Ophthalmol 4:592, 1987.
209. Berger WE: Betaxolol in patients with glaucoma and asthma. Am J Ophthalmol 4:600, 1987.
210. Harris LS, Greenstein SH, Bloom AF: Respiratory difficulties with betaxolol. Am J Ophthalmol 102:274, 1986.
211. Roholt PC: Betaxolol and restrictive airway disease. Arch Ophthalmol 105:1172, 1987.
212. Goldberg I: Betaxolol. Aust N Z J Ophthalmol 17:9, 1989.
213. Doyle WJ, Weber PA, Meeks RH: Effect of topical timolol maleate on exercise performance. Arch Ophthalmol 102:1517, 1984.
214. Leier CV, Baker ND, Weber PA: Cardiovascular effects of ophthalmic timolol. Ann Intern Med 104:197, 1986.
215. Atkins JM, Pugh BR Jr, Timewell RM: Cardiovascular effects of topical β-blockers during exercise. Am J Ophthalmol 99:173, 1985.
216. Ball S: Congestive heart failure from betaxolol. Arch Ophthalmol 105:320, 1987.
217. Zabel RW, MacDonald IM: Sinus arrest associated with betaxolol ophthalmic drops. Am J Ophthalmol 104:431, 1987.
218. Dorigo MT, Crivellari MP, Fracasso G, et al: Valutazione della frequenza cardiaca mediante registrazione elettrocardiografica (Holter) dopo instillazione di befunololo. Boll Ocul 67:309, 1988.
219. Bonomi L, Orcelli P, Luraschi M, et al: Lack of systemic metabolic effects of treatment with timolol eyedrops. Glaucoma 8:41, 1986.
220. Coleman AL, Diehl DLC, Jampel HD, et al: Topical timolol decreases plasma high-density lipoprotein cholesterol level. Arch Ophthalmol 108:1260, 1990.
221. Fraunfelder FT, Meyer SM, Ore P, et al: Alopecia possibly secondary to topical ophthalmic β-blockers. JAMA 263:1493, 1990.
222. Lustgarten JS: Topical timolol-induced arthropathy. Am J Ophthalmol 105:687, 1988.
223. Herishanu Y, Rosenberg P: β-Blockers and myasthenia gravis. Ann Intern Med 83:834, 1975.
224. Shaivitz SA: Timolol and myasthenia gravis. JAMA 242:1611, 1979.
225. Verkijk A: Worsening of myasthenia gravis with timolol maleate eyedrops. Ann Neurol 17:211, 1985.
226. Lynch MG, Whitson JT, Brown RH, et al: Topical β-blocker therapy and central nervous system side effects. Arch Ophthalmol 106:908, 1988.
227. Waal HJ: Propranolol-induced depression. BMJ 2:50, 1967.
228. Hinshelwood RD: Hallucinations in propranolol. BMJ 1:445, 1969.
229. Petrie WM, Maffucci RJ, Woosley RL: Propranolol and depression. Am J Psychiatry 139:92, 1982.
230. Cove-Smith JR, Kirk CA: CNS-related side-effects with metoprolol and atenolol. Eur J Clin Pharmacol 28:69, 1985.
231. Westerlund A: Central nervous system side-effects with hydrophilic and lipophilic β-blockers. Eur J Clin Pharmacol 28:73, 1985.
232. Betts TA, Alford C: β-Blockers and sleep: A controlled trial. Eur J Clin Pharmacol 28:65, 1985.
233. Davidorf FH: Did I tell you the story about Jim the neurologist? Contemp Ophthalmic Forum 5:4, 1987.
234. de Vries J, van de Merwe SA, Jan de Heer L: From timolol to betaxolol. [Letter] Arch Ophthalmol 107:634, 1989.
235. Orlando RG: Clinical depression associated with betaxolol. Am J Ophthalmol 102:275, 1986.
236. Abel EA, DiCicco LM, Orenberg EK, et al: Drugs in exacerbation of psoriasis. J Am Acad Dermatol 15:1007, 1986.
237. Arntzen N, Kavli G, Volden G: Psoriasis provoked by β-blocking agents. Acta Derm Venereol (Stockh) 64:346, 1984.
238. Savola J, Vehviäinen O, Äääinen NJ: Psoriasis as a side effect of β-blockers. BMJ 295:637, 1987.
239. Gold MH, Holy AK, Roenigk HH: β-Blocking drugs and psoriasis: A review of cutaneous side effects and retrospective analysis of their effects on psoriasis. J Am Acad Dermatol 19:837, 1988.

240. Puig L, Goni FJ, Roque AM, et al: Psoriasis induced by ophthalmic timolol preparations. Am J Ophthalmol 108:455, 1989.
241. Schneeweiss A: Drug Therapy in Cardiovascular Diseases. Philadelphia, Lea & Febiger, 1986, pp 793–794.
242. Harrison R, Kaufmann CS: Clonidine: Effects of a topically administered solution on intraocular pressure and blood pressure in open-angle glaucoma. Arch Ophthalmol 95:1368, 1977.
243. Hodapp E, Kolker AE, Kass MA: The effect of topical clonidine on intraocular pressure. Arch Ophthalmol 99:1208, 1981.
244. Kaskel D, Becker H, Rudolf H: Fühwirkungen von Clonidin Adrenalin und Pilocarpin auf den Augennendruck und Episkleralvenendruck des gesunden menschlichen Auges. Graefes Arch Clin Exp Ophthalmol 213:251, 1980.
245. Krieglstein GK, Langham ME, Leydhecker W: The peripheral and central neural actions of clonidine in normal and glaucomatous eyes. Invest Ophthalmol Vis Sci 17:149, 1978.
246. Ralli R: Clonidine effect on the intraocular pressure and eye circulation. Acta Ophthalmol 125:37, 1975.
247. Lee DA, Topper JE, Brubaker RF: Effect of clonidine on aqueous humor flow in normal human eyes. Exp Eye Res 38:239, 1984.
248. Mittag TW, Tormay A: Drug responses of adenylate cyclase in iris–ciliary body determined by adenine labelling. Invest Ophthalmol Vis Sci 26:396, 1985.
249. Abrams DA, Robin AL, Pollack IP, et al: The safety and efficacy of topical 1% ALO 2145 (*p*-aminoclonidine hydrochloride) in normal volunteers. Arch Ophthalmol 105:1205, 1987.
250. Gharagozloo NZ, Relf SJ, Brubaker RF: Aqueous flow is reduced by α-adrenergic agonist apraclonidine hydrochloride (ALO 2145). Ophthalmology 95:1217, 1988.
251. Robin AL, Pollack IP, de Faller JM: Effects of topical 1% ALO 2145 (*p*-aminoclonidine hydrochloride) on the acute intraocular pressure rise after argon laser iridotomy. Arch Ophthalmol 105:1208, 1987.
252. Brown RH, Stewart RH, Lynch MG, et al: ALO 2145 reduces the intraocular pressure elevation after anterior segment laser surgery. Ophthalmology 95:378, 1988.
253. Robin AL, Pollack IP, House B, et al: Effects of ALO 2145 on intraocular pressure following argon laser trabeculoplasty. Arch Ophthalmol 105:646, 1987.
254. Pollack IP, Brown RH, Crandall AS, et al: Prevention of the rise in intraocular pressure following neodymium-YAG posterior capsulotomy using topical 1% apraclonidine. Arch Ophthalmol 106:754, 1988.
255. Jampel HD, Robin AL, Quigley HA, et al: Apraclonidine hydrochloride: A one-week dose response study. Arch Ophthalmol 106:1069, 1988.
256. Morrison JC, Robin AL: Adjunctive glaucoma therapy: A comparison of apraclonidine and dipivefrin when added to timolol maleate. Ophthalmology 96:3, 1989.
257. Alphagan (Brimonidine Tartrate Ophthalmic Solution). Product monograph. Irvine, CA, Allergan, Inc., 1996, pp 1–42.
258. Baurmann H, Jankolovitz M, Wirmer M, et al: Simultaneous observation of ocular vessels in the anterior and posterior segments of normotonic and hypertensive experimental animals after administration of clonidine and propranolol. Klin Monatsbl Augenheilkd 189:467, 1986.
259. Marquardt R, Pillunat LE, Stodtmeister R: Ocular hemodynamics following local application of clonidine. Klin Monatsbl Augenheilkd 193:637, 1988.
260. Iopidine (Apraclonidine Ophthalmic Solution, 0.5%). Product monograph. Ft. Worth, TX, Alcon Ophthalmic, Alcon Laboratories, Inc., 1996, pp 3–27.
261. Schuman JS: Clinical experience with brimonidine 0.2% and timolol 0.5% in glaucoma and ocular hypertension. Surv Ophthalmol 41(Suppl 1):S26–S37, 1996.
262. Nordlund JR, Pasquale LR, Robin AL, et al: The cardiovascular, pulmonary and ocular hypotensive effects of 0.2% brimonidine. Arch Ophthalmol 113:77, 1995.
263. Burke JA, Schuman JS, Serle JB, et al: New approaches in glaucoma management: A clinical profile of brimonidine. Surv Ophthalmol 113:77, 1995.
264. Allergan, Inc. Final Report: The long-term safety and ocular hypertensive efficacy of brimonidine tartrate 0.2% in subjects with open-angle glaucoma or ocular hypertension. Study No. A342-104-7831 (1 year). Irvine, CA, Allergan, March 1996.
265. Walters TR: Development and use of brimonidine in treating acute and chronic elevations in intraocular pressure: A review of safety, efficacy, dose response, and dosing studies. Surv Ophthalmol 41(Suppl 1):S19, 1996.
266. Wilensky JT: The role of brimonidine in the treatment of open-angle glaucoma. Surv Ophthalmol 41(Suppl 1):S3, 1996.
267. Corneli HM, Banner WW, Vernon DD, et al: Toddler eats clonidine patch and nearly quits smoking for life. JAMA 261:42, 1989.
268. Abrams DA, Robin AL, Pollack IP, et al: The safety and efficacy of topical 1% ALO 2145 (*p*-aminoclonidine monohydrochloride) in normal volunteers. Arch Ophthalmol 105:1205, 1987.
269. Robin AL: Short-term effects of unilateral 1% ALO 2145 (*p*-aminoclonidine hydrochloride) therapy. Arch Ophthalmol 106:912, 1988.
270. Trusopt (Dorzolamide Hydrochloride Ophthalmic Solution). Product insert. West Point, PA, Merck & Co, 1994.
271. Kass MA: Topical carbonic anhydrase inhibitors. Am J Ophthalmol 107:280, 1989.
272. Podos SM, Serle JB: Topically active carbonic anhydrase inhibitors for glaucoma. Arch Ophthalmol 109:38, 1991.
273. Buclin T, Lippa EA, Biollaz J, et al: Absence of metabolic effects of the novel topically active carbonic anhydrase inhibitor MK-927 and its *S*-isomer during a two-week ocular administration. Eur J Clin Pharmacol 36:A188, 1989.
274. Maren TH, Bar-llan A, Conroy CW, et al: Chemical and pharmacological properties of MK-927 a sulfonamide carbonic anhydrase inhibitor that lowers intraocular pressure by the topical route. Exp Eye Res 50:27, 1990.
275. Sugrue MF, Gautheron P, Grove J, et al: MK-927: A topically active ocular hypotensive carbonic anhydrase inhibitor. J Ocul Pharmacol 6:9, 1990.
276. Wang RF, Serle JB, Podos SM, et al: The effect of MK-927, a topical carbonic anhydrase inhibitor, on IOP in glaucomatous monkeys. Curr Eye Res 9:163, 1990.
277. Wang RF, Serle JB, Podos SM, et al: The ocular hypotensive effect of the topical carbonic anhydrase inhibitor L-671 152 in glaucomatous monkeys. Arch Ophthalmol 108:511, 1990.
278. Lippa EA, Von Denffer HA, Hofmann HM, et al: Local tolerance and activity of MK-927: A novel topical carbonic anhydrase inhibitor. Arch Ophthalmol 106:1694, 1988.
279. Bron AM, Lippa EA, Hofmann HM, et al: MK-927: A topically effective carbonic anhydrase inhibitor in patients. Arch Ophthalmol 107:1143, 1989.
280. Pfeiffer N, Hennekes R, Lippa EA, et al: MK-927: A single-dose efficacy of a novel topical carbonic anhydrase inhibitor. Br J Ophthalmol 74:405, 1990.
281. Higginbotham EJ, Kass MA, Lippa EA, et al: MK-927: A topical carbonic anhydrase inhibitor: Dose response and duration of action. Arch Ophthalmol 108:65, 1990.
282. Serle JB, Lustgarten JS, Lippa EA, et al: MK-927: A topical carbonic anhydrase inhibitor. Arch Ophthalmol 108:838, 1990.
283. Bron A, Lippa EA, Gunning F, et al: Multiple-dose efficacy comparison of the two topical carbonic anhydrase inhibitors sezolamide and MK-927. Arch Ophthalmol 109:50, 1991.
284. Sugrue MF, Mallorga P, Schwam H, et al: A comparison of L-671 152 and MK-927: Two topically effective ocular hypotensive carbonic anhydrase inhibitors in experimental animals. Curr Eye Res 108:607, 1990.
285. Berson FG: Carbonic anhydrase inhibitors of the eye: A review. J Toxicol Cutan Ocul Toxicol 1:169, 1982.
286. Stanescu B, Michels J: The effects of acetazolamide on the human electroretinogram. Invest Ophthalmol Vis Sci 14:935, 1975.
287. Yonemura D: Susceptibility of the standing potential of the eye to acetazolamide and its clinical application. Folia Ophthalmol Jpn 29:408, 1978.
288. Missotten L, Van Tornout I, et al: The effect of β-blocking drugs and carboxyanhydrase inhibitors on the standing potential of the eye. Bull Soc Belge Ophtalmol 191:65, 1980.
289. Epstein DL, Grant WM: Management of carbonic anhydrase inhibitor side effects. Symp Ocul Ther 11:51, 1979.
290. Goodfield M, Davis J, Jeffcoate W: Acetazolamide and symptomatic metabolic acidosis in mild renal failure. BMJ 284:422, 1982.
291. Maisey DN, Brown RD: Acetazolamide and symptomatic metabolic acidosis in mild renal failure. BMJ 283:1527, 1981.
292. Fraunfelder FT, Meyer SM, Bagby GC Jr, Dreis MW: Hematologic reactions to carbonic anhydrase inhibitors. Am J Ophthalmol 100:79, 1986.
293. Mogk LG, Cyrlin MN: Blood dyscrasias and carbonic anhydrase inhibitors. Ophthalmology 95:768, 1988.
294. Goh Y: The metabolism and actions of prostaglandins in the eye. Folia Ophthalmol Jpn 40:2589, 1989.

295. Bito LZ: Prostaglandins and other eicosanoids: Their ocular transport pharmacokinetics and therapeutic effects. Trans Ophthalmol Soc 105:162, 1986.
296. Yamane A, Tokura T, Sano T, et al: Experimental studies on the relationship of prostaglandin to the occurrence of corneal edema and neovascularization in anterior segmental ischemia in the rabbit eyes. Folia Ophthalmol Jpn 38:1579, 1987.
297. Kaufman PL: Effects of intracamerally infused prostaglandins on outflow facility in cynomolgus monkey eyes with intact or retrodisplaced ciliary muscle. Exp Eye Res 43:819, 1986.
298. Crawford K, Kaufman PL: Pilocarpine antagonizes prostaglandin $F_{2\alpha}$-induced ocular hypotension in monkeys. Evidence for enhancement of uveoscleral outflow by prostaglandin $F_{2\alpha}$. Arch Ophthalmol 105:1112, 1987.
299. Kerstetter JR, Brubaker RF, Wilson SE, et al: Prostaglandin $F_{2\alpha}$-1-isopropylester lowers intraocular pressure without decreasing aqueous humor flow. Am J Ophthalmol 105:30, 1988.
300. Crawford K, Kaufman PL, Gabelt BT: Effects of topical $PGF_{2\alpha}$ on aqueous humor dynamics in cynomolgus monkeys. Curr Eye Res 6:1035, 1987.
301. Nilsson SFE, Samuelsson M, Bill A, et al: Increased uveoscleral outflow as a possible mechanism of ocular hypotension caused by prostaglandin $F_{2\alpha}$-1-isopropylester in the cynomolgus monkey. Exp Eye Res 48:707, 1989.
302. Gabelt BT, Kaufman PL: Prostaglandin $F_{2\alpha}$ increases uveoscleral outflow in the cynomolgus monkey. Exp Eye Res 49:389, 1989.
303. Camras CB, Friedman AH, Rodrigues MM, et al: Multiple dosing of prostaglandin $F_{2\alpha}$ or epinephrine on cynomolgus monkey eyes. Invest Ophthalmol Vis Sci 29:1428, 1988.
304. Lee PY, Shao H, Xu L, Qu CK: The effect of prostaglandin $F_{2\alpha}$ on intraocular pressure in normotensive human subjects. Invest Ophthalmol Vis Sci 29:1474, 1988.
305. Villumsen J, Alm A: Prostaglandin $F_{2\alpha}$-isopropylester eye drops: Effects in normal human eyes. Br J Ophthalmol 73:419, 1989.
306. Villumsen J, Alm A, Öderstöm M: Prostaglandin $F_{2\alpha}$-isopropylester eye drops: Effect on intraocular pressure in open-angle glaucoma. Br J Ophthalmol 73:975, 1989.
307. Flach AJ, Eliason JA: Topical prostaglandin E_2 effects on normal human intraocular pressure. J Ocul Pharmacol 4:13, 1988.
308. Fujiwara H, Fukutomi T, Katayama T, et al: Study on the pharmacological effects of prostaglandin E_1 (PGE_1) on human eye. Report 2: Analysis of effect of PGE_1 on human retinal vessels. Acta Soc Ophthalmol Jpn 90:393, 1986.
309. Xalatan (Latanoprost Solution 0.005%). A New Direction in Glaucoma Therapy. Product monograph. Kalamazoo, MI, Pharmacia & Upjohn, 1996, pp 1–11.
310. Watson P, Stjernschantz J: A six month, randomized, double-masked study comparing latanoprost with timolol on open-angle glaucoma and ocular hypertension. Ophthalmology 103:126, 1996.

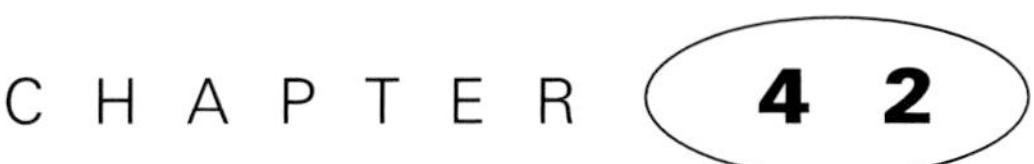

Ocular Toxicity of Systemic Medications

Sarkis H. Soukasian and Michael B. Raizman

The eye with its associated adnexal tissues is a highly specialized sensory-motor organ system. The composition includes a combination of diverse tissues: secretory and resorption organs, permeable and semipermeable membranes, and pigment layers, as well as striated and smooth muscles. Each may react to toxic influences with morphologic and functional changes that may result in potential visual impairment. Metabolic variations, affinities, and storage characteristics account for the response of different tissues to specific drugs and toxic substances. The ability to visualize intraocular structures makes it possible to detect many pathologic changes directly and noninvasively. Because of this, subtle ocular toxicity may be detected in the absence of or before the onset of symptoms.

The intermittent or chronic administration of certain oral, transdermal, and parenteral (including intrathecal and intracarotid) medications may produce a variety of side effects in one or more areas in the eye and visual system. It is important to recognize the ocular effects following the systemic application of drugs. Although adverse effects are frequently encountered within the first 2 weeks of therapy, they may be delayed. The ophthalmologist may not initially relate the ocular side effects to the systemically applied drugs. This is especially true if there is a long latent period between drug intake and the pathologic eye changes or if the toxic effects of the drug are persistent or even progressive after withdrawal of the drug, as with phenothiazine.

The toxic effect of certain drugs may be cumulative and dose dependent. For example, the retinopathy associated with chloroquine therapy may appear years into therapy. Therefore, the daily dose and duration need to be monitored. The toxic effect of other drugs may be idiosyncratic and occur after a single dose, as in Stevens-Johnson syndrome (in which a variety of ingested drugs such as sulfonamides, barbiturates, salicylates, phenylbutazone, penicillin, phenytoin, and others have been implicated) or with ibuprofen-induced optic neuritis.

Toxicity may depend on the solubility characteristics of the drug and its ability to gain access through certain barriers such as the blood-brain barrier or the blood-ocular barrier. The route of administration becomes critically important, since such barriers may be bypassed (as in the case of intrathecal administration of certain chemotherapeutic agents). Massive concentrations of a drug may be locally delivered in a fashion that bypasses the hepatic metabolism to limit systemic toxicity, but with significant local toxic

Text continued on page 464

TABLE 42–1. **Ocular Toxicity and Side Effects of Systemic Medications**

Drug	Class	Uses	Route	Side Effects	Dose Relationship	Comments
Anesthetic (Inhalation)						
Methoxyflurane	Methyl ether	Inhalation anesthetic	Inhalation	Crystalline retinopathy[6, 7]	Prolonged anesthesia	Calcium oxalate crystals in retinal pigment epithelium and retina[6, 7]
Antianginal						
Atenolol (including labetalol, metoprolol, nadolol, and pindolol)	β-Adrenergic–blocking agent	Antianginal and antihypertensive	Oral, IV	Sicca syndrome,[8] visual hallucinations,[1] myasthenic neuromuscular-blocking effect (may worsen myasthenia gravis)[9]	Yes	Work-up myasthenia if patient exhibits extraocular muscle paresis[1]
Diltiazem (also nifedipine, verapamil)	Calcium channel blocker	Antianginal	Oral, sublingual, IV	Rare; ocular irritation with periorbital edema and blurred vision,[10, 11] retinal ischemia,[12] and transient blindness[1]	Yes	Reversible
Practolol	β-Adrenergic–blocking agent	Antianginal and antihypertensive	Oral, IV	Keratoconjunctivitis sicca, conjunctival cicatrization, keratitis with opacities,[1, 13–16] and myasthenic neuromuscular-blocking effect[17]	Duration related	Side effects reversible in early stages, but decreased tear production may persist.[1] This drug for general use has been withdrawn from the market. Mechanism of toxicity may be related to production of antibodies to practolol metabolite.[18, 19] Oculomucocutaneous findings not seen with other β-adrenergic–blocking agents
Propranolol	β-Adrenergic–blocking agent	Antianginal and antihypertensive	Oral, IV	Sicca syndrome,[20] myasthenic neuromuscular-blocking effect,[1] visual hallucinations, and ? inflammatory orbital pseudotumor[21]	Yes	Reversible
Antianxiety						
Alprazolam (including clonazepam, flurazepam, triazolam)	Benzodiazepine	Antianxiety	Oral, IV, IM	Decreased corneal reflex, accommodation, and depth perception,[1] abnormal extraocular muscle movement,[22] allergic conjunctivitis,[1] ?mydriasis precipitating narrow-angle glaucoma[1]	No	Side effects reversible
Antiarrhythmic						
Amiodarone	Benzofuran derivative	Antiarrhythmic (ventricular)	Oral, IV	Whorl-like (vortex pattern) epithelial keratopathy (98%), resulting in photophobia (3%), halos (2%), and blurred vision (1%),[23–29] sicca syndrome,[30] lens opacities,[31] skin pigmentation,[32, 33] papillopathy and optic neuropathy,[34, 35] pseudotumor cerebri,[36, 37] ?retinopathy (hypopigmentation)[1, 38, 39]	Dosage and duration related (keratopathy) with minimal corneal deposits with dosages <200 mg/day but in nearly all patients with >400 mg/day[28, 40, 41]; unclear for papillopathy[34, 35]	Keratopathy due to cationic amphophilic properties of drug that binds to polar lipids and produces a lysosomal disorder, as in Fabry's disease.[26, 42] Onset of keratopathy as early as 6 days but usually by 6 wk; usually resolves in 3 mos after discontinuation but may have prolonged effect owing to long half-life.[29, 35, 40] Keratopathy not indication to discontinue drug, but papillopathy is a relative indication[35]
Digitalis	Digitalis glycoside	Antiarrhythmic and for congestive heart failure	Oral, IV	11–25% side effects with toxic doses.[1] Color vision abnormalities (yellow-blue),[43, 44] visual sensations and hallucinations,[45] scotomas,[46] retinal toxicity with abnormal ERG amplitudes[47]	Yes	Reversible. Toxicity may be made worse with concomitant quinidine therapy (ERG may be helpful). Color testing (yellow-blue) may be helpful in adjusting dosage[1]
Disopyramide	Anticholinergic	Antiarrhythmic	Oral, IV	Blurry vision, decreased accommodation and lacrimation; mydriasis may precipitate narrow-angle glaucoma[1, 48, 49]	Yes	Side effects due to anticholinergic effects, which are reversible
Procainamide	Procaine hydrochloride analog	Antiarrhythmic	Oral, IV	Rare; lupus-like syndrome with scleritis[50]	No	
Anticonvulsant						
Phenytoin	Hydantoin	Anticonvulsant	Oral, IV, IM	Nystagmus, lens opacities,[51, 52] benign intracranial hypertension,[53] ocular teratogenic effects[54]	Yes	Nystagmus may persist for months after discontinuation. Fine nystagmus at therapeutic doses; coarse nystagmus in toxic states[1]

Antidepressant						
Amitriptyline (including desipramine, imipramine, nortriptyline)	Tricyclic antidepressant	Antidepressant	Oral	Mydriasis and cycloplegia (may precipitate narrow-angle glaucoma), aggravate keratoconjunctivitis sicca owing to anticholinergic effects,[55, 56] oculomotor abnormalities[57, 58]	Yes	Reversible
Carbamazepine	Iminostilbene derivative	Antidepressant, pain associated with trigeminal neuralgia	Oral	Blurred vision, extraocular muscle abnormalities with diplopia,[60, 61] downbeat nystagmus,[62, 63] sluggish pupil and papilledema with toxic doses,[64] retinal pigmentary changes[65]	Yes; side effects with dosages >1.2 g	Reversible with decrease in dosage
Doxepin (including amoxapine, clomipramine)	Tricyclic antidepressant	Antidepressant (also for psychoneurotic anxiety)	Oral, IV	Blurred vision, mydriasis, accommodation disturbances, and aggravation of keratoconjunctivitis sicca due to anticholinergic effects.[1] Nystagmus and ophthalmoplegia with toxic states[59]	Yes	Reversible
Methylphenidate	Piperidine derivative	Antidepressant and for hyperkinetic syndrome in children	Oral, IV (see Comments)	Rare; mydriasis. Talc retinopathy (see Comments)[67, 68]	Yes, usually with overdose	Illicit IV use of crushed tablets is responsible for talc and cornstarch (used as fillers) retinopathy
Phenelzine	Monoamine oxidase inhibitor	Antidepressant	Oral	Rare; mydriasis, miosis, anisocoria,[1] nystagmus,[1] diplopia, and myasthenic neuromuscular blockade[66]	Yes, usually with overdose	MAO inhibitor activity increased with concomitant use of other MAO inhibitors and tricyclic antidepressants
Antihistamine						
Brompheniramine (also chlorpheniramine, dexbrompheniramine, dimethindene, triprolidine)	Alkylamine	See Cyproheptadine	Oral	See Pyrilamine.[70] Facial dyskinesia with chronic use[71–73]	See Pyrilamine	Alkylamine has the lowest incidence of ocular side effects[1]
Cyproheptadine (Periactin) (also azatadine)	Phenothiazine analog	Antihistamine used in allergic or vasomotor rhinitis, allergic conjunctivitis	Oral	Rare. Atropine-like effects causing mydriasis and decreased secretions aggravating keratoconjunctivitis sicca[1]		Side effects usually disappear even with continued use.[1] May precipitate narrow-angle glaucoma
Diphenhydramine (Benadryl)	Ethanolamine	See Cyproheptadine	Oral	See Pyrilamine		Toxic doses responsible for visual hallucinations and nystagmus[1]
Pyrilamine (also tripelennamine)	Ethylenediamine	See Cyproheptadine	Oral	See Cyproheptadine. With long-term use, anisocoria, decreased accommodation, and blurred vision.[1] Facial dyskinesia (blepharospasm),[1] visual hallucinations[69]	Visual hallucinations with overdose[65]	See Cyproheptadine
Antihyperlipidemic						
Niacin (nicotinic acid)	Vitamin	Antihyperlipidemic	Oral	Metamorphopsia, blurring, central or paracentral scotoma, maculopathy, "atypical CME" with no accumulation of fluorescein on angiogram[74, 75]	Yes, >1.5/day	Symptoms precede findings. Amsler grid may demonstrate central visual change Reversible
Antihypertensive						
Clonidine	α-Adrenergic agonist	Antihypertensive	Oral	Miosis and mydriasis (toxic doses), ?retinal abnormalities (depigmentation, degeneration, tears)[1]	Yes	Reversible; unclear if retinal findings coincidental or drug related[1]
Hydralazine	Phthalazine derivative	Antihypertensive	Oral, IV	Nonspecific ocular irritation, lupus-like syndrome with episcleritis, retinal vasculitis, and exophthalmos[1, 76–79]	Transient	Reversible
Antiinflammatory						
Ibuprofen (Motrin, Advil)	Nonsteroidal antiinflammatory drug that inhibits cyclooxygenase (propionic acid)	Antiinflammatory, analgesic, antipyretic Osteoarthritis, rheumatoid arthritis, gout, ankylosing spondylitis, cystoid macular edema, ?ocular inflammation[102]	Oral	Rare. With rechallenge refractive error changes, diplopia, photophobia, dry eyes, decrease in color vision,[1, 96–98] optic neuritis with central scotomas, toxic amblyopia[99–100]	Optic neuritis and toxic amblyopia are idiosyncratic	Optic neuritis and toxic amblyopia are reversible with visual acuity returning to normal in 1–3 mo but color vision not returning for up to 8 mo.[1] May be irreversible if drug not discontinued

Table continued on following page

TABLE 42–1. **Ocular Toxicity and Side Effects of Systemic Medications** *Continued*

Drug	Class	Uses	Route	Side Effects	Dose Relationship	Comments
Indomethacin (Indocin)	See Ibuprofen (indole)	See Ibuprofen	Oral	Decreased vision, diplopia, color vision defects, hypersensitivity reactions, including Stevens-Johnson syndrome,[1] corneal deposits, including whorl-like epithelial deposits,[103, 104] papilledema secondary to orbital pseudotumor[105, 106]	?	Corneal deposits is not an indication to discontinue the drug
Ketoprofen (Orudis)	See Ibuprofen (propionic acid)	See Ibuprofen	Oral	Nonspecific conjunctivitis and dermatologic reactions,[1, 107] cholinergic crisis,[108] and papilledema secondary to orbital pseudotumor[109]		In general, nonsteroidal antiinflammatories are photosensitizers
Naproxen (Naprosyn)	See Ibuprofen (propionic acid)	See Ibuprofen	Oral	Whorl-like corneal opacities,[110] optic neuritis[1]	Optic neuritis is idiosyncratic	This drug is a photosensitizer; ?role in maculopathy or necrotizing vasculitis[1, 111, 112]
Piroxicam (Feldene)	See Ibuprofen (oxicam and enolic acid)	See Ibuprofen	Oral	Rare and insignificant[1]	Idiosyncratic	Most widely prescribed nonsteroidal antiinflammatory worldwide[1]
Prednisone	Corticosteroids	Antiinflammatory Adrenocortical insufficiency replacement	Oral	Cataracts (PSC),[80–83] ocular hypertension and glaucoma,[84, 85] pseudotumor cerebri and papilledema with withdrawal,[86, 87] exophthalmos with long-term use,[88, 89] decreased tear lysozyme,[90] ?decreased resistance to infection,[1] myasthenic neuromuscular-blocking effect (extraocular muscle paresis, ptosis[1]), delayed wound healing[1]	Cataracts usually dose related,[81, 82] increased risk of pressure elevation with ocular hypertension, glaucoma, or family history of glaucoma and diabetes[91]	Exophthalmos may not completely reverse.[86] Increase, then slowly taper dose in pseudotumor cerebri.[92] Pressure may rarely remain elevated after discontinuation.[93] Cataracts may rarely progress after discontinuation;[94] may be reversible in children[95]
Sulindac (Clinoril)	See Ibuprofen (indene)	See Ibuprofen	Oral	Rare and insignificant[1]	Idiosyncratic	
Antimalarial						
Chloroquine (see also hydroxychloroquine)	Quinoline	Antimalarial and antirheumatic Rheumatoid arthritis, lupus erythematosus	Oral	Whorl-like corneal epithelial deposits, Hudson-Stähli line,[1, 113–115] accommodation, motility, subcapsular cataracts,[1] central and paracentral scotoma, photophobia, nyctalopia, photopsia, macular pigmentation, loss of macular reflex,[115, 116] macular edema,[113, 117] bull's-eye maculopathy,[118] bone spicule formation, optic disc pallor, vascular attenuation (end stage),[119, 120] ERG[116, 119, 120] and EOG abnormalities[116, 121, 122]	Yes (cumulative dose); little toxicity if 3.5 mg/kg/day, <250 mg/day for small patients, <100 g total <1 year[84, 85]	Toxicity greater with chloroquine than with hydroxychloroquine.[115] Corneal changes reversible. Retinal changes may be irreversible or progressive after discontinuation.[114, 119, 121, 125–128] Since early changes are nonspecific and patients with toxicity may be asymptomatic, routine testing is required. Every 6 mo: vision, history, Amsler grid,[129–131] central visual field with red target,[116, 121] color testing,[119, 132, 133] ?ERG,[116, 119, 120] ?EOG[115, 134]
Dapsone	Sulfone	Antimalarial and antiinflammatory	Oral	Rare. Optic atrophy[135]	Dose related	With massive doses
Hydroxychloroquine (see also chloroquine)	Quinoline	See Chloroquine	See Chloroquine	See Chloroquine. Safe <6.5 mg/kg/day or 400 mg/day for smaller patients[123, 124]	See Chloroquine[137]	
Quinine	Alkaloid	Antimalarial Nocturnal leg cramps, myotonia congenita, myokymia, attempted abortions	Oral	Toxic amblyopia, sudden vision loss, retinal arterial constriction, venous congestion, retinal edema, macular pigmentary changes, disc edema, optic nerve hypoplasia,[1, 136, 138] myasthenic neuromuscular blockade (extraocular muscle paralysis, ptosis)[66]	Dose related (massive); occasionally with low chronic administration	Use on rise, especially in "street drugs." Vision loss may be acute or progressive with usually some return of vision.[1] Prenatal maternal ingestion may cause optic nerve hypoplasia. Acute therapy unclear[1]
Antimicrobial						
Atovaquone	Analog of ubiquinone	Antiparasitic and *Pneumocystis carinii* in AIDS	Oral	Vortex keratopathy[141]		
Cefazolin (including first, second, and third generations)	Cephalosporin	Antibacterial	Oral, IM, IV	Rare. Allergic reactions, including Stevens-Johnson syndrome,[142, 143] ?retinopathy (cephaloridine)[1]	No	Side effects reversible

Chloramphenicol	Dichloracetic acid derivative	Antibacterial	Oral, IV	Rare. Decreased vision, optic neuritis, optic atrophy, toxic amblyopia,[1, 147] retinopathy[148]	Dose related; total >100 g or duration >6 wk	Findings most often in children.[1] Most feared side effect is aplastic anemia, which is most likely idiosyncratic
Ciprofloxacin	Fluoroquinolone	Antibacterial	Oral, IM, IV	Rare. Blurred vision, photophobia, altered color vision, toxic optic neuropathy[144–146]	Dose related[146]; ?duration related	Quinolone group common to quinine and chloroquine may be responsible for optic nerve toxicity.[146] Optic neuropathy is slowly reversible[146]
Clofazimine	Phenazine derivative	Antibacterial used for leprosy	Oral	Eyelid and conjunctival pigmentation, corneal epithelial changes[1, 163, 164]	Yes	Side effects are reversible
Doxycycline (also tetracycline, minocycline)	Polycyclic naphthacene carboxamide	Antibacterial	Oral	Eyelid skin conjunctival hyperpigmentation,[149] hyperpigmented conjunctival cysts,[150] blue-gray scleral pigmentation (minocycline),[151] orbital pseudotumor,[152, 153] extraocular muscle paralysis, aggravation of myasthenia gravis[66]	Orbital pseudotumor not dose related; pigmentation dose related	Most side effects are reversible. Orbital pseudotumor mostly seen with tetracycline and minocycline ?due to greater lipid solubility. Scleral pigmentation (minocycline) frequently associated with pigmentary changes elsewhere
Ethambutol		Tuberculostatic	Oral	Color vision abnormalities, visual field changes (scotomas), axial and paraaxial optic neuritis[167, 168]	Dose related. Infrequent with doses ≤15 mg/kg/day[169]	Optic neuritis symptoms usually noted at 3–6 mo. Increased toxicity with renal disease. With regular doses, home visual acuity and color vision testing recommended. With higher doses, screen patient at 2- to 4-wk intervals[1] Visual-evoked response helpful in detecting subclinical toxic effects.[171] Visual recovery variable. ?Treat optic nerve toxicity with zinc sulfate or parenteral hydroxycobalamin[1]
Gentamicin (including tobramycin, streptomycin)	Aminoglycoside	Antibacterial	IV, IM, intrathecal	Papilledema secondary to pseudotumor cerebri,[1] myasthenic neuromuscular blockade (paralysis of extraocular blockade and ptosis),[154] blindness and optic atrophy with intrathecal administration	No	Most side effects are reversible after discontinuation
Isoniazid	Hydrazide of isonicotinic acid	Antitubercular	Oral	Rare. Optic and retrobulbar neuritis[172–174] with visual field and color vision abnormalities	No	Side effects usually seen in malnourished or chronically ill patients. Many side effects can be prevented by daily administration of pyridoxine[1]
Nalidixic acid	Naphthyridine	Antibacterial	Oral	Visual disturbances, color vision defects, papilledema due to increased intracranial pressure,[105, 155, 156] lupoid skin changes[157]	Most not dose related	Side effects reversible if dosage is decreased or drug discontinued.[1] Increased intracranial pressure reported in persons younger than age 20[1]
Penicillin (including semisynthetic penicillins)	Penicillin	Antibacterial	Oral, IM, IV	Rare. Allergic reactions, including Stevens-Johnson syndrome.[139] Aggravation of ocular signs of myasthenia gravis (ampicillin), including paralysis of extraocular muscles, diplopia, and ptosis,[66, 140] pseudotumor cerebri[105]		
Rifabutin	Synthetic rifamycin	Antitubercular and prophylaxis against *Mycobacterium avium* complex in AIDS	Oral	Anterior uveitis, hypopyon uveitis,[175–182] white-yellow vitreous opacities[178]	May be dose related with increased incidence with 600 mg/day, less common with 300 mg/day[177, 179, 180]	Occurs with concomitant use of rifabutin with clarithromycin and fluconazole. Immunologically mediated process rather than direct drug toxicity; resolves with topical corticosteroid therapy frequently without discontinuation of rifabutin
Rifampin	Hydrazone derivative of rifamycin B	Antitubercular and antibacterial	Oral	Conjunctival hyperemia, conjunctivitis (may be exudative), orange staining of contact lenses[183–185]	Yes	Reversible ocular side effects in 5–15% of patients and more frequently seen with intermittent use[1]
Sulfamethoxazole (including other sulfa-containing medications such as sulfadiazine and sulfasalazine)	Sulfonamide	Antibacterial, ?antiinflammatory	Oral	Myopia due to lens thickening from ciliary body edema,[158–160] allergic reactions, including Stevens-Johnson syndrome,[161] anterior uveitis,[162] optic neuritis[1]	No	Side effects rare and reversible

Table continued on following page

TABLE 42–1. **Ocular Toxicity and Side Effects of Systemic Medications** *Continued*

Drug	Class	Uses	Route	Side Effects	Dose Relationship	Comments
Suramin	Nonmetallic polyanion	Antiprotozoan used for adjuvant therapy in AIDS patients (inhibitor of reverse transcriptase of HTLV-III)	Oral	Vortex-like epithelial keratopathy,[165] ocular irritation, optic atrophy[1, 166]	Dose related	Side effects usually depend on nutritional status. Optic atrophy secondary to inflammatory response to dead microfilariae.[1] Keratopathy due to lysosomotropic properties that inhibit lysosomal enzymes. Reversibility of keratopathy unclear at present owing to prolonged half-life[165]
Antineoplastic or Immunosuppressive						
Busulfan	Alkylating agent	Cancer chemotherapy Chronic leukemia Polycythemia vera Myelofibrosis		Keratoconjunctivitis sicca,[199] posterior subcapsular cataract with polychromatic sheen 10–30%[200–203]	Yes, 2–6 mg/day for months to years	
Chlorambucil	Alkylating agent	Cancer chemotherapy Chronic leukemia Immunosuppression Vasculitis with RA Behçet's disease Autoimmune hemolytic anemia	Oral	Rare but includes keratitis, hemorrhagic retinopathy, and oculomotor disturbances[198]	Yes	
cis-Platinum (cisplatin)	Alkylating agent	Cancer chemotherapy Testicular cancer Breast cancer Bladder cancer Lung cancer Gastrointestinal cancer Lymphoma Osteogenic sarcoma	IV, intracarotid	Blurred vision (62%),[191] impaired color vision (23%),[191] retinal toxicity (ERG) (84%),[191] macular pigmentation (46%),[191] disc edema, retrobulbar neuritis,[192, 193] cortical blindness.[194] With intracarotid administration, ipsilateral vision loss due to retinal and optic nerve ischemia (15–60%)[195–197]	Yes, >600 mg/m²	Blurred and color vision abnormalities are reversible
Cyclophosphamide	Alkylating agent	Cancer chemotherapy Lymphoma Breast cancer Immunosuppressive Rheumatoid arthritis Wegener's granulomatosis Mooren's ulcer Cicatricial pemphigoid Behçet's disease Graves' disease ophthalmopathy	Oral, IM, IV	Blurred vision (17%),[188] keratoconjunctivitis sicca (50%),[189] pinpoint pupil due to parasympathomimetic effect[190]	Yes	
Cytosine arabinoside	Pyrimidine analog	Cancer chemotherapy Acute leukemia Refractory lymphoma	IV	Keratoconjunctivitis, central punctate opacities with subepithelial granular deposits, microcysts, reversible superficial punctate keratitis (38–100%)[220–223]	Yes	Resolution of symptoms in weeks, prednisolone phosphate or 2-deoxycytidine prophylaxis[222, 225]
			Intrathecal	Optic neuropathy (may be potentiated by cranial irradiation)[224]		
Doxorubicin (Adriamycin)	Antimicrobial anthracycline that binds DNA	Cancer chemotherapy Sarcoma Leukemia Lymphoma		Lacrimation (25%), red discoloration of tears[198, 245]		

Fludarabine	Purine analog	Cancer chemotherapy Leukemia		Decreased vision due to optic neuritis or cortical blindness, encephalopathy[226]	Yes	
5-Fluorouracil	Pyrimidine analog	Cancer chemotherapy Breast cancer GI cancer GU cancer	IV	Blurred vision, ocular pain, photophobia, lacrimation, conjunctivitis, blepharitis, keratitis (25–38%),[5, 210, 211] cicatricial ectropion,[212] punctal and canalicular stenosis,[213, 214] blepharospasm,[215] oculomotor disturbance,[216] nystagmus,[217] optic neuropathy[218]	Most are reversible 6–14 mo for cicatricial changes[214, 277]	Massage, topical corticointubation[213, 219]
		Actinic keratosis	Topical	Systemic absorption may cause similar corneal and external disease findings[1]		
Methotrexate	Folic acid analog	Cancer chemotherapy Leukemia Solid tumors Immunosuppressive Rheumatoid arthritis Psoriasis Uveitis	Oral, IM, IV Intrathecal, intracarotid	Periorbital edema, photophobia, ocular pain and burning, blepharitis, conjunctivitis, and decreased tear production (25%),[1, 233, 234] optic neuropathy,[235] macular edema and pigment epithelial changes[236]	Yes (IV)	Resolves off therapy; artificial tears[51]
Mitomycin C	Antimicrobial that cross-links DNA	Cancer chemotherapy Solid tumors		Blurred vision[245]		
Mitotane	Antimicrobial DDT derivative	Cancer chemotherapy Adrenocortical cancer		Neuroretinopathy, disc edema, retinal hemorrhages, retinal edema, cataracts (3–16%)[248, 249]		
Nitrogen mustard	Alkylating agent	Cancer chemotherapy Lymphoma Brain tumor	IV, intracarotid	Necrotizing uveitis and vasculitis (intracarotid)[186, 187]	Most likely	
Nitrosoureas (BCNU, CCNU, methyl-CCNU)	Alkylating agent	Cancer chemotherapy Primary CNS tumor Lymphoma Multiple myeloma Colon and gastric cancer	Oral, IV, intracarotid	Usually benign. Conjunctival hyperemia and blurred vision (4%),[204] ?optic neuritis,[205] ipsilateral periorbital edema, orbital pain and congestion, conjunctivitis, chemosis, neuroretinal toxicity (70%) (NFL infarcts, intraretinal hemorrhages, and disc edema,[204, 206, 207] with intracarotid administration)	Yes (dose and rapidity of infusion)[204, 206, 207] with intracarotid administration	ERG; pressure on eye during infusion or Honan's balloon[208, 209] to limit toxicity
Plicamycin (mithramycin)	Antimicrobial Inhibits RNA synthesis by binding DNA	Cancer chemotherapy Testicular cancer Hypercalcemia		Periorbital pallor[245]		
Tamoxifen	Antihormonal estrogen antagonist	Cancer chemotherapy Breast cancer	Oral	Whorl-like epithelial keratopathy,[237] maculopathy with superficial white refractile opacities associated with cystoid macular edema,[237, 238] optic disc edema,[239, 240] posterior subcapsular cataracts[241]	Yes (120–200 mg/m² for >1 yr; cumulative dose of 90–230 g)	May be irreversible Toxicity unlikely with standard doses[242] but has been reported.[243, 244] Presence of a few intraretinal crystals in absence of macular edema or vision loss or presence of posterior subcapsular opacities does not warrant discontinuation of drug[241]
Vincristine	Vinca alkaloid	Cancer chemotherapy Leukemia Lymphoma Solid tumors	IV	Cranial nerve palsy (50%), internuclear ophthalmoplegia, corneal hypesthesia,[227] optic neuropathy–demyelination,[228] night blindness,[229] and cortical blindness[230, 231]	Yes	Increased toxicity with hepatic dysfunction. Resolves in 3 mo[227] ?Irreversible[221, 228, 231, 232] Reversible in 1–14 days
Antipsychotic						
Chlorpromazine	Phenothiazine	Antipsychotic	Oral, IM, IV	Similar to thioridazine. Pigmentation of skin, conjunctiva, and cornea,[257–259] pigmentary retinopathy (fine)[42, 260]		Pigmentary changes may be reversible[260]
Haloperidol	Buterophenone derivative	Antipsychotic	Oral, IM	Decrease or paralysis of accommodation, mydriasis that may precipitate narrow-angle glaucoma[1] and ?cataracts[261]	Yes	Transient and reversible side effects
Lithium carbonate	Lithium salt	Antipsychotic	Oral	Ocular irritation and photophobia,[1, 262] blurred vision, extraocular muscle abnormalities, exophthalmos,[263] papilledema due to pseudotumor cerebri[264]	Yes	Reversible; toxic drug response related to blood levels (>2 mEq/L);[37] exophthalmos may be seen at normal levels owing to effect on thyroid[263]

Table continued on following page

TABLE 42–1. **Ocular Toxicity and Side Effects of Systemic Medications** *Continued*

Drug	Class	Uses	Route	Side Effects	Dose Relationship	Comments
Thioridazine	Phenothiazine	Antipsychotic	Oral, IM, IV	Decreased vision, paralysis of accommodation, mydriasis due to anticholinergic properties,[1] corneal pigment deposits (epithelium and Descemet's membrane), corneal edema, lens surface deposits.[250, 251] Granularity of posterior pole, transient disc and retinal edema,[252–254] nummular retinopathy,[255] paracentral and ring scotoma,[254] abnormal ERG and EOG,[255, 256] myasthenic neuromuscular blockade, extraocular muscle paralysis, diplopia, ptosis[1, 66]	Dose and duration related. Rare, <1000 mg/day[93] Recommended dose <300 mg/day; maximum 800 mg/day	Symptoms improve after discontinuation, but fundus changes may progress[259]
Antiparkinsonism						
Amantadine	Tricyclic amine	Parkinson's disease Antiviral used in prophylaxis of influenza A2	Oral	Rare. Transient decreased vision, superficial punctate keratitis,[1] sudden vision loss,[265] visual hallucinations[266]	Dose related	Side effects reversible with discontinuation
Benztropine (also biperiden, chlorphenoxamine)	Anticholinergic	Parkinson's disease Control of extrapyramidal disorders	Oral	Decreased accommodation; rarely mydriasis may precipitate narrow-angle glaucoma, hallucinations[1]	Dose related	Ocular side effects more common with benztropine versus biperiden
Levodopa	β-Adrenergic–blocking agent	Parkinson's disease	Oral	Mydriasis may precipitate narrow-angle glaucoma, miosis, ptosis, blepharospasm, visual hallucinations, oculogyric crisis[1, 267]	Dose related	Side effects reversible
Antirheumatic (see also Antiinflammatory and Antineoplastic or Immunosuppressive)						
Allopurinol	Xanthine oxidase inhibitor	Chronic hyperuricemia, gout	Oral	?Cataract,[268–270] ?macular edema and hemorrhage,[271] toxic epidermal necrolysis (Lyell's syndrome)[272–274]	Unclear with cataracts and maculopathy, not dose-related toxic epidermal necrolysis	
Gold	Heavy metal	Rheumatoid arthritis, lupus erythematosus	IM	Conjunctival and corneal deposition, occasionally lens deposition, rarely ptosis, diplopia, nystagmus[275–277]	Yes, >1 g, 1 g/day for years for lenticular deposition	Cornea and lens deposits do not affect visual acuity and are not an indication for discontinuing therapy Deposits reversible after discontinuation
Antispasmodic						
Dicyclomine	Anticholinergic	Antispasmodic	Oral	Rare. Decreased vision, mydriasis (rarely may precipitate narrow-angle glaucoma), decreased accommodation, and photophobia[1]	Yes	Due to mild antichoinergic activity. Side effects reversible and not indication to discontinue drug

Dermatologic						
Canthaxanthine	Carotenoid (non–provitamin A)	Tanning agent for vitiligo, photosensitive dermatitis	Oral	Metamorphopsia, decreased vision,[278, 279] yellow, refractile inner retinal deposits surrounding fovea[278, 279]	Yes; total 30–40 g, >50% retinopathy; total >60 g, >55–100% retinopathy	Increased retinopathy with ingestion of other carotenoids[279, 280]
Chrysarobin		Keratinolytic	Topical	Keratoconjunctivitis[278, 279]	Yes	Symptoms rarely last for weeks after discontinuation
Methoxsalen (also trioxsalen)	Psoralen	Vitiliginous lesions	Oral, topical	?Cataracts[281, 282]		Used in conjunction with ultraviolet light for photochemotherapy (PUVA). Patient requires adequate UV-blocking goggles after therapy
Immunosuppressive (see Antineoplastic or Immunosuppressive)						
Industrial						
Methanol	Alcohol (rubbing, wood)	Industry	Oral, inhalation	Decreased vision, nystagmus, mydriasis, disc and retinal edema, central and cecocentral scotoma, optic atrophy and excavation[283–286]	Variable, as low as 1 oz[287]	Primary site of injury is the optic nerve.[288, 289] Emergency medical therapy (respiratory support, dialysis, ethanol) is required. Vision may improve, usually in 6 days[283]
Stimulant (Gastrointestinal and Urinary Tracts)						
Bethanechol	Quaternary ammonium parasympatho-mimetic	Gastrointestinal and urinary tract stimulant	Oral, subcutaneous	Rare. Occular irritation with lacrimation, decreased accommodation, and miosis[1]		Side effects may continue long after the drug is discontinued
Miscellaneous						
Deferoxamine mesylate	Chelating agent	Removal of excess systemic iron	IV, subcutaneous	Cataracts, visual loss, optic neuropathy, retinal pigmentary degeneration[290–294]	Duration related	Toxicity may be rapid in onset and irreversible.[291–293] Retinopathy reported with single subcutaneous dose[294]
Pamidronate	Biphosphonate	Inhibitor of bone resorption used in hypercalcemia of malignancy, painful bone metastases, and Paget's disease	IV	Mild to severe anterior uveitis and nonspecific conjunctivitis[290, 295]		Anterior uveitis frequently bilateral and may require topical therapy[296]

Abbreviations: AIDS, acquired immunodeficiency syndrome; BCNU, carmustine; CCNU, lomustine; CME, cystoid macular edema; CNS, central nervous system; DDT, chlorophenothane; EOG, electrooculogram; ERG, electroretinogram; GI, gastrointestinal; GU, genitourinary; HTLV, human T-cell lymphotrophic virus; MAO, monoamine oxidase; NFL, nerve fiber layer; PSC, posterior subcapsular cataract; PUVA, psoralen ultraviolet light application; RA, rheumatoid arthritis; UV, ultraviolet.

manifestations (as in the case of intracarotid administration of nitrosoureas, such as bischloroethylnitrosourea [BCNU], for the treatment of primary central nervous system tumors).

The route of drug delivery to the eye and its specific characteristics influence the type of toxicity. Drugs that gain access to the eye through tears may manifest ocular surface abnormality in the form of toxic conjunctivitis or epithelial keratitis (e.g., certain antimetabolites such as methotrexate). Drug access into the eye via the aqueous humor may produce lenticular or posterior corneal changes (e.g., the pigmentary deposits on the anterior lens capsule and posterior cornea seen with chronic phenothiazine use or the formation of posterior subcapsular cataracts due to lens epithelial toxicity from antimetabolites such as busulfan). A variety of drugs used for a diverse range of medical conditions may manifest a similar pattern of toxicity if they possess similar chemical-physical properties. A whorl-pattern epithelial keratopathy may be produced by the group of drugs that possess cationic amphiphilic properties (e.g., amiodarone used for cardiac arrhythmias, chloroquine used as an antimalarial and in collagen vascular disease, indomethacin used as an analgesic and antiinflammatory, and suramin used as an antiprotozoal and as a reverse transcriptase inhibitor of human T-cell lymphotrophic virus III. By binding to polar lipids and thus accumulating in the lysosomes of epithelial cells, these agents produce a "lysosomal disorder" similar to the lysosomal enzyme disorder seen in Fabry's disease and with a similar clinical pattern. Drugs that have affinity for particular chemical components often manifest their toxicity in areas where high concentrations of these components are present. Since the uvea has the highest melanin content of any tissue in the body, it is not surprising that drugs with a high affinity for melanin (e.g., chloroquine and hydroxychloroquine) induce retinal-uveal toxicity.

Not all ocular changes due to systemic drugs require discontinuation of the drug, since some may be inconsequential and ultimately reversible, as with the whorl-like corneal epithelial deposits seen with the cardiac antiarrhythmic amiodarone or the ocular hypotensive effects of orally administered β-blockers used for the therapy of hypertension or angina pectoris. However, other adverse ocular reactions may be irreversible, as with ethambutol-associated optic neuropathy. Thus, it is critical to be aware of the nature of the toxicity and the prognosis in order to plan the appropriate strategies for patient monitoring and management.

Side effects caused by one member of a given chemical family are often, but not always, caused by other members of the same drug group. Therefore, knowledge of side effects of one drug should alert one to monitor for side effects when drugs from a similar family are used. Experimental trials of new agents must include monitoring for the side effects anticipated by the chemical family.

The ophthalmologist must be familiar with the appropriate visual tests and monitoring requirements appropriate for particular drug regimens. It is critical to

1. Identify the toxic agent and know its chemical family
2. Know if the effects are reversible or irreversible in order to determine the appropriate plan of action
3. Be aware if a drug toxicity is cumulative or dose dependent and monitor the specific parameters carefully
4. Be familiar with the appropriate diagnostic tests

Comprehensive reviews of ocular toxicity exist.[1–5] Table 42–1 summarizes important side effects with practical information for recognizing and managing toxicity along with appropriate references.

REFERENCES

1. Fraunfelder FT, Meyer SM: Drug-Induced Ocular Side Effects and Their Drug Interactions, 3rd ed. Philadelphia, Lea & Febiger, 1989.
2. Grant WM: Toxicology of the Eye, 3rd ed. Springfield, IL, Charles C Thomas, 1986.
3. Pavan-Langston D, Dunkel EC: Handbook of Ocular Drug Therapy and Ocular Side Effects of the Systemic Drugs. Boston, Little, Brown. 1991.
4. Physicians' Desk Reference. Oradell, NJ, Medical Economics, 1991.
5. Imperia PS, Lazarus HM, Lass JH: Ocular complications of systemic cancer chemotherapy. Surv Ophthalmol 34:209, 1989.
6. Bullock JD, Albert DM: Flecked retina. Appearance secondary to oxalate crystals from methoxyflurane anesthesia. Arch Ophthalmol 93:26, 1975.
7. Albert DM, Bullock JD, Lahav M, et al: Flecked retina secondary to oxalate crystals from methoxyflurane anesthesia: Clinical and experimental studies. Trans Am Acad Ophthalmol Otolaryngol 79:817, 1975.
8. Almog Y, Monselise M, Almog C: The effect of oral treatment with beta-blockers on the tear secretion. Metab Pediatr Syst Ophthalmol 6:343, 1982.
9. Weber JCP: Beta-adrenoreceptor antagonists and diplopia. Lancet 2:826, 1982.
10. Silverstone PH: Periorbital edema caused by nifedipine. BMJ 288:1654, 1984.
11. Tordjam K, Rosenthal T, Bursztyn M: Nifedipine-induced periorbital edema. Am J Cardiol 55:1445, 1985.
12. Pitlik S, Manor RS, Lipshitz I, et al: Transient retinal ischaemia induced by nifedipine. BMJ 287:1845, 1983.
13. Felix RH, Ive FA, Dahl MDC: Cutaneous and ocular reactions to practolol. BMJ 4:321, 1974.
14. Rahi AHS, Chapman CM, Garner A, et al: Pathology of practolol-induced ocular toxicology. Br J Ophthalmol 60:312, 1976.
15. Van Joost T, Crone RA, Overdijk AD: Ocular cicatricial pemphigoid associated with practolol therapy. Br J Dermatol 94:447, 1976.
16. Wright P: Untoward effects associated with practolol administration: Oculomucocutaneous syndrome. BMJ 1:595, 1975.
17. Hughes RO, Zacharias FJ: Myasthenic syndrome during treatment with practolol. BMJ 1:460, 1976.
18. Amos HE, Brigden WD, McKerron RA: Untoward effects associated with practolol: Demonstration of antibody binding to epithelial tissue. BMJ 1:598, 1975.
19. Amos HE, Lake BG, Artis J: Possible role of antibody specific for a practolol metabolite in the pathogenesis of oculomucocutaneous syndrome. BMJ 1:402, 1978.
20. Singer L, Knobel B, Romem M: Influence of systemic administered beta-blockers on tear secretion. Ann Ophthalmol 16:728, 1984.
21. Yeomans SM, Knox DL, Green WR, Murgatroyd GW: Ocular inflammatory pseudotumor associated with propranolol therapy. Ophthalmology 90:1422, 1983.
22. Sandyk R: Orofacial dyskinesia associated with lorazepam therapy. Clin Pharm 5:419, 1986.
23. Joseph E, Rouselie JE: Cited by Francois J: Cornea verticillata. Doc Ophthalmol 27:235, 1969.
24. Francois J: Cornea verticillata. Doc Ophthalmol 27:235, 1969.
25. Bron AJ: Vortex patterns of the corneal epithelium. Trans Ophthalmol Soc UK 43:455, 1973.
26. D'Amico DJ, Kenyon KR. Ruskin JN: Amiodarone keratopathy. Drug-induced lipid storage disease. Arch Ophthalmol 99:257, 1981.
27. Ingram DV, Jakggarao NSV, Chamberlin DA: Ocular changes resulting from therapy with amiodarone. Br J Ophthalmol 66:676, 1982.
28. Ingram DV: Ocular effects of long-term amiodarone therapy. Am Heart J 99:257, 1983.
29. Orlando RG, Dangel ME, Schaal SG: Clinical experience and grading of amiodarone keratopathy. Ophthalmology 91:1184, 1984.
30. Dickerson EJ, Wolman RL: Sicca syndrome associated with amiodarone therapy. BMJ 293:510, 1986.
31. Flach AJ, Dolan BJ, Sudduth B, et al: Amiodarone-induced lens opacities. Arch Ophthalmol 101:1554, 1983.
32. Delage C, Lagace T, Huard H: Pseudocyanotic pigmentation of the

skin induced by amiodarone: A light and electron microscopic study. Can Med Assoc J 112:1205, 1975.
33. Trimble JW, Mendelson DS, Fetter BF, et al: Cutaneous pigmentation secondary to amiodarone therapy. Arch Dermatol 119:914, 1983.
34. Gittinger JW Jr, Asdourian GK: Papillopathy caused by amiodarone. Arch Ophthalmol 105:349, 1987.
35. Feiner LA, Younge BR, Kazmier FJ, et al: Optic neuropathy and amiodarone therapy. Mayo Clin Proc 62:702, 1987.
36. Fikkers BG, Bogousslavsky J, Regli F, et al: Pseudotumor cerebri with amiodarone. J Neurol Neurosurg Psychiatry 49:606, 1986.
37. Lopez AC, Lopez AM, Jimenez SF, et al: Acute intracranial hypertension during amiodarone infusion. Crit Care Med 13:688, 1985.
38. Ghosh M, McMulloch C: Amiodarone-induced ultrastructural changes in human eyes. Can J Ophthalmol 19:178, 1984.
39. Francois H: Cornea verticillata. Bull Soc Belge Ophthalmol 150:656, 1968.
40. Amiodarone. Med Lett Drugs Ther 28:49, 1986.
41. Kaplan LJ, Cappaert WE: Amiodarone keratopathy. Correlation to dosage and duration. Arch Ophthalmol 100:601, 1982.
42. D'Amico DJ, Kenyon KR: Drug-induced lipidosis of the cornea and conjunctiva. Int Ophthalmol 4:67, 1981.
43. LeSage JM: Color vision deficiencies in people taking digoxin. Invest Ophthalmol Vis Sci 24(Suppl):59, 1983.
44. Ritebrock N, Alken RG: Color vision deficiencies: A common sign of intoxication in chronically digoxin-treated patients. J Cardiovasc Pharmacol 2:93, 1983.
45. Closson RG: Visual hallucinations as the earliest symptom of digoxin intoxication. Arch Neurol 40:386, 1983.
46. Massaro FJ, Moulton JS, Linkewich JA, Major DA: Scotomas secondary to digoxin intoxication. Drug Intell Clin Pharm 17:368, 1983.
47. Weleber RG, Shults WT: Digoxin retinal toxicity. Clinical and electrophysiologic evaluation of a cone dysfunction syndrome. Arch Ophthalmol 99:1568, 1981.
48. Frucht J, Freimann I, Merlin S: Ocular side effects of disopyramide. Br J Ophthalmol 68:890, 1984.
49. Trope GE, Hind VMD: Closed-angle glaucoma in patients on disopyramide. Lancet 1:329, 1981.
50. Turgeon T, Salmovits P: Scleritis as the presenting manifestation of procainamide induced lupus. Ophthalmology 96:68, 1989.
51. Bar S, Feller N, Savir H: Presenile cataracts in phenytoin-treated epileptic patients. Arch Ophthalmol 101:422, 1983.
52. Mathers W, Kattan H, Earll J, Lemp M: Development of presenile cataracts in association with high serum levels of phenytoin. Ann Ophthalmol 19:291, 1987.
53. Kalanie H, Niakan E, Horati Y, Rolak LA: Phenytoin-induced intracranial hypertension. Neurology 36:443, 1986.
54. Bartoshesky LE, Bhan I, Naqpaul K, Pashayan H: Severe cardiac and ophthalmologic malformations in an infant exposed to diphenylhydantoin in utero. Pediatrics 69:209, 1982.
55. Von Knorring L: Changes in saliva secretion and accommodation width during short-term administration of imipramine and zimelidine in healthy volunteers. Int Pharmacopsychiatry 16:69, 1981.
56. Blackwell B, Stefopoulos A, Enders P, et al: Anticholinergic activity of two tricyclic antidepressants. Am J Psychiatry 135:722, 1978.
57. Beal MF: Amitriptyline ophthalmoplegia. Neurology 32:1409, 1982.
58. Delaney P, Light R: Gaze paresis in amitriptyline overdose. Ann Neurol 9:513, 1981.
59. Donhoe SP: Bilateral internuclear ophthalmoplegia from doxepin overdose. Neurology 34:259, 1984.
60. Mullally WJ: Carbamazepine-induced ophthalmoplegia. Arch Neurol 39:64, 1982.
61. Noda S, Umezaki H: Carbamazepine-induced ophthalmoplegia. Neurology 32:1320, 1982.
62. Chrouso's GA, Cowdry R, Schuelein M, et al: Two cases of downbeat nystagmus and oscillopsia associated with carbamazepine. Am J Ophthalmol 103:221, 1987.
63. Wheller SD, Ramsey RE, Weiss J: Drug induced downbeat nystagmus. Ann Neurol 12:227, 1982.
64. Sullivan JB, Rumack BH, Peterson RG: Acute carbamazepine toxicity resulting from overdose. Neurology 31:621, 1981.
65. Neilsen N, Syversen K: Possible retinotoxic effect of carbamazepine. Acta Ophthalmol 64:287, 1986.
66. Kaeser HE: Drug-induced myasthenic syndromes. Acta Neurol Scand 70(Suppl 100):39, 1984.
67. Gumby P: Methylphenidate abuse produces retinopathy. JAMA 241:546, 1979.
68. Tse DT, Ober RR: Talc retinopathy. Am J Ophthalmol 90:624, 1980.
69. Hays DP, Johnson BF, Perry R: Prolonged hallucinations following a modest overdose of tripelennamine. Clin Toxicol 16:331, 1980.
70. Farber AS: Ocular side effects of antihistamine-decongestant combinations. Am J Ophthalmol 94:565, 1982.
71. Granacher RP Jr: Facial dyskinesia after antihistamines. N Engl J Med 296:516, 1977.
72. Sovner RD: Dyskinesia associated with chronic antihistamine use. [Letter] N Engl J Med 294:113, 1976.
73. Davis WA: Dyskinesia associated with chronic antihistamine use. [Letter] N Engl J Med 294:113, 1976.
74. Gass JDM: Nicotinic acid maculopathy. Am J Ophthalmol 76:500, 1953.
75. Millay RH, Klein ML, Illingworth DR: Niacin maculopathy. Ophthalmology 95:930, 1988.
76. Doherty M, Maddison PJ, Grey RHB: Hydralazine induced lupus syndrome with eye disease. BMJ 290:675, 1985.
77. Johansson M, Manhem P: SLE-syndrome with exophthalmos after treatment with hydralazine. Lakartidningen 72:153, 1975.
78. Mansilla-Tinoco R, Harland SJ, Ryan PJ, et al: Hydralazine, antinuclear antibodies, and lupus syndrome. BMJ 284:936, 1982.
79. Peacock A, Weatherall D: Hydralazine-induced necrotizing vasculitis. BMJ 282:1121, 1981.
80. Loredo A, Rodriguez RS, Murillo L: Cataracts after short term corticosteroid treatment. N Engl J Med 286:160, 1972.
81. Kennedy I: Cortisone-induced opacities of the crystalline lens. Trans Aust Coll Ophthalmol 73:236, 1972.
82. Pfefferman R, Gombos GM, Kountz SL: Ocular complications after renal transplantation. Ann Ophthalmol 9:467, 1967.
83. Black RL, Oglesby RB, von Sallman L, Bunimm JJ: Posterior subcapsular cataracts induced by corticosteroids in patients with rheumatoid arthritis. JAMA 174:150, 1960.
84. McDonnell PJ, Muir MGK: Glaucoma associated with systemic corticosteroid therapy. Lancet 2:386, 1985.
85. Williamson J, Peterson RW, McGavin DD, et al: Posterior subcapsular cataracts and glaucoma associated with long-term oral corticosteroid therapy: In patients with rheumatoid arthritis and related conditions. Br J Ophthalmol 53:361, 1969.
86. Walker AE, Adamkiewicz JT: Pseudotumor cerebri associated with prolonged corticosteroid therapy. JAMA 188:779, 1964.
87. Ivey KJ, Denbesten L: Pseudotumor cerebri associated with corticosteroid therapy in an adult. JAMA 208:1698, 1969.
88. Sloansky HH, Kolbert G, Gartner S: Exophthalmos induced by steroids. Arch Ophthalmol 77:579, 1967.
89. Cohen BA, Som PM, Haffner PH, Friedman AH: Case report: Steroid exophthalmos. J Comput Assist Tomogr 5:907, 1981.
90. Nassif KF: Ocular surface defense mechanisms. *In* Tabbara KF. Hyndiuk RA (eds): Infections of the Eye. Boston, Little, Brown, 1986, p 37.
91. Becker B: Diabetes mellitus and primary open angle glaucoma. Am J Ophthalmol 71:1, 1971.
92. Havener WH: Corticosteroid therapy. *In* Havener WH (ed): Ocular Pharmacology. St. Louis, CV Mosby, 1983, p 433.
93. Spaeth GL, Rodrigues MM, Weinreb S: Steroid induced glaucoma: A. Persistent elevation of intraocular pressure. B. Histopathological aspects. Trans Am Ophthalmol Soc 75:353, 1977.
94. Polansky JR, Weinreb RN: Anti-inflammatory agents—Steroids as anti-inflammatory agents. *In* Sears ML (ed): Pharmacology of the Eye. New York, Springer-Verlag, 1984, p 459.
95. Forman AR, Loreto JA, Tina LU: Reversibility of corticosteroid-associated cataracts in children with nephrotic syndrome. Am J Ophthalmol 84:75, 1977.
96. Asherov J, Schoenberg A, Weinberger A: Diplopia following ibuprofen administration. [Letter] JAMA 248:649, 1982.
97. Tullio CJ: Ibuprofen-induced visual disturbance. Am J Hosp Pharm 38:1962, 1981.
98. Fraunfelder FT: Interim report: National registry of possible drug-induced ocular side effects. Ophthalmology 87:87, 1980.
99. Palmer CAL: Toxic amblyopia from ibuprofen. BMJ 3:765, 1972.
100. Callum LMT, Bowen DI: Ocular side effects of ibuprofen. Br J Ophthalmol 55:472, 1971.
101. Hamburger HA, Beckman H, Thompson R: Visual evoked potentials and ibuprofen (Motrin) toxicity. Ann Ophthalmol 16:328, 1984.
102. Foster CS: Nonsteroidal anti-inflammatory drugs and immunosuppressives. *In* Lamberts DN, Potter DE (eds): Clinical Ophthalmic Pharmacology. Boston, Little, Brown, 1987, p 173.

103. Burns CA: Indomethacin, reduced retinal sensitivity, and corneal deposits. Am J Ophthalmol 66:825, 1968.
104. Tillmann W, Keitel L: Indomethacin-induced corneal deposits. Klin Monatsbl Augenheilkd 170:756, 1977.
105. Katzman B, Lu LW, Tiwari RP, Bansal R: Pseudomotor cerebri: An observation and review. Ann Ophthalmol 13:887, 1981.
106. Konomi H, Imai M, Nihei K, et al: Indomethacin causing pseudomotor cerebri in Bartter's syndrome. N Engl J Med 298:855, 1978.
107. Umez-Eronini EM: Conjunctivitis due to ketoprofen. Lancet 2:737, 1978.
108. McDowell IFW, McConnell JB: Cholinergic crisis in myasthenia gravis precipitated by ketoprofen. BMJ 291:1094, 1985.
109. Larizza D, Colombo A, Lorini R, Severi F: Ketoprofen causing pseudotumor cerebri in Bartter's syndrome. N Engl J Med 300:796, 1979.
110. Szmyd L Jr, Perry HD: Keratopathy associated with the use of naproxen. Am J Ophthalmol 99:598, 1985.
111. Mordes JP, Johnson MW, Soter NA: Possible naproxen-associated vasculitis. Arch Intern Med 140:985, 1980.
112. Shelley WB, Elpern DJ, Shelley ED: Naproxen photosensitization demonstrated by challenge. Cutis 38:169, 1986.
113. Hobbs HE, Eadie SP, Somerville F: Ocular lesions after treatment with chloroquine. Br J Ophthalmol 45:284, 1961.
114. Henkind P, Rothfield NF: Ocular abnormalities in patients treated with synthetic antimalarial drugs. N Engl J Med 269:433, 1963.
115. Bernstein HN: Ophthalmic considerations and testing in patients receiving long-term antimalarial therapy. Am J Med 75(1A):25, 1983.
116. Henkind P, Carr RE, Siegel IM: Early chloroquine retinopathy: Clinical and functional findings. Arch Ophthalmol 71:157, 1964.
117. Ellsworth RJ, Zeller RW: Chloroquine (Aralen)–induced retinal damage. Arch Ophthalmol 66:269, 1961.
118. Hart WM, Burde RM, Johnston GP, Drews RC: Static perimetry in chloroquine retinopathy. Perifoveal patterns of visual field depression. Arch Ophthalmol 102:377, 1984.
119. Okun E, Gouras P, Berstein H, Von Sallman L: Chloroquine retinopathy: A report of eight cases with ERG and dark-adaptation findings. Arch Ophthalmol 69:59, 1963.
120. Nylander U: Ocular damage in chloroquine therapy. Acta Ophthalmol 44:335, 1966.
121. Percival SPB, Behrman J: Ophthalmological safety of chloroquine. Br J Ophthalmol 53:101, 1969.
122. Arden GB, Kolb H: Antimalarial therapy and early retinal changes in patients with rheumatoid arthritis. BMJ 29:270, 1966.
123. MacKenzie AH: Dose refinements in long-term therapy of rheumatoid arthritis with antimalarials. Am J Med 75(1A):40, 1983.
124. Johnson MW, Vine AK: Hydroxychloroquine therapy in massive total doses without retinal toxicity. Am J Ophthalmol 104:139, 1987.
125. Burns RP: Delayed onset of chloroquine retinopathy. N Engl J Med 275:693, 1966.
126. Carr RE, Henkind P, Rothfield N, et al: Ocular toxicity of antimalarial drugs, long-term follow-up. Am J Ophthalmol 66:738, 1968.
127. Brinkley JR, Dubois EL, Ryan SJ: Long-term course of chloroquine retinopathy after cessation of medication. Am J Ophthalmol 88:1, 1979.
128. Sassani JW, Brucker AJ, Cobbs W, Campbell C: Progressive chloroquine retinopathy. Ann Ophthalmol 15:19, 1983.
129. Easterbrook M: The use of Amsler grids in early chloroquine retinopathy. Ophthalmology 91:1368, 1984.
130. Easterbrook M: The sensitivity of Amsler grid testing in early chloroquine retinopathy. Trans Ophthalmol Soc UK 104:204, 1985.
131. Wolfe KA, Sadun AA, Kitridou RC: The detection of hydroxychloroquine maculopathy with threshold Amsler grid testing. Invest Ophthalmol Vis Sci 31(Suppl):136, 1990.
132. Nozik RA, Weinstock FJ, Vignos PJ: Ocular complications of chloroquine, a series and case presentation with a simple method for early detection of retinopathy. Am J Ophthalmol 58:774, 1969.
133. Van Lith GHM, Mak GTM, Wijnands H: Clinical importance of the electrooculogram with special reference to the chloroquine retinopathy. Bibl Ophthalmol 85:2, 1976.
134. Van Lith GHM: Electro-ophthalmology and side effects of drugs. Doc Ophthalmol 58:774, 1969.
135. Daneshmend TK, Homeida M: Dapsone-induced optic atrophy and motor neuropathy. BMJ 283:311, 1981.
136. Brinton GS, Norton EW, Zahn JR, Knighton JW: Ocular quinine toxicity. Am J Ophthalmol 90:403, 1980.
137. Dyson EH, Proudfoot AT, Prescott LF, Heyworth R: Death and blindness due to overdose of quinine. BMJ 291:31, 1985.
138. Friedman L, Rothkoff L, Zaks U: Clinical observations on quinine toxicity. Ann Ophthalmol 12:641, 1980.
139. Davidson NJ, Windebank WJ: Stevens-Johnson syndrome and amoxycillin. BMJ 292:380, 1986.
140. Argov Z, Brenner T, Abramsky O: Ampicillin may aggravate clinical and experimental myasthenia gravis. Arch Neurol 43:255, 1986.
141. Shah GK, Cantrill HL, Holland EJ: Vortex keratopathy associated with atovaquone. Am J Ophthalmol 120:669, 1995.
142. Green ST, Natarajan S, Campbell JC: Erythema multiforme following cefotaxime therapy. Postgrad Med J 62:415, 1986.
143. Kannangara DW, Smith B, Cohen K: Exfoliative dermatitis during cefoxitin therapy. Arch Intern Med 142:1031, 1982.
144. Arcieri G, Griffith E, Gruenwaldt G, et al: Ciprofloxacin: An update on clinical experience. Am J Med 82(Suppl 4A):381, 1987.
145. Rahm V, Schacht P: Safety of ciprofloxacin: A review. Scand J Infect Dis 60(Suppl):120, 1989.
146. Vrabec TA, Sergott RC, Jaeger EA, et al: Reversible visual loss in a patient receiving high-dose ciprofloxacin hydrochloride (Cipro). Ophthalmology 97:707, 1990.
147. Godel V, Nemet P, Lazar M: Chloramphenicol optic neuropathy. Arch Ophthalmol 98:1417, 1980.
148. Lambda PA, Sood NN, Moorthy SS: Retinopathy due to chloramphenicol. Scot Med J 13:166, 1968.
149. Brothers DM, Hidayat AA: Conjunctival pigmentation associated with tetracycline medication. Ophthalmology 88:1212, 1981.
150. Messmer E, Font RL, Sheldon G, Murphy D: Pigmented conjunctival cysts following tetracycline/minocycline therapy. Histochemical and electron microscopic observations. Ophthalmology 90:1462, 1983.
151. Fraunfelder FT, Randall JA: Minocycline-induced scleral pigmentation. Ophthalmology 104:936, 1997.
152. Meacock DJ, Hewer RL: Tetracycline and benign intracranial hypertension. BMJ 282:1240, 1981.
153. Walters B, Gubbay S: Tetracycline and benign intracranial hypertension. Report of five cases. BMJ 282:19, 1981.
154. Argov Z, Mastaglia FL: Disorders of neuromuscular transmission caused by drugs. N Engl J Med 301:409, 1979.
155. Gedroyc W, Shorvon SD: Acute intracranial hypertension and nalidixic acid therapy. Neurology 32:212, 1982.
156. Kilpatrick C, Ebeling P: Intracranial hypertension in nalidixic acid therapy. Med J Aust 1:252, 1982.
157. Rubinstein A: LE-like disease caused by nalidixic acid. N Engl J Med 301:1288, 1979.
158. Bovino JA, Marcus DF: The mechanism of transient myopia induced by sulfonamide therapy. Am J Ophthalmol 94:99, 1982.
159. Chirls IA, Norris JW: Transient myopia associated with vaginal sulfanilamide suppositories. Am J Ophthalmol 98:120, 1984.
160. Hook SR, Holladay JT, Praeger TC, Goosey JD: Transient myopia induced by sulfonamides. Am J Ophthalmol 101:495, 1986.
161. Genvert GI, Cohen EJ, Donnenfeld ED, Blecher MH: Erythema multiforme after use of topical sulfacetamide. Am J Ophthalmol 99:465, 1985.
162. Tilden ME, Rosenbaum JT, Fraunfelder FT: Systemic sulfonamides as a cause of bilateral, anterior uveitis. Arch Ophthalmol 109:67, 1991.
163. Ohman L, Wahlberg I: Ocular side effects of clofazimine. Lancet 2:933, 1975.
164. Walinder PE, Gip L, Stempa M: Corneal changes in patients treated with clofazimine. Br J Ophthalmol 60:526, 1976.
165. Teich SA, Handwerger S, Mathur-Wagh U, et al: Toxic keratopathy associated with suramin therapy. N Engl J Med 314:1455, 1986.
166. Thylefors B, Rolland A: The risk of optic atrophy following suramin treatment of ocular onchocerciasis. Bull WHO 57:479, 1979.
167. Joubert PH, Strobele JG, Ogle CW, van der Merwe CA: Subclinical impairment of colour vision in patients receiving ethambutol. Br J Clin Pharmacol 21:213, 1986.
168. Arruga J: Test of subjective desaturation of color in diagnosis of effect of ethambutol on anterior optic pathway. Bull Soc Ophthalmol Fr 82:182, 1982.
169. Chatterjee VK, Buchanan DR, Friedmann AI, Green M: Ocular toxicity following ethambutol in standard dosage. Br J Dis Chest 80:288, 1986.
170. Leibold, JE: The ocular toxicity of ethambutol and its relation to dose. Ann N Y Acad Sci 135:904, 1966.
171. Yiannikas C, Walsh JC, McLeod JG: Visual evoked potentials in the detection of subclinical optic toxic effects secondary to ethambutol. Arch Neurol 40:645, 1983.

172. Böke W: Untersuchungen zur Frage der Sehnervenschäden unter INH-Behandlung. Ber Ophthal Ges 59:282, 1955.
173. Kiyosawa M, Ishikawa S: A case of isoniazid-induced optic neuropathy. Neuroophthalmology 2:67, 1981.
174. Renard G, Morax PV: Optic neuritis in the course of treatment of tuberculosis. Ann Oculist 210:53, 1977.
175. Saran BR, Maguire AM, Nichols C, et al: Hypopyon uveitis in patients with acquired immunodeficiency syndrome treated for systemic *Mycobacterium avium* complex infection with rifabutin. Arch Ophthalmol 112:1159, 1994.
176. Jacobs DS, Piliero PJ, Kuperwaser MG, et al: Acute uveitis associated with rifabutin use in patients with human immunodeficiency virus infection. Am J Ophthalmol 118:716, 1994.
177. Shafran SD, Singer J, Zarowny DB, et al: A comparison of two regimens for the treatment of *Mycobacterium avium* complex bacteremia in AIDS: rifabutin, ethambutol, and clarithromycin versus rifampin, ethambutol, clofazimine, ciprofloxacin. Canadian HIV Trials Network Protocol 010 Study Group. N Engl J Med 335:377, 1996.
178. Chaknis MJ, Brooks SE, Mitchell KT, Marcus DM: Inflammatory opacities of the vitreous in rifabutin-associated uveitis. Am J Ophthalmol 122:580, 1996.
179. Lowe SH, Kroon FP, Bollemeyer JG, et al: Uveitis during treatment of disseminated *Mycobacterium avium-intracellulare* complex infection with the combination of rifabutin, clarithromycin and ethambutol. Neth J Med 48:P211, 1996.
180. Tseng AL, Walmsley SL: Rifabutin-associated uveitis. Ann Pharmacother 29:1149, 1995.
181. Dunn AM, Tizer K, Cervia JS: Rifabutin-associated uveitis in a pediatric patient. Pediatr Infect Dis J 14:246, 1995.
182. Karbassi M, Nikou S: Acute uveitis in patients with acquired immunodeficiency syndrome receiving prophylactic rifabutin. Arch Ophthalmol 113:699, 1995.
183. Girling DJ: Ocular toxicity due to rifampicin. BMJ 1:585, 1976.
184. Fraunfelder FT: Orange tears: Am J Ophthalmol 89:752, 1980.
185. Lyons RW: Orange contact lenses from rifampin. N Engl J Med 300:372, 1979.
186. Anderson B, Anderson B Jr: Necrotizing uveitis incident to perfusion of intracranial malignancies with nitrogen mustard or related compounds. Trans Am Ophthalmol Soc 58:95, 1960.
187. Sullivan RD, Jones R Jr, Schnabel TG Jr, et al: The treatment of human cancer with intra-arterial nitrogen mustard. Cancer 6:121, 1953.
188. Kende G, Sirkin SR, Thomas PRM, et al: Blurring of vision. A previously undescribed complication of cyclophosphamide therapy. Cancer 44:69, 1979.
189. Jack MK, Hicks JD: Ocular complications in high-dose chemoradiotherapy and marrow transplantation. Ann Ophthalmol 13:709, 1981.
190. Fraunfelder FT, Meyers SM: Ocular toxicity of antineoplastic agents. Ophthalmology 90:1, 1983.
191. Wilding G, Caruso R, Lawrence TS, et al: Retinal toxicity after high-dose cisplatin therapy. J Clin Oncol 3:1683, 1985.
192. Becher R, Schutt P, Osieka R, et al: Peripheral neuropathy and ophthalmologic toxicity after treatment with cis-dichlorodiamminoplatinum. II: J Cancer Res Clin Oncol 96:219, 1980.
193. Ostrow S, Hahn D, Wiernick PH, et al: Ophthalmologic toxicity after cis-dichlorodiammineplatinum (II) therapy. Cancer Treat Rep 62:1592, 1978.
194. Berman IJ, Mann MP: Seizures and transient cortical blindness associated with cis-platinum (II) diamminedichloride (PDD) therapy in a thirty year old man. Cancer 45:764, 1980.
195. Feun LG, Wallace S, Feun L, et al: Intracarotid infusion of cis-diamminedichloroplatinum in the treatment of recurrent malignant intracerebral tumors. Cancer 54:794, 1984.
196. Lass JH, Lazarus HM, Reed MD, Herzig RH: Topical corticosteroid therapy for corneal toxicity from systemically administered cytarabine. Am J Ophthalmol 94:617, 1982.
197. Stewart DJ, Wallace S, Feun L, et al: A phase I study of intracarotid artery infusion of cis-diamminedichloroplatinum (II) in patients with recurrent malignant intracerebral tumors. Cancer Res 42:2059, 1982.
198. Vizel M, Oster MW: Ocular side effects of cancer chemotherapy. Cancer 49:1999, 1982.
199. Sidi Y, Douer D, Pinkhas J: Sicca syndrome in a patient with toxic reaction to busulfan. JAMA 238:1951, 1977.
200. Dahlgren S, Holm G, Svanborg N, Watz R: Clinical and morphological side-effects of busulfan (Myleran) treatment. Acta Med Scand 192:129, 1972.
201. Podos SM, Canellos GP: Lens changes in chronic granulocytic leukemia. Possible relationship to chemotherapy. Am J Ophthalmol 68:500, 1969.
202. Ravindranathan MP, Paul VJ, Kuriakose ET: Cataract after busulphan treatment. BMJ 1:218, 1972.
203. Podos SM, Canellos GP: Ocular toxicity of busulfan. Am J Ophthalmol 68:500, 1969.
204. Shingelton BJ, Bienfang DC, Albert DM, et al: Ocular toxicity associated with high dose carmustine. Arch Ophthalmol 100:1766, 1982.
205. Louie AC, Turrisi AT, Muggia FM, et al: Visual abnormalities following nitrosourea treatment. Med Pediatr Oncol 5:245, 1978.
206. Grimson BS, Maheley MS Jr, Dubey HD, et al: Ophthalmic and central nervous system complications following intracarotid BCNU (carmustine). J Clin Neuroophthalmol 1:261, 1981.
207. McLennan R, Taylor JR: Optic neuroretinitis in association with BCNU and procarbazine therapy. Med Pediatr Oncol 4:43, 1978.
208. Gebarski SS, Greenberg HS, Gabrielsen TO, et al: Orbital angiographic changes after intracarotid BCNU chemotherapy. Am J Neuroradiol 5:55, 1984.
209. Miller DF, Bay JW, Lederman RJ, et al: Ocular and orbital toxicity following intracarotid injection of BCNU (carmustine) and cisplatinum for malignant gliomas. Ophthalmology 92:402, 1985.
210. Hammersley J, Luce JK, Florent TR, et al: Excessive lacrimation from fluorouracil treatment. JAMA 225:747, 1973.
211. Horio T, Murai T, Ikai K: Photosensitivity due to a fluorouracil derivative. Arch Dermatol 114:1498, 1978.
212. Straus DJ, Mausolf FA, Ellerby RA, et al: Cicatricial ectropion secondary to 5-fluorouracil therapy. Med Pediatr Oncol 3:15, 1977.
213. Caravella LP, Burns JA, Zangmeister M: Punctual-canalicular stenosis related to systemic fluorouracil therapy. Arch Ophthalmol 99:284, 1981.
214. Haidal DJ, Hurwitz BS, Yeung KY: Tear-duct fibrosis (dacrostenosis) due to 5-fluorouracil. [Letter] Ann Intern Med 88:657, 1978.
215. Salminen L, Jantti V, Bronross M: Blepharospasm associated with tegafur combination chemotherapy. [Letter] Am J Ophthalmol 97:649, 1984.
216. Bixenamn WW, Nicholls JVV, Warwick OH: Oculomotor disturbances associated with 5-fluorouracil chemotherapy. Am J Ophthalmol 83:789, 1977.
217. Weiss HD, Walker MD, Wierni PH: Neurotoxicity of commonly used antineoplastic agents. N Engl J Med 291:75, 1974.
218. Adams JW, Bofenkamp TM, Kobrin J, et al: Recurrent acute toxic optic neuropathy secondary to 5-FU. [Letter] Cancer Treat Rep 68:565, 1984.
219. Straus DJ, Mausolf FA, Ellerby RA, et al: Cicatricial ectropion secondary to 5-fluorouracil therapy. Med Pediatr Oncol 3:15, 1977.
220. Castleberry RP, Crist WM, Holbrook T, et al: The cytosine arabinoside (Ara C) syndrome. Med Pediatr Oncol 9:257, 1981.
221. Hopen G, Mondino BJ, Johnson BL, et al: Corneal toxicity with systemic cytarabine. Am J Ophthalmol 91:500, 1981.
222. Lass JH, Lazarus HM, Reed MD, Herzig RH: Topical corticosteroid therapy for corneal toxicity from systemically administered cytarabine. Am J Ophthalmol 94:617, 1982.
223. Ritch PS, Hansen RM, Heuer DK: Ocular toxicity from high dose cytosine arabinoside. Cancer 51:430, 1983.
224. Margileth DA, Poplack DG, Tizzo PA, et al: Blindness during remission in two patients with acute lymphoblastic leukemia: A possible complication of multimodality therapy. Cancer 39:58, 1977.
225. Lazarus HM, Hartnett ME, Reed MD, et al: Comparison of the prophylactic effects of 2-deoxycytidine and prednisolone for high-dose intravenous cytarabine-induced keratitis. Am J Ophthalmol 104:476, 1987.
226. Chung JG, Leyland-Jones BR, Caryk SM, et al: Central nervous system toxicity of fludarabine phosphate. Cancer Treat Rep 70:1225, 1986.
227. Albert DM, Wong VG, Henderson ES: Ocular complications of vincristine therapy. Arch Ophthalmol 78:709, 1967.
228. Sanderson PA, Kuwabara T, Cogan DG: Optic neuropathy presumably caused by vincristine therapy. Am J Ophthalmol 81:146, 1976.
229. Ripps H, Carr RE, Siegel IM, et al: Functional abnormalities in vincristine-induced night blindness. Invest Ophthalmol Vis Sci 25:787, 1984.
230. Byrd RL, Rohrbaugh TM, Raney RB Jr, et al: Transient cortical blindness secondary to vincristine therapy in childhood malignancies. Cancer 47:37, 1981.

231. Awidi AS: Blindness and vincristine. [Letter] Ann Intern Med 93:781, 1980.
232. Shurin SB, Rekate HL, Annable W: Optic atrophy induced by vincristine. Pediatrics 70:288, 1982.
233. Doroshow JH, Locker GY, Gasterland DE, et al: Ocular irritation from high-dose methotrexate therapy: Pharmokinetics of drug in the tear film. Cancer 48:2158, 1981.
234. Johnson DR, Burns RP: Blepharoconjunctivitis associated with cancer chemotherapy. Trans Pac Coast Otoophthalmol Soc Annu Mt 46:43, 1965.
235. Christophidis N, Vajda FJE, Lucas I, et al: Ocular side effects with 5-fluorouracil. Aust N Z J Med 9:143, 1979.
236. Millay RH, Klein ML, Shults WT, et al: Maculopathy associated with combination chemotherapy and osmotic opening of the blood-brain barrier. Am J Ophthalmol 102:626, 1986.
237. Kaiser-Kupfer MI, Lippman ME: Tamoxifen retinopathy. Cancer Treat Rep 62:315, 1978.
238. McKeown CA, Swartz M, Blom J, et al: Tamoxifen retinopathy. Br J Ophthalmol 65:177, 1981.
239. Ashford AR, Donev I, Tiwari RP, et al: Reversible ocular toxicity related to tamoxifen therapy. Cancer 61:33, 1988.
240. Pugesgaard T, von Eiben FE: Bilateral optic neuritis evolved during tamoxifen treatment. Cancer 58:383, 1986.
241. Gorin BM: An update regarding chronic, low-dose tamoxifen administration and ocular toxicity. National Surgical Adjuvant Breast and Bowel Program (NSABP) letter to oncologist and eye care professionals. Attachment E, p 12; 1997.
242. Beck M, Mills PV: Ocular assessment of patients treated with tamoxifen. Cancer Treat Rep 63:1833, 1979.
243. Vinding T, Nielson NV: Retinopathy caused by treatment with tamoxifen in low dosage. Acta Ophthalmol 61:45, 1983.
244. Griffiths MFP: Tamoxifen retinopathy at low dosage. Am J Ophthalmol 104:185, 1987.
245. Vizel M, Oster MW: Ocular side effects of cancer chemotherapy. Cancer 49:1999, 1982.
246. Weiss JN, Weinberg RS, Regelson W: Keratopathy after oral administration of tilorone hydrochloride. Am J Ophthalmol 89:46, 1980.
247. Weiss JN, Ochs AL, Abedi S, et al: Retinopathy after tilorone hydrochloride. Am J Ophthalmol 90:846, 1980.
248. Hoffman DL, Mattox VR: Treatment of adrenocortical carcinoma with *o,p′*-DDD. Med Clin North Am 56:999, 1972.
249. Hutter A, Kayhoe D: Adrenal cortical carcinoma: Results of treatment with *op*-DDD in 138 patients. Am J Med 41:583, 1966.
250. Deluise VP, Flynn JT: Asymmetric anterior segment changes induced by chloropromazine. Ann Ophthalmol 13:953, 1981.
251. May RH, Selymes P, Weekley RD, et al: Thioridazine therapy: Results and complications. J Nerv Ment Dis 130:230, 1960.
252. Weekley RD, Potts AM, Reboton J, et al: Pigmentary retinopathy in patients receiving high doses of a new phenothiazine. Arch Ophthalmol 64:64, 1960.
253. Cameron ME, Lawrence JM, Olrich JG: Thioridazine (Mellaril) retinopathy. Br J Ophthalmol 56:131, 1972.
254. Kozy D, Doft BH, Lipkowitz J: Nummular thioridazine retinopathy. Retina 4:253, 1984.
255. Davidorf FH: Thioridazine pigmentary retinopathy. Arch Ophthalmol 90:251, 1973.
256. De Margerie J: Ocular changes produced by a phenothiazine drug: Thioridazine. Trans Can Ophthalmol Soc 25:160, 1962.
257. Zelickson AS, Zeller HC: A new and unusual reaction to chlorpromazine. JAMA 188:144, 1964.
258. DeLong SL, Poley BJ, McFarlane JR: Ocular changes associated with long-term chlorpromazine therapy. Arch Ophthalmol 73:611, 1965.
259. Siddall JR: The ocular toxic findings with prolonged and high dosage chlorpromazine intake. Arch Ophthalmol 74:460, 1965.
260. Siddall JR: Ocular and toxic changes associated with chlorpromazine and thioridazine. Can J Ophthalmol 190:190, 1966.
261. Honda S: Drug-induced cataract in mentally ill subjects. Jpn J Clin Ophthalmol 28:521, 1974.
262. Caplan RP, Fry AH: Photophobia in lithium intoxication. BMJ 285:1314, 1982.
263. Thompson CH, Baylis PH: Asymptomatic Graves' disease during lithium therapy. Postgrad Med J 62:295, 1986.
264. Saul RF, Hamburger HA, Selhorst JB: Pseudotumor cerebri secondary to lithium carbonate. JAMA 253:2869, 1985.
265. Pearlman JT, Kadish AH, Ramseyer JC: Vision loss associated with amantadine hydrochloride use. JAMA 237:1200, 1977.
266. Postma JU, Van Tilburg W: Visual hallucinations and delirium during treatment with amantadine (Symmetrel). J Am Geriatr Soc 23:212, 1975.
267. Shimizu N, Cohen B, Bala SP, et al: Ocular dyskinesias in patients with Parkinson's disease treated with levodopa. Ann Neurol 1:167, 1977.
268. Fraunfelder FT, Lerman S: Allopurinol and cataracts. Am J Ophthalmol 99:215, 1985.
269. Lerman S, Megaw JM, Gardner K: Allopurinol therapy and human cataractogenesis. Am J Ophthalmol 94:141, 1982.
270. Jick H, Brandt DE: Allopurinol and cataracts. Am J Ophthalmol 98:355, 1984.
271. Laval J: Allopurinol and macular lesions. Arch Ophthalmol 80:415, 1968.
272. Singer JZ, Wallace SL: The allopurinol hypersensitivity syndrome. Unnecessary morbidity and mortality. Arthritis Rheum 29:82, 1986.
273. Dan M, Jedwab M, Peled M, Shibolet S: Allopurinol-induced toxic epidermal necrolysis. Int J Dermatol 23:142, 1984.
274. Aubock J, Fritsch P: Asymptomatic hyperuricemia and allopurinol induced toxic epidermal necrolysis. BMJ 290:1969, 1985.
275. Kincaid MC, Green WR, Hoover RE, Schenck PH: Ocular chrysiasis. Arch Ophthalmol 100:1791, 1982.
276. McCormick SA, DeBartolomeo AG, Rajie VK, Schwab IR: Ocular chrysiasis. Ophthalmology 92:1432, 1985.
277. Weidle EG: Lenticular chrysiasis in oral chrysotherapy. Am J Ophthalmol 103:240, 1987.
278. Cortin P, Corriveau LA, Rousseau AP, et al: Maculopathie en paillettes d'or. Can J Ophthalmol 17:103, 1982.
279. Cortin P, Boudreault G, Rousseau AP, et al: La rétinopathie à la canthaxanthine. 2: Facteurs prédisposants. Can J Ophthalmol 19:215, 1984.
280. Boudreault G, Cortin P, Corriveau LA, et al: La rétinopathie à la canthaxanthine. 1: Etude clinique de 51 consommateurs. Can J Ophthalmol 18:325, 1983.
281. Lafond G, Roy PE, Grenier R: Lens opacities appearing during therapy with methoxsalen and long-wavelength ultraviolet radiation. Can J Ophthalmol 19:173, 1984.
282. Woo TY, Wong RC, Wong JM, et al: Lenticular psoralen photoproducts and cataracts of a PUVA treated psoriatic patient. Arch Dermatol 121:1307, 1985.
283. Benton CD, Calhoun FP: The ocular effects of methyl alcohol poisoning: Report of a catastrophe involving three hundred and twenty persons. Trans Am Acad Ophthalmol Otolaryngol 56:875, 1952.
284. McGregor IS: A study in the histopathological changes in the retina and late changes in the visual field in acute methyl alcohol poisoning. Br J Ophthalmol 27:523, 1943.
285. Krohlman GM, Pidde WJ: Acute methyl alcohol poisoning. Can J Ophthalmol 3:270, 1968.
286. Benton CD, Calhoun FP: The ocular effects of methyl alcohol poisoning: Report of a catastrophe involving 320 persons. Am J Ophthalmol 36:1677, 1953.
287. Bennett IL, Carey FH, Mitchell GL, et al: Acute methyl alcohol poisoning: A review based on experiences in an outbreak of 323 cases. Medicine 32:431, 1953.
288. Hayreh MS, Hayreh SS, Baumbach GL, et al: Methyl alcohol poisoning. III: Ocular toxicity. Arch Ophthalmol 95:1851, 1977.
289. Baumbach GL, Cancilla PA, Martin-Amat G, et al: Methyl alcohol poisoning. IV: Alterations of the morphological findings of the retina and optic nerve. Arch Ophthalmol 95:1859, 1977.
290. Bloomfiled SE, Markenson AL, Mill DR, Peterson CM: Lens opacities in thalassemia. J Pediatr Ophthalmol Strabismus 15:154, 1978.
291. Orton RB, de Veber LL, Sulh HM: Ocular and auditory toxicity of long-term, high-dose subcutaneous deferoxamine therapy. Can J Ophthalmol 20:153, 1982.
292. Lakhanpal V, Schocket SS, Jiji R: Deferoxamine (Desferal)–induced toxic retinal pigmentary degeneration and presumed optic neuropathy. Ophthalmology 91:443, 1984.
293. Olivieri NF, Buncic JR, Chew E, et al: Visual and auditory neurotoxicity in patients receiving subcutaneous deferoxamine infusions. N Engl J Med 314:869, 1986.
294. Mehta AM, Engstrom RE, Kreiger AE: Deferoxamine-associated retinopathy after subcutaneous injection. Am J Ophthalmol 118:260, 1994.
295. Siris ES: Biphosphonates and iritis. Lancet 341:436, 1993.
296. Fraunfelder FT, Macarol V: Pamifronate disodium and possible ocular adverse drug reaction. Am J Ophthalmol 118:220, 1994.

CHAPTER 43

Toxicology of Surgical Solutions and Drugs

James W. Slack and Robert A. Hyndiuk

In this chapter, we review the toxicity of agents often used during ophthalmic surgery including antiseptics, irrigating solutions, viscoelastics, mydriatics and miotics, vitreous substitutes, tissue adhesives, and other miscellaneous agents. The proprietary names are often used to discuss specific products because the toxicity of many solutions is due to some component of the vehicle rather than the active ingredient.

Antiseptics

Presurgical skin antiseptics are commonly used to reduce periorbital skin flora prior to ophthalmic surgery. Potential corneal and conjunctival toxicity may result from inadvertent exposure to an antiseptic via the tear film during facial skin preparation. The toxicity of several commonly used skin antiseptics, including alcohol, iodine, povidone-iodine solution (without detergent), povidone-iodine surgical scrub (with detergent), Hibiclens (4% chlorhexidine gluconate and 4% isopropyl alcohol with detergent), and pHisoHex (3% hexachlorophene with detergent) are discussed (Table 43–1). Of the commonly used preoperative skin antiseptics, only povidone-iodine solution (without detergent) has been demonstrated to be nontoxic to the cornea and can be recommended for presurgical preparation for ocular surgery.

ALCOHOLS

A 70% ethanol (ethyl alcohol) solution produces corneal epithelial sloughing and corneal edema in rabbit studies[1] and similar changes clinically, but recovery is generally complete.[2] Isopropanol (isopropyl alcohol) has a greater bactericidal effect than ethanol but with a greater expected toxicity.[3, 4]

TABLE 43–1. **Toxicity of Antiseptics**

Agent	Toxicity	References
Alcohol	Deepithelialization, edema	1, 2
Iodine	Deepithelialization, edema, sensitization (prevalence 15%)	1, 2, 5
Povidone-iodine solution	5% Solution tolerated well	5, 8–11
Povidone-iodine scrub	Deepithelialization, edema	1
Hibiclens	Deepithelialization, edema, endothelial cell loss, bullous keratopathy, corneal neovascularization, opacification, ectasia	13, 16–19
pHisoHex	Conjunctivitis, deepithelialization, edema, deep keratitis, persistent irritation, photophobia	1, 30

IODINE

Tincture of iodine (2% iodine, 2.35% sodium iodine, and 44 to 50% ethyl alcohol) causes epithelial sloughing and corneal edema when applied topically and may sensitize 15% of treated patients.[1, 2, 5]

POVIDONE-IODINE

The iodophor povidone-iodine (polyvinylpyrrolidone-iodine [PVP-I]) is a water-soluble complex of approximately 85% povidone (polyvinylpyrrolidone [PVP]), 10% available iodine, and 5% iodide ion.[6] A 10% aqueous solution of povidone-iodine, therefore, contains 1% available iodine. The povidone-iodine complex retains the germicidal activity of iodine but without the irritating or sensitizing characteristics.[5] Its reddish brown color helps delineate the area treated, but it can be washed off easily without staining as tincture of iodine does.[6, 7]

In 1966, Kiffney and Hattaway[8] evaluated povidone-iodine as an ophthalmic antiseptic using New Zealand White rabbits. Eyes that received drops of undiluted PVP-I hourly for 8 hours exhibited inflamed conjunctivas, absence of corneal epithelium, stromal edema, and anterior keratitis; eyes that received a 1:1 dilution of PVP-I with sterile water showed no gross effects or histologic changes. They also found that half-strength solution of PVP-I was twice as effective in sterilizing the cul de sac of rabbits as were solutions of saline, 20% silver proteinate, aqueous penicillin, and chloramphenicol.[8]

Hale used a 5% povidone-iodine solution in 2000 cases and Azar in 50 cases with no untoward complications.[9, 10] Shepard[11] used a 5% povidone-iodine solution to prepare the periocular region and irrigate the cul de sac without subsequent washout in 929 eyes. There were no cases of external infection or endophthalmitis, but four cases of mild transient conjunctival irritation were attributed to the povidone-iodine solution.

It is important to distinguish povidone-iodine solution from povidone-iodine surgical scrub. Betadine Solution (Purdue Frederick, Norwalk, CT) is a 10% solution of povidone-iodine without detergent, whereas Betadine Surgical Scrub (Purdue Frederick) is a 7.5% solution of povidone-iodine with a detergent.[1, 12] A case of a 33-year-old man who developed conjunctival chemosis, an epithelial defect, and corneal edema after accidental instillation of povidone-iodine scrub into his tear film, despite prompt irrigation with balanced salt solution, encouraged MacRae, Brown, and Edelhauser to conduct a study comparing the corneal toxicity of several commonly used skin antiseptics.[1] Using rabbits, they showed that instillation of 30 mL of povidone-iodine solution (without detergent) caused no deepithelialization or increase in corneal thickness compared with the saline control. However, povidone-iodine surgical scrub, 70% ethanol, tincture of iodine, Hibiclens, and pHisoHex all caused 30 to 100% corneal deepithelialization and a significant increase in corneal thickness. They did not find significant corneal toxicity if they irrigated the povidone-iodine scrub from the eye with saline at 30 seconds or diluted it 1:2 with normal saline. Healing studies after the creation of an epithelial defect showed that eyes treated with povidone-iodine scrub had more deepithelialization and swelled more than eyes treated with povidone-iodine solution or balanced salt solution. Electron microscopy demonstrated that 3 hours after exposure, only the first cell layer of the epithelium was sloughing in eyes treated with povidone-iodine solution, whereas the epithelium sloughed to Bowman's zone in eyes treated with povidone-iodine scrub, Hibiclens, or pHisoHex.[1]

HIBICLENS

Hibiclens (Zeneca Pharmaceuticals, Wilmington, DE) contains 4% chlorhexidine gluconate with inactive ingredients, fragrance, isopropyl alcohol (4%), purified water, red 40, and other ingredients in a sudsing base adjusted to a pH of 5.0 to 6.5.[13] Chlorhexidine has several advantages as a topical antiseptic, including lack of absorption through intact skin, effectiveness that is not significantly reduced by the presence of organic matter such as blood, and persistence of antimicrobial activity due to protein binding.[13–15] However, Hibiclens should not be used as a preoperative skin preparation for the face or head, because of the potential for serious ocular toxicity.[13, 16]

Case reports of accidental exposure to Hibiclens have described variable corneal toxicity.[16–18] Stott[17] described a surgeon who developed multiple corneal epithelial defects and decreased vision for 1 week after accidentally splashing Hibiclens in his eye while scrubbing for surgery. Of the five cases reported by Phinney,[16] all patients experienced ocular pain and had conjunctival inflammation, corneal epithelial defects, and corneal edema. Corneal edema cleared in 6 to 7 months in most cases but progressed to bullous keratopathy and eventually required penetrating keratoplasty in two patients. Specular microscopy showed endothelial cell loss in the patients who did not require keratoplasty. All patients developed corneal neovascularization. Hamed[19] described two patients with severe Hibiclens keratitis who developed chronic epithelial defects, dense corneal opacification, vascularization, thinning, and ectasia (Fig. 43–1).

Several studies have evaluated the toxicity of the active germicide in Hibiclens, chlorhexidine gluconate, which is also used as a preservative and contact lens disinfectant. Scanning electron microscopic evidence of epithelial toxicity has been described after exposure to concentrations of chlorhexidine as low as 0.005%.[20–22] Green and associates[23] demonstrated that corneal swelling occurred with endothelial perfusions of chlorhexidine 0.002% or greater in a protein-free bathing solution. Perfusion of the epithelium with chlorhexidine at concentrations likely to be found with contact lens wear and with protein in the bathing solution, however, revealed no significant toxicity. Gasset and Ishii[24] found no endothelial toxicity in rabbits dosed with one drop of 2% chlorhexidine twice daily for 1 week. Using a wound-healing study, Hamill, Osato, and Wilhelmus[25] showed that 40 mL of a 1% or smaller concentration of chlorhexidine did not delay healing, whereas 2 and 4% concentrations delayed it significantly.

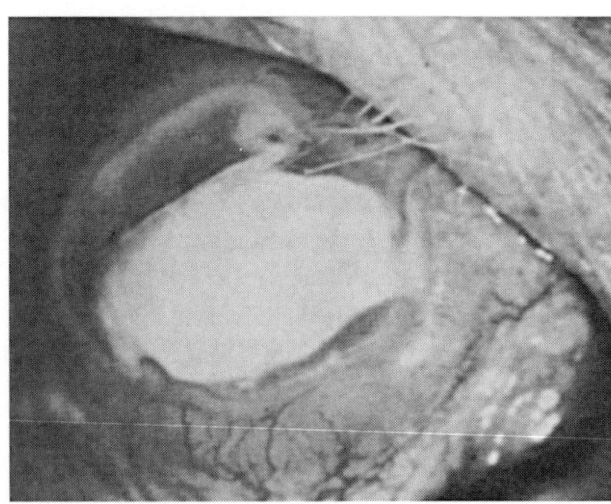

FIGURE 43–1. Four months after exposure to Hibiclens there is peripheral vascularization, thinning, and central necrotic sequestrum. (Reprinted from Hamed LM, Ellis FD, Boudreault G, et al: Hibiclens keratitis. Am J Ophthalmol 104:50, 1987. With permission from Elsevier Science.)

The detergent in Hibiclens is a nonionic poloxamer.[26] Marsh and Maurice[27] showed that single drops of nonionic detergents increased corneal permeability to fluorescein, thus it is likely that the presence of detergent enhances the tissue penetration and toxicity of chlorhexidine. The progression of stromal edema, which is sometimes seen in Hibiclens keratitis, may be caused by a slow release of protein-bound chlorhexidine.[16, 23] The combination of a high chlorhexidine concentration, protein binding, and epithelial disruption due to the detergent probably all contribute to the clinical toxicity seen with Hibiclens.[16]

The manufacturer warns that Hibiclens should not be used as a preoperative skin preparation for the face or head and should be thoroughly and promptly irrigated if the eyes are exposed.[13]

PHISOHEX

pHisoHex (Sanofi Winthrop, New York, NY)[28] is a sudsing bacteriostatic skin cleanser that contains the active ingredient hexachlorophene (3%) in an emulsion of entsufon sodium (a synthetic detergent), petrolatum, lanolin cholesterols, methylcellulose, polyethylene glycol, polyethylene glycol monostearate, lauryl myristyl diethanolamide, sodium benzoate, and water. Hexachlorophene is effective against gram-positive (but not gram-negative) organisms.[29] Rapid absorption of hexachlorophene may occur with toxic blood levels when preparations are applied to burns or to skin involved with a generalized dermatologic condition.

Browning and Lippas[30] reported two cases of pHisoHex

keratitis characterized by acute chemical conjunctivitis, deepithelialization, deep keratitis, and corneal edema that resolved in 5 to 8 weeks. Photophobia and intermittent superficial irritation persisted for months after the incident in both cases, but vision returned to normal. Animal studies confirmed epithelial and endothelial toxicity to one drop of topically applied pHisoHex.[1, 30]

Dormans and van Logten showed that hexachlorophene (0.3%) has a cytotoxic effect on rabbit epithelium, as demonstrated by scanning electron microscopy.[22] However, Browning and Lippas[30] found minimal clinical epithelial toxicity in rabbit eyes treated with one drop of 3% hexachlorophene. The toxicity of pHisoHex is probably related to the detergent, entsufon sodium. The study that evaluated this, however, used trinitrotoluene,[30] which, according to a representative for the manufacturer, is not equivalent to entsufon sodium and is not a component of pHisoHex (Gottlieb, personal communication, December 3, 1990).[31]

PARACHLOROMETAXYLENOL

Parachlorometaxylenol is a topical antimicrobial agent used as a hand scrub preparation as well as in electrocardiogram paste and over-the-counter products. It is a more potent sensitizer than iodine or chlorhexidine[32] with several reports of contact dermatitis.[33–35] It has not been associated with or specifically tested for ocular toxicity to our knowledge.

Irrigating Solutions

Intraocular irrigating solutions are an integral component of current surgical techniques for cataract extraction, phacoemulsification, filtration surgery, penetrating keratoplasty, and pars plana vitrectomy. An irrigating solution functions to keep the globe formed and maintain normal pressure-volume relationships during surgery. Since an intraocular irrigating solution comes in contact with the cornea, lens, trabecular meshwork, uvea, and retina, an ideal irrigant should preserve the biologic function and structural integrity of these tissues. Past studies have confirmed the intuitive view that these tissues are best protected with a solution that is similar in chemical composition to aqueous and vitreous humor (Table 43–2).[36–39] To avoid adverse effects of intraocular irrigating solutions, we recommend using a more "complete" solution (e.g., BSS Plus [Alcon Laboratories, Fort Worth, TX]) when a moderate to large volume of irrigant is expected to be used and for patients with a low endothelial cell count (e.g., below 2000/mm^2), abnormal endothelial morphometry, guttate, corneal thickness greater than 0.6 mm, Waite-Beetham (corneal stress) lines, or diabetes, because these patients may be more susceptible to surgical trauma.[40–42]

COMPONENTS

Electrolytes

Sodium is the major extracellular ion of aqueous humor and serves to maintain cellular tonicity. It is the major ion transported by cells for volume regulation, and it is necessary for the metabolic pump to function in the corneal endothelium.[43]

TABLE 43–2. **Chemical Composition of Human Aqueous and Vitreous Humor, BSS Plus, and BSS***

	Human Aqueous Humor	Human Vitreous Humor	BSS Plus	BSS
Sodium	162.9	144	160.0	155.7
Potassium	2.2–3.9	5.5	5.0	10.1
Calcium	1.8	1.6	1.0	3.3
Magnesium	1.1	1.3	1.0	1.5
Chloride	131.6	177.0	130.0	128.9
Bicarbonate	20.15	15.0	25.0	—
Phosphate	0.62	0.4	3.0	—
Lactate	2.5	7.8	—	—
Glucose	2.7–3.7	3.4	5.0	—
Ascorbate	1.06	2.0	—	—
Glutathione	0.0019	—	0.3	—
Citrate	—	—	—	5.8
Acetate	—	—	—	28.6
pH	7.38	—	7.4	7.6
Osmolality (mOsm)	304		305	298

*All concentrations expressed in mm/L or mEq/L of solution.
From McDermott ML, Edelhauser HF, Hack HM, et al: Ophthalmic irrigants: A current review and update. Ophthalmic Surg 19:724, 1988.

Potassium is the major intracellular cation in cells. The inward transport of K^+ is coupled with the outward transport of Na^+ by the enzyme Na^+, K^+-ATPase. A low potassium ion concentration is needed in an irrigating solution to maintain the normal physiologic relationship.

Magnesium is a cofactor for some ATPases and for many cellular biochemical reactions. It should be present in an intraocular irrigating solution in a concentration similar to that found in aqueous humor.[44]

Calcium is essential to maintain the barrier function and apical junctions of the corneal endothelium.[45, 46] An irrigating solution that lacks calcium can result in endothelial junction breakdown and corneal edema.[36] Calcium is also an essential ion for retinal metabolism.[47]

pH and Osmolality

Perfusion studies of rabbit and human corneas showed toxicity, including direct cell damage, disruption of junctional complexes, and increased swelling rate when a solution with a pH outside the range of 6.5 to 8.5 was used.[48] Normal saline (0.9% NaCl) and lactated Ringer (LR) solution can both fall below this pH tolerance range. It should also be noted that the addition of antibiotics or epinephrine may change the pH of an irrigating solution.[49]

If the essential ions are present, the corneal endothelium can tolerate a fairly wide range of solution osmolality (200 to 400 mOsm) without exhibiting marked endothelial cell breakdown.[50] However, an ideal irrigating solution should be isoosmotic with the intracellular tissues (i.e., 305 mOsm) and have a pH of 7.4.[51] In practice, solutions with a pH of 6.8 to 8.2 are considered safe for intraocular use.

Modification of the irrigating solution may solve a different type of osmotic problem. Lens opacification may occur during vitrectomy in diabetic patients, presumably because of the osmotic stress caused by trapped polyols within the lens.[52, 53] Glucose fortification of the irrigant BSS Plus to 335 mOsm has been shown to reduce the lens opacification that can occur during diabetic vitrectomy.[54, 55]

Bicarbonate

Bicarbonate is a major component of aqueous humor and is the principal buffer in aqueous and cerebrospinal fluid, which lack the buffering effects of proteins.[44] Active transport of bicarbonate across the corneal endothelium is thought to contribute to the endothelial pump function that keeps the cornea from becoming edematous.[56, 57] However, some researchers have been unable to locate a bicarbonate-transporting ATPase in the cornea endothelial cell membrane to confirm this.[58, 59] Several studies have revealed a beneficial effect of bicarbonate in maintaining corneal endothelial cell potential[60, 61] and corneal thickness.[62, 63] Bicarbonate has also been shown to support normal retinal function.[39, 64, 65]

Although bicarbonate is the most physiologic buffer for intraocular irrigating solutions, its use requires a closed system, because the pH increases as the solution's partial pressure of CO_2 (P_{CO_2}) equilibrates with the atmosphere.[66] Acetate-citrate and HEPES (a synthetic organic buffer) buffered systems are also used. Some solutions with HEPES buffer have been shown to reversibly decrease the endothelial short-circuit potential to zero[67] and cause increased swelling or decreased deturgescence in rabbit and human corneas and also a reduction in endothelial Na^+, K^+-ATPase activity.[68]

Glucose

Glucose (dextrose) is present in aqueous humor in concentrations of 2.7 to 3.7 mM/L (see Table 43–2) and provides ocular tissues with an energy source for the production of adenosine triphosphate to maintain normal cellular functions. Glycolysis probably accounts for 63 to 93% of glucose metabolism in the endothelium, and the pentose shunt accounts for the rest.[43, 69] The presence of glucose is also considered to be important in order to maintain the normal electroretinogram (ERG) amplitude.[65, 70]

Glutathione

Glutathione is a tripeptide with a reactive sulfhydryl group that exists in oxidized (GSSH) and reduced (GSH) forms. Its exact role is unclear, but it has been suggested that it may function as a redox buffer to detoxify free radicals produced during intraocular surgery.[63, 71]

Dikstein and Maurice first demonstrated glutathione's influence on fluid transport in the isolated cornea.[72] Anderson and coworkers[73, 74] suggested that the disulfide of the oxidized form interacted with membrane thiol groups, resulting in a conformational change that would reduce membrane permeability and thus increase net fluid transport. Edelhauser and coworkers[75] found that endothelial cells lost their barrier functions and apical junctions became disrupted when intracellular endothelial glutathione was completely oxidized. This suggested a need for both the oxidized and reduced forms. Further studies showed disruption of endothelial fluid transport when total intracellular glutathione fell below one third of the normal value in vivo.[76, 77] The addition of glutathione to irrigants was also shown to allow maintenance of the transendothelial electrical potential.[78]

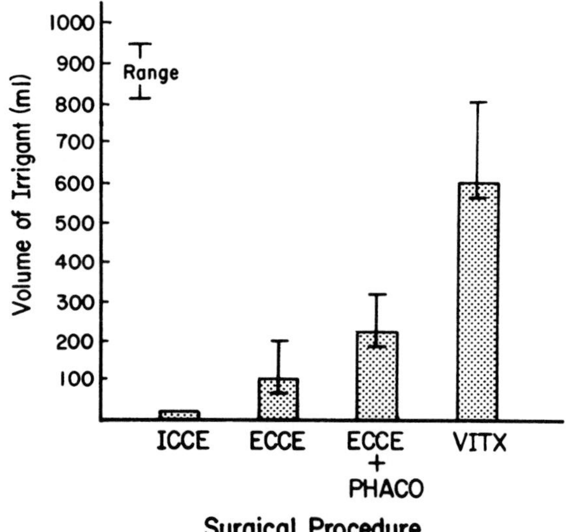

FIGURE 43–2. Comparative estimates of irrigant volume for a particular surgical procedure. (From McDermott ML, Edelhauser HF, Hack HM, et al: Ophthalmic irrigants: A current review and update. Ophthalmic Surg 19:724, 1988.)

SOLUTIONS

With the change to extracapsular cataract extraction and the emergence of phacoemulsification and vitrectomy, the volume (and potential toxicity) of irrigants used during surgery has increased (Fig. 43–2). Several irrigants have been evaluated for potential toxicity (Table 43–3).

Normal Saline

Normal saline solution (0.9% NaCl) was once the predominant irrigant, but it lacks essential ions and has been shown

TABLE 43–3. **Toxicity of Irrigating Solutions**

Solution	Toxicity	Mechanism	References
Normal saline	Corneal endothelium	Lack of essential ions	79, 80
	lens opacification [↓]		55
	ERG B-wave amplitude		39
Plasmalyte 148	Corneal endothelium	Lack of calcium	36, 81–83
Lactated Ringer solution	Corneal endothelium	Acidic, hypotonic	80, 84, 85
BSS	Corneal endothelium	Acetate-citrate buffer (?), lack of glutathione (?)	79, 86, 88
SMA_2	Corneal endothelium	Calcium chelation with acetate-citrate buffer (?)	51, 65, 88–93
GBR	Tolerated well		37, 60, 65, 66, 72, 94–98
BSS Plus	Tolerated well		84–86, 99–101

to be toxic to the cornea.[79, 80] Complete endothelial destruction has been observed within 1 hour of infusion.[80] Intravitreal irrigation with 0.9% NaCl has been associated with a decrease in ERG B-wave amplitude[39] and development of a progressive posterior subcapsular cataract.[55]

Plasmalyte 148

Plasmalyte 148 was the standard solution used during phacoemulsification in the early 1970s. Several initial animal studies using short-duration exposure did not reveal corneal endothelial damage.[81–83] Later studies, however, revealed endothelial cell disruption and corneal edema,[36] findings consistent with the solution's lack of calcium.

Lactated Ringer Solution

LR solution was formulated as an intravenous solution. The solution is hypotonic and acidic compared with aqueous, and the pH may vary from one batch to another. Comparison of perfusion of rabbit corneas in vitro has shown that corneal swelling occurs at a rate higher than that seen with balanced salt solution (BSS) but less than with Plasmalyte 148 and normal saline. Ultrastructural changes observed after prolonged perfusion include vacuolization of the cytoplasm, dilatation of the rough endoplasmic reticulum, and pyknotic changes in the nuclei.[80]

A clinical trial comparing LR solution and BSS Plus for vitrectomy reported significantly increased corneal thickness in eyes treated with LR solution.[84] A more recent comparison of irrigating solutions for vitrectomy showed a 31% endothelial cell loss with LR solution versus a 7% loss with BSS Plus.[85]

Balanced Salt Solution

Balanced salt solution (BSS) is an acetate-citrate-buffered solution that contains sodium, potassium, chloride, and calcium. BSS is currently the most widely used intraocular irrigant in the United States and is marketed commercially by many companies. Short-term application to tissue culture preparations of rabbit endothelium showed no morphologic damage; perfusion in vivo produced transient corneal edema.[79] Comparison with BSS Plus for cat perfusion in vivo revealed a significant increase in corneal thickness, increased coefficient of variation of cell area (polymegathism), and a decrease in the percentage of hexagonal cells (pleomorphism).[86] Comparison with BSS Plus for transendothelial electrical potential difference (TEPD) across isolated rabbit corneal endothelium showed a more rapid decrease in the TEPD for the BSS group if the solutions were gassed with an air-CO_2 mixture.[87] Morphologic changes, including disruption of intercellular junctions, have been noted on electron microscopy of perfused human corneas in vitro.[88]

SMA_2

The Japanese formulation SMA_2 (Senju Pharmaceutical Co., Osaka, Japan) is similar to BSS but is buffered by both acetate-citrate and bicarbonate. It was found to protect the corneal endothelium, prevent corneal edema, preserve ERG amplitude in rabbit studies,[65, 89, 90] and prevent corneal complications after pars plana vitrectomy.[91] The use of SMA_2, however, has also been associated with an increase in polymegathism and pleomorphism in a cat model in vivo[88] and with increased endothelial permeability.[92] A human perfusion study in vitro showed a higher swelling rate and breakdown of the endothelial cell junctions with SMA_2 than with BSS.[88] This is similar to what occurs with a calcium-free solution, and it has been suggested that the citrate in this solution may chelate the calcium.[51, 93]

Glutathione Bicarbonate Ringer Solution

Glutathione bicarbonate Ringer (GBR) solution contains sodium bicarbonate, glucose, glutathione, and adenosine in addition to the basic electrolytes. Based on studies by Dikstein and Maurice[72] and McCarey and coworkers,[94] it has become the standard by which to evaluate other solutions, using rabbit cornea-perfusion studies. In other animal studies in vitro GBR has been shown to preserve endothelial electrical potentials,[60] crystalline lens function,[95] lens clarity in primates,[37] and ERG B-wave amplitudes,[65] better than normal saline, LR solution, or Ringer solution supplemented with glucose and bicarbonate. One study suggested that glutathione and adenosine could be omitted without increasing corneal toxicity.[96]

Clinically, GBR resulted in fewer corneal complications and less endothelial cell damage than did LR solution for vitrectomy in one study,[97] whereas another study found no significant difference between the GBR and LR solutions.[98]

A commercial preparation of this solution was difficult to produce because of the unstable compounds, reduced glutathione, adenosine, and bicarbonate. The solution must be prepared just prior to use, with aeration with 95% air and 5% carbon dioxide to adjust the pH to 7.4.[66] To circumvent these problems, the commercial irrigant BSS Plus was formulated to closely resemble GBR and human aqueous but also to be pharmacologically stable.

BSS Plus

BSS Plus is a two-component system that is mixed to give a bicarbonate-buffered electrolyte solution containing glucose and oxidized glutathione. Laboratory studies have shown that it maintains corneal endothelial structure and function.[86, 99] A perfusion study of preserved human corneas in vitro demonstrated less swelling and a tendency for better endothelial surface morphology in eyes perfused with BSS Plus solution compared with BSS.[100] Clinical studies using BSS Plus have shown less corneal edema and less endothelial cell loss after vitrectomy compared with LR solution,[84, 85] and its safety has been demonstrated in pediatric intraocular surgery.[101] AMO Endosol EXTRA (Allergan Medical Optics, Irvine, CA) is an alternative enriched irrigating solution that should be bioequivalent to BSS Plus.

CONTAMINATION

Contamination of an intraocular irrigant may lead to ocular toxicity. In 1983, 500-mL bottles of a BSS-type solution were recalled following reports of corneal decompensation that resulted from the solution's interaction with the glass container that caused an alkaline shift in pH.[102] Fungal contamination, a recurrent problem, has resulted in numerous cases of endophthalmitis.[103–107] Nonmicrobial particulate matter may also contaminate irrigating solutions.[108, 109] Toxic keratopathy requiring penetrating keratoplasty has been reported from chlorhexidine, centrimide, and cialit when bottles were mixed up in irrigating solutions prepared by a hospital pharmacy.[110]

The addition of adjunctive solutions such as mydriatics,[111] miotics,[112] and antibiotics[113] raises the potential for toxicity. The vehicle rather than the drug itself may be the toxic component.[49, 114] Benzalkonium chloride, for example, can result in corneal endothelial toxicity even at concentrations as low as 0.0001%.[115] The pH of antibiotic vitreous infusion combinations is a potential cause of retinal toxicity. The bicarbonate buffer in BSS Plus protects better against acid shifts in pH caused by common intravitreal antibiotics.[116]

Viscoelastics

Viscoelastic solutions are often used in anterior segment surgery, principally for protection of the corneal endothelium and tissue manipulation. Although there has been some concern about potential corneal toxicity and inflammatory properties, the main clinical problem with the viscoelastics has been postoperative elevation of intraocular pressure (Table 43–4). While the use of viscoelastics for drug delivery has been suggested, a study by McDermott and Edelhauser showed that viscoelastic solutions do not exhibit significant drug binding, thus enhanced toxicity from other intraocular agents via an adsorptive mechanism is not expected.[117] The rheologic properties (e.g., viscosity, coatability) of each agent are important in determining its suitability for specific applications in ocular surgery but are not discussed in detail in this section (see Chap. 31, Viscoelastics.).

SODIUM HYALURONATE

Sodium hyaluronate (hyaluronic acid)[118] is a naturally occurring glycosaminoglycan (mucopolysaccharide) consisting of a long, unbranched chain of alternating *N*-acetyl-glucosamine and sodium gluconate (Fig. 43–3). In the eye, sodium hyaluronate is normally present in high concentrations in the vitreous humor and in the connective tissue of the trabecular meshwork,[119] where it may influence aqueous outflow.[120] The cornea endothelium is naturally covered with a layer of sodium hyaluronate, and endothelial cells have the capacity to bind high molecular weight hyaluronate.[121 122]

Healon (Pharmacia & Upjohn, Kalamazoo, MI) is a 10 mg/mL sodium hyaluronate solution manufactured from rooster combs. Amvisc (Chiron Vision, Claremont, CA) was previously available from MedChem, Woburn, Massachusetts, as a 10 mg/mL sodium hyaluronate solution made from rooster combs but slightly less viscous than Healon because of its lower molecular weight.[123] One study found this version of Amvisc to be associated with greater inflammation and ocular hypertension than Healon,[124] but a subsequent investigation found no clinical differences between the two solu-

TABLE 43–4. **Toxicity of Viscoelastic Agents**

Agent	Toxicity	References
Sodium hyaluronate (Healon, Amvisc)	Elevated IOP	119, 123–125, 143, 155, 171–180
	Inflammatory potential	124, 125, 130–133
	Potential endothelial Cellular toxicity	138–141
Chondroitin sulfate (Viscoat)	Elevated IOP	143, 155, 178–180
	Potential endothelial Cellular toxicity	123, 143, 144
	Band keratopathy with early formulations	145–147
HPMC (Occucoat)	Elevated IOP	143, 150, 155
	Inflammatory potential	160
	Potential endothelial Cellular toxicity	139, 143, 161, 162
	Less protective in phacoemulsification (?)	163
Polyacrylamide (Orcolon)	Delayed (microgel-associated) glaucoma	166

Abbreviation: IOP, intraocular pressure.

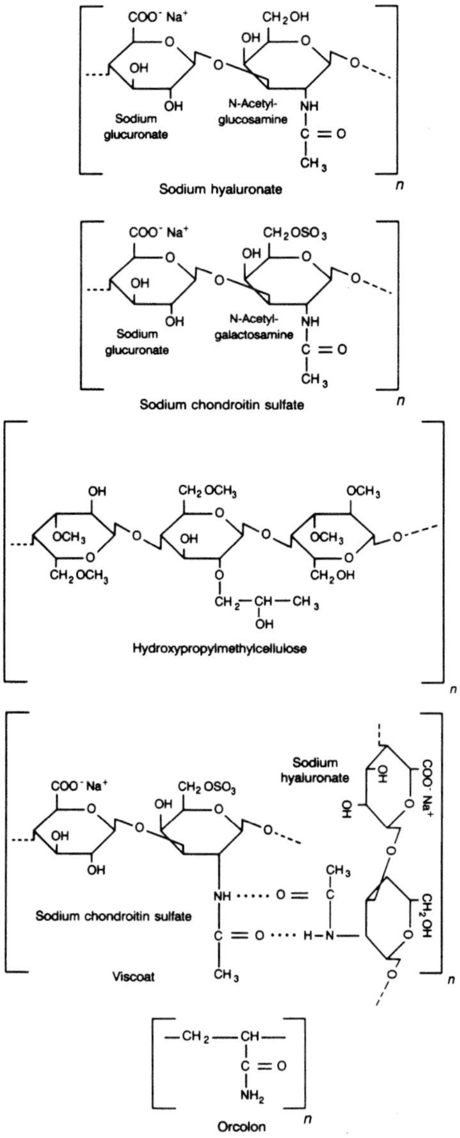

FIGURE 43–3. Chemical structures of some viscoelastic substances. (From Liesegang TJ: Viscoelastic substances in ophthalmology. Surv Ophthalmol 34:268, 1990.)

tions.[125] Amvisc is now supplied as a 12 mg/mL solution adjusted to yield a viscosity of approximately 40,000 centistokes.[126] Amvisc Plus (Chiron Vision) is a 16 mg/mL solution of sodium hyaluronate adjusted to yield approximately 55,000 centistokes.[126] Healon GV (Pharmacia & Upjohn) is a 14 mg/mL high molecular weight sodium hyaluronate solution that is the most viscous of the commercially available agents. One report noted potentially visually significant crystalline deposits on intraocular lens' surfaces associated with the use of Healon GV.[127] AMO Vitrax (Allergan, Irvine, CA), a 30 mg/mL sodium hyaluronate solution with a viscosity of approximately 40,000 centipoise, was rated less transparent and less easy to evacuate than Healon in one study.[128] Other companies have developed methods to manufacture sodium hyaluronate using microbial fermentation derived from genetic engineering technology, but there is disagreement as to whether the sodium hyaluronate produced from microbial fermentation or from rooster combs is more consistently refined without protein by-products. A prospective randomized multicenter clinical trial reported Provisc (Alcon Laboratories, Fort Worth, TX) 10 mg/mL sodium hyaluronate to be clinically equivalent to Healon.[129]

The inflammatory potential of sodium hyaluronate, which is reproducibly determined by injection into owl monkey vitreous, may vary from one batch to another and is independent of origin or concentration.[130, 131] Intraocular inflammation and subsequent bullous keratopathy associated with the reuse of injection cannulas was initially attributed to sodium hyaluronate that had been denatured by disinfectants or autoclaving.[132, 133] More recent reports demonstrate that heat-denatured sodium hyaluronate itself is not toxic,[134] but contamination by a detergent residue inside reusable cannulas[135] and 0.2% chlorhexidine digluconate, sometimes used as a sterilizing solution, can be toxic to the endothelium. Several companies now routinely supply disposable cannulas with their viscoelastic syringes.

Although sodium hyaluronate does not decrease corneal wound strength[136] and is well tolerated in routine cataract surgery,[137] several reports suggest that in certain situations sodium hyaluronate may have toxic effects on corneal endothelial cells using a cell culture model. McCulley[138] and Meyer and McCulley[139] found that Healon exhibited greater cytotoxicity than Viscoat (Alcon Surgical, Fort Worth, TX) or hydroxypropylmethylcellulose, whereas using another cell culture model, Nguyen and associates[140] found that Healon was less toxic than Viscoat or Amvisc Plus. Regardless of any chemical toxicity, the physical effects of a viscoelastic agent, by creating a mechanical barrier between endothelial cells and nutrient aqueous humor or by transmission of shearing forces to cell membranes, may play a role in clinically observed toxicity. After keratoplasty, we have observed sectoral corneal edema associated with residual Healon in the anterior chamber remaining overnight in contact with the corneal endothelium. Lindstrom[141] has noted that human donor corneas covered with Healon demonstrate significant endothelial cell death after 30 minutes and almost complete cell death after 2 hours. To avoid this problem, we routinely use corneal preservation media, rather than viscoelastic material, to cover the endothelial surface of trephined donor corneas during penetrating keratoplasty.

CHONDROITIN SULFATE

Chondroitin sulfate is a naturally occurring glycosaminoglycan that consists of repeating disaccharide subunits of *N*-acetyl-galactosamine and sodium gluconate. Unlike sodium hyaluronate, it is sulfated and negatively charged, which may allow it to better coat positively charged implant surfaces and reduce electrostatic interaction between an intraocular lens and the endothelium.[142] Although 20% chondroitin sulfate is useful in coating tissue, it cannot maintain space or separate tissue well because of its low viscosity (Table 43–5) and may cause dehydration because of its high osmolality.[143, 144] Increasing the viscosity by increasing the concentration to 50% results in endothelial cell damage because of hyperosmolarity.[123]

Viscoat is a mixture of 3% sodium hyaluronate produced by bacterial fermentation and 4% chondroitin sulfate from shark fin cartilage. An early formulation with a high phosphate concentration was associated with several cases of acute band keratopathy,[145–148] but reformulation appears to have solved that problem. In 1987, a recall of Viscoat related to the presence of endotoxins, which resulted in postoperative inflammation, has also been resolved. A rabbit eye model of phacoemulsification and traumatic lens implantation showed that Viscoat was more protective to the corneal endothelium and remained in the anterior chamber compared with Healon.[149]

HYDROXYPROPYLMETHYLCELLULOSE

Methylcellulose solutions are well known in ophthalmology for use as artificial tears and gonioscopic solutions. Hydroxypropylmethylcellulose (HPMC) is a synthetic modification of methylcellulose that consists of long chains of glucose molecules in which methoxy and hydroxypropyl side chains

TABLE 43–5. **Physical Properties of Viscoelastic Substances**

	Healon*	Amvisc*	Amvisc Plus*	Chondroitin Sulfate	Viscoat	Occucoat	Orcolon	Cellugel
Dynamic viscosity, cps*	40,000–64,000	40,000–42,000	55,000	30 at 20% 1000 at 50%	40,000	4000	40,000	12,000–15,000 at 25°C
Color	Clear	Clear	Clear	Yellow	Clear	Clear	Clear	Clear
Pseudoplasticity	+ + +	+ + +	+ + +	No	+ +	+	No	†
Contact angle, degrees	60	60	†	†	52	50	20	†

*At shear rate of 2/sec, 25°C.
†Not available.
From Liesegang TJ: Viscoelastic substances in ophthalmology. Surv Ophthalmol 34:268, 1990.

substitute for the hydrogen of the hydroxyl groups, resulting in increased hydrophilicity.[123] Numerous investigators have reported that HPMC is a safe and effective viscoelastic.[143, 150–157] However, some have questioned the wisdom of using HPMC intraocularly,[158] because it is a wood pulp product that is not a natural component of humans or other animals and its fate in the body is unknown.[159]

The formulations produced by individual hospital pharmacies are inconsistent and may contain vegetable matter particulate contaminants.[158] Vitreous replacement has resulted in severe inflammation in animal studies of some preparations.[160] The introduction of OcuCoat (Storz Ophthalmics, St. Louis, MO), a dual-filtered commercial preparation of 2% HPMC, has alleviated some of these concerns.

HPMC and Viscoat both caused less endothelial cell toxicity than Healon in a cell culture model[139] but caused more mitochondrial changes in another study.[161] When used as they would be clinically (i.e., if they do not remain for hours in contact with the corneal endothelium), HPMC, sodium hyaluronate, and chondroitin sulfate all appear to be tolerated well by the corneal endothelium.[143, 162] In comparative clinical trials, HPMC was associated with greater corneal thickness than sodium hyaluronate on the first postoperative day after phacoemulsification[163] but offered similar corneal protection using standard extracapsular techniques.[157, 164]

OTHER VISCOELASTICS

Orcolon (Optical Radiation Corporation, Azusa, CA) is a synthetic viscoelastic solution that consists of 0.5% polyacrylamide. Polyacrylamide has long been used in chromatography and electrophoresis and was found to be safe and comparable with sodium hyaluronate with regard to intraocular pressure elevation and postoperative electron microscopy of the endothelium in an animal study.[165] The report of several cases of "Orcolon glaucoma,"[166] occurring days to weeks postoperatively, forced the recall of the product from the market in late 1991. The manufacturer claimed that microgels associated with preparation and delivery of the product caused the rise in pressure and that a change in the preparation of Orcolon would eliminate the potential for this unique glaucoma.

Although potential problems should be considered when any protein is used in the eye,[167] there has been interest in using human collagen as a viscoelastic agent.[168, 169] Collagel (Domilens, Quebec, Canada), made of collagen type IV derived from human placenta, was comparable with Healon in one clinical study.[170]

INTRAOCULAR PRESSURE ELEVATION

Besides their cost, the biggest drawback to the use of viscoelastic solutions has been their tendency to cause a postoperative elevation of intraocular pressure. The mechanism involved is probably mechanical obstruction to outflow. Studies on human and animal eyes have shown decreased outflow facility with sodium hyaluronate that is relieved with hyaluronidase.[171–174] The viscosity, chain length, molecular volume, molecular rigidity, and charge of a viscoelastic may all contribute to outflow obstruction.[123, 175] Interaction with fibrin probably plays a role, because intracameral administration of low molecular weight heparin in rabbit eyes inhibits the hyaluronic acid–induced intraocular pressure elevation.[174]

The bulk of intraocular viscoelastic left in the eye after surgery leaves unchanged through the trabecular meshwork as a large molecule,[171] but some of the agent may leave through the iris and ciliary body.[176] Individual variation in postoperative pressure elevation may be explained by the variation in trabecular pore size and charge and by the amount of fibrin, albumin, and inflammatory products that are produced during surgery.[123] It is interesting that even after the intraocular pressure returns to normal, the aqueous humor can be 3500 times more viscous than normal and have 370 times the normal concentration of sodium hyaluronate.[175] Animal studies have shown that if 1% sodium hyaluronate replaces less than half the aqueous humor volume, no significant increase in intraocular pressure results.[119]

Some studies have suggested a lower risk for increased postoperative intraocular pressure elevation with Amvisc Plus,[177] Viscoat,[178, 179] or methylcellulose,[150] whereas other studies found no significant difference between intraocular pressures with Viscoat and Healon[180] and Healon GV and Healon.[181] Glasser and coworkers[155] demonstrated in a cat model that Healon, Viscoat, and 2% methylcellulose all cause an increase in intraocular pressure that is reduced when the agent is washed out (Fig. 43–4). This study and others illustrate the importance of early postoperative measurements in certain patients, because the pressure tends to peak at 2 to 7 hours and often returns to preoperative levels by 24 hours.[119, 143, 155]

Although further investigation may clarify which viscoelastic agents are safest, it should be assumed that any viscoelastic solution may significantly elevate postoperative intraocular pressure, even if theoretically all of the viscoelastic was removed intraoperatively. When it is difficult or risky to remove the viscoelastic agent (e.g., with corneal transplantation associated with anterior chamber intraocular lens), careful monitoring and the use of topical or systemic ocular pressure–lowering agents can blunt the ocular hypertensive response, thus increasing the safety of using a viscoelastic agent. This is especially important for patients who have ocular hypertension or glaucoma preoperatively, because these patients are at increased risk of developing dangerously high intraocular pressure elevations after cataract or corneal transplant surgery and viscoelastic use. We recommend removal of the viscoelastic solution at the end of surgery whenever feasible and anticipation of possible inordinate elevation of intraocular pressure postoperatively, especially in patients at increased risk.

Mydriatics and Miotics

Intraoperative control of pupillary diameter is often desired to ease certain surgical maneuvers during intraocular surgery. A large pupil facilitates extracapsular cataract extraction, phacoemulsification, aspiration of cortical material, and insertion of posterior chamber intraocular lenses. Even with adequate preoperative pupillary dilatation, a supplemental intraocular mydriatic is often helpful in counteracting the pupillary constriction that can occur with mechanical stimulation of the iris.[182] A small pupil, on the other hand, may help protect the vitreous face, prevent iris incarceration in the wound, facilitate anterior chamber intraocular lens

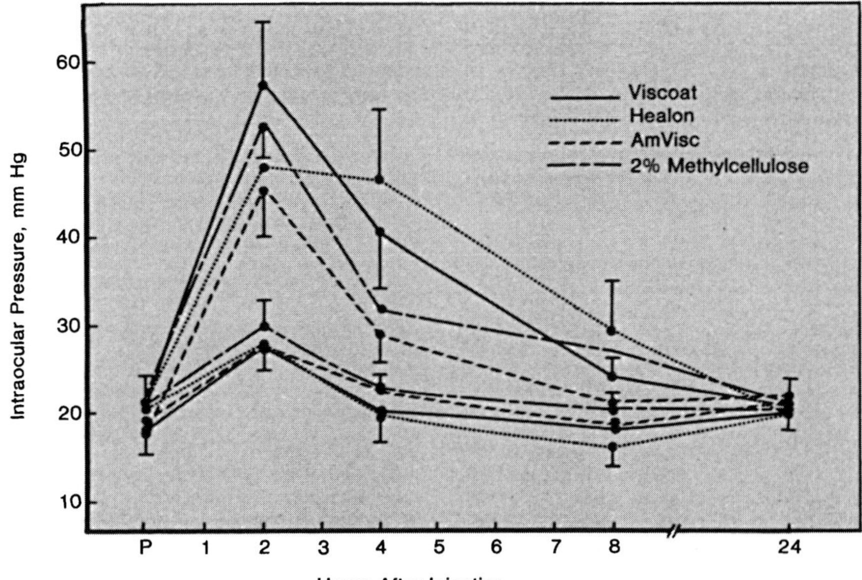

FIGURE 43–4. Intraocular pressure after anterior injection of viscous solutions. The upper four curves indicate values without washout. The lower four curves indicate values with anterior chamber washout; bar gauge, mean ± SE; P, preoperative values. (N = 5 for each measurement.) (From Glasser DB, Matsuda M, Edelhauser HF: A comparison of the efficacy and toxicity of and intraocular pressure response to viscous solutions in the anterior chamber. Arch Ophthalmol 104:1819, 1986.)

insertion, and prevent pupillary capture of a posterior chamber intraocular lens.

MYDRIATICS

Dilutions of commercially prepared epinephrine solutions are commonly used intracamerally to maintain pupillary dilatation during ocular surgery. The first clinical report of postoperative corneal edema after intraocular epinephrine use[183] led to animal studies that showed that the corneal endothelial toxicity of commercial epinephrine preparations was related to the presence of sodium bisulfite used as a preservative, rather than to a direct toxic effect from the epinephrine.[114] Whereas one cell culture model indicated a toxic effect on human trabecular cells with epinephrine at concentration of 10(−6) M or higher,[184] another study showed that the preservative benzalkonium chloride alone was responsible for the inhibitory effects on trabecular cells.[185] Even solutions marked "no preservatives" may contain sodium bisulfite that the manufacturer regards as an antioxidant, which may produce corneal edema.[49] Edelhauser and associates[49] further demonstrated that endothelial toxicity is related to the low pH and high buffer capacity of commercially available epinephrine solutions, which in turn is related to the concentration of the antioxidant sodium bisulfite as well as to the vehicle formulation.

One study demonstrated that a preservative-free, sulfite-free epinephrine 1:1000 sterile solution for injection (American Regent Laboratories) may offer an extra margin of safety for intraocular use.[186] When this solution was injected undiluted into the anterior chamber of rabbits' eyes, negligible corneal toxicity was observed compared with the marked corneal edema and endothelial toxicity seen in previous studies using epinephrine solutions that contained sodium bisulfite and a higher buffer capacity.[186]

We routinely use 0.5 mL of 1:1000 epinephrine added to 500 mL of irrigating solution, for a final dilution of 1:1,000,000. When a more concentrated solution is necessary, 1 mL of 1:1000 epinephrine may be added to 30 mL of irrigating solution (1:30,000), and 0.2 mL of this mixture is injected into the anterior chamber.[187] Plasma concentrations of adrenaline and noradrenaline do not rise significantly after intraocular irrigation with a solution of epinephrine 1:500,000.[188] With the use of more concentrated solutions and preoperative phenylephrine for dilatation, however, ocular surgical personnel should remain alert for signs of potential systemic epinephrine toxicity, such as headache, palpitations, tachycardia, and blood pressure elevation.

Acute macular neuroretinopathy has been reported in association with intravenous epinephrine [189, 190] but not with intracameral use to date. Topical phenylephrine 2.5% has been shown to cause cellular vacuolation within keratocytes and endothelial cells, with corneal edema after removal of the epithelium in rabbits [191] and sloughing of the endothelial cell monolayer in a cell culture model.[192] Clinically, intraocular phenylephrine has been associated with corneal edema[193] and a reduced endothelial cell count (Table 43–6).[194]

MIOTICS

Although one early study noted no ocular toxicity after injection of pilocarpine into the anterior chamber of rabbits,[195] Coles demonstrated that pilocarpine concentrations in excess of 0.25% produce dose-related corneal endothelial toxicity, including corneal swelling, margination of nuclear chromatin, and cytoplasmic vacuolization during rabbit corneal perfusions.[196] Jay and MacDonald reported two cases of severe corneal edema following the use of intraocular pilocarpine but found toxicity only in a cell culture model when the pilocarpine vehicle lacked calcium or was not isotonic.[197] Although sympatholytic agents such as thymoxamine and dapiprazole have been proposed as intraocular miotics,[112] they are not commercially available as such and have not undergone the rigorous toxicity testing used to evaluate other intraocular solutions.[187] The two currently available intraocular miotics are the parasympathomimetic agents acetylcholine, which has a direct action on the iris sphincter muscle and is rapidly broken down by acetylcholinesterase,

TABLE 43–6. **Toxicity of Mydriatics and Miotics**

Agent	Toxicity	Mechanism	References
Mydriatics			
Epinephrine	Corneal endothelium	Sodium bisulfite preservative, acid pH	49, 114, 183, 185, 186
Phenylephrine	Corneal endothelium, keratocytes		191–194
Miotics			
Pilocarpine	Corneal endothelium		195–197
Acetylcholine (Miochol)	Corneal endothelium (?)	Nonphysiologic vehicle	194, 195, 199–205
	Transient cataract with early formulation	Osmotic	198
	Systemic hypotension, bradycardia, breathing difficulties		207–211
Carbachol (Miostat)	Corneal endothelium (?)		195, 200–206

and carbachol, which has both a direct and an indirect action on the iris sphincter and is not destroyed by acetylcholinesterase.

Miochol (formerly Iolab Pharmaceuticals; now CIBA Vision Ophthalmics, Duluth, GA) was available for years as a 1% solution of acetylcholine in a vehicle containing 3% mannitol in water, whereas MIOSTAT (Alcon Laboratories, Fort Worth, TX) is a 0.01% carbachol in a BSS. Miochol-induced transient cataract was reported due to the hyperosmotic effect of an early preparation of Miochol that contained 5% mannitol.[198]

In clinical studies, Lang and Hassard did not find a difference in endothelial cell loss 20 days after intracapsular cataract extraction when Miochol, as opposed to air, was instilled to reconstitute the anterior chamber.[194] Menchini and coworkers, however, demonstrated increased mean endothelial cell area, endothelial folds, and corneal edema at various intervals following extracapsular cataract surgery in patients receiving intraocular Miochol compared with topical pilocarpine.[199]

Animal studies of corneal toxicity have reported mildly conflicting results. Some have shown no toxicity with either acetylcholine or carbachol injections into the anterior chamber of rabbits[195, 200] or cats,[201] whereas two perfusion studies of rabbit eyes in vitro observed an initial increase in the corneal swelling rate in eyes perfused with carbachol but demonstrated no endothelial cell alterations by electron microscopy.[201, 203]

Yee and Edelhauser performed human corneal perfusions in vitro, which showed increased swelling rate and corneal thickness in eyes perfused with Miochol compared to MIOSTAT, as well as electron microscopic evidence of vacuolation and loss of the normal endothelial cell mosaic.[204] A similar study was presented by one of us (JWS) at the 1990 ASCRS symposium, which confirmed these findings (unpublished data). Yee and associates further demonstrated, using bovine endothelial cell cultures, that the mechanism of toxicity from Miochol is not related to the active ingredient acetylcholine or the mannitol but to the lack of a physiologic buffered salt vehicle.[205, 206] Miochol has been reformulated since these studies and is currently available in an electrolyte diluent as Miochol-E.

Rare adverse systemic effects, including hypotension, bradycardia, and breathing difficulty, have been reported from intraocular acetylcholine,[207–211] but to our knowledge these effects have not been reported with carbachol.

Decreased intraocular pressure is a potentially beneficial secondary ocular effect of intraocular miotics that may mitigate viscoelastic-induced pressure elevation. A number of studies have examined the ocular hypotensive effect of intraocular miotics.[212–223] This pressure-lowering effect persists approximately 48 to 72 hours after intraocular instillation of carbachol[214, 216, 217] but only 6 hours after acetylcholine.[218, 219] One study found more prolonged cell and flare inflammation following cataract surgery with carbachol compared with acetylcholine,[224] but there has not been evidence of clinically significant differences in long-term outcomes, such as visually significant cystoid macular edema or glaucomatous visual field loss.

Vitreous Substitutes

Air, sulfur hexafluoride, the perfluorocarbon gases and liquids, and silicone oil are often used to maintain intraocular volume and provide mechanical tamponade while preserving visualization during ophthalmic surgery. Although it may seem out of place to discuss agents such as air and the chemically inert perfluorocarbon gases in a toxicology section, all of these materials may cause adverse effects in conjunction with ocular surgery (Table 43–7).

AIR

Air may be used to maintain the anterior chamber, prevent corneal touch during intraocular lens insertion, and facilitate the identification of corneal astigmatism and the presence of vitreous in the anterior chamber. Air is also used during posterior segment procedures, either alone or in combination with other gases, to promote closure of retinal breaks.

Although we could find no reports of endophthalmitis specifically attributed to the instillation of air, aspiration of air through a millipore filter (e.g., Millex-GS 0.22-mm filter unit) has been recommended to ensure sterility.[225]

Several investigations have found evidence of corneal endothelial cell damage or loss[194, 226–229] and corneal edema[229] when air is allowed to remain in contact with the corneal endothelium. A study using human eye bank eyes also noted increased endothelial cell damage when phacoemulsification was performed in the presence of air bubbles and demonstrated a protective effect with the viscoelastic agent Viscoat.[230]

Experimental studies have demonstrated that instillation of air in the anterior chamber increases vascular permeability[231, 232] and can cause mild to fibrinous iritis with synechia formation.[229, 233, 234] Lens opacification has been demonstrated with both anterior chamber[187] and intravitreal[235] air injection. Intraocular air has been associated with the development of pupillary and angle-block glaucoma in phakic and aphakic

TABLE 43–7. **Toxicity of Vitreous Substitutes**

Agent	Toxicity	Mechanism	References
Air	Corneal endothelium		194, 226–230
	Uveitis		229, 231–234
	Lens opacification		229, 235
	Elevated IOP/pupillary block	Mechanical barrier	236–238
	Retina	Traumatic injection	236, 242, 243
Gas	Corneal endothelium	Mechanical barrier	226, 247, 248
	Uveitis		249
	Lens opacification		229, 232, 235, 242, 250–253
	Lens displacement with endothelial touch and decompensation		265
	Elevated IOP/pupillary block	Expansive properties	232, 239, 249–252, 254–262
	Retina	Traumatic injection	235, 245, 249, 263, 264
Perfluorocarbon liquids	Corneal endothelium, vascularization		247, 274, 286, 287
	Uveitis		274, 278, 281, 285
	Lens opacification		276
	Elevated IOP		272, 274, 285
	Hypotony		272
	Retina	Oxidative/Mechanical barrier	275, 277, 279, 280–284, 288, 289
Silicone	Corneal endothelium, opacification, vascularization, thinning, retrocorneal membrane, bullous keratopathy	Mechanical barrier	291, 292, 296–314, 320
	Band keratopathy		315–319
	Uveitis		356
	Lens opacification	Mechanical barrier	298, 299, 308, 309, 315, 316, 321–330
	Elevated IOP/pupillary block glaucoma	Outflow obstruction Intraneural migration (?)	295, 298, 299, 309–311, 315, 316, 322, 325, 328, 331–338
	Retina	Lipid extraction (?)	298, 300, 312, 313, 315, 327, 331, 332, 339–354

Abbreviation: IOP, intraocular pressure.

patients.[236–238] Applanation tonometry is preferred to Schiøtz tonometry for assessing intraocular pressure in gas-filled eyes, because the latter can give false-low measurements.[239–241]

The retina appears to tolerate vitreous replacement by air.[242] Traumatic or misplaced injection of air may result in lens opacification, retinal tears or dialysis, hemorrhage at the injection site, and avulsion of the vitreous base.[236, 243]

GAS

As early as 1911, Ohm reported the use of intraocular gas for the treatment of retinal detachment.[244] Interest in the clinical use of sulfur hexafluoride (SF_6) and the perfluorocarbon gases (Cn F^{2n+2}) has grown because of the expansile qualities and greater duration of mechanical tamponade that these agents provide (Table 43–8). Indications include giant retinal tears, large retinal breaks with fish-mouth phenomenon, posterior breaks, macular holes, total retinal detachment with multiple breaks and large meridional folds, restoration of intraocular volume after the drainage of subretinal fluid,[245] and reformation of a persistently flat chamber after filtration surgery.[246]

Corneal endothelial degeneration and corneal edema have resulted from sulfur hexafluoride and other perfluorocarbon gases in several experimental studies.[226, 247, 248] Van Horn and associates suggested that it is a mechanical barrier effect that limits the access of nutrients to the endothelium rather than a direct toxic reaction to the gas that is responsible for the damage to the corneal endothelium.[226]

In one clinical study, transient fibrinous iritis occurred in 26 of 101 patients who underwent vitrectomy with sulfur hexafluoride gas, suggesting that the gas may be an iris irritant or may simply act as a scaffold for the deposition of the fibrinous membrane in the pupil.[249] Lens opacification has been reported by numerous investigators.[229, 232, 235, 242, 250–253] There appears to be greater potential for cataract formation with longer-lasting agents,[252] and partial clearing of the lens opacification may occur if the gas is removed.[229]

The incidence of elevated intraocular pressure after fluid-gas exchange or retinal detachment surgery ranges from 26 to 59%[254] and has been described in numerous studies.[249–252, 255–257] Owing to the expansile properties of the perfluorocarbon gases, and because the traditional signs and symptoms of elevated intraocular pressure may be difficult to interpret in postoperative patients, careful and regular monitoring of postoperative intraocular pressure is particularly important, with the release of gas by paracentesis for pressures over 40 mm Hg.[232] Soluble general anesthetic agents like nitrous oxide can increase intraocular bubble volume and may produce a concomitant rise in intraocular pressure.[239, 258, 259] If nitrous oxide is used in a patient with an intraocular gas bubble, the intraocular pressure should be closely monitored during the first 10 to 30 minutes.[260] Nitrous oxide should also be discontinued at least 15 minutes prior to injection of intraocular gas.[254] Rapid atmospheric decompression with air or other high-altitude travel may result in bubble expansion with concomitant elevation of intraocular pressure and potential compromise of central retinal artery blood flow.[261, 262]

Retained intraocular gas appears to cause minimal retinal

TABLE 43–8. **Physical Characteristics of Gases Used in Vitreoretinal Surgery**

	Molecular Weight	Purity (mole %)	Expansion	Longevity* (days)	Nonexpanding Concentration (%)
Air	29	—	0	5–7	
Xenon	131	99.995	0	1	
Sulfur hexafluoride	146	99.9	1.9–2.0	10–14	18
Perfluoromethane	88	99.7	1.9	10–14	
Perfluoroethane	138	99.9	3.3	30–35	16†
Perfluoropropane	188	99.7	4	55–65	14

*Based on 1 ml of pure gas.
†Estimated.
From Chang S: Intraocular gases. *In* Ryan SJ (ed): Retina. St. Louis, CV Mosby, 1989.

toxicity;[235, 245] however, as with air, injection site hemorrhage, iatrogenic retinal breaks, and subretinal injection may occur.[249, 263, 264] In addition, anterior displacement of an intraocular lens with endothelial touch and corneal decompensation has been described.[265]

PERFLUOROCARBON LIQUIDS

Perfluorocarbon liquids have been used medically as blood substitutes and in organ perfusion.[266,267] Haidt and associates[268] first reported on experimental use of perfluorocarbon liquids as a vitreous substitute in 1982. They have been used to facilitate surgery involving dislocated intraocular and crystalline lenses, retinal detachments, giant retinal tears, proliferative retinopathy, trauma, and drainage of suprachoroidal hemorrhages and their use in ophthalmology was reviewed by Peyman and associates.[269]

Pure perfluorocarbon liquids are generally considered biologically inert, but impurities including compounds with nitrogen bonds and hydrogen-fluoride bonds found in the liquids may be toxic.[266, 270, 271] Although several studies have shown potential for short-term tamponade with perfluorophenanthrene,[247, 272, 273] numerous reports have demonstrated poor long-term tolerance with this and other perfluorocarbon liquids.[274–289]

SILICONE OIL

Silicone oils are viscous hydrophobic fluid synthetic polymers that have a common repetitive backbone of siloxane (Si-O-Si) units. The physicochemical properties of silicone fluids are determined by the chemical structure of radical side groups, radical termination of the chain, and the chain's length.[290] The most commonly used silicone oil in ophthalmology is polydimethylsiloxane (Fig. 43–5), but the term "silicone oil" is often loosely used to designate any of the silicone fluids, without regard to the exact chemical composition.

No international purity standard defines "medical grade" silicone oil. A certain amount of low molecular weight constituents and chemical impurities contaminate clinically used silicone oils and may unfavorably affect biocompatibility and accelerate bubble emulsification.[290–292] The variation in chemical composition and lack of standards make comparison of clinical results subject to uncertainty. Early studies reported silicone fluids to be tolerated well by ocular tissues,[293–295] but later investigations have demonstrated adverse effects, including keratopathy, cataract formation, glaucoma, and retinopathy.

Corneal changes range from mild haze[296] to progressive stromal opacification, vascularization, and bullous keratopathy.[291, 292, 297–313] Sternberg and coworkers[314] found retrocorneal membrane formation, corneal thinning, and a 40% reduction in the endothelial density in rabbits and cats after anterior chamber instillation of silicone oil. They also found ultrastructural changes that suggested the mechanism of damage was the barrier to the nutrition supplied by the aqueous rather than a specific toxic effect. Many studies have reported band keratopathy,[315–319] which may occur in as

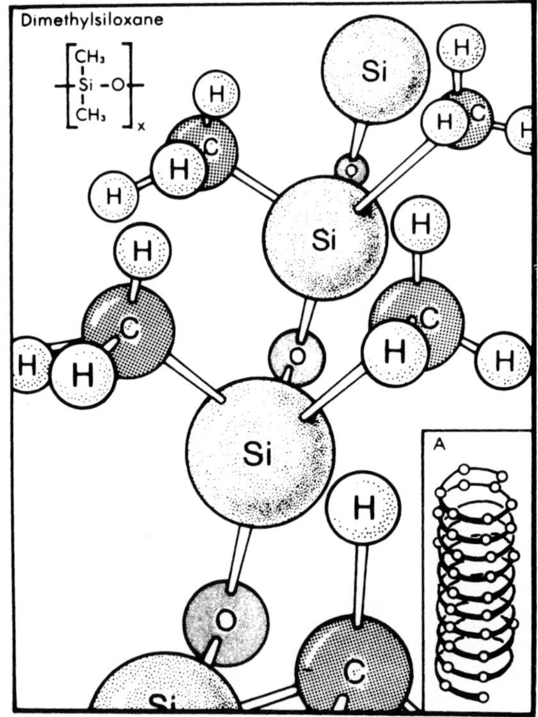

FIGURE 43–5. Graphic representation of the molecular structure of the most commonly used silicone oil, dimethylsiloxane. The linear chain coils into a helix, composed of six (Si-O) units per turn. For a molecular weight of 28,000 (1000 cS), the helix will have 63 turns in average. Interdigitation of the helices is known to occur for helices with more than 100 turns (5000 cS). The siloxane chain termination is not represented. *A,* Siloxane helix. (From Parel JM: Silicone oils: Physicochemical properties. *In* Glaser BM, Michels RG [eds]: Retina. St. Louis, CV Mosby, 1989.)

many as 100% of patients within 6 months if oil touches the endothelium.[316] Patients noted to have a layered area of emulsified silicone oil in the superior chamber angle (hyperoleum) may be at increased risk for band keratopathy.[319] The overall incidence of corneal abnormalities at 24 months in the Silicone Study was 27%.[320]

Cataract formation is the most common complication of injecting silicone into the human eye,[321] and it is well documented.[298, 299, 308, 309, 315, 316, 322–330] The effect is thought to result from prevention of normal metabolic exchange due to contact of the silicone globule with the posterior lens capsule.[315]

Acute pupillary block and chronic glaucoma are well recognized complications of silicone oil injection.[295, 298, 299, 309, 310, 315, 316, 322, 325, 331–336] Ando pointed out that a large inferior iridectomy is almost always effective in preventing pupillary block.[333] Silicone-laden macrophages demonstrated in the trabecular meshwork suggest that the likely mechanism of chronic elevated intraocular pressure is obstruction to outflow from the cellular reaction to the silicone.[298, 315] Histologic evidence also suggests that intraneural migration of silicone may contribute to optic nerve damage.[337, 338]

It is uncertain whether silicone oil produces functional retinopathy. Electrophysiologic studies are difficult to interpret because of the preoperative effect of the detachment itself and the insulating effect of silicone fluids,[315] but the degree of recovery following removal of silicone suggests that any toxicity is probably small.[339, 340] Although some investigators have documented good retinal tolerance,[341, 342] other studies have demonstrated toxic effects of intravitreal silicone oil,[311–313, 331, 332, 343, 344] and the removal of silicone oil after temporary tamponade has been recommended.[327, 328] Refojo and associates[345] showed that silicone fluids are not inert and can extract lipids such as retinol and cholesterol from intraocular tissues. Histologic examination has revealed intraretinal silicone vacuoles[298, 300, 315, 332, 346, 347] and marked thinning of the outer plexiform layer.[348] Silicone oil has also been shown to increase the mitogenic activity of retinal pigmented epithelial cells[349] and is associated with proliferative vitreoretinopathy.[350–353] Retinoic acid in silicone oil appears to have an inhibitory effect on the proliferative vitreoretinopathy in an animal model.[354, 355] Anterior segment ischemia,[346] fibrous ingrowth,[297] and excessive postoperative inflammation[356] have also been associated with injection of silicone oil.

Tissue Adhesives

Tissue adhesives offer the attraction of sutureless surgery and provide a mechanism for repairing potentially difficult surgical wounds like perforated corneal ulcers and leaking filtering blebs. The ideal properties of a tissue adhesive depend on the specific application, but in general they include rapid binding, high tensile strength, biodegradability, and no toxicity. Fibrin and thrombin have been evaluated as tissue glues,[357] but they lack significant tensile strength.[358] Interest continues in developing biologically derived tissue adhesives with materials like collagen[359] and muscle-activated protein,[360] but currently, the most practical tissue adhesives are the synthetic cyanoacrylates.

Coover and associates first reported the adhesive action of alkyl-2-cyanoacrylates in 1959.[361] The first commercially available product, methyl-2-cyanoacrylate (Eastman 910 adhesive, Krazy Glue), is still widely available but is regarded as too toxic for most clinical applications.[362] Currently, *N*-butyl-2-cyanoacrylate (Histoacryl blau) is commonly used in practice to seal small corneal perforations.

Unlike most other adhesives the cyanoacrylate monomers harden by anionic polymerization initiated by water or weak bases on the adherent surfaces, thus no additional heat, solvent, evaporation, or catalyst is required.[363, 364] In an aqueous medium, all polycyanoacrylates degrade by the cleavage of carbon to carbon bonds in the polymer backbone with the release of formaldehyde and an alkylcyanoacetate.[365, 366] The lower alkylcyanoacrylates break down more rapidly than the higher alkyl derivatives.[365] The increased release of formaldehyde from the more rapidly degraded lower alkylcyanoacrylates is thought to be at least partially responsible for the higher level of toxicity that has been reported with these products.[365, 367–370] Tissue culture studies have confirmed the greater toxicity of lower molecular weight cyanoacrylate derivatives[369, 370] and have found decreased toxicity following several washings of the polymerized adhesive,[370] suggesting that impurities may contribute to the toxic effects.

Several different studies of corneal toxicity after topical or intralamellar application of cyanoacrylates report variable results (Table 43–9).[371–374] The smaller amount of tissue adhesive applied probably accounts for the relatively inert behavior described by Gasset and associates[373] compared with the marked toxicity noted by Girard and coworkers.[372] An early polymorphonuclear inflammatory response is followed by foreign body granulomatous keratitis,[371, 375] and corneal neovascularization may follow.[374] The tissue reaction is localized, and there is no significant penetration of the monomer or its degradation products into the stroma, aqueous, or surrounding ocular tissues,[376] but giant papillary conjunctivitis and symblephara formation have been associated with use of cyanoacrylates.[377, 378]

Bloomfield and coworkers[379] noted no significant inflam-

TABLE 43–9. **Toxicity of Cyanoacrylate Tissue Adhesive**

Agent	Toxicity	Mechanism	References
Methyl-2-cyanoacrylate (Krazy Glue)	Too toxic for most clinical uses	Relatively rapid release of formaldehyde	362, 365–370
n-Butyl-2-cyanoacrylate (Histoacryl blau)	Inflammatory response	Release of formaldehyde	365–370
	Conjunctival symblepharon/GPC		377, 378
	Corneal neovascularization/failed graft		371–376
	Cataract (?)		383
	Intramuscular loss of cell nuclei		372, 385
	Coagulative retinal necrosis vs. well tolerated		386, 387, 389–392
	Stymied neurite growth		388

matory reaction after instillation of cyanoacrylates into the anterior chamber of rabbits, whereas Gasset and associates[373] reported iritis that lasted for 1 week and histologic evidence of fibrous or fibrovascular plaques on the adjacent cornea or iris and of endothelial cell injury. A similar inflammatory response was reported by Macsai and associates.[380] The marked reaction reported by Girard and coworkers, including opacification, vascularization, and deformation of the cornea with obliteration of the chamber angle structures, probably relates to the large volume (0.5 mL) that was injected.[372] Accidental instillation of cyanoacrylate glue into the anterior chamber during repair of a dehiscent corneal graft wound resulted in failure of the corneal graft, but no permanent ocular damage was observed following repeat penetrating keratoplasty with surgical removal of the adhesive.[381] In another report, inadvertent instillation of cyanoacrylate into the anterior chamber resulted in iridocorneal and iridolenticular adhesion.[382]

Despite the occurrence of cataract formation following tissue adhesive repair of corneal perforations, this complication should not necessarily be attributed to the chemical toxicity of the cyanoacrylate adhesive. It is probably due mainly to the mechanical effect, when polymerization of the adhesive occurs over the lens in a perforated cornea with a flat anterior chamber.[383] This can be prevented by using a tiny corneal or scleral tissue patch in the bed when closing a large corneal perforation with adhesive.[383] Intramuscular injection of cyanoacrylate derivatives has produced an inflammatory response[372] and histologic evidence of loss of muscle cell nuclei, fibroblastic invasion, giant cell formation, and an acute inflammatory response.[385]

Severe, localized coagulative retinal necrosis[386, 387] and stymied neurite growth[388] have been demonstrated experimentally. Other clinical and experimental studies have found cyanoacrylate tissue adhesives to be tolerated fairly well when used for transvitreal retinopexy[389] or scleral buckle procedures;[390] they cause only minimal localized inflammation.[391] The higher cyanoacrylate analogs may be advantageous for retina surgeons because of their slower polymerization time and reduced toxicity.[392] Human[393] and animal[394] studies have shown good tolerance to butyl 2-cyanoacrylate used for plastic surgery wounds, but it is not advised for punctal occlusion.[395] Dermatitis has been associated with cyanoacrylates,[396, 397] and inadvertent lid adhesion and corneal abrasion may occur.[398, 399]

Miscellaneous Agents (Table 43–10)

α-CHYMOTRYPSIN

α-Chymotrypsin, previously available as Catarase 1:5000 (IOLAB Pharmaceuticals) and Zolyse (Alcon Surgical), is a proteolytic pancreatic enzyme capable of breaking peptide bonds that has been used to facilitate intracapsular cataract extraction since the discovery of enzymatic zonulolysis in 1957 by Joaquin Barraquer.[400] Systemic anaphylaxis has been described but, to our knowledge, has not been reported with intraocular use.[401]

Although several case reports[402, 403] and early clinical[404] and animal[405] studies suggested that corneal endothelial toxicity might be a problem, later investigations revealed that corneal edema or opacification was associated with extreme elevation in intraocular pressure[406, 407] and specific corneal toxicity was not a significant problem with routine posterior chamber instillation of α-chymotrypsin.[408] Intralamellar injection of α-chymotrypsin, however, can cause corneal edema, opacification, and necrosis.[408, 409] Early studies also suggested that corneoscleral wound healing was inhibited by α-chymotrypsin,[404, 410] but this has been discounted by later studies, which found no reduction in wound strength.[408, 411]

Kirsch[412] was the first to recognize the temporary postoperative elevation of intraocular pressure that can be caused by α-chymotrypsin, which has been called "transient enzymatic glaucoma." Further investigation showed that the glaucoma is dose related[407, 413] and associated with temporarily decreased outflow facility.[414, 415] Anderson,[416] using electron microscopy, demonstrated obstruction of the trabecular meshwork by zonular fragments. The obstructive mechanism is supported by another study that reproduced the elevation of intraocular pressure in owl monkeys by intracameral injec-

TABLE 43–10. **Toxicity of Miscellaneous Agents**

Agent	Toxicity	Mechanism	References
α-Chymotrypsin (Catarase, Zolyse)	Corneal edema in early reports	Elevated IOP	402–408
	Corneal edema, opacification, neovascularization	Intralamellar injection	408, 409
	Inhibition of wound healing (?)		404, 408, 410, 411
	Elevated IOP	Decreased outflow facility by zonular fragments, possible inflammatory component	406, 407, 412–419
	Retinopathy (?)		406, 407, 419–422
Thrombin	Inflammatory reaction		426, 428, 429, 430
	[↓] Rabbit ERG sensitivity		431
	Corneal endothelium (?)	Hypertonicity, particulates	431–434
t-PA	Tolerated well by retina		449–452
	Rebleeding/AC hemorrhage	Dose related	455–460, 464, 465
	Transient periocular pain		460, 464
	Fibrin recurrence		460, 461
Detergent	Delayed epithelial healing		1, 16
	Corneal edema	Breakdown of endothelial barrier	467, 468

Abbreviation: IOP, intraocular pressure.

tion of unfiltered aqueous humor from other animals previously treated with α-chymotrypsin.[417] The ability to inhibit pressure elevation with indomethacin in rabbits, however, suggests that prostaglandin-mediated disruption of the blood-ocular barrier by α-chymotrypsin may also play a role.[418] Glaucomatous optic nerve cupping and optic atrophy have been described, but they appear to be due to elevated intraocular pressure rather than to any specific neurotoxicity.[406, 407, 419] Severe vitritis may occur if α-chymotrypsin is used and the vitreous face is not intact.

There are also reports of retinopathy associated with the injection of α-chymotrypsin;[406, 407, 419–422] however, many of the described changes may have been due to intercurrent glaucoma. Clinically, α-chymotrypsin appears to be well tolerated by the retina when used routinely for intracapsular cataract extraction.

THROMBIN

Thrombin has been used as an intraocular hemostatic agent since the mid-1940s.[423–425] More recently, its application during vitrectomy for stage V retinopathy of prematurity or diabetic vitrectomy requiring dissection of vascularized epiretinal membranes has sparked renewed interest.[426, 427]

Thompson and associates[426] treated patients with 100 U/mL of thrombin in the vitreous infusate and reported an incidence of excessive postoperative inflammatory reaction of at least 20%, prompting them to suggest washing out the thrombin infusate before the end of surgery. Aaberg[428] noted that the inflammatory reaction was seen principally in diabetic eyes and may have been related to both the fibrin and the diabetes process. He pointed out techniques, such as intermittent therapy, to minimize the inflammatory response. Maxwell and coworkers[429] reported no significantly increased inflammation when intermittent boluses of 100 U/mL of thrombin were used in 20 patients. Olsen and associates reported postvitrectomy hypopyon in 5 of 60 patients after intravitreal bovine thrombin for macular hole surgery.[430]

Animal studies have demonstrated no evidence of corneal toxicity in rabbits[431] or sheep.[432] Decreased electroretinographic sensitivity in rabbits was reported in one study that did not note any histologic evidence of retinal damage.[431]

McDermott and associates[433] evaluated the toxicity of two commercially available preparations of thrombin: Thrombostat (Parke-Davis, Morris Plains, NJ) and Thrombinar (Armour Pharmaceutical, now Jones Medical Industries, St. Louis, MO) with human corneal endothelial perfusions in vitro. Corneas perfused with 100 U/mL showed significant attenuation in the rate of detumescence but no structural alterations. Corneas perfused with 1000 U/mL showed intracellular and intercellular vacuole formation and altered junctional complexes that were likely due to the solution's hypertonicity. McDermott and coworkers emphasized that thrombin preparations are based on topical use. The more demanding requirements of an intracameral solution—purity, pH, osmolality, and vehicle—were not considered.[433] Indeed, McDermott's group measured a large quantity of particulate contamination in one of the thrombin preparations and noted a high concentration of glycine 2.5 times the serum level previously associated with retinal toxicity.[433]

TISSUE PLASMINOGEN ACTIVATOR

Genetic engineering technology has allowed the production of recombinant human tissue plasminogen activator (t-PA), available as Activase (Genentech, South San Francisco, CA) and best known for its use in promoting lysis of thrombi in acute myocardial infarction.[435] Snyder and associates[436] first reported on the use of t-PA to clear intraocular fibrin in an experimental rabbit model. Other plasminogen activators such as streptokinase and urokinase previously had been used intraocularly to treat hyphema and vitreous hemorrhage, but they were associated with a large inflammatory response and corneal toxicity,[437–443] although one study found no direct corneal toxicity with urokinase, 1000 to 5000 U/mL.[444] Snyder and associates have addressed several reasons why t-PA is theoretically preferable for intraocular use, including its preferential activation of plasminogen at the site of the clot and the potential for increased purity.[445]

Several animal and in vitro studies produced encouraging results showing minimal or no ocular toxicity.[445–448] Later studies with rabbits' eyes have noted retinal toxicity with intravitreal injection of over approximately 25-μg doses of t-PA[449–451] that may be due to the vehicle rather than to the t-PA itself.[449] Lensectomy and vitrectomy appear to widen the therapeutic window, whereas the addition of a large gas bubble may potentiate toxicity.[451] Tractional retinal detachments were more frequent in eyes treated with t-PA in one rabbit model of induced vitreous hemorrhage.[452] In a cat model, an irreversible toxic reaction was seen with subretinal infusion of 1000 mg/L of t-PA that was attributable to the carrier vehicle, while concentrations from 2.5 to 200 mg/L were well tolerated.[453] Investigators have also reported on intravitreal t-PA for experimental subretinal hemorrhage in a rabbit model.[454]

Intraocular hemorrhage has been noted in traumatic hyphema models,[455, 456] experimental filtration surgery,[457] and in a retinal bleeding model.[458]

Clinically, Williams and coworkers[459] reported no complications from the use of 25 μg of t-PA for postvitrectomy fibrin formation. Jaffe and coworkers[460] noted transient periocular pain in three patients and anterior chamber hemorrhage in 2 of 23 eyes treated for severe fibrin formation following vitrectomy surgery for complicated proliferative retinopathy, diabetic tractional retinal detachment, or endophthalmitis. They also noted recurrence of fibrin formation in 10 of 23 eyes, which characteristically was less severe but required repeat injection in four patients. Dabbs and associates[461] found no direct evidence of toxicity due to t-PA but did note recurrence of fibrin accumulation in six of seven eyes after t-PA treatment for massive fibrin deposition following diabetic vitrectomy surgery and evidence of intraocular bleeding in all seven eyes. Williams and colleagues[462] demonstrated that doses of intraocular t-PA smaller than 25 μg are effective in treating postvitrectomy fibrin formation and appear to minimize the risk of intraocular hemorrhage and potential retinal toxicity. They noted no bleeding complications in 17 eyes after the administration of t-PA doses ranging from 3 to 12.5 μg.

Snyder and associates used intracameral t-PA for excessive fibrin response after penetrating keratoplasty and had good results.[463] Moon and associates showed no evidence of toxicity from t-PA in the treatment of postcataract fibrinous

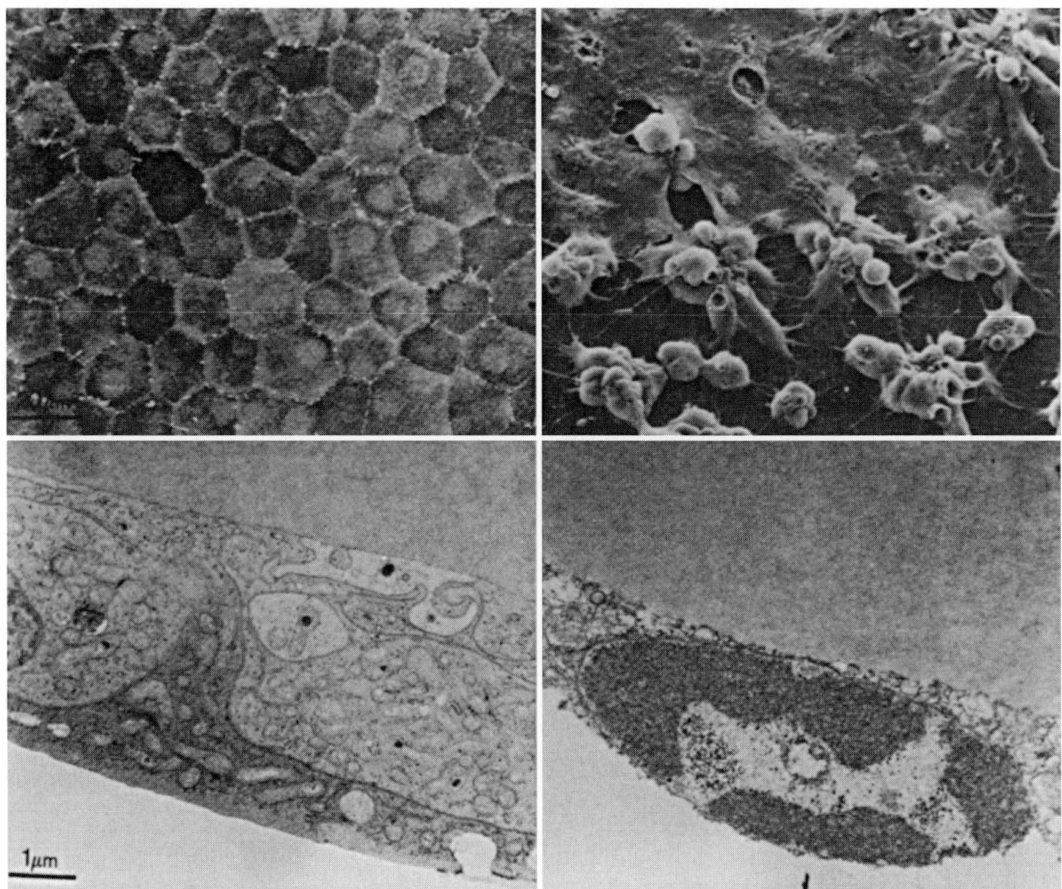

FIGURE 43–6. *Top left,* Scanning electron micrograph of human corneal endothelium after 3 minutes of perfusion with balanced salt solution plus. The mosaic pattern of endothelial cells is intact. *Top right,* Scanning electron micrograph of human corneal endothelium after 3 minutes of perfusion with a 1% detergent solution. Many endothelial cells are detached from Descemet's membrane. Remaining cells show degenerative changes, such as cell shrinkage, junctional separation, and gaps between cells. *Bottom left,* Transmission electron micrograph of human corneal endothelium after 3 minutes of perfusion with balanced salt solution plus. There is a smooth posterior surface with normal intracellular organelles and a few cytoplasmic vacuoles. *Bottom right,* Transmission electron micrograph of human corneal endothelium after 3 minutes of perfusion with a 1% detergent solution. Only remnants of endothelial cells are attached to Descemet's membrane. The outer plasma membrane is ruptured with extensive dilatation of the endoplasmic reticulum, cytoplasmic vacuolization, and severe mitochondrial swelling. Note the pyknotic nucleus with the clumping of the nuclear chromatin. (From Nuyts RMMA, Edelhauser HF, Pels E, Breebaart AC: Toxic effects of detergents on the corneal endothelium. Arch Ophthalmol 108:1158, 1990.)

membranes in 52 eyes as measured by slit-lamp biomicroscopy, intraocular pressure, and corneal endothelial cell density, size, and morphology; however, complications did include periorbital pain (4 eyes) and anterior chamber hemorrhage (four eyes).[464] This drug (t-PA) has also been used following glaucoma surgery intracamerally to clear aqueous outflow obstruction by blood/fibrin clot and subconjunctivally to release adherent trabeculectomy flaps.[465, 466]

DETERGENTS

In the section on antiseptics, we mentioned that topical detergents have been associated with epithelial toxicity, delayed healing, and corneal edema.[1, 16] The corneal endothelium tends to be much more sensitive than the epithelium to the toxic effects of solutions, as illustrated by the extremely low (0.0001%) benzalkonium chloride toxicity threshold demonstrated by Green and associates.[115] Although one might not expect the corneal endothelium to be exposed to detergent clinically, the following cases and investigation described by Breebaart and coworkers[467] and Nuyts and associates[468] deserve special mention and consideration by ophthalmic surgeons.

Breebaart's group[467] described 18 patients who developed acute corneal decompensation following uncomplicated intraocular surgery (mean endothelial cell loss of 72%) and coined the term "toxic endothelial cell destruction" for the syndrome. Epidemiologic evaluation revealed that the syndrome was caused by a detergent residue inside reusable irrigating cannulas that probably were not flushed well enough after exposure to ultrasonic cleaning solution. Nuyts and associates[468] identified the toxic component to be an ethoxylated fatty alcohol with a C_{10} chain length, a nonionic detergent. They confirmed the endothelial toxicity using Janus green photometry, corneal perfusions in vitro, and endothelial permeability studies that demonstrated the toxic effects to result from endothelial barrier breakdown (Fig. 43–6). The importance of maintaining vigilance for similar occurrences cannot be overemphasized.

Acknowledgment

Supported in part by an unrestricted grant from Research to Prevent Blindness, Inc., and Core Center Grant EY01931.

REFERENCES

1. MacRae SM, Brown B, Edelhauser HF: The corneal toxicity of presurgical skin antiseptics. Am J Ophthalmol 97:221, 1984.
2. Grant MW: Toxicology of the Eye, 3rd ed. Springfield, IL, Charles C Thomas, 1986.
3. Tanner FW, Wilson FL: Germicidal actions of aliphatic alcohols. Proc Soc Exp Biol Med 52:138, 1943.
4. Morgan JP III, Haug RH, Kosman JW: Antimicrobial skin preparations for the maxillofacial region. J Oral Maxillofac Surg 54:89, 1996.
5. Zintel HA: Asepsis and antisepsis. Surg Clin North Am 36:257, 1956.
6. Gershenfeld L: Povidone-iodine as a topical antiseptic. Am J Surg 94:938, 1957.
7. Joress SM: A study of disinfection of the skin: A comparison of povidone-iodine with other agents used for surgical scrubs. Ann Surg 155:296, 1962.
8. Kiffney GT, Hattaway AC: Povidone-iodine as an ophthalmic antiseptic. Surg Forum 17:434, 1966.
9. Hale LM: Povidone-iodine in ophthalmic surgery. Ophthalmic Surg 5:9, 1970.
10. Azar RF: Control of infection in eye surgery. Proceedings of the 2nd World Congress on Antisepsis. New York, HP Pub., 163, 1980.
11. Shepard DD: [cited by Betadine 5% Sterile Ophthalmic Prep Solution (Product information guide).] Skillman, NJ, Escalon Ophthalmics, 1990.
12. Physicians' Desk Reference, 51st ed. [Product information.] Montvale, NJ, Medical Economics, 1997.
13. Physicians' Desk Reference, 51st ed. [Product information.] Montvale, NJ, Medical Economics, 1997.
14. Lowbury JL, Lilly HA: The effect of blood on disinfection of surgeons' hands. Br J Surg 64:19, 1974.
15. Peterson AF, Rosenberg A, Alatary SD: Comparative evaluation of surgical scrub preparations. Surg Gynecol Obstet 146:63, 1978.
16. Phinney RB, Mondino BJ, Hofbauer JD, et al: Corneal edema related to accidental Hibiclens exposure. Am J Ophthalmol 106:210, 1988.
17. Stott WG: Antiseptic (Hibiclens) and eye injuries. Med J Aust 2:456, 1980.
18. Shore JW: Hibiclens keratitis. [Letter] Am J Ophthalmol 104:670, 1987.
19. Hamed LM, Ellis FD, Boudreault G, et al: Hibiclens keratitis. Am J Ophthalmol 104:50, 1987.
20. Burstein NL: Preservative cytotoxic threshold for benzalkonium chloride and chlorhexidine digluconate in cat and rabbit corneas. Invest Ophthalmol Vis Sci 19:308, 1980.
21. Pfister RR, Burstein NL: The effects of ophthalmic drugs, vehicles, and preservatives on corneal epithelium: A scanning electron microscope study. Invest Ophthalmol 15:246, 1976.
22. Dormans JAMA, van Logten MJ: The effects of ophthalmic preservatives on corneal epithelium of the rabbit: A scanning electron microscope study. Toxicol Appl Pharmacol 62:251, 1982.
23. Green K, Livingston V, Bowman K, Hull DS: Chlorhexidine effects on corneal epithelium and endothelium. Arch Ophthalmol 98:1273, 1980.
24. Gasset AR, Ishii Y: Cytotoxicity of chlorhexidine. Can J Ophthalmol 10:98, 1975.
25. Hamill MB, Osato MS, Wilhelmus KR: Experimental evaluation of chlorhexidine gluconate for ocular antisepsis. Antimicrob Agents Chemother 26:793, 1984.
26. Bryant CA, Rodeheaver GT, Reem EM, et al: Search for a nontoxic surgical scrub solution for periorbital lacerations. Ann Emerg Med 13:317, 1984.
27. Marsh RJ, Maurice DM: The influence of non-ionic detergents and other surfactants on human corneal permeability. Exp Eye Res 11:43, 1971.
28. Physicians' Desk Reference, 51st ed. [Product information.] Montvale, NJ, Medical Economics, 1997.
29. Topical antiseptics and antibiotics. Med Lett 19:83, 1977.
30. Browning CW, Lippas L: pHisoHex keratitis. Arch Ophthalmol 53:817, 1955.
31. Griffiths MC (ed): USAN and the USP Dictionary of Drug Names. Rockville, MD, United States Pharmacopeial Convention, 1984.
32. Goh CL: Contact sensitivity to topical antimicrobials. II: Sensitizing potentials of some topical antimicrobials. Contact Dermatitis 21:166, 1989.
33. Storrs FJ: Parachlorometaxylenol allergic contact dermatitis in seven individuals. Contact Dermatitis 1:211, 1975.
34. Ranchoff RE, Steck WD, Taylor JS, et al: Electrocardiography electrode and hand dermatitis from parachlorometaxylenol. J Am Acad Dermatol 15:348, 1986.
35. Myatt AD, Beck MH: Contact sensitivity to parachlorometaxylenol (PCMX). Clin Exp Dermatol 10:491, 1985.
36. Edelhauser HF, Van Horn DL, Schultz RO, Hyndiuk RA: Comparative toxicity of intraocular irrigating solutions on the corneal endothelium. Am J Ophthalmol 81:473, 1976.
37. Christiansen JM, Kollarits CR, Fukui H, et al: Intraocular irrigating solutions and lens clarity. Am J Ophthalmol 82:594, 1976.
38. Kahn MG, Giblin FJ, Epstein DL: Glutathione in calf trabecular meshwork and its relation to aqueous humor outflow facility. Invest Ophthalmol Vis Sci 24:1283, 1983.
39. Moorhead LC, Redburn DA, Merritt J, et al: The effects of intravitreal irrigation during vitrectomy on the electroretinogram. Am J Ophthalmol 88:239, 1979.
40. Rao GN, Shaw EL, Arthur EJ, et al: Endothelial cell morphology and corneal deturgescence. Ann Ophthalmol 11:885, 1979.
41. Rao GN, Aquavella JV, Goldberg SH, et al: Pseudophakic bullous keratopathy: Relationship to preoperative corneal endothelial status. Ophthalmology 91:1135, 1984.
42. Hyndiuk RA: Intraocular Solutions and the Corneal Endothelium. American Academy of Ophthalmology North Central Regional Update Course. Chicago, Syllabus, 1988.
43. Riley MV: Transport of ions and metabolites across the corneal endothelium. *In* McDevitt DS (ed): Cell Biology of the Eye. New York, Academic Press, 1982.
44. Edelhauser HF, MacRae SM: Irrigating and viscous solutions. *In* Sears ML, Tarkkanen A (eds): Surgical Pharmacology of the Eye. New York, Raven, 1985.
45. Kaye GI, Mishima S, Cole JD, et al: Studies on the cornea. VII: Effects of perfusion with a Ca^{++}-free medium on the corneal endothelium. Invest Ophthalmol Vis Sci 7:53, 1968.
46. Stern ME, Edelhauser HF, Pederson HJ, et al: Effects of ionophores X537A and A23187 and calcium free medium on corneal endothelial morphology. Invest Ophthalmol Vis Sci 20:497, 1981.
47. Lolley RN: Metabolism of retinal rod outer segment. *In* Anderson RE (ed): Biochemistry of the Eye. San Francisco, American Academy of Ophthalmology, 1983.
48. Gonnering R, Edelhauser HF, Van Horn DL, et al: The pH tolerance of rabbit and human corneal endothelium. Invest Ophthalmol Vis Sci 18:373, 1979.
49. Edelhauser HF, Hyndiuk RA, Zeeb A, et al: Corneal edema and the intraocular use of epinephrine. Am J Ophthalmol 93:327, 1982.
50. Edelhauser HF, Hanneken AM, Pederson HJ, et al: Osmotic tolerance of rabbit and human corneal endothelium. Arch Ophthalmol 99:1281, 1981.
51. Edelhauser HF: Intraocular irrigating solutions. *In* Lamberts DW, Potter DE (eds): Clinical Ophthalmic Pharmacology. Boston, Little, Brown, 1987.
52. Jacob TJC, Duncan G: Glucose induced membrane permeability changes in the lens. Exp Eye Res 37:445, 1982.
53. Kinoshita JH, Kador P, Catiler M: Aldose reductase in diabetic cataracts. JAMA 246:257, 1981.
54. Haimann MH, Abrams GW: Prevention of lens opacification during diabetic vitrectomy. Ophthalmology 91:116, 1984.
55. Haimann MH, Abrams GW, Edelhauser HF, et al: The effect of intraocular irrigating solutions on lens clarity in normal and diabetic rabbits. Am J Ophthalmol 94:594, 1982.
56. Hodson S, Miller F: The bicarbonate ion pump in the endothelium which regulates the hydration of rabbit cornea. J Physiol 263:563, 1976.
57. Hull DS, Green K, Boyd M, et al: Corneal endothelial bicarbonate

transport and the effect of carbonic anhydrase inhibitors on endothelial permeability and fluxes in cornea thickness. Invest Ophthalmol Vis Sci 16:883, 1977.
58. Riley MV, Peters MI: The localization of the anion-sensitive ATPase activity in corneal endothelium. Biochem Biophys Acta 644:251, 1981.
59. Whikehart DR, Soppet DR: Activities of transport enzymes located in the plasma membranes of corneal endothelial cells. Invest Ophthalmol Vis Sci 21:819, 1981.
60. Wiederholt M, Koch M: Effect of intraocular irrigating solutions in intracellular membrane potentials and swelling rate of isolated human and rabbit cornea. Invest Ophthalmol Vis Sci 18:313, 1979.
61. Hodson S, Wigham C, Williams L, et al: Observations on the human cornea in vitro. Exp Eye Res 32:353, 1981.
62. Hodson S: Evidence for a bicarbonate-dependent sodium pump in corneal endothelium. Exp Eye Res 11:20, 1971.
63. Hodson S: The regulation of corneal hydration by a salt pump requiring the presence of sodium and bicarbonate ion. J Physiol 236:271, 1974.
64. Winkler BS, Simson V, Benner J: Importance of bicarbonate in retinal function. Invest Ophthalmol Vis Sci 16:766, 1977.
65. Negi A, Honda Y, Kawano S: Effects of intraocular irrigating solutions on the electroretinographic B-wave. Am J Ophthalmol 92:28, 1981.
66. McDermott ML, Edelhauser HF, Hack HM, et al: Ophthalmic irrigants: A current review and update. Ophthalmic Surg 19:724, 1988.
67. Graham MV, Hodson S: Intraocular irrigating and replacement fluid. Trans Ophthalmol Soc U K 100:282, 1980.
68. Geroski DH, Grosserode RS, Edelhauser HF: A comparison of HEPES and bicarbonate buffered intraocular irrigating solutions: Effects on endothelial function in human and rabbit corneas. J Toxicol Cutan Ocul Toxicol 1:299, 1983.
69. Geroski DH, Edelhauser HF, O'Brien WJ: Hexose-monophosphate shunt response to diamide in component layers of the cornea. Exp Eye Res 26:611, 1978.
70. Textorious O, Nilsson SEG, Anderson BE: Effects of intraocular perfusion with two alternating irrigation solutions on the simultaneously recorded electroretinogram of albino rabbits. Doc Ophthalmol 63:349, 1986.
71. Riley MV: The chemistry of aqueous humor. *In* Anderson RE (ed): Biochemistry of the Eye. San Francisco, American Academy of Ophthalmology, 1983.
72. Dikstein S, Maurice DM: The metabolic basis to the fluid pump in the cornea. J Physiol 221:29, 1972.
73. Anderson EI, Fischbarg J, Spector A: Fluid transport, ATP level and ATPase activities in isolated rabbit corneal endothelium. Biochem Biophys Acta 307:557, 1973.
74. Anderson EI, Fischbarg J, Spector A: Disulfide stimulation of fluid transport and effect on ATP level in rabbit corneal endothelium. Exp Eye Res 19:1, 1974.
75. Edelhauser HF, Van Horn DL, Miller P, et al: Effect of thiol-oxidation of glutathione with diamide on corneal endothelial function, junctional complexes, and microfilaments. J Cell Biol 68:567, 1976.
76. Whikehart DR, Edelhauser HF: Glutathione in rabbit corneal endothelia: The effects of selected perfusion fluids. Invest Ophthalmol Vis Sci 17:455, 1978.
77. Ng MC, Riley MV: Relation of intracellular levels and redox state of glutathione to endothelial function in the rabbit cornea. Exp Eye Res 30:511, 1980.
78. Hodson SA, Wigham CG: Effect of glutathione on human corneal transendothelial potential difference. J Physiol 301:34, 1980.
79. Merrill DL, Fleming TC, Girard LJ: The effects of physiologic balanced salt solutions and normal saline on intraocular and extraocular tissues. Am J Ophthalmol 49:895, 1960.
80. Edelhauser HF, Van Horn DL, Hyndiuk RA, Schultz RO: Intraocular irrigating solutions: Their effect on the corneal endothelium. Arch Ophthalmol 93:648, 1975.
81. Emery JM, Landes DJ, Bendken RM: The phacoemulsifier: An evaluation of performance safety margins. *In* Emery JM, Paton D (eds): Current Concepts in Cataract Surgery. Selected Proceedings of the Third Biennial Cataract Surgical Congress. St Louis, CV Mosby, 1974.
82. Polack FM, Sugar A: The phacoemulsification procedure. II: Corneal endothelial changes. Invest Ophthalmol Vis Sci 15:458, 1976.
83. McCarey BD, Polack FM, Marshall W: The phacoemulsification procedure. I: The effect of intraocular irrigating solutions on the corneal endothelium. Invest Ophthalmol Vis Sci 15:449, 1976.
84. Benson WE, Diamond JG, Tasman W: Intraocular irrigating solutions for pars plana vitrectomy. Arch Ophthalmol 99:1013, 1981.
85. Matsuda M, Tano Y, Edelhauser HF: Comparison of intraocular irrigating solutions used for pars plana vitrectomy and prevention of endothelial cell loss. Jpn J Ophthalmol 28:230, 1984.
86. Glasser DB, Matsuda M, Ellis JG, et al: Effects of intraocular irrigating solutions on the corneal endothelium after in vivo anterior chamber irrigation. Am J Ophthalmol 99:321, 1985.
87. Li J, Akiyama R, Kuang K, et al: Effects of BSS and BSS+ irrigation solutions on rabbit corneal transendothelial electrical potential difference. Cornea 12:199, 1993.
88. Glasser DB, Matsuda M, Edelhauser HF: Comparison of corneal endothelial structural and functional integrity after irrigation with bicarbonate-buffered and acetate-citrate-buffered solutions. *In* Cavanagh HD (ed): The Cornea: Transactions of the World Congress on the Cornea III. New York, Raven, 1988.
89. Otori Y, Hohki T, Yamamoto Y, et al: Physiological studies on the intraocular irrigating solution for ophthalmic surgery: A preliminary report. Acta Soc Ophthalmol Jpn 84:1272, 1980.
90. Otori Y, Hohki T, Nakao Y, et al: Studies on the intraocular irrigating solution for ophthalmic surgery. Report 2: Reappraisal of the role of bicarbonate concentration. Acta Soc Ophthalmol Jpn 85:1237, 1981.
91. Matsuda M, Tano Y, Inaba M: Corneal complications after pars plana vitrectomy using SMA_2 for an intraocular irrigating solution. Folia Ophthal Jpn 34:1424, 1983.
92. Araie M: Barrier function of corneal endothelium and the intraocular irrigating solutions. Arch Ophthalmol 104:435, 1986.
93. Kaye G, Tice L: Studies on the cornea. V: Electron microscopic localization of adenosine triphosphate activity in the rabbit cornea in relation to transport. Invest Ophthalmol 5:22, 1966.
94. McCarey BE, Edelhauser HF, Van Horn DL: Functional and structural changes in the corneal endothelium during in vitro perfusion. Invest Ophthalmol Vis Sci 12:410, 1973.
95. Sanders DR, Peyman GA, McEnerney JK, et al: In vitro evaluations of intraocular infusion fluids: Effects on the lens and cornea. Ophthalmic Surg 8:63, 1977.
96. McEnerney JK, Peyman GA: Simplification of glutathione-bicarbonate-Ringer's solution: Its effect on corneal thickness. Invest Ophthalmol Vis Sci 16:657, 1977.
97. Waltman SR, Carroll D, Schemmelpfenning W, et al: Intraocular irrigating solutions for clinical vitrectomy. Ophthalmic Surg 6:90, 1975.
98. de Jong PTVM, Strous C, Fiedt Kok JP: Glutathione bicarbonate Ringer's intraocular irrigating fluid: Prospective double blind study. Ophthalmologica 186:35, 1983.
99. Edelhauser HF, Gonnering R, Van Horn DL: Intraocular irrigating solutions: A comparative study of BSS Plus and lactated Ringer's solution. Arch Ophthalmol 96:516, 1978.
100. McDermott M, Snyder R, Slack J, et al: Effects of intraocular irrigants on the preserved human corneal endothelium. Cornea 10:402, 1991.
101. Burke MJ, Parks MM, Calhoun JH, et al: Safety evaluation of BSS Plus in pediatric intraocular surgery. J Pediatr Ophthalmol Strabismus 18:45, 1981.
102. Kraff MC [cited by McDermott ML, Edelhauser HF, Hack HM, et al]: Ophthalmic irrigants: A current review and update. Ophthalmic Surg 19:724, 1988.
103. Pettit TH, Olson RJ, Foos RY, et al: Fungal endophthalmitis following intraocular lens implantation. Arch Ophthalmol 98:1025, 1980.
104. O'Day DM, Sommer A: Clinical Alert 1/1. Fungal Contamination from Balanced Salt Solution. San Francisco, American Academy of Ophthalmology, October 18, 1984.
105. Isenberg RA, Weiss RL, Apple DJ, et al: Fungal contamination of balanced salt solution. J Am Intraocul Implant Soc 11:485, 1985.
106. Stern WH, Tamura E, Jacobs RA, et al: Epidemic postsurgical *Candida parapsilosis* endophthalmitis: Clinical findings and management of 15 consecutive cases. Ophthalmology 92:1701, 1985.
107. Samples JR, Binder PS: Contamination of irrigating solution used for cataract surgery. Ophthalmic Surg 15:66, 1984.
108. Winding O, Gregerson E: Particulate contamination in eye surgery. Acta Ophthalmol 63:629, 1985.
109. Neumann AC: Particulate and microbial contamination of intraocular irrigating solutions. J Cataract Refract Surg 12:485, 1986.
110. van Rij G, Beekhuis WH, Eggink CA, et al: Toxic keratopathy due to the accidental use of chlorhexidine, cetrimide and cialit. Doc Ophthalmol 90:7, 1995.
111. Freeman JM, Gettlfinger TC: Maintaining pupillary dilation during lens implant surgery. J Am Intraocul Implant Soc 7:172, 1981.
112. Grehn F: Intraocular thymoxamine for miosis during cataract surgery. Am J Ophthalmol 103:709, 1987.

113. Gills JP: Prevention of endophthalmitis by intraocular solution filtration and antibiotics. J Am Intraocul Implant Soc 11:185, 1985.
114. Hull DS, Chemotti MT, Edelhauser HF, et al: Effect of epinephrine on the corneal endothelium. Am J Ophthalmol 79:245, 1975.
115. Green K, Hull DS, Vaughn ED, et al: Rabbit endothelial response to ophthalmic preservatives. Arch Ophthalmol 95:2218, 1977.
116. Winkler BS, Trese MT: The pH of antibiotic vitreous infusion combinations: A potential cause of retinal toxicity. Ophthalmic Surg 23:622, 1992.
117. McDermott ML, Edelhauser HF: Drug binding of ophthalmic viscoelastic agents. Arch Ophthalmol 107:261, 1989.
118. Goa KL, Benfield P: Hyaluronic acid: A review of its pharmacology and use as a surgical aid in ophthalmology, and its therapeutic potential in joint disease and wound healing. Drugs 47:536, 1994.
119. Balazs EA: Sodium hyaluronate and viscosurgery. *In* Miller D, Stegmann R (eds): Healon: A Guide To Its Use In Ophthalmic Surgery. New York, Wiley Medical, 1983.
120. Barany EH: The action of different kinds of hyaluronidase on the resistance to flow through the angle of the anterior chamber. Acta Ophthalmol 34:397, 1956.
121. Madsen K, Schenholm M, Jahnke G, et al: Hyaluronate binding to intact corneas and cultured endothelial cells. Invest Ophthalmol Vis Sci 30:2132, 1989.
122. Harfstrand A, Molander N, Stenevi U, et al: Evidence of hyaluronic acid and hyaluronic acid binding sites on human corneal endothelium. J Cataract Refract Surg 18:265, 1992.
123. Liesegang TJ: Viscoelastic substances in ophthalmology. Surv Ophthalmol 34:268, 1990.
124. Alpar JJ: Comparison of Healon and Amvisc. Ann Ophthalmol 17:647, 1985.
125. Sharpe ED, Simmons RJ: A prospective comparison of Amvisc and Healon in cataract surgery. J Cataract Refract Surg 12:47, 1986.
126. Physicians' Desk Reference for Ophthalmology, 25th ed. [Product information.] Montvale, NJ, Medical Economics, 1997.
127. Jensen MK, Crandall AS, Mamalis N, et al: Crystallization on intraocular lens surfaces associated with the use of Healon GV. Arch Ophthalmol 112:1037, 1994.
128. Colin J, Durand L, Mouillon M, et al: Comparative clinical trial of AMO Vitrax and Healon use in extracapsular cataract extraction. J Cataract Refract Surg 21:196, 1995.
129. Lehmann R, Brint S, Stewart R, et al: Clinical comparison of Provisc and Healon in cataract surgery. J Cataract Refract Surg 21: 543, 1995.
130. Hultsch E: The scope of hyaluronic acid as an experimental intraocular implant. Ophthalmology 87:706, 1980.
131. Balazs EA: Viscosurgery: Features of a true viscosurgical tool and its role in ophthalmic surgery. *In* Miller D, Stegmann R (eds): Treatment of Anterior Segment Ocular Trauma. Montreal, Medicopea, 1986.
132. Kim JH: Intraocular inflammation of denatured viscoelastic substance in cases of cataract extraction and lens implantation. J Cataract Refract Surg 13:537, 1987.
133. Sutphin JE, Papadimus TJ: Post-cataract extraction corneal edema: Epidemiological intervention and control. Invest Ophthalmol Vis Sci 30 (Suppl):165, 1989.
134. Ohguro N, Matsuda M, Kinoshita S: The effects of denatured sodium hyaluronate on the corneal endothelium in cats. Am J Ophthalmol 112:424, 1991.
135. Nuyts RMMA, Boot N, van Best JA, et al: Long term changes in human corneal endothelium following toxic endothelial cell destruction: A specular microscopic and fluorophotometric study. Br J Ophthalmol 80:15, 1996.
136. Arzeno A, Miller D: Effect of sodium hyaluronate on corneal wound healing. Arch Ophthalmol 100:152, 1982.
137. McKnight SJ, Gianiacomo J, Adelstein E: Inflammatory response to viscoelastic materials. Ophthalmic Surg 18:804, 1987.
138. McCulley J: Evaluating clinical properties of viscoelastics. Presented at the Eighth Annual Royal Hawaiian Eye Meeting, January 1987.
139. Meyer DR, McCulley JP: Different prospects of risk management from in vitro toxicology and its relevance to the evolution of viscoelastic formulations. *In* Rosen ES (ed): Viscoelastic Materials: Basic Science and Clinical Applications. New York, Pergamon, 1989.
140. Nguyen LK, Yee RW, Sigler SC, et al: Use of in vitro models of bovine corneal endothelial cells to determine the relative toxicity of viscoelastic agents. J Cataract Refract Surg 18:7, 1992.
141. Lindstrom RL: Personal communication, 1991.
142. Harrison SE, Soll DB, Shayegan M, et al: Chondroitin sulfate: A new and effective protective agent for intraocular lens insertion. Ophthalmology 89:1254, 1982.
143. MacRae SM, Edelhauser HF, Hyndiuk RA, et al: The effects of sodium hyaluronate, chondroitin sulfate, and methylcellulose on the corneal endothelium and intraocular pressure. Am J Ophthalmol 95:332, 1983.
144. Soll DB, Harrison SE, Arturi FC, et al: Evaluation and protection of corneal endothelium. J Am Intraocul Implant Soc 6:239, 1980.
145. Binder PS, Deg JK, Kohl FS: Calcific band keratopathy after intraocular chondroitin sulfate. Arch Ophthalmol 105:1243, 1987.
146. Nevyas AS, Raber IM, Eagle RC Jr, et al: Acute band keratopathy following intraocular Viscoat. Arch Ophthalmol 105:958, 1987.
147. Coffman MR, Mann PM: Corneal subepithelial deposits after use of sodium chondroitin. Am J Ophthalmol 102:279, 1986.
148. Ullman S, Lichtenstein SB, Heerlein K: Corneal opacities secondary to Viscoat. J Cataract Refract Surg 12:489, 1986.
149. Glasser DB, Katz HR, Boyd JE, et al: Protective effects of viscous solutions in phacoemulsification and traumatic lens implantation. Arch Ophthalmol 107:1047, 1989.
150. Aron-Rosa D, Cohn HC, Aron JJ, et al: Methylcellulose instead of Healon in extracapsular surgery with intraocular lens implantation. Ophthalmology 90:1235, 1983.
151. Fechner PU, Fechner MU: Methylcellulose and lens implantation. Br J Ophthalmol 67:259, 1983.
152. Bigar F, Gloor B, Schimmelpfennig B, et al: The tolerance of hydroxypropylmethylcellulose in implantation of posterior chamber lenses. Klin Monatsbl Augenheilkd 193:21, 1988.
153. Robert Y, Gloor B, Wachsmuth ED, et al: Evaluation of the tolerance of the intraocular injection of hydroxypropylmethylcellulose in animal experiments. Klin Monatsbl Augenheilkd 192:337, 1988.
154. Hazariwala K, Mortimer CB, Slomovic AR: Comparison of 2% hydroxypropyl methylcellulose and 1% sodium hyaluronate in implant surgery. Can J Ophthalmol 23:259, 1988.
155. Glasser DB, Matsuda M, Edelhauser HF: A comparison of the efficacy and toxicity of and intraocular pressure response to viscous solutions in the anterior chamber. Arch Ophthalmol 104:1819, 1986.
156. Kerr Muir MG, Sherrard ES, Andrews V, et al: Air, methylcellulose, sodium hyaluronate and the corneal endothelium; endothelial protective agents. Eye 1:480, 1987.
157. Liesegang TJ, Bourne WM, Ilstrup DM: The use of hydroxypropyl methylcellulose in extracapsular cataract extraction with intraocular lens implantation. Am J Ophthalmol 102:723, 1986.
158. Rosen ES, Gregory RPF, Barnett F: Is 2% hydroxypropyl methylcellulose a safe solution for intraoperative clinical applications? J Cataract Refract Surg 12:679, 1986.
159. Smith SG, Lindstrom RL, Muller RA, et al: Safety and efficacy of 2% methylcellulose in cat and monkey cataract implant surgery. J Am Intraocul Implant Soc 10:160, 1984.
160. Koster R, Stilma JS: Comparison of vitreous replacement with Healon and with HPMC in rabbit eyes. Doc Ophthalmol 61:247, 1986.
161. Condon PJ, Gillan J, Mullaney J, et al: Ultrastructural studies of the effect of viscoelastic substances on the endothelium of human donor corneae: A pilot study. *In* Rosen ES (ed): Viscoelastic Materials: Basic Science and Clinical Applications. New York, Pergamon, 1989.
162. Graue EL, Polack FM, Balazs EA: The protective effect of Na-hyaluronate to corneal endothelium. Exp Eye Res 31:119, 1980.
163. Pederson OO: Comparison of the protective effects of methylcellulose and sodium hyaluronate on corneal swelling following phacoemulsification of senile cataracts. J Cataract Refract Surg 16:594, 1990.
164. Thomsen M, Simonsen AH, Andreassen TT: Comparison of sodium hyaluronate and methylcellulose in extracapsular cataract extraction. Acta Ophthalmol 65:400, 1987.
165. Roberts B, Peiffer RL Jr: Experimental evaluation of a synthetic viscoelastic material on intraocular pressure and corneal endothelium. J Cataract Refract Surg 15:321, 1989.
166. Siegel MJ, Spiro HJ, Miller JA, et al: Secondary glaucoma and uveitis associated with Orcolon. Arch Ophthalmol 109:1496, 1991.
167. Balazs EA: The introduction of elastoviscous hyaluron for viscosurgery. *In* Rosen ES (ed): Viscoelastic Materials: Basic Science and Clinical Applications. New York, Pergamon, 1989.
168. Charleux J, Dupont D, Charleux M, et al: Human placental collagen type IV: An alternative as viscoelastic solution in ocular microsurgery. *In* Proceedings of the XXV International Congress of Ophthalmology, Rome, 1986. Amsterdam, Kugler and Ghedini, 1987.
169. Bothner H, Wik O: Rheology of intraocular solutions. *In* Rosen ES

(ed): Viscoelastic Materials: Basic Science and Clinical Applications. New York, Pergamon, 1989.

170. Bleckmann H, Vogt R, Garus HJ: Collagel: A new viscoelastic substance for ophthalmic surgery. J Cataract Refract Surg 18:20, 1992.
171. Berson FG, Patterson MM, Epstein DL: Obstruction of aqueous outflow by sodium hyaluronate in enucleated human eyes. Am J Ophthalmol 95:668, 1983.
172. Calder IG, Smith VH: Hyaluronidase and sodium hyaluronate in cataract surgery. Br J Ophthalmol 70:418, 1986.
173. Hein SR, Keates RH, Weber PA: Elimination of sodium hyaluronate-induced decrease in outflow facility with hyaluronidase. Ophthalmic Surg 17:731, 1986.
174. Kondo H, Hayashi H, Oshima K: Low molecular weight heparin inhibits raised intraocular pressure following intracameral administration of sodium hyaluronate. Nippon Ganka Gakkai Zasshi 98:423, 1994.
175. Denlinger JL, Balazs EA: The fate of exogenous viscoelastic hyaluron solutions in the primate eye. *In* Rosen ES (ed): Viscoelastic Materials: Basic Science and Clinical Applications. New York, Pergamon, 1989.
176. Miyauchi S, Iwata S: Biochemical studies on the use of sodium hyaluronate in the anterior eye segment. II: The molecular behavior of sodium hyaluronate injected into anterior chamber of rabbits. Curr Eye Res 3:611, 1984.
177. Levy NS, Boone L: Effect of hyaluronic acid viscosity on IOP elevation after cataract surgery. Glaucoma 11:82, 1989.
178. Embriano PJ: Postoperative pressure after phacoemulsification: Sodium hyaluronate vs. sodium chondroitin sulfate-sodium hyaluronate. Ann Ophthalmol 21:85, 1989.
179. Lane SS, Naylor DW, Kullerstrand LJ, et al: Prospective comparison of the effects of OcuCoat, Viscoat, and Healon on intraocular pressure and endothelial cell loss. J Cataract Refract Surg 17:21, 1991.
180. Barron BA, Busin M, Page C, et al: Comparison of the effects of Viscoat and Healon on postoperative intraocular pressure. Am J Ophthalmol 100:377, 1985.
181. Kohnen T, von Ehr M, Schutte E, et al: Evaluation of intraocular pressure with Healon and Healon GV in sutureless cataract surgery with foldable lens implantation. J Cataract Refract Surg 22:227, 1996.
182. Corbett MC, Richard AB: Intraocular adrenaline maintains mydriasis during cataract surgery. Br J Ophthalmol 78:95, 1994.
183. Dohlman C, Hyndiuk RA: Subclinical and manifest corneal edema after cataract extraction. *In* Transactions of the New Orleans Academy of Ophthalmology. St Louis, CV Mosby, 1972.
184. Tripathi JB, Tripathi RC, Millard CB: Epinephrine induced toxicity of human trabecular cells in vitro. Lens Eye Toxic Res 6:141, 1989.
185. Samples JR, Binder PS, Nayak S: The effect of epinephrine and benzalkonium chloride on cultured corneal endothelial and trabecular meshwork cells. Exp Eye Res 49:1, 1989.
186. Slack JW, Edelhauser HF, Helenek MJ: A bisulfite-free epinephrine solution. Am J Ophthalmol 110:77, 1990.
187. Glasser DB, Edelhauser HF: Toxicity of surgical solutions. Int Ophthalmol Clin 29:179, 1989.
188. Fell D, Watson AP, Hindocha N: Plasma concentrations of catecholamines following intraocular irrigation with adrenaline. Br J Anaesth 62:573, 1989.
189. Desai UR, Sudhamathi K, Natarajan S: Intravenous epinephrine and acute macular neuroretinopathy. Arch Ophthalmol 111:1026, 1993.
190. O'Brien DM, Farmer SG, Kalina RE, et al: Acute macular neuroretinopathy following intravenous sympathomimetics. Retina 9:281, 1989.
191. Edelhauser HF, Hine JE, Pederson H, et al: The effect of phenylephrine on the cornea. Arch Ophthalmol 97:937, 1979.
192. Lapalus P, Ettaiche M, Fredj-Reygrobellet D, et al: Cytotoxicity studies in ophthalmology. Lens Eye Toxic Res 7:231, 1990.
193. Machemer R [cited by Woog JJ, Albert DM]: Toxicology of intraoperative pharmacologic agents. *In* Sears ML, Tarkkanen A (eds): Surgical Pharmacology of the Eye. New York, Raven, 1985.
194. Lang RM, Hassard DTR: Effects on corneal endothelium of anterior chamber reconstituents instilled during intracapsular cataract extraction. Can J Ophthalmol 16:70, 1981.
195. McDonald TO, Beasley C, Borgmann A, et al: Intraocular administration of carbamylcholine chloride. Ann Ophthalmol 1:232, 1969.
196. Coles WH: Pilocarpine toxicity: Effects on the rabbit corneal endothelium. Arch Ophthalmol 93:36, 1975.
197. Jay JL, MacDonald M: Effects of intraocular miotics on cultured bovine corneal endothelium. Br J Ophthalmol 62:815, 1978.
198. Lazar M, Rosen N, Nemet P: Miochol-induced transient cataract. Ann Ophthalmol 9:1142, 1977.
199. Menchini U, Scialdone A, Fantaguzzi S, et al: Clinical evaluation of the effect of acetylcholine on the corneal endothelium. J Cataract Refract Surg 15:421, 1989.
200. McDonald TO, Roberts MD, Borgman AR: Intraocular safety of carbamylcholine chloride (carbachol) in rabbit eyes. Ann Ophthalmol 2:878, 1970.
201. Olson RJ, Kolodner H, Riddle P, et al: Commonly used intraocular medications and the corneal endothelium. Arch Ophthalmol 98:2224, 1980.
202. Vaughn ED, Hull DS, Green K: Effect of intraocular miotics on corneal endothelium. Arch Ophthalmol 96:1897, 1978.
203. Birnbaum DB, Hull DS, Green K, et al: Effect of carbachol on rabbit corneal endothelium. Arch Ophthalmol 105:253, 1987.
204. Yee RW, Edelhauser HF: Comparison of intraocular acetylcholine and carbachol. J Cataract Refract Surg 12:18, 1986.
205. Yee RW, Wallace G, Yu HS: Effects of the components of miochol and miostat on bovine corneal endothelial cells. Invest Ophthalmol Vis Sci 30 (Suppl):335, 1989.
206. Yee RW, Meenakshi S, Yu HS, et al: Effects of acetylcholine and carbachol on bovine corneal endothelial cells in vitro. J Cataract Refract Surg 22:591, 1996.
207. Rongey KA, Weisman H: Hypotension following intraocular acetylcholine. Anesthesiology 36:412, 1972.
208. Babinski M, Smith B, Wickerham EP: Hypotension and bradycardia following intraocular acetylcholine injection. Arch Ophthalmol 94:675, 1976.
209. Gombos GM: Systemic reactions following intraocular acetylcholine instillation. Ann Ophthalmol 14:529, 1982.
210. Brinkley JR, Henrick A: Vascular hypotension and bradycardia following intraocular injection of acetylcholine during cataract surgery. Am J Ophthalmol 97:40, 1984.
211. Rasch D, Holt J, Wilson M, et al: Bronchospasm following intraocular injection of acetylcholine in a patient taking metoprolol. Anesthesiology 59:583, 1983.
212. McKinzie JW, Boggs MB: Comparison of postoperative intraocular pressures after use of Miochol and Miostat. J Cataract Refract Surg 15:185, 1989.
213. Ruiz RS, Rhem MN, Prager TC: Effects of carbachol and acetylcholine on intraocular pressure after cataract extraction. Am J Ophthalmol 107:7, 1989.
214. Wood TO: Effect of carbachol on postoperative intraocular pressure. J Cataract Refract Surg 14:654, 1988.
215. Hesse RJ, Smith AD, Roberts AD, et al: The effect of carbachol combined with intraoperative viscoelastic substances on postoperative IOP response. Ophthalmic Surg 19:224, 1988.
216. Linn DK, Zimmerman TJ, Nardin GF, et al: Effect of intracameral carbachol on intraocular pressure after cataract extraction. Am J Ophthalmol 107:133, 1989.
217. Hollands RH, Drance SM, Schulzer M: The effect of intracameral carbachol on intraocular pressure after cataract extraction. Am J Ophthalmol 104:225, 1987.
218. Hollands RH, Drance SM, Schulzer M: The effect of acetylcholine on early postoperative intraocular pressure. Am J Ophthalmol 103:749, 1987.
219. Kim JY, Sohn JH, Youn DH: Effects of intracameral carbachol and acetylcholine on early postoperative intraocular pressure after cataract extraction. Korean J Ophthalmol 8:61, 1994.
220. Wedrich A, Menapace R: Intraocular pressure following small incision cataract surgery and polyHEMA posterior chamber lens implantation: A comparison between acetylcholine and carbachol. J Cataract Refract Surg 18:500, 1992.
221. Hollands RH, Drance SM, House PH, et al: Control of intraocular pressure after cataract extraction. Can J Ophthalmol 25:128, 1990.
222. McKinzie JW, Boggs MB Jr: Comparison of postoperative intraocular pressures after use of Miochol and Miostat. J Cataract Refract Surg 15:185, 1989.
223. Ruiz RS, Rhem MN, Prager TC: Effects of carbachol and acetylcholine on intraocular pressure after cataract extraction. Am J Ophthalmol 107:7, 1989.
224. Roberts CW: Intraocular miotics and postoperative inflammation. J Cataract Refract Surg 19:731, 1993.
225. Foulks GN: Drugs used in cataract surgery. *In* Lamberts DW, Potter DE (eds): Clinical Ophthalmic Pharmacology. Boston, Little, Brown, 1987.
226. Van Horn DL, Edelhauser HF, Aaberg TM, et al: In vivo effects of

air and sulfur hexafluoride gas on rabbit corneal endothelium. Invest Ophthalmol 11:1028, 1972.
227. Olson RJ: Air and the corneal endothelium: An in vivo specular microscopy study in cats. Arch Ophthalmol 98:1283, 1980.
228. Leibowitz HM, Laing RA, Sandstrom M: Corneal endothelium: The effect of air in the anterior chamber. Arch Ophthalmol 92:227, 1974.
229. Brubaker S, Peyman GA, Vygantas C: Toxicity of octafluorocyclobutane after intracameral injection. Arch Ophthalmol 92:324, 1974.
230. Craig MT, Olson RJ, Mamalis N, et al: Air bubble endothelial damage during phacoemulsification in human eye bank eyes: The protective effects of Healon and Viscoat. J Cataract Refract Surg 16:597, 1990.
231. Constable IJ, Swann DA: Vitreous substitution with gases. Arch Ophthalmol 93:416, 1975.
232. Machemer R, Allen AW: Retinal tears 180° and greater: Management with vitrectomy and intravitreal gas. Arch Ophthalmol 94:1340, 1976.
233. Von Sallman L [cited by Woog JJ, Albert DM]: Toxicology of intraoperative pharmacologic agents. *In* Sears ML, Tarkkanen A (eds): Surgical Pharmacology of the Eye. New York, Raven, 1985.
234. Stallard HB [cited by Woog JJ, Albert DM]: Toxicology of intraoperative pharmacologic agents. *In* Sears ML, Tarkkanen A (eds): Surgical Pharmacology of the Eye. New York, Raven, 1985.
235. Fineberg E, Machemer R, Sullivan P, et al: Sulfur hexafluoride in owl monkey vitreous cavity. Am J Ophthalmol 79:67, 1975.
236. Chawla HB, Birchall CH: Intravitreal air in retinal detachment surgery. Br J Ophthalmol 57:60, 1973.
237. Chawla HB: Intravitreal air in aphakic retinal detachment. Br J Ophthalmol 57:58, 1973.
238. Scheie HG, Frayer W: Ocular hypertension induced by air in the anterior chamber. Trans Am Ophthalmol Soc 48:88, 1950.
239. Aronowitz JD, Brubaker RF: Effect of intraocular gas on intraocular pressure. Arch Ophthalmol 94:1191, 1976.
240. Moses RA: Schiotz tonometry with an air bubble in the eye. Am J Ophthalmol 62:281, 1966.
241. Poliner LS, Schoch LH: Intraocular pressure assessment in gas-filled eyes following vitrectomy. Arch Ophthalmol 105:200, 1987.
242. Peyman GA, Vygantas CM, Bennett TO, et al: Octafluorocyclobutane in vitreous and aqueous humor replacement. Arch Ophthalmol 93:514, 1975.
243. Norton EW, Aaberg T, Fung W, et al: Giant retinal tears. I: Clinical management with intravitreal air. Am J Ophthalmol 68:1011, 1969.
244. Ohm J [cited in Chang S: Intraocular gases]: *In* Glaser BM, Michels RG (eds): Retina. St Louis, CV Mosby, 1989.
245. Norton EWD: Intraocular gases in the management of selected retinal detachments. Trans Am Acad Ophthalmol Otolaryngol 77:85, 1973.
246. Wilson MR, Yoshizumi MO, Lee DA, et al: Use of intraocular gas in flat anterior chamber after filtration surgery. Arch Ophthalmol 106:1345, 1988.
247. Nabih M, Peyman GA, Clark LC Jr, et al: Experimental evaluation of perfluorophenanthrene as a high specific gravity vitreous substitute: A preliminary report. Ophthalmic Surg 20:286, 1989.
248. Foulks GN, de Juan E, Hatchell DL, et al: The effect of perfluoropropane on the cornea in rabbits and cats. Arch Ophthalmol 105:256, 1987.
249. Abrams GW, Swanson DE, Sabates WI, et al: The results of sulfur hexafluoride gas in vitreous surgery. Am J Ophthalmol 94:165, 1982.
250. Lincoff H, Coleman J, Kreissig I, et al: The perfluorocarbon gases in the treatment of retinal detachment. Ophthalmology 90:546, 1983.
251. Sabates WI, Abrams GW, Swanson DE, et al: The use of intraocular gases: The results of sulfur hexafluoride gas in retinal detachment surgery. Ophthalmology 88:447, 1981.
252. Chang S, Lincoff HA, Coleman DJ, et al: Perfluorocarbon gases in vitreous surgery. Ophthalmology 92:651, 1985.
253. O'Connor PR: Intravitreous air injection and the Custodis procedure. Ophthalmic Surg 7:86, 1976.
254. Chang S: Intraocular gases. *In* Glaser BM, Michels RG (eds): Retina. St. Louis, CV Mosby, 1989.
255. Constable IJ: Perfluoropentane in experimental ocular surgery. Invest Ophthalmol 13:627, 1974.
256. Killey FP, Edelhauser HF, Aaberg TM: Intraocular sulfur hexafluoride and octofluorocyclobutane: Effects on intraocular pressure and vitreous volume. Arch Ophthalmol 96:511, 1978.
257. Schepens CL, Freeman HM, Thompson RF: A power driven multipositional operating table. Arch Ophthalmol 73:671, 1965.
258. Smith RB, Carl B, Linn JG Jr, et al: Effect of nitrous oxide on air in vitreous. Am J Ophthalmol 78:314, 1974.
259. Wolf GL, Capuano C, Hartung J: Effect of nitrous oxide on gas bubble volume in the anterior chamber. Arch Ophthalmol 103:418, 1985.
260. Stinson TW III, Donlon JV: Interaction of intraocular air and sulfur hexafluoride with nitrous oxide: A computer simulation. Anesthesiology 56:385, 1982.
261. Dieckert JP, O'Connor PS, Schacklett DE, et al: Air travel and intraocular gas. Ophthalmology 93:642, 1986.
262. Hanscom TA, Diddie KR: Mountain travel and intraocular gas bubbles. Am J Ophthalmol 104:546, 1987.
263. Lincoff H, Kreissig I, Jakobiec F: The inadvertent injection of gas beneath the retina in a pseudophakic eye. Ophthalmology 93:408, 1986.
264. Chang S, Reppucci V, Zimmerman NJ, et al: Perfluorocarbon liquids in the management of traumatic retinal detachments. Ophthalmology 96:785, 1989.
265. Diddie KR, Smith RE: Intraocular gas injection in the pseudophakic patient. Am J Ophthalmol 89:659, 1980.
266. Clark LC, Jr, Gollan F: Survival of mammals breathing organic fluids equilibrated with oxygen at atmospheric pressure. Science 152:1755, 1966.
267. Biro GP, Blais P: Perfluorocarbon blood substitutes. Crit Rev Oncol Hematol 6:311, 1987.
268. Haidt SJ, Clark LC Jr, Ginsberg J: Liquid perfluorocarbon replacement of the eye. [Abstract] Invest Ophthalmol Vis Sci 22 (Suppl):223, 1982.
269. Peyman GA, Schulman JA, Sullivan B: Perfluorocarbon liquids in ophthalmology. Surv Ophthalmol 39:375, 1995.
270. Berrocal MH, Chang S: Perfluorocarbon liquids in vitreous surgery. Ophthalmol Clin N Am 7:67, 1994.
271. Sparrow JR, Ortiz R, MacLeish PR, et al: Fibroblast behavior at aqueous interfaces with perfluorocarbon, silicone and fluorosilicone liquids. Invest Ophthalmol Vis Sci 31:638, 1990.
272. Adile SL, Peyman GA, Greve MDJ, et al: Postoperative chronic pressure abnormalities in the Vitreon study. Ophthalmic Surg 25:584, 1994.
273. Peyman GA, Conway MD, Soike KF, et al: Long term vitreous replacement in primates with intravitreal Vitreon or Vitreon plus silicone. Ophthalmic Surg 22:657, 1991.
274. Viebahn M, Buettner H: Perfluophenanthrene unsuitable for postoperative retinal tamponade. Am J Ophthalmol 118:124, 1994.
275. de Queiroz JM, Jr, Blanks JC, Ozler SA, et al: Subretinal perfluorocarbon liquids: An experimental study. Retina 12 (Suppl 3):S33, 1992.
276. Flores-Aguilar M, Munguia D, Loeb E, et al: Intraocular tolerance of perfluorooctylbromide (perflubron). Retina 15:446, 1995.
277. Sparrow JR, Matthews GP, Iwamoto T, et al: Retinal tolerance to intravitreal perfluoroethylcyclohexane liquid in the rabbit. Retina 13:56, 1993.
278. Conway MD, Peyman GA, Karacorlu M, et al: Perfluorooctylbromide (PFOB) as a vitreous substitute in non-human primates. Int Ophthalmol 17:259, 1993.
279. Velikay M, Stolba U, Wedrich A, et al: The effect of chemical stability and purification of perfluorocarbon liquids in experimental extended term vitreous substitution. Graefes Arch Clin Exp Ophthalmol 233:26, 1995.
280. Eckardt C, Nicolai U: Clinical and histologic findings after several weeks of intraocular tamponade with perfluorodecalin. Ophthalmologe 90:443, 1993.
281. Augustin AJ, Spitznas M, Koch FH, et al: Local effects of different perfluorochemical agents. Graefes Arch Clin Exp Ophthalmol 233:45, 1995
282. Berglin L, Ren J, Algvere PV: Retinal detachment and degeneration in response to subretinal perfluorodecalin in rabbit eyes. Graefes Arch Clin Exp Ophthalmol 231:233, 1993.
283. Devin F, Jourdan T, Saracco JB, et al: Experimental tolerance to perfluorodecalin used in prolonged intraocular tamponade. Ophthalmologica 209:306, 1995.
284. Velikay M, Wedrich A, Stolba U, et al: Experimental long-term vitreous replacement with purified and nonpurified perfluorodecalin. Am J Ophthalmol 116:565, 1993.
285. Foster RE, Smiddy WS, Alfonso EC, et al: Secondary glaucoma associated with retained perfluorophenanthrene. Am J Ophthalmol 118:253, 1994.
286. Wilbanks GA, Apel AJG, Jolly SS, et al: Perfluorodecalin corneal toxicity: Five case reports. Cornea 15:329, 1996.
287. Moreira H, de Queiroz JM, Liggett PE, et al: Corneal toxicity study of two perfluorocarbon liquids in rabbit eyes. Cornea 11:376, 1992.

288. Chang S, Sparrow JR, Iwamoto T, et al: Experimental studies of tolerance to intravitreal perfluoro-*N*-octane liquid. Retina 11:367, 1991.
289. Eckardt C, Nicolai U, Winter M, et al: Experimental intraocular tolerance to liquid perfluorooctane and perfluoropolyether. Retina 11:375, 1991.
290. Parel JM: Silicone oils: Physicochemical properties. *In* Glaser BM, Michels RG (eds): Retina. St Louis, CV Mosby, 1989.
291. Nakamura K, Refojo MF, Crabtree DV, et al: Ocular toxicity of low-molecular-weight components of silicone and fluorosilicone oils. Invest Ophthalmol Vis Sci 32:3007, 1991.
292. Green K, Cheeks L, Stewart DA, et al: Role of toxic ingredients in silicone oils in the induction of increased corneal endothelial permeability. Lens Eye Toxic Res 9:377, 1992.
293. Stone W Jr: Alloplasty in surgery of the eye. N Engl J Med 258:486, 1958.
294. Armaly MF: Ocular tolerance to silicones. I: Replacement of aqueous and vitreous by silicone fluids. Arch Ophthalmol 68:390, 1962.
295. Cibis PA, Becker B, Okun E, et al: The use of liquid silicone in retinal detachment surgery. Arch Ophthalmol 68:590, 1962.
296. Labelle P, Okun E: Ocular tolerance to liquid silicone: An experimental study. Can J Ophthalmol 7:199, 1972.
297. Cibis PA: Vitreoretinal Pathology and Surgery in Retinal Detachment. St Louis, CV Mosby, 1965.
298. Okun E [cited by Woog JJ, Albert DM]: Toxicology of intraoperative pharmacologic agents. *In* Sears ML, Tarkkanen A (eds): Surgical Pharmacology of the Eye. New York, Raven, 1985.
299. Grey RHB, Leaver PK [cited by Woog JJ, Albert DM]: Toxicology of intraoperative pharmacologic agents. *In* Sears ML, Tarkkanen A (eds): Surgical Pharmacology of the Eye. New York, Raven, 1985.
300. Scott JD [cited by Woog JJ, Albert DM]: Toxicology of intraoperative pharmacologic agents. *In* Sears ML, Tarkkanen A (eds): Surgical Pharmacology of the Eye. New York, Raven, 1985.
301. Setala K, Ruusuvaara P, Punnonen E, et al: Changes in corneal endothelium after treatment of retinal detachment with intraocular silicone oil. Acta Ophthalmol (Copenh) 67:37, 1989.
302. Liu KR, Peyman GA, Miceli MV: Experimental evaluation of low-viscosity fluorosilicone oil as a temporary vitreous substitute. Ophthalmic Surg 20:720, 1989.
303. Legler U, Seiberth V, Knorz MC, et al: Loss of corneal endothelial cells following pars plana vitrectomy and silicone oil implantation. Fortschr Ophthamol 87:290, 1990.
304. Gao RL: Specular microscopy of the corneal endothelium after entry of silicone oil into the anterior chamber. Chung Hua Yen Ko Tsa Chih 26:267, 1990.
305. Nawricki J, Rydzynski K, Nawrocka Z, et al: Study on the influence of silicone oils of various viscosities on anterior eye structures. Klin Oczna 94:173, 1992.
306. Choi WC, Choi SK, Lee JH: Silicone oil keratopathy. Korean J Ophthalmol 7:65, 1993.
307. Desatnik H, Ashkenazi I, Hirsh A, et al: Silicone oil-induced corneal hydrops? Ann Ophthalmol 24:288, 1992.
308. Pang MP, Peyman GA, Kao GW: Early anterior segment complications after silicone oil injection. Can J Ophthalmol 21:271, 1986.
309. Casswell AG, Gregor ZJ: Silicone oil removal. I: The effect on the complications of silicone oil. Br J Ophthalmol 71:893, 1987.
310. Gao RL, Neubauer L, Tang S, et al: Silicone oil in the anterior chamber. Graefes Arch Clin Exp Ophthalmol 227:106, 1989.
311. Suzuki M, Okada T, Takeuchi S, et al: Effect of silicone oil on ocular tissues. Jpn J Ophthalmol 35:282, 1991.
312. Doi M, Refojo MF: Histopathology of rabbit eyes with silicone-fluorosilicone copolymer oil as six months internal retinal tamponade. Exp Eye Res 61:469, 1995.
313. Knorr HL, Seltsam A, Holbach L, et al: Intraocular silicone oil tamponade: A clinico-pathologic study of 36 enucleated eyes. Ophthalmologe 93:130, 1996.
314. Sternberg P Jr, Hatchell DL, Foulks GN, et al: The effect of silicone oil on the cornea. Arch Ophthalmol 103:90, 1985.
315. Leaver PK, Grey RHB, Garner A: Silicone oil injection in the treatment of massive preretinal retraction. II: Late complications in 93 eyes. Br J Ophthalmol 63:361, 1979.
316. Haut J, Ullern M, Chermet M, et al: Complications of intraocular injections of silicone combined with vitrectomy. Ophthalmologica 180:29, 1980.
317. Federman JL, Schubert HD: Complications associated with the use of silicone oil in 150 eyes after retina-vitreous surgery. Ophthalmology 95:870, 1988.
318. Beekhuis WH, van Rij G, Zivojnovic R: Silicone oil keratopathy: Indications for keratoplasty. Br J Ophthalmol 69:247, 1985.
319. Bennett SR, Abrams GW: Band keratopathy from emulsified silicone oil. Arch Ophthalmol 108:1387, 1990.
320. Abrams GW, Azen SP, Barr CC, et al: The incidence of corneal abnormalities in the silicone study. Arch Ophthalmol 113:764, 1995.
321. Leaver PK: Complications of intraocular silicone oil. *In* Glaser BM, Michels RG (eds): Retina. St Louis, CV Mosby, 1989.
322. Watzke RC: Silicone retinopoiesis for retinal detachment: A long-term clinical evaluation. Arch Ophthalmol 77:185, 1967.
323. Lucke KH, Foerster MH, Laqua H: Long-term results of vitrectomy and silicone oil in 500 cases of complicated retinal detachments. Am J Ophthalmol 104:624, 1987.
324. Cockerham WD, Schepens CL, Freeman HM: Silicone injection in retinal detachment. Arch Ophthalmol 83:704, 1970.
325. Kanski JJ, Daniel R: Intravitreal silicone injection in retinal detachment. Br J Ophthalmol 57:542, 1973.
326. Chan C, Okun E: The question of ocular tolerance to intravitreal liquid silicone: A long-term analysis. Ophthalmology 93:651, 1986.
327. Gonvers M: Temporary silicone oil tamponade in the management of retinal detachment with proliferative vitreoretinopathy. Am J Ophthalmol 100:239, 1985.
328. Ando F: Usefulness and limit of silicone in management of complicated retinal detachment. Jpn J Ophthalmol 31:138, 1987.
329. Yamasaki A, Nagata M, Takagi S, et al: Time-course of lens opacity and morphological changes in rabbit lens epithelial cells after intravitreal silicone oil injection. Jpn J Ophthalmol 38:116, 1994.
330. Borislav D: Cataract after silicone oil implantation. Doc Ophthalmol 83:79, 1993.
331. Lee PF, Donovan RH, Mukai N, et al: Intravitreous injection of silicone: An experimental study. I: Clinical picture and histology of the eye. Ann Ophthalmol 1:15, 1969.
332. Mukai N, Lee PF, Schepens CL: Intravitreous injection of silicone: An experimental study. II: Histochemistry and electron microscopy. Ann Ophthalmol 4:273, 1972.
333. Ando F: Intraocular hypertension resulting from pupillary block by silicone oil. Am J Ophthalmol 99:87, 1985.
334. de Corral LR, Cohen SB, Peyman GA: Effect of intravitreal silicone oil on intraocular pressure. Ophthalmic Surg 18:446, 1987.
335. Slezak H, Haddad R, Scholda C: Pathogenesis of secondary glaucoma after intraocular silicone oil administration. Klin Monatsbl Augenheilkd 205:298, 1994.
336. Nowack C, Lucke K, Laqua H: Removal of silicone oil in treatment of so-called emulsification glaucoma. Ophthalmologe 89:462, 1992.
337. Ni C, Wang WJ, Albert DM, et al: Intravitreous silicone injection: Histopathologic findings in a human eye after 12 years. Arch Ophthalmol 101:1399, 1983.
338. Shields CL, Eagle RC: Pseudo-Schnabel's cavernous degeneration of the optic nerve secondary to intraocular silicone oil. Arch Ophthalmol 107:714, 1989.
339. Foerster MH, Esser J, Laqua H: Silicone oil and its influence on electrophysiologic findings. Am J Ophthalmol 99:201, 1985.
340. Frumar KD, Gregor ZJ, Carter RM, et al: Electroretinographic changes after vitrectomy and intraocular tamponade. Retina 5:16, 1985.
341. Ober RR, Blanks JC, Ogden TE, et al: Experimental retinal tolerance to liquid silicone. Retina 3:77, 1983.
342. Soheilian M, Peyman GA, Moritera T, et al: Experimental retinal tolerance to very low viscosity silicone oil (100 cs) as a vitreous substitute compared to higher viscosity silicone oil (5000 cs). Int Ophthalmol 19:57, 1995.
343. Mukai N, Lee PF, Oguri M, et al: A long-term evaluation of silicone retinopathy in monkeys. Can J Ophthalmol 10:391, 1975.
344. Eckhardt C, Schmidt D, Czank M: Intraocular tolerance to silicone oils of different specific gravities: An experimental study. Ophthalmologica 201:133, 1990.
345. Refojo MF, Leong FL, Chung H, et al: Extraction of retinol and cholesterol by intraocular silicone oils. Ophthalmology 95:614, 1988.
346. Sugar HS, Okamura ID: Ocular findings six years after intravitreal silicone injection. Arch Ophthalmol 94:612, 1976.
347. Blodi FC: Injection and impregnation of liquid silicone into ocular tissues. Am J Ophthalmol 71:1044, 1971.

348. Gonvers M, Hornung JP, de Courten C: The effect of liquid silicone on the rabbit retina. Histologic and ultrastructural study. Arch Ophthalmol 104:1057, 1986.
349. Lambrou FH, Burke JM, Aaberg TM: Effect of silicone oil on experimental traction retinal detachment. Arch Ophthalmol 105:1269, 1987.
350. Lewis H, Burke JM, Abrams GW, Aaberg TM: Perisilicone proliferation after vitrectomy for proliferative vitreoretinopathy. Ophthalmology 95:583, 1988.
351. Pastor JC, Lopez MI, Saornil MA, et al: Intravitreal silicone and fluorosilicone oils: Pathologic findings in rabbit eyes. Acta Ophthalmol (Copenh) 70:651, 1992.
352. Eckardt C, Nicolai U, Czank M, et al: Ocular tissue after intravitreous silicone oil injection: Histologic and electron microscopy studies. Ophthalmologe 90:250, 1993.
353. Nicolai U, Eckardt C: Immunohistochemical findings of epiretinal membranes after silicone oil injection. Fortschr Ophthalmol 88:660, 1991.
354. Nakagawa M, Refojo MJ, Marin JF, et al: Retinoic acid in silicone and silicone-fluorosilicone copolymer oils in a rabbit model of proliferative vitreoretinopathy. Invest Ophthalmol Vis Sci 36:2388, 1995.
355. Araiz JJ, Refojo MF, Arroyo MH, et al: Antiproliferative effect of retinoic acid in intravitreous silicone oil in an animal model of proliferative vitreoretinopathy. Invest Ophthalmol Vis Sci 34:522, 1993.
356. Johnson RN, Flynn HW Jr, Parel JM, et al: Transient hypopyon with marked anterior chamber fibrin following pars plana vitrectomy and silicone oil injection. Arch Ophthalmol 107:683, 1989.
357. Zauberman H, Hemo I: Use of fibrin glue in ocular surgery. Ophthalmic Surg 19:132, 1988.
358. Khodadoust AA: Tissue adhesives in ophthalmology. *In* Sears M, Tarkkanen A (eds): Surgical Pharmacology of the Eye. New York, Raven, 1985.
359. De Toledo AR, Witlock DR, Kaminski LA, et al: Preliminary evaluation of a new collagen-derived bioadhesive. [Abstract] Invest Ophthalmol Vis Sci 31:317, 1990.
360. Liggett PE, Cano M, Green RL, et al: Intraocular inflammatory and toxic effects of a new tissue adhesive for retinopexy: Muscle-activated protein. [Abstract] Invest Ophthalmol Vis Sci 28:206 1987.
361. Coover HW, Joyner FB, Shearer HN, et al: Chemistry and performance of cyanoacrylate adhesives. Soc Plastic Eng 15:413, 1959.
362. Refojo MF, Dohlman CH, Koliopoulos J: Adhesives in ophthalmology: A review. Surv Ophthalmol 15:217, 1971.
363. Leonard F: The *N*-alkylalphacyanoacrylate tissue adhesives. Ann N Y Acad Sci 146:203, 1968.
364. Priluck IA, Doughman DJ, Harris JE: Tissue adhesives. *In* Leopold H, Burns RP (eds): Symposium on Ocular Therapy, vol 9. New York, John Wiley, 1976.
365. Leonard F, Kulkarni RK, Brandes G, et al: Synthesis and degradation of poly (alkyl alpha-cyanoacrylates). J Appl Polymer Sci 10:259, 1966.
366. Cameron JL, Woodward SC, Pulaski EJ, et al: The degradation of cyanoacrylate tissue adhesive. I. Surgery 58:424, 1965.
367. Lehman RAW, Hayes GJ, Leonard F: Toxicity of alkyl-2-cyanoacrylates. I: Peripheral nerve. Arch Surg 93:441, 1966.
368. Woodward SC, Herrman JB, Cameron JL, et al: Histotoxicity of cyanoacrylate tissue adhesive in the rat. Ann Surg 162:113, 1965.
369. DeRenzis FA, Aleo JJ: An in vitro bioassay of cyanoacrylate cytotoxicity. Oral Surg 30:803, 1970.
370. Nesburn AB, Ziniti P: Cell culture toxicity of two cyanoacrylate adhesives. [Abstract] Invest Ophthalmol 8:648, 1969.
371. Aronson SB, McMaster PRB, Moore TE Jr, et al: Toxicity of the cyanoacrylates. Arch Ophthalmol 84:342, 1970.
372. Girard LJ, Cobb S, Reed T, et al: Surgical adhesives and bonded contact lenses: An experimental study. Ann Ophthalmol 1:65, 1969.
373. Gasset AR, Hood CI, Ellison ED, Kaufman HE: Ocular tolerance to cyanoacrylate monomer tissue adhesive analogues. Invest Ophthalmol 9:3, 1970.
374. Hanna C, Shibley S: Tissue reaction to intracorneal silicone rubber (Silastic RTV 382) and methyl-2-cyanoacrylate (Eastman 910 adhesive). Am J Ophthalmol 60:323, 1965.
375. Ferry AP, Barnert AH: Granulomatous keratitis resulting from use of cyanoacrylate adhesive for closure of perforated corneal ulcer. Am J Ophthalmol 72:538, 1971.
376. Sani BP, Refojo MF: ^{14}C-isobutyl 2-cyanoacrylate adhesive: Determination of absorption in the cornea. Arch Ophthalmol 87:216, 1972.
377. Carlson AN, Wilhelmus KR: Giant papillary conjunctivitis associated with cyanoacrylate glue. Am J Ophthalmol 104:437, 1987.
378. Leahey AB, Gottsch JD: Symblepharon associated with cyanoacrylate tissue adhesive. Arch Ophthalmol 111:168, 1993.
379. Bloomfield S, Barnert AH, Kanter PD: The use of Eastman 910 monomer as an adhesive in ocular surgery. I: Biologic effects on ocular tissue. Am J Ophthalmol 55:742, 1963.
380. Macsai M, Kuczak J, Robin JB: Scanning electron microscopic evaluation of the effects of intracameral injection of cyanoacrylate in the rabbit. Refract Corneal Surg 6:193, 1990.
381. Siegal JE, Zaidman GW: Surgical removal of cyanoacrylate adhesive after accidental instillation in the anterior chamber. Ophthalmic Surg 20:179, 1989.
382. Markowitz GD, Orlin SE, Frayer WC, et al: Corneal endothelial polymerization of Histoacryl adhesive: A report of a new intraocular complication. Ophthalmic Surg 26:256, 1995.
383. Hyndiuk RA, Hull DS, Kinyoun JL: Free tissue patch and cyanoacrylate in corneal perforations. Ophthalmic Surg 5:50, 1974.
384. Gudas PP, Altman B, Nicolson DH, et al: Corneal perforations in Sjögren syndrome. Arch Ophthalmol 90:470, 1973.
385. Munton CGF: Tissue adhesive in ocular surgery: A prospective study. Exp Eye Res 11:1, 1971.
386. Hida T, Sheta SM, Proia AD, et al: Retinal toxicity of cyanoacrylate tissue adhesive in the rabbit. Retina 8:148, 1988.
387. Seelenfreund MH, Refojo MF, Schepens CL: Sealing choroidal perforations with cyanoacrylate adhesives. Arch Ophthalmol 83:619, 1970.
388. Jaffe MJ, Von Fricken MA, Silberstein L, et al: A screening method using tissue culture for evaluation of potential retinal adhesives. Retina 9:328, 1989.
389. McCuen BW II, Hida T, Sheta SM: Transvitreal cyanoacrylate retinopexy in the management of complicated retina detachment. Am J Ophthalmol 104:127, 1987.
390. Vygantas MC, Kanter PJ: Experimental buckling with homologous sclera and cyanoacrylate. Arch Ophthalmol 91:126, 1974.
391. Spitznas M, Lossagh H, Vogel M, et al: Intraocular use of butyl-2-cyanoacrylate in retinal detachment surgery: A preliminary report. Mod Probl Ophthalmol 12:183, 1974.
392. Hyndiuk RA: Discussion of paper by McCuen BW II, Hida T, Sheta SM, Machemer R: Transvitreal cyanoacrylate retinopexy in the management of complicated retinal detachment. Trans Am Ophthalmol Soc 84:206, 1987.
393. Kamer FM, Joseph JH: Histoacryl: Its use in aesthetic facial plastic surgery. Arch Otolaryngol Head Neck Surg 115:193, 1989.
394. Veloudios A, Kratky V, Heathcote JG, et al: Cyanoacrylate tissue adhesive in blepharoplasty. Ophthalmic Plast Reconstr Surg 12:89, 1996.
395. Kohler U: Complications following temporary occlusion of the nasolacrimal duct with tissue adhesive (Histoacryl). Klin Monatsbl Augenheilkd 189:486, 1986.
396. Shelley ED, Shelley WB: Chronic dermatitis simulating small-plaque parapsoriasis due to cyanoacrylate adhesive used on fingernails. JAMA 252:2456, 1984.
397. Calnan CD: Cyanoacrylate dermatitis. Contact Dermatitis 5:165, 1979.
398. Fisher AA: Reactions to cyanoacrylate adhesives: "Instant glue." Cutis 35:18, 1985.
399. Dean BS, Krenzelok EP: Cyanoacrylates and corneal abrasion. Clin Toxicol 27:169, 1989.
400. Barraquer J, cited in Barraquer RI and Barraquer J: Useful enzymes. *In* Sears ML, Tarkkanen A (eds): Surgical Pharmacology of the Eye. New York, Raven, 1985.
401. Howell IL: Anaphylactic reaction of chymotrypsin. JAMA 175:322, 1961.
402. Hogan MJ: Alpha yes? or alpha no? [Editorial] Arch Ophthalmol 76:3, 1966.
403. Ray PK: Use of 200 times the recommended dose of alpha-chymotrypsin without complications. Br J Ophthalmol 48:230, 1964.
404. Townes CD: Unfavorable effects of alpha-chymotrypsin in cataract surgery. Arch Ophthalmol 64:108, 1960.
405. von Sallman L: Experimental studies of some ocular effects of alpha-chymotrypsin. Trans Am Acad Ophthalmol Otolaryngol 64:25, 1960.
406. Lessell S, Kuwabara T: Experimental alpha-chymotrypsin glaucoma. Arch Ophthalmol 81:853, 1969.
407. Kalvin NH, Hamasaki DI, Gass JDM: Experimental glaucoma in monkeys. I: Relationship between intraocular pressure and cupping of the optic disc and cavernous atrophy of the optic nerve. Arch Ophthalmol 76:82, 1966.

408. Bedrossian RH, Calli RA: Clinical application of new laboratory data on alpha-chymotrypsin. Arch Ophthalmol 67:616, 1962.
409. Radnot M, Pazor R: Effect of alpha-chymotrypsin on the cornea. Am J Ophthalmol 51:598, 1961.
410. Munich W, cited by Woog JJ, Albert DM: Toxicology of intraoperative pharmacologic agents. *In* Sears ML, Tarkkanen A (eds): Surgical Pharmacology of the Eye. New York, Raven, 1985.
411. Fink A, Bernstein HN, Binkhorst D: Effect of alpha-chymotrypsin on corneal wound healing. Arch Ophthalmol 67:616, 1961.
412. Kirsch RE: Use of alpha-chymotrypsin in cataract extraction followed by transient glaucoma. Arch Ophthalmol 72:612, 1964.
413. Kirsch RE: Dose relationship of alpha-chymotrypsin in production of glaucoma after cataract extraction. Arch Ophthalmol 75:774, 1966.
414. Galin MA, Barasch KR, Harris LS: Enzymatic zonulolysis and intraocular pressure. Am J Ophthalmol 61:690, 1966.
415. Kirsch RE: Further studies on glaucoma following cataract extraction associated with the use of alpha-chymotrypsin. Trans Am Acad Ophthalmol Otolaryngol 69:1011, 1965.
416. Anderson DR: Experimental alpha-chymotrypsin glaucoma studied by scanning electron microscopy. Am J Ophthalmol 71:470, 1971.
417. Chee P, Hamasaki T: The basis of chymotrypsin-induced glaucoma. Arch Ophthalmol 85:103, 1971.
418. Sears D, Sears M: Blood aqueous barrier and alpha-chymotrypsin glaucoma in rabbits. Am J Ophthalmol 77:378, 1974.
419. Zimmerman LE, DeVenecia G, Hamasaki DI: Pathology of the optic nerve in experimental acute glaucoma. Invest Ophthalmol 6:109, 1967.
420. O'Malley C, Moskovitz M, Straatsma BR: Experimentally induced adverse effects of alpha-chymotrypsin. Arch Ophthalmol 66:539, 1961.
421. Kalvin HN, Hamasaki DI, Gass JDM: Experimental glaucoma in monkeys. II: Studies of intraocular vascularity during glaucoma. Arch Ophthalmol 76:94, 1966.
422. Leydhecker W, Dardenne U, cited by Woog JJ, Albert DM: Toxicology of intraoperative pharmacologic agents. *In* Sears ML, Tarkkanen A (eds): Surgical Pharmacology of the Eye. New York, Raven, 1985.
423. Parry TGW, Laszlo GC: Thrombin technique in ophthalmic surgery. Br J Ophthalmol 30:176, 1946.
424. Savory W: Some uses of thrombin and fibrinogen in ophthalmic surgery. Trans Ophthalmol Soc U K 67:323, 1947.
425. Hughes WL [cited in McDermott ML, Edelhauser HF, Mannis MJ]: Intracameral thrombin and the corneal endothelium. Am J Ophthalmol 106:414, 1988.
426. Thompson JT, Glaser BM, Michels RG, et al: The use of thrombin to control hemorrhage during vitrectomy. Ophthalmology 93:279, 1986.
427. Blacharski PA, Charles ST: Thrombin infusion to control bleeding during vitrectomy for stage V retinopathy of prematurity. Arch Ophthalmol 105:203, 1987.
428. Aaberg TM: Balancing the benefits and risks of intracameral thrombin. [Editorial] Am J Ophthalmol 106:485, 1988.
429. Maxwell DP Jr, Orlick ME, Diamond JG: Intermittent intraocular thrombin as an adjunct to vitrectomy. Ophthalmic Surg 20:108, 1989.
430. Olsen TW, Sternberg P, Martin DF, et al: Postoperative hypopyon after intravitreal bovine thrombin for macular hole surgery. Am J Ophthalmol 121:575, 1996.
431. DeBustros S, Glaser BM, Johnson MA: Thrombin infusion for the control of intraocular bleeding during vitreous surgery. Arch Ophthalmol 103:837, 1985.
432. Mannis MJ, Sweet E, Landers MB, et al: Uses of thrombin in ocular surgery. Effect on the corneal endothelium. Arch Ophthalmol 106:251, 1988.
433. McDermott ML, Edelhauser HF, Mannis MJ: Intracameral thrombin and the corneal endothelium. Am J Ophthalmol 106:414, 1988.
434. Creel DJ, Wang JM, Wong KC: Transient blindness associated with transurethral resection of the prostate. Arch Ophthalmol 105:1537, 1987.
435. Van de Werf F, Bergmann SR, Fox KA, et al: Coronary thrombolysis with intravenously administered human tissue-type plasminogen activator produced by recombinant DNA technology. Circulation 69:605, 1984.
436. Snyder RW, Williams GA, Lambrou FH: Clearance of intraocular fibrin using recombinant human tissue plasminogen activator. [Abstract] Invest Ophthalmol Vis Sci 28(Suppl):210, 1987.
437. Horven I, Opsahl R, cited by Woog JJ, Albert DM: Toxicology of intraoperative pharmacologic agents. *In* Sears ML, Tarkkanen A (eds): Surgical Pharmacology of the Eye. New York, Raven, 1985.
438. Podos S, Liebman S, Pollen A: Treatment of experimental total hyphemas with intraocular fibrinolytic agents. Arch Ophthalmol 71:537, 1964.
439. Kozial J, Peyman GA, Sanders DR, et al: Urokinase in experimental vitreous hemorrhage. Ophthalmic Surg 6:79, 1975.
440. Chapman-Smith JS, Crock GW: Urokinase in the management of vitreous haemorrhage. Br J Ophthalmol 61:500, 1977.
441. Friedman MW: Streptokinase in ophthalmology. Am J Ophthalmol 35:1184, 1952.
442. Rakusin W: Urokinase in the management of traumatic hyphema. Br J Ophthalmol 55:826, 1971.
443. Leet DM: Treatment of total hyphemas with urokinase. Am J Ophthalmol 84:79, 1977.
444. Hull DS, Green K: Effect of urokinase on corneal endothelium. Arch Ophthalmol 98:1285, 1980.
445. Snyder RW, Lambrou FH, Williams GA: Intraocular fibrinolysis with recombinant human tissue plasminogen activator: Experimental treatment in a rabbit model. Arch Ophthalmol 105:1277, 1987.
446. Lambrou FH, Snyder RW, Williams GA, et al: Treatment of experimental intravitreal fibrin with tissue plasminogen activator. Am J Ophthalmol 104:619, 1987.
447. Johnson RN, Olsen K, Hernandez E: Tissue plasminogen activator treatment of postoperative intraocular fibrin. Ophthalmology 95:592, 1988.
448. McDermott ML, Edelhauser HF, Hyndiuk RA, Koenig SB: Tissue plasminogen activator and the corneal endothelium. Am J Ophthalmol 108:91, 1989.
449. Johnson MW, Olsen KR, Hernandez E, et al: Retinal toxicity of recombinant tissue plasminogen activities in the rabbit. Arch Ophthalmol 108:259, 1990.
450. Min WK, Kim YB, Resolution of experimental intravitreal fibrin by tissue plasminogen activator. Korean J Ophthalmol 4:58, 1990.
451. Irvine WD, Johnson MW, Hernandez E, et al: Retinal toxicity of human tissue plasminogen activator in vitrectomized rabbit eyes. Arch Ophthalmol 109:718, 1991.
452. Johnson RN, Olsen KR, Hernandez E: Intravitreal tissue plasminogen activator treatment of experimental vitreous hemorrhage. Arch Ophthalmol 107:891, 1989.
453. Benner JD, Morse LS, Toth CA, et al: Evaluation of a commercial recombinant tissue-type plasminogen activator preparation in the subretinal space of the cat. Arch Ophthalmol 109:1731, 1991.
454. Coll GE, Sparrow JR, Marinovic A, et al: Effect of intravitreal tissue plasminogen activator on experimental subretinal hemorrhage. Retina 15:319, 1995.
455. Williams DF, Han DP, Abrams GW: Rebleeding in experimental traumatic hyphema treated with intraocular tissue plasminogen activator. Arch Ophthalmol 108:264, 1990.
456. Howard GR, Vukich J, Fiscella RG, et al: Intraocular tissue plasminogen activator in a rabbit model of traumatic hyphema. Arch Ophthalmol 109:272, 1991.
457. Ozment RR, Liaw ZL, Krug J, et al: Use of experimental tissue plasminogen activator in experimental filtration surgery. [Abstract] Invest Ophthalmol Vis Sci (Suppl)30:418, 1989.
458. Sternberg P, Aquilar HE, Drews C, at al: The effect of tissue plasminogen activator on retinal bleeding. Arch Ophthalmol 108:720, 1990.
459. Williams GA, Lambrou FH, Jaffe GA, et al: Treatment of postvitrectomy fibrin formation with intraocular tissue plasminogen activator. Arch Ophthalmol 106:1055, 1988.
460. Jaffe GJ, Abrams GW, Williams GA, Han DP: Tissue plasminogen activator for postvitrectomy fibrin formation. Ophthalmology 97:184, 1990.
461. Dabbs CK, Aaberg TM, Aguilar HE, et al: Complications of tissue plasminogen activator therapy after vitrectomy for diabetes. Am J Ophthalmol 110:354, 1990.
462. Williams DF, Bennett SR, Abrams GW, et al: Low-dose intraocular tissue plasminogen activator for treatment of postvitrectomy fibrin formation. Am J Ophthalmol 109:606, 1990.
463. Snyder RW, Sherman MD, Allinson RW: Intracameral tissue plasminogen activator for treatment of excessive fibrin response after penetrating keratoplasty. Am J Ophthalmol 109:483, 1990.
464. Moon J, Chung S, Myong Y, et al: Treatment of postcataract fibrinous membranes with tissue plasminogen activator. Ophthalmology 99:1256, 1992.

465. Lundy DC, Sidoti P, Winarko T, et al: Intracameral tissue plasminogen activator after glaucoma surgery: Indications, effectiveness, and complications. Ophthalmology 103:274, 1996.
466. Piltz JR, Starita RJ: The use of subconjunctivally administered tissue plasminogen activator after trabeculectomy. Ophthalmic Surg 25:51, 1994.
467. Breebaart AC, Nuyts RMMA, Pels E, et al: Toxic endothelial cell destruction of the cornea after routine extracapsular cataract surgery. Arch Ophthalmol 108:1121, 1990.
468. Nuyts RMMA, Edelhauser HF, Pels E, Breebaart AC: Toxic effects of detergents on the corneal endothelium. Arch Ophthalmol 108:1158, 1990.

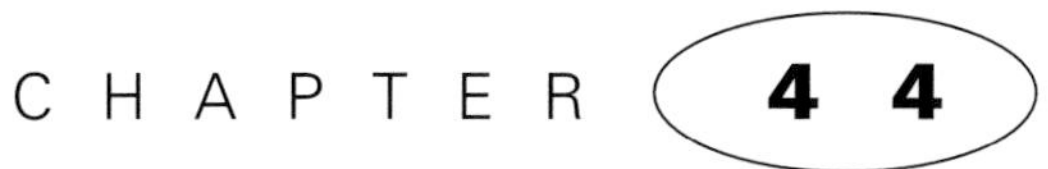

Toxicology of Over-the-Counter Ophthalmic Medications

Jeffrey P. Gilbard

A major consideration in the formulation of over-the-counter ophthalmic medications has been to maximize safety. Toward this goal, strict guidelines have been published regarding the physical characteristics of these solutions and the ingredients that may be included.[1] Nevertheless, the potential for side effects or toxicity should be kept in mind by the physician who prescribes them and the patient who uses them. Frequently patients are described as being "allergic" to an eye drop. In the absence of itching, most of these patients are actually experiencing some form of toxicity.

As we examine the potential for side effects of over-the-counter medications, we first consider eyewashes and the ionic composition of ophthalmic medications. We then turn our attention to preservatives and, finally, to the active ingredients themselves.

Eyewashes and Aqueous Ophthalmic Vehicles

Eyewashes contain water along with tonicity agents to establish isotonicity and buffering agents to establish a neutral pH. In a multidose delivery system, eyewashes are also required to contain a preservative.[1] Except for the requirement for a preservative, the description of an eyewash describes the foundation for all ophthalmic solutions. The effects of deviating from a neutral pH range are widely recognized. The effect of ionic composition has been the subject of more recent study.

IONIC COMPOSITION

It has become clear that the ocular surface requires more than sodium and chloride for the maintenance of cellular integrity and health. Pfister and Burstein could not demonstrate toxicity to the corneal epithelium after the instillation of a single drop of 0.9% sodium chloride.[2] Sussman and Friedman, however, found that the instillation of 0.9% sodium chloride solution in the rabbit eye every 15 minutes resulted in hyperemia and photophobia.[3] They did not state how many drops were required to observe these effects. Merrill and coworkers studied the effect of 0.9% sodium chloride on conjunctival epithelium in tissue culture and demonstrated toxicity beginning 3 to 5 minutes after the initial exposure.[4] Toxicity was not observed after exposure to a 35-minute perfusion with Hanks balanced salt solution or a commercial balanced salt solution. Bachman and Wilson observed differences in specular reflectance of rabbit corneas based on the bathing solution tested.[5] They concluded that 0.9% sodium chloride alone resulted in increased cell desquamation, and that the addition of certain electrolytes to the sodium chloride solution diminished this effect.

These experiments and others show that with continued use and exposure, traditional solutions without the proper electrolyte composition and balance alter the ocular surface. Ultimately, it has been shown that the electrolyte requirements of the surface of the eye coincide with the unique electrolyte balance of the normal tear film. This electrolyte balance is different from that of both aqueous humor and serum.[6, 7] Of key importance are the levels of sodium, chloride, potassium, and bicarbonate and, to a lesser extent, the presence of trace amounts of calcium, magnesium, and phosphate.[8, 9] In retrospect it seems obvious that the ocular surface would have specific electrolyte requirements. There is a blood-tear barrier, and as a result the living cells on the ocular surface have no blood supply. All living cells depend on oxygen and electrolytes to function. In the case of the eye surface these electrolytes come from the tear film. Currently there is only one eye drop, a treatment for dry eye, that provides these electrolytes in a patented formula.[8–10]

PRESERVATIVES

Preservatives are required in all ophthalmic preparations packaged in multidose containers. Although these preservatives reduce the risk of bacterial contamination, they also increase the potential for toxicity. Preservatives can cause loss of cell surface microvilli; plasma membrane disruption;

and desquamation.[2] The most commonly used preservatives in ophthalmic medications are benzalkonium chloride, chlorobutanol, and chlorhexidine digluconate. Mercurial compounds such as phenylmercuric nitrate and thimerosal have lost favor.

Various studies have demonstrated that currently used preservatives are toxic to the corneal epithelium,[2, 11–13] the corneal endothelium,[14–16] and the stroma.[17] The frequency and duration of use at which toxicity from solutions with preservatives becomes clinically relevant is unclear. When eye drop use is frequent (i.e., more than three or four times a day) and the intention of eye drop use is the treatment of an ocular surface, the trend has been to use preservative-free formulations packaged in unit-dose or single-use containers.

A new preservative system based on sodium perborate has been introduced. Sodium perborate reacts with water to form hydrogen peroxide. In this system sodium perborate is used in very low concentrations, yielding in turn very low concentrations of hydrogen peroxide. On the eye catalase and other peroxidative enzymes in the conjunctival epithelium break down the hydrogen peroxide to water and oxygen. This system appears to be a significant advance in preservative technology.[18]

Ophthalmic Lubricant Solutions

Ophthalmic lubricant solutions, or lubricating eye drops, contain an ophthalmic demulcent (or demulcents) as their active ingredient. Although the U.S. Food and Drug Administration does not formally permit ophthalmic lubricant eye drops to be labeled as an artificial tear solution, the term *artificial tear solution* has gained widespread use.

The demulcents in these solutions are water-soluble polymers that can be categorized into four types:

1. Polyethers, including polyethylene glycol
2. Polyvinyls, including polyvinyl alcohol and povidone
3. Cellulose derivatives, including methylcellulose, hydroxypropyl methylcellulose, and carboxymethylcellulose
4. Dextrans

These water-soluble polymers can be synthesized to different molecular weights to alter the viscosity. Increased viscosity of the solution is associated with increased ocular retention time[19] and a prolongation of the time of the tear film's breakup.[20] In addition to altering the solution's viscosity, these polymers, singly or in combination, can decrease as well as increase the wetting angle of saline on a mucin-free but polymer-coated cornea. In in vitro systems, a decreased wetting angle is sometimes resistant to saline rinsing, suggesting adsorption of polymers by the corneal surface.[21, 22]

There are relatively few data regarding the effect of these agents on ocular surface epithelial cell morphology or function. Of note is one study that suggests that epithelial defects in rabbit eyes may heal more slowly when treated topically with methylcellulose or polyvinyl alcohol than when treatment is withheld.[23]

With careful use, lubricating eye drops may reduce dry eye symptoms by decreasing friction between irritated tissues. Nevertheless, there are data indicating that excessively frequent use of traditional lubricating eye drops may have adverse effects.[24, 25] Wilson reported that the inappropriate use of traditional lubricating eye drops is the second most common cause of medicamentosa.[24] In vivo, it has been shown that all lubricating eye drops except one have the potential to decrease corneal epithelial glycogen levels and conjunctival goblet cell density with prolonged use.[10] All these studies indicate that lubricating eye drop use should be monitored carefully by the physician. Schwab and Abbott have published their findings in a series of patients in whom side effects from lubricating eye drops, including corneal ulceration, went unrecognized.[25]

It has been recommended that solutions containing polyvinyl alcohol not be used in conjunction with other eye drops containing borates, as borates precipitate polyvinyl alcohol out of solution.[26]

Ocular Decongestants

Ocular decongestants contain a vasoconstrictor as their active ingredient.[1] The most commonly used vasoconstrictors are naphazoline hydrochloride 0.012 to 0.1%, tetrahydrozoline hydrochloride 0.5%, and phenylephrine 0.12%. Ocular decongestants are commonly used to treat conjunctival hyperemia secondary to ocular allergies and nonspecific conjunctivitis. Ocular decongestants are not specific treatment for bacterial or viral infection, dry eye, or ocular inflammation. Decongestants may mask these problems and delay specific treatment. Patients should be alerted to this potential consequence of self-treatment with over-the-counter decongestant therapy.

When applied to the conjunctiva, sympathomimetic agents act directly on α-adrenergic receptors in the eye, producing contraction of the dilator muscle of the pupil and constriction of arterioles in the conjunctiva. It has been reported that α-adrenergic stimulation may cause sufficient pupil dilatation to produce angle-closure glaucoma and in rare instances may exacerbate angina or hypertension.[27]

NAPHAZOLINE AND TETRAHYDROZOLINE

Naphazoline and tetrahydrozoline are generally well tolerated by patients, aside from an occasional complaint of a mild, transient, burning sensation.[28, 29] Naphazoline 0.05% applied topically four times a day has been reported to cause punctate epithelial keratitis.[30] Concerns have been raised with respect to using naphazoline in patients with abnormally shallow anterior chambers with critically narrow chamber angles.[31]

PHENYLEPHRINE

Phenylephrine 0.125% has been reported to cause sufficient mydriasis to result in angle-closure glaucoma.[32] Phenylephrine has little or no effect on intraocular pressure in normal eyes but may precipitate an angle-closure attack in eyes with plateau iris syndrome or narrow angles.[33] Chronic use of phenylephrine can result in rebound vasodilatation that can lead to dependence and overuse.[33]

Ocular Astringents

Zinc sulfate 0.25% is the only astringent approved for over-the-counter ophthalmic use.[1] It is thought to clear mucus from the outer surface of the eye by precipitating proteins. Zinc sulfate is generally considered safe up to concentrations of 1%.

Ophthalmic Lubricating Ointments

The active ingredients in lubricating ointments include lanolin, light mineral oil, mineral oil, paraffin, petrolatum, white ointment, white petrolatum, white wax, and yellow wax.[1]

Taniwaki has studied 16 ointment bases and their toxic effects on the cornea in rabbits.[34, 35] The ointment bases were divided into three categories:

1. Hydrophilic bases (Propeto [white petroleum jelly] and 10% lanolin; Propeto and 1% Tween 20 [polysorbate 20]; camellia oil and 1% Tween 20; and carbowax)
2. Hydrophobic bases (yellow petrolatum; white petrolatum Propeto; and Plastibase [polyethylene resin 5%, liquid paraffin 95%])
3. Oils (liquid paraffin; camellia oil; salad oil; and sesame oil)

Taniwaki concluded that all 16 agents impeded healing of the corneal epithelium, with hydrophilic ointments having the greatest effect.[34, 35] His findings conflict with those of Hanna and coworkers, who found that unpreserved bland ointments do not inhibit corneal wound-healing rates.[36]

Currently available ophthalmic ointments no longer use unwashed lanolin or the stiffer more viscous grades of petrolatum. Petrolatum-based ointments can be made less viscous by the addition of mineral oil.

Hyperosmolar Agents

The active agent and ingredient of hyperosmolar agents is sodium chloride in a concentration of 2 to 5%.[1] We have already discussed the potential effects of sodium chloride on the ocular surface. Formulations of 2 and 5% sodium chloride have osmolarities of 680 and 1720 mOsm/L, respectively.[37]

There is now considerable evidence to support the theory that elevated tear film osmolarity is the link between decreased tear secretion and the ocular surface disease of dry eye, and this is discussed in great length in Chapter 15 (Fungal Infections of the Eye).[38–46] This does not appear to have any bearing on the clinical use of hyperosmolar agents. For clinical effects to be observed, it appears that a prolonged increase in tear osmolarity is required, and it is doubtful if such an increase could be sustained given the usual dosing frequency for these medications.

Obviously, hyperosmolar agents would not be a recommended treatment for dry eye disease. However, hyperosmolar agents are clinically useful for the treatment of corneal edema[37] and recurrent erosion syndrome.[47] For corneal edema, a common dosing frequency is four or five times a day. For recurrent erosion syndrome, a 5% sodium chloride ointment is usually prescribed at bedtime. At these dosing frequencies, toxicity, aside from stinging or burning on instillation, has not been observed or reported clinically.

Conclusions

It is important to recognize that all ophthalmic medications, even those available over the counter, have the potential for side effects. It is the role of the physician to supervise the use of these medications so that patients can use them to optimal effect.

REFERENCES

1. Department of Health and Human Services, Food and Drug Administration: 21 CFR Parts 349 and 369. Ophthalmic drug products for over-the-counter human use; final monograph; final rule. Fed Reg March 4, 1988.
2. Pfister RR, Burstein N: The effects of ophthalmic drugs, vehicles, and preservatives on corneal epithelium. A scanning electron microscope study. Invest Ophthalmol 15:246, 1976.
3. Sussman JD, Friedman M: Irritation of rabbit eye caused by contact-lens wetting solution. Am J Ophthalmol 68:703, 1969.
4. Merrill DL, Fleming TC, Girard LJ: The effects of physiologic balanced salt solution and normal saline on intraocular and extraocular tissues. Am J Ophthalmol 49:895, 1960.
5. Bachman WG, Wilson GS: Essential ions for maintenance of the corneal epithelial surface. Invest Ophthalmol Vis Sci 26:1484, 1985.
6. Van Haeringen NJ: Clinical biochemistry of tears. Surv Ophthalmol 26:84, 1981.
7. Gilbard JP: Human tear film electrolyte concentrations in health and dry-eye disease. Int Ophthalmol Clin 34:27, 1994.
8. Gilbard JP: Non-toxic ophthalmic preparations. US Patent October 4, 1988, pp 4,775, 531.
9. Gilbard JP, Rossi SR, Gray Heyda K: Ophthalmic solutions, the ocular surface, and a unique therapeutic artificial tear formulation. Am J Ophthalmol 107:348, 1989.
10. Gilbard JP, Rossi SR. An electrolyte-based solution that increases corneal glycogen and conjunctival goblet cell density in a rabbit model for keratoconjunctivitis sicca. Ophthalmology 99:600, 1992.
11. Green K, Livingston V, Bowman K, Hull DS: Chlorhexidine effects on corneal epithelium and endothelium. Arch Ophthalmol 98:1273, 1980.
12. Burstein NL: Preservative cytotoxic threshold for benzalkonium chloride and chlorhexidine digluconate in cat and rabbit corneas. Invest Ophthalmol 19:308, 1980.
13. Neville R, Dennis P, Sens D, Crouch R: Preservative cytotoxicity to cultured corneal epithelial cells. Curr Eye Res 5:367, 1986.
14. Gasset AR, Ishii Y, Kaufman HE, Miller T: Cytotoxicity of ophthalmic preservatives. Am J Ophthalmol 78:98, 1974.
15. Collin HB, Grabsch BE: The effect of ophthalmic preservatives on the shape of corneal endothelial cells. Acta Ophthalmol 60:93, 1982.
16. Collin HB, Carroll N: Ultrastructural changes to the corneal endothelium due to benzalkonium chloride. Acta Ophthalmol 64:226, 1986.
17. Collin HB: Ultrastructural changes to corneal stromal cells due to ophthalmic preservatives. Acta Ophthalmol 64:72, 1986.
18. Chalmers RL, Tsao M, Scott G: The rate of in vivo neutralization of residual H_2O_2 from hydrogel lenses. Contact Lens Spectrum 4(7):21, 1989.
19. Benedetto DA, Shah DO, Kaufman HE: The instilled fluid dynamics and surface chemistry of polymers in the preocular tear film. Invest Ophthalmol 14:887, 1975.
20. Norn MS, Opauszki A: Effects of ophthalmic vehicles on the stability of the precorneal film. Acta Ophthalmol 55:23, 1977.
21. Lemp MA, Szymanski ES: Polymer adsorption at the ocular surface. Arch Ophthalmol 93:134, 1975.
22. Hecht G, Hively CD: Ophthalmic solution. US Patent 4,039,662, August 2, 1977.
23. Krishna N, Brow F: Polyvinyl alcohol as an ophthalmic vehicle: Effect of regeneration of corneal epithelium. Am J Ophthalmol 57:99, 1964.
24. Wilson FM II: Adverse external ocular effects of topical ophthalmic therapy: An epidemiologic, laboratory, and clinical study. Trans Am Ophthalmol Soc 81:854, 1983.
25. Schwab IR, Abbott RL: Toxic ulcerative keratopathy. An unrecognized problem. Ophthalmology 96:1187, 1989.
26. Kralian LM: What's artificial in artificial tears? Am J Optom Physiol Opt 63:304, 1986.
27. Kersten RC: Ophthalmic drugs. Prim Care 9:743, 1984.
28. Abelson MB, Yamamoto GK, Allansmith MR: Effects of ocular decongestants. Arch Ophthalmol 98:856, 1980.
29. Abelson MB, Butrus SI, Weston JH, Rosner B: Tolerance and absence of rebound vasodilation following topical ocular decongestant usage. Ophthalmology 91:1364, 1984.

30. Komi T, Maeda I, Uno Y, Otsuka H: Inhibitory effect of sodium chondroitin sulfate on epithelial keratitis induced by naphazoline. Acta Soc Ophthalmol Jpn 68:154, 1964.
31. Grant WM: Toxicology of the Eye. Springfield, IL, Charles C Thomas, 1974, p 733.
32. Weiss DI, Shaffer RN: Mydriatic effects of one-eighth percent phenylephrine. Arch Ophthalmol 68:727, 1962.
33. Meyer SM, Fraunfelder FT: Phenylephrine hydrochloride. Ophthalmology 87:1177, 1980.
34. Taniwaki T: Experimental studies on corneal damage due to ophthalmic ointments and oils. Acta Soc Ophthalmol Jpn 69:809, 1965.
35. Taniwaki T: Experimental studies on the corneal damage by the ophthalmic ointment and oil. Jpn J Ophthalmol 10:9, 1966.
36. Hanna C, Fraunfelder FT, Cable M, Hardberger R: The effect of ophthalmic ointments on corneal wound healing. Am J Ophthalmol 76:193, 1973.
37. Insler MS, Benefield DW, Ross EV: Topical hyperosmolar solutions in the reduction of corneal edema. CLAO J 13:149, 1987.
38. Gilbard JP, Carter JB, Verges C, et al: Effect of hyperosmolarity on ocular surface epithelium in vivo. *In* Metabolic Eye Diseases. Proceedings of the VIIth Congress of the European Society of Ophthalmology. Helsinki, May 21–25, 1984. European Society of Ophthalmology, 1985, pp 354–358.
39. Huang AJW, Belldegrun R, Hanninen L, et al: Effects of hypertonic solutions on conjunctival epithelium and mucinlike glycoprotein discharge. Cornea 8:15, 1989.
40. Gilbard JP, Carter JB, Sang DN, et al: Morphologic effect of hyperosmolarity on rabbit corneal epithelium. Ophthalmology 91:1205, 1984.
41. Gilbard JP, Rossi SR, Azar DT, et al: Effect of punctal occlusion by Freeman silicone plug insertion on tear osmolarity in dry eye disorders. CLAO J 15:216, 1989.
42. Gilbard JP, Rossi S, Gray K: A new rabbit model for keratoconjunctivitis sicca. Invest Ophthalmol Vis Sci 28:225, 1987.
43. Gilbard JP, Rossi SR, Gray KL, et al: Tear film osmolarity and ocular surface disease in two rabbit models for keratoconjunctivitis sicca. Invest Ophthalmol Vis Sci 29:374, 1988.
44. Gilbard JP, Rossi SR, Gray KL, Hanninen LA: Natural history of disease in a rabbit model for keratoconjunctivitis sicca. Acta Ophthalmol 67 (Suppl 192):95, 1989.
45. Gilbard JP, Rossi SR, Gray Heyda K: Tear film and ocular surface changes after closure of the meibomian gland orifices in the rabbit. Ophthalmology 96:1180, 1989.
46. Gilbard JP, Rossi SR: Tear film and ocular surface changes in a rabbit model of neurotrophic keratitis. Ophthalmology 97:308, 1990.
47. Gilbard JP, Cohen GR, Baum J: Decreased tear osmolarity and absence of the inferior marginal tear strip following sleep. Cornea 11:231, 1992.

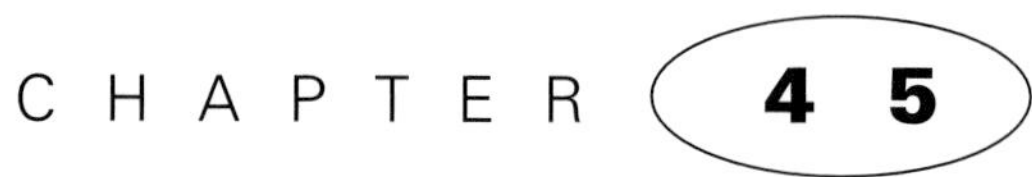

Table of Toxicology

Cynthia Mattox

The following table is a compilation of the information in the preceding chapters in the Toxicology Section. The information has been limited to effects seen in humans. Please see the appropriate chapter for more information on animal studies and references. The information has been divided into clinically useful categories of anterior segment, posterior segment, and clinically relevant systemic toxicities.

Drug	Anterior Segment	Posterior Segment	Systemic Toxic Effects
	Antiglaucoma Agents		
Cholinergic Agents **Anticholinesterases** Echothiophate iodide Demecarium bromide Physostigmine **Direct-Acting Agonists** Pilocarpine Carbachol (also has indirect action)	Conjunctival hyperemia Pemphigoid-like changes Follicular conjunctivitis Tear duct stenosis (rare) Miosis Gradual shallowing of anterior chamber (anticholinesterases) Iritis Pupillary border cysts (anticholinesterases, especially in phakic patients) Induce accommodation Temporary functional myopia Reduce outflow resistance Anterior and posterior subcapsular lens changes Breakdown of blood aqueous barrier	Possible association with retinal detachment Acute ERG alterations	**Acute Poisoning: Anticholinesterases** Cholinergic crisis—sweating, GI disturbances, defecation, bradycardia, respiratory paralysis **Acute Poisoning: Direct-Acting Agents** Sweating, salivation, nausea, tremor, hypotension Potential bronchoconstriction in asthmatics

Drug	Anterior Segment	Posterior Segment	Systemic Toxic Effects
	***Antiglaucoma Agents** Continued*		
Adrenergic Agonists: Nonselective Epinephrine Dipivefrin	Allergic contact sensitivity of conjunctiva and lids Adrenochrome deposits in conjunctiva and sclera Dacryoliths Pemphigoid-like changes Follicular conjunctivitis Reduce blood flow to the ciliary processes but not to the ciliary muscle	Cystoid macular edema (especially in patients with aphakia) Increase prostaglandin E levels in aqueous and vitreous (rabbits)	Hypertension, dysrhythmias
Adrenergic α_2-Agonists Apraclonidine Brimonidine	Decrease aqueous production (apraclonidine); vasoconstriction of conjunctival and episcleral vessels Mild mydriasis Upper lid elevation Reduces aqueous inflow Topical discomfort Hyperemia (brimonidine) Blurred vision Follicular conjunctivitis Contact dermatitis		Dry mouth Fatigue, somnolence Headache Gastrointestinal complaints Others: see Table 41–3
Adrenergic (β-Blockers) Betaxolol—selective for β_1-receptors Timolol, levobunolol, and metipranolol—nonselective Carteolol—nonselective, with intrinsic sympathomimetic activity	Transient topical discomfort Corneal anesthesia Reduce tear secretion Potential corneal epithelial and endothelial changes Decrease aqueous production	Changes in retinal blood flow Cystoid macular edema	Bronchoconstriction in patients with chronic obstructive pulmonary disease (COPD), asthma, or bronchospasem (β_1-selective agents may have milder effects) Cardiac: decrease contractility and heart rate, and prolong atrioventricular (AV) conduction Aggravate congestive heart failure, bradycardia, and high-grade AV block (β-blockers with ISA may have fewer cardiovascular side effects) Depression Impotence Lower high-density lipoproteins and raise triglycerides Alopecia Arthropathy (rare) Exacerbation of myasthenia gravis (rare) Psoriasis
Oral or Intravenous Carbonic Anhydrase Inhibitors Acetazolamide Methazolamide Dichlorphenamide *Topical Carbonic Anhydrase Inhibitors (CAIs)* Dorzolamide Brinzolamide	Induce myopia (rare) Lower IOP by decreasing aqueous production Topical CAIs: Topical discomfort Punctate keratopathy Blurred vision Follicular conjunctivitis, allergy		(Much less common with topical CAIs) Paresthesias—transient Malaise syndrome: fatigue, weight loss, anorexia, impotence, depression Metabolic acidosis (especially in patients with COPD and renal disease) Severe acidosis when taking salicylates Blood dyscrasias: thrombocytopenia, agranulocytosis, aplastic anemia Rarely osteomalacia, skin rashes, hair loss, or hirsutism Renal lithiasis Sensitivity in patients with sulfa allergy **Topical CAIs** Bitter taste Headache Nausea

Table continued on following page

Drug	Anterior Segment	Posterior Segment	Systemic Toxic Effects
	***Antiglaucoma Agents** Continued*		
Prostaglandins Latanoprost	Transient eye ache Topical discomfort Conjunctival and episcleral vasodilatation Lower IOP by increasing uveoscleral outflow Blurred vision Punctate epitheliopathy Photophobia Increase iris and periorbital skin pigmentation Lengthen and darken lashes		
	Antiinflammatory Agents		
Topical or Periocular Corticosteroids	Topical irritation Punctate keratitis Mechanical epithelial keratitis from aggregates in suspension Granulomas May aggravate corneal "melting" syndromes and scleromalacia perforans, enhance lytic action of collagenases May aggravate Behçet's disease Paralysis of accommodation Anterior uveitis Subconjunctival scarring (after subconjunctival injection) Cataract Glaucoma (decrease in outflow facility) Mydriasis (due to vehicle) Ptosis (due to vehicle) Delay wound healing Alter defense against infection	Retinal/choroidal emboli (after injection) Optic atrophy May aggravate Eales' disease May aggravate toxoplasmosis	Fat atrophy (retrobulbar or subcutaneous injection) Skin atrophy or depigmentation (subcutaneous injection) May lower plasma cortisol levels after prolonged use
Systemic Corticosteroids Ocular Effects	Myopia Diplopia Exophthalmos Decrease tear lysozyme Cataract Glaucoma Alter defense against infection Delay wound healing	— Pseudotumor cerebri/papilledema (usually after abrupt withdrawal) Central serous chorioretinopathy	Visual hallucinations
Systemic Nonsteroidal Antiinflammatory Agents Ocular Toxicity	Potential for photoxicity Changes in refractive error Diplopia Superficial corneal crystalline deposits Increase risk of rebleeding in hyphema patients	Diminish color vision Optic neuritis Reversible toxic ambylopia Pseudotumor cerebri	
Topical Nonsteroidal Antiinflammatory Agents Flurbiprofen Suprofen Diclofenac Ketorolac	Prevent intraoperative miosis Mild antiinflammatory effects Transient topical discomfort Inhibit corneoscleral wound healing Exacerbate epithelial herpes simplex virus keratitis May promote bleeding intraoperatively		Potential for asthma exacerbation
Topical Antihistamines and Decongestants	Stinging, burning Epithelial erosions Punctal stenosis Corneal pigment deposits Iris pigment release Iritis Blurred vision Mydriasis May precipitate acute angle closure in susceptible patients Increase IOP		Headache Dizziness Nervousness Cardiac dysrhythmias Hypertension Hypotension Possible hypertensive crisis when used in combination with monoamine oxidase inhibitors

Drug	Anterior Segment	Posterior Segment	Systemic Toxic Effects
	***Antiinflammatory Agents** Continued*		
Oral Antihistamines	Increase dry eye symptoms Occasional blurred vision or diplopia Mydriasis Precipitate acute angle closure in susceptible patients Reduce accommodation		Rarely hallucinations, temporary blindness, and absence of pupillary light reflexes from overdosage
Mast Cell Stabilizing Agents	Transient burning or stinging Conjunctival hyperemia and chemosis		
Disodium cromoglycate Cromolyn sodium Lodoxamide			
Topical Lubricant Solutions and Ointments	Most cause decreased corneal epithelial glycogen Decreased goblet cell density		
Preservatives Used in Topical Ophthalmic Solutions	Toxic to corneal epithelium, stroma, and endothelium		
Benzalkonium chloride Chlorobutanol Chlorhexidine Digluconate Thimerosal			
Sodium perborate	Much less toxic		
	Immunosuppressive Agents		
Alkylating Agents			
Busulfan	Keratoconjunctivitis sicca Posterior subcapsular cataract with polychromatic sheen		
Chlorambucil	Diplopia Keratoconjunctivitis sicca	Pseudotumor cerebri Rare hemorrhagic retinopathy	Bone marrow suppression Gonadal suppression Carcinogenic, mutagenic, and teratogenic potential
Cisplatin	Blurred vision Alters color vision	ERG abnormalities Macular pigmentation Disc edema Retrobulbar neuritis Retinal and optic nerve ischemia after intracarotid use	Cortical blindness
Cyclophosphamide (Cytoxan)	Blurred vision Blepharoconjunctivitis Keratoconjunctivitis sicca		Bone marrow suppression Hemorrhagic cystitis and increased risk of urinary bladder malignancies Gonadal suppression Increased risk of leukemia, lymphomas, and solid tumors Renal and hepatic toxicity Alopecia Interstitial fibrosis
Nitrogen mustard		Necrotizing uveitis and vasculitis after intracarotid use	
Nitrosoureas BCNU, CCNU, methyl-CCNU	Blurred vision Conjunctival hyperemia Ipsilateral periorbital edema Pain and congestion Conjunctivitis and chemosis	Neuroretinal toxicity, nerve fiber layer infarcts, hemorrhages, and disc edema with intracarotid use Possible optic neuritis	
Antimetabolites			
Azathioprine (Imuran)			Bone marrow suppression Hepatotoxicity GI symptoms—anorexia, nausea, vomiting, diarrhea Fever and arthralgias
Cyclosporine	Systemic therapy: decreased vision Eyelid or conjunctival erythema Nonspecific conjunctivitis Urticaria Topical therapy: eyelid irritation Punctate keratitis		Nephrotoxicity Systemic hypertension in 25% of patients Normochromic, normocytic anemia in 25% of patients Increases erythrocyte sedimentation rate in 40% of patients Hirsutism

Table continued on following page

Drug	Anterior Segment	Posterior Segment	Systemic Toxic Effects
	***Immunosuppressive Agents** Continued*		
			Gingival hyperplasia Central nervous system toxicity Increases incidence of viral infections
Cytosine arabinoside	Keratoconjunctivitis Central punctate corneal opacities with subepithelial granular deposits Microcysts Superficial punctate keratitis	Optic neuropathy	
Fludarabine		Optic neuritis	Cortical blindness Encephalopathy
5-Fluorouracil	Systemic therapy: 25% of patients develop mild blepharitis and conjunctival irritation Cicatricial changes in lids, conjunctiva, and lacrimal drainage system Oculomotor disturbance Nystagmus Topical therapy for skin lesions around the eye: burning, irritation, tearing Cicatricial changes in lids and conjunctiva Subconjunctival injection: corneal epithelial defects Inhibition of corneal and conjunctival epithelial proliferation and healing Subconjuctival hemorrhage Late: corneal ulceration, perforation, scarring in patients with underlying corneal disease Wound leaks, bleb leaks with late endophthalmitis	Systemic therapy: optic neuropathy	Neurotoxicity with brain stem involvement may produce oculomotor disturbances
Methotrexate	Burning and itching from high levels in tears 25% of patients: periorbital edema, blepharitis, conjunctival hyperemia, epiphora, photophobia Decreases tear production	Optic neuropathy Macular edema Retinal pigment epithelial changes	Acute and chronic pneumonitis (felt to be an idiosyncratic or hypersensitivity reaction) Hepatotoxicity Mucosal ulcerations GI symptoms Bone marrow depression Teratogenic Interaction with nonsteroidal antiinflammatory agents: severe bone marrow and renal toxicity
Vincristine	Corneal hypoesthesia	Optic neuropathy Nyctalopia	Cranial nerve palsy Internuclear ophthalmoplegia Cortical blindness
Antimicrobial Antineoplastic Agents			
Doxorubicin (Adriamycin)	Lacrimation Red discoloration of tears		
Mitomycin	Topical use: conjunctival irritation Tearing Mild superficial punctate keratitis with high dose Topical after pterygium surgery: Secondary glaucoma Corneal perforation Corneal edema Scleral calcification Sudden cataract Iritis Photophobia After intraoperative use in glaucoma filtering surgery: Inhibition of wound healing Bleb leaks Hypotony Systemic use: blurred vision		

Drug	Anterior Segment	Posterior Segment	Systemic Toxic Effects
	***Immunosuppressive Agents** Continued*		
Mitotane	Cataracts	Neuroretinopathy Retinal hemorrhages	
Plicamycin (Mithramycin)	Periorbital pallor		
Other Antineoplastic Agents			
Tamoxifen	Decreased visual acuity White, whorl-like subepithelial corneal deposits Posterior subcapsular cataracts	Small, white refractile deposits in sensory retina, perimacular Macular edema on fluorescein angiography	
Thiotepa	Ocular irritation and allergy Eyelid depigmentation Keratitis and conjunctivitis with prolonged use Lacrimal punctal occlusion		
Tilorone	Whorl-like keratopathy Visual field constriction	Retinal arteriolar narrowing and fine pigment mottling ERG and EOG attenuation	
	Systemic Medications		
Anesthetic—inhalant Methoxyflurane		Yellow-white punctate lesions in posterior pole and midperiphery of retina Cotton-wool spots Calcium oxalate crystals found in retinal pigment epithelium, retina, and retinal vessels	Renal failure Calcium oxalate crystals
Antianginal and Antihypertensive Agents			
Atenolol, labetalol, metoprolol, nadolol, pindolol	Sicca syndrome Visual hallucinations Decreased IOP		May worsen myasthenia gravis
Clonidine	Miosis and mydriasis in toxic doses	Possible association with retinal abnormalities (depigmentation, degeneration, tears)	
Diltiazem, nifedipine, verapamil	Ocular irritation with periorbital edema and blurred vision Transient blindness	Retinal ischemia	
Hydralazine	Nonspecific ocular irritation Lupus-like syndrome with episcleritis and exophthalmos	Lupus-like syndrome with retinal vasculitis	
Practolol	Keratoconjunctivitis sicca Conjunctival cicatrization Keratitis with opacities		May worsen myasthenia gravis
Propranolol	Sicca syndrome Visual hallucinations Inflammatory orbital psuedotumor		May worsen myasthenia gravis
Antianxiety Agents			
Alprazolam, clonazepam, flurazepam, triazolam	Allergic conjunctivitis Decreased corneal reflex Decreased accommodation and depth perception Abnormal extraocular muscle movement Possible mydriasis precipitating angle-closure glaucoma		
Antiarrhythmic Agents			
Amiodarone	Whorl-like epithelial keratopathy (occasionally symptomatic) Sicca syndrome Lens opacities	Optic neuropathy Pseudotumor cerebri Possible hypopigmentation in retina	Skin pigmentation
Digitalis	Color vision abnormalities (yellow-blue) Visual sensations and hallucinations Scotomas	Retinal toxicity with abnormal ERG amplitudes	
Disopyramide	Blurred vision Decreased lacrimation Decreased accommodation and mydriasis May precipitate angle-closure glaucoma		

Table continued on following page

Drug	Anterior Segment	Posterior Segment	Systemic Toxic Effects
	***Systemic Medications** Continued*		
Procainamide	Rare lupus-like syndrome with scleritis		
Anticonvulsant Agent			
Phenytoin	Nystagmus Lens opacities	Pseudotumor cerebri	Ocular teratogenic effects
Antidepressants			
Amitriptyline Desipramine Imipramine Nortriptyline	Keratoconjunctivitis sicca Mydriasis and cycloplegia that may precipitate angle-closure glaucoma Oculomotor abnormalities		
Doxepin, amoxapine, clomipramine	Blurred vision Mydriasis and decreased accommodation Keratoconjunctivitis sicca Nystagmus and ophthalmoplegia with toxic doses		
Carbamazepine	Blurred vision Extraocular muscle abnormalities with diplopia Downbeat nystagmus Sluggish pupil reaction with toxic doses	Papilledema with toxic doses Retinal pigmentary changes	
Phenelzine	Rarely mydriasis, miosis, anisocoria, nystagmus		May aggravate myasthenia gravis
Methylphenidate	Rarely mydriasis	Illicit IV use may cause talc retinopathy	
Antihistamines			
Brompheniramine Chlorpheniramine Dexbrompheniramine Dimethindene Triprolidine Diphenhydramine Pyrilamine Tripelennamine Cyproheptadine	Keratoconjunctiviis sicca Mydriasis and decreased accommodation May precipitate angle-closure glaucoma Facial dyskinesia and blepharospasm Visual hallucinations		
Antihyperlipidemic Agent			
Niacin (nicotinic acid, vitamin B_6)	Metamorphopsias, blurring Central scotomas or halos Mildly decreased vision	Bilateral maculopathy that mimics cystoid macular edema appearance clinically No accumulation of fluorescein on angiography	
Antimalarial/Antirheumatic Agents			
Allopurinol	Possibly cataractogenic	Possible macular edema and hemorrhage	Toxic epidermal necrolysis
Chloroquine (C) Hydroxychloroqine (HC)	Reversible corneal opacities (C) Motility and accommodation disturbances (C) Central or paracentral scotomas Photophobia Nyctalopia Photopsias	Early: irregularity of macular pigmentation Loss of foveal reflex Later: increased pigmentary irregularity, especially in inferior macula "Bull's-eye" maculopathy End-stage: peripheral pigmentary irregularity and bone spicule formation Vascular attenuation Optic disc pallor Incidence of retinopathy increases with both dose and duration of treatment: Low risk—chloroquine ≤250 mg/day, or cumulative dose ≤100 g, or ≤1 yr of treatment Hydroxychloroquine—≤400 mg/day	
Dapsone		Rare optic atrophy with massive doses	

Drug	Anterior Segment	Posterior Segment	Systemic Toxic Effects
	***Systemic Medications** Continued*		
Gold	Conjunctival and corneal deposition Rarely ptosis, diplopia, nystagmus		
Quinine	Sudden vision loss	Massive doses: toxic amblyopia Retinal arterial constriction and venous congestion Disc and retinal edema Macular pigmentary changes	
Antipsychotic Agents			
Phenothiazines:			
Thioridazine—rare cases of retinopathy with current recommended dose	Blurring nyctalopia, brown discoloration of vision Irregular paracentral scotomas or ring scotomas	Late: more coarse pigmentation Large plaques of hyperpigmentation Areas of depigmentation and loss of choriocapillaris Variation: nummular retinopathy Multiple large, round areas of depigmentation and atrophy posterior to equator; relative sparing of macula	
Chlorpromazine	Pigmentation of conjunctiva Pigmented changes of cornea and lens	Rare retinopathy: round depigmented spots in posterior pole, or fine pigmentary clumping	Pigmentation of sun-exposed skin
Haloperidol	Decrease or paralysis of accommodation Mydriasis that may precipitate angle-closure glaucoma Possible cataract changes		
Lithium carbonate	Blurred vision Irritation and photophobia Extraocular muscle abnormalities Exophthalmos	Pseudotumor cerebri	
Antiparkinsonian Agents			
Amantadine	Rarely sudden vision loss Transient decreased vision Superficial punctate keratopathy Visual hallucinations		
Benztropine, biperiden, chlorphenozamine	Decreased accommodation Mydriasis may precipitate angle-closure glaucoma Hallucinations		
Levodopa	Blepharospasm Miosis and ptosis Mydriasis may precipitate angle-closure glaucoma Visual hallucinations Oculogyric crisis		
Antispasmodic Agent			
Dicyclomine	Blurred vision Mydriasis and decreased accommodation May precipitate angle-closure glaucoma		
Dermatologic Agents			
Canthaxanthine	Metamorphopsia Mildly decreased vision Reduced sensitivity to static perimetry in central 10 degrees	Refractile, yellow deposits in innermost layers of the retina, usually in a ring around the fovea Dose related	Bronzing of skin
Chrysarobin	Keratoconjunctivitis		
Methoxsalen, trioxsalen	Possibly cataractogenic		
Gastrointestinal Stimulant			
Bethanechol	Irritation and tearing Decreased accommodation and miosis		

Table continued on following page

Drug	Anterior Segment	Posterior Segment	Systemic Toxic Effects
	***Systemic Medications** Continued*		
Industrial Agents			
Methanol	Nystagmus Dilated, poorly reactive pupils Central or centrocecal scotoma	Early: edema of disc and peripapillary retina Later: spreading of retinal edema, dilatation of retinal vessels Optic atrophy and cupping become apparent in 1–2 mo	Metabolic acidosis Depressed level of consciousness that may progress to coma and death
	Antiseptic Agents		
Alcohol	Corneal epithelial sloughing Corneal edema		
Iodine	Epithelial sloughing and corneal edema May sensitize 15% of treated patients		
Povidone-iodine	5% solution—rare transient conjunctival irritation Scrub—corneal deepithelialization and increased corneal thickness		
Hibiclens	Corneal epithelial defects Corneal edema that may progress to bullous keratopathy from endothelial cell loss Corneal neovascularization		
pHisoHex	Acute chemical conjunctivitis Deepithelialization Deep keratitis and corneal edema Endothelial toxicity		Toxic blood levels of hexachlorophene when applied to burns or generalized dermatologic conditions
	Intraocular Surgical Solutions and Drugs		
Intraocular Irrigating Solutions			
Normal saline	Endothelial toxicity Progressive posterior subcapsular cataract	Decrease in ERG B-wave amplitude	
Plasmalyte-148	Endothelial cell disruption and corneal edema		
Lactated Ringer's solution	Corneal edema with endothelial cell loss		
Balanced salt solution	Transient corneal edema Morphologic endothelial cell changes		
SMA 2	Breakdown of endothelial cell junctions		
BSS Plus	Maintains corneal endothelial structure		
Viscoelastic Agents			
Sodium hyaluronate (Healon, Healon GV, Amvisc, Amvisc Plus, AMO Vitrax, Provisc)	Corneal endothelial toxicity after prolonged contact Endothelial cell death after 30 min of contact with human donor corneas Increased IOP postoperatively		
Chondroitin sulfate (Viscoat = 3% sodium hyaluronate + 4% chondroitin sulfate)	Well tolerated by corneal endothelium over short periods of contact time Postoperative IOP rise		
Hydroxypropyl-methyl cellulose (HPMC, Occucoat)	May contain vegetable matter contaminants if prepared by individual pharmacies Postoperative IOP rise		
Orcolon (polyacrylamide)	Delayed severe, uncontrollable IOP elevations		
Intraocular Mydriatics			
Epinephrine	Endothelial toxicity related to preservatives or antioxidants Preservative-free, sulfite-free 1:1000 sterile solution for injection is nontoxic to corneal endothelium		
Phenylephrine	Corneal edema and reduced endothelial cell counts		

Drug	Anterior Segment	Posterior Segment	Systemic Toxic Effects
	Intraocular Surgical Solutions and Drugs *Continued*		
Intraocular Miotics			
Acetylcholine (Miochol, Miochol-E)	In vitro: increased swelling rate and corneal thickness related to lack of buffered salt vehicle in Miochol; Miochol-E has electrolyte diluent Ocular hypotensive effect for 6 hr		Rare hypotension, bradycardia, and breathing difficulties reported
Carbachol (Miostat)	Ocular hypotensive effect for 48–72 hr		
Intraocular Gases			
Air	Corneal endothelial cell damage or loss Increases vascular permeability, iritis Lens opacification Pupillary block angle-closure glaucoma in phakic and aphakic patients	Misplaced injections may result in retinal tears, hemorrhage, and avulsion of vitreous base	Nitrous oxide anesthesia can increase bubble volume
Sulfur hexafluoride Other perfluorocarbon gases	Corneal endothelial degeneration and corneal edema Fibrinous iritis Lens opacification IOP elevation	Misplaced injection complications, as earlier	Nitrous oxide can increase bubble volume
Intraocular Liquids			
Perfluorocarbon liquids	***Long-term retention is toxic***		
Silicone oil	***Corneal endothelial toxicity*** ***Band keratopathy*** ***Cataract*** ***Glaucoma—outflow obstruction*** ***Anterior segment ischemia*** ***Fibrous ingrowth*** ***Excessive inflammation***	***Intraneural migration may cause optic nerve damage*** ***Intraretinal silicone vacuoles*** ***Thinning of outer plexiform layer*** ***Associated with periretinal proliferation***	
Tissue Adhesives			
Cyanoacrylates	Localized tissue reaction: polymorphonuclear neutrophil inflammatory response, foreign body granulomatous keratitis, and corneal neovascularization		Intramuscular injection produces an inflammatory response Higher molecular weight cyanoacrylates show less tissue toxicity
Alpha-chymotrypsin	Postoperative elevation of IOP obstruction of trabecular meshwork by zonular fragments	Severe vitritis if used when vitreous face is not intact	
Thrombin	Excessive postoperative inflammation in diabetic patients when used as continuous infusion		
Tissue plasminogen activator	Rebleeding in experimental traumatic hyphema model Anterior chamber hemorrhage in experimental filtration surgery	Recurrence of fibrin formation Intraocular hemorrhage seen in diabetic eyes after vitrectomy and 25-μg dose	
Detergents	Epithelial toxicity Delayed healing Corneal edema from severe endothelial cell loss if intraocular exposure occurs		
	Ocular Antiinfective Agents		
Antibiotics			
Aminoglycosides Amikacin, gentamicin, tobramycin, neomycin	Topical gentamicin, tobramycin, neomycin: bulbar injection, toxic conjunctivitis Chemosis and erythema of eyelids Punctate keratopathy Subconjunctival gentamicin: mydriasis, conjunctival paresthesia, acute toxic myopathy of extraocular muscle	Macular infarction with severe retinal vascular nonperfusion on fluorescein angiography—gentamicin more commonly than amikacin	See general toxicology texts for systemic toxicities

Table continued on following page

Drug	Anterior Segment	Posterior Segment	Systemic Toxic Effects
	***Ocular Antiinfective Agents** Continued*		
	Macular infarction reported following postoperative injection of gentamicin and tobramycin		
Cephalosporins	Cefazolin: well-tolerated topically and subconjunctivally		
Penicillins	Carbenicillin: burning pain and chemosis with subconjunctival injection Methicillin: mild chemosis and injection with subconjunctival use Penicillin: nontoxic to external eye, made with distilled water		
Bacitracin	Topical and subconjunctival dosing: results in therapeutic aqueous levels only when epithelial defect or inflammation is present		
Chloramphenicol	Nontoxic to external eye		
Clindamicin	Nontoxic externally, increased intraocular levels in the presence of an epithelial defect		
Erythromycin	Topical: nontoxic Low-dose subconjunctival doses well tolerated Intracameral toxic		
Fluoroquinolones			
Ciprofloxacin, norfloxacin, ofloxacin	Topical ciprofloxacin: nontoxic, occasional white crystalline precipitate in the superficial portion of the corneal defect		
Polymyxin B	Topical: nontoxic		
Sulfonamides	Sulfadiazine ointment: topical use for 1 yr caused concretions in the palpebral conjunctiva Transient myopia		
Vancomycin	Fortified: irritation, conjunctival injection, superficial punctate keratopathy Subconjunctival: conjunctival necrosis and sloughing reported Safe in corneal storage media		
Antifungal Agents			
Natamycin	Superficial punctate keratopathy with prolonged use Conjunctival necrosis reported after subconjunctival injection		
Amphotericin B	Topical 0.15% solution: well tolerated Subconjunctival: severe pain, chemosis, and conjunctival necrosis At higher dose, subconjunctival nodule reported Anterior chamber injection: no clinical evidence of corneal decompensation	Case reports of 5–10 μg intravitreal injections: no evidence of toxicity	
Flucytosine	Topical: well tolerated but less effective		
Miconazole	Topical: occasional superficial punctate keatopathy	Case report of multiple intravitreal injections of 25 μg with good result	
Antiviral Agents			
Idoxuridine	Conjunctival injection, follicular conjunctivitis, allergic blepharoconjunctivitis, and cicatrization, punctal scarring		

Drug	Anterior Segment	Posterior Segment	Systemic Toxic Effects
	***Ocular Antiinfective Agents** Continued*		
	Perilimbal filaments, superficial punctate keratopathy, delayed corneal healing, and corneal edema		
Vidarabine	Conjunctival injection, follicular conjunctivitis, punctal scarring or occlusion Delay in stromal wound healing Significant conjunctival inflammation with subconjunctival injection		
Trifluridine	Conjunctival injection, superficial punctate keratopathy, filamentary keratitis, and punctal occlusion Cicatrization and corneal epithelial dysplasia have been reported Reversible crystalline epithelial keratitis reported		
Acyclovir	Mild superficial punctate keratopathy and follicular conjunctivitis	2 cases of intravitreal infusions without toxicity	
Ganciclovir		200-μg intravitreal doses tolerated without evidence of ocular toxicity seen with multiple injections Sustained delivery systems without clinical evidence of toxicity	Bone marrow depression
Foscarnet		Report of intravitreal injection without toxicity	
Cidofivir		Intravitreal doses of <40 μg not toxic clinically	
	Other Systemic Antiinfective Agents		
Cephalosporins		Possible retinopathy with cephaloridine	
Chloramphenicol	Rarely, decreased vision	Rarely, optic neuritis and optic atrophy Rarely, toxic amblyopia Retinopathy	Aplastic anemia—idiosyncratic reaction
Ciprofloxacin	Blurred vision and photophobia Altered color vision	Toxic optic neuropathy	
Clofazimine	Conjunctival pigmentation Corneal epithelial changes		Eyelid skin pigmentation
Doxycyline, tetracycline, minocycline	Conjunctival hyperpigmentation and cysts Orbital psuedotumor Extraocular muscle paralysis	Pseudotumor cerebri	Eyelid skin pigmentation May aggravate myasthenia gravis
Ethambutol	Color vision abnormalities Scotomas	Axial and paraaxial optic neuritis	
Gentamicin, tobramycin, streptomycin		Pseudotumor cerebri Blindness and optic atrophy with intrathecal use	May aggravate myasthenia gravis
Isoniazid		Rare optic and retrobulbar neuritis	
Nalidixic acid	Visual disturbances Color vision defects	Papilledema from increased intracranial pressure	Lupoid-like skin changes
Penicillin, including some synthetic penicillins		Pseudotumor cerebri	May aggravate myasthenia gravis
Rifampin	Conjunctival hyperemia Conjunctivitis Orange staining of contact lenses		
Sulfa drugs	Myopia due to lens thickening from ciliary body edema Anterior uveitis	Optic neuritis	
Suramin	Vortex-like epithelial keratopathy Irritation	Optic atrophy	

Abbreviations: GI, gastrointestinal; ERG, electroretinogram; ISA, intrinsic sympathomimetic activity; IOP, intraocular pressure; BCNU, carmustine (bis-chloroethyl-nitrosourea); CCNU, lomustine N-(2-chloroethyl-N′cyclohexyl-N-nitrosourea); EOG, electrooculogram.

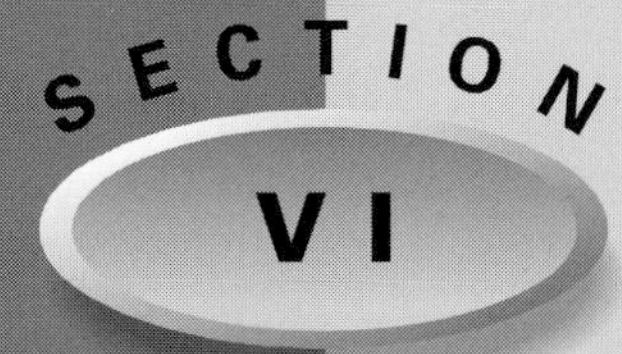

Epidemiology

Edited by

JOHANNA M. SEDDON

CHAPTER 46

Epidemiology of Age-Related Cataract

Susan E. Hankinson

The function of the lens is to transmit and focus light rays on the retina. To function optimally, the lens must remain transparent, a characteristic imparted by the high degree of spatial order and unvarying density of the lens cells.[1] The lens is composed of only two cell types, epithelial and fiber cells. The epithelial cells, which form a single layer on the anterior surface of the lens, differentiate into fiber cells. As the fiber cells form, they are compressed inward toward the center of the lens.[2] They eventually lose their nuclei and organelles such that virtually no protein synthesis occurs in the inner region of the lens. In contrast with protein in other organs, that in the lens exists for many years.

In a cataractous lens, transparency is reduced and changes in the index of refraction cause light scattering and opacification, which in turn cause a decrease in visual acuity.[2] Opacities are proposed to form through several mechanisms, including protein oxidation and precipitation and osmotic stress.[3] An opacity may form in one or more areas of the lens; a cortical cataract results from deterioration of the younger fiber cells, whereas a nuclear cataract results from deterioration of older fiber cells in the center of the lens. In posterior subcapsular (PSC) cataract, epithelial cells migrate to the posterior pole, where they form irregularities that scatter light. It has been suggested that these different types of cataracts have differing etiologies.[3–5]

Cataract has several established causes: intraocular trauma or surgery, chronic intraocular inflammation, long-term steroid use, and congenital cataract.[6] However, most cataracts in adults are of unknown etiology and are called senile or age-related cataracts.[6] In essence, senile cataract is a diagnosis of exclusion: It is made in adults 45 years of age or older who have a cataract with no known cause.

Public Health Significance

Cataract is an important cause of visual impairment worldwide: More than 50 million people are affected.[7] Cataract has been estimated to cause more than 55% of cases of blindness in countries such as Nepal and India.[8] In the United States, cataract is responsible for more than 43,000 cases of legal blindness and for 3.3 million cases of visual impairment.[9] In developed countries such as the United States, cataract surgical procedures are both successful and widely available, yet they carry a significant cost. For example, in 1989, cataract extraction was the most commonly reimbursed surgical procedure in persons over 65 years of age in the United States, accounting for 12% of the Medicare budget.[10] It has been estimated that if cataract formation were delayed by 10 years, the need for cataract extraction surgery might be reduced by 45%.[9] Identifying the factors that influence the risk of cataract formation is therefore highly important.

Prevalence and Incidence of Age-Related Cataract

A major advance in cataract research in the last two decades has been to document the prevalence of cataract in several different populations. Cataract prevalence is defined as the number of persons with cataract (or aphakia) in a population divided by the total number of persons in the population and is generally expressed as a percentage. Prevalence data help define the magnitude of the disease burden and, if collected for a number of countries with different cultural and environmental conditions, can be helpful in generating hypotheses regarding the etiology of cataract formation. Cataract incidence (or cumulative incidence), on the other hand, is defined as the number of new cases of cataract that occur over a specified period of time divided by the total number of persons in the population who are free from cataract at baseline. Incidence data are collected by examining a population at least twice (at baseline, to determine who does not have cataract, and later, to determine who in the baseline population has since developed cataract).

NATIONAL HEALTH AND NUTRITION EXAMINATION SURVEY

Two large studies have been conducted in the United States to determine the prevalence of senile cataract. In 1971 and 1972, the National Health and Nutrition Examination Survey (NHANES) was conducted among more than 10,000 persons between the ages of 1 and 74 years.[11] The participants were chosen to represent the noninstitutionalized civilian population in the United States at that time. In addition, the sampling scheme was weighted toward preschool children, women of child-bearing age, the elderly (ages 65 to 74 years), and persons with a low income. The participation rate in this study was approximately 72%.

Prevalence data have been reported for the 3056 persons (ages 45 to 74 years) who underwent a complete ophthalmic examination, including slit-lamp biomicroscopy and direct ophthalmoscopy. Lens changes were considered present only if they were detected with both the ophthalmoscope and the slit lamp. Cataract was defined as either aphakia or an opacity resulting in visual acuity of 20/25 or worse; separate prevalence rates for senile cataract have not been reported. Cataract was found in approximately 4.9% of participants aged 45 to 64 years and 27.6% of those aged 65 to 75 years[12] (Table 46–1). This study also assessed the prevalence of cataract by race. Prevalence was higher among African American men and women in each age category.

FRAMINGHAM EYE STUDY

The Framingham Heart Study was begun in 1948 among approximately 5000 adult residents of Framingham, Massachusetts. In 1973, the surviving members of the cohort, then aged 52 to 85 years, were invited to participate in the Framingham Eye Study.[13] Eighty-four percent of the 2940 participants still living in the local area and 19% of the 1037 participants living elsewhere were examined. The overall response rate was 67%.

TABLE 46–1. **Prevalence (%) of Cataract by Age and Gender in Five Population-Based Surveys**

NHANES (n = 3056)*			
	Age (Years)		
Gender		**45–64**	**65–75**
Males		6.2	25.6
Females		3.6	29.5
Total		4.9	27.6
Framingham Eye Study (n = 2477)†			
	Age (Years)		
Gender	**52–64**	**65–74**	**75–84**
Males	4.3	16.0	40.9
Females	4.7	19.3	48.9
Total	4.5	18.0	45.9
Punjab Study (n = 527)‡			
	Age (Years)		
Gender	**52–64**	**65–74**	**75–85**
Males	26.2	35.7	79.3
Females	32.7	52.6	84.6
Total	29.4	43.3	81.8
Tibet Eye Study (n = 782)§			
	Age (Years)		
Gender	**50–59**	**60–69**	**70+**
Males	4.2	23.3	32.4
Females	5.7	27.6	65.6
Total	5.0	26.0	53.1
Beaver Dam Eye Study (n = 3304)¶			
	Age (Years)		
Gender	**55–64**	**65–74**	**75–84**
Males	3.9	14.3	38.8
Females	10.0	23.5	45.9
Total	7.2	19.6	43.4

*Aphakia or cataract resulting in a visual acuity of 20/25 or worse.
†Aphakia or senile cataract resulting in a visual acuity of 20/30 or worse.
‡527 participants aged 50 or older. Aphakia or senile cataract resulting in a visual acuity of 20/60 or worse.
§Aphakia or senile cataract resulting in a visual acuity of 20/40 or worse.
¶Cataract resulting in a visual acuity of 20/32 or worse.

Data were reported for both senile lens changes and senile cataract. Senile lens changes were defined as vacuoles, water clefts, lamellar separations, cortical or posterior subcapsular opacities, nuclear sclerosis, aphakia, or other miscellaneous changes in the lens. Senile cataract was defined as aphakia or an opacity resulting in a best-corrected visual acuity of 20/30 or worse and not attributable to congenital or other secondary causes. The prevalence of senile cataract was 4.5% among adults 52 to 64 years of age, 18% among those 65 to 74 years of age, and 45.9% among those 75 to 85 years of age (see Table 46–1). In each age category, the prevalence of age-related cataract was higher in women than in men. Although these data are useful, several limitations of the study must be considered before these prevalences are generalized to the U.S. population as a whole. The participants were all white residents of a single suburban town in the United States, and prevalence estimates were based on the 84% of the surviving members of the original cohort who still resided in the local area.

POPULATION-BASED PREVALENCE STUDY IN INDIA

A population-based prevalence study was conducted in the Punjab of northwest India in 1976 and 1977.[14] All adults over the age of 30 years residing in one of three districts in the Punjab were invited to participate. Overall, 76% of the 796 eligible men and 91% of the 733 eligible women participated, for a total of 1269 participants. The ophthalmic examination was conducted by distant direct ophthalmoscopy through an undilated pupil. A senile cataract was defined as either aphakia or an opacity occurring in at least one eye resulting in a best-corrected visual acuity of 20/60 or worse and not considered congenital or due to a secondary cause. The prevalence of cataract was 0.2% among persons aged 30 to 39 years, 2.2% among those aged 40 to 49 years, 14.7% among those aged 50 to 59 years, 42.0% among those aged 60 to 69 years, 55.7% among those aged 70 to 78 years, and 87.8% among those 79 years and older (see Table 46–1). Interestingly, the age-adjusted prevalence of senile cataract was almost three times higher than that in the Framingham Study or the NHANES, even though the visual acuity criteria were considerably stricter.[4]

TIBET EYE STUDY

The prevalence of cataract in Tibet was determined in a population-based survey conducted in 1987.[15] The survey was conducted among 27 villages in Duilong-Deqing County, near Lhasa, China, and included 2660 participants, of whom 782 were aged 50 years or older. The participation rate was approximately 92%. The cataract status of each participant was assessed using a slit-lamp; senile cataract was defined as aphakia or cataract resulting in a visual acuity of 20/40 or worse that could not be attributed to a known cause of cataract. The prevalence of senile cataract was 5% among persons 50 to 59 years of age, 26% among those 60 to 69 years of age, and 53.1% among those 70 years of age or older (see Table 46–1). In each age category, women had a higher prevalence of cataract.

POPULATION-BASED PREVALENCE STUDY IN SAUDI ARABIA

A population-based survey of eye disease was conducted in Saudi Arabia among 14,577 persons who were chosen to represent the settled population of Saudi Arabia.[16] (Another small, nonstatistically selected sample was also examined to assess eye disease among the nonsettled, or Bedouin, population.) In all, 1127 men and 1117 women over the age of 40 years participated in the survey. Examinations were performed with a ×4 magnifying loupe and a hand-held flashlight, and direct ophthalmoscopy was attempted for all persons over the age of 40. In this study, the severity of cataracts was graded as minimal, moderate, or advanced rather than by the degree of decrease in visual acuity. An advanced cataract was a mature cataract, and a moderate cataract was one in which the fundus could still be visualized, although not clearly.

The prevalence of any opacity (a minimal cataract with or without a decrease in visual acuity, a moderate or advanced cataract, or aphakia) was 21% among men and 30% among women aged 40 to 59 years and 72% among men and 74% among women aged 60 or older. For cataract resulting in a loss of visual acuity (degree of loss unspecified), the prevalence in the 40- to 59-year age group was 14.6% for men and 21.7% for women; in the over-60-year age group, the prevalence was 60.5% for men and 68.6% for women.

BEAVER DAM EYE STUDY

Another population-based prevalence survey of cataract was conducted in Beaver Dam, Wisconsin.[17] The study was conducted in 1990 to 1992 among approximately 4900 adults who were 43 to 84 years of age. Both slit-lamp and retroillumination photographs were taken of the lenses using a Topcon SL5 Photoslit Lamp and Neitz CR-T camera, respectively; photographs were later graded using a standardized protocol. Overall, the prevalence of opacities appeared comparable with that reported in the Framingham Eye Study (see Table 46–1). Again, in each age category, women had a higher prevalence of cataract than men.

Comparison of prevalences across studies is limited by the different assessment techniques and different definitions of cataract. The prevalence in Tibet does not appear to be higher than that in the United States; again, however, the comparison is complicated by the different age categories and different visual acuity criteria used in the respective studies. Similarly, it is not possible to determine if the prevalence of cataract is higher in Saudi Arabia because of how cataract was defined. The prevalence of cataract in India does seem considerably higher than that in the United States.

GENDER DIFFERENCES IN CATARACT PREVALENCE

Several studies have assessed cataract prevalence by gender. The NHANES study,[11] the Framingham Eye Study,[13] and the Punjab study[14] all noted a higher prevalence of cataract among women. Using data from these three studies, Hiller and associates[11] calculated that the age-adjusted relative risk for women was 1.13 (95% confidence interval [CI] of 1.02 to 1.25); that is, women had a significantly (13%) higher prevalence of age-related cataract than men. The reason for these apparent differences is not known.

INCIDENCE OF CATARACT

To date, only one study has evaluated the cumulative incidence of cataract in a large group of adults.[18] In a case-control study begun in 1987,[5] 1193 adults were reexamined at least twice at approximately 6-month intervals starting in 1989. Both at baseline and each follow-up visit, slit-lamp and retroillumination lens photographs were taken and graded using the Lens Opacities Classification System (LOCS) II. An incident cataract was defined as a new opacity noted in at least one eye on two consecutive visits. The 3-year cumulative incidence rates for persons 55 to 64 years of age were 16.6%, 2.1%, and 3% for cortical, nuclear, and posterior subcapsular cataract, respectively. Comparable incidence rates for adults 65 to 74 years of age were 18.1%, 6.5%, and 6.4%. Cataract progression among participants with preexisting cataract also was evaluated, and as might be expected, was much greater than the cumulative incidence for each of the three types of opacity.

Medical Care Utilization Data: National Hospital Discharge Survey and National Ambulatory Medical Care Survey

The National Hospital Discharge Survey, conducted by the National Center for Health Statistics, collects medical record data on patients admitted to noninstitutional hospitals in the United States (excluding military and Veterans Administration hospitals).[19] Although only hospitals with six or more beds and those in which the average length of stay is less than 30 days are included in this survey, these hospitals account for approximately 95% of all hospital discharges.[6] In 1984, data were collected from approximately 192,000 medical records from 407 hospitals.

Data are tallied by both first-listed diagnosis and all-listed diagnoses. The all-listed diagnoses category includes the diagnosis of cataract from the medical record if it was listed as one of the first seven diagnostic codes. In 1979, 79,000 persons (18.3 per 10,000) aged 45 to 64 years and 289,000 (121.8 per 10,000) aged 65 years or older had a first-listed diagnosis of cataract.[20] Cataract was included under all-listed diagnoses in 92,000 records (21.2 per 10,000) for the former age group and in 349,000 records (149.3 per 10,000) for the latter. In 1984, the numbers were slightly lower in the younger group and somewhat higher in the older (Table 46–2).[21] In this survey, cataract is the most common cause of hospitalization for eye diseases.

The National Ambulatory Medical Care Survey supplies data on the number of office visits made to ambulatory care physicians for the diagnosis of cataract.[22, 23] In 1975, approximately 2 million visits were made to physicians' offices for cataract; by 1991, this number had more than tripled to 7.5 million visits. These data help to quantity the impact of cataract on the medical care system.

TABLE 46–2. **Number (in Thousands) and Rate (Per 10,000) of First-Listed and All-Listed Cataract Diagnoses from the 1979 and 1984 National Hospital Discharge Survey, Utilization of Short-Stay Hospitals**

	First-Listed				All-Listed			
	45–64		*65+*		*45–64*		*65+*	
Year	*No.*	*Rate*	*No.*	*Rate*	*No.*	*Rate*	*No.*	*Rate*
1979	79	18.3	289	121.8	92	21.2	349	149.3
1984	74	16.6	395	140.7	89	19.9	464	165.5

Definition of Cataract in Epidemiologic Research

End-points used in the epidemiologic study of cataract have included all cataracts as a single group, cataract extraction, and specific cataract subtype (e.g., nuclear, cortical, posterior subcapsular, and mixed). The choice of what end-point to use depends on the size and design of the study, the population studied, and the hypotheses addressed.

Screening of the entire study population for cataract, with a standardized assessment of specific cataract types, is ideal and should be performed if possible. This approach allows all cases to be identified and properly classified and permits an assessment of risk factors by specific cataract type. Several classification systems, such as LOCS,[24] give reproducible results when used by specifically trained ophthalmologists. Cataracts can be assessed at the time of examination or later from lens photographs. The advantage of the latter option is that the researcher can use the photographs to assess the opacities by several different grading schemes.[25]

In large studies (e.g., the Nurses' Health Study with 121,700 participants or the Physician's Health Study with 22,071 participants), screening of the entire population for cataract is not feasible; yet these studies, because of their size, can detect weaker but still important associations and can provide more precise estimates of effect than small studies can. Therefore, an alternative definition of disease status is needed, such as the study participant reporting either a cataract or a cataract extraction with later confirmation by the diagnosing physician. Because detection of an early cataract depends on whether a patient is screened, the validity of the study is compromised if the end-point of cataract is used and screening is associated with the exposure of interest. For this reason, the use of self-reported cataract, without requiring an associated decrease in visual acuity, can be recommended only when essentially all participants undergo routine eye examinations. Requiring a decrease in visual acuity due to the cataract as part of the case definition decreases the chance of this bias.

The use of cataract extraction as the disease end-point is generally the best option in large studies, in which direct examination is not feasible. If the analysis is restricted to cataract extraction, few, if any, false-positive cases will be identified, and the chance for variation in diagnostic thresholds is minimized. Although rates of cataract extraction vary with the ophthalmologist, and participants may have different thresholds for undergoing surgery, the results of a study will not be biased if these factors are not associated with the exposure of interest. The validity of this assumption should be assessed, because it may vary according to the study population. For example, the investigators may examine the correlation between exposure and either frequency of visual screening or visual acuity at the time of cataract extraction (in the latter, to determine if those with the exposure of interest are more or less likely to undergo extraction early in the natural history of the cataract).

If cataract extraction is used as an end-point and information is not available on the type of cataract involved, several points must be considered. Because PSC cataracts cause visual changes early in their development, they are disproportionately represented in the total requiring surgery.[26] Studies that include opacities not yet requiring extraction are likely to have a mix of cataract types different from that in studies that assess only persons who have undergone cataract extraction. If different types of cataracts truly have different etiologies,[3, 4] the associations found in studies including early opacities may be different from those found in studies based on extractions. Although a study assessing all cataracts combined precludes etiologic analyses for specific types, appropriate public health recommendations can nevertheless be made if a particular factor is found to increase the risk of cataract in general.

Possible Risk Factors for Cataract Formation

DIABETES

The role of diabetes in the development of cataract has been controversial. In the past, some investigators thought that cataracts did not occur more often in diabetics but rather were simply diagnosed more often because of the increased frequency of visual examinations in this group. Diabetics may also be more likely to undergo cataract extraction because of the need to visualize the retina clearly in order to monitor the development and progression of retinopathy. Thus, it is important to evaluate the association of diabetes and cataract in population-based surveys and not by studies of persons undergoing screening or cataract extraction. Both the Framingham Eye Study and the NHANES, the two largest and most comprehensive prevalence studies to date, found a threefold to fourfold excess risk of cataract among diabetics less than 65 years of age.[27] Because of the relatively strong association indicated by these data (and the biologic plausibility of the association), it is now generally accepted that diabetics have a higher risk of cataract.

Diabetes may increase the risk of cataract formation by several possible mechanisms. For example, when glucose levels are high, aldose reductase is converted to the sugar alcohol sorbitol[3]; sorbitol accumulates in the lens, creating osmotic stress that can result in swelling and rupture of the lens fibers and eventual opacification. A second mechanism is the glycosylation of lens proteins. Glycosylation may increase a protein's susceptibility to oxidation, eventually leading to cataract formation.[3]

DIET

The possible effects of dietary intake on cataract development have only recently been assessed in epidemiologic studies. A number of hypotheses have been suggested; for example, that high dietary intake of antioxidant vitamins may decrease the risk of cataract and that low protein intake or high lactose or galactose intake may increase the risk. Although few studies have addressed these issues to date, our knowledge in this area is increasing rapidly because of a recent expansion of research efforts.

OXIDATION AND THE EFFECTS OF ANTIOXIDANTS

Free radicals are highly reactive molecules that can cause serious injury to cells by random oxidative reactions.[3] These molecules occur both naturally (produced by the mitochondria during the electron transport cycle) and through exposure to radiation. It has been hypothesized that dietary antioxidants may decrease the risk of cataract by preventing oxidation of the lens proteins.[3] Such protection by vitamins C and E, riboflavin, and more recently carotene has been hypothesized. Vitamins C and E and carotene are effective antioxidants, whereas riboflavin, though not an antioxidant, is integral to the function of an antioxidant enzyme.[28]

Vitamin C

Vitamin C has been found in relatively high concentrations in the lens[29]; levels are reduced in the cataractous lens.[30] Levels of ascorbic acid in the lens have been reported to increase with vitamin C supplementation in patients scheduled for cataract extraction.[31] Ascorbate prevents opacity formation in rat lenses exposed to light[29] and prevents glucocorticoid-induced cataract formation in chick embryos.[32]

Jacques and colleagues[33] collected blood samples from 77 case-patients and 35 controls and noted an inverse association of plasma vitamin C with risk of cataract, although this association was statistically significant only among persons with PSC cataract. Although these results were suggestive, the small size of the study limited the authors' ability to control for factors that may have distorted the results. In a case-control study conducted in India, Mohan and coworkers[34] noted no association of plasma ascorbate with most cataract types but found a positive association with combined nuclear-PSC cataract (relative risk [RR] = 1.87; 95% CI = 1.29 to 2.69). A limitation of using plasma vitamin C to define exposure is that plasma levels reflect only recent intake[35] and therefore may not accurately reflect long-term intake. A decreased risk of cataract has been reported among consumers of 3.5 or more servings of fruits and vegetables per day,[36] although this is an index not only of vitamin C intake but also of carotene intake. Leske and colleagues[4] assessed dietary intake of vitamin C in a large study with 945 case-patients and 435 controls and noted a decreased risk of nuclear cataract among those in the top 20% of intake.

The NHANES study showed no association with cataract prevalence when either vitamin C intake (calculated from a 24-hour dietary recall) or usual frequency of fruit consumption was assessed.[37] Recently, in a large study of 1008 cases and 469 controls in Italy,[5] participants completed a semiquantitative food-frequency questionnaire. Again, no association was noted between any of the cataract types and dietary vitamin C intake. In the Nurses' Health Study, the first large prospective study to assess this relationship, more than 90,000 female registered nurses completed a semiquantitative dietary questionnaire in 1980; from 1980 to 1988, 493 of these women reported extraction of a senile cataract.[38] This study found no association between dietary vitamin C intake and cataract.

Vitamin E

Vitamin E (tocopherol), a fat-soluble antioxidant, breaks the chain reaction of lipid peroxidase formation in cell membranes and may help maintain the integrity of cell membranes in the lens.[39] Tocopherol has been found to reduce lens damage in rabbits exposed to the oxidant aminotriazol[40] and is known to prevent cataracts in rats made diabetic with streptozotocin.[41] However, tocopherol did not prevent galactose cataract in rats fed a diet of 50% galactose, although the cataracts in the tocopherol-treated group may have been somewhat less severe.[42] Vitamin E is found in the human lens, but it is not known whether supplementation increases levels in the lens. It has been reported that vitamin E levels in the rat lens do not increase with dietary supplementation.[43]

Several studies have found no association between dietary vitamin E intake and cataract formation.[5, 33, 34, 38] One case-control study revealed a statistically significant decrease in cortical and mixed cataract among persons in the highest quintile of vitamin E intake.[4] The same study found an inverse association between plasma vitamin E and nuclear cataract.[44] A similar inverse association was reported in the Baltimore Longitudinal Study of Aging.[45] A prospective evaluation of opacity progression noted an inverse association between plasma vitamin E levels and progression of cortical, but not nuclear, opacities.[46]

Carotenoids

Although carotenoids are effective antioxidants at a partial pressure of oxygen present in the lens,[47] no published animal or in vitro studies have addressed their possible relation to cataract. Although the antioxidant activity of carotene is well established and probably the best known, other carotenoids (e.g., lycopene, lutein) are also effective antioxidants[48, 49] and could serve that function in the lens.

Five studies have assessed the association between either carotene or retinol and cataract. Jacques and associates[33] found that total plasma carotenoids were protective (odds ratio [OR] = 0.18 in the highest tertile of plasma levels, $P < .10$), although the Baltimore Study on Aging reported no substantial association with plasma β-carotene.[45] Leske and coworkers[4] reported that total vitamin A was protective for cortical, nuclear, and mixed cataracts, whereas in the large Italian case-control study,[5] retinol intake was not associated with risk of cataract. Associations with specific foods were not evaluated in any of these studies.

In the Nurses' Health Study, carotenoid and total vitamin A intake without supplements were inversely associated with the risk of cataract extraction.[38] Women in the highest quintile of carotene intake experienced a 25% reduction in cataract risk relative to those in the lowest category of intake, and those in the highest quintile of total vitamin A intake (excluding supplements) experienced a 40% reduction in risk. When foods containing carotene were examined, the richest source of β-carotene—carrots—was not related to cataract extraction. Intake of spinach was consistently associated with a decreased risk of cataract on all three dietary questionnaires, perhaps indicating a protective role for a carotenoid other than β-carotene.

Riboflavin

Riboflavin is required for the synthesis of flavin adenine dinucleotide, a cofactor for the antioxidant enzyme glutathione reductase.[28] In several animal species, a deficiency in riboflavin results in cataract formation.[3] No increase in cataract was noted in rats fed a riboflavin-deficient diet only, although in rats fed a high-galactose/riboflavin-deficient diet, cataracts formed sooner and were more severe than in rats fed a high-galactose diet only.[50]

Leske and associates noted a 40% decrease in the risk of cortical cataract among persons in the highest quintile of dietary riboflavin intake[4] and found an inverse association of the highest levels of plasma riboflavin with both nuclear and PSC cataract. The Nurses' Health Study noted a slight, nonsignificant decrease in risk among women in the highest quintile of riboflavin intake.[38] A number of other studies, including those by Jacques and colleagues,[33] Mohan and coworkers,[34] and the Italian-American Cataract Study group,[5] have found no association of riboflavin with cataract. In a clinical trial conducted in China among adults with multiple chronic nutrient deficiencies, a combination of riboflavin and niacin resulted in a 41% lower prevalence of nuclear cataract,[51] suggesting that cataract risk is increased at or near deficiency levels.

Vitamin Supplement Use

A case-control study conducted in Canada[52] noted a 70% reduction in cataract among persons who had used vitamin C supplements over the previous 5 years and a 55% reduction among those who had used vitamin E supplements. The Nurses' Health Study noted a 45% reduction in risk among women who used vitamin C supplements for 10 years or more.[38] The latter study did not report a reduction in cataract risk among short-term users of vitamin E supplements (because few members of the cohort used vitamin E supplements for more than 5 years, the ability of the study to detect an effect with long-term use was limited). Several studies have reported an inverse association between multivitamin and cataract,[4, 53] including one prospective study.[54] In contrast, Robertson and associates[52] found no such association among users of multivitamins, even though a strong inverse association had been noted among users of specific vitamin C and E supplements. Similarly, Hankinson and colleagues[38] observed no decrease in risk even among persons who used multivitamins regularly for 10 years or more.

Glucose-6-Phosphate Dehydrogenase

The effect of a deficiency in glucose-6-phosphate dehydrogenase has been addressed in several studies. Such deficiency decreases the supply of nicotinamide adenine dinucleotide needed for the protection of reduced glutathione. Orzalesi and coworkers[55] reported that glucose-6-phosphate dehydrogenase deficiency was almost three times more common among men with cataracts than among male controls (unadjusted OR = 2.9; 95% CI = 1.9 to 4.3). Yurigir and colleagues[56] also found a higher incidence of this red blood cell deficiency in persons with cataracts than in those without (33.3% in case = patients versus 8.2% in controls; $P < .001$).

Antioxidant Scores

Most,[4, 31, 57] but not all,[5] studies have found a combined antioxidant score to be inversely associated with cataract. These index variables are created under the assumption that the different antioxidants may function cumulatively to protect the lens. A number of different scores, using a range of antioxidant nutrients, have been evaluated; these differences have made it difficult to compare results among studies.

Although overall, epidemiologic studies to date lend support to the hypothesis that antioxidants reduce the risk of cataract formation, the specific nutrient or nutrients involved and the magnitude of the associations remain uncertain. Reasons for these inconsistencies include different ranges of nutrient intake in different study populations, varying case definitions, varying degrees of measurement error in assessing nutrient levels, incomplete control for confounding, interactions among nutrient intake and other variables (e.g., smoking), and chance. Several strategies to resolve these inconsistencies include conducting large (preferably prospective) studies with comprehensive assessments of both dietary intake and other cataract risk factors, presenting the dietary ranges for all nutrients evaluated in published papers, evaluating more than one nutrient in a single statistical model, and assessing these relationships in randomized clinical trial settings (which can sometimes be efficiently accomplished by piggy-backing onto ongoing clinical trials of other disease end-points). Further data examining these associations are needed before any public health recommendations can be made.

LOW-PROTEIN OR AMINO-ACID–DEFICIENT DIETS

Both low-protein diets and specific amino acid deficiencies have been proposed as risk factors for cataract. In 1932, Curtis and colleagues first noted that a diet deficient in tryptophan causes cataracts in young rats, a finding that other studies have well documented.[3] Diets deficient in phenylalanine and histidine were also found to be cataractogenic in rats.[3] Ratnakar[58] found that the addition of even 5% galactose to the feed of rats on a protein-deficient diet resulted in a high rate of cataract formation, a result indicating that protein deficiency may increase the lens' susceptibility to other insults.

Two studies, both conducted in India, have examined low-protein diets as a risk factor for cataract. In a cross-sectional study, Chatterjee and colleagues[14] found that persons with the lowest reported intake of beans, lentils, meat, milk, eggs, and curd had a 1.5- to 2.5-fold increased risk of cataract when controlled for age, caste, marital status, education, and weight.

In a case-control study, Mohan and colleagues[34] collected information on usual monthly consumption of foods containing protein, thiamine, riboflavin, vitamin A, ascorbic acid, vitamin E, and calcium. Because they found each of these dietary constituents to be highly correlated, protein intake alone was entered in their statistical model to represent general nutritional status. For each one standard deviation increase in protein intake (the amount in grams was not reported), the risk of cataract decreased by approximately 20%, a statistically significant change. Unfortunately, it was not possible to discern whether the nutrient associated with risk of cataract was protein or another dietary constituent.

GALACTOSEMIA AND GALACTOSE INTAKE

Three enzymes are required for the metabolism of galactose: galactokinase, galactose-1-phosphate uridyl transferase, and galactose-4-epimerase.[58, 59] A deficiency of any one of these three enzymes results in cataracts, usually within the first few months of life. In all three deficiency disorders, galactose builds up in the blood and a fraction of it is converted to galactitol by the enzyme aldose reductase. The accumulation of this sugar alcohol within cells of the lens results in hyperosmosis, which causes an influx of water into the lens. The lens fibers swell and eventually rupture, forming vacuoles and resulting in opacification.[60]

Homozygous galactokinase deficiency is rare (1:153,000 to 1:286,000); however, approximately 1 in 309 persons is estimated to be a heterozygous carrier.[59] One study found an increased prevalence of heterozygosity in patients with senile cataracts,[60] although at least one other study has not.[61]

Because decreased lactase activity results in reduced lactose absorption, several investigators have hypothesized that lactose absorbers who also have a decreased ability to metabolize galactose (homozygous galactosemics and perhaps heterozygous carriers) should be at an increased risk of cataract. Simoons[62] correlated cataract prevalence with the geographic distribution of lactose absorbers. Rinaldi and colleagues[63] reported a significantly higher frequency of lactose absorbers in a group of patients with cataracts than in a group of controls. In contrast, Lisker and coworkers[64] found 45% of 64 cataract patients and 71% of control subjects to be lactose absorbers. The influence, if any, of lactose intake and both lactose and galactose metabolism on cataract risk remains uncertain.

ALCOHOL INTAKE

Several recent epidemiologic studies have evaluated the relationship between alcohol intake and risk of cataract. Three studies, one of which was prospective,[65] found a positive association between either moderate[65, 66] or heavy[67] alcohol consumption and cataract. The data from these studies were generally most consistent for an association between alcohol use and posterior subcapsular cataract.[65, 66] Two other studies noted a U-shaped relation with a lower risk of cataract among moderate alcohol consumers.[68, 69] Additional assessments of this association are warranted. Several biologic mechanisms have been proposed for a positive association, including a direct toxic effect of alcohol or its metabolites (e.g., acetaldehyde)[70] and an indirect effect of alcohol mediated through changes in carbohydrate metabolism or antioxidant levels.

SUN EXPOSURE

Sun exposure is known to be damaging to a number of tissues in the eye. Ultraviolet (UV) radiation makes up approximately 5% of the sun's energy and is the most important part of the sun's rays in terms of disease risk in humans.[71] UV radiation could increase the risk of cataract through several different mechanisms: stimulation of photosynthetic processes involving oxygen radicals, disruption of the membrane-cation transport system, or injury to nucleic acids in the epithelial cells of the lens.[71] Both cortical and PSC cataract have been induced by UV irradiation in animal studies.[71] Yet, surprisingly few epidemiologic studies have assessed the relation between sun exposure and cataract despite the strong biologic plausibility and supportive evidence from animal studies.

Several ecologic studies have been conducted to assess the association between sun exposure and cataract formation. An ecologic study is one in which disease frequency is compared in two or more populations, with exposure information being assigned by group or population rather than by individual.[72] The advantage of such a study is that it can be performed quickly and at a low cost and can generate important hypotheses concerning exposure-disease relationships. However, because of the limited exposure information, it is not possible to know whether persons developing the disease of interest were indeed exposed. In addition, information is generally not available on other potentially important variables that might serve to distort the relationship between exposure and disease.

In an ecologic study conducted in Australia by Hollows and Moran,[73] the cataract status of 64,307 aborigines and 41,254 nonaborigines was examined. The continent of Australia was divided into five different zones, each defined by its level of UV light exposure. Cataract prevalence, controlling for age in rather wide categories, was higher in the higher UV light zones. A second study was conducted among 30,565 lifelong residents of Nepal.[74] Altitude and seasonally adjusted average sunlight in 87 villages were assessed. Sites with an average of 12 hours of daily sunlight had an almost fourfold higher prevalence of cataract than those with 7 hours of sunlight. Surprisingly, altitude and cataract were inversely associated; this was attributed to the blockage of sunlight at higher altitudes by neighboring mountains. Neither of these studies was able to control for potentially important variables, such as smoking status and diet.

Data from the NHANES have also been used to assess the association between sunlight and cataract. Sunlight exposure at the 35 NHANES sites was defined by the total number of hours of sunshine annually (data generated by the U.S. Weather Bureau).[75] Persons with cataract were compared with those who had no disease, those who had benign eye tumors, and those who had optic nerve disease in each area. After controlling for age, the prevalence of cataract increased with increasing annual hours of sunlight exposure (categories of 2400, 2400 to 2800, and 3000+ hours). In a second assessment of sun exposure using these data, UV radiation was measured.[11] Estimates of average daily ultraviolet B (UVB) counts were calculated at each site using data on latitude, elevation, and cloud cover. To decrease the effects of migration, the study included only the 2225 persons aged 45 to 74 years who had resided at least half of their lifetime in the state in which the examination was conducted. A statistically significant 14% increase in cataract prevalence was associated with a 1000-count increase in UVB exposure. For example, controlling for age, education, diabetes, race, and urban/rural residence, the prevalence of cataract for those exposed to UVB at a level similar to that in Tucson, Arizona, was 58% higher than for those exposed to UVB levels similar to those in Albany, New York—a statistically significant increase.

Several observational studies have also assessed the association between sunlight and cataract. In a case-control study conducted in North Carolina, Collman and associates[76] collected information on lifetime sun exposure from 113 patients and 160 age- and sex-matched controls. Lifetime sun exposure was assessed by multiplying the intensity of solar radiation near a subject's residence by the number of years at the residence and the estimated number of hours spent outdoors. The authors noted a weak positive association of lifetime sun exposure with both cortical and PSC cataract, although the number of cases of each was very small (9 and 13 cases, respectively) and these findings were not statistically significant. No association with nuclear cataract was found. Dolezal and colleagues[77] examined 160 patients admitted to the hospital for cataract extraction and 160 controls who were primarily friends and relatives of the patients. No difference in lifetime sun exposure was noted, although the range of sun exposure may have been rather limited because of the choice of the controls.

To date, the most detailed study of sun exposure and cataract was of 838 Chesapeake Bay watermen in Maryland.[78] A detailed questionnaire was administered to participants to assess sun exposure since adolescence, the use of eyeglasses and hats, medical history, smoking, and diet. Using the questionnaire data, laboratory data on the effectiveness of eyeglass and hat use in blocking sun exposure of the lens and data from UV monitors worn by a number of workers, the investigators calculated annual and cumulative sun exposure for each individual. The risk of cortical cataract was 60% greater (RR = 1.60; 95% CI = 1.01 to 2.64) with a doubling of cumulative sun exposure. Assessment of average annual sun exposure in four categories showed an increase in risk with increasing exposure for those with cortical cataract, although this increase was not statistically significant. No association was noted with nuclear cataract. Bochow and colleagues[26] examined 160 persons with posterior subcapsular cataract and 160 controls, matched by age, sex, and referral pattern. Sun exposure, both annual and cumulative, was calculated as it was in the Watermen Study, and as in that study, the positive association between cataract and sun exposure was statistically significant.

The results of animal studies and ecologic studies, in conjunction with the strength of the proposed biologic mechanism, all support an association between sun exposure and cataract, although the exact nature and strength of the association remains uncertain. Difficulties in quantifying exposure—"collecting data on time spent outdoors in the sun, the level of UV radiation in specific locales, and the use of eyeglasses and hats"—make such studies complex.

SMOKING

Several epidemiologic studies have assessed the association between cataract and smoking. Although the mechanism by which smoking may increase cataract risk is not known, one hypothesis is that smoking increases oxidative stress in the lens. In support of this hypothesis, several studies have found that smokers have lower plasma levels of β-carotene than nonsmokers at the same level of dietary carotenoid intake.[79]

Most epidemiologic studies have noted an increased risk of cataract among smokers. In a cross-sectional study, Klein and associates[12] assessed smoking and cataract among diabetics and found a positive association in those who were diagnosed with diabetes after age 30. Flaye and coworkers[80] found that nuclear cataracts were 2.5 times more common among current smokers than among nonsmokers; however, the increase in risk was constant across the three smoking categories (i.e., 1 to 14, 15 to 24, and 25+ cigarettes per day). Among ex-smokers, cataracts were more common in those who had smoked heavily, whereas no increase in risk was noted in past light or moderate smokers. In a third cross-sectional study, conducted among 838 male Chesapeake Bay watermen, the increased risk of nuclear opacities among 40-pack-year smokers (i.e., 1 pack per day for 40 years) relative to nonsmokers was a statistically significant 40%.[81] A marginally significant increase in risk (P = .06) also was noted for PSC. In a recent prospective evaluation of this cohort, the risk of progression of nuclear opacities was about 2.5 times higher in current smokers compared with those who had never smoked or past smokers.[82] In a case-control study, current smokers, defined as those who had smoked at least one cigarette per day for at least 1 year and still smoked, had a 70% increased risk of nuclear cataract.[4] The association between cataract and cigarette smoking was assessed prospectively among 21, 316 U.S. male physicians.[83] Current smokers of 20 or more cigarettes per day had a statistically significant twofold increase in cataract risk relative to nonsmokers. Among past smokers, those with predominantly PSC cataract were at a slightly increased risk, whereas no association was noted with nuclear cataract. Similarly, in a prospective study of women, those who smoked 35 or more cigarettes per day had a significant 63% increased risk of cataract extraction relative to those who had never smoked.[84]

Three case-control studies, one conducted in India,[34] a second in Italy,[5] and the third in an ophthalmology practice in Maryland,[26] reported no association between smoking and cataract; unfortunately, however, neither the prevalence of the exposure in the study population nor the associated relative risks were presented. In general, results are most consistent for a relationship between smoking and nuclear cataract. An increase in risk has not been noted for cortical cataract and, except for the reports by Bochow and associates,[26] Christen and coworkers,[83] and Hankinson and colleagues,[84] most studies have had a limited ability to assess the effect of smoking on PSC cataract, because this group made up a very small subset of their cases. Although findings have not been entirely consistent, smoking does appear to be one of the best confirmed risk factors for cataract.

ASPIRIN USE

Experimental evidence supports a possible relation between aspirin use and decreased risk of cataracts. Acetylation of lens proteins by aspirin protects them from chemical agents such as cyanate, glucose, glucose-6-phosphate, and other sugars.[85] Aspirin also inhibits aldose reductase, an enzyme that converts glucose into sorbitol, a lens-damaging agent.[3]

Cotlier and Sharma[86] first reported a protective effect of aspirin on cataract. They found that chronic aspirin consumers had approximately one-third the prevalence of cataracts as had controls ($P < .005$). In a case-control study, the odds ratio associated with aspirin use was 0.25 (95% CI = 0.10 to 0.66).[87]

In contrast, Klein and colleagues[12] assessed aspirin use among 1370 diabetic patients and found no association with cataract. Harding and van Heyningen[88] found a 50% decrease in risk among users of aspirin-like analgesics but no association among those who used aspirin specifically. Among 838 men, neither dose nor duration of past analgesic use was associated with the presence of ocular opacities.[78] In a case-control study, aspirin exposure, assessed by the number of aspirin purchases at a Health Maintenance Organization pharmacy, was not associated with cataract extraction.[89] In a large prospective study among women,[90] no association was noted even for women who consumed 7 or more tablets per week for at least 20 years. In a nonmasked clinical trial of the effect of 500 mg of aspirin/day on heart disease, rates of self-reported cataract among participants in the aspirin group were comparable with the control group.[91]

In the Physician's Health Study, a randomized, placebo-controlled trial, 22, 071 U.S. physicians aged 40 to 84 years were assigned to either 325 mg aspirin every other day or placebo (alternating every other day with β-carotene or placebo).[92] No association was noted when all cataracts were assessed, whereas there was a small, although not statistically significant, decrease in the risk of cataract extraction among aspirin users (cataract: RR = 0.95; 95% CI = 0.74 to 1.22; cataract extraction: RR = 0.80; 95% CI = 0.56 to 1.15). A second randomized trial, wherein the use of 625 mg/day of aspirin for up to 5 years was evaluated among adults with diabetic retinopathy, noted no decrease in the development of visually significant cataract among aspirin users.[93] These randomized trials indicate that using low to moderate doses of aspirin over a period of 5 years would not result in a substantial decrease in cataract risk, if any. Whether there is an effect at the same or higher doses over a longer period of time is unknown, although current observational studies overall do not support such an association.

POSTMENOPAUSAL HORMONE USE

Two recent cross-sectional studies have noted an inverse relationship between current postmenopausal hormone use and cataract. However, the studies were somewhat inconsistent in that the inverse association was noted for nuclear cataract in one[94] and cortical cataract in the other.[95] The biologic plausibility of such an association is unclear but could relate to the antioxidant properties of exogenous estrogen.[96] Given the increasing prevalence of postmenopausal hormone use, further evaluations of this association are clearly warranted.

SEVERE DIARRHEA

Harding and Rixon[97] have proposed that the dehydration and uremia associated with severe diarrhea could increase the levels of cyanate in the body and that cyanate-associated carbamylation of lens proteins would result in cataract formation. They showed that carbamylation of lens proteins can occur in vitro and can induce conformational changes in the lens proteins, making them susceptible to cataract formation. Harding and colleagues have proposed that bouts of severe diarrhea in the more tropical Third World countries, rather than increased exposure to sun, account for the higher prevalence of cataract.[8] To date, few studies have addressed this association. In a matched case-control study conducted in India, case-patients were four times more likely than controls to have reported at least one episode of diarrhea severe enough to render the person seriously ill for at least 3 days (95% CI = 2.2 to 10.2) and were 21 times more likely to have reported two or more bouts of diarrhea (95% CI = 8.9 to 31.0).[98] Harding and van Heyningen, in a case-control study of cataract conducted in Oxford, England, found that case-patients were twice as likely to have suffered from severe diarrhea as controls.[99] However, studies conducted in Southern India[100] and Bangladesh[101] noted no association.

REFERENCES

1. Young RW: Age-related deterioration of the lens. *In* Young RW (ed): Age-Related Cataract. New York, Oxford University Press, 1991, pp 33–56.
2. Luntz MH: Clinical types of cataract. *In* Tasman W (ed): Duane's Clinical Ophthalmology. Philadelphia, JB Lippincott, 1990.
3. Bunce GE, Kinoshita J, Horwitz J: Nutritional factors in cataract. Annu Rev Nutr 10:233, 1990.
4. Leske MC, Chylack LT, Suh-Yuh W, et al: The lens opacities case-control study: Risk factors for cataract. Arch Ophthalmol 109:244, 1991.
5. The Italian-American Study Group: Risk factors for age-related cortical, nuclear, and PSC cataracts. Am J Epidemiol 133:541, 1991.
6. Leske MC, Sperduto R: The epidemiology of senile cataracts: A review. Am J Epidemiol 118:152, 1983.
7. International Agency for the Prevention of Blindness: World Blindness and Its Prevention. New York, Oxford University Press, 1980.
8. Harding JJ, van Heyningen R: Epidemiology and risk factors for cataract. Eye 1:537, 1987.
9. Report of the Cataract Panel: Vision Research: A National Plan, 1983–1987. U.S. Department of Health and Human Services, NIH Publication No. 83-2473, vol 2, part 3.
10. Stark WJ, Sommer A, Smith RE: Changing trends in intraocular lens implantation. Arch Ophthalmol 107:1441, 1989.
11. Hiller R, Sperduto RD, Ederer F: Epidemiologic associations with cataract in the 1971–1972 National Health and Nutrition Examination Survey. Am J Epidemiol 118:239, 1983.
12. Klein BE, Klein R: Cataracts and macular degeneration in older Americans. Arch Ophthalmol 100:571, 1982.
13. Kahn HA, Leibowitz HM, Ganley JP, et al: The Framingham Eye Study. I. Outline and major prevalence findings. Am J Epidemiol 106:17, 1977.
14. Chatterjee A, Milton RC, Thyle S: Prevalence and aetiology of cataract in Punjab. Br J Ophthalmol 66:35, 1982.
15. Hu TS, Zhen Q, Sperduto RD, et al: Age-related cataract in the Tibet Eye Study. Arch Ophthalmol 107:666, 1989.
16. Tabbara KF, Ross-Degnan D: Blindness in Saudi Arabia. JAMA 255:3378, 1986.
17. Klein BEK, Klein R, Linton KLP: Prevalence of age-related lens opacities in a population: The Beaver Dam Eye Study. Ophthalmology 99:546, 1992.
18. The Italian-American Cataract Study Group: Incidence and progression of cortical, nuclear and posterior subcapsular cataract. Am J Ophthalmol 118:623, 1994.
19. US Department of Health and Human Services: Current estimates from the National Health Interview Survey, 1988. Hyattsville, MD, National Center for Health Statistics, 1982. (DHHS Publication No. [PHS] 89-1501; National Health Survey Series 10, No. 173.)
20. US Department of Health and Human Services: Inpatient utilization of short-stay hospitals by diagnosis, United States, 1984. Hyattsville,

MD, National Center for Health Statistics, 1987. (DHHS Publication No. [PHS] 87-1750; National Health Survey Series 13, No. 89.)
21. US Department of Health and Human Services: Inpatient utilization of short-stay hospitals by diagnosis, United States, 1979. Hyattsville, MD, National Center for Health Statistics, 1982. (DHHS Publication No. [PHS] 83-1730; National Health Survey Series 13, No. 69.)
22. US Department of Health and Human Services: The national ambulatory medical care survey. United States, 1975. Tuesday August 5, 1997–1981 and 1985 trends. Hyattsville, MD, National Center for Health Statistics, 1988. (DHHS Publication No. [PHS] 88-1754; National Health Survey Series 13, No. 93.)
23. US Department of Health and Human Services: The national hospital ambulatory medical care survey: 1992 emergency department summary. Hyattsville, MD, National Center for Health Statistics, 1996. (DHHS Publication No. [PHS] 96-1786; National Health Survey Series 13, No. 125.)
24. Leske MC, Chylack LT, Sperduto R, et al: Evaluation of a lens opacities classification system. Arch Ophthalmol 106:327, 1988.
25. West SK, Taylor HR: The detection and grading of cataract: An epidemiologic perspective. Surv Ophthalmol 31:175, 1986.
26. Bochow TW, West SK, Emmet EA, et al: Ultraviolet light exposure and risk of posterior subcapsular cataracts. Arch Ophthalmol 107:369, 1989.
27. Ederer F, Hiller R, Taylor HR: Senile lens changes and diabetes in two population studies. Am J Ophthalmol 91:381, 1981.
28. Draper HH: Nutritional modulation of oxygen radical therapy. Adv Nutr Res 8:119, 1990.
29. Varma SD: Ascorbic acid and the eye with special reference to the lens. Ann N Y Acad Sci 498:280, 1987.
30. Taylor A: Associations between nutrition and cataract. Nutr Rev 47:225, 1989.
31. Taylor A, Jacques PF, Nadler D, et al: Relationship in humans between ascorbic acid consumption and levels of total and reduced ascorbic acid in lens, aqueous humor and plasma. Curr Eye Res 10:751, 1991.
32. Nishigori H, Hayashi R, Lee JW, et al: Preventive effect of ascorbic acid against glucocorticoid-induced cataract formation of developing chick embryos. Exp Eye Res 40:445, 1985.
33. Jacques PF, Hartz SC, Chylack LT, et al: Nutritional status in persons with and without senile cataract: Blood vitamin and mineral levels. Am J Clin Nutr 48:152, 1988.
34. Mohan M, Sperduto RD, Angra SK, et al: India-US case-control study of age-related cataracts. Arch Ophthalmol 107:670, 1989.
35. Jacob RA, Skalka JH, Omaye ST: Biochemical indices of human vitamin C status. Am J Clin Nutr 46:818, 1987.
36. Jacques PF, Chylack LT: Epidemiologic evidence of a role for the antioxidant vitamins and carotenoids in cataract prevention. Am J Clin Nutr 53:352S, 1991.
37. Goldberg J, Flowerdew G, Tso MOM, et al: Age-related macular degeneration and cataract: Are dietary antioxidants protective? Am J Epidemiol 128:904, 1988.
38. Hankinson SE, Stampfer MJ, Seddon JM, et al: Nutrient intake and cataract extraction in women: A prospective study. BMJ 305:335, 1992.
39. Bunce GE, Hess JL: Cataract—What is the role of nutrition in lens health? Nutr Today 6:6, 1988.
40. Bhuyan KC, Bhuyan DK: Molecular mechanism of cataractogenesis. III. Toxic metabolites of oxygen as initiators of lipid peroxidation and cataract. Curr Eye Res 3:67, 1984.
41. Trevithick JR, Linklater HA, Mitton KP, et al: Modelling cortical cataractogenesis: Activity of vitamin E and esters in preventing cataracts and gamma-crystallin leakage from lenses in diabetic rats. Ann N Y Acad Sci 570:358, 1989.
42. Creighton MO, Ross WM, Stewart-DeHaan PJ, et al: Modelling cortical cataractogenesis. VII: Effects of vitamin E treatment on galactose-induced cataracts. Exp Eye Res 40:213, 1985.
43. Stephens RJ, Negi DS, Short SM, et al: Vitamin E distribution in ocular tissues following long-term dietary depletion and supplementation as determined by microdissection and gas chromatography–mass spectrometry. Exp Eye Res 47:237, 1988.
44. Leske MC, Wu SY, Hyman L, et al: The Lens Opacities Case-Control Study Group. Arch Ophthalmol 113:1113, 1995.
45. Vitale S, West S, Hallfrisch J, et al: Plasma antioxidants and risk of cortical and nuclear cataract. Epidemiology 4:195, 1993.
46. Rouhiainen P, Rouhiainen H, Salonen JT: Association between low plasma vitamin E concentration and progression of early cortical lens opacities. Am J Epidemiol 144:496, 1996.
47. Burton GW, Ingold KU: β-Carotene: An unusual type of lipid antioxidant. Science 224:569, 1984.
48. DiMascio P, Kaiser S, Sies H: Lycopene as the most efficient biological carotenoid singlet oxygen quencher. Arch Biochem Biophys 274:532, 1989.
49. Krinsky NI: Antioxidant function of carotenoids. Free Radic Biol Med 7:617, 1989.
50. Srivastana SK, Beutler E: Galactose cataract in riboflavin deficient rats. Biochem Med 6:372, 1972.
51. Sperduto RD, Hu TS, Milton RC, et al: The Linxian Cataract Studies: Two nutrition intervention trials. Arch Ophthalmol 111:1246, 1993.
52. Robertson JM, Donner AP, Trevithick JR: Vitamin E intake and risk of cataracts in humans. Ann N Y Acad Sci 503:372, 1990.
53. Mares-Perlman JA, Klein BEK, Klein R, et al: Relation between lens opacities and vitamin and mineral supplement use. Ophthalmology 101:316, 1994.
54. Seddon JM, Christen WG, Manson JE, et al: The use of vitamin supplements and the risk of cataract among US male physicians. Am J Public Health 84:788, 1994.
55. Orzalesi N, Sorcinelli R, Guiso G: Increased incidence of cataracts in male subjects deficient in glucose-6-phosphate dehydrogenase. Arch Ophthalmol 99:69, 1981.
56. Yurigir G, Varinli I, Donma O: Glucose-6-phosphate dehydrogenase deficiency both in red blood cells and lenses of the normal and cataractous native population of Cukurova, the southern part of Italy. Ophthalmic Res 21:155, 1989.
57. Jacques PF, Chylack LT, McGandy RB, et al: Antioxidant status in persons with and without senile cataract. Arch Ophthalmol 106:337, 1988.
58. Ratnakar KS: Interaction of galactose and dietary protein deficiency on rat lens. Ophthalmic Res 17:344, 1985.
59. Stambolian D: Galactose and cataract. Surv Ophthalmol 32:333, 1988.
60. Skalka HW, Prchal JT: Presenile cataract formation and decreased activity of galactosemic enzymes. Arch Ophthalmol 98:269, 1980.
61. Magnani M, Cucchiarini L, Ctocchi V, et al: Red blood cell galactokinase activity and presenile cataracts. Enzyme 29:58, 1983.
62. Simoons FJ: A geographic approach to senile cataracts: Possible links with milk consumption, lactase activity, and galactose metabolism. Dig Dis Sci 27:257, 1982.
63. Rinaldi E, Albini L, Costagliola C, et al: High frequency of lactose absorbers among adults with idiopathic senile and presenile cataracts in a population with a high prevalence of primary adult lactose malabsorption. Lancet 1:355, 1984.
64. Lisker R, Cervantes G, Perez-Briceno R, et al: Lack of relationship between lactose absorption and senile cataracts. Ann Ophthalmol 20:436, 1988.
65. Manson JE, Christen WG, Seddon JM, et al: A prospective study of alcohol consumption and risk of cataract. Am J Prev Med 10:156, 1994.
66. Munoz B, Tajchman U, Bochow T, et al: Alcohol use and risk of posterior subcapsular opacities. Arch Ophthalmol 111:110, 1993.
67. Ritter LL, Klein BEK, Klein R, et al: Alcohol use and lens opacities in the Beaver Dam Eye Study. Arch Ophthalmol 111:113, 1993.
68. Clayton RM, Cuthbert J, Duffy J, et al: Some risk factors associated with cataract in SE Scotland. Trans Ophthalmol Soc UK 102:331, 1982.
69. Phillips CI, Clayton RM, Cuthbert J, et al: Human cataract risk factors: Significance of abstention from and high consumption of, ethanol (u-curve) and non-significance of smoking. Ophthalmic Res 28:237, 1996.
70. Harding JJ: Physiology, biochemistry, pathogenesis, and epidemiology of cataract. Curr Opin Ophthalmol 2:3, 1991.
71. Taylor HR: Ultraviolet radiation and the eye: An epidemiologic study. Trans Am Ophthalmol Soc 87:802, 1989.
72. Rothman KJ: Modern Epidemiology. Boston, Little Brown, 1986.
73. Hollows F, Moran D: Cataract—the ultraviolet factor. Lancet 1:1249, 1981.
74. Brilliant LB, Grasset NC, Pokhrel RP, et al: Associations among cataract prevalence, sunlight hours, and altitude in the Himalayas. Am J Epidemiol 118:250, 1983.
75. Hiller R, Giacometti L, Yuen K: Sunlight and cataract: An epidemiologic investigation. Am J Epidemiol 105:450, 1977.
76. Collman GW, Shore DL, Shy CM, et al: Sunlight and other risk factors for cataracts: An epidemiologic study. Am J Public Health 78:1459, 1988.
77. Dolezal JM, Perkins ES, Wallace RB: Sunlight, skin sensitivity, and senile cataract. Am J Epidemiol 129:559, 1989.

78. Taylor HR, West SK, Rosenthal FS, et al: Effect of ultraviolet radiation on cataract formation. N Engl J Med 319:1429, 1988.
79. Stryker WS, Kaplan LA, Stein EA, et al: The relation of diet, cigarette smoking and alcohol consumption to plasma beta-carotene and alpha-tocopherol levels. Am J Epidemiol 127:283, 1988.
80. Flaye DE, Sullivan KN, Cullinan TR, et al: Cataracts and cigarette smoking. Eye 3:379, 1989.
81. West S, Munoz B, Emmett EA, et al: Cigarette smoking and risk of nuclear cataracts. Arch Ophthalmol 107:1166, 1989.
82. West S, Munoz B, Schein OD, et al: Cigarette smoking and risk for progression of nuclear opacities. Arch Ophthalmol 113:1377, 1995.
83. Christen WG, Manson JE, Seddon JM, et al: A prospective study of cigarette smoking and risk of cataract in men. JAMA 268:989, 1992.
84. Hankinson SE, Willett WC, Colditz GA, et al: A prospective study of smoking and risk of cataract in women. JAMA 268:994, 1992.
85. Rao GN, Lardis MP, Cotlier E: Acetylation of lens crystallins: A possible mechanism by which aspirin could prevent cataract formation. Biochem Biophys Res Commun 128:1125, 1985.
86. Cotlier E, Sharma YR: Aspirin and senile cataracts in rheumatoid arthritis. Lancet 1:338, 1981.
87. Chen TT, Hockwin RD, Knowles W, et al: Cataract and health status: A case-control study. Ophthalmic Res 20:1, 1988.
88. Harding JJ, van Heyningen R: Epidemiology and risk factors for cataract. Eye 1:537, 1987.
89. Walker AM, Jick H, Gorman MR, et al: Steroids, diabetes, analgesics, and the risk of cataract. Lessons from the epidemiology of cataract extraction. J Clin Res Drug Dev 2:227, 1988.
90. Hankinson SE, Seddon JM, Colditz GA, et al: A prospective study of aspirin use and cataract extraction in women. Arch Ophthalmol 111:503–508, 1993.
91. Peto R, Gray R, Collins R, et al: Randomized trial of prophylactic daily aspirin in British male doctors. Br Med J 296:313, 1988.
92. Seddon JM, Christen WG, Manson JE, et al: Low-dose aspirin and risks of cataract in a randomized trial of US physicians. Arch Ophthalmol 109:252, 1991.
93. Chew EY, Williams GA, Burton TC, et al: Early Treatment Diabetic Retinopathy Study Research Group. Aspirin effects on the development of cataracts in patients with diabetes mellitus. Arch Ophthalmol 110:339, 1992.
94. Klein BEK, Klein R, Ritter LL: Is there evidence of estrogen effect on age-related lens opacities? The Beaver Dam Eye Study. Arch Ophthalmol 112:85, 1994.
95. Cumming RG, Mitchell P: Hormone replacement therapy, reproductive factors and cataract: The Blue Mountains Eye Study. Am J Epidemiol 145:242, 1997.
96. Subbiah MTR, Kessel B, Agrawal M, et al: Antioxidant potential of specific estrogens on lipid peroxidation. J Clin Endocrin Metab 313:1095, 1993.
97. Harding JJ, Rixon KC: Carbamylation of lens proteins: A possible factor in cataractogenesis in some tropical countries. Exp Eye Res 31:567, 1980.
98. Minassian DC, Mehra V, Jones BR: Dehydrational crises from severe diarrhea or heatstroke and risk of cataract. Lancet 1:751, 1984.
99. Harding JJ, van Heyningen R: Case-control study of cataract in Oxford. Dev Ophthalmol 15:99, 1987.
100. Bhatnager R, West KP Jr, Vitale S, et al: Risk of cataract and history of severe diarrheal disease in southern India. Arch Ophthalmol 109:696, 1991.
101. Kahn MU, Kahn MR, Sheikh AK: Dehydrating diarrhoea and cataract in rural Bangladesh. Ind J Med Res 85:311, 1987.

CHAPTER 47

Epidemiology of Age-Related Macular Degeneration

Johanna M. Seddon

Age-related macular degeneration (AMD) is the leading cause of irreversible blindness in older individuals in all developed countries around the world.[1, 2] Patients with the mild or moderate forms of this disease can develop metamorphopsia and visual impairment, whereas those with the advanced stages often develop loss of central vision leading to legal blindness. This impairment adversely affects activities of daily living, rendering it more difficult to read, write, and drive, and thus forcing many individuals in their retirement years to lose their independence. The prevalence of this disease is increasing as the proportion of our elderly population rises, which underscores the growing impact of this problem on our society.

We have no treatment available for the dry or nonexudative forms of this disease, which comprise about 85% of the cases. For the remaining 15% of cases, laser treatment is the only known proven treatment, and other experimental therapies under investigation have not yet proved to be beneficial in randomized clinical trials. The only possible method to decrease the incidence of this disease to date is to refrain from cigarette smoking.[3] Although several potential protective or aggravating factors have been suggested in one or more studies, the only other established associated risk factors are increasing age and a family history of the disease, neither of which can be modified. Dietary measures may also be helpful,[4–6] but this is not definitive and results of ongoing prospective studies and clinical trials are needed.[7] Measures to halt the progression of this disease also remain elusive. Thus, the challenge facing clinical scientists into the next decade and the new millenium is to find the causes and mechanisms of this disease in order to develop preventive measures and better treatments.

This chapter reviews the classification and definition of macular degeneration, its frequency, and the known and potential factors associated with the occurrence of this prevalent condition.

Classification and Definition

Macular degenerative changes have typically been classified into two clinical forms: dry or wet; and the latter form is also called exudative. Both types can lead to visual loss. In the dry form, visual loss is usually gradual. Ophthalmoscopy reveals yellow, subretinal deposits called drusen or retinal pigment irregularities including hyperpigmentation or hypopigmentation changes. Drusen, which become confluent, can evolve into drusenoid retinal pigment epithelial detachments; some of these lesions progress to atrophic areas or to exudative disease. Geographic atrophy involving the center of the macula may occur through other routes of progression, from drusen and pigment changes or as a separate entity. Each of these signs can be further subdivided into various categories according to the number and size of the lesions. In the wet or exudative form, vision loss can appear to occur suddenly, when a choroidal neovascular membrane leaks fluid or blood into the subpigment epithelial or subretinal space. Serous retinal pigment epithelial detachments, with or without coexisting choroidal neovascularization, are also subclassified into the wet stage of the disease. Exudative serous retinal pigment epithelial detachments often, but not always, advance to the neovascular stage. This phenotypic heterogeneity, or wide range of clinical findings, has led to the use of various definitions of AMD, and, as a result, difficulties with comparisons among studies.

It is important for investigators to standardize definitions of a disease and its subtypes in order to enhance comparability and to promote collaborative efforts.[8] Toward this goal, an international classification and grading system for AMD was developed.[9] In this system, early age-related maculopathy (ARM) is defined as the presence of drusen and retinal pigment epithelial (RPE) irregularities, and the terms late ARM or AMD are limited to the occurrence of geographic atrophy and neovascular disease, the forms most often associated with greater visual loss.

Other systems subcategorize the clinical manifestations even further according to the specific type of early ARM and AMD, which, for example, can yield a 4- or 5-step grading system.[7, 10] Alternative and more detailed systems have been used in some of the population-based studies described later.[11, 12] The classification of age-related maculopathy will no doubt change in the future as genetic and epidemiologic studies provide further insight into the pathogenesis of this disease, and subcategories of AMD are better defined.

Prevalence

Several population-based studies have provided information on the prevalence of AMD: The National Health and Nutrition Examination Survey (NHANES)[13, 14] the Framingham Eye Study (FES),[15] the Chesapeake Bay Watermen Study,[12] the Beaver Dam Eye Study,[16] as well as studies outside the United States including the Rotterdam Study in the Netherlands,[17] the Blue Mountains Study in Australia,[18] and a study in rural southern Italy.[19]

The first NHANES was a national survey conducted between 1971 and 1973 to provide data on the civilian noninstitutionalized population between the ages of 1 and 74.[13] Ophthalmic examinations were done at 35 centers across the United States by ophthalmologists according to a standardized protocol. Although 14,000 were selected for participation, only 10,000 were examined. The diagnosis of AMD was made if there were drusen or pigmentary changes present and if the vision was 20/25 or worse. Drusen were common after middle age, and the presence of AMD increased substantially after age 64.

The FES was conducted from 1973 to 1975 and provided data on 2631 persons aged 52 to 85.[15] In the FES, the macula was evaluated for pigment disturbance; drusen; perimacular circinate exudates; and serous fluid, hemorrhage, or fibrovascular proliferation. If an eye had any of these lesions, and the etiology of these lesions was thought to be age-related, and if the vision in that eye was 20/30 or worse, the eye was classified as having AMD. The prevalence of exudative macular degeneration in persons 52 years of age or older was 1.5%. The dry type accounted for 90% of all cases of AMD.

The Watermen Study, based on fundus photographs of 777 participants from the eastern shore of Maryland, described the earliest changes in macular degeneration and the changes associated with exudative maculopathy.[12] The prevalence of large, confluent, or soft drusen was age related; by the eighth decade, 26% of all participants had large or soft drusen. Late AMD (atrophy or neovascular disease) occurred in 1.8% of subjects overall and in 6% of individuals 70 years of age or older.

The Beaver Dam Eye Study was a National Eye Institute–sponsored census of the population of Beaver Dam, Wisconsin.[16] Eligible persons between the ages of 43 and 84 years of age were examined between 1987 and 1988. Stereoscopic 30-degree fundus photographs were taken of the disc, macula, and temporal to the macula. The photographs were graded according to the Wisconsin Age-Related Maculopathy Grading System.[11] Table 47–1 shows the prevalence of early and late AMD in the Beaver Dam Eye Study according to age and gender. Early ARM was defined as the presence of any drusen, except for hard indistinct, with RPE degeneration or increased retinal pigment in the macular area. Late ARM or AMD was defined as the presence of geographic

TABLE 47–1. **Prevalence of Age-Related Maculopathy According to Age and Gender**

	Females		Males	
Age (yr)	***Early ARM (%)***	***Late ARM (%)***	***Early ARM (%)***	***Late ARM (%)***
43–54	6.6	0.1	10.5	0
55–64	12.2	0.5	15.6	0.8
65–74	18.3	1.5	17.5	1.1
75+	29.7	7.8	29.6	5.6

Abbreviation: ARM, age-related maculopathy.
Adapted from Klein R, Klein BEK, Linton KLP: Prevalence of age-related maculopathy. Ophthalmology 99:933–943, 1992.

atrophy or exudative disease, or both. The early forms are much more common than are the late stages of ARM, and both types increase in frequency with increasing age. The prevalence of late age-related maculopathy was 1.6% overall (not shown), and exudative maculopathy was present in at least one eye in 1.2% and geographic atrophy in 0.6% of the population. The prevalence of late ARM rose to 7.1% in persons 75 years of age or older.

The third NHANES was conducted in 1988 to 1991. NHANES III sampled approximately 40,000 persons and used a complex, multistage area probability design.[20] Americans older than 60 years of age were sampled at a higher rate. Unlike other studies, a nonmydriatic camera was used to photograph the retina of one eye. The photograph was centered on a point midway between the temporal arcades and between the fovea and optic nerve. A total of 7412 persons 40 years of age or older were eligible, of whom 4540 persons had fundus photographs. Of these photographs, 4007 could be graded for AMD. Photographs were graded for any drusen, soft drusen, retinal pigment epithelial degeneration, increased retinal pigment, geographic atrophy, signs of exudative macular degeneration (subretinal hemorrhage, subretinal fibrous scar, retinal pigment epithelial detachment, or serous detachment of the sensory retina), using a modification of the Wisconsin Age-Related Maculopathy Grading System.[11]

Total prevalence of AMD in the United States was estimated from NHANES III, after adjusting for sampling weights, examination weights, selection probability, nonresponse rates, and poststratification.[14] The estimated total prevalence of any AMD in the 1991 civilian noninstitutionalized population of the United States 40 years or older was 9.2% (8.5 million people), and 417,000 people were estimated to have the late stage of AMD.

The large population-based studies conducted outside the United States have revealed similar or lower rates of maculopathy. In the Rotterdam Study in the Netherlands, fundus photographs of 6251 participants aged 55 to 98 years were reviewed for drusen, pigmentary changes, and atrophic or neovascular AMD.[17] The prevalence of AMD was observed to be slightly lower in that study compared with the Beaver Dam Study in Wisconsin. The authors used a different photographic technique, but other reasons for the differences are unclear. In the Blue Mountains Eye Study in Australia, in which a fundus photographic technique similar to that in the Beaver Dam Study was used, the authors also found lower prevalence of all lesions related to AMD in each age strata.[18] After an adjustment for age, differences were significant for both soft drusen and retinal pigmentary abnormalities and lower but not significantly different for geographic atrophy and exudative disease.

In a population-based study of 354 participants in rural southern Italy who had clinical or photographic assessment of the macula, the prevalence rates of ARM and AMD were also lower than those found in the United States.[19] Although technical differences among studies cannot be ruled out, the lower prevalence rates found outside the United States may also reflect genetic or environmental influences.

Incidence

There have been very few studies evaluating the incidence of AMD. The FES used the age-specific prevalence data to estimate 5-year incidence rates of AMD according to the definition of AMD in that study as described earlier. These estimates were 0.9, 0.9, 2.5, 6.7, and 10.8% for individuals who were 55, 60, 65, 70, and 75 years of age, respectively.[21]

The Beaver Dam Eye Study determined the 5-year cumulative incidence of developing early and late AMD in a population of 3583 adults (age range of 43 to 86 years).[22] Patients examined in 1987 and 1988 were reexamined in 1993. Incidence of early AMD was defined as the development of either soft indistinct drusen or the presence of any type of drusen associated with retinal pigment epithelial depigmentation or increased retinal pigment at follow-up, when none of the lesions were present at baseline. Incidence of late AMD was defined as the development of either exudative macular degeneration or pure geographic atrophy at follow-up, when none of these were present at baseline. Incidence of early AMD increased from 3.9% in individuals aged 43 to 54 years to 22.8% in persons 75 years of age and older. The overall 5-year incidence of late AMD was 0.9%; exudative changes in 0.6%; and pure geographic atrophy in 0.3%. Persons 75 years of age or older had a 5.4% incidence rate of late AMD. Eyes with soft indistinct drusen and larger areas of involvement by drusen were at higher risk of developing pigmentary abnormalities and late AMD. Eyes with increased retinal pigment or retinal pigment epithelial depigmentation were also more likely to develop geographic atrophy and exudative macular degeneration.

Psychosocial Impact

Patients with visual loss due to AMD and other medical problems often report AMD as their worst medical problem. Patients with visual loss due to AMD have a diminished quality of life.[23, 24] In a study of well-being, patients with AMD had lower scores than did those with chronic obstructive pulmonary disease and acquired immune deficiency syndrome.[25] Among these elderly patients, worse quality of life was related to greater emotional distress, worse self-reported general health, and more difficulty carrying out daily activities.[25] Such an impact on the patient's psychosocial well-being and activities of daily living underscores the growing importance of this disease on the expanding elderly population.

Sociodemographic Risk Factors

AGE

All studies demonstrate that the prevalence, incidence, and progression of all forms of AMD rise steeply with increasing age. There was a 17-fold increased risk of AMD comparing the oldest to the youngest age group in the Framingham Study.[15] In the Watermen Study, the prevalence of moderate to advanced AMD doubled with each decade after age 60.[12] In the Beaver Dam Study, approximately 30% of individuals 75 years of age or older had early ARM; of the remainder, 23% developed early ARM within 5 years.[16, 22] By 75 years of age and older in that study, 7.1% had late ARM or AMD compared with 0.1% in the age group of 43 to 54 years and 0.6% among people aged 55 to 64.

SEX

In the Beaver Dam Eye Study, while controlling for age, there was no overall difference in the frequency of AMD between men and women.[16] However, exudative macular degeneration was more frequent in women 75 years or older compared with men of that age (6.7% vs. 2.6%, $P = .02$).[16] A similar finding was observed in the FES.[15] In NHANES III, men, regardless of race and age, had a lower prevalence of AMD than did women.[14] Incidence rates within the Beaver Dam population also suggest a gender difference. After adjusting for age, women 75 years of age or older had approximately twice the incidence of early ARM compared with men of that age.[22] In the Blue Mountains Eye Study, there were consistent, although not significant, sex differences in prevalence for most lesions of ARM, with women having higher rates for AMD and soft indistinct drusen but no retinal pigmentary abnormalities.[18] No gender differences were seen in the Rotterdam Study.[17] Residual confounding by age in the broad age category "75 and older" may partially explain these differences. However, true gender differences may exist, and further research is needed to confirm and expand these findings.

RACE/ETHNICITY

Mexican Americans, and non-Hispanic blacks, were sampled at a higher rate in NHANES III.[14] Race/ethnicity was based on self- or surrogate response. Other Hispanics, Asians, and Native Americans were included but were not reported due to inadequate sample sizes. A higher frequency of ARM was reported in whites compared with blacks.[14] Rates for late ARM were too low to make statistical comparisons. In the Baltimore Eye Survey, AMD accounted for 30% of bilateral blindness among whites and for 0% among blacks.[26]

Data from a population-based study in Barbados, West Indies,[27] revealed that age-related macular changes occurred commonly but at a lower frequency than in predominantly white populations in other studies. These changes increased with age and were observed with similar frequency among men and women.

The prevalence of ARM was also compared by geographic region and ethnicity in Southern Colorado and Central Wisconsin.[28] Late stage ARM (or AMD) was significantly less frequent among Hispanics in Colorado compared with non-Hispanic whites in Beaver Dam (odds ratio [OR] of 0.07; 95% confidence interval [CI] of 0.01 to 0.49). Among non-Hispanic whites, the prevalence of any ARM was significantly lower in Colorado than Wisconsin, after controlling for various potential risk factors. These non-Hispanic white groups in the two regions also reported different European heritages.

Overall, the literature to date suggests that early ARM is common among blacks and Hispanics, although less common than among non-Hispanic whites, whereas late ARM or AMD is much less frequent in these groups compared with non-Hispanic whites. These observations provide support for a potential genetic component to this disease. Furthermore, differences in prevalence rates between non-Hispanic whites in different regions of the United States suggest that ethnicity may be an important determinant of AMD.

SOCIOECONOMIC STATUS

The Eye Disease Case Control Study (EDCCS) was a National Eye Institute–sponsored multicenter study involving five academic medical centers and was designed to study risk factors for neovascular AMD, central retinal vein occlusion, rhegmatogenous retinal detachments, and idiopathic macular holes.[29] Cases with AMD were individuals with angiographically documented exudative disease. Controls were patients seen in the same local clinical areas who were 55 to 80 years of age and did not have any of the five diseases under study. Persons with higher levels of education had a slightly reduced risk of neovascular AMD, but the association did not remain statistically significant after multivariate modeling.[29] In the Beaver Dam Eye Study, no association was found between education, income, employment status, marital status, and the incidence of maculopathy.[30] Furthermore, no associations were noted in another case-control study[31] or in the FES,[15] although different definitions of macular degeneration were used in those reports, compared with the more recent studies.

Ocular Risk Factors

IRIS COLOR

Investigators have postulated that higher levels of ocular melanin may be protective against light-induced oxidative damage to the retina. To date, the literature is inconclusive about the relationship between iris color and AMD. Darker irides have been found to be protective in some[31–34] but not other studies.[29, 35–38] Differences in studies may be related partly to the use of different definitions of disease, different number and types of other factors evaluated simultaneously, and perhaps residual confounding by ethnicity in some studies.

REFRACTIVE ERROR

Several case-control studies have shown an association between AMD and hyperopia.[29, 31, 39] The potential problem with some of these studies is the setting (ophthalmology practices) in which they were conducted. Because ophthalmology practices tend to contain higher percentages of myopic patients, controls selected from such practices would tend to have a higher prevalence of myopia than would the general population.

CUP:DISC RATIO

The EDCCS demonstrated that eyes with larger cup:disc ratios had a reduced risk of exudative AMD. This effect persisted even after multivariate modeling,[29] adjusting for known and potential confounding factors. Whether this finding, which is consistent with the association with hyperopic refractive error mentioned earlier, is meaningful in terms of the mechanisms associated with the development of AMD, awaits further study.

LENS OPACITIES

The literature has not shown a consistent relationship between the presence of cataract and AMD. FES investigators found no relationship,[40] whereas data from the NHANES Study did support a relationship between AMD and lens opacities.[41] In the Beaver Dam Eye Study, in which photographs of the lens and macula were studied, nuclear sclerosis was associated with increased odds of early ARM (OR of 1.96; 95% CI of 1.3 to 3), but not of late ARM. Neither cortical nor posterior subcapsular cataracts were related to ARM.[42]

On the other hand, investigators have postulated that cataract surgery may increase the risk for AMD, perhaps because the cataractous lens can block damaging ultraviolet light. Inflammatory changes after cataract surgery may also cause progression of early to late ARM. In the NHANES, aphakia was associated with a twofold increased risk of AMD (OR of 2; 95% CI of 1.44 to 2.78).[13] Another study evaluated 47 patients with bilateral, symmetric, early AMD, who underwent extracapsular cataract extraction with intraocular lens implantation in one eye. Progression of AMD occurred more often in the surgical eyes compared with the fellow eyes.[43] In the Beaver Dam Eye Study, previous cataract surgery at baseline was associated with a statistically significant increased risk for progression of ARM (OR of 2.7) and for development of late ARM (OR of 2.8; 95% CI of 1.03 to 7.6).[38] A study of postmortem eyes was suggestive of an increase in disciform scars in eyes with cataract extraction and implantation of an intraocular lens, but no differences in occurrence of choroidal neovascularization or other signs of maculopathy other than hard drusen were seen compared with phakic eyes.[44]

Environmental and Medical Factors

SMOKING

The preponderance of epidemiologic evidence indicates a strong positive association between both wet and dry AMD and smoking. Two large prospective cohort studies have evaluated the relationship between smoking and wet AMD and dry AMD associated with visual loss.[3, 45, 46] In the Nurses' Health Study, women who currently smoked 25 or more cigarettes per day had a relative risk (RR) of 2.4 (95% CI of 1.4 to 4), and women who were past smokers had an RR of 2 (95% CI of 1.2 to 3.4) for AMD compared with women who never smoked.[3] Risk increased as pack-years of smoking increased indicating a dose-dependent relationship. Risk for AMD remained elevated for many years after smoking cessation. Results were consistent for various definitions of AMD, including wet AMD, dry AMD with different levels of visual loss, and for different definitions of smoking. Among women, it was estimated that 29% of the AMD cases in that study could be attributed to smoking.[3] These results were supported by a later study among men participating in the Physicians' Health Study,[46] suggesting that smoking is an important, independent, avoidable cause of AMD.

Several cross-sectional and case-control studies have also shown an increased risk for wet AMD among smokers.[29, 31, 47–51] Some studies, however, have found no relationship,[39, 52–54] or an inverse relationship.[55] Despite inconsistent results in these types of studies, the strong positive relationship between smoking and AMD seen in large prospective studies is persuasive.[3, 45, 46] AMD appears to be yet another smoking-related condition.

Mechanisms by which smoking may increase risk of developing macular degeneration include its adverse effect on blood lipids by decreasing levels of HDL and increasing platelet aggregability and fibrinogen, increasing oxidative stress and lipid peroxidation, and reducing plasma levels of antioxidants.[3]

CARDIOVASCULAR-RELATED FACTORS

Cardiovascular Diseases

Some studies have suggested an association between AMD and clinical manifestations of cardiovascular disease. The presence of atherosclerotic lesions, determined by ultrasound, was examined in relation to risk of macular degeneration in a large population-based study conducted in the Netherlands.[56] Results obtained from this cross-sectional study showed a 4.5-fold increased risk of late macular degeneration (defined as geographic atrophy or neovascular macular degeneration as determined by grading of fundus photographs) associated with plaques in the carotid bifurcation and a twofold increased risk associated with plaques in the common carotid artery. Lower-extremity arterial disease (as measured by the ratio of the systolic blood pressure level [SBP] of the ankle to SBP of the arm) was also associated with a 2.5 times increased risk of AMD. In addition, a case-control study found a relationship between AMD and history of one or more cardiovascular diseases.[31] The NHANES-I study reported a positive association between AMD and cerebrovascular disease, but positive associations with other vascular diseases did not reach statistical significance.[57] A Finnish study reported a significant correlation between the occurrence of AMD and the severity of retinal arteriosclerosis.[53] However, other studies found that persons who reported a history of CVD did not have a significantly greater risk of AMD.[29, 58, 59]

Blood Pressure and Hypertension

The role of blood pressure in the etiology of AMD remains unclear. There was a small and consistent statistically significant relationship between AMD and systemic hypertension in two cross-sectional population-based studies.[57, 60] One small case-control study found that persons with AMD were significantly more likely to be taking antihypertensive medication.[61] Also, a significant relationship was found between AMD and diastolic blood pressure measured several years before the eye examination in the FES,[52] and in a small Israeli study.[62] The Beaver Dam Study reported that systolic blood pressure was associated with incidence of RPE depigentation.[58] In the Macular Photocoagulation Study, there was an increased incidence of exudative AMD associated with hypertension, in the second eye of individuals with exudative AMD in one eye at baseline (relative risk of 1.7; 95% CI of 1.2 to 2.4).[63]

Cross-sectional[56, 58] and case-control studies,[29] as well as one prospective study[59] in which duration of hypertension was not taken into account, did not show an increased risk of late AMD associated with current hypertension or systolic or diastolic blood pressure. However, in the EDCCS, a trend for an increased risk associated with higher systolic blood pressure was evident.[29]

Taken together, the evidence suggests a possible mild to moderate association between elevated blood pressure and AMD. Assessment of this relationship could be enhanced by evaluating the duration of hypertension and its subsequent effects on onset and progression of maculopathy.

Cholesterol Levels and Dietary Fat Intake

There is some evidence linking cholesterol level to AMD, but not all results are consistent. The EDCCS reported a statistically significant fourfold increased risk of exudative AMD associated with the highest serum cholesterol level (>4.88 mmol/L), and a twofold increased risk in the middle cholesterol level group, compared with the lowest cholesterol level group, controlling for other factors.[29] No significant association was noted between AMD and cholesterol level in the FES[52] and in a few small studies.[64, 65] A study of plasma cholesterol and fatty acid levels found no difference between 65 cases of exudative AMD and control pairs.[66] The Beaver Dam Study found that early AMD was related to low total serum cholesterol levels in women and men older than age 75. Furthermore, men with early AMD had higher high-density lipoprotein-cholesterol (HDL-C) and lower total cholesterol/HDL-C ratios.[58, 67] Slightly, but not significantly, increased risk of wet AMD was seen with increasing triglyceride level in the EDCCS,[29] but this finding was not confirmed in the Rotterdam Study[56] or the Beaver Dam Study[58] (both of which had small numbers of exudative AMD cases and therefore limited power).

In a preliminary study, dietary fat intake was associated with a slightly elevated risk of exudative AMD in the EDCCS. This association was primarily due to vegetable fat rather than animal fat. For omega-3 fatty acid intake, an inverse association was found in the multivariate model.[68] In the Beaver Dam Study, persons in the highest quintile of saturated fat and cholesterol intake compared with the lowest quintile had 80% and 60% increased risk, respectively, for early AMD. Results for advanced AMD regarding total fat intake were in the same direction, but were not statistically significant.[69]

In summary, serum cholesterol levels may be related to exudative AMD.[29] The possible association between AMD and dietary fat and cholesterol intake may indicate a relationship with atherosclerosis.[70] Longitudinal follow-up studies are necessary to delineate the effects of serum lipid levels and dietary lipid intake on subsequent development and progression of AMD.

Diabetes and Hyperglycemia

Many studies have investigated the relationship between diabetes and/or hyperglycemia and AMD, and most have found no significant relationships.[29, 31, 52–54, 63] Three studies suggested a possible positive association. A small case-control study found a nonsignificant increased risk of AMD related to a history of diabetes.[39] Another small study reported a positive association between serum glucose levels and the mean area affected by drusen only in women who did not have diabetes.[62] The Beaver Dam Study found no overall association between early or late AMD and diabetes or glycosylated hemoglobin, a measure of glycemia, although a positive association was found between glycosylated hemoglobin and exudative AMD only in older men. However, sample sizes in these subgroup analyses were very small.[71] Based on the scant literature to date, the association between hyperglycemia or diabetes and AMD, if any, is probably weak. One difficulty with these studies is the uncertainty of diagnosing AMD in the presence of diabetic retinopathy. Also, many studies of AMD exclude persons with diabetic retinopathy. This could result in attenuated relationships between AMD and diabetes in published studies.

REPRODUCTIVE AND RELATED FACTORS

The suggestion that cardiovascular disease may increase risk of AMD has led to some interest in the effect of estrogen-related variables on risk of AMD in women. The EDCCS showed a marked decrease in the risk of neovascular AMD among postmenopausal women who used estrogen therapy.[29] The odds of neovascular AMD were 0.3 (95% CI of 0.1 to 0.8) in current users of estrogen therapy. Former use of estrogen therapy was also associated with reduced risk (OR of 0.6; 95% CI of 0.3 to 1), although the magnitude of the effect was not as large as that for current use of estrogen therapy. No relationship was found in the Beaver Dam Study between years of estrogen therapy and exudative AMD (OR of 0.9 [per 1 year of therapy], 95% CI of 0.8 to 1.1) or any of the less severe forms of AMD among women.[72] However, the Beaver Dam Eye Study had limited power to detect a potential effect of estrogen therapy because there were few cases of exudative AMD (n = 40) and late AMD (n = 49). The Blue Mountains Eye Study reported no relationship between AMD and hormone replacement therapy or early menopause, although there was a small but significant decrease in risk of early ARM with increasing number of years between menarche and menopause.[73]

The EDCCS found that women with one or more pregnancies were twice as likely to have exudative AMD as were nulliparous women (OR of 2.2; 95% CI of 1.3 to 3.9).[29] The Beaver Dam Eye Study found no relation between the number of pregnancies and the risk of exudative or late AMD; however, the study had limited power to detect an effect.[72]

A nested case-control study of age at menopause and risk of atrophic or neovascular AMD was conducted with data obtained from the Rotterdam Study.[74] Risk of AMD was almost twice that among women who had undergone menopause before 45 years of age compared with those who had their menopause at 45 years of age or later (OR of 1.9; 95% CI of 1 to 3.8). Compared with age at menopause at or after age 45 years, menopause induced by oophorectomy before 45 years of age was associated with an OR of 3.8 (95% CI of 1.1 to 12.6). This result, however, was based on only five cases of AMD who underwent oophorectomy before 45 years of age. Although the evidence is sparse, a protective effect of estrogen on AMD cannot be ruled out, and further research is warranted.

SUNLIGHT

The literature to date regarding the association between sunlight exposure and AMD is conflicting. Overall, the data do not support a strong association between ultraviolet (UV) radiation exposure and risk of AMD, although a small effect as well as an adverse effect of blue light exposure is possible.

In a study of 838 Maryland Watermen,[75] sunlight exposure was assessed by detailed interview and field measurements. Statistical models were used to estimate average annual ocular exposure to UV-A, UV-B, and blue light. A modest, positive relationship between blue light or visible light exposure over the preceding 20 years and risk of advanced AMD was seen, with an odds ratio of 1.36 (95% CI of 1 to 1.85) for each 0.1 increase in "Maryland Sun-Years." No adverse effects were observed for UV-A or UV-B exposure. However, only eight men had advanced AMD (geographic atrophy or exudative disease).

In the Beaver Dam Eye Study,[76] no relationship was seen between advanced AMD or early ARM and UV-B exposure, but the effects of UV-A or blue light were not assessed. However, a twofold increased risk of advanced AMD was associated with increased time spent outdoors in the summer. The odds ratio was 2.19 (95% CI of 1.12 to 4.25) for spending 75% or more time outdoors compared with less than 25% leisure time spent outdoors in the summer.

The EDCCS also evaluated crude measures of sunlight exposure.[29] In contrast to the Beaver Dam Study results, no association was seen between exudative AMD and leisure time spent outdoors in summer (OR of 1.1; 95% CI of 0.7 to 1.7, for great amount of time versus none or very little time spent outdoors in the summer). Advanced AMD was not associated with leisure time spent outdoors in the winter, occupational sunlight exposure, or the use of sunglasses or hats with brims, similar to the previous study.[76]

In an Australian case-control study,[77] a greater proportion of people with advanced AMD reported higher sensitivity to sunburn compared with the control group. The controls actually had greater median hours of sun exposure than did the case-control group; however, when results were stratified by sun sensitivity, the difference in median hours of sun exposure was diminished among those who tanned poorly. The authors suggested that sun-sensitive individuals may be at increased risk of AMD, although they tend to avoid sun exposure.

Conflicting results in these studies exemplify the difficulties encountered with studying this complex exposure. These include challenges in measurement of acute and chronic lifetime exposure and the effect of potential confounding variables, such as sun sensitivity and sun-avoidance behaviors. Furthermore, different populations with different stages of AMD as well as people with varying intensity of exposures have been evaluated.

Nutritional Factors

ANTIOXIDANTS

The possible role of antioxidant vitamins in the pathogenesis of AMD has received a great deal of attention. Many remain hopeful that a dietary intervention with increased consumption of antioxidant nutrients could become a primary preventive method for controlling oxidative damage that may lead to AMD. However, results of prospective studies and randomized clinical trials are needed before firm conclusions can be drawn.

Antioxidants including vitamin C (ascorbic acid); vitamin E (alpha-tocopherol); and the carotenoids, including alpha-carotene, beta-carotene, cryptoxanthin, lutein, and zeaxanthin may be relevant to AMD due to their physiologic functions and the location of some of these nutrients in the retina. Trace minerals like zinc, selenium, copper, and manganese may also be involved in antioxidant functions of the retina.[78] Theoretically, antioxidants could prevent oxidative damage to the retina, which could, in turn, prevent development of AMD.[79, 80] Damage to retinal photoreceptor cells could be caused by photo-oxidation or by free radical–induced lipid peroxidation.[81, 82] This could lead to impaired function of the retinal pigment epithelium and, eventually, to degeneration involving the macula. The deposit of oxidized compounds in healthy tissue may result in cell death because they are indigestible by cellular enzymes.[80, 83] Antioxidants may scavenge, decompose, or reduce the formation of harmful compounds.

The EDCCS reported that persons with higher serum levels of carotenoids (sum of serum lutein/zeaxanthin, beta-carotene, alpha-carotene, cryptoxanthin, and lycopene levels) had greatly reduced the risk of exudative AMD.[29] Persons with higher individual serum levels of lutein/zeaxanthin, beta-carotene, alpha-carotene, and crypotxanthin had reduced risks of exudative AMD. The study did not find a statistically significant protective effect for serum levels of vitamin C, vitamin E, or selenium individually, but when these were combined into an antioxidant index with carotenoids, there was a significant reduction in risk of exudative AMD with increasing levels of the index.[5] In the Dietary Intake Study of the EDCCS, an inverse association between exudative AMD and dietary intake of carotenoids from foods was observed.[4] A high intake of green leafy vegetables containing the carotenoids lutein and zeaxanthin was associated with a reduction in the risk of exudative AMD. Intake of vitamin C was associated with a small but nonsignificant reduction in risk. Intake of vitamin A or vitamin E was not associated with a reduction in risk.[4]

A cross-sectional study using NHANES-I data examined the relationship between the prevalence of any AMD and vitamins A and C intake. A weak protective effect was seen with increased consumption of fruits and vegetables rich in vitamin A (which are also rich in carotenoids).[57] The Beaver Dam Study found no effect of supplemental antioxidant vitamins alone or in combination on risk of early or late ARM.[84] However, in a case-control study nested within that study, a low serum level of one carotenoid, lycopene, was associated with presence of any AMD.[6] Another study reported a protective effect for any AMD among those who had higher serum vitamin E and among those who had higher values for an antioxidant index of vitamins C, E, and beta-carotene, but no protective effect was seen for vitamin supplementation.[85] A study of plasma levels of vitamins A and E and five carotenoids found no relationship with exudative AMD in 65 case-control pairs.[66]

A small randomized trial demonstrated less visual loss due to AMD and less accumulation of drusen in the group of 97 patients assigned to high-dose zinc supplementation, compared with 84 patients in the placebo group.[86] However, another small randomized trial found that zinc supplementation had no short-term effect on the course of disease in 112 patients with wet AMD.[87] The Beaver Dam Study found a weak protective effect of zinc intake on early ARM.[84] The

EDCCS did not find any significant relationships between serum zinc levels or zinc supplementation and risk of exudative AMD.[29]

Overall, results suggest that diets rich in antioxidant-rich fruits and vegetables may be related to a lower risk of exudative AMD. Increased blood levels of carotenoids and antioxidant vitamins were also related to decreased risk of exudative AMD in some reports. However, these relationships need to be confirmed with prospective studies. The effect of dietary antioxidants on the incidence or progression of early AMD has not yet been sufficiently evaluated. Supplementation with antioxidant vitamins or minerals has not yet been shown to reduce the risk of AMD. The important potential benefits of foods and supplements are currently under investigation in a large randomized clinical trial among subjects with and without AMD at baseline, the Age-Related Eye Disease Study, sponsored by the National Eye Institute.[88] This study is evaluating whether supplementation with a high dose of zinc or antioxidant vitamins C and E and beta-carotene can reduce the incidence and progression of AMD as well as lens opacities.

ALCOHOL INTAKE

Studies that have examined the relationship between AMD and alcohol consumption have yielded mixed results. In the EDCCS, no significant relationship between alcohol intake and exudative AMD was noted in univariate analyses.[29] In a separate multivariate analysis, alcohol intake appeared to be associated with a decreased risk of disease in the highest quartile of intake compared with nondrinkers.[89] Another case-control study found a nonsignificant association between current daily alcohol intake and AMD, with a suggestion of a nonlinear trend of higher risk of AMD in persons who had five drinks or more per day and a slightly lower risk in persons who had one or two drinks per day compared with nondrinkers.[47] In a case-control study using NHANES-I data, moderate wine consumption was associated with decreased risk of developing AMD, although the analysis did not control for the potential confounding effects of smoking.[90] In two population-based cross-sectional studies, evidence for an association between alcohol and AMD was weak. The Beaver Dam Study found a slightly increased risk for retinal pigment degeneration in persons who consumed beer in the past year,[91] whereas the Blue Mountains Eye Study found increased risk of early ARM only in current "spirits" drinkers.[92] Neither study found increased risk for AMD related to total alcohol intake.

In summary, the evidence suggests that alcohol intake has little effect on AMD. Evaluation of this relationship would be enhanced by determining lifetime alcohol intake rather than current intake, distinguishing between specific beverage intake and total alcohol intake, and using prospective follow-up methods to estimate the effects of alcohol intake on the development and progression of AMD. The role of dietary fats was considered in the previous section.

Genetics of Age-Related Macular Degeneration

There is increasing evidence that genetic or familial factors may play a role in the etiology of AMD. The evidence includes the demonstration of familial aggregation,[93–95] a few twin case reports,[96, 97] a case-control study,[31] and a segregation analysis.[98] Most recently, mutations in a gene associated with Stargardt's disease, *ABCR*,[99] have also been reported to occur in some cases of AMD.[100] The degree of heritability and the relative role of genetic and environmental factors, however, are still unknown. This is currently under investigation.

Several difficulties are associated with evaluating the genetics of this disease. AMD occurs late in life and usually only one generation in the appropriate age range is available for study. The parents are often deceased, and the children are too young to manifest the disease. The phenotype is heterogeneous, with potentially all stages of AMD represented within families. Furthermore, this disease is likely complex, involving multiple genes, as well as environmental factors. These challenges can be addressed partially by applying genetic epidemiologic methods of analyses, involving affected siblings and other affected and unaffected relatives in addition to evaluation of large families and twins.

Familial aggregation of this disease has been demonstrated.[93–95] In one study,[93] first-degree relatives of cases with AMD were compared with first-degree relatives of control subjects without AMD. The prevalence of medical record confirmed age-related maculopathy was significantly higher among first-degree relatives of all case probands (23.7%) compared with first-degree relatives of control probands (11.6%) with an age- and sex-adjusted OR of 2.4 (95% CI of 1.2 to 4.7). When relatives of cases with exudative disease were evaluated, the OR was 3.1 (95% CI of 1.5 to 6.7) for relatives of cases compared with relatives of controls. These results suggest that macular degeneration has a familial component and that genetic or shared environmental factors, or both, contribute to its development. In another study,[94] 20 of 81 siblings of affected patients had AMD compared with only 1 of 78 siblings of control subjects. An adjustment for age differences was not mentioned in that study. When siblings and spouses of cases were compared in another study,[95] there was a trend for concordance of drusen characteristics between siblings but not between spouses. These data also support the familial aggregation of this disease. Additional evidence for a genetic component was suggested by a segregation analysis involving the Beaver Dam population.[98] Complex analyses with assumptions suggested that 55 to 57% of the variability in AMD could be attributed to single gene segregation. Also, in a case-control study, cases were twice as likely to report a family history of this disease.[31] A few small twin studies also suggest a genetic predisposition to the disease.[96, 97]

Collectively, the evidence supports the search for a genetic component. For this reason, several studies are underway to accomplish this goal. For example, we launched a large population-based twin study in 1992 after a pilot study to determine the heritable component of this disease and to dissect its genetic and environmental components. Applying standardized protocols and forms, which we developed for this twin study,[10] we also launched a family study to conduct linkage analyses, search for candidate genes, and conduct a genomic screen. From this effort, we reported on the lack of association or linkage with AMD for two candidate genes.[101, 102] One of these genes, tissue inhibitor of metalloproteinase-3 (*TIMP-3*) was found to be mutated in Sorsby's fundus dystrophy, a rare hereditary macular dystrophy that phenotypically resembles AMD.[103] For the other gene we studied, apolipoprotein E, allelic variation is related to cardiovascular disease and some forms of retinal degenerations, but we did not find an association or linkage with advanced AMD in our study.[102] More recently, a decreased frequency of the E4 allele was reported among cases with primarily soft drusen compared with controls.[104]

Evidence for a genetic component, at least in some families, was suggested by pursuing the gene associated with Stargardt's disease.[99] This gene, a retina-specific ATP binding cassette transporter (*ABCR* gene), is expressed exclusively in the retina in the rod photoreceptors.[105] Investigators at four major institutions reported that mutations in this gene are also associated with AMD, primarily the dry form.[100] Corroboration of this finding and the exploration of the function of this gene are active areas of investigation. Genotype-phenotype correlations are also being evaluated in probands and their families.[106]

The recent increased interest in the genetic component of AMD underscores the need to determine more definitively the degree of heritability of various forms of this disease; the exact role of *ABCR* mutations as well as the potential role of mutations in other genes; and the relative contributions of genetic, lifestyle, and environmental factors.

REFERENCES

1. Statistics on blindness in the model reporting area, 1969–70. National Institute for Neurological Diseases and Blindness, Section on Blindness Statistics, US Department of Health Education, and Welfare. Washington, DC, US GPO, 1973. (DHEW publication no. [NIH] 73-427.)
2. National Advisory Eye Council (US): Vision research: A national plan 1994–98. Bethesda, MD, US Department of Health and Human Services, 1993. (NIH publication 93-3186.)
3. Seddon JM, Willett WC, Speizer FE, Hankinson SE: A prospective study of cigarette smoking and age-related macular degeneration in women. JAMA 276:1141–1146, 1996.
4. Seddon JM, Ajani UA, Sperduto RD, et al: Dietary carotenoids, vitamins A, C, and E, and advanced age-related macular degeneration. JAMA 272:1413–1420, 1994.
5. Eye Disorders Case-Control Study Group: Antioxidant status and neovascular age-related macular degeneration. Arch Ophthalmol 111:104–109, 1993.
6. Mares-Perlman JA, Brady WE, Klein R, et al: Serum antioxidants and age-related macular degeneration in a population-based case-control study. Arch Ophthalmol 113:1518–1512, 1995.
7. Age-Related Eye Disease Study Manual of Procedures: Bethesda, MD, National Eye Institute, 1992.
8. Seddon J, Gragoudas E, Egan K: Standardized data collection and coding in eye disease epidemiology: The uveal melanoma data system. Opthalmic Surg 22:127–136, 1991.
9. Bird AC, Bressler NM, Bressler SB, et al: An international classification and grading system for age-related maculopathy and age-related macular degeneration. Surv Ophthalmol 39:367–374, 1995.
10. Seddon JM, Samelson LJ, Page WF, et al: Twin study of macular degeneration: Methodology and application to genetic epidemiologic studies. Invest Ophthalmol Vis Sci 38:S676, 1996.
11. Klein R, Davis MD, Magli YL, et al: The Wisconsin age-related maculopathy grading system. Ophthalmology 98:1128–1134, 1991.
12. Bressler NM, Bressler SB, West SK, et al: The grading and prevalence of macular degeneration in Chesapeake Bay Watermen. Arch Ophthalmol 107:847–852, 1989.
13. Ganley J, Roberts J: Eye conditions and related need for medical care among persons 1–74 years of age, United States, 1971–72. Vital and Health Statistics, Series 11. No. 228. Washington, DC, DHHS Publication No. (PHS) 83-1678, March 1983.
14. Klein R, Rowland ML, Harris MI: Racial/ethnic differences in age-related maculopathy. Third National Health and Nutrition Examination Survey. Ophthalmology 102:371–381, 1995.
15. Leibowitz HM, Krueger DE, Maunder LR, et al: The Framingham Eye Study Monograph. Surv Ophthalmol 24(S):335–610, 1980.
16. Klein R, Klein BEK, Linton KLP: Prevalence of age-related maculopathy. Ophthalmology 99:933–943, 1992.
17. Vingerling JR, Dielemans I, Hofman A, et al: The prevalence of age-related maculopathy in the Rotterdam Study. Ophthalmology 102:205–210, 1995.
18. Mitchell P, Smith W, Attebo K, Wang JJ: Prevalence of age-related maculopathy in Australia: The Blue Mountains Eye Study. Ophthalmology 102:1450–1060, 1995.
19. Pagliarini S, Moramarco A, Wormald RPL, et al: Age-related macular disease in rural southern Italy. Arch Ophthalmol 115:616–622, 1997.
20. National Center for Health Statistics: Plan and operation of the NHANES III. United States 1988–1994. Vital Health Stat 1(32), 1994.
21. Podgor MJ, Leske MC, Ederer F: Incidence estimates for lens changes, macular changes, open-angle glaucoma and diabetic retinopathy. Am J Epidemiol 118:208–212, 1983.
22. Klein R, Klein BEK, Jensen C, et al: The five-year incidence and progression of age-related maculopathy. Ophthalmology 104:7–21, 1997.
23. Davis C, Lovie-Kitchin J, Thompson B: Psychosocial adjustment to age-related macular degeneration. J Vis Impair Blind 1:16–27, 1995.
24. Alexander MF, Maguire MG, Lietman TM, et al: Assessment of visual function in patients with age-related macular degeneration and low visual acuity. Arch Ophthalmol 105:1543–1547, 1988.
25. Williams RA, Brody BL, Thomas RG, et al: The psychosocial impact of macular degeneration. Arch Ophthalmol 116:514–520, 1998.
26. Sommer A, Tielsch JM, Katz J, Quigley HA, et al: Racial differences in the cause-specific prevalence of blindness in East Baltimore. N Engl J Med 325:1412–1417, 1991.
27. Schachat AP, Hyman L, Leske C, Connell AMS, et al: Features of age-related macular degeneration in a black population. Arch Ophthalmol 113:728–735, 1995.
28. Cruickshanks KJ, Hamman RF, Klein R, Nondahl DM, et al: The prevalence of age-related maculopathy by geographic region and ethnicity. Arch Ophthalmol 115:242–250, 1997.
29. The Eye Disease Case-Control Study Group: Risk factors for neovascular age-related macular degeneration. Arch Ophthalmol 110:1701–1708, 1992.
30. Klein R, Klein BEK, Jensen SC, et al: The relation of socioeconomic factors to age-related cataract, maculopathy and impaired vision. Ophthalmology 101:1969–1979, 1994.
31. Hyman LG, Lilienfeld AM, Ferris FL, et al: Senile macular degeneration: A case-control study. Am J Epidemiol 118:213–227, 1983.
32. Weiter JJ, Delori FC, Wing GL, et al: Relationship of senile macular degeneration to ocular pigmentation. Am J Ophthalmol 99:185–187, 1985.
33. Holz FG, Piguet B, Minassian DC, et al: Decreasing stromal iris pigmentation as a risk factor for age-related macular degeneration. Am J Ophthalmol 117:19–23, 1994.
34. Sandberg MA, Gaudio AR, Miller S, et al: Iris pigmentation and extent of disease in patients with neovascular age-related macular degeneration. Invest Ophthalmol Vis Sci 35:2734–2740, 1994.
35. Blumenkranz MS, Russell SR, Robey MG, et al: Risk factors in age-related maculopathy complicated by choroidal neovascularization. Ophthalmology 93:552–558, 1986.
36. Gibson JM, Shaw DE, Rosenthal AR: Senile cataract and senile macular degeneration: An investigation into possible risk factors. Trans Ophthalmol Soc UK 105:463–468, 1986.
37. West SK, Rosenthal FS, Bressler NM, et al: Exposure to sunlight and other risk factors for age-related macular degeneration. Arch Ophthalmol 107:875–879, 1989.
38. Klein R, Barbara BEK, Jensen SC, Cruikshanks KJ: The relationship between ocular factors to the incidence and progression of age-related maculopathy. Arch Ophthalmol 116:506–513, 1998.
39. Maltzman BA, Mulvihill MN, Greenbaum A: Senile macular degeneration and risk factors: A case-control study. Ann Ophthalmol 11:1197–1201, 1979.
40. Sperduto R, Hiller R, Seigel D: Lens opacities and senile maculopathy. Arch Ophthalmol 99:1004–1008, 1981.
41. Liu IY, White L, LaCroix AZ: The association between age-related macular degeneration and lens opacities in the aged. Am J Public Health 79:765–769, 1989.

42. Klein R, Klein BE, Wang Q, et al: Is age-related maculopathy associated with cataracts? Arch Ophthalmol 112:191–196, 1994.
43. Pollack A, Marcovich A, Bukelman A, et al: Age-related macular degeneration after extracapsular cataract extraction with intraocular lens implantation. Ophthalmology 103:1546–1554, 1996.
44. van der Schaft TL, Mooy CM, de Brujin WC, et al: Increased prevalence of disciform macular degeneration after cataract extraction with implantation of an intraocular lens. Br J Ophthalmol 78:441–445, 1994.
45. Seddon J, Hankinson S, Speizer F, et al: A prospective study of smoking and age-related macular degeneration. [Abstract] Am J Epidemiol 241:136, 1995.
46. Christen WG, Glynn RJ, Manson JE, et al: A prospective study of cigarette smoking and risk of age-related macular degeneration in men. JAMA 276:1147–1151, 1996.
47. Vinding T, Appleyard M, Nyboe J, et al: Risk factor analysis for atrophic and exudative age-related macular degeneration: An epidemiologic study of 1000 aged individuals. Acta Ophthalmol 70:66–72, 1992.
48. Klein R, Klein BEK, Linton KLP, et al: The Beaver Dam Eye Study: The relation of age-related maculopathy to smoking. Am J Epidemiol 137:190–200, 1993.
49. Holz FG, Wolfensberger TJ, Piguet B, et al: Bilateral macular drusen in age-related degeneration. Ophthalmology 101:1522–1528, 1994.
50. Smith W, Mitchell P, Leeder SR: Smoking and age-related maculopathy. The Blue Mountains Eye Study. Arch Ophthalmol 114:1518–1523, 1996.
51. Vingerling JR, Hofman A, Grobbee DE, et al: Age-related macular degeneration and smoking: The Rotterdam Study. Arch Ophthalmol 114:1193–1196, 1996.
52. Kahn HA, Leibowitz HM, Ganley JP, et al: The Framingham Eye Study II: Association of ophthalmic pathology with single variables previously measured in the Framingham Heart Study. Am J Epidemiol 106:33–41, 1977.
53. Hirvela H, Luukinen H, Laara E, et al: Risk factors of age-related maculopathy in a population 70 years of age or older. Ophthalmology 103:871–877, 1996.
54. Pauleikhoff D, Wormald RP, Wright L, et al: Macular disease in an elderly population. Ger J Ophthalmol 1:12–15, 1992.
55. West SK, Rosenthal FS, Bressler NM, et al: Exposure to sunlight and other risk factors for age-related macular degeneration. Arch Ophthalmol 107:875–879, 1989.
56. Vingerling JR, Dielemans I, Bots ML, et al: Age-related macular degeneration is associated with atherosclerosis: The Rotterdam Study. Am J Epidemiol 142:404–409, 1995.
57. Goldberg J, Flowerdew G, Smith E, et al: Factors associated with age-related macular degeneration: An analysis of data from the first National Health and Nutrition Examination Survey. Am J Epidemiol 128:700–710, 1988.
58. Klein R, Klein BEK, Franke T: The relationship of cardiovascular disease and its risk factors to age-related maculopathy. Ophthalmology 100:406–414, 1993.
59. Vinding T: Age-related macular degeneration: An epidemiological study of 1000 elderly individuals. With reference to prevalence, funduscopic findings, visual impairment and risk factors. Acta Ophthalmol Scand 217 Suppl:1–32, 1995.
60. Sperduto RD, Hiller R: Systemic hypertension and age-related macular degeneration in the Framingham Eye Study. Arch Ophthalmol 104:216, 1986.
61. Delaney WV, Oates RP: Senile macular degeneration: A preliminary study. Ann Ophthalmol 14:21–24, 1982.
62. Vidaurri JS, Peter J, Halfon ST, et al: Association between drusen and some of the risk factors for coronary artery disease. Ophthalmologica 188:243–247, 1984.
63. Macular Photocoagulation Study Group: Risk factors for choroidal neovascularization in the second eye of patients with juxtafoveal or subfoveal choroidal neovascularization secondary to age-related macular degeneration. Arch Ophthalmol 151:741–747, 1997.
64. Albrink MJ, Fasanella RM: Serum lipids in patients with senile macular degeneration. Am J Ophthalmol 55:709–713, 1963.
65. Landolfo V, DeSimone S: Senile macular degeneration and alteration of the metabolism of the lipids. Ophthalmologica Basel 177:248–253, 1978.
66. Sanders TAB, Haines AP, Wormald R, et al: Essential fatty acids, plasma cholesterol, and fat-soluble vitamins in subjects with age-related maculopathy and matched control subjects. Am J Clin Nutr 57:428–433, 1993.
67. Klein R, Klein BEK, Jensen SC: The relation of cardiovascular disease and its risk factors to the 5-year incidence of age-related maculopathy: The Beaver Dam Eye Study. Ophthalmology 104:1804–1812, 1997.
68. Seddon J, Ajani U, Sperduto R, et al: Dietary fat intake and age-related macular degeneration. Invest Ophthalmol Vis Sci 25:2003, 1994.
69. Mares-Perlman JA, Brady WE, Klein R: Dietary fat and age-related maculopathy. Arch Ophthalmol 113:743–748, 1995.
70. Friedman E: Dietary fat and age-related maculopathy. Arch Ophthalmol 114:235–236, 1996.
71. Klein R, Klein BEK, Moss SE: Diabetes, hyperglycemia and age-related maculopathy: The Beaver Dam Eye Study. Ophthalmology 99:1527–1534, 1992.
72. Klein BEK, Klein R, Jensen SC, et al: Are sex hormones associated with age-related maculopathy in women? The Beaver Dam Eye Study. Trans Am Ophthalm Soc 92:285–289, 1994.
73. Smith W, Mitchell P, Wang JJ: Gender estrogen, hormone replacement and age-related macular degeneration: Results from the Blue Mountains Eye Study. Aus N Z J Ophthalmol 25 (Suppl 1):S13–S15, 1997.
74. Vingerling JR, Dielemans I, Witteman JC, et al: Macular degeneration and early menopause: A case-control study. BMJ 310:1570–1571, 1995.
75. Taylor HR, West S, Munoz B, et al: The long-term effects of visible light on the eye. Arch Ophthalmol 110:99–104, 1992.
76. Cruickshanks KJ, Klein R, Klein BEK: Sunlight and age-related macular degeneration: The Beaver Dam Eye Study. Arch Ophthalmol 111:514–518, 1993.
77. Darzins P, Mitchell P, Heller RF: Sun exposure and age-related macular degeneration: An Australian case-control study. Ophthalmology 104:770–776, 1997.
78. Hung S, Seddon JM: The relationship between nutritional factors and age-related macular degeneration. *In* Bendich A, Deckelbaum R (eds): Preventive Medicine: The Comprehensive Guide for Health Professionals. Totowa, NJ, Humana Press, 1997, pp 245–265.
79. Seddon JM, Hennekens CH: Vitamins, minerals and macular degeneration. Arch Ophthalmol 112:176–179, 1994.
80. Sperduto RD, Ferris FL, Kurinij N: Do we have a nutritional treatment for age-related cataract or macular degeneration? Arch Ophthalmol 108:1403–1405, 1990.
81. Anderson RE, Rapp LM, Wiegand RD: Lipid peroxidation and retinal degeneration. Curr Eye Res 3:223–227, 1984.
82. Anderson RE, Kretzer FL, Rapp LM: Free radicals and ocular disease. Adv Exp Med Biol 366:73–86, 1994.
83. Young RW: Pathophysiology of age-related macular degeneration. Surv Ophthalmol 31:291–306, 1987.
84. Mares Perlman JA, Brady WE, Klein R, et al: Association of zinc and antioxidant nutrients with age-related maculopathy. Arch Ophthalmol 114:991–997, 1996.
85. West S, Vitale S, Hallfrisch J, et al: Are antioxidants or supplements protective for age-related macular degeneration? Arch Ophthalmol 112:222–227, 1994.
86. Newsome DA, Swartz M, Leone NC, et al: Oral zinc in macular degeneration. Arch Ophthalmol 106:192–198, 1988.
87. Stur M, Titti M, Reitner A, et al: Oral zinc and the second eye in age-related macular degeneration. Invest Ophthalmol Vis Sci 37:1225–1235, 1996.
88. Age-Related Eye Disease Study Group: Age-Related Eye Disease Study (AREDS) Phase II Manual of Operations. Potomac, MD, The Emmes Corporation, 1992.
89. Ajani UA, Willett W, Miller D, et al: Alcohol consumption and neovascular age-related macular degeneration. [Abstract] Am J Epidemiol 138:646, 1993.
90. Obisesan TO, Hirsch R, Kosoko O, et al: Moderate wine consumption is associated with decreased odds of developing age-related macular degeneration in NHANES-1. J Am Geriatr Soc 46:1–7, 1998.
91. Ritter LL, Klein R, Klein BE, et al: Alcohol use and age-related maculopathy in the Beaver Dam Eye Study. Am J Ophthalmol 120:190–196, 1995.
92. Smith W, Mitchell P: Alcohol intake and age-related maculopathy. Am J Ophthalmol 122:743–745, 1996.
93. Seddon JM, Ajani UA, Mitchell BD: Familial aggregation of age-related maculopathy. Am J Ophthalmol 123:199–206, 1997.
93a. Seddon J, Cho E, Stamfer M, et al: Prospective study of alcohol consumption and the risk of age-related macular degeneration. Invest Ophthalmol Vis Sci 40:S568, 1999.
94. Silvestri G, Johnston PB, Hughes AE: Is genetic predisposition an important risk factor in age-related macular degeneration? Eye 8:564–568, 1994.

95. Piguet B, Wells JA, Palmvang IB, et al: Age-related Bruch's membrane change: A clinical study of the relative role of heredity and environment. Br J Ophthalmol 77:400–403, 1993.
96. Meyers SM, Greene T, Gutman FA: A twin study of age-related macular degeneration. Am J Ophthalmol 120:757–766, 1995.
97. Klein ML, Mauldin WM, Stoumbos VD: Heredity and age-related macular degeneration: Observations in monozygotic twins. Arch Ophthalmol 112:932–937, 1994.
98. Heiba IM, Elston RC, Klein BEK, et al: Sibling correlations and segregation analysis of age-related maculopathy: The Beaver Dam Eye Study. Genet Epidemiol 11:51–67, 1994.
99. Allikmets R, Singh N, Sun H, et al: A photoreceptor cell-specific ATP-binding transporter gene (ABCR) is mutated in recessive Stargardt macular dystrophy. Nat Genet 124:331–343, 1997.
100. Allikmets R, Shroyer NF, Singh N, et al: Mutation of the Stargardt disease gene (ABCR) in age-related macular degeneration. Science 277:1805–1807, 1997.
101. De La Paz MA, Pericak-Vance MA, Lennon F, et al: Exclusion of TIMP3 as a candidate locus in age-related macular degeneration. Invest Ophthalmol Vis Sci 38:1060–1065, 1997.
102. Seddon JM, De La Paz M, Clements K, et al: No association between apolipoprotein E and advanced age-related macular degeneration. Am J Hum Genet S59:A388, 1996.
103. Weber BHF, Vogt G, Pruett RC, et al: Mutations in the tissue inhibitor of metalloproteinases-3 (TIMP3) in patients with Sorsby's fundus dystrophy. Nat Genet 8:352–356, 1994.
104. Souied EH, Benlian P, Amouyel P, et al: The E4 allele of the apolipoprotein E gene as a potential protective factor for exudative age-related macular degeneration. Am J Ophthalmol 125:353–359, 1998.
105. Sun H, Nathans J: Stargardt's ABCR is localized to the disc membrane of retinal rod outer segments. Nat Genet 17:15–16, 1997.
106. Seddon J, Bernstein P, Lewis R, et al: Evaluation of the association between phenotypic characteristics and ABCR genetic mutations in age-related macular degeneration. Invest Ophthalmol Vis Sci 39:S962, 1998.

CHAPTER 48

Epidemiology of Glaucoma

M. Roy Wilson

The ultimate goal in the management of a chronic disease such as primary open-angle glaucoma (POAG) is to design intervention programs that can prevent, or at least control, the debilitating outcomes associated with the disease. This requires a linking of knowledge derived from epidemiology to that derived from the basic and clinical sciences. The major contributions from the basic and clinical sciences are relatively clear-cut: a better understanding of the pathophysiologic mechanisms in the development and progression of the disease and treatment strategies aimed at influencing disease progression. Most of the other glaucoma-related chapters in this book are devoted to these topics.

Until recently, contributions to glaucoma knowledge derived from epidemiology were not widely recognized. Implicit in the definition of "epidemiology" is the fact that disease is not randomly distributed throughout a population; instead, the frequency differs among subgroups. Knowledge of this uneven distribution, and of the factors that influence this distribution, may provide valuable clues as to what factors are important in pathogenesis and development. Epidemiology is also an analytic tool that can be used to aid judgments about the relevance of such factors in clinical decision making.

The contributions of epidemiology to a better understanding of glaucoma are thus inexorably linked to contributions from the basic and clinical sciences. This chapter provides a synthesis of the current state of the epidemiology-derived knowledge of POAG. However, glaucoma epidemiology is still in its infancy, and much remains unknown or controversial. Each major topic thus includes a discussion of what is not yet understood.

Primary Open-Angle Glaucoma as a Public Health Problem

From reviews of various sources of data, it can be estimated that 2.25 million Americans 40 years of age and older have POAG.[1] Worldwide, about 104,650,000 people have elevated intraocular pressure (intraocular pressure [IOP] >21 mm Hg) and that 2,400,000 develop POAG yearly. Between 84,000 and 116,000 persons are estimated to be bilaterally blind (visual acuity <20/200) from POAG in the United States. This figure increases to more than 3 million globally.[2]

The societal costs of these figures are staggering. The estimated expenditures for glaucoma treatment total at least $1.6 billion for direct costs alone. Income transferred from the federal government to assist persons blind from glaucoma via a number of mechanisms (e.g., Social Security disability income, automatic Medicare and Medicaid eligibility, and income tax credits) amount to at least $1.05 billion per year.[3] Indirect costs, including lost earnings and requirements for caretaking services because of blindness, are difficult to estimate but are undoubtedly substantial.

Even so, the entire impact of the problem of glaucoma from a public health perspective is not fully appreciated. Remarkably little attention has been focused on issues related to having the disease or to treating it. Thus, information related to the possible psychologic effects of having a potentially blinding chronic disease, the qualitative functional loss associated with diminished visual fields, or the debilitating side effects of treatment is scarce. A clinical trial assessing quality of life in persons undergoing initial surgical versus medical treatment for glaucoma is ongoing (1998). Results of this trial will likely address some of these important issues.

Prevalence

Interpretation of prevalence studies must consider the various methodologies and definitions of glaucoma used. Any prevalence study should meet a number of basic requirements: (1) there should be a well-defined population to which the prevalence estimate corresponds, (2) every effort should be made to examine all of the defined population or a specified sample of the defined population, (3) the proportion of the population or of the sample that was actually examined should be reported, (4) if sampling is used, sampled subjects should represent the population, with no subgroup systematically excluded from examination, and (5) the diagnostic criteria for glaucoma should be specified and consistently applied. Studies based on self-selected or small nonrepresentative segments of the population are particularly susceptible to bias. A population-based study design is preferable. Yet, even among studies using this design, methodologic shortcomings are often present, and study results must be compared with caution. Major differences among studies have been the diagnostic criteria used for glaucoma and the thoroughness of case-finding. Studies have used elevated IOPs, optic nerve pathology, and visual-field defects, either singularly or in various combinations, to define glaucoma. More recent studies have uniformly required the presence of visual-field defects. However, study criteria for deciding which subjects undergo visual-field examinations have differed. Ideally, this diagnostic test should be offered to all study subjects.

Historically, population-based glaucoma prevalence surveys performed in Ferndale (Wales),[4] Dalby (Sweden),[5] and Framingham, Massachusetts,[6] have often been cited and deserve mention. Glaucoma prevalences were 0.47% (Ferndale), 0.86% (Dalby), and 1.6% (Framingham). The diagnostic criteria for POAG in the two European studies were based on abnormal disc cupping and loosely defined visual-field defects, whereas the Framingham study relied solely on rigorously defined visual-field criteria. Thus, the Welsh and Swedish studies would have excluded subjects with high IOPs and field defects only; conversely, subjects not suspected of having glaucoma did not undergo perimetric examinations in the Framingham study and would have been excluded from an opportunity to be diagnosed as having glaucoma. These methodologic flaws would be expected to underestimate true prevalence.

More recently, population-based prevalence studies have been performed in Tierp, Sweden (1984 to 1986),[7] Baltimore (1985 to 1988),[8] Beaver Dam, Wisconsin (1987 to 1988),[9] County Roscommon, Ireland (1988 to 1990),[10] Japan (1988 to 1989),[11] St. Lucia, West Indies (1985 to 1986),[12] Barbados, West Indies (1988 to 1989),[13] Rotterdam, The Netherlands (1991 to 1993),[14] and Blue Mountains, Australia (1992 to 1993).[15] Table 48–1 summarizes some of the major features and the prevalence results obtained. The diagnostic criteria used in these studies differed slightly, but all required evidence of glaucomatous damage by disc cupping or visual-field abnormalities and were independent of IOP. Of considerable interest is the finding of much higher POAG prevalences among the black populations of the West Indies.[12, 13] Intermarriages among different racial and ethnic groups have occurred much less frequently in the West Indies than in the United States. Thus, the hypothesis of an inherently higher rate of disease among the more genetically homogeneous black populations of the West Indies must be considered. Alternatively, the differences in prevalence among these black populations may be a result of differences in study design.

Population-based data on POAG prevalence in other racial populations are few and of variable quality. One of the better-designed studies was a nationwide survey conducted throughout seven regions of Japan.[11] However, a low participation rate of only 51% was a major limitation of this study, and the potential for selection bias must be considered. This

TABLE 48–1. **Population-Based Glaucoma Surveys**

	N	Age Range (years)	Prevalence (%)	Ethnicity
United States				
Baltimore, MD[8]	5308	≥40	1.7	White American
			5.6	African American
Beaver Dam, WI[9]	4926	43–84	2.1	White American
Europe				
Tierp, Sweden[7]	760	65–74	5.7*	White Swedish
County Roscommon, Ireland[10]	2186	≥50	1.9	White Irish
Rotterdam, The Netherlands[14]	3062	≥55	1.1	White Dutch
Caribbean				
St. Lucia[12]	1679	≥30	8.8	Black West Indian
Barbados[13]	4314	≥40	7.0	Black West Indian
Asia/Other				
Japan[11]	8126	≥40	2.6	Japanese
Australia[15]	3654	≥49	3.0	White Australian

*Included a large population of subjects with diagnosis of pseudo exfoliation glaucoma.

study classified the various types of glaucoma and found prevalences of 2.62% for POAG (including normal tension glaucoma) and 0.34% for primary angle-closure glaucoma (PACG). This prevalence for PACG is much lower than that reported from among other Asian populations.[16–18] One well-performed population-based study in the Hövsgöl Province of Northern Mongolia found a prevalence of 1.4% for PACG and only 0.5% for POAG.[19] These results underscore the fact that Asia is composed of heterogeneous groups of people, and one cannot use results obtained from specific regions to generalize about all Asians.

A population-based general ophthalmic prevalence survey among Alaska's Northwestern Eskimos found a glaucoma prevalence of 0.65%, but most were of the angle-closure variety.[20] This study suffered from the fact that the diagnosis of open-angle glaucoma was based on the tangent screen visual-field defects in the presence of either an elevated IOP (>21 mm Hg) or a cup:disc ratio of more than 0.5. Because a substantial proportion of persons with glaucoma present with normal IOPs and many have cup:disc ratios of less than 0.5, the reported prevalence of POAG (0.06%) was undoubtedly underestimated. Nonetheless, it is probably safe to conclude that the prevalence of POAG in this population is very low.

Reliable population-based data among Hispanics and among Africans are lacking. Although data from the West Indies[12, 13] and from Baltimore[8] would suggest a very high POAG prevalence for Africans, anecdotal evidence indicates that prevalences among the various regions are extremely wide—even among various tribes within the same region of Africa.

Incidence

Prevalence data do not permit estimates of risk of disease over time, nor do they permit etiologic inference. Incidence data provide a direct measure of the rate at which individuals in a given population develop disease and can thus provide a basis for statements about probability or risk of disease. Despite their desirability, reliable POAG incidence data are scarce.

Studies attempting to measure open-angle glaucoma incidence can be divided into two types: (1) those that are population-based and (2) those that target a specific "high-risk" subpopulation. Because of the relatively low incidence, large cohorts and long follow-up periods are necessary to obtain a sufficient number of newly diagnosed glaucoma cases to ensure valid estimates. These study-design limitations greatly increase the difficulty of conducting true population-based incidence studies; only a few such studies have been attempted.

Both the Barbados Eye Study[13] and the Baltimore Eye Study[8] were designed to yield incidence data, and final results are expected to be published in 1998. Preliminary results from Barbados were presented at the 1997 Annual Meeting of the Association for Research in Vision and Ophthalmology; a 4-year incidence of 2.2% (95% CI: 1.7 to 2.8) was reported for the black West Indian population. Although issues related to study design preclude making a direct comparison, a glaucoma annual incidence of between 0.19% and 0.24% was reported in the white population of Dalby, Sweden.[21]

Because of difficulties in performing population-based incidence studies for a disease with low incidence, various investigators have attempted to determine incidence rates for glaucoma in selected high-risk subpopulations. Such was the case with the Collaborative Glaucoma Study,[22] which was a prospective study conducted in five centers during a 13-year period to identify factors that influence the development of glaucomatous visual-field defects. The sample consisted of relatives of patients with open-angle glaucoma augmented with a group of persons with IOPs greater than 20 mm Hg. Glaucomatous visual-field defects developed in 1.7% of the 5886 eyes included in the analysis, with the last defect detected at 7 years of follow-up. Annual incidence rates can be calculated from the data and range from 0.25 to 0.54%. Higher incidence rates were obtained during the latter years of follow-up, but the denominators, representing eligible persons, were small, and these estimates are thus unstable. Notably, mortality tables were constructed for eyes with different levels of IOPs. The 5-year survival (free of visual-field defects) rate for eyes with IOPs greater than or equal to 20 mm Hg was 93.3%, whereas it was 98.5% for eyes with lower IOPs.

In a number of other studies, cohorts of subjects with higher-than-normal IOPs were followed for variable time periods.[23–26] Their data do not permit the calculation of incidence rates because cases lost to follow-up were not reported or appropriate analytic methods were not used. Comparison of the results of these studies is difficult because of varying subject inclusion criteria and varying diagnostic criteria employed by their multiple investigators. The major finding of this entire group of studies is twofold: (1) visual-field defects develop infrequently, even in subjects with higher-than-normal IOPs, and (2) the higher the baseline IOP, the greater the risk of subsequently developing visual-field defects. The currently ongoing Ocular Hypertension Treatment Study is expected to yield reliable data on POAG incidence for persons with various levels of elevated IOP.

The lack of good population-based incidence data has prompted the derivation of incidence estimates from age-specific prevalence data.[27] Such estimates are regarded as gross approximations, and their use is usually restricted to certain specific purposes such as the planning of epidemiologic studies.

Risk Factors for Disease Development

Epidemiologic studies have identified subgroups of people with high or low prevalences of POAG. Differences in occurrence of disease among subgroups lead to hypotheses that can be investigated through more searching analytic studies. Ultimately, the goal is to identify risk factors and design intervention trials to ascertain whether modification of such factors reduces the amount of disease. Some factors—for example, age, gender, race, and family history—are not amenable to modification. If they are major determinants of disease, however, their identification would be useful in developing screening strategies.

It would be desirable to be able to predict glaucoma risk potential based on an individual's specific characteristics, traits, and habits. Unfortunately, our knowledge in glaucoma epidemiology is yet inadequate for such prediction. Aside from the important role of elevated IOP in disease development, much of what is known of factors related to glaucoma risk is in the realm of demographic characteristics and broad categories of systemic factors. Currently, the data concerning the possible relevance of personal habits, general toxic exposures, or eye exposures to the onset of glaucoma are minimal.

There is general agreement that IOP is the most important known risk factor for glaucoma development. Evidence clearly indicates that increased IOP can cause glaucoma. Experimentally induced high IOP in animals results in typical glaucomatous cupping.[28, 29] Acute angle closure and many cases of unilateral secondary glaucoma support a cause-effect relationship between high IOP and glaucomatous damage. Even at normal IOP levels, asymmetric IOP has been noted to correlate with asymmetric cupping and field loss, with greater damage occurring on the side with higher pressure.[30, 31]

Additional support is obtained from population surveys that have shown an increase in prevalence of POAG with increasing levels of IOP.[4, 5, 16, 30] However, many subjects with elevated IOP do not have glaucoma, and follow-ups of subjects with elevated IOP have demonstrated that they may never develop glaucoma. Thus, elevated IOP is frequently not sufficient and is, in fact, not a necessary condition for glaucomatous damage. Population surveys have consistently demonstrated that one-third to one-half of subjects did not have elevated IOP at the time of diagnosis.[5, 6, 8, 9, 10] Even if elevated IOP could probably have been demonstrated for most of these subjects had multiple testings been performed, a proportion would have remained in which IOP was never elevated.

The fact that some eyes with high IOP do not develop glaucomatous damage and some eyes with low IOP suffer definite glaucomatous damage indicates that other factors contribute to pathogenesis. Other ocular factors that have been implicated as risk factors include myopia, large cup:disc ratio, asymmetric cupping, and disc hemorrhages.

Data regarding the possible role of myopia are conflicting. A number of studies have demonstrated an association between myopia and POAG.[32, 33] However, these studies were clinic-based studies, and the potential for selection bias must be considered, because persons with refractive errors are more likely to seek eye care and have a higher probability of being diagnosed with glaucoma. Additional studies are necessary to clarify the relationship between myopia and POAG before this factor can unequivocally be considered a glaucoma risk factor.

Discs with large cup:disc ratios also tend to be larger with proportionately more neural rim tissue.[34] Thus, whether larger cup:disc ratios, per se, predispose to glaucomatous damage is unclear. An enlarged cup:disc ratio, as well as asymmetric cupping, may be a sign of early disease, however. From a practical standpoint, subjects with "suspicious" discs must be observed closely for development of signs of clinically significant glaucoma, and the question of whether these disc parameters are true risk factors may be moot.

The transient nature of disc hemorrhages makes it difficult to assess the importance of this factor for subsequent glaucomatous damage. Fairly consistent evidence indicates a poorer prognosis in glaucomatous eyes with disc hemorrhages compared with those without hemorrhages.[35, 36] Disc hemorrhages suggest microinfarctions and thus vascular pathology at the anterior optic nerve head. It seems reasonable to assume that this same pathophysiologic process may place a nonglaucomatous eye at increased risk for glaucomatous damage. Although disc hemorrhages have been shown to precede retinal nerve fiber layer defects, glaucomatous changes of the optic nerve head, and glaucomatous visual-field defects, it is not known how frequently this occurs.[37–40] An extreme view, one that is not well supported or accepted, proposes that disc hemorrhages precede all cases of open-angle glaucoma.[41]

Good evidence supports race, age, and family history as nonocular factors related to glaucoma risk. As indicated earlier, blacks have a disproportionately high prevalence of POAG. Although race-specific incidence data are not yet available, it is reasonable to assume that incidence data will reflect a similar racial disparity. Precisely why blacks are at increased risk of developing glaucoma is not known. Higher IOPs and large cup:disc ratios among blacks have been suggested as possible causal mechanisms. However, data conflict as to whether blacks have higher IOPs than do whites,[42, 43] and as discussed previously, the relevance of larger cup:disc ratios is uncertain.

Nearly every population-based study has demonstrated that the prevalence of glaucoma increases with advancing age.[5–15] Prevalence estimates have generally been three to eight times higher in the oldest age groups as compared with persons in their 40s. Further, the Collaborative Glaucoma Study identified age as the major predictor of glaucoma incidence.[22] As with race, the exact causal mechanisms are unknown, and underlying susceptibility factors must be investigated. The higher IOPs noted with increased age in most studies were not found among the Japanese.[11] Yet, glaucoma prevalence increased with age, suggesting that the optic nerves of the elderly are more susceptible to damage for reasons other than just higher IOPs.

There is little doubt that familial factors are important in the underlying susceptibility to POAG. Several ocular parameters associated with POAG, such as IOP and size of cup, are known to be influenced by heredity.[38, 44] Relatives of glaucoma patients would thus be expected to exhibit abnormalities of these parameters more often and to more likely be diagnosed as having glaucoma. Accurate estimates of the exact risk of POAG in relatives are lacking, however. Most studies that have attempted to determine this risk had the potential for selection and recall bias because of incomplete ascertainment of relatives.

Juvenile-onset glaucoma has been traced over generations,[45, 46] and an autosomal dominant inheritance pattern has been found.[46] Genetic linkage analysis has successfully identified the location of genes for many simple mendelian disorders, including some associated with glaucoma, such as juvenile open-angle glaucoma[46, 47] and Axenfeld-Rieger's syndrome.[48] Although twin studies have confirmed a genetic influence in POAG,[49] a definite mendelian inheritance pattern has not been established.

The genetic factors influencing POAG appear to be multifactorial and complex. Recently, glaucoma was associated with one of three mutations found in a gene encoding a trabecular meshwork protein (TIGR).[50] It is believed that these mutations account for approximately 3% of POAG cases. The search for other genetic markers associated with

POAG promises to be an intensive area of investigation for the near future.

Broad categories of systemic factors constitute the other major nonocular area of information on POAG risk. Diabetes,[51] systemic hypertension,[52] and various other vascular abnormalities such as migraines[53] have been implicated as risk factors for glaucoma. Much of the data regarding possible associations between these factors and glaucoma are contradictory, however.

Evidence that any of these disorders is a glaucoma risk factor is perhaps strongest for diabetes. The Baltimore Eye Survey did not detect an association between diabetes and glaucoma overall but did find an association among persons in whom glaucoma had been diagnosed prior to the survey examination.[54] This finding suggested selection bias, because a person with diabetes is more likely to be in the health care system and thus to have glaucoma detected. The Blue Mountain Eye Study explored the possible relationship between diabetes and glaucoma and differed from the Baltimore Eye Study in that fasting plasma glucose levels, in addition to historical information, were used in the ascertainment of diabetes.[55] This study found a substantial and consistent association between diabetes and glaucoma.

Although the evidence that systemic hypertension is a risk factor for glaucoma is not as strong as that for diabetes, the hypothesis that microcirculatory effects on the optic disc may lead to increased glaucoma susceptibility is biologically plausible. The Rotterdam Study reported an association of systemic hypertension with high-tension glaucoma but not with normal-tension glaucoma.[14] The Baltimore Eye Survey reported modest, positive associations of increased systolic and diastolic blood pressure with POAG, but the 95% confidence intervals of the odds ratio for these associations included 1.00, the value of no association. However, lower perfusion pressure (blood pressure − IOP) was strongly associated with an increased prevalence of POAG.[56] Although not yet clearly documented, these results suggest that POAG may be associated with a change in factors related to ocular blood flow.

Though the data conflict, migraine and peripheral vasospasm may be important in the development of some cases of glaucoma, particularly those in which IOP is in the normal or low range.[57] Investigations of other systemic factors for association with POAG have been scant, and the results have been inconclusive. One interesting observation has been that among Japanese, IOP has not been found to increase with age as it does in Western populations.[58] One explanation for this apparent discrepancy is that IOP is related to body build, and that Japanese typically do not get obese with age as do many Americans and Europeans. Another interesting finding has been the relationship between lean body mass and increased prevalence of POAG among the participants of the Barbados Eye Study.[59] These results suggest that anthromorphologic considerations may warrant further study.

Data conflict as to whether POAG is more frequently associated with men or with women. A higher prevalence among women was reported in Dalby (Sweden),[5] a higher prevalence among men in Tierp (Sweden),[7] Framingham,[6] and Barbados,[13] and no difference in St. Lucia,[12] Wales,[4] Baltimore,[8] and Beaver Dam.[9]

Treatment Issues

Thus far, treatments for POAG have focused exclusively on lowering IOP. The efficacy of medications, laser, and incisional surgery in lowering IOP has been extensively documented. The value of these treatments, however, in reducing the occurrence or progression of visual-field damage has been questioned.[60]

Whether elevated IOP alone, in the absence of glaucomatous damage, should be treated is highly controversial. Published trials of medical versus no treatment of eyes with elevated pressure have yielded conflicting results.[61–63] The Ocular Hypertension Treatment Study, a multicenter clinical trial, was thus designed to definitively resolve this issue and is currently in the follow-up stage. Despite uncertainties surrounding the treatment of IOP alone, it is generally well accepted that patients with definite glaucoma, regardless of disease stage, should be treated. An overwhelming amount of evidence indicates that prognosis depends largely on the level of IOP. A number of studies have suggested that lowering IOP decreases the rate of visual-field damage progression.[64–66] Improvement of optic disc and visual-field appearance and changes in retinal nerve fiber layer thickness have even been correlated with the degree of IOP reduction.[67, 68] Skeptics remain who are not convinced of the efficacy of lowering IOP in retarding progressive glaucomatous damage, however. This skepticism is partly based on the fact that the benefits of lowering IOP have not been demonstrated through controlled, randomized, clinical trials. Thus, the Early Manifest Glaucoma Trial, a study designed to investigate the effectiveness of medical treatment of early open-angle glaucoma in influencing progression of visual-field damage, is under way in Sweden.

Screening Issues

Guidelines for determining whether a disease is screenable have been well summarized. According to the United States Congressional Office of Technology Assessment, a screenable disease must satisfactorily address the following major issues:[69]

1. The disease sought must have a recognizable latent or early stage, during which persons with the disease can easily be identified before symptoms develop.
2. There must be an accepted and effective treatment that must be more effective when initiated in the early (asymptomatic) stage than when begun in the later, symptomatic stages of the disease.
3. There must be an appropriate, acceptable, and reasonably accurate screening test.

At first glance, glaucoma is a strong candidate disease for screening programs. It is a leading cause of blindness and consequent disability; it is asymptomatic in the early stages; and though not unequivocably proven, treatment is probably more effective if begun early in the disease process. Unfortunately, an objective assessment of the most commonly used techniques for screening demonstrates that none of them is effective.

Tonometry has been used as a screening test for glaucoma for more than 40 years. However, we have yet to identify a set of tonometric criteria that adequately classify persons in terms of their disease status. Data from a number of studies have demonstrated the futility of using the widely accepted cutoff of 21 mm Hg for screening purposes.[70] Moreover, no matter what IOP level is chosen, the balance of sensitivity and specificity is unacceptable.

Ophthalmoscopic evaluation of the optic nerve has been proposed as a screening tool, but this technique suffers from poor reliability, the need for trained personnel, and the possible need to dilate the pupils for adequate visualization. Technologic advances in optic nerve imaging permit more objective measurements of various optic disc parameters,[71] but the high cost and lack of portability of these instruments render their use in large-population screenings impractical.

Visual-field testing with computerized bowl perimetry remains the standard for glaucoma case-finding. Lack of portability and the extended time required for patient instruction and testing limit its use for general-population screenings. Smaller, faster machines are currently being manufactured, and alternative perimetric devices such as Oculokinetic Perimetry[72] and laptop computer techniques[73] have been introduced. These techniques require validation and evaluation of their utility in population-based screening settings.

Another issue to consider is that the prevalence of glaucoma in the unselected, general population is relatively low. Thus, the predictive power of a positive test result will be low. In other words, only a small proportion of those identified as glaucomatous by the screening test—even with a highly valid and suitable test—will actually have the disease; the remainder will nonetheless undergo costly, unproductive diagnostic work-ups. The higher the prevalence of disease, the more likely it is that a positive test result will predict the disease. Thus, focus has gradually shifted from widespread population-based screening to case-finding in high-risk individuals to obtain a high yield of true cases.

Summary

Much of our knowledge of glaucoma epidemiology has come from population-based prevalence studies. These studies have documented the relatively common occurrence of higher-than-normal IOP without evidence of glaucomatous damage, glaucomatous damage with normal IOP, and the influence of age and race on disease prevalence. Research is now focusing on determining glaucoma incidence, investigating possible risk factors for disease development, and examining factors that influence glaucoma progression and outcome. As epidemiologic data addressing these issues are collected, our understanding of glaucoma will grow and will greatly influence our clinical management of this blinding disease.

REFERENCES

1. Wilson MR: Primary open-angle glaucoma: Magnitude of the problem in the United States. J Glaucoma 1:64, 1992.
2. World Development Report 1993: Investing in Health. The International Bank for Reconstruction and Development/The World Bank. New York, Oxford University, 1993.
3. Tielsch JM: Therapy for glaucoma: Costs and consequences in glaucoma and therapy. *In* Ball SS, Franklin RM (eds): Transactions of New Orleans Academy of Ophthalmology. Amsterdam, Kugler, 1993.
4. Hollows FC, Graham PA: Intraocular pressure, glaucoma, and glaucoma suspects in a defined population. Br J Ophthalmol 50:570, 1986.
5. Bengtsson B: The prevalence of glaucoma. Br J Ophthalmol 65:46, 1981.
6. Kahn HA, Milton RC: Revised Framingham Eye Study: Prevalence of glaucoma and diabetic retinopathy. Am J Epidemiol 111:769, 1989.
7. Ekström C: Prevalence of open-angle glaucoma in central Sweden: The Tierp Glaucoma Survey. Acta Ophthalmol Scand 74:107, 1996.
8. Tielsch JM, et al: Racial variations in the prevalence of primary open-angle glaucoma: The Baltimore Eye Survey. JAMA 266:369, 1991.
9. Klein BEK, et al: Prevalence of glaucoma: The Beaver Dam Eye Study. Ophthalmology 99:1499, 1992.
10. Coffey M, et al: Prevalence of glaucoma in the West of Ireland. Br J Ophthalmol 77:17, 1993.
11. Shiose Y, et al: Epidemiology of glaucoma in Japan: A nationwide glaucoma survey. Jpn J Ophthalmol 35:133, 1991.
12. Mason RP, et al: National survey of the prevalence and risk factors of glaucoma in St. Lucia, West Indies. Part I: Prevalence findings. Ophthalmology 65:1363, 1989.
13. Leske MC, et al: The Barbados Eye Study: Prevalence of open-angle glaucoma. Arch Ophthalmol 112:821, 1994.
14. Dielemars I, et al: The prevalence of primary open-angle glaucoma in a population-based study in the Netherlands: The Rotterdam Study. Ophthalmology 101:1851, 1994.
15. Mitchell P, et al: Prevalence of open-angle glaucoma in Australia. Ophthalmology 103:1661, 1996.
16. Guo BK, et al: A survey of ocular disease in a residential district of Shanghai. Chin J Ophthalmol 19:43, 1983.
17. Hu Z, et al: An epidemiologic investigation of glaucoma in Beijing City and Shun-yi County. Chin J Ophthalmol 25:115, 1989.
18. Lim ASM: PACG in Singapore. Aust J Ophthalmol 7:23, 1979.
19. Foster P, et al: Glaucoma in Mongolia: A population-based survey in Hövsgöl Province, Northern Mongolia. Arch Ophthalmol 114:1235, 1996.
20. Arkell SM, et al: The prevalence of glaucoma among Eskimos of Northwest Alaska. Arch Ophthalmol 105:482, 1987.
21. Bengtsson B: Incidence of manifest glaucoma. Br J Ophthalmol 73:483, 1989.
22. Armaly MF, et al: Biostatistical analysis of the Collaborative Glaucoma Study. I: Summary report of the risk factors for glaucomatous visual field defects. Arch Ophthalmol 98:2163, 1980.
23. David R, Livingston DG, Luntz MH: Ocular hypertension—A long-term follow-up of treated and untreated patients. Br J Ophthalmol 61:688, 1977.
24. Hovding G, Aasved H: Prognostic factors in the development of manifest open-angle glaucoma. A long-term follow-up study of hypertensive and normotensive eyes. Acta Ophthalmol (Copenh) 64:601, 1986.
25. Shappert-Kimmijser J: A five-year follow-up of subjects with intraocular pressure of 22–30 mm Hg without anomalies of optic nerve and visual field typical for glaucoma at first investigation. Ophthalmologica 162:289, 1979.
26. Walker WM: Ocular hypertension: Follow-up of 109 cases from 1963 to 1974. Trans Ophthalmol Soc UK 94:525, 1974.
27. Leske MC, Ederer F, Podgor M: Estimating incidence from age-specific prevalence in glaucoma. Am J Epidemiol 113:606, 1981.
28. Gaasterland O, Tanashima T, Kuwabara T: Axoplasmic flow during chronic experimental glaucoma. I: Light and electron microscopic studies of the monkey optic nerve-head during development of glaucomatous cupping. Invest Ophthalmol Vis Sci 17:838, 1978.
29. Quigley HA, Addicks EM: Chronic experimental glaucoma in primates. II: Effect of extended intraocular pressure elevation on optic nerve head and axonal transport. Invest Ophthalmol Vis Sci 19:137, 1980.
30. Cartwright MJ, Anderson DR: Correlation of asymmetric damage with asymmetric intraocular pressure in normal-tension glaucoma (low-tension glaucoma). Arch Ophthalmol 106:898, 1988.
31. Crighton A, et al: Unequal intraocular pressure and its relation to asymmetric visual field defects in low-tension glaucoma. Ophthalmology 46:1312, 1989.
32. Lotufo D, et al: Juvenile glaucoma, race, and refraction. JAMA 261:249, 1989.
33. Perkins ES, Phelps CS: Open-angle glaucoma, ocular hypertension, low tension glaucoma, and refraction. Arch Ophthalmol 100:1464, 1982.
34. Quigley HA, Brown ME, Morrison JD, Drance SM: The size and shape of the optic disc in normal human eyes. Arch Ophthalmol 100:135, 1982.
35. Airaksinen PJ, Tuulonen A: Early glaucoma changes in patients with and without an optic disc hemorrhage. Acta Ophthalmol (Copenh) 62:197, 1984.
36. Shiab ZM, Lee PH, Hay P: The significance of disc hemorrhage in open-angle glaucoma. Ophthalmology 89:211, 1982.

37. Airaksinen PJ, Mustanen E: Optic nerve hemorrhages precede retinal nerve fiber defects in ocular hypertension. Acta Ophthalmol 59:627, 1981.
38. Armaly MF: Genetic determination of cup/disc ratio of the optic nerve. Arch Ophthalmol 78:35, 1967.
39. Drance SM, Gegg IS: Sector hemorrhage—A probable ischemic disc change in chronic simple glaucoma. Can J Ophthalmol 5:137, 1970.
40. Bengtsson SB, Krakau CET: Observations concerning the course of glaucoma. Acta Ophthalmol (Copenh) 67:261, 1989.
41. Krakau T: Disc hemorrhages and the etiology of glaucoma. Acta Ophthalmol (Copenh) 65:31, 1989.
42. Coulehan JL, et al: Racial differences in intraocular tension and glaucoma surgery. Am J Epidemiol 111:759, 1980.
43. Sommer A, et al: Relationship between intraocular pressure and primary open-angle glaucoma among white and black Americans. Arch Ophthalmol 109:1090, 1991.
44. Armaly MF: The genetic determination of ocular pressure in the normal eye. Arch Ophthalmol 78:187, 1967.
45. Dorozynski A: Privacy rules blindside French glaucoma effort. Science 252:369, 1991.
46. Johnson AT, et al: Clinical features and linkage analysis of a family with autosomal dominant juvenile glaucoma. Ophthalmology 100:524, 1993.
47. Sheffield VC, et al: Genetic linkage of familial open-angle glaucoma to chromosome 1q21-q31. Nature Genet 336:164, 1993.
48. Vaux C, et al: Evidence that Rieger syndrome maps to 4q25 or 4q27. J Med Genet 29:256, 1992.
49. Teikari JM: Genetic factors in open-angle (simple and capsular) glaucoma. A population-based twin study. Acta Ophthalmol (Copenh) 65:715, 1987.
50. Stone EM, et al: Identification of a gene that causes primary open-angle glaucoma. Science 275:668, 1997.
51. Katz J, Sommer A: Risk factors for primary open-angle glaucoma. Am J Prev Med 4:110, 1988.
52. Leighton DA, Phillips CI: Systemic blood pressure in glaucoma. Br J Ophthalmol 52:447, 1972.
53. Phelps CD, Corbett JJ: Migraine and low-tension glaucoma: A case-control study. Invest Ophthalmol Vis Sci 26:1105, 1985.
54. Tielsch JM, et al: Diabetes, intraocular pressure and primary open-angle glaucoma in the Baltimore Eye Survey. Ophthalmology 102:48, 1995.
55. Mitchell P, et al: Open-angle glaucoma and diabetes: The Blue Mountains Eye Study, Australia. Ophthalmology 104:712, 1997.
56. Tielsch JM, et al: Hypertension, perfusion pressure, and primary open-angle glaucoma: A population-based assessment. Arch Ophthalmol 113:216, 1995.
57. Corbett JJ, et al: The neurologic evaluation of patients with low-tension glaucoma. Invest Ophthalmol Vis Sci 26:1101, 1985.
58. Shiose Y: Intraocular pressure: New perspectives. Surv Ophthalmol 34:413, 1980.
59. Leske MC, et al: Risk factors for open-angle glaucoma: The Barbados Eye Study. Arch Ophthalmol 113:918, 1995.
60. Eddy DM, Billings J: The quality of medical evidence and medical practice: Report prepared for the National Leadership Commission on Health Care, 1988.
61. Epstein DL, et al: A long-term clinical trial of timolol therapy vs no treatment in the management of glaucoma suspects. Ophthalmology 96:1460, 1989.
62. Kass MA, et al: Topical timolol administration reduces the incidence of glaucomatous damage in ocular hypertensive individuals: A randomized, double-masked, long-term clinical trial. Arch Ophthalmol 107:1590, 1989.
63. Schulzer M, Drance SM, Gordon DR: A comparison of treated and untreated glaucoma suspects. Ophthalmology 98:301, 1991.
64. Mao LK, Stewart WC, Shields MB: Correlation between intraocular pressure control and progressive glaucomatous damage in primary open-angle glaucoma. Am J Ophthalmol 111:51, 1991.
65. Quigley HA, Maumenee AE: Long-term follow-up of treated open-angle glaucoma. Am J Ophthalmol 87:519, 1979.
66. Stewart WC, Chorak RP, Hunt HH, Sethuraman G: Factors associated with visual loss in patients with advanced glaucomatous changes in the optic nerve head. Am J Ophthalmol 116:176, 1993.
67. Katz LJ, et al: Reversible optic disc cupping and visual field improvement in adults with glaucoma. Am J Ophthalmol 107:485, 1989.
68. Sogano S, Tomita G, Kitazawa Y: Changes in retinal nerve fiber layer thickness after reduction of intra-ocular pressure in chronic open-angle glaucoma. Ophthalmology 100:1253, 1993.
69. Foreman J: OTA investigating glaucoma screening for the elderly. Arch Ophthalmol 108:25, 1990.
70. Tielsch JM: Screening for primary open-angle glaucoma: Alternative strategies and future directions. J Glaucoma 1:214, 1992.
71. Weinreb RN, Dreher AW, Billie J: Quantitative assessment of the optic nerve head with the laser tomographic scanner. Int J Ophthalmol 13:25, 1989.
72. Damato BE, et al: A hand-held OKP chart for the screening of glaucoma: Preliminary evaluation. Eye 4:632, 1990.
73. Wu X, et al: Laptop computer perimetry for glaucoma screening. Invest Ophthmol Vis Sci 32 (Suppl):810, 1991.

CHAPTER 49

Epidemiology of Diabetic Retinopathy

Donald S. Fong

Diabetic retinopathy is the leading cause of blindness among Americans between the ages of 20 and 74 years.[1] Blindness is 25 times more common in diabetic than in nondiabetic patients.[2, 3] Knowing the demographic distribution of this disease and understanding the clinical risk factors will direct laboratory research toward solving this immense public health problem and aid us in the management of diabetic patients. This chapter presents descriptive and analytic epidemiologic data for diabetic retinopathy in the United States.

There are two common types of diabetes mellitus: insulin-dependent diabetes mellitus (IDDM) and non–insulin-dependent diabetes mellitus (NIDDM). The latter is more common than IDDM and constitutes 90 to 95% of all diagnosed cases of diabetes in the United States. These two types of diabetes differ in their clinical characteristics, causes, and pathophysiologic basis for disease. The main clinical difference is in their propensity to develop diabetic ketoacidosis in the basal metabolic state; insulin is required in

IDDM to prevent ketoacidosis, whereas in NIDDM, ketoacidosis is unlikely even when the glycemic control is poor. IDDM occurs in younger patients, whereas NIDDM usually presents in older patients. Typically, IDDM presents acutely and manifests the typical symptoms of polyphagia, polydipsia, and polyuria. In contrast, NIDDM is insidious and may be present for years before being diagnosed; in the United States, there may be as many undiagnosed cases of NIDDM as diagnosed cases.

From the ophthalmic standpoint, patients with IDDM have a higher risk of developing severe proliferative diabetic retinopathy (PDR) than those with NIDDM. However, a greater percentage of cases of severe PDR is caused by NIDDM, because the prevalence of NIDDM is so much higher in the general population.[4]

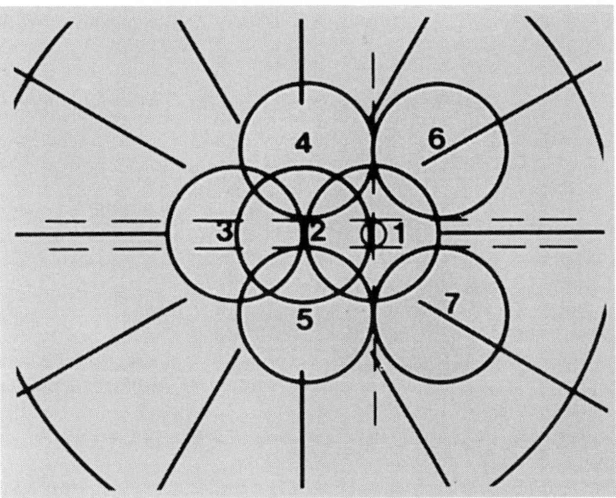

FIGURE 49–1. Seven standard fields of the modified Airlie House classification (shown for a right eye). Field 1 is centered on the optic disc, field 2 is centered on the macula, and field 3 is just temporal to the macula. Fields 4 through 7 are tangential to horizontal lines passing through the upper and lower poles of the disc and to a vertical line passing through its center.

Clinical Studies and Diabetic Retinopathy

Studies of diabetic retinopathy should specify the type of diabetes included in the analysis, because IDDM and NIDDM are different diseases, and risk factors for the development of diabetic retinopathy may be different for each type of diabetes. Studies estimating the prevalence of retinopathy require a sensitive method to detect even the lowest grade of retinopathy. Fundus photography is more sensitive than ophthalmoscopy in detecting the lower grades of retinopathy and should be used in studies of incidence and prevalence.

In one study of the diagnosis of diabetic retinopathy by ophthalmoscopy, general ophthalmologists and retinal specialists had correct diagnosis rates of only 52 and 70%, respectively.[5] The possible diagnoses were normal, maculopathy, background retinopathy, preproliferative retinopathy, proliferative retinopathy, or other. General ophthalmologists did not diagnose PDR in 9% of patients with PDR. In another study with fewer diagnostic possibilities, ophthalmoscopy agreed with fundus photography 85.7% of the time.[6] The disagreements occurred in eyes with less severe forms of retinopathy. When more severe stages of retinopathy are studied, less sensitive but repeated measures may be sufficient.

The fundus photographs should be classified in a clinically useful and standard grading system to ensure validity and enable comparisons between studies. The classification system should be graduated to reflect the progression of retinopathy. One commonly used grading system is the modification of the Airlie House classification of diabetic retinopathy.[7] The Early Treatment of Diabetic Retinopathy Study (ETDRS) used a further modification that may reflect more precisely the natural progression of diabetic retinopathy.[8] Both systems involve grading the retinopathy from photographs of the seven standard fields of the retina (Fig. 49–1).

Definitions

Diabetic retinopathy has been traditionally divided into nonproliferative and proliferative categories. The nonproliferative category can be subdivided into background, transitional, and preproliferative retinopathy. Although there is no evidence to suggest that the characteristics of retinopathy are different between the IDDM and NIDDM forms, it is unusual to see isolated maculopathy in IDDM, a common finding in NIDDM.

The definition of retinopathy has varied among studies. The most recent National Eye Institute–sponsored clinical trial, the ETDRS, has identified certain retinal lesions to be followed (Table 49–1).[9] The ETDRS was a randomized clinical trial of photocoagulation versus deferral of photocoagulation that had 7 years of careful follow-up and allowed the observation of the natural history of diabetic retinopathy. From the ETDRS, three retinal factors have been identified that are predictive of progression during follow-up. These factors are the severity of: (1) intraretinal microvascular abnormality, (2) hemorrhages and microaneurysm, and (3) venous beading. A classification that considers the natural history of diabetic retinopathy as well as the orderly progression of risk of severe visual loss was also determined (Table 49–2).

In addition to the severity of retinopathy, diabetic macular edema also can be diagnosed and graded. Macular edema is defined as thickening in the macula as seen by biomicroscopy or fundus photography. The ETDRS has demonstrated that clinically significant macular edema (Table 49–3) is an entity that can lead to moderate visual loss if not treated by focal photocoagulation.

Incidence and Prevalence

There are no national data on the prevalence or incidence of diabetic retinopathy in the United States. Population studies have been performed on select populations such as inhabitants of Rochester, Minnesota; Framingham, Massachusetts; and Pittsburgh, Pennsylvania; Mexican Americans in San Antonio, Texas; and Pima Indians.[10–14] Some of these studies have used only ophthalmoscopic diagnosis of diabetic retinopathy. The only large population-based study using fundus photography to document diabetic retinopathy is the Wisconsin Epidemiologic Study of Diabetic Retinopathy (WESDR).

TABLE 49–1. **Lesions Characteristic of Diabetic Retinopathy**

Fundus Characteristic Graded in Multiple Fields (Fields 1–7)
New vessels on or within 1 disc diameter (DD) of the disc
Microaneurysms
Hemorrhages and microaneurysms
Drusen
Hard exudates
Soft exudates
Intraretinal microvascular abnormalities
Venous abnormalities
Venous beading
Venous narrowing
Venous loops and reduplication
Arteriolar abnormalities
Arteriolar narrowing
Arteriolar sheathing
Arteriovenous nicking
New vessels elsewhere
Dilated tips of new vessels elsewhere
Fibrous proliferations elsewhere
Plane of proliferation elsewhere
Preretinal hemorrhage
Vitreous hemorrhage
Retinal elevation
Scars of prior photocoagulation
Characteristics Graded Only in Field 1
New vessels on or within 1 DD of disc
Dilated tips of new vessels of disc
Fibrous proliferations on or within 1 DD of disc
Plane of proliferation on or within 1 DD of disc
Papillary swelling
Characteristics Graded Only in Field 2
Hard exudate rings
Posterior vitreous detachment
Retinal thickening
Hard exudate in macular area
Cystoid spaces
Clinically significant macular edema

In the WESDR, previously diagnosed diabetic patients were identified in 11 counties in Wisconsin. Because the determination of insulin dependency in previously diagnosed diabetic patients can be difficult, the WESDR investigators chose to divide the patients into two cohorts according to the age of diagnosis. The first cohort comprised the entire sample of diabetic patients whose disease was diagnosed before 30 years of age. The second cohort was a stratified random sample of diabetic patients whose diagnosis was made after the age of 30 years. The first group comprises predominantly IDDM patients and is referred to as the *younger-onset group*. The second cohort, the *older-onset group*, comprises both individuals who use and those who do not use insulin. The subgroup of insulin-using patients in the older-onset group comprises both patients with IDDM and those with NIDDM, whereas the subgroup not using insulin comprises primarily patients with NIDDM.

The prevalence of diabetic retinopathy determined in the WESDR between 1980 and 1982 was 50.1%. The prevalence of PDR with high-risk characteristics (Diabetic Retinopathy Study high-risk characteristics for severe visual loss of 5/200 or worse)[15] was 2.2%. Younger-onset patients with diabetes had the highest prevalence of any retinopathy, PDR, and macular edema, whereas the older-onset group had the lowest incidence (Table 49–4).

The 4-year incidence of retinopathy in the entire WESDR cohort was 40.3%, whereas the incidence of PDR with high-risk characteristics was 2.4%. The younger-onset group had the highest incidence of progression and progression to PDR, whereas the older-onset group not using insulin had

TABLE 49–2. **ETDRS Retinopathy Severity Scale**

Diabetic retinopathy (DR) absent
Microaneurysms (MAs) and other characteristics absent
DR questionable
Hard exudate (HE), soft exudate (SE), or intraretinal microvascular abnormalities (IRMAs) definitely present
MAs absent
Hemorrhage(s)—definite
Microaneurysms only
MAs definitely present
Other characteristics absent
Mild nonproliferative diabetic retinopathy (mild NPDR)
One or more of the following:
Venous loops definitely present
SE, IRMAs, or venous beading (VB) questionable
Retinal hemorrhages present
HE definitely present
SE definitely present
Moderate NPDR
One of the following:
Hemorrhages or microaneurysms (H/MAs) moderate
IRMAs definite
Moderately severe NPDR
Moderate NPDR and one of the following:
IRMAs definite
H/MA severe
VB definite
Severe NPDR
One or more of the following:
Two of three of the moderately severe NPDR characteristics
H/MA severe
IRMAs moderate
VB definite
Mild proliferative diabetic retinopathy (PDR)
Fibrous proliferation at the disc (FPD) or fibrous proliferation elsewhere (FPE) present with
Neovascularization of the disc (NVD) and neovascularization elsewhere (NVE) absent *or*
NVE—definite
Moderate PDR
Either of the following:
NVE moderate or NVD definite; vitreous hemorrhage (VH) and preretinal hemorrhage (PRH) absent or questionable
VH or PRH definite; NVE moderate; NVD absent
High-risk PDR
Any of the following:
VH or PRH moderate
NVE moderate; VH or PRH definite
NVD definite; VH or PRH definite
NVD moderate

From ETDRS Report Number 12: Fundus photographic risk factors for progression of diabetic retinopathy. Ophthalmology 98:823–833, 1991.
Abbreviation: ETDRS, Early Treatment Diabetic Retinopathy Study.

TABLE 49–3. **Clinically Significant Macular Edema**

Thickening at or within 500 μm from the center of the macula
Hard exudates at or within 500 μm from the center of the macula, if there is thickening of the adjacent retina
An area or areas of thickening at least 1 disc area in size, at least part of which is within 1 disc diameter of the center of the macula

From Early Treatment Diabetic Retinopathy Study Group: Report 1: Photocoagulation for diabetic macular edema. Arch Ophthalmol 103:1796–1806, 1985.

TABLE 49–4. **Retinopathy Status at Baseline Examination in WESDR**

Retinopathy	Younger Onset Using Insulin (%)	Older Onset Using Insulin (%)	Older Onset Not Using Insulin (%)
No	29	30	61
Nonproliferative			
Mild	30	31	27
Moderate or severe	18	26	9
Proliferative			
No HRC	13	9	1
HRC	10	5	1
CSME	44	11	4

From Klein R, Klein BE, Moss SE: The Wisconsin epidemiologic study of diabetic retinopathy: A review. Diabetes Metab Rev 5:559, 1989.
Abbreviations: WESDR, Wisconsin Epidemiologic Study of Diabetic Retinopathy; HRC, high-risk characteristics as defined in Diabetic Retinopathy Study, report No. 4; CSME, clinically significant macular edema as defined in Early Treatment Diabetic Retinopathy Study; report No. 1.

the lowest rates. The older-onset patients with diabetes had the highest incidence of macular edema (Table 49–5).

One clinical impression that was confirmed in the WESDR is that in the younger-onset group (IDDM), the first lesion that develops is retinal microaneurysms, whereas in the older-onset group, the first lesion may be of higher severity.

Although the WESDR provides the only population-based data for calculating rates, there are caveats common to this epidemiologic study: The population in Wisconsin is relatively homogeneous ethnically, consisting of few African Americans, Hispanics, and Asians. Since the study was based on previously diagnosed individuals with diabetes, NIDDM rates may be skewed, because up to one-half of all persons with NIDDM are undiagnosed.[16]

Generalizing the WESDR data to the U.S. population, 11,000 new cases of diabetic macular edema, 22,000 cases of new PDR, and 5000 new cases of blindness are estimated to occur each year.[17]

Risk Factors

Many risk factors have been identified for the development and progression of diabetic retinopathy. Although fundus photography is the preferable method to document diabetic retinopathy, ophthalmoscopy by an ophthalmologist probably has enough sensitivity to be valid when the end-point is PDR. Although NIDDM is more common and NIDDM accounts for more cases of PDR, the number of studies examining retinopathy risk factors in NIDDM is small. Most of the studies involve IDDM patients.

DURATION

Of the multitude of risk factors, the strongest predictor for the development and progression of retinopathy is the duration of diabetes. In IDDM, as among younger-onset patients with diabetes in the WESDR, the prevalence of any retinopathy was 8% at 3 years, 25% at 5 years, 60% at 10 years, and 80% at 15 years. The prevalence of proliferative diabetic retinopathy was 0% at 3 years and increased to 25% at 15 years.[18] In the Pittsburgh Epidemiology of Diabetes Complications Study (PEDCS), patients with IDDM were divided into three age groups: those currently younger than 18 years, those 18 to 29 years, and those older than 30 years.[19] In both the 18- to 29- and the 30-year-old age groups, a longer duration of diabetes was observed in those with PDR than in those with no retinopathy. The odds ratio calculated for the duration from a stepwise logistic regression model was 1.60 ($P < .01$) for those patients 18 to 29 years of age and 1.30 ($P < .01$) for those older than 30 years.

Among groups comprising mostly NIDDM patients, e.g., the older-onset individuals in the WESDR, retinopathy was more prevalent sooner after the diagnosis; 23% had retinopathy at 3 years and 2% had PDR.[20] However, after 20 years of disease, fewer older-onset individuals had any PDR than in the younger-onset group.

The incidence of retinopathy also increases with an in-

TABLE 49–5. **Four-Year Cumulative Incidence of Any Retinopathy, Progression of Retinopathy, Progression to Proliferative Retinopathy, and Incidence of CSME in WESDR**

Status	No. at Risk (%)		
	Younger Onset Using Insulin	***Older Onset Using Insulin***	***Older Onset Not Using Insulin***
Incidence of any retinopathy	271 (59.0)	194 (47.4)	320 (34.4)
Progression	713 (41.2)	418 (34.0)	486 (24.9)
Progression to PDR	719 (10.5)	418 (7.4)	418 (2.3)
Incidence of CSME	610 (4.3)	278 (5.1)	379 (1.3)

Data from Klein R, Klein BEK, Moss SE, et al: The Wisconsin epidemiologic study of diabetic retinopathy. IX: Four-year incidence and progression of diabetic retinopathy when age at diagnosis is less than 30 years. Arch Ophthalmol 107:273–243, 1989; and Klein R, Klein BEK, Moss SE, et al: The Wisconsin epidemiologic study of diabetic retinopathy. X: Four-year incidence and progression of diabetic retinopathy when age at diagnosis is 30 years or more. Arch Ophthalmol 107:244–249, 1989.
Abbreviations: PDR, proliferative diabetic retinopathy; CSME, clinically significant macular edema; WESDR, Wisconsin Epidemiologic Study of Diabetic Retinopathy.

creasing duration of disease. The 4-year incidence of PDR in the WESDR younger-onset group increased from 0% during the first 5 years to 27.9% during the years 13 to 14 of diabetes. After 15 years, the incidence of PDR remained stable. In a cohort study of patients with IDDM from the Joslin Diabetes Center, the incidence (cases of PDR per 1000 person-years) for the development of PDR was 1.5 in patients with less than 10 years of diabetes, rose to 30 during the second decade of diabetes, and remained at this level for the next 25 years.[21]

In the WESDR older-onset group, the 4-year incidence of PDR in those with less than 5 years of follow-up was 2%. In the Rochester study, the 20-year cumulative incidence of PDR was 4 and 2% in obese and nonobese NIDDM patients,[22] respectively. Among Mexican American patients with NIDDM in the San Antonio study, the duration of disease was significantly associated with the development of retinopathy. Comparing those patients with a duration of diabetes less than 10 years to those with a duration greater than 10 years, the odds ratio is 3.31 ($P < .001$) for any retinopathy and 5.51 ($P < .001$) for severe retinopathy (preproliferative and severe retinopathy).[13]

Although the duration of diabetes has been noted as an important variable, the effect of the duration over 20 years has not been great. Duration is likely a surrogate variable representing exposure to some factor or factors yet to be understood.

HYPERGLYCEMIA

The relationship between hyperglycemia and retinopathy has also been noted in many epidemiologic studies. In the WESDR, the level of glycemic control was measured by the level of hemoglobin A_{1c}, a measure of blood glucose control during the preceding 8 to 12 weeks.[23] Among the WESDR younger-onset patients (IDDM), subjects in the highest quartile were 1.5 times as likely to have any retinopathy when the duration of disease was less than 10 years.

A 4-year cohort study of IDDM patients with background diabetic retinopathy at the Joslin Clinic calculated the 4-year risk of severe progression of background diabetic retinopathy to be 5.3, 16.4, and 26.1 ($P < .001$) for the highest three quartiles of hemoglobin A_{1c} compared with the lowest quartile.[24] A similar finding was noted in an earlier study at the Joslin Clinic.[21]

Among IDDM patients younger than 18 years in the PEDCS, those who developed retinopathy had higher levels of glycosylated hemoglobin than those who did not develop retinopathy (10.4% versus 12.1%, $P < .001$).[19] No association was found in the older age groups between the hemoglobin A_{1c} level and the development of any retinopathy or PDR, however. In the Pittsburgh Prospective Insulin-Dependent Diabetes Cohort Study, 7 of 62 newly diagnosed patients with IDDM developed retinopathy.[25] Those who developed retinopathy had a higher level of hemoglobin A_{1c} than those who did not (13% versus 11.7%, $P < .05$).

Among the WESDR older-onset patients with diabetes, those in the highest quartile of glycosylated hemoglobin were 2.5 times as likely to have retinopathy as those in the lowest quartile. This relationship existed even after controlling for the duration of diabetes. In the Rochester study of NIDDM, after other factors were controlled for, an elevated fasting blood sugar level was associated with an increased risk of developing diabetic retinopathy and PDR. In the San Antonio study of NIDDM in Mexican Americans, the severity of glycemia was assessed by glucose sum (the sum of the fasting, 1-hour, and 2-hour glucose values during the oral glucose tolerance test).[13] The odds ratio for having any retinopathy was calculated to be 2.12 ($P < .5$) and 4.23 ($P < .01$) for the second and highest tertile, using the lowest tertile as the reference. The odds ratio for developing either preproliferative retinopathy or PDR was 2.02 ($P < .05$) and 3.42 ($P < .01$) for the second and highest quartile, using the lowest quartile as reference. In the 2-hour glucose tolerance tests, Pima Indians with NIDDM have an incidence ratio of 1.3 (confidence interval: 0.9 to 1.7) for PDR.[26]

A number of clinical trials have been performed to examine the effects of blood glucose control and retinopathy. These trials are discussed in the Clinical Trials section. Briefly, no study has shown that control of blood sugar levels prevents the development of retinopathy.

PROTEINURIA AND RENAL DISEASE

Diabetic nephropathy has also been strongly associated with diabetic retinopathy. Among WESDR younger-onset patients with 10 years or more of diabetes, those patients with gross proteinuria were three times as likely to have proliferative retinopathy as those with absent or trace proteinuria ($P < .001$). The Joslin Diabetes Center's 40-year cohort study also showed the association between persistent proteinuria and proliferative retinopathy. In PEDCS, nephropathy was associated with the development of PDR in the 18- to 29-year age group and in the older-than-30-year age group. An association with background retinopathy was found only in those in the 18- to 29-year age group but not in those in the younger-than-18-year age group.

Among WESDR older-onset patients with diabetes, proteinuria was associated with a higher prevalence of retinopathy even after controlling for the duration of disease, glycosylated hemoglobin levels, systolic blood pressure, the age at diagnosis, and the body mass index. In Pima Indians with NIDDM, proteinuria also was predictive of PDR (incidence ratio of 2.5, 95% confidence interval, 1.1 to 5.8).[26] However, the association with proteinuria was not observed in the Rochester patients with NIDDM.[22]

BLOOD PRESSURE

Epidemiologic studies have not consistently confirmed elevated blood pressure as a risk factor for the development or progression of diabetic retinopathy. Among the WESDR younger-onset patients (IDDM), the relative risk of elevated systolic blood pressure for developing retinopathy was 1.8, and for elevated diastolic blood pressure it was 1.2.[27] For progression of diabetic retinopathy, the relative risk was 1.1 and 1.3 for systolic and diastolic blood pressures. In the Joslin Diabetes Center patients with IDDM, higher diastolic, but not systolic, blood pressure was predictive of progression of diabetic retinopathy.[24] Comparing the highest tertile to the lowest reference tertile, the odds ratio was 14.1 ($P < .0005$). This study is more compatible with a hypothesis that low blood pressure is protective than that high pressures increase the risk. In the PEDCS younger-than-18-year age group, neither diastolic nor systolic blood pressure was associated with the development of background retinopathy. In the 18- to 29-year-old group, elevated blood pressure was not associated with the development of background retinopathy, but both elevated systolic and diastolic blood pressures were associated with PDR. Similarly, among IDDM patients older than 30 years, both systolic and diastolic blood pressures were associated with PDR. After excluding nephropathy, diastolic blood pressure was still associated with PDR.

Among older-onset patients in the WESDR, neither systolic nor diastolic blood pressure was related to the incidence or progression of diabetic retinopathy. Similarly, no association was detected in Mexican Americans in San Antonio or in those with NIDDM in Rochester. Among Pima Indian patients with NIDDM, the presence of either systolic blood pressure greater than 140 mm Hg or diastolic blood pressure greater than 90 mm Hg was associated with an incidence ratio of 2.2, but this was not found to be statistically significant.

SEX

The prevalence of PDR is higher in young male diabetic patients than in young female patients, but there is no difference in the incidence of progression between the sexes.[18] Among older diabetic patients, there is no sex differential. The explanation for the difference in prevalence of proliferative changes in young male diabetic patients may relate to the observation that young male diabetic patients with proliferative changes are more likely to participate in studies.

RACE

Pima Indians have the highest prevalence and incidence of NIDDM in the world. The 20-year cumulative incidence of PDR was 14%.[26] Mexican Americans also have a high prevalence of NIDDM and diabetic retinopathy when compared with non-Hispanic whites from San Antonio and from the WESDR. Compared with non-Hispanic whites, Mexican Americans have three to five times the prevalence of NIDDM and are more likely to develop any retinopathy and severe retinopathy (preproliferative and proliferative retinopathy). The odds ratio, calculated by multiple logistic regression, is 3.18 (95% confidence interval, 1.32 to 7.66).[13] Another study of Hispanics in the San Luis Valley, Colorado, showed no increased prevalence of diabetes.[28] The failure to detect an association may be due to the increased Hispanic admixture in the whites used for controls in the San Luis Valley study.

The epidemiology of diabetic retinopathy in Asian Americans is limited; only Japanese Americans have been studied. In one study of Japanese Americans living in Seattle, the prevalence of diabetic retinopathy was reported to be only 11.5%.[29] Additional epidemiologic studies need to be performed on Asian Americans.

There are no population-based data available on diabetic retinopathy in African Americans. One non–population-based report of West Indians who immigrated to Great Britain showed no racial differences when compared with whites in England.[30]

GENETICS

Genetic factors probably play a role in the development of diabetic retinopathy. In studies of identical twins who have diabetes, the retinopathy was observed to have a similar onset and severity.[31, 32]

HLA-DR antigens have been examined in the WESDR and at the Joslin Clinic. After controlling for the duration of diabetes, diastolic blood pressure, proteinuria, and a history of hypertension, the DR4 allele was associated with an increased risk of PDR in the WESDR. The Joslin Clinic study showed an increased risk of PDR in DR3 and DR4 homozygotes that was neutralized in the presence of myopia. DR3 and DR4 heterozygotes showed decreased risk.[33] Other studies have shown no association between HLA antigens and diabetic retinopathy.[34, 35]

AGE AT EXAMINATION

In the WESDR younger-onset group, children 10 to 12 years old compared with those younger than 10 years have a 4-year relative risk of 3.6 (95% confidence interval, 1.4 to 9.1). This increased risk is believed to be due to the 10- to 12-year-old children's passing through puberty during the 4-year period of follow-up. Before puberty, children rarely develop diabetic retinopathy regardless of the duration of diabetes. The changes that predispose diabetic children at puberty is uncertain, but during puberty elevations of levels of growth hormone, insulin-like growth factors, and sex hormones have all been considered as causes.

At the Joslin Diabetes Center, the severity of diabetes was correlated with a younger age at examination.[24] In each of three groups in the PEDCS (younger than 18 years, 18 to 29 years, older than 30 years), the presence of any retinopathy and PDR was associated with an older age at examination.[19]

Among patients with NIDDM, e.g., WESDR older-onset subjects, a younger age at examination was a strong risk factor for the 4-year progression of diabetic retinopathy. PDR was not seen in those older than 75 years at examination. No association was detected among Mexican American NIDDM patients.

AGE AT DIAGNOSIS

Among the WESDR younger-onset patients, the age at diagnosis was associated with the presence of diabetic retinopathy. In the 40-year cohort study of Joslin Diabetes Center IDDM patients, there was a suggestion that the age at diagnosis (12 to 20 years versus 0 to 11 years) was a risk factor; the relative risk was 1.78 ($P < .051$).[21]

Among WESDR insulin-using older-onset people, retinopathy was more frequent among those diagnosed at an earlier age.[20] However, after controlling for other risk factors, the age at diagnosis was not found to be an independent risk factor. Likewise, no association was detected in the Rochester study.

BODY WEIGHT

Among WESDR younger-onset subjects, the body mass index (body mass in kilograms per surface area in square meters) was associated with retinopathy in those with diabetes of less than 10 years' duration.[18] After multivariate analysis, no association was detected, however. Similarly, at the Joslin Diabetes Center, no difference in body mass index was detected in those subjects with progressing retinopathy.

In the WESDR, body mass was associated with the presence or severity of diabetic retinopathy in older-onset patients not using insulin, but it has not been found to be predictive of the incidence or progression of retinopathy.[20] Other studies have shown either no, positive, or negative association between body mass index in older patients and retinopathy. Among those with NIDDM in Rochester, the relative weight was deemed to be a predictor ($P < .05$) in a multivariate analysis for development of any retinopathy.[22] No association between the body mass index and PDR was found among Pima Indian NIDDM patients.[26]

LIPIDS

The relationship between cholesterol and diabetic retinopathy is not clear. In the PEDCS, compared with those without retinopathy, subjects in the younger-than-18-year age group with background retinopathy had higher levels of low-density lipoprotein cholesterol and lower levels of high-density lipoprotein cholesterol. A similar association existed in the 18- to 29-year and older-than-30-year age groups. In the stepwise logistic regression analysis using background retinopathy as the end-point, the only association detected was low-density lipoprotein cholesterol in the group composed of 18- to 29-year-olds; the calculated odds ratio for low-density lipoprotein cholesterol was 1.86 (95% confidence interval, 1.32 to 2.62). However, the association with PDR did not persist in the stepwise logistic regression analysis.

Among NIDDM patients, elevated cholesterol levels were found to be a risk factor among Pima Indians, but not among Indians from Oklahoma or Mexican Americans in the San Luis Valley.[26, 36]

PREGNANCY

There are few epidemiologic studies on the effect of pregnancy on the progression of diabetic retinopathy.[37–40] One review reported that 8% of women with minimal to no retinopathy had progression during their pregnancy; if PDR was present, 25% progressed.[41]

In one prospective study, the risk of progression of retinopathy was 2.3 higher during pregnancy compared with controls during a similar time period.[42]

SMOKING

Although some epidemiologic studies have shown a relationship between smoking and retinopathy, most studies have not. Among patients with IDDM, for example, the WESDR younger-onset subjects, neither the presence, the severity, nor the progression of retinopathy was association with cigarette smoking.[43] Among Joslin Diabetes Center patients with IDDM, smoking was not correlated with progression of retinopathy.[24] Smoking was not examined as a risk factor in the PEDCS.

In neither WESDR older-onset subjects, Mexican American patients with NIDDM in San Antonio, nor Pima Indians with NIDDM was an association between cigarette smoking and retinopathy detected. However, one study did show an association with smoking.[28]

ACETYLSALICYLIC ACID

Among IDDM patients from the Joslin Diabetes Center and WESDR, aspirin usage was not found to be a risk factor for diabetic retinopathy.[33, 44] In the ETDRS patients, aspirin did not affect the natural history of nonproliferative diabetic retinopathy.[45] In addition, the risk of vitreous hemorrhage in people with proliferative disease was also not increased. A more in-depth discussion is presented in the Clinical Trials section of this chapter.

ALCOHOL

There are few epidemiologic studies examining the relationship between alcohol and retinopathy. In a case-control study of IDDM from the Joslin Diabetes Center, the percentage of subjects consuming alcohol was similar in those subjects with and without PDR.[33] In a prospective study of 296 diabetic men, in heavy drinkers the relative risk of developing severe retinopathy was 3.5 (95% confidence interval, 1.2 to 8.4).[46]

SOCIOECONOMIC STATUS

There are few studies on the relationship between socioeconomic status and diabetic retinopathy. One case-control study reported an association between PDR and working-class occupational status and lower income in patients with IDDM.[47] Among Mexican Americans in San Antonio, the socioeconomic status determined by Duncan's socioeconomic index, education, and income was not associated with the retinopathy status.[48] Similarly, in Oklahoma Indians socioeconomic factors were also not found to be a risk factor for retinopathy.[36]

Clinical Trials

Of all the predictors of retinopathy reviewed, the only important risk factor that can be modified is the level of hyperglycemia. Hyperglycemia may only be a marker for the severity of the diabetic process, and if this is the case, there is little to affect the severity of the diabetes. On the other hand, if hyperglycemia represents the level of control, modification of the insulin regimen may affect the course of diabetic retinopathy. Evidence for the role of hyperglycemia in the development of retinopathy is also present in experimental studies in animals; poorly controlled diabetic animals are more likely to develop diabetic retinopathy.[49] Several clinical studies have attempted to demonstrate the effect of tight glycemic control.

GLYCEMIC CONTROL

The Kroc Collaborative Study Group randomized 70 patients with IDDM with mild nonproliferative diabetic retinopathy into two groups: tight control (continuous subcutaneous insulin infusion) and conventional insulin therapy.[50, 51] The investigators were able to achieve a difference of 2% ($P < .0001$) in the level of glycosylated hemoglobin between the tight control group and the conventional management group. At 8 months of follow-up, both treatment groups had worsening of their retinopathy level ($P < .0001$), evidenced primarily by an increase in the number of soft exudates. This progression in retinopathy was worse in the continuous subcutaneous insulin infusion group, but the change was not statistically significant. Between the 8- and 24-month follow-up visits, patients randomized to one treatment group had the option to switch groups. Of 34 subjects assigned to continuous subcutaneous insulin infusion, 23 continued, and 24 of 34 subjects assigned to conventional insulin therapy continued with assigned therapy. After 24 months, the difference in retinopathy between the two groups of patients who chose to stay with the assigned therapy was not different.

The Steno group randomized 30 IDDM patients with background diabetic retinopathy to tight and conventional management.[52, 53] The difference in glycosylated hemoglobin levels between tight and conventional management was 1.6 ($P < .01$). After 3 years, 3 of 14 patients in the tight control group and 8 of 14 in the conventional management group progressed. Again, the most common lesion cited by the authors for diagnosing progression in retinopathy was the appearance of soft exudates.

The Oslo study enrolled 45 patients with IDDM and randomized 15 patients to either continuous subcutaneous infusion of insulin, multiple injections of insulin, or conventional therapy.[54, 55] Glycemic control was better in the two intensive therapy groups between baseline and 2 years after randomization ($P < .01$). At 12 months, the investigators noted that the control group showed steady worsening of their retinopathy when assessed by fluorescein angiography; the multiple injection group showed no changes in retinopathy stage; and the continuous subcutaneous insulin infusion group showed worsening of the average retinopathy status at 3 months and improvement between 6 and 12 months. The most common change in retinopathy was the appearance of cotton-wool spots, noted only in the intensive therapy group. By 1 year, most of the cotton-wool spots had regressed. The investigators also examined the severity of microaneurysms and hemorrhages. At 2 years, the continuous subcutaneous insulin infusion group and the multiple injection group had fewer microaneurysms and hemorrhages ($P < .01$).

Evaluating the results from the three trials, we find equivocal evidence for the beneficial effect of tight control on the progression of retinopathy. One consistent observation was the increased incidence of cotton-wool spots soon after the initiation of intensive control. One interpretation is that the retina over years of hyperglycemia became accustomed to the high levels of glucose, and the rapid tightening of serum glucose levels resulted in relative retinal glucose ischemia. Recently, however, the significance of the increased number of cotton-wool spots has become uncertain because results from the ETDRS suggest that cotton-wool spots do not have prognostic value.

The results of the individual trials also are difficult to interpret, because all three of the studies had small sample sizes, had short follow-ups, and did not adjust for patients with different levels of retinopathy. Finally, the control of the serum glucose level may have its most powerful effect on the prevention of retinopathy but not on the progression of preexistent retinopathy. None of the trials included patients with no retinopathy. To address these issues, the Diabetes Control and Complications Trial (DCCT) was designed and executed.[56] The DCCT asked whether intensive treatment of glycemia would prevent or delay the progression of early nonproliferative diabetic retinopathy (primary prevention), and whether intensive glycemic control would prevent the progression of early retinopathy to more advanced forms of retinopathy (secondary intervention).

Patients eligible for the primary prevention cohort had to have had IDDM for 1 to 5 years, have no retinopathy as detected by seven-field photography, and have urinary albumin excretion of less than 200 mg per 24 hours. For the secondary intervention cohort, patients had to have had IDDM for 1 to 15 years, have very mild to moderate nonproliferative diabetic retinopathy, and have urinary albumin excretion of less than 200 mg per 24 hours. These patients from 29 clinical centers were randomized to either conventional treatment or intensive treatment.

Conventional treatment was one to two daily injections of insulin, without daily adjustment in insulin dosage. The goals of the treatment were an absence of symptoms from glycosuria or hyperglycemia; an absence of ketonuria or frequent serious hypoglycemia; normal growth and development; and development of ideal body weight. Women who became pregnant received intensive treatment until delivery. Because the goals were not a specific glycosylated hemoglobin target, physicians taking care of these patients were masked to the patients' glycosylated hemoglobin levels, unless the level of glycosylated hemoglobin A_{1c} was 2 SDs above the mean, when the physicians were notified. Patients assigned to intensive treatment received more than three injections of insulin or insulin by external pump. The goal was achieving monthly glycosylated hemoglobin and preprandial, postprandial, and weekly 3 AM glycemic measurements that were within normal limits. Dosages of insulin were adjusted by self-monitoring of blood glucose (more than four times per day), diet, and exercise.

The main outcome measure was a three-step change in retinopathy level on fundus photography that was sustained for 6 months. The strength of the study was that nonophthalmic end-points were also examined. The DCCT looked at nephropathic, neuropathic, neuropsychologic, macrovascular, and quality-of-life end-points.

The 1441 patients in the DCCT were followed for a mean of 6.5 years. Of these patients, 99% completed the study, and 95% of all scheduled examinations were completed. Although 95 women originally assigned to conventional treatment were switched to intensive therapy during their pregnancies, 97% of the time was spent in the assigned therapy.

Although the goal was euglycemia for the intensive group, only 5% were able to maintain a normal average glycosylated hemoglobin value. However, 44% in the intensive group achieve the normal glycosylated goal at least once. Furthermore, the intensive group did achieve a clinically significant and statistically significant difference ($P < .001$) in their levels of glycosylated hemoglobin.

In the primary prevention cohort, the cumulative incidence of a three-step increase in retinopathy level sustained over 6 months was quite similar between the two groups during the first 36 months. From that point on, there was a persistent decrease in the intensive group. From 5 years onward, the cumulative incidence was approximately 50% less in the intensive group. During a mean follow-up of 6 years, retinopathy developed in 23 patients in the intensive group and 91 in the conventional group. Intensive therapy reduced the mean risk of retinopathy by 76% (95% confidence interval: 62 to 85). There were too few patients who developed PDR, severe nonproliferative diabetic retinopathy, clinically significant macular edema, and conditions requiring the use of laser to look for differences between the two therapies.

In the secondary intervention cohort, the intensive group had a higher cumulative incidence of sustained progression during the first year. However, by 36 months, the intensive group had lower risks of progression. Intensive therapy reduced the risk of progression by 54% (95% confidence interval: 39 to 66). In addition, the risk of PDR, severe nonproliferative diabetic retinopathy, and laser photocoagulation was lower in the intensive group.

The protective effect of intensive therapy for retinopathy was found to be consistent in all subgroups (e.g., groups divided by age, sex, duration of disease, percentage of ideal body weight, level of retinopathy, blood pressure, clinical neuropathy, baseline glycosylated hemoglobin level, and albuminuria). Intensive therapy was protective against neuropathy. There were too few patients with advanced nephropathy, but intensive treatment was protective against microalbuminuria and albuminuria. Because the subjects enrolled in the study were young, there were very few macrovascular end-points such as myocardial infarction and strokes, but intensive therapy reduced the development of hypercholesterolemia.

Mortality did not differ between the conventional and intensive treatment groups; there were seven deaths in the intensive and four in the conventional treatment groups. However, the incidence of severe hypoglycemia was three times higher in the intensive group ($P < .001$). There were 62 hypoglycemic episodes per 100 patient-years in the intensive group and 19 in the conventional group. There were 54 hospitalizations for treatment of severe hypoglycemia in 40 patients in the intensive group and 36 in 27 patients in the conventional treatment group.

This increased risk of hypoglycemia is a significant problem. Although protection against retinopathy and other vascular complications is beneficial, the risk of death from severe hypoglycemic episodes must be considered. At present, there does not appear to be any optimal glycemic target that both maximizes protection against vascular complications and minimizes the risk of hypoglycemic episodes. Because there is no universal glycemic goal, the DCCT recommends that therapy should be individualized. Therapy should be directed toward achieving the lowest glycemic level that is the safest in terms of the hypoglycemic risk for each patient.

Weight gain was another problem with intensive treatment. There was a 33% increased risk of becoming 120% over ideal body weight. At 5 years, patients receiving intensive therapy gained an average of 4.6 kg more than those in the conventional group. Weight gain is another problem that may offset the benefit of tight control. Weight gain often leads to hyperinsulinemia, a known risk factor for macrovascular diseases such as myocardial infarction. Although young patients such as those enrolled in the DCCT are not at high risk, older patients may be more susceptible to macrovascular events. Whether intensive therapy is beneficial for older patients and those with NIDDM was not addressed by the DCCT. However, given all the benefits, tight control is probably beneficial for older patients. The method of control for older patients may not be multiple injections of insulin. Rather, intensive therapy may be exercise and diet control instead of insulin.

In summary, intensive treatment of IDDM delays the onset and slows the progression of diabetic retinopathy. In addition, intensive treatment protects against nephropathy, neuropathy, and macrovascular disease. The DCCT also confirmed the early worsening of retinopathy with intensive glycemic control seen in the early treatment. However, early worsening still leads to a reduction in retinopathy.

TREATMENT OF DIABETIC RETINOPATHY

The current management of diabetes does not prevent the development of retinopathy. Because diabetic retinopathy is a significant source of visual loss among diabetic patients, three National Eye Institute multicenter clinical trials to determine the optimal management regimen for patients with diabetic retinopathy have been completed. These trials are the Diabetic Retinopathy Study (DRS), the ETDRS, and the Diabetic Retinopathy Vitrectomy Study (DRVS).

Diabetic Retinopathy Study

The DRS was the first multicenter randomized controlled clinical trail in ophthalmology.[57] The study addressed the question of whether photocoagulation therapy was beneficial in patients with diabetic retinopathy. More than 1700 patients with severe nonproliferative or proliferative diabetic retinopathy at 15 medical centers were randomized to either indefinite deferral of treatment or scatter treatment with either argon laser or xenon arc. Eligible patients had to have: (1) diabetic retinopathy in both eyes, either proliferative in one eye or severe nonproliferative in both eyes, (2) visual acuity of at least 20/100 in both eyes, and (3) both eyes suitable for photocoagulation.

The study showed a reduction, after only 2 years, in the cumulative event rate (visual acuity less than 5/200 at two consecutive 4-month follow-up visits) from 16.3% in untreated eyes to 6.4% in treated eyes ($z = 5.5$). This early demonstration of efficacy prompted the operating committee to change the protocol to allow those in the control group with "high-risk characteristics" (see later) to receive photocoagulation. This early benefit persisted at 5 years; the difference between the treated group compared with the control group was even greater ($z = 11.0$). In addition, argon laser compared with xenon arc photocoagulation was found to cause fewer side effects (e.g., visual field loss).

The study further identified eyes that were at high risk for severe visual loss and for which photocoagulation was of particular benefit. The features of these eyes are described in DRS report No. 4 as "high-risk characteristics" and can be summarized as follows: (1) neovascularization of the disc, severity greater than standard photo 10A, (2) any neovascularization of the disc if accompanied by vitreous or preretinal hemorrhage, and (3) vitreous hemorrhage accompanied by one-half disc area of neovascularization elsewhere.[58] Although the DRS showed convincingly that photocoagulation was beneficial, the study only addressed the question of treatment versus indefinite deferral. The optimal time in the course of diabetic retinopathy when photocoagulation therapy should be applied was not addressed.

Early Treatment Diabetic Retinopathy Study

The ETDRS was designed to evaluate photocoagulation and aspirin treatment in patients with nonproliferative and early proliferative diabetic retinopathy. The ETDRS was designed to determine when in the course of diabetic retinopathy it is most effective to initiate panretinal photocoagulation, whether photocoagulation is effective in the treatment of diabetic macular edema, and whether aspirin treatment is effective in altering the course of diabetic retinopathy.

Eligible patients were required to have diabetic retinopathy in both eyes, and each eye had to meet one of the two following criteria: (1) no macular edema; visual acuity of 20/40 or better; and moderate, severe nonproliferative, or early proliferative retinopathy; or (2) macular edema; visual acuity of 20/200 or better; and mild, moderate, or severe nonproliferative retinopathy, or early PDR. Patients were assigned randomly to aspirin (650 mg/day) or placebo. One eye of each patient was assigned to early photocoagulation and the other eye to deferral of photocoagulation. Both eyes were examined at intervals of 4 months or less, and photocoagulation was initiated when the eye assigned to deferral developed high-risk characteristics. Eyes chosen for early photocoagulation were assigned randomly to either full or mild panretinal photocoagulation techniques. In addition, eyes with macular edema were assigned randomly to either immediate or delayed focal photocoagulation.

The results from the ETDRS showed that early treatment compared with deferral or photocoagulation until high-risk characteristics were observed is associated with a small reduction in the incidence of severe visual loss. The 5-year rates of severe visual loss were 2.6% in the early treatment group versus 3.7% in the deferral-of-treatment group. The relative risk of severe visual loss in eyes randomized to early photocoagulation compared with eyes assigned to deferral was 0.77 (99% confidence interval, 0.56 to 1.06). Furthermore, scatter laser photocoagulation is probably not beneficial for eyes with mild or moderate nonproliferative diabetic retinopathy.

Regarding the management of diabetic macular edema, the ETDRS demonstrated that eyes with clinically significant macular edema should be considered for treatment. Eyes assigned to immediate focal photocoagulation were about half as likely to double their visual angle (12% in those treated versus 24% in those assigned to deferral, $z = 2.58$) at 3 years.[59]

The ETDRS showed that aspirin did not affect the course of retinopathy in those patients with nonproliferative or early proliferative diabetic retinopathy. The study enrolled 3711 patients and assigned 1855 to placebo. There was a 40% 5-year rate of developing high-risk proliferative retinopathy, and the study was designed to detect a 25% treatment effect. The power in the design was greater than 99% but with decreased compliance, the net power to demonstrate a difference was 89%. The relative risk of developing high-risk PDR in patients assigned to aspirin compared with those assigned to placebo was 0.97 with a 99% confidence interval of 0.85 to 1.11. The interpretation of this tight confidence interval is that aspirin probably has no beneficial effects on the progression of retinopathy. When other end-points are examined, there also did not appear to be any harmful effects for diabetic patients with retinopathy. These findings led to the conclusion that aspirin does not modify the natural history of diabetic retinopathy.

Dipyridamole Aspirin Micro Angiopathie Diabetique

The Dipyridamole Aspirin Micro Angiopathie Diabetique study is a placebo-controlled randomized trail that randomized 420 persons with "early" diabetic retinopathy to either aspirin (330 mg three times a day), aspirin (same dosage) plus dipyridamole (75 mg three times a day), or placebo.[60] In contrast to the ETDRS, more patients with lower grades of retinopathy were enrolled and a higher dose of aspirin was studied. The subjects were followed over 3 years, and worsening was assessed by microaneurysm counts on fluorescein angiograms. Those assigned to aspirin and aspirin plus dipyridamole had similar counts, whereas those assigned to placebo had an increase in microaneurysm count. The results of this study suggests that aspirin may be protective against a progression in retinopathy, but one problem affecting the interpretation is the use of a nonstandard grading system of retinopathy.

Diabetic Retinopathy Vitrectomy Study

The DRVS was a National Eye Institute–supported multicenter, randomized clinical trial that addressed the risks and benefits of performing pars plana vitrectomy in eyes with severe PDR. The DRVS was divided into three studies. The first study, DRVS–Group N, was a natural history study to examine the course of severe PDR managed by conventional therapy. The second study, DRVS–Group H, examined the timing of vitrectomy in eyes with severe vitreous hemorrhage of less than 6 months' duration. The third study, DRVS–Group NR, was a randomized clinical trial comparing early vitrectomy with conventional management in eyes with extensive, active neovascular, or fibrovascular proliferations and useful vision.

In DRVS–Group N, 747 eyes with very severe PDR were followed with conventional management over a 2-year period.[61] Decreases in visual acuity were more likely during the first year than the second year of follow-up. After 2 years, visual acuity was less than 5/200 in 45% of eyes with more than four disc areas of new vessels and visual acuity of 10/30 and 10/50 at baseline, and in only 14% of eyes with traction retinal detachment not involving the macula and without active new vessels or fresh vitreous hemorrhage at baseline. Vitrectomy was only performed when the retinal detachment involved the center of the macula and if severe vitreous hemorrhage failed to clear after a 1-year period. Vitrectomy was performed in 25% of eyes after 2 years of follow-up.

In DRVS–Group H, 1616 eyes with recent severe diabetic vitreous hemorrhage reducing visual acuity to 5/200 or less for at least 1 month were randomly assigned to either early vitrectomy or deferral of vitrectomy for 1 year.[62] After 2 years of follow-up, 25% of the early vitrectomy group had visual acuity of 10/20 or better compared with 15% in the deferral group ($P = .01$). The benefit was demonstrated for patients with IDDM (36% versus 12% in the deferral group, $P = .0001$) but not for patients with NIDDM (16% versus 18% in the deferral group). Initially, the proportion of patients with no light perception visual acuity was higher in patients assigned to early vitrectomy than in those assigned to deferral. After 2 and 3 years of follow-up, the differences between the groups were not significant.

Four-year follow-up again showed that the proportion of eyes with visual acuity of 10/20 or better was higher ($P < .05$) in the early vitrectomy group than in the deferral group.[63] The benefit of early vitrectomy to patients with IDDM, but not to patients with NIDDM, remained after 4 years of follow-up. This difference between types of diabetic patients may be due to the higher percentage of younger patients with more severe PDR in the IDDM group. Conversely, patients with NIDDM tend to be older and have maculas that may have undergone some aging changes, thereby limiting the potential benefit of early vitrectomy.

In DRVS–Group NR, 370 eyes with advanced, active PDR and visual acuity of 10/200 or better were randomly assigned to either early vitrectomy or conventional management.[64] After 4 years of follow-up, the percentage of eyes with visual acuity of 10/20 or better was 44% in the early vitrectomy group and 28% in the conventional management group ($P < .05$). The proportion with a very poor visual outcome was similar in the two groups. The advantage of early vitrectomy tended to increase with increasing severity of new vessels. In the group with the least severe new vessels, no advantage of early vitrectomy was apparent. The decision to perform early vitrectomy on eyes with severe PDR and good vision remains a complex clinical decision.

Summary

Diabetic retinopathy is a major cause of blindness in the United States. Diabetic retinopathy occurs in both IDDM and NIDDM. Because NIDDM accounts for 90% of diagnosed cases of diabetes, most cases of PDR are due to NIDDM even though the retinopathy is more severe in IDDM.

Many risk factors for diabetic retinopathy have been studied. The most important risk factors are the duration of diabetes and hyperglycemia. Hyperglycemia is the one risk factor that can be modified with therapy. The DCCT convincingly showed that glycemic control can reduce the risk of retinopathy.

Three National Eye Institute, multicenter randomized controlled clinical trials have looked at the role of laser photocoagulation and vitrectomy surgery on the management of diabetic retinopathy. The DRS showed that laser photocoagulation versus indefinite deferral was beneficial in patients with PDR. The ETDRS answered three questions: (1) The study demonstrated that photocoagulation is efficacious for clinically significant macular edema. (2) Aspirin does not affect the natural history of diabetic retinopathy; specifically, aspirin does not increase the risk of vitreous hemorrhage. (3) Early photocoagulation compared with deferral until the appearance of high-risk characteristics is associated with only a small reduction in severe visual loss. The DRVS showed that vitrectomy surgery is efficacious in the management of certain eyes with vitreous hemorrhage and in certain eyes with active fibrovascular proliferation.

REFERENCES

1. National Society to Prevent Blindness: Vision Problems in the US: Facts and Figures. National Society to Prevent Blindness, Schaumberg, IL, 1980.
2. Kahn HA, Hiller R: Blindness caused by diabetic retinopathy. Am J Ophthalmol 78:58, 1974.
3. Palmberg PF: Diabetic retinopathy. Diabetes 26:703, 1977.
4. Klein R, Klein BEK, Moss SE: Visual impairment in diabetes. Ophthalmology 91:1, 1984.
5. Sussman EJ, Tsiaras WG, Soper KA: Diagnosis of diabetic eye disease. JAMA 247:3231, 1982.
6. Moss SE, Klein R, Kessler SD, Richie KA: Comparison between ophthalmoscopy and fundus photography in determining severity of diabetic retinopathy. Ophthalmology 92:62, 1985.
7. Diabetic Retinopathy Study Research Group: Report 7: A modification of the Airlie House classification of diabetic retinopathy. Invest Ophthalmol Vis Sci 21:210, 1981.
8. Early Treatment Diabetic Retinopathy Study Research Group: Report 10: Grading diabetic retinopathy from stereoscopic color fundus photographs—An extension of the modified Airlie House classification. Ophthalmology 98:786, 1991.
9. Early Treatment Diabetic Retinopathy Study Research Group: Fundus photographic risk factors for progression of diabetic retinopathy. ETDRS report number 12. Ophthalmology 98:823, 1991.
10. Dwyer MS, Melton LG, Ballard DJ, et al: Incidence of diabetic retinopathy and blindness: A population-based study in Rochester, Minnesota. Diabetes Care 8:316, 1985.
11. Kahn HA, Leibowitz HM, Ganley JP, et al: The Framingham Eye Study. I: Outline and major prevalence findings. Am J Epidemiol 106:17, 1977.
12. Orchard TJ, Dorman JS, Maser RE, et al: Prevalence of complications in IDDm by sex and duration. Pittsburgh Epidemiology of Diabetes Complications Study II. Diabetes 39:1116, 1990.
13. Haffner SM, Fong D, Stern MP, et al: Diabetic retinopathy in Mexican Americans and non-Hispanic whites. Diabetes 37:878, 1988.
14. Bennett PH, Rushforth NB, Miller M, et al: Epidemiologic studies of diabetes in the Pima Indians. Recent Prog Horm Res 32:333, 1976.
15. Diabetic Retinopathy Study Research Group: Four risk factors for severe visual loss in diabetic retinopathy: The third report from the Diabetic Retinopathy Study. Arch Ophthalmol 97:654, 1979.
16. Harris MI, Hadden WC, Knowler WC, Bennett PH: Prevalence of diabetes and impaired glucose tolerance and plasma glucose levels in the U.S. population aged 20–74 yr. Diabetes Care 36:523, 1987.
17. Javitt JC, Canner JK, Sommer A: Cost effectiveness of current approaches to the control of retinopathy in Type 1 diabetics. Ophthalmology 96:255, 1989.
18. Klein R, Klein BE, Moss SE, et al: The Wisconsin Epidemiologic Study of Diabetic Retinopathy. II: Prevalence and risk of diabetic retinopathy when age at diagnosis is less than 30 years. Arch Ophthalmol 102:520, 1984.
19. Kostraba JN, Klein R, Dorman JS, et al: The Epidemiology of Diabetes Complications Study. IV: Correlates of diabetic background and proliferative retinopathy. Am J Epidemiol 133:381, 1991.
20. Klein R, Klein BEK, Moss SE, et al: The Wisconsin Epidemiologic Study of Diabetic Retinopathy. III: Prevalence and risk of diabetic retinopathy when age at diagnosis is 30 or more years. Arch Ophthalmol 102:527, 1984.
21. Krolewski AS, Warram JH, Rand LI, et al: Risk of proliferative diabetic retinopathy in juvenile-onset type I diabetes: A 40-year follow-up study. Diabetes Care 9:443, 1986.
22. Ballard DJ, Melton LJ, Dwyer MS, et al: Risk factors for diabetic retinopathy: A population-based study in Rochester, Minnesota. Diabetes Care 9:334, 1986.
23. Klein R, Klein BEK, Moss SE, et al: Glycosylated hemoglobin predicts the incidence and progression of diabetic retinopathy. JAMA 250:2864, 1988.
24. Janka HU, Warram JH, Rand LI, Krolewski AS: Risk factors for progression of background retinopathy in long-standing IDDM. Diabetes 38:460, 1989.

25. D'Antonio JA, Ellis D, Doft BH, et al: Diabetes complications and glycemic control. The Pittsburgh Prospective Insulin-Dependent Diabetes Cohort Study Status Report after 5 yr of IDDM. Diabetes Care 12:694, 1989.
26. Nelson RG, Wolfe JA, Horton MB, et al: Proliferative retinopathy in NIDDM. Incidence and risk factors in Pima Indians. Diabetes 38:435, 1989.
27. Klein R, Klein BEK, Moss SE, et al: Is blood pressure a predictor of the incidence or progression of diabetic retinopathy? Arch Intern Med 149:2427, 1989.
28. Hamman RF, Mayer EJ, Moo-Young GA, et al: Prevalence and risk factors of diabetic retinopathy in non-Hispanic whites and Hispanics with NIDDM. San Luis Valley Diabetes Study. Diabetes 38:1231, 1989.
29. Fujimoto WY, Leonetti DL, Kinyoun JL, et al: Prevalence of complications among second-generation Japanese-American men with diabetes, impaired glucose tolerance, or normal glucose tolerance. Diabetes 36:730, 1987.
30. Cruickshank JK, Alleyne SA: Black West Indian and matched white diabetics in Britain compared with diabetics in Jamaica: Body mass, blood pressure, and vascular disease. Diabetes Care 10:170, 1987.
31. Lelie RDG, Pyke DA: Diabetic retinopathy in identical twins. Diabetes 31:19, 1982.
32. Tattersall RB, Pyke DA: Diabetes in identical twins. Lancet 2:1120, 1972.
33. Rand LT, Krolewski AS, Aiello LM, et al: Multiple factors in the prediction of risk of proliferative diabetic retinopathy. N Engl J Med 113:1433, 1985.
34. Cove DH, Walker JM, Mackintosh P, et al: Are HLA types or *Bf* alleles markers for diabetic retinopathy? Diabetologica 19:402, 1980.
35. Jervell J. Solheim B: HLA-antigens in long standing insulin dependent diabetics with terminal nephropathy and retinopathy with and without loss of vision. Diabetologia 17:391, 1979.
36. West KM, Erdreich LJ, Stober JA: A detailed study of risk factors for retinopathy and nephropathy in diabetes. Diabetes 19:501, 1980.
37. Dibble CM, Kochenour NK, Worley RJ, et al: Effect of pregnancy on diabetic retinopathy. Obstet Gynecol 59:699, 1982.
38. Soubrane G, Canivet J, Coscas G: Influence of pregnancy on the evolution of background retinopathy. Int Ophthalmol 8:249, 1985.
39. Moloney JBM, Drury IM: The effect of pregnancy on the natural course of diabetic retinopathy. Am J Ophthlamol 93:745, 1982.
40. Phelps RK, Sakol P, Metzger BE, et al: Changes in diabetic retinopathy during pregnancy correlates with regulation of hyperglycemia. Arch Ophthalmol 104:1806, 1986.
41. Rodman HM, Singerman LJ, Aiello LM, et al: Diabetic retinopathy and its relationship to pregnancy. *In* Merkatz ER, Adams PAJ (eds): The Diabetic Pregnancy—A Perinatal Perspective. New York, Grune & Stratton, 1979, pp 73–91.
42. Klein BEK, Moss SE, Klein R: Effect of pregnancy on progression of diabetic retinopathy. Diabetes Care 12:34, 1990.
43. Klein R, Klein BEK, Davis MD: Is cigarette smoking associated with diabetic retinopathy? Am J Epidemiol 118:228, 1983.
44. Klein BEK, Klein R, Moss SE: Is aspirin usage associated with diabetic retinopathy? Diabetes Care 10:495, 1987.
45. ETDRS Research Group: Effects of aspirin treatment on diabetic retinopathy: ETDRS report number 8. Ophthalmology 98:757, 1991.
46. Young RJ, McCulloch DK, Prescott RJ, Clarke BF: Alcohol: Another risk factor for diabetic retinopathy? BMJ 288:1035, 1984.
47. Hanna AK, Roy M, Zinman B, et al: An evaluation of factors associated with proliferative diabetic retinopathy. Clin Invest Med 8:109, 1985.
48. Haffner SM, Hazuda HP, Stern MP, et al: Effect of socioeconomic status on hyperglycemia and retinopathy levels in Mexican Americans with NIDDM. Diabetes Care 12:128, 1989.
49. Engerman RL, Bloodworth JMB, Nelson SL: Relationship of microvascular disease in diabetes to metabolic control. Diabetes 26:760, 1977.
50. The Kroc Collaborative Study Group: Blood glucose control and the evolution of diabetic retinopathy and albuminuria: A preliminary multicenter trial. N Engl J Med 311:365, 1984.
51. The Kroc Collaborative Study Group: Diabetic retinopathy after two years of intensified insulin treatment: Follow-up of the Kroc Collaborative Study JAMA 260:37, 1988.
52. Lauritzen T, Frost-Larsen K, Larsen HW, et al: Effect on one year of near-normal blood glucose levels on retinopathy in insulin-dependent diabetics. Lancet 1:200, 1983.
53. Lauritzen T, Frost-Larsen K, Larsen HW, et al: Two year experience with continuous subcutaneous insulin infusion in relation to retinopathy and neuropathy. Diabetes 34 (Suppl 3):74, 1985.
54. Dahl-Jorgensen K, Brinchmann-Hansen O, Hansen KF, et al: Rapid tightening of blood glucose control leads to transient deterioration of retinopathy in insulin-dependent diabetes mellitus: The Oslo Study. BMJ 290:811, 1985.
55. Dahl-Jorgensen K, Brinchmann-Hasen O, Hansen KF, et al: Effect of near normoglycaemia for two years on progression of early diabetic retinopathy, nephropathy, neuropathy: The Oslo Study. BMJ 293:1195, 1986.
56. Diabetes Control and Complications Trial Research Group: The effect of intensive treatment of diabetes on the development and progression of long-term complications in insulin-dependent diabetes mellitus. N Engl J Med 329:977, 1993.
57. The Diabetic Retinopathy Study Research Group: Preliminary report on effects of photocoagulation therapy. Am J Ophthalmol 81:1, 1976.
58. DRS Research Group: Four risk factors for severe visual loss in diabetic retinopathy. Arch Ophthalmol 97:654, 1979.
59. Early Treatment Diabetic Retinopathy Study Research Group: Photocoagulation for diabetic macular edema. ETDRS report number 1. Arch Opthalmol 103:1796, 1985.
60. The DAMAD Study Group: Effect of aspirin alone and aspirin plus dipyridamole in early diabetic retinopathy. A multicenter randomized controlled clinical trial. Diabetes 38:491, 1989.
61. The Diabetic Retinopathy Vitrectomy Study Research Group: Two year course of visual acuity in severe proliferative diabetic retinopathy with conventional management. DRVS report 1. Ophthalmology 92:492, 1985.
62. The DRVS Research Group: Early vitrectomy for severe vitreous hemorrhage in diabetic retinopathy. DRVS report 2. Arch Ophthalmol 103:1644, 1985.
63. DRVS Research Group: Early vitrectomy for severe vitreous hemorrhage in diabetic retinopathy. Four year results of a randomized trial. DRVS report 5. Arch Ophthalmol 108:958, 1990.
64. The DRVS Study Group: Early vitrectomy for severe proliferative diabetic retinopathy in eyes with useful vision. DRVS report 3. Ophthalmology 95:1307, 1988.

Lasers in Ophthalmology

Edited by

DIMITRI T. AZAR

JOAN W. MILLER

CHAPTER 50

Ophthalmic Laser-Tissue Interactions

Jeffrey W. Berger

In parallel and nearly synchronous with the development of the laser, medical scientists and practitioners have been exploring potential applications of laser technology for diagnosis and treatment of ophthalmic diseases. Since the report of the first laser,[1] the applicability of newly developed laser sources to ophthalmology—offering novel wavelengths, power, pulse energies, and spatial and temporal pulse characteristics—has received much attention. In part, ophthalmic laser investigation has been technology-driven. As new technology became available, applications were sought.

Laser technology has been applied successfully in many problem-driven applications in which existing methods for diagnosis and treatment were inadequate or unacceptable. For example, panretinal photocoagulation for proliferative diabetic retinopathy (PDR) has prevented blindness in great numbers of patients with diabetes mellitus; neodymium:yttrium-aluminum-garnet (Nd:YAG) laser capsular photodisruption obviates the need for invasive surgical management for posterior capsular opacification following cataract surgery. Moreover, experimental studies relevant to excimer laser ablative photodecomposition of the cornea were reported in the mid-1980s, and subsequent United States Food and Drug Administration (FDA) approval has stimulated great interest in laser refractive surgery in this country. Ongoing investigational studies suggest that fiberoptic delivery of mid-infrared erbium laser energy may offer heretofore unattainable precision in intraocular microsurgery; laser-assisted, photosensitizer-mediated photodynamic therapy (PDT) of choroidal neovascularization may offer tissue-damage selectivity not possible with conventional laser retinal photocoagulation. Accordingly, the wide range of laser-tissue interactions is relevant to current and future ophthalmic practice.

The first ophthalmic laser applications relied on the pulsed (~600 msec) ruby laser[2–4] coupled to a monocular direct ophthalmoscopic delivery system. Investigators reported interesting and provocative results relevant to laser treatment for retinal breaks and PDR. However, the development of the argon laser presented several advantages. Continuous-wave pulses were more readily delivered by fiberoptics, permitting slit-lamp–based, high-magnification binocular delivery. In addition, the blue and green argon laser light is better absorbed by melanin, yielding predictable, uniform coagulation burns with pulse lengths of 0.1 to 0.2 seconds. The differences in laser-tissue interactions were readily identified and served to drive the development of a clinically useful tool.

Q-switching the ruby laser produces high-power, short laser pulses. Krasnov[5] postulated that laser-induced mechanical effects would facilitate laser goniopuncture, increasing outflow facility in eyes with open-angle glaucoma. These early applications of photodisruption were extended with the development of ultrashort-pulse, small-spot-size, stable Nd:YAG lasers. Accordingly, even the earliest ophthalmologic studies recognized the significance of laser-tissue interactions.

In order to characterize and understand laser-tissue interactions, it is necessary to consider the fundamental properties of both the laser and the tissue.

Laser Fundamentals

First introduced as the optical MASER following rediscovery of the scientific principles in the microwave portion of the electromagnetic spectrum and development of corresponding enabling technologies,[1, 2] the LASER (*l*ight *a*mplification by the *s*timulated *e*mission of *r*adiation) can be viewed as a source of photons with specific features. Unlike conventional light sources, laser light is monochromatic and spatially and temporally coherent. The coherence properties facilitate diagnostic applications wherein geometric or velocimetric data can be obtained by analysis of laser light interferometry. Monochromaticity permits application-specific wavelength selection.

The potential for light amplification follows directly from Einstein's description of absorption, spontaneous emission, and stimulated emission (Fig. 50–1). On traversing a medium that is characterized by two energy levels, a photon may be absorbed, raising the electron energy from E_0 to E_1. In competition with this process, a photon may be emitted

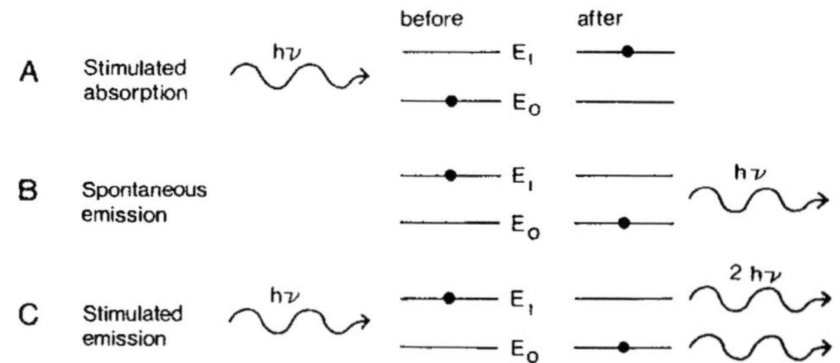

FIGURE 50–1. Schematic depiction of absorption *(A)*, spontaneous emission *(B)*, and stimulated emission *(C)*. The photon energy hν is equivalent to the energy difference between the ground (E_0) and excited (E_1) electronic states. (From Steinert RF, Puliafito CA: The Neodymium:YAG Laser in Ophthalmology. Principles and Clinical Applications of Photodisruption. Philadelphia, WB Saunders, 1985.)

following spontaneous relaxation from the excited to the ground state. Alternately, a passing photon may "tickle" the electron in the excited state, resulting in the emission of a photon with electronic relaxation from E_1 to E_0. Importantly, the emitted photon is of equal energy and *in phase* (spatially and temporally coherent) with the stimulating photon. This process is called *stimulated emission* and is required for laser action.

If the photons traverse a medium largely populated by ground-state electrons, absorption is favored. Photon intensity decreases exponentially with path length. However, if the excited state is heavily populated, stimulated emission is favored with respect to absorption, and there is a net gain in photon intensity during transit—that is, *light amplification*.

Under normal circumstances, the ground-state lowest energy configuration is strongly preferred and preferentially populated as determined by fundamental laws of statistical mechanics. Therefore, light intensity is reduced during passage through media. However, if *population inversion* is achieved—that is, if the excited electronic state is more populated than the ground state—light may be amplified. Population of the excited state requires energy input or *pumping*.

Light amplification is a function of pathlength. If population inversion exists, longer passes through the active medium yield greater amplification. The length of a laser cavity is limited by practical considerations. Ordinarily, the laser cavity is bounded by totally reflecting and partially reflecting mirrors (Fig. 50–2). The partially reflecting mirror allows a small fraction of the light to escape from the cavity, providing a source for laser photons.[6]

In practice, it is difficult to achieve population inversion in a two-level system. The ground state is highly preferred. The ruby laser employs a three-level system wherein pumping to the higher excited state is followed by relaxation to an intermediate excited state, and laser action is between the intermediate state and the ground state (Fig. 50–3). The Nd:YAG laser is a four-level laser with laser action between the intermediate energy states (Fig. 50–4). Because the lower laser level is much less populated than a typical ground state, laser action is potentiated with less energy input, and stimulated emission is more favorable when compared with a three-level laser.

Therefore, the necessary elements for a laser include an active medium with appropriate energy levels facilitating population inversion, a mechanism for energy input into the system to stimulate and support population inversion, optical feedback to maximize light amplification, and a mechanism for photon delivery as a laser beam.[6]

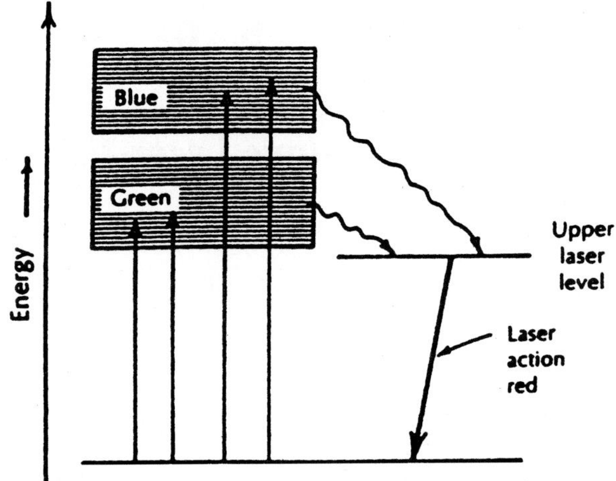

FIGURE 50–3. Energy level diagram for the ruby laser, a typical three-level laser system. (From L'Esperance FA: Ophthalmic Lasers. St. Louis, CV Mosby, 1989.)

As described, laser action continues as long as pumping is provided, resulting in continuous wave emission. To achieve higher peak powers, the laser energy can be compressed in time by *Q-switching* or *mode locking*.

In Q-switched systems, a fast-switch, time-variable absorber is incorporated into the laser cavity. A rotating mirror, saturable dye, or acousto-optical modulator is rapidly switched, favoring or inhibiting optical feedback (Fig. 50–5). When a saturable dye is opaque, optical feedback is inhibited. Pumping serves to maximize population inversion. When the dye is made transparent, oscillation and stimulated emission are favored, and a single high-power laser pulse is emitted from the cavity.

Mode locking capitalizes on the summation of peaks from a large number of axial laser modes. Again, saturable dyes are often used and most easily understood. These dyes bleach when exposed to high laser powers but are opaque to lower powers. Therefore, when axial modes are out of phase, oscillation is not permitted and population inversion

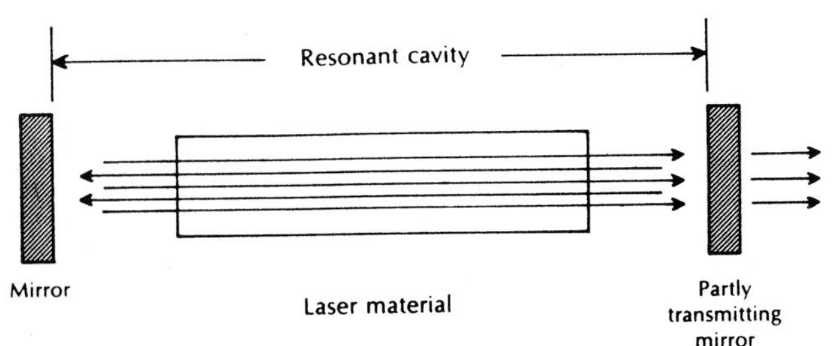

FIGURE 50–2. Schematic depiction of a laser. The partly transmitting mirror allows for amplification, with a fraction of the photons escaping on each pass. (From L'Esperance FA: Ophthalmic Lasers. St. Louis, CV Mosby, 1989.)

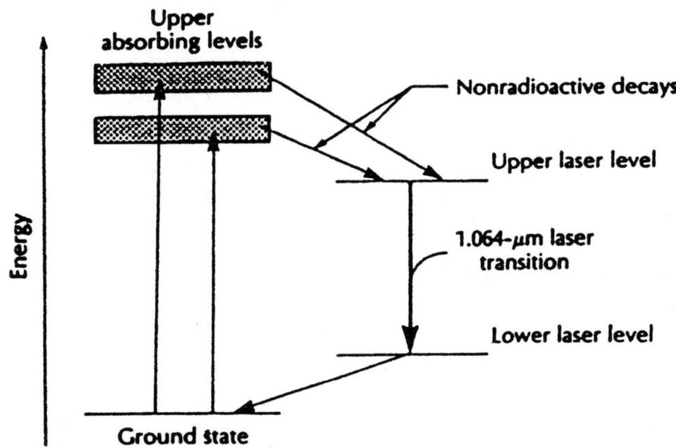

FIGURE 50–4. Energy level diagram for the Nd:YAG laser, a typical four-level laser system. (From L'Esperance FA: Ophthalmic Lasers. St. Louis, CV Mosby, 1989.)

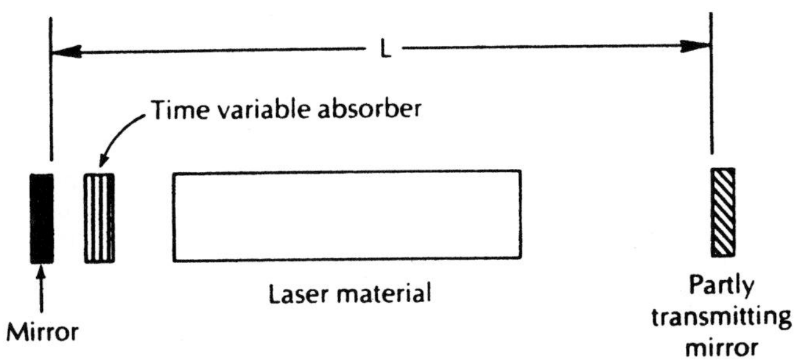

FIGURE 50–5. Schematic configuration for a Q-switched laser. (From L'Esperance FA: Ophthalmic Lasers. St. Louis, CV Mosby, 1989.)

is maximized. When axial modes are in phase, the dye bleaches, and oscillation and amplification occur with laser emission from the cavity.

The laser, then, is a source for high-power, directional, monochromatic light with high spatial and temporal coherence, and these properties can be exploited to achieve specific laser-tissue interactions.

Light-Tissue Interactions

The electromagnetic spectrum specifies the wavelengths of radiant energy on a continuum, from ultrashort wavelengths less than 1 nm (cosmic rays) to very long radio waves with wavelengths of greater than 1 km. *Laser-tissue interactions* simply correspond to a subset of the interactions of radiant energy with biomaterials. The ultraviolet, visible, and infrared portions of the electromagnetic spectrum are relevant to ophthalmic laser-tissue interactions. Table 50–1 presents a summary of the wavelengths of commonly used and selected investigational laser sources.

Although both wave theory and particle theory are required to account for the various physical properties of light, laser photobiology can be understood by considering the radiant energy to be composed of particles, or energy packets, called *photons*. The energy of a photon is proportional to the frequency of electromagnetic oscillation and inversely proportional to its wavelength:

$$E = hc/\lambda$$

where h is Planck's constant, c is the speed of light, and λ is the laser wavelength and is inversely proportional to the laser frequency.

It is axiomatic that all laser-tissue interactions follow absorption of photons by biologic tissue molecules. Following absorption, photons may: (1) be reradiated without loss of energy as scattering ("elastic"), (2) be reradiated with loss of energy ("inelastic") and shift toward longer wavelengths such as fluorescence or phosphorescence, (3) increase the molecular translational, rotational, or vibrational kinetic energies, resulting in a rise in tissue temperature, or (4) initiate photochemical reactions. The energy of the photon absorbed and the physical chemical properties of the tissue chromophore determine the favored interaction. As a rule of thumb, ultraviolet photons may be of sufficient energy to break molecular bonds, visible light induces electronic excited states with subsequent interactions mediated by radiative and nonradiative decay to the ground state, and infrared light increases rotational and vibrational kinetic energy, inducing rise in tissue temperature.

Laser-tissue interactions may be divided into photothermal, photochemical, and photomechanical effects (Fig. 50–6).

TABLE 50–1. **Commonly Used Clinical and Investigational Laser Sources in Ophthalmology***

ArF	193 nm	Ablative decomposition (AD)
Nd:YLF×5	211 nm	AD
Nd:YAG×5	213 nm	AD
KrF	247 nm	AD
Argon ion	488/514 nm	Coagulation
Nd:YAG×2	532 nm	Coagulation
Organic dye	570–630 nm	Coagulation
Krypton red	647 nm	Coagulation
Ruby	694 nm	Coagulation
Diode	780–850 nm	Coagulation
Nd:YLF	1053 nm	Disruption
Nd:YAG	1064 nm	Disruption
Ho:YAG	2120 nm (2.1 μm)	Ablation
Er:YSGG	2.79 μm	Ablation
Er:YAG	2.94 μm	Ablation
Carbon dioxide	10.6 μm	Ablation

*The laser source is listed with its most common wavelength and mechanism used. Note that each laser may interact with more than one mechanism. For example, the Nd:YAG laser is a coagulator in transscleral application, but when Q-switched, is a photodisruptor for capsulotomy. Note also that only the most common wavelength is listed. For the diode laser, most applications have used 810-nm GaAl As, but other diode materials support visible and mid-infrared wavelengths.

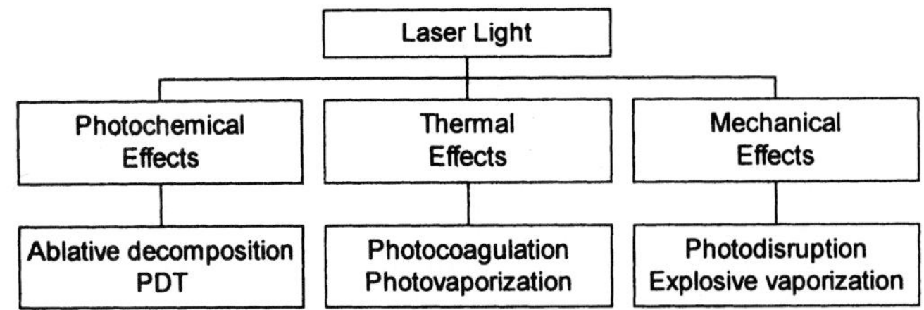

FIGURE 50–6. Laser-tissue interactions may be divided into photochemical, photothermal, and photomechanical interactions.

PHOTOTHERMAL EFFECTS

The magnitude of the tissue-temperature rise is critical to the nature of the photothermal laser-tissue interaction. With a low temperature rise, the tissue effect may be transient; reparative mechanisms may restore the tissue to its normal state. With a very high rise in tissue temperature, the tissue water is boiled and removed (photovaporization). Between these two extremes, a moderate temperature rise may be associated with irreversible protein denaturation and cellular injury.

Following a temperature rise of at least 10°C, weak bonds stabilizing tertiary and quaternary structural features of proteins and nucleic acids are broken; these biomolecules are irreversibly denatured. Concomitant with molecular alteration is a loss of biologic activity for cell maintenance molecules, such as respiratory, synthetic, or degradative enzymes, and an alteration in structural integrity mediated by damage to cell membrane moieties. The ability of a laser pulse to denature tissue is a function of the time-temperature profile as quantified by the Arrhenius integral of the target tissue[7]

$$\Omega(t) = \int q(T(t'))\, dt'$$

where q is the denaturation rate dependent on the absolute temperature T expressed as a function of time. A modest temperature rise requires more time to induce tissue coagulation. As a clinical example, the time-temperature profile influences the visibility of a retinal photocoagulation lesion; "hotter" burns are immediately visible, whereas less "hot" burns may not be visible immediately following laser application but are rendered visible by subsequent inflammatory and repair processes.

The tissue temperature rise depends on laser pulse characteristics and tissue thermal and optical properties. The tissue-temperature rise increases with increasing laser power, and because dissipative mechanisms such as convective and conductive cooling are minimized during short laser pulses, the maximum tissue temperature rise is greater for shorter laser pulses. Indeed, for just-detectable retinal photocoagulative lesions, the total energy required is not constant but increases with laser exposure time.[8]

The tissue optical properties are a major determinant of the laser-tissue interaction. Tissue heating increases as the concentration of absorbers increases, and as the convolution between the spectral content of the laser light and the absorption spectrum of the chromophores increases. For example, retinal pigment epithelium (RPE) melanin strongly absorbs argon-green laser light (514 nm), resulting in retinal photocoagulation, but the cornea is essentially devoid of species absorbing green light. Therefore, the cornea transmits green light with high efficiency.

Photovaporization results from a laser-tissue interaction in which the tissue temperature exceeds the boiling point of the tissue water. On a microscopic scale, for example, the local temperature rise of an irradiated RPE melanosome may exceed the tissue boiling point with the production of a small but visible vapor bubble, whereas the surrounding bulk tissue is coagulated. Alternatively, if the absorbing species is more homogeneously distributed such that the irradiated volume is brought beyond its boiling point, the target tissue is vaporized. For example, the tissue water itself is the absorbing chromophore for erbium:YAG laser application. Following adequate laser application, the tissue water is boiled, and the tissue is ablated.

PHOTOCHEMICAL EFFECTS

Photochemistry may follow light interaction with native or exogenous chromophores. Photons of ultraviolet light may have enough energy to break chemical bonds. The photon energy in excess of that needed to break the bond is partly converted to the kinetic energy associated with fragment-ejection velocity.[9]

Photochemistry can also be initiated after absorption of visible or infrared light, particularly after administration of exogenous chromophores. Photosensitizers, including hematoporphyrin derivative, benzoporphyrin derivative, and chloroaluminum sulfonated phthalocyanine, absorb red or near-infrared light and are promoted to their excited triplet state. The excited triplet state may then directly mediate photochemistry by electron abstraction and free-radical production. More favorable is the triplet-triplet interaction with ground-triplet-state molecular oxygen leading to the production of highly reactive oxygen species including singlet oxygen. These highly reactive oxygen species then mediate subsequent oxidation reactions, leading to local molecular and cellular injury.

Unlike photothermal processes, photochemical reactions are favored with long exposure times at irradiance levels too low to mediate photothermal injury. Moreover, although high-intensity light exposure may mediate prompt photochemical injury, long exposures to ambient light have been implicated as contributors to cataractogenesis and age-related macular degeneration. Near-ultraviolet and blue light incident on the lens, and blue light incident on the retina and subretinal structures, may interact with native chromophores, resulting in cumulative photooxidative injury.

PHOTOMECHANICAL EFFECTS

Following laser radiation, acoustomechanical sequelae are mediated by thermoelastic waves associated with tissue heating to subevaporative temperatures, electrostrictive stresses arising from the very high electric field at the focal point of a high-power laser, explosive photovaporization, optical breakdown, stimulated Brillouin scattering arising from laser-generated pressure waves, and recoil pressure associated with material ejection.[10]

Although most laser-tissue interactions are associated with at least a minor mechanical effect, the magnitude of this effect varies greatly. For example, laser photocoagulation with a moderate temperature rise produces thermoelastic waves, usually without tissue-altering sequelae. Photovaporization results in vapor-bubble production with potential tissue disruption; tissue removal is a photothermal ablative process, but local tissue injury is partly mediated by the acoustomechanical sequelae of bubble production, expansion, and collapse. Finally, for some lasers, photomechanical effects mediate the principal laser-tissue interaction.

In ophthalmic applications, optical breakdown is important. The "transparent" media of the eye weakly absorb Nd:YAG laser 1064-nm radiation. Similarly, an opaque posterior capsule does not contain chromophores to directly absorb near-infrared laser light. However, by Q-switching the laser output of the Nd:YAG laser, very short (nanoseconds or shorter) high-power pulses can be focused to irradiate a small tissue volume. The high laser irradiance ionizes the target volume, producing a "soup" of ions called *plasma*. The plasma absorbs subsequent photons, the temperature of the plasma increases, and the plasma expands at supersonic velocity with shock-wave production.[6] These shock waves mechanically disrupt tissue adjacent to the target volume.

Optical Properties of the Eye and Adnexa

Laser-tissue interactions depend on the absorbing *chromophores* and nonabsorbing tissue species, as well as the spectral content of the incident light. Depending on the wavelength, absorbing species in ophthalmic applications include obvious chromophores such as melanin, photopigments, hemoglobin, and xanthophyll, as well as nonpigmented moieties such as tissue water (for infrared-mediated photoablation), and peptide bonds (for ultraviolet ablative photodecomposition). Photoionization, as a precursor for photodisruption, is least intuitive. The medium is otherwise transparent (nonabsorbing) to the incident light, but the light is of sufficient intensity with an associated large electric field such that electrons are split from target molecules resulting in the production of a plasma. The plasma may then absorb photons mediating subsequent laser-tissue interactions.

The major function of the anterior structures of the eye is to transmit light to the retina for phototransduction with minimal attenuation and distortion. Accordingly, the cornea, aqueous, lens, and vitreous are essentially nonabsorbing in the visible part of the spectrum (Fig. 50–7*A* and *B*). Laser-tissue interactions for these tissues must therefore capitalize on chromophores absorbing outside of the visible range, or nonlinear processes. For example, in these tissues, water is the principal chromophore for absorption of mid- and far-infrared laser light as delivered by holmium, erbium, or carbon dioxide sources. In addition, high-power lasers may photoionize otherwise transparent biomolecules, mediating tissue disruption.

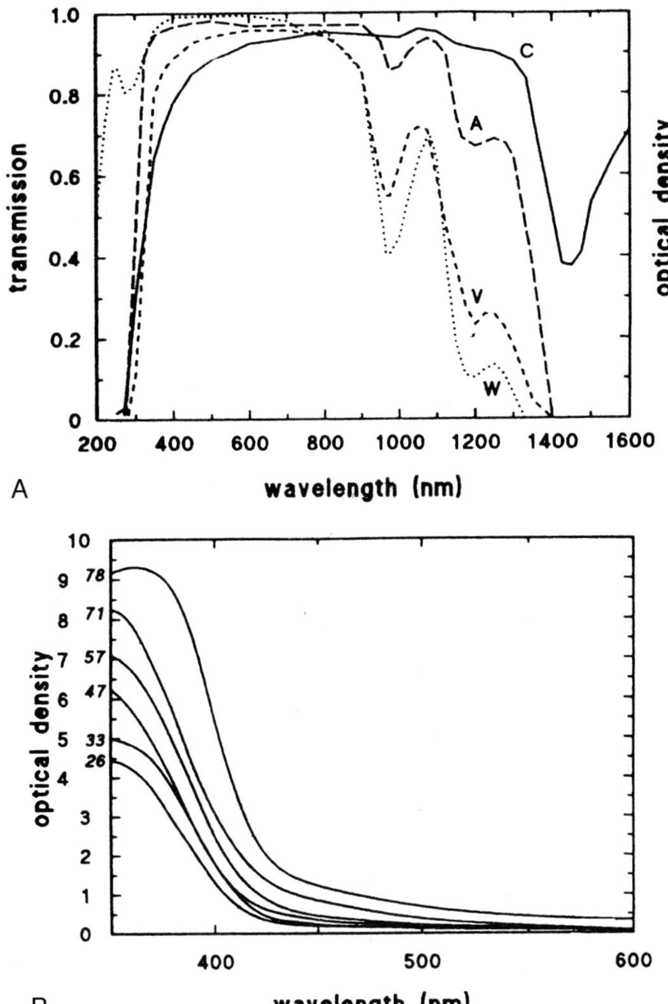

FIGURE 50–7. *A*, Spectral transmission curves of rhesus monkey ocular media for cornea *(C)*, aqueous *(A)*, and vitreous *(V)*. For comparison, the transmission of distilled water is depicted *(W)*. *B*, Optical density through the lens for six lenses as specified by the italic ordinate. (From Mellerio J: Light effects on the retina. *In* Albert DM, Jakobiec FA [eds]: Principles and Practice of Ophthalmology. Philadelphia, WB Saunders, 1994.)

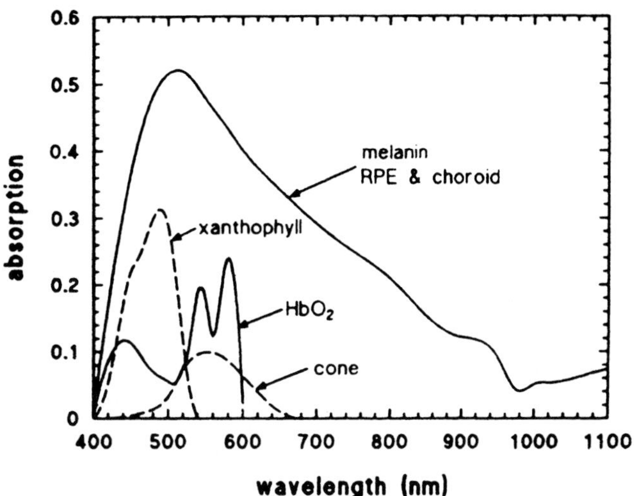

FIGURE 50–8. Absorption curves for ocular pigments. Transmission through a 52-year-old lens is assumed. The hemoglobin is assumed to be in a retinal vessel 10 μm in diameter. RPE, retinal pigment epithelium. (From Mellerio J: Light effects on the retina. *In* Albert DM, Jakobiec FA [eds]: Principles and Practice of Ophthalmology. Philadelphia, WB Saunders, 1994.)

The pigmented eye and adnexal structures, including the iris, angle, ciliary body, RPE, and choroid, directly absorb incident photons as determined by the spectral content of the incident light and the absorption spectrum of the resident chromophores. In theory, all resident chromophores, including cytochromes, photopigments, xanthophyll, hemoglobin, proteins, and melanin, contribute to light absorption (Fig. 50–8). However, the melanin contribution greatly overwhelms that of other absorbing species.

The optical properties of the sclera are perhaps least well understood and profoundly influence the efficacy of transscleral laser application. The careful studies of Vogel and associates[11] provide insight into the absorption, scattering, and transmission properties of sclera. At the blue end of the spectrum, absorption is considerable, perhaps because of scleral melanin, β-carotene, and low transmission associated with light scattering resulting from the refractive index mismatch between collagen fibrils ($n = 1.47$) and surrounding ground substance ($n = 1.36$). With longer wavelength, absorption and scattering are minimized, and transmission increases from less than 10% at 400 nm to greater than 50% at 1064 nm (Fig. 50–9*A*). In addition, scattering is further minimized by scleral compression. Firm pressure greatly increases scleral transmission, particularly at shorter wavelengths (Fig. 50–9*B*).

Photocoagulation

Within a year of the development of the ruby laser by Maiman,[1] Zaret and coworkers[2] investigated iris and retinal photocoagulation in rabbits. The development of delivery systems for intraocular application permitted laser retinopexy for retinal breaks. The application of the ruby laser for retinal scatter photocoagulation in PDR by Beetham and coworkers[12] laid the foundations for what is arguably the single most important ophthalmic laser application, panretinal photocoagulation for PDR.

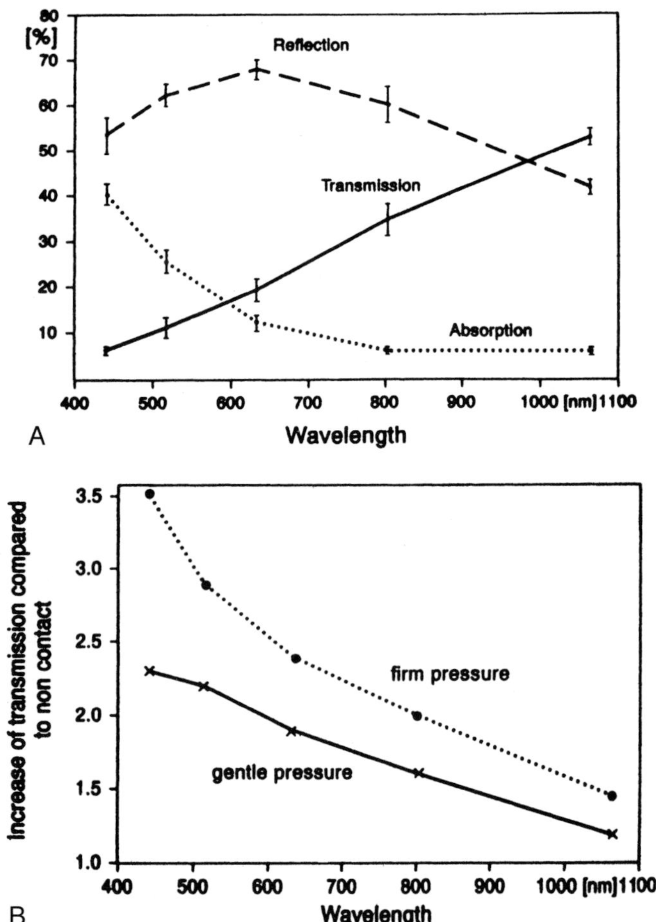

FIGURE 50–9. *A*, Reflection, absorption, and transmission of human sclera as a function of wavelength. *B*, Ratio of scleral transmission with pressure when compared with transmission without pressure. (From Vogel A, et al: Optical properties of the human sclera and their consequences for transscleral laser application. Lasers Surg Med 11:331, 1991.)

Modern photocoagulation originated with Meyer-Schwickerath, who published his observations regarding focused-sunlight–mediated retinal photocoagulation in 1949. For dosimetric repeatability and technical simplicity, he later developed a retinal photocoagulator based on the xenon-arc lamp.[13] The development of the laser offered greater wavelength selectivity, smaller spot sizes, and greater focusing precision, making arc-lamp systems obsolete.

The benefits of scatter photocoagulation for PDR were first demonstrated with the ruby laser. L'Esperance's development of an ophthalmic argon laser in 1968[14] offered technical superiority; since then, it has been shown that retinal photocoagulation can be achieved with many wavelengths, though none has supplanted argon green in popularity.

Photocoagulative applications in ophthalmology include photocoagulation for neovascular retinal and macular diseases, macular edema, trabeculoplasty, iridoplasty, iridotomy, cyclophotocoagulation/cyclophotodestruction, destruction of pigmented skin lesions, and other less common or investigational applications. As a paradigm for other laser applications, laser-tissue interactions relevant to retinal laser photocoagulation are discussed in the following paragraphs.

Retinal photocoagulation relies on transmission of light through the anterior eye structures and the absorption of incident light by native fundus chromophores.[15] Absorption with resulting temperature rise coagulates the adjacent retina. Therefore, retinal photocoagulation depends sensitively on the transmission spectrum of the cornea, aqueous humor, lens, and vitreous, as well as the absorption spectrum, concentration, and anatomic localization of potential absorbing moieties. The high concentration and broad absorption spectrum of RPE and uveal melanin overwhelm the potential contributions of less concentrated fundus chromophores; absorption by xanthophyll, hemoglobin, photopigments, and cellular constituents such as cytochromes contributes little, if at all, to the laser-tissue interaction (see Fig. 50–8).[15] Accordingly, retinal photocoagulation may be induced by wavelengths transmitted by the ocular media and absorbed by melanin, and the wavelength of the tissue photocoagulation depends on the differential transmission and absorption.

The transmission of the ocular media plateaus at greater than 90% for wavelengths from 500 to 900 nm (see Fig. 50–7*A* and *B*), whereas melanin absorption falls sharply over this range (see Fig. 50–8). Therefore, longer wavelength application requires greater laser intensities for equivalent biologic effect and results in deeper tissue penetration, because longer wavelengths are less efficiently absorbed by RPE and choroidal melanin. Although the mechanism of action for the beneficial effects of scatter laser photocoagulation for PDR has not been established, it is thought that retinal destruction may be central to blunting the production of angiogenic moieties.[16] Moreover, because pain is mediated by deep choroidal neurons, confinement of absorption to the RPE is theoretically advantageous, and shorter wavelengths may be preferred. To minimize potentially injurious sequelae of blue light, argon-green light at 514 nm is the most commonly used wavelength for retinal photocoagulation.

Recently, commercial systems have become available using frequency-doubled Nd:YAG (1064 nm) laser output at 532 nm. When compared with argon green at 514 nm, this laser has the advantage of offering less absorption by macular xanthophyll and greater absorption by hemoglobin. In addition, this laser offers solid-state dependability and low maintenance. In clinical studies, this wavelength appears to be as efficacious as argon-green laser therapy.[17]

For macular applications, dye yellow at 577 nm presents theoretical advantages. This wavelength is not well absorbed by macular xanthophyll and is relatively well absorbed by tissue hemoglobin (see Fig. 50–8), maximizing absorption by microaneurysms and choroidal neovascular membranes while minimizing retinal absorption by macular xanthophyll. The practical benefit for this theoretical advantage is not well established. Moreover, because light scattering is greater with shorter wavelengths, yellow and red light penetrate through cataractous lenses more efficiently than green light does, again presenting a theoretical advantage for clinical laser application.

Diode lasers offer the benefits of low cost, low maintenance, high efficiency, standard electrical requirements, and portability.[18, 19] However, the deeper penetration of near-infrared light results in less visible burns and potentially more pain.[20] Histologic studies have demonstrated that although argon laser lesions result in both inner and outer retinal damage, 810-nm diode laser lesions, because of greater tissue penetration, result in outer retinal and choroidal injury[21, 22] (Fig. 50–10). Conversely, the increased penetration of near-infrared light through blood is advantageous for the treatment of retinal lesions partially obscured by overlying hemorrhage. For age-related macular degeneration, it may be that if a neovascular lesion can be identified by indocyanine green (ICG) angiography with excitation and emission at 805 and 835 mm, respectively, it can be treated with 810-nm diode laser radiation.[23, 24]

Vogel and Birngruber[21] modeled the laser-tissue interactions in the fundus following laser irradiation with 514- to 810-nm radiation. They found a much higher temperature rise in the middle and outer choroid following longer wavelength irradiation secondary to deeper penetration of the incident light (see Fig. 50–10). Although the absorption coefficient for RPE melanin is 1500/cm at 514 nm, it drops to 150/cm at 810 nm. These authors concluded that "argon green laser wavelengths are best suited for most clinical applications of photocoagulation." However, their conclusion is predicated on achieving equivalent levels of retinal photodestruction, which might be critical for the efficacy of panretinal photocoagulation in PDR.[16] Specifically, argon-green irradiation is associated with a lower choroidal temperature rise for a given rise in temperature at the RPE. Conversely, deeper penetration with minimal photoreceptor injury may be useful for other macular laser applications, including treatment for diabetic macular edema and age-related macular degeneration; this notion has driven investigations toward sub–ophthalmoscopically visible retinal photocoagulation with short-pulse visible and diode lasers.[25–27]

Although light gray/white burns are appropriate for most argon laser photocoagulative applications, the optimal near-infrared diode laser interaction may be associated with invisible or nearly visible lesions, presenting obvious difficulties for power titration. Pulse shape modulation has been investigated to achieve better thermal localization and more selective tissue injury (Fig. 50–11) with mixed results.[25, 26] The technical advantages of these laser sources are substantial, but more widespread use may await the development of moderate-power, *visible*, compact diode laser sources. Alternatively, the deep penetration of infrared light permits transscleral application for cyclophotodestruction and laser retinopexy. The former is now a well-accepted arrow in the quiver of the glaucoma specialist for otherwise intractable glaucoma, whereas the latter is now being evaluated for treatment of retinal tears in the clinical setting and in the operating room.[28]

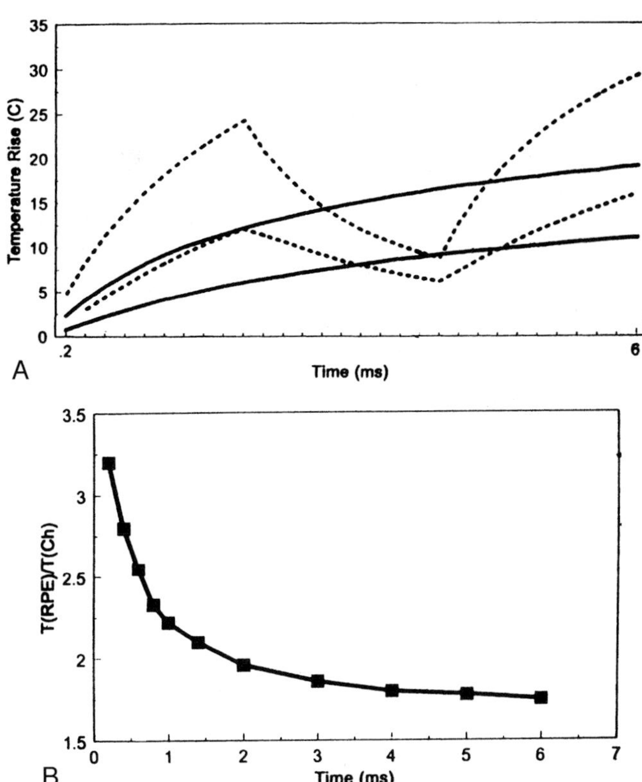

FIGURE 50–11. *A*, Calculated temperature rise following micropulsed *(broken line)* and continuous *(solid line)* 100-msec 810-nm diode laser application for the retinal pigment epithelium (RPE) *(upper curves)* and deep choroid (Ch) *(lower curves)*. Micropulsed application depicts 2-W, 2 msec on/2 msec off application, whereas continuous mode reflects 1 W of continuous power. *B*, The calculated ratio of the temperature rise at the RPE to the temperature rise in the deep choroid during a 6-msec, 1-W, 810-nm laser pulse. Equivalently, the data reflect the temperature ratio following single-micropulse laser application in which the abscissa corresponds to the duration of the micropulse. (From Berger JW: Thermal modeling of micropulsed diode laser retinal photocoagulation. Lasers Surg Med 20:411, 1997.)

As with diode laser micropulsing,[25, 26] short-duration visible laser pulses—for example, 5-μs argon laser pulses—have been shown to selectively damage the RPE while sparing the choriocapillaris and photoreceptors.[27] It has been demonstrated that short pulse lengths and low duty factors (laser "on" time divided by total pulse length) allow for maximum thermal localization with greatest tissue selectivity.[26] The logistical difficulties in titrating sub–ophthalmoscopically visible laser pulses notwithstanding, this approach may offer advantages compared with conventional retinal photocoagulation. However, these advantages have not been proven in clinical studies.

Aside from retinal applications, photocoagulation mediates both laser trabeculoplasty as performed with visible (most commonly argon) and near-infrared (diode) lasers and argon

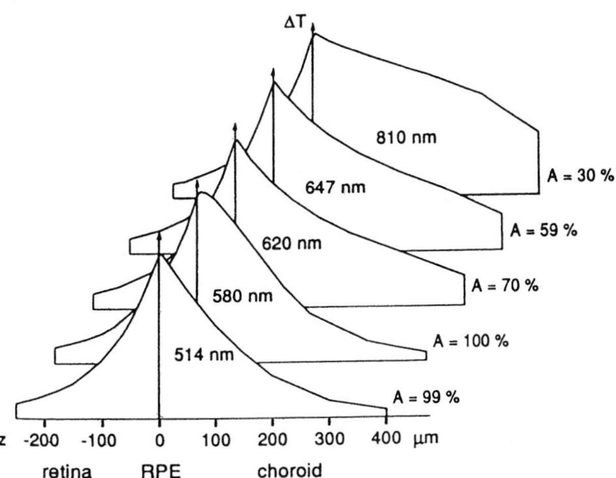

FIGURE 50–10. Temperature profiles in retina and choroid as calculated by Vogel and Birngruber[21] for a 500-μm spot size at a duration of 100 msec. The curves are normalized to the same temperature elevation at the retinal pigment epithelium (RPE). *A* represents the fraction of incident light absorbed by the RPE and choroid.

laser iridotomy. Although the initial laser-tissue interactions are virtually identical to retinal applications—specifically, the absorption of laser light by uveal melanin—the subsequent biologic response differs. For laser trabeculoplasty, a mechanical theory was initially postulated whereby local shrinkage allowed for expansion of Schlemm's canal and the trabecular meshwork.[29] However, it may be that laser absorption stimulates trabecular meshwork cells, leading to turnover of trabecular extracellular matrix.[30]

Photodisruption

Photodisruption follows nonlinear laser-tissue interactions at the target volume of a high-power laser pulse. For example, the transparent media of the eye, including the cornea, aqueous humor, lens, and vitreous, are nearly transparent to 1064-nm Nd:YAG laser radiation. However, in Q-switched or mode-locked operation, very-high-intensity electric fields are present near the focal volume. The electric field is powerful enough to strip electrons from the irradiated molecules, creating a *plasma* of positively and negatively charged species. This plasma then absorbs subsequent photons with a rise in temperature.[6] Plasma temperatures may reach 20,000 K. The plasma expands at supersonic velocities, producing shock waves and acoustic waves. Tissue disruption is mediated by the acoustomechanical sequelae of the laser-tissue interaction.

The first application of photodisruption to the eye was trabecular laser goniopuncture in 1972. Using a Q-switched ruby laser, Krasnov[5] attempted to augment outflow facility in eyes with open-angle glaucoma. Since then, the development of Q-switched and mode-locked neodymium laser sources combined with the increasing popularity of extracapsular cataract extraction (which frequently requires subsequent posterior capsulotomy) has stimulated the development of efficient, practical Nd:YAG lasers for capsular photodisruption.[6] This application has greatly facilitated visual rehabilitation in eyes otherwise requiring open surgical capsulotomy.

Laser powers of greater than 10^{10} W/cm^2 are required to initiate optical breakdown. Nominal laser energies, such as the 1 mJ commonly used for Nd:YAG laser capsulotomy, would ordinarily not initiate nonlinear processes. However, by confining this energy in space to a focal point on the order of 50 μm, and in time to a pulse length of several nanoseconds or less, very high peak laser powers are achieved.

Plasma formation begins by impurity-accentuated focal heating as thermionic emission or multiphoton absorption. For example, with molecular ionization energies on the order of 10 electron volts (eV), eight or nine 1064-nm (1.2-eV) photons would be required to initiate ionization.[6] Short (20- to 30-picosecond) mode-locked pulses are powerful enough to favor this mechanism; longer Q-switch pulses probably rely on thermionic emission.

Once initiated, ionization continues and grows by *cascade*. Newly produced, high-energy ions accelerate and ionize adjacent molecules, with the total population of ionized species growing as each ion ionizes two or more neighbors. Amplification continues as long as the laser irradiance overwhelms loss mechanisms such as diffusion out of the focal volume and inelastic collisions. Once created, the plasma scatters and absorbs incident light, prohibiting laser propagation distal to the focal volume.

Elegant experiments have demonstrated that Nd:YAG laser–induced optical breakdown is associated with plasma formation on the subnanosecond time scale. The plasma has a lifetime of several nanoseconds.[31] Although a number of mechanisms may contribute to the generation of mechanical stress waves, shock-wave production with plasma expansion is by far the most important interaction. Following 10-mJ, 10-ns frequency-doubled Nd:YAG laser application, the shock wave travels at 2100 m/sec for the first 100 μm, slowing to 1700 m/sec thereafter.[31] With 5-mJ, 7-ns Q-switched Nd:YAG laser application, an acoustic transient on the order of 9 to 16 bar is measured 18 mm from the focal point, with pressures exceeding 200 bar 1 mm from the focal point.[32] Under these conditions, the maximum bubble size is 1.5 to 2.3 mm.

Unlike photocoagulative applications, thermal interactions are limited in photodisruption. For nominal pulse energies, thermal denaturation arising from contact with the very hot plasma is probably limited to a region within 100 μm of the focal point,[33] and mechanical interactions determine the tissue response to laser application. For example, iridotomy may be performed with either argon or Q-switched Nd:YAG lasers. In the former, coagulation and necrosis results in tissue removal. In the latter, the iris is disrupted through mechanical interactions.

By compressing the pulse energy to a shorter pulse duration, a greater peak laser power is achieved. With this approach, optical breakdown is initiated with picosecond laser pulses at pulse energies two orders of magnitude less than that required for nanosecond pulses.[34, 35] Picosecond pulses with lower pulse energies are associated with smaller bubbles and reduced mechanical effects, offering much greater precision in tissue disruption[35–37] (Figs. 50–12 and 50–13). Using an in vitro model, Lin and colleagues[34] demonstrated that 100-picosecond photodisruption with pulse energies from 40 to 110 μJ cuts tissue while not damaging adjacent structures within 100 μm of the target. Efficiency was achieved with repetition rates up to 200 Hz.

Vogel and associates[35] noted qualitatively similar results,

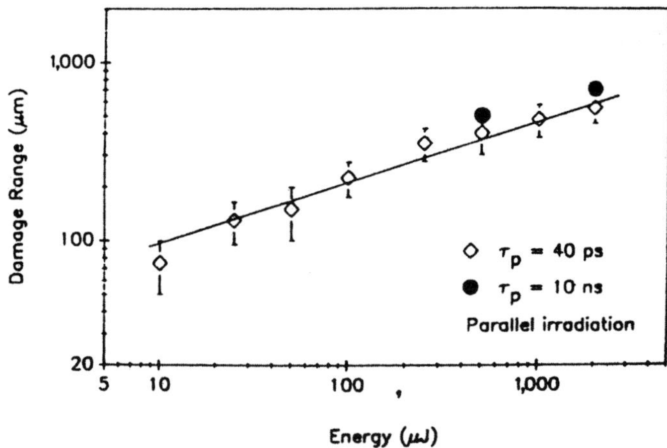

FIGURE 50–12. Damage range versus pulse energy for laser-induced optical breakdown adjacent to corneal endothelium in a model system. (From Zyesset B, et al: Time-resolved measurement of picosecond optical breakdown. Appl Physics [B] 48:139, 1989.)

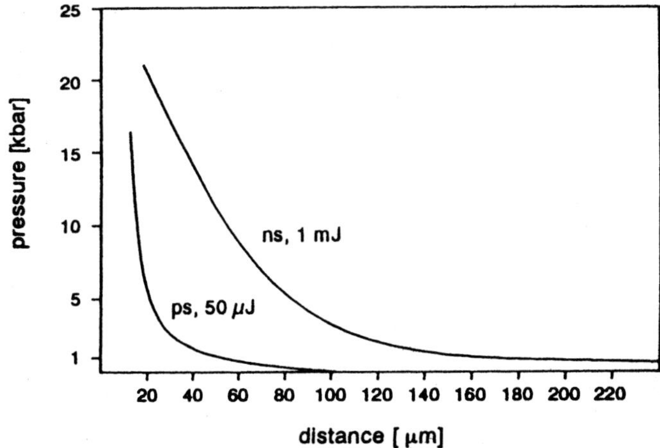

FIGURE 50–13. Shock wave pressure after optical breakdown for a 30-picosecond versus a 6-nanosecond laser pulse plotted as a function of distance from the emission center. (From Vogel A, et al: Mechanisms of intraocular photodisruption with picosecond and nanosecond laser pulses. Lasers Surg Med 15:32, 1994.)

demonstrating that the shock-wave pressure falls sharply at a distance of 20 μm for a 30-picosecond, 50 μJ laser pulse when compared with the less localized effects of nanosecond pulses (see Fig. 50–13). Juhasz and coworkers[38] extended these observations to the femtosecond regimen. With 150-femtosecond, 620-nm pulses, the magnitude of the shock wave and cavitation bubbles generated in water and corneal tissue was smaller than those measured following nanosecond or picosecond pulses.

Exploiting this precision, investigators have explored the application of picosecond photodisruption to corneal and vitreoretinal surgical maneuvers. Puliafito and colleagues[36] and Little and Jack[39] investigated transcorneal Nd:YAG-laser vitreous surgery, but their technique was limited by the imprecision of nanosecond-pulse sequelae. When they cut membranes between 1.5 and 3 mm from the retinal surface, injury was documented in five of seven cases.[36] Cohen and associates[40] reported their results using an Nd:yttrium lithium fluoride (YLF) picosecond laser for segmentation of PDR membranes in an FDA-approved phase-I protocol. In selected cases, this laser—operating at 60 picoseconds/pulse, 100 μJ/pulse, and 1000 pulses/sec—safely disrupted proliferative tissue near the retinal surface. Similarly, several groups are investigating short-pulse neodymium lasers for highly precise intrastromal corneal ablation for refractive surgery.[41]

Clearly, tissue response depends on the contributions of all mechanisms as determined by pulse length, pulse energy, and pulse geometry. Moreover, the elegant studies of Juhasz and coworkers[42] demonstrated the differences in shock-wave and cavitation-bubble dynamics in water versus corneal tissue. Although the contribution of tissue micromechanics to the effect of short-duration stress transients has not been explored methodically, mechanical tissue properties may profoundly influence the laser-tissue interaction.

Photoablation

Laser-mediated tissue removal follows bond-breaking with tissue ejection as in excimer photorefractive keratectomy, or thermoablation as mediated by mid-infrared tissue photovaporization. Ultraviolet laser ablative decomposition is discussed later.

Tissue photovaporization depends on water absorption. The tissue water serves as the chromophore; material is vaporized (ablated) when sufficient energy is delivered to both raise the local temperature beyond the boiling point *and* provide for the heat of vaporization. The development of the CO_2 laser, with an output at 10.6 μm and a very high water absorption coefficient (950/cm), offered possibilities for surface ablation and tissue removal with local cauterization—bloodless surgery. Much later, mid-infrared laser systems with greater water absorption—especially erbium-based laser systems—were developed and evaluated for highly precise tissue removal.

The infrared water absorption spectrum is depicted in Figure 50–14. Greater absorption coefficients are associated with shorter tissue penetration depths and, at least theoretically, greater microsurgical precision. In transection of experimental vitreous membranes, the Er:YAG laser (water absorption coefficient of 13,000/cm) was much more precise in tissue ablation[43] when compared with the CO_2 laser (950/cm)[44] or the holmium laser (23/cm).[45] However, experimental observations and predictions based on ablation depth do not agree completely. For the Er:YAG laser, calculations based on absorption coefficient imply ablation depths and surgical precision on the order of several micrometers, whereas experimental and modeling studies suggest penetration depths on the order of tens of micrometers for moderate values of radiant exposure.[46, 47] In addition, bubbles generated during the ablation process achieve sizes on the millimeter scale. For example, Lin and colleagues[48] measured a bubble size of 1 mm following 1-mJ, free-running Er:YAG laser application in water. Berger and associates noted similar results and used experiment and modeling studies to demonstrate further that the bubble size increases as the cube root of the incident pulse energy.[49, 50]

Because damage zones are usually much smaller than 1 mm (5 to 10 μm in Q-switched application and 10 to 50 μm in free-running application[51]), the generated vapor bubbles

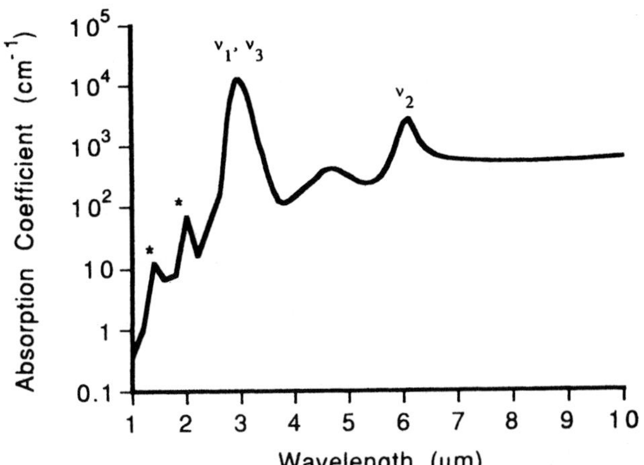

FIGURE 50–14. Infrared water absorption spectrum. ν_1, ν_2, and ν_3 are the vibrational symmetric stretch, symmetric bend, and asymmetric stretch modes. The overtones are designated by an asterisk. (From Walsh JT, Cummings JP: Effect of the dynamic optical properties of water on mid-infrared laser absorption. Lasers Surg Med 15:295, 1994.)

must be "gentle."[50] Moreover, these modeling studies suggest that low pulse energies delivered at a high repetition rate maximizes ablation efficiency while minimizing the maximum bubble size and pressure amplitude.

The tissue thermal relaxation time is defined by the equation

$$\tau = 1/(4\kappa\alpha^2)$$

where α is the absorption coefficient and κ is the tissue thermal diffusivity. For pulses shorter than the thermal relaxation time, the energy is spatially confined; thermal diffusion out of the target volume during longer laser pulses results in less localized effects. This phenomenon contributes to the extreme precision of tissue ablation mediated by the Q-switched Er:YAG laser.

Because tissue removal is thermally mediated, heat deposition with unintentional tissue thermal injury is a concern. However, the temperature rise has been moderate in model systems for anterior and posterior segment applications (Fig. 50–15).[52, 53]

In part because of concerns regarding the mutagenicity of ultraviolet radiation and the toxic gases associated with excimer lasers, investigators have explored solid-state, mid-infrared laser keratectomy. Although results thus far have demonstrated less precision when compared with ultraviolet laser ablation (see later), several centers are pursuing this line of research as an alternative to excimer-laser keratectomy.[54] In accordance with predictions based on laser-tissue interactions, cutting in cornea is least precise with the CO_2 laser, followed by the normal-mode Er:YAG laser and the Q-switched Er:YAG laser; excimer-laser ablation is the most precise.

Corneal reshaping with the holmium laser has been explored to correct hyperopia.[55, 56] Although not ablative, mid-infrared pulses at 2.1 μm heat the peripheral corneal tissue to subablative temperatures, resulting in a steepening of the central cornea and a myopic shift.

The development of flexible, durable fiberoptics permitting the delivery of mid-infrared laser pulses has stimulated

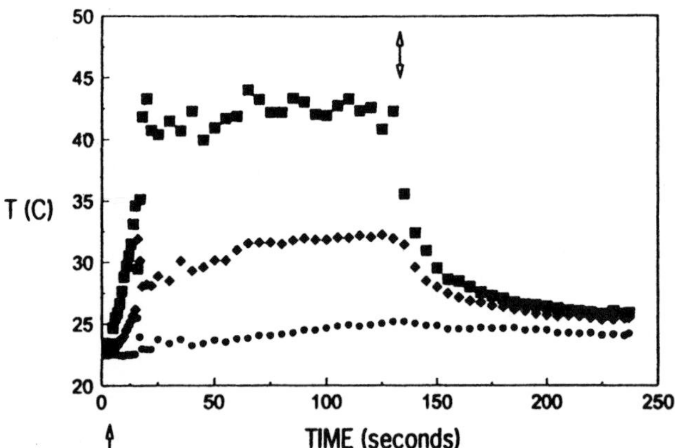

FIGURE 50–15. Experimental measurement of thermal transients in bovine vitreous. The temperature is depicted 0.5 mm *(squares),* 2.5 mm *(diamonds),* and 6 mm *(circles)* from the laser tip in response to 10-Hz, 6-mJ, free-running Er:YAG laser irradiation. The laser is turned on *(arrow)* and off *(double-headed arrow)* at 3 seconds and 125 seconds, respectively. (From Berger JW, et al: Measurement and modeling of thermal transients during Er:YAG laser irradiation of vitreous. Lasers Surg Med 19:388, 1996.)

work toward intraocular, laser-assisted microsurgery.[43, 46, 49, 50, 53, 57–59] Delivery of Er:YAG laser 2.94-μm pulses facilitates tissue ablation and removal, and a number of systems are in various stages of research and development for cataract extraction, glaucoma filtration surgery, and vitreoretinal surgery.

The recently developed semiconductor continuous-wave, 1.94-μm diode laser offers attractive features. It emits at the local water absorption peak near 1.93 μm and offers the reliability, portability, and economy characteristic of solid-state diode sources. Further, fiberoptic delivery is technically more straightforward for the 1.94-μm diode laser pulses when compared with the 2.94-μm Er:YAG laser pulses. The water absorption coefficient of 1.94-μm radiation is 80 times lower than that of 2.94-μm radiation; the penetration depth is 80 times higher.[60] Therefore, on a per-pulse basis, the diode laser is more efficient for tissue removal. Conversely, the erbium laser, in theory, offers a nearly twofold increase in precision for tissue removal.

Azzolini and coworkers[61] described their initial experience with the 1.94-μm diode laser in performing vitreoretinal surgical maneuvers in rabbit eye. Cutting efficiency was limited by low available powers. Retinotomy was performed with thermal damage zones ranging from 50 to 200 μm, but experimentally induced epiretinal membranes were only superficially ablated.

Cutaneous laser resurfacing has received extraordinary attention in both the popular and the scientific literature.[62] Although the CO_2 laser has been available for many years, ablation of skin with limited charring of adjacent and subjacent tissue requires pulse durations on the order of, or less than, the tissue thermal relaxation time.[63] This requirement serves to limit thermal diffusion and localize the deposited thermal energy. The combination of short pulses with scanning delivery systems has resulted in a clinically useful tool.

Ross and colleagues[64] showed that CO_2 laser ablation caused adjacent char in pig skin only with pulse lengths greater than 1 msec. For 10-msec pulses, thermal diffusion outpaced ablation velocity, resulting in deposition of thermal energy and tissue temperature increase to subablation levels associated with thermal damage. For pulses shorter than 1 msec, the ablation velocity exceeds thermal diffusion, with confinement of tissue damage. Thermal damage zones in guinea pig skin were 750 μm for 50-msec CO_2-laser pulse widths, 170 μm for 2-msec pulses, and 50 μm for 2-μsec pulses.[63]

These authors[64] also suggest a reevaluation of current wisdom regarding laser resurfacing and wrinkle removal. Typically, wrinkle removal is explained by noting that wrinkle "shoulders" are treated by a laser pass, but the troughs are left untreated. In fact, because average visible periorbital wrinkles are 300 μm thick and typical ablation depths are on the order of 30 to 50 μm, 7 to 10 passes would be required for smoothing. However, only 2 or 3 passes yield clinical improvement; therefore, nonablative tissue contraction may contribute to clinical efficacy.

Compared with 1-msec CO_2 laser pulses, free-running Er:YAG laser pulses offer shorter duration (typically 300 μsec), limiting thermal diffusion and greatly reducing penetration depth corresponding to a water absorption coefficient of 13,000/cm for the Er:YAG laser versus 950/cm for the CO_2 laser. Greater precision is theoretically possible. Kaufmann and Hibst[65] demonstrated extreme precision in their studies of pulsed Er:YAG laser cutaneous surgery in pig skin and human patients. Hohenleutner and associates[66] reported similar results. However, bleeding limited the utility of this technique for treatment of deeper lesions. Erbium may indeed supplant CO_2 lasers for skin resurfacing, but it appears that cutting precision is but one of many aspects of the laser-tissue interaction that make for a clinically useful tool.

Ablative Decomposition

By combining excited inert gas atoms with rare gas halogens, excited dimer rare gas halide *excimers* are produced. Ultraviolet photon emission characteristic of the transition energy causes decay to a weakly bound or unbound ground state. Argon fluoride, krypton fluoride, and xenon chloride emit laser wavelengths of 193, 247, and 308 nm, respectively. Nucleic acid and protein molecular bonds absorb in this regime and serve as the tissue chromophores. Since the development of these laser sources, investigators have studied the interaction of excimer laser radiation with ocular tissues. Excimer laser-tissue applications are discussed elsewhere in more detail. The principles of ablative decomposition are reviewed here briefly.

Photons in the deep ultraviolet (on the order of 200 nm or shorter) have enough energy to break molecular bonds. Energy in excess of that required to break bonds is imparted to molecular fragments, leading to high-velocity particle ejection. Whereas photovaporization-mediated tissue removal depends on tissue ejection subsequent to tissue water boiling, tissue removal mediated by the ultraviolet laser follows direct breaking of molecular bonds.

Besides bond breaking, there is an acoustic effect with shock-wave production and significant mechanical sequelae.[67–69] Explosive material ejection is associated with the production of intense pressure transients. Siano and colleagues[69] measured pressure transients in porcine eyes subjected to conditions of clinical argon fluoride excimer laser photorefractive keratectomy. They measured maximal compression and rarefaction amplitudes of 90 and −40 bar, respectively. These results support the notion that considerable mechanical energy is imparted to the eye during excimer photorefractive keratectomy and may be relevant to optimal energy delivery in clinical applications.

Interestingly, ablation at 193 nm with the excimer laser—although commonly called a "cold" laser—deposits thermal energy. Under clinically relevant conditions, Feld and associates[70] measured a bulk tissue temperature rise, suggesting that approximately 25% of incident energy is converted to heat. The origin of this phenomenon is unclear and may reflect direct tissue heating as well as dissipative, nonradiative deactivation pathways after the absorption event. The implications of this effect for corneal healing and haze have not been methodically explored.

Untoward nonmechanical effects from excimer laser sources received early attention. In theory, ultraviolet light carries significant mutagenic potential. However, argon fluoride excimer laser irradiation of human skin led to no unscheduled DNA synthesis activity, suggesting that DNA repair mechanisms are not activated by 193-nm radiation as they are following krypton fluoride 248-nm irradiation.[71] Moreover, Ediger[72] calculated a minute lens exposure to excimer laser–induced ultraviolet fluorescence, suggesting that the risk for cataractogenicity is extremely low. Recently, aerosolization of infectious virus by excimer laser,[73] particularly herpes simplex virus and adenovirus, has been demonstrated. This finding warrants further investigation concerning surgical team safety during ultraviolet-laser application.

Keratectomy has received the greatest attention for excimer-laser applications. Therefore, excimer laser–corneal tissue interactions have been most intensely studied. However, the potential for tissue removal with extreme precision has prompted investigation of excimer-laser applications for lens removal[74] and vitreous surgery.[75] Because ultraviolet light cannot be delivered to the intraocular target tissues with a transpupillary approach owing to strong absorption by the otherwise transparent ocular media, fiberoptic delivery is required. Lewis and coworkers[75] presented their method for needle-guided excimer laser delivery and demonstrated ultra-precise retinal tissue ablation with minimal adjacent tissue injury. Further development of delivery systems for intraocular application of ultraviolet light as derived from excimer and nonexcimer, solid-state laser sources may yield heretofore unachievable precision for intraocular surgical maneuvers.

Similarly, although the excimer laser is most widely used for ultraviolet-laser applications, solid-state laser sources, such as the Novatec and the fifth harmonic of the Nd:YAG or Nd:YLF lasers (at 213 and 211 nm, respectively), may eventually supplant excimer lasers in ultraviolet applications.[76] Laser-tissue interactions do not depend on the laser medium; therefore, experience and understanding accumulated in excimer-laser ophthalmic applications are readily transferable to nonexcimer, ultraviolet-laser applications.

Laser-Tissue Interactions Mediated by Exogenous Chromophores

Although the laser-tissue interactions described earlier depend on the interaction of laser light with native tissue moieties, exogenous agents may be administered to achieve high concentrations in the target volume to mediate photochemical reactions. The fundamentals of laser-tissue interactions in PDT are briefly described here.

PDT has received considerable attention for treatment of ocular tumors and choroidal neovascularization.[77–82] For example, results in phase I and II clinical trials demonstrate that PDT using benzoporphyrin-derivative achieves short-term closure of choroidal neovascularization in age-related macular degeneration (AMD).[80–82]

Following light absorption, the excited singlet state may decay nonradiatively, decay with photon emission (fluorescence), or undergo intersystem crossing to the excited triplet state.[83] The excited triplet state may then interact directly with the substrate, resulting in production of free radicals and ions, which may subsequently mediate local tissue injury (type I mechanism). Alternatively, because ground-state molecular oxygen exists in a triplet state, the production of chromophore excited triplet states (^{3}Sens*) favors triplet-triplet annihilation with the production of highly reactive singlet oxygen (type II mechanism):

$$h\nu + {}^1\text{Sens} \Rightarrow {}^3\text{Sens}^*$$

$$ {}^3\text{Sens}^* + {}^3\text{O}_2 \Rightarrow {}^1\text{Sens} + {}^1\text{O}_2$$

It is thought that this pathway mediates the major portion of photodynamic action.[78, 84] Singlet oxygen ($^1O_2$), other generated reactive oxygen species (including superoxide anion [O_2^-] and hydroxyl radicals [·OH]), and the excited triplet state of the photosensitizer (^{3}Sens*) may then mediate local tissue injury through electron abstraction, free-radical chemistry, and oxidative reactions.

At least theoretically, the choice of photosensitizer does not influence the details of the laser-tissue interaction.[85] However, the photosensitizer properties, including triplet quantum yield, absorption maximum, systemic toxicity, and metabolism, greatly influence practical considerations for photodynamic applications.

Photodynamic vascular thrombosis is predicated on vascular endothelial cell damage following light activation of intravenously injected photosensitizer.[86] The production of reactive oxygen species leads to localized endothelial cell injury, with platelet aggregation and vascular occlusion. Phthalocyanine dyes have received much attention because of high photodynamic efficiency and very low systemic toxicity. Excitation at 675 nm has previously required high-cost, high-maintenance dye lasers, but the development of visible-wavelength diode lasers could increase affordability and convenience.[87]

Indocyanine green (ICG) is a potentially attractive exogenous chromophore because it absorbs close to the emission maximum of the most commonly available diode lasers at 810 nm.[88, 89] It is demonstrably safe as a diagnostic tool in posterior segment angiography, and its localization can be identified by commercially available imaging systems. Naturally, investigators have questioned the utility of ICG-guided and ICG-enhanced photodestruction of neovascular lesions, especially those associated with macular degeneration.[88–90]

It is important to clarify the potential role for ICG in this application; confusion is considerable. Although the benefit of photocoagulation for neovascular lesions in AMD as identified by ICG angiography has not been proven in a large, well-designed, randomized, prospective clinical trial, ICG angiography may have a role in identifying lesions amenable to laser treatment that are otherwise ineligible for treatment based on fluorescein angiography characteristics. This approach is called *ICG-guided* photocoagulation.

In contrast, one might speculate that ICG acts as an exogenous chromophore mediating photochemical or photothermal tissue injury (*ICG-enhanced* laser therapy). If ICG acts merely as an absorber to potentiate photocoagulation, exogenous dye administration may confer little benefit; selectivity is lost because native ocular chromophores including melanin readily absorb infrared light. As Vogel and Birngruber[21] noted, injection of typical ICG doses of 3 to 4 mg/kg of body weight yields a corresponding absorption coefficient of 20/cm at 810 nm, which is small compared with the absorption coefficient of the RPE melanin (150/cm). Therefore, at least theoretically, ICG is not likely to greatly enhance thermally mediated laser photocoagulation. Moreover, because ICG-mediated photodynamic action has not been demonstrated, the role for this agent in enhancing tissue injury is not well established.

A novel application of chromophore-enhanced laser absorption involves tissue welding.[91] Several groups have investigated irradiation of ICG or other chromophores linked to albumin to mediate sutureless tissue welding. This technique is still in development but may be applicable to corneal and cutaneous surgery.

The Future

Almost exclusively, the application of laser technology to ophthalmic diagnosis and treatment has been empirical. As new lasers are developed, interested clinicians and scientists explore the possible application of these novel laser systems to investigative ophthalmology and clinical practice. As laser sources covering the wide spectrum of possible pulse characteristics, including pulse energy/power, wavelength, and temporal and spatial pulse profiles, are developed and become available, selectivity increases; desirable interactions may be enhanced while untoward tissue injury is minimized, leading to greater safety and efficacy in ophthalmic laser applications.

REFERENCES

1. Maiman TH: Stimulated optical radiation in ruby. Nature 187:493, 1960.
2. Zaret MM, Breinin GM, Schmidt H, et al: Ocular lesions produced by an optical maser (laser). Science 134:1525, 1961.
3. Zweng HC, Flocks M, Kapany NS, et al: Experimental laser photocoagulation. Am J Ophthalmol 58:353, 1964.
4. Campbell CJ, Rittler MC, Koester CJ: The optical maser as a retinal photocoagulator: An evaluation. Trans Am Acad Ophthalmol Otolaryngol 67:58, 1963.
5. Krasnov MM: Laser puncture of the anterior chamber angle in glaucoma. Vestn Oftalmol 3:27, 1972.
6. Steinert RF, Puliafito CA: The Neodymium:YAG Laser in Ophthalmology. Principles and Clinical Applications of Photodisruption. Philadelphia, WB Saunders, 1985.
7. Birngruber R: Thermal modelling in biological tissues. *In* Hillenkamp F, Pratesi R, Sacchi CA (eds): Lasers in Biology and Medicine. New York, Plenum, 1980, pp 777–790.
8. Sliney DH: New chromophores for ophthalmic laser surgery. Lasers Light Ophthalmol 2:53, 1988.
9. Krauss JM, Puliafito CA, Steinert RF: Photoablation. *In* Albert DM, Jakobiec FA (eds): Principles and Practice of Ophthalmology. Philadelphia, WB Saunders, 1994.
10. Sigrist MW: Laser generation of acoustic waves in liquids and gases. J Appl Physics 60:R83–R121, 1986.
11. Vogel A, Dlugos C, Nuffer R, Birngruber R: Optical properties of the human sclera and their consequences for transscleral laser application. Lasers Surg Med 11:331–340, 1991.
12. Beetham WP, Aiello LM, Balodimos M, Koncz L: Ruby laser photocoagulation of early diabetic retinopathy. Arch Ophthalmol 83:261, 1970.
13. Meyer-Schwickerath G: Light Coagulation. St. Louis, CV Mosby, 1960.
14. L'Esperance FA: Ophthalmic Lasers. St. Louis, CV Mosby, 1989.
15. Mainster MA: Wavelength selection in macular photocoagulation. Tissue optics, thermal effects and laser systems. Ophthalmology 93:952–958, 1986.
16. Wolbarsht ML, Landers MB III: The rationale of photocoagulation therapy for proliferative diabetic retinopathy: A review and a model. Ophthalmic Surg 11:235–245, 1980.
17. Bandello F, Brancato R, Lattanzio R, et al: Double-frequency Nd:YAG laser vs argon green laser in the treatment of proliferative diabetic retinopathy: Randomized study with long term follow up. Lasers Surg Med 19:173–176, 1996.
18. Puliafito CA, Deutsch TF, Boll J, To K: Semiconductor laser endophotocoagulation of the retina. Arch Ophthalmol 105:424–427, 1987.
19. Smiddy WE, Hernandez LAT: Histologic results of retinal diode laser photocoagulation in rabbit eyes. Ophthalmology 110:693–698, 1992.
20. Balles MW, Puliafito CA, D'Amico DJ, et al: Semiconductor diode laser photocoagulation in retinal vascular disease. Ophthalmology 97:1553–1561, 1990.
21. Vogel A, Birngruber R: Temperature profiles in human retina and choroid during laser coagulation with different wavelengths ranging from 514 to 810 nm. Lasers Light Ophthalmol 5:9–16, 1992.

22. Brancato R, Pratesi R, Leoni G, et al: Histopathology of diode and argon laser lesions in rabbit retina. Inv Ophthalmol Vis Sci 30:1504–1510, 1989.
23. Cohen SM, Shen JH, Smiddy WE: Laser energy and dye fluorescence transmission through blood in vitro. Am J Ophthalmol 119:452–457, 1995.
24. Berger JW: Laser energy and dye fluorescence transmission through blood in vitro. [Letter] Am J Ophthalmol 120:404–405, 1995.
25. Friberg TR, Venkatesh S: Alteration of pulse shape configuration affects the pain response during diode laser photocoagulation. Lasers Surg Med 16:380–383, 1995.
26. Berger JW: Thermal modelling of micropulsed diode laser retinal photocoagulation. Lasers Surg Med 20:411–417, 1997.
27. Roider J, Michaud NA, Flotte TJ, Birngruber R: Response of the retinal pigment epithelium to selective photocoagulation. Arch Ophthalmol 110:1786–1792, 1992.
28. Haller J, Blair N, DeJuan E, et al: A multicenter trial of transcleral diode retinopexy in retinal detachment surgery. Inv Ophthalmol Vis Sci ARVO Abstracts 38:4321, 1997.
29. Wise JB: Glaucoma treatment by trabecular tightening with the argon laser. Int Ophthalmol Clin 21:69–78, 1981.
30. Van Buskirk EM, Pond V, Rosenquist RC, et al: Argon laser trabeculoplasty: Studies of mechanism of action. Ophthalmology 91:1005–1010, 1984.
31. Fujimoto JG, Lin WZ, Ippen EP, et al: Time-resolved studies of Nd:YAG laser-induced breakdown. Inv Ophthalmol Vis Sci 26:1771–1777, 1985.
32. Vogel A, Hentschel W, Holzfuss J, Lauterborn W: Cavitation bubble dynamics and acoustic transient generation in ocular surgery with pulsed Nd:YAG lasers. Ophthalmology 93:1259–1269, 1986.
33. Hu CL, Barnes FS: The thermal-chemical damage in biological material under laser irradiation. IEEE Trans Biomed Eng 17:220, 1970.
34. Lin CP, Weaver YK, Birngruber R, et al: Intraocular microsurgery with a picosecond Nd:YAG laser. Lasers Surg Med 15:44–53, 1994.
35. Vogel A, Busch S, Jungnickel K, Birngruber R: Mechanisms of intraocular photodisruption with picosecond and nanosecond laser pulses. Lasers Surg Med 15:32–43, 1994.
36. Puliafito CA, Wasson PJ, Steinert RF, Gragoudas ES: Neodynium YAG laser surgery on experimental vitreous membranes. Arch Ophthalmol 102:843–847, 1984.
37. Zyesset B, Fujimoto JG, Deutsch TF: Time-resolved measurements of picosecond optical breakdown. Appl Physics [B] 48:139–147, 1989.
38. Juhasz T, Kastis GA, Suarez C, et al: Time-resolved observations of shock waves and cavitation bubbles generated by femtosecond laser pulses in corneal tissue and water. Lasers Surg Med 19:23–31, 1996.
39. Little HL, Jack RL: Q switched Nd:YAG laser surgery of the vitreous. Graefes Arch Clin Exp Ophthalmol 224:240–246, 1986.
40. Cohen BZ, Wald KJ, Toyoma K: Nd:YLF picosecond laser segmentation for retinal traction associated with proliferative diabetic retinopathy. Am J Ophthalmol 123:515–523, 1997.
41. Nienz MH, Hoppeler TP, Juhasz T, et al: Intrastromal ablation for refractive corneal surgery using picosecond infrared laser pulses. Lasers Light Ophthalmol 5:149–155, 1993.
42. Juhasz T, Hu XH, Turi L, Bor Z: Dynamics of shock waves and cavitation bubbles generated by picosecond laser pulses in corneal tissue and water. Lasers Surg Med 15:91–98, 1994.
43. Brazitikos PD, D'Amico DJ, Bernal MT, Walsh AW: Erbium:YAG laser surgery of the vitreous and retina. Ophthalmology 102:278–290, 1995.
44. Meyers S, Bonner RF, Rodrigues MM, Ballintine EJ: Phototransection of vitreal membranes with the carbon dioxide laser in rabbits. Ophthalmology 90:563–568, 1983.
45. Borirakchanyavat S, Puliafito CA, Kliman GH, et al: Ho:YAG laser surgery on experimental vitreous membranes. Arch Ophthalmol 110:1605–1609, 1991.
46. Berger JW, Kim SH, LaMarche KJ, et al: Er:YAG laser drilling of cataractous lens: Predicting the ablation rate with a simple model. Proc SPIE 2393:148–159, 1995.
47. Walsh JT, Cummings JP: Effect of the dynamic optical properties of water on mid-infrared laser ablation. Lasers Surg Med 15:295–305, 1994.
48. Lin CP, Stern D, Puliafito CA: High speed photography of Er:YAG laser ablation in fluid. Implications for laser vitreous surgery. Inv Ophthalmol Vis Sci 31:2546–2550, 1990.
49. Berger JW, Bochow TW, Kim RY, D'Amico DJ: Biophysical considerations for optimizing energy delivery during Er:YAG laser vitreoretinal surgery. Proc SPIE 2673:146–156, 1996.
50. Berger JW, D'Amico DJ: Modeling of erbium:YAG laser mediated explosive photovaporization: Implications for vitreoretinal surgery. Ophthalmic Surg Lasers 28:133–139, 1997.
51. Walsh JT, Flotte TJ, Deutsch TF: Er:YAG laser ablation of tissue: Effect of pulse duration and tissue type on thermal damage. Lasers Surg Med 9:314–326, 1989.
52. Berger JW, Bochow TW, Talamo JH, D'Amico DJ: Measurement and modelling of thermal transients during Er:YAG laser irradiation of vitreous. Lasers Surg Med 19:388–396, 1996.
53. Berger JW, Talamo JH, Kim SH, et al: Temperature measurements during phacoemulsification and Er:YAG laser phacoablation in model systems. J Cat Refr Surgery 22:372–378, 1996.
54. Cubeddu R, Brancato R, Sozzi C, et al: Study of photoablation of rabbit corneas by Er:YAG laser. Lasers Surg Med 19:32–39, 1996.
55. Seiler T, Matallaner M, Bende T: Laser thermokeratoplasty by means of a pulsed holmium YAG laser for hyperopic correction. J Refractive Corneal Surg 6:99–102, 1990.
56. Tutton MK, Cherry PMH: Holmium:YAG laser thermokeratoplasty to correct hyperopia: Two years follow up. Ophthalmic Surg Lasers 27:S521–S524, 1996.
57. Bochow TW, Kim RY, Berger JW, D'Amico DJ: Photovitrectomy. A novel approach for vitreous removal. Inv Ophthalmol Vis Sci ARVO Abstracts 36:S384, 1995.
58. Kim RY, Bochow TW, Berger JW, et al: Ab externo subconjunctival sclerostomy in rabbits with an erbium:YAG laser and a side firing probe. Acute clinical and histologic observations. Inv Ophthalmol Vis Sci ARVO Abstracts 38:S167, 1997.
59. McHam ML, Eisenberg DL, Schuman JS, Wang N: Erbium:YAG laser sclerectomy with a sapphire optical fiber. Ophthalmic Surg Lasers 28:55–58, 1997.
60. Hale GM, Querry MR: Optical constants of water in the 200 nm to 200 micron wavelength region. Appl Optics 12:555–563, 1973.
61. Azzolini C, Gobbi PG, Brancato R, et al: New semiconductor laser for vitreoretinal surgery. Laser Surg Med 19:177–183, 1996.
62. Biesman BS: Cutaneous facial resurfacing with the carbon dioxide laser. Ophthalmic Surg Lasers 27:685–698, 1996.
63. Walsh J, Flotte T, Anderson R, Deutsch T: Pulsed CO_2 laser ablation: Effect of tissue type and pulse duration on thermal damage. Lasers Surg Med 8:108–118, 1988.
64. Ross EV, Domankevitz Y, Skrobal M, Anderson RR: Effects of CO_2 laser pulse duration in ablation and residual thermal damage: Implications for skin resurfacing. Lasers Surg Med 19:123–129, 1996.
65. Kaufmann R, Hibst R: Pulsed erbium:YAG laser ablation in cutaneous surgery. Lasers Surg Med 19:324–330, 1996.
66. Hohenleutner V, Hohenleutner S, Baumler W, Landthaler W: Fast and effective skin ablation with an erbium:YAG laser: Determination of ablation rates and thermal damage zones. Lasers Surg Med 20:242–247, 1997.
67. Srinivasan R, Dyre PE, Braren B: Far ultraviolet laser ablation of the cornea. Photoacoustic studies. Lasers Surg Med 6:514–519, 1987.
68. Bor Z, Hopp B, Racz B, et al: Plume emission, shock wave and surface wave formation during excimer laser ablation of the cornea. Refractive Corneal Surg 9:S111–S115, 1993.
69. Siano S, Pini R, Gobbi PG, et al: Intraocular measurements of pressure transients induced by excimer laser radiation. Lasers Surg Med 20:416–425, 1997.
70. Feld JR, Lin CP, Puliafito CA: Energy balance studies help explain the mechanism of excimer laser ablation of the cornea. Inv Ophthalmol Vis Sci ARVO Abstracts 35:2011, 1994.
71. Green HA, Margolis R, Boll J, et al: Unscheduled DNA synthesis in human skin after in vitro ultraviolet excimer laser ablation. J Invest Dermatol 89:201–204, 1987.
72. Ediger MN: Excimer laser induced fluorescence of rabbit cornea: Radiometric measurement through the cornea. Lasers Surg Med 11:93–98, 1991.
73. Moreira LB, Sanchez D, Trousdale MD, et al: Aerosolization of infectious virus by excimer laser. Am J Ophthalmol 123:297–302, 1997.
74. Puliafito CA, Steinert RF, Deutsch TF, et al: Excimer laser ablation of the cornea and lens. Ophthalmology 92:741, 1985.
75. Lewis A, Palanker D, Hemo I, et al: Microsurgery of the retina with a needle-guided 193 nm excimer laser. Inv Ophthalmol Vis Sci 33:2377–2381, 1992.
76. Ren Q, Simon G, Legeais JM, et al: UV solid state laser (213 nm) photorefractive keratectomy: In vivo study. Ophthalmology 101:883–889, 1994.

77. Hill RA, Reddi S, Kenney ME, et al: Photodynamic therapy of ocular melanoma with bis silicon 2,3 naphthocyanine in a rabbit model. Inv Ophthalmol Vis Sci 36:2476–2481, 1995.
78. Dougherty TJ: Photodynamic therapy of malignant tumors. Crit Rev Oncol Hematol 2:83–116, 1984.
79. Kim RY, Hu LK, Foster BS, et al: Photodynamic therapy of pigmented choroidal melanomas of greater than 3-mm thickness. Ophthalmology 103:2029–2036, 1996.
80. Gragoudas ES, Schmidt-Erfurth U, Sickenberg M, et al: Results and preliminary dosimetry of PDT for choroidal neovascularization in AMD in a phase I/phase II study. Inv Ophthalmol Vis Sci ARVO Abstracts 38:S17, 1997.
81. Husain D, Miller JW, Michaud N, et al: Intravenous infusion of liposomal benzoporphyrin derivative for photodynamic therapy of experimental choroidal neovascularization. Arch Ophthalmol 114:978–985, 1996.
82. Miller JW, Walsh AW, Kramer M, et al: Photodynamic therapy of experimental choroidal neovascularization using lipoprotein-delivered benzoporphyrin. Arch Ophthalmol 113:810–818, 1995.
83. Vanderkooi JM, Berger JW: Review: Excited triplet states used to study biological macromolecules at room temperature. Biochim Biophys Acta 976:1–27, 1990.
84. Henderson BW, Dougherty TJ: How does photodynamic therapy work? Photochem Photobiol 155:145–157, 1992.
85. Gomer CJ, Rucker N, Ferrario A, Wong S: Properties and applications of photodynamic therapy. Radiation Res 120:1–18, 1989.
86. Nanda SK, Hatchell DL, Tiedeman JS, et al: A new method for vascular occlusion: Photochemical initiation of thrombosis. Arch Ophthalmol 105:1121–1124, 1987.
87. Iliaki OE, Naoumidid II, Tsilimbaris MK, Palikaris IG: Photothrombosis of retinal and choroidal vessels in rabbit eyes using chloroaluminum sulfonated phthalocyanine and a diode laser. Lasers Surg Med 19:3111–3123, 1996.
88. Slakter JS, Yannuzzi LA, Sorenson JA, Guyer DR: A pilot study of indocyanine green videoangiography-guided laser photocoagulation of occult choroidal neovascularization in age-related macular degeneration. Arch Ophthalmol 112:465–472, 1994.
89. Guyer DR, Yannuzzi LA, Ladas I, et al: Indocyanine green-guided laser photocoagulation of focal spots at the edge of plaques of choroidal neovascularization. Arch Ophthalmol 114:693–697, 1996.
90. Reichel E, Puliafito CA: Indocyanine green dye enhanced diode laser photocoagulation of well-defined subfoveal choroidal neovascular membranes. Inv Ophthalmol Vis Sci ARVO Abstracts 34:1164, 1993.
91. Poppas DP, Wright EJ, Guthrie PD, et al: Human albumin solders for clinical application during laser tissue welding. Lasers Surg Med 19:2–8, 1996.

CHAPTER 51

Erbium:YAG Laser Photothermal Ablation: Applications for Vitreoretinal, Lens, Scleral, Corneal, and Iris Surgery

Periklis D. Brazitikos, Donald J. D'Amico, and George R. Marcellino

Laser technology has multiple applications in current ocular therapy. Since the construction of the first laser in 1960[1] and the introduction of photocoagulation for treating retinal vascular diseases,[2, 3] photocoagulation has become highly developed and widely used for the treatment of numerous ocular conditions. Many photocoagulative lasers and delivery systems are available to the clinician. Nevertheless, other laser-tissue interactions are possible with various laser wavelengths and technologies, and surgeons are increasingly using these interactions in ophthalmic and other fields of surgery with success.

Photocoagulation is the most commonly used ocular lesion created by a laser and has been produced by various lasers, including argon, krypton,[4, 5] ruby,[6] tunable dye,[7] diode,[8] and frequency-doubled neodymium:yttrium aluminum garnet (YAG).[9] In photocoagulation, chromophores within the eye, including melanin, hemoglobin, and xanthophyll, absorb light energy in a wavelength-dependent fashion and convert the energy to heat. Adjustment of the energy in order to increase tissue temperature to a level of 50°C to 100°C results in denaturation of proteins and coagulation.

Photodisruption is defined as the use of high-peak-power ionizing laser pulses to disrupt tissue. Concentration of light energy in an ultrashort period of time and in a small space achieves high irradiance or density of power and creates optical breakdown. During optical breakdown, the target medium is ionized because of dissociation of the electrons from their atoms, and a plasma is created that leads to tissue disruption.[10] In photodisrupting lasers, the high-peak–power pulses are produced by sharply reducing the energy delivery time with techniques such as Q-switching or mode locking the laser.[11] Q-switched pulses last 2 to 30 nsec, whereas mode-locked pulses typically last 20 to 30 psec. The most widely used laser photodisruptor in ophthalmic surgery is the 1064-nm Nd:YAG laser. Major ophthalmic applications of the Nd:YAG laser include posterior capsulotomy,[12] anterior vitreolysis,[13] and iridotomy.[14]

Ablative photodecomposition[15] is the laser-tissue interaction produced by the argon-fluoride (193 nm) excimer laser and the xenon-chloride (308 nm) excimer laser. In this process, the energy is absorbed by tissue proteins with resultant disruption of chemical bonds. The driving forces for ablative photodecomposition are the ultraviolet photons emitted by the laser and the energy of the broken chemical bonds, which result in small volatile tissue fragments that are ablated from the irradiated surface.[16] The excimer laser has gained wide clinical application in corneal and refractive surgery.[17, 18]

Lasers emitting at the infrared portion of light ablate tissue through the laser-tissue interaction of *photothermal ablation*. In this process, infrared laser energy is absorbed by tissue water and converted to heat, inducing volatilization with subsequent tissue ejection and ablation.[19, 20] This is the mechanism by which the erbium (Er):YAG and other infrared lasers operate.

Characteristics of the Er:YAG Laser

TISSUE INTERACTIONS OF INFRARED LASERS

Infrared lasers emit in the nonvisible portion of the light spectrum, with wavelengths greater than 750 nm. The laser-tissue interactions of infrared lasers use the water in tissue as the principal chromophore that absorbs energy, which in turn is converted to heat. With sufficient heat deposition and a rise in temperature to more than 100°C, boiling and volatilization occur with consequent high-pressure tissue expansion and ablation in a process known as photothermal ablation or photovaporization.[19, 20] Between the ablated, photovaporized area and the normal tissue is an intermediate zone of thermal photocoagulation damage due to a temperature rise sufficient for coagulation but not vaporization at the margins of the central vaporization zone. This intermediate zone of thermal damage is highly significant, because its size relative to the central ablative zone has important implications for the precision and, conversely, the coagulation attainable with a given infrared wavelength. Photothermal ablation has been produced in a variety of tissues, including skin, bone, aorta, cornea, sclera, retina, lens, and iris.[19–30] Infrared lasers have been used in ophthalmology as cutting or ablating devices and include the 10.6-μm CO_2 laser,[22] the 2.94-μm Er:YAG laser,[19–21, 23–26] the 2.7- to 3-μm hydrogen fluoride laser,[21, 27] the 2.79-μm Er:YSGC laser,[21] the 2.12-μm holmium:YAG laser,[28] the 2.02-μm thulium:YAG,[29] and the 1.8- to 2.1-μm Co:MgF_2 laser.[30] The extent of the collateral thermal damage induced by these lasers mainly depends on the absorption of the infrared wavelength in water. The maximum absorption peak of water is at approximately 2.9 μm, which coincides with the Er:YAG laser emission wavelength. This high water absorbance indicates that the 2.94-μm wavelength permits the most precise confinement of the laser energy deposition.[19] With an absorption coefficient for water of 13.000 cm^{-1} at 2.94 μm[31–33] in tissue, which is typically 70% water, the optical penetration depth, $1/\alpha$, is approximately 1 μm.[19] Experimental studies have confirmed the sharpness and accuracy of the ablations or incisions performed by the Er:YAG laser in a variety of biologic tissues compared with the other infrared lasers. The Er:YAG laser–induced thermal damage at the margins of the vaporized zone is at the level of 10 to 60 μm,[21, 26] compared with the 150- to 450-μm coagulated zone induced by the holmium:YAG laser[28] and the several hundred micrometers of thermally coagulated tissue at the cut edge of incisions performed by the CO_2 laser.[22] Conversely, the minimal coagulation zone surrounding the vaporized or transected tissue indicates that the Er:YAG laser produces minimal hemostatic coagulation in the margins of the transected tissue, compared with the heavy surrounding coagulation observed with the CO_2 laser.

RATIONALE FOR Er:YAG LASER USE IN INTRAOCULAR SURGERY

Despite enormous technical advances in intraocular surgery, surgical approaches remain limited to mechanical methods. The investigation of lasers as instruments for intraocular surgical maneuvers is attractive because laser technology may offer advantages such as sharper, tractionless cutting and ablation; finer control; and greater ease of surgical approach compared with conventional instruments. Conversely, the extent of collateral thermal damage induced by a given wavelength, the technical complexity of various lasers and delivery systems, and cost are the major disadvantages that will also influence eventual clinical use. Infrared lasers, through the laser-tissue interaction of photothermal ablation,[19, 20] as well as excimer lasers through ablative photodecomposition,[15, 16] are currently the best candidates for incision and ablation of biologic tissues. Among the infrared lasers, the most promising laser is the 2.94-μm Er:YAG laser; its use in ocular surgery is presented in detail in the remainder of this chapter. Ultraviolet excimer lasers also have promise as surgical instruments and are the most precise at tissue removal. This extreme sharpness of ultraviolet irradiation has been demonstrated in intraocular surgery for retinal ablation and transection of vitreous strands.[34, 35] However, ultraviolet lasers have substantial disadvantages for intraocular use, including technical complexity, high costs,[36] potential mutagenicity,[37–40] cataractogenesis,[41] limited transmission through optical fibers, and the absence of any practical delivery system for intraocular surgery.[34, 35]

INSTRUMENTATION

The 2.94-μm Er:YAG laser is a solid-state laser that uses an yttrium-aluminum-garnet host and the erbium as a dopant or element within the crystal. This crystal is excited by means of a xenon flash lamp, but diode-pumped Er:YAG lasers of moderate energy also have been developed. The maximal tissue absorption of the Er:YAG laser, with a theoretical short penetration depth of 1 μm,[19] precludes delivery across any distance in water. Consequently, although corneal surgery can be accomplished with direct propagation of the laser beam in air, intraocular use of this wavelength requires a delivery system consisting of a fiberoptic attached to handheld endoprobes. The 2.94-μm wavelength of the Er:YAG laser can be transmitted effectively through very few fibers, including low hydroxyl-fused silica, zirconium fluoride, and new proprietary materials. Low hydroxyl-fused silica fiberoptics display high-energy attenuation and are limited to 40 cm in length. Zirconium-fluoride fibers, although they have high throughput efficiencies, are hygroscopic and rapidly degraded in a wet field and are prone to damage at higher radiant exposures.[42] Recent technologic advances have yielded a long, flexible, midinfrared fiber with excellent transmission and durability.[43–49] Fiberoptics are connected to handpieces made of sapphire or quartz rods tapered to a diameter of 600 to 50 μm and fashioned into 20-G endoprobes.[42–49]

Most Er:YAG laser systems operate in the pulsed mode, generating pulses lasting 100 to 300 μsec. This pulse duration greatly exceeds the thermal relaxation time of the irradiated tissue, which is approximately 1 μsec.[19] Therefore, the ablation crater is surrounded by a 10- to 60-μm zone of thermal coagulation in histologic specimens.[21, 26, 42, 43] Q-switched Er:YAG lasers have been also developed with pulses lasting less than 1 μsec, well below the thermal relaxation time of tissue, and these lasers induce less thermal damage, typically 5 to 10 μm.[19, 21] However, current fiberoptic technology does not satisfactorily transmit high-peak–power Q-switched pulses, which limits Q-switched laser applications to tissues that can be treated directly, such as the cornea.

Er:YAG Laser Vitreoretinal Surgery

EXPERIMENTAL STUDIES

Peyman and Katoh[24] performed full-thickness retinotomies in an enucleated eye with an Er:YAG laser. However, they did not provide histologic measurements and fluences in their report. Margolis and associates[42] reported results on the Er:YAG laser used for transection of experimental vitreous membranes in rabbit eyes. They performed 34 effective membrane transections at distances of 500 to 3600 μm from the retina. They used a low hydroxyl-fused silica or a zirconium-fluoride fiberoptic connected to a 200-μm sapphire tip and operated in a fluid-filled eye in contact with the target tissue. They observed that a threshold radiant exposure or fluence of approximately 4.5 J/cm² is required for visible effect on the membranes after 10 pulses. Histology of transected membranes showed a narrow zone of coagulated tissue of 10 to 60 μm. In the same study, they noted a high rate of retinal complications (53%), consisting of small retinal burns and hemorrhages, when the laser was used close to the retina. They also determined the retinal damage thresholds. With the sapphire probe 1 mm from the retina and using 10 pulses, they produced retinal lesions with 3.6 mJ per pulse. Ellsworth and coworkers[51] performed Er:YAG laser full-thickness retinotomies in human autopsy eyes with a 400-μm sapphire probe and multiple 14-mJ pulses and observed a collateral thermal damage zone of 20 μm or less.

D'Amico and colleagues[26] used an Er:YAG laser with a repetition rate up to 30 Hz, connected to a midinfrared-transmitting fiberoptic attached to a sapphire 375-μm probe, to create lesions of various depths in the retina of enucleated rabbit eyes. The point of the study was to examine the potential applicability of this laser in making discrete lesions of graded depth in the retinal surface as a model of retinotomies and epiretinal membrane removal during vitrectomy. Experiments were performed in a noncontact fashion in an air-retina interface, as well as in a near-contact fashion with the retina and laser probe submerged in fluid. With the probe at 0.4 mm from the retina in an air environment, the inner retina underwent graded ablation, with the depth of the crater proportional to the fluence. The crater was 30 μm deep after a single pulse with a radiant exposure of 1.3 J/cm²; a full-thickness retinotomy was performed with a pulse of 3.9 J/cm². When 20 pulses were delivered at a rate of one pulse per second, a fluence of 2.6 J/cm² permitted full-thickness retinotomy (Fig. 51–1). The adjacent zone of coagulated tissue was 15 to 50 μm. With the probe in close contact with the retina in a nontransmitting fluid (saline) environment, 20 pulses of 3.6 J/cm² permitted full-thickness retinotomy. The authors concluded that the Er:YAG laser is capable of controlled, gradual ablation of the retinal surface and therefore could be applied to vitreoretinal surgery, particularly for the removal of membranes lying on the retina.

Using the same Er:YAG laser system and highly transmitting midinfrared fiberoptic, Brazitikos and coworkers[43] further explored the applicability of the Er:YAG laser in vitreoretinal surgery. In living rabbit eyes, they performed retinotomies on detached retina, transections of elevated vitreous membranes, incisions and surface ablations of traumatically induced epiretinal membranes, and retinal threshold studies. They also introduced new 20-G probe designs with quartz tips 75 to 175 μm in diameter, permitting laser use via sclerotomy in a manner analogous to laser endophotocoagulation. The newly developed midinfrared fiber showed excellent transmission and durability. Linear retinotomies on detached retina, as a model for relaxing retinotomies, were easily performed. In a fluid medium with the probe tip in close contact with the target tissue, a single complication was noted in 25 transections of elevated membranes (Fig. 51–2). Histology of the cut edges revealed a collateral thermal damage zone of 10 to 60 μm. Vessels coagulated within vascularized membranes if the vessels fell within the thermal damage zone (Fig. 51–3). Epiretinal membrane ablation was performed in nontransmitting aqueous media and in transmitting media including air and perfluoro-*N*-octane; with the latter, transmission was approximately 95% for this wavelength. The authors noted no macroscopic retinal damage during membrane ablation in aqueous media. Light microscopy showed partial (Fig. 51–4) to full-thickness (Fig. 51–5) membrane ablation with a maximum collateral thermal damage of 50 μm or less. In contrast with fluid media, air (Fig. 51–6) and perfluoro-*N*-octane (Fig. 51–7) lent a chalky appearance to the target tissue during laser irradiation. In perfluoro-*N*-octane media, con-

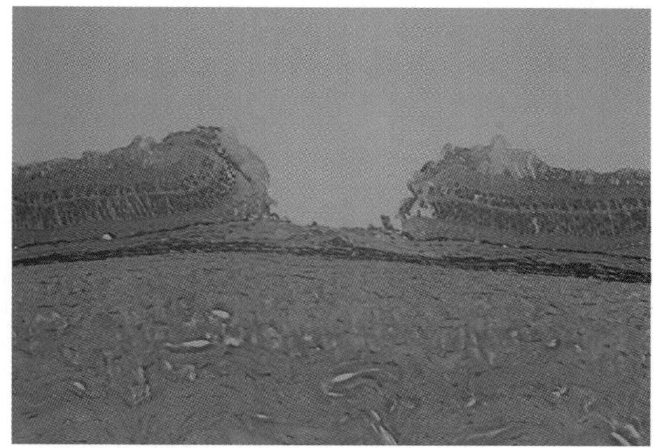

FIGURE 51–1. Photomicrograph of a full-thickness retinotomy created in an air environment with 20 pulses at a fluence of 2.6 J/cm² with the probe 0.4 mm from the retinal surface. One can see an intermediate zone of coagulation for approximately 40 μm (toluidine blue, original magnification ×31.25).

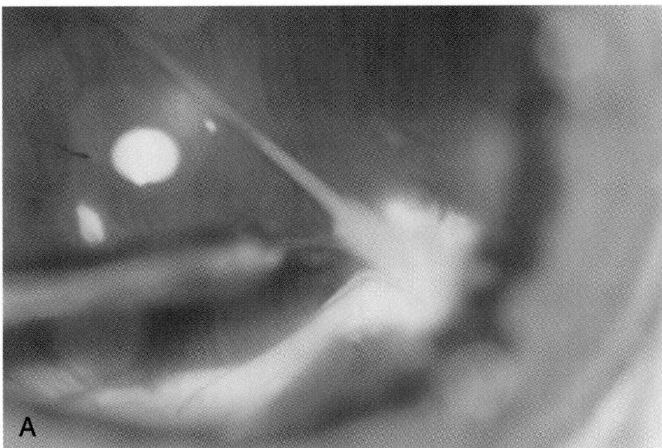

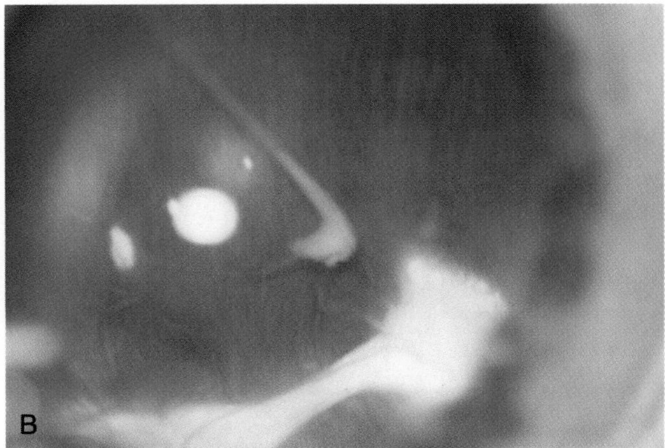

FIGURE 51–2. Erbium:YAG laser vitreous membrane transection that developed around a suture tract in a rabbit eye. *A,* The transection is performed at the thickest part of the vitreous membrane at a distance of approximately 0.5 mm from the retina. Exit scar is close to the medullary ray. The 75-μm quartz tip used during surgery can be seen emerging from the stainless steel shaft. Energy during transection was 1 mJ at 10 Hz. *B,* Postoperative photograph showing the complete transection of the membrane. Ablated tissue debris is seen in the surrounding vitreous. The underlying retina does not show any macroscopic damage.

tinuous bubble formation and progressive clouding of the perfluoro-*N*-octane during surgery compromised visualization. Histology revealed that the visible whitening of the irradiated tissue was due to an increased thermal damage with pronounced desiccation (Figs. 51–8 and 51–9). These observations suggest that the laser-tissue interaction in nontransmitting aqueous media differs from that in eyes filled with transmitting air and perfluoro-*N*-octane. In aqueous medium, continuous rehydration of treated tissue had a cooling effect, and the ejection of dessicated debris occurred more readily because of the lower surface tension of water compared with air or perfluoro-*N*-octane.

Brazitikos and coworkers[43] also successfully performed epiretinal membrane incisions in saline (Fig. 51–10). Nonhemorrhagic retinal damage occurred in 2 eyes and small hemorrhage in 5 in a total of 18 successful incisions. Histology showed sharp margins of the cut edges with lateral damage of 50 μm or less (Fig. 51–11). These authors also determined retinal threshold studies and found they depended on the tip diameter. Smaller endoprobe tips permitted the use of higher radiant exposures (J/cm^2) without damaging the underlying retina. At 1 mm from the retina, the retinal damage threshold was 14.5 J/cm^2 (3.5 mJ) with a 175-μm probe compared with 47.5 J/cm^2 (2.1 mJ) with a 75-μm probe. At 0.5 mm from the retina, energy levels up to 1.3 mJ—energies typically used for epiretinal membrane surgery—were safe. Brazitikos and associates[43] concluded that the Er:YAG laser coupled with the flexible and durable fiberoptic system attached to interchangeable 20G endoprobes could be applied to intraocular surgery with considerable sharpness and safety.

In order to understand the process of Er:YAG laser re-

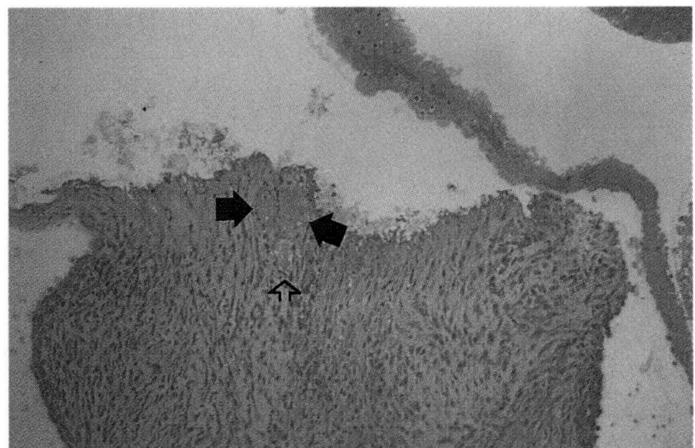

FIGURE 51–3. Photomicrograph of the transection site of a preretinal membrane proliferating in a rabbit eye. Erbium:YAG laser transection was performed with a 175-μm quartz probe with 1.9 mJ at 10 Hz. Note the regular margin of the cut edge. The thermal damage, evident by the decrease in fibroblast nuclei, extends approximately 60 μm and has induced coagulation of two small vessels *(arrows)*; another vessel beyond the damage zone is not coagulated *(arrowhead)* (toluidine blue; original magnification ×31). (From Brazitikos PD, D'Amico DJ, Bernal M-T, Walsh AW: Erbium:Yag laser surgery of the vitreous and retina. Ophthalmology 102:278, 1995.)

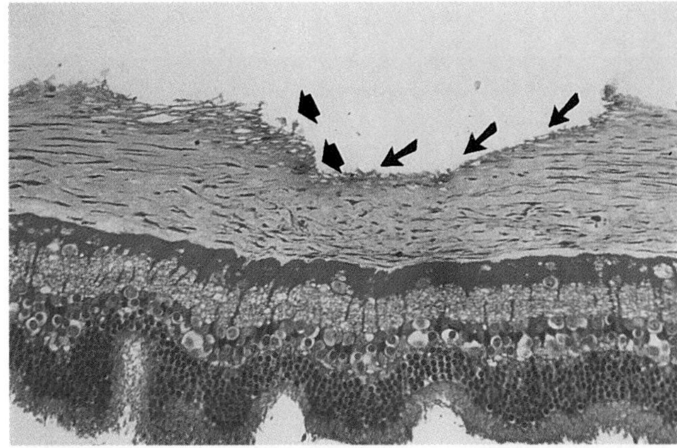

FIGURE 51–4. Photomicrograph showing erbium:YAG laser epiretinal membrane ablation extending to a depth of 70 μm in the center. The incidental beam was delivered obliquely from right to left in an aqueous-filled rabbit eye with a 75-μm endoprobe with an energy of 0.5 mJ at 10 Hz. Thermal damage ranges from 10 μm in the tissue oblique to the laser beam *(long arrows)* to 40 μm in the tissue perpendicular to the beam *(large arrows)*. Retinal detachment is an artifact, and retinal folds are secondary to tangential contraction of the epiretinal membrane (toluidine blue; original magnification ×62.5).

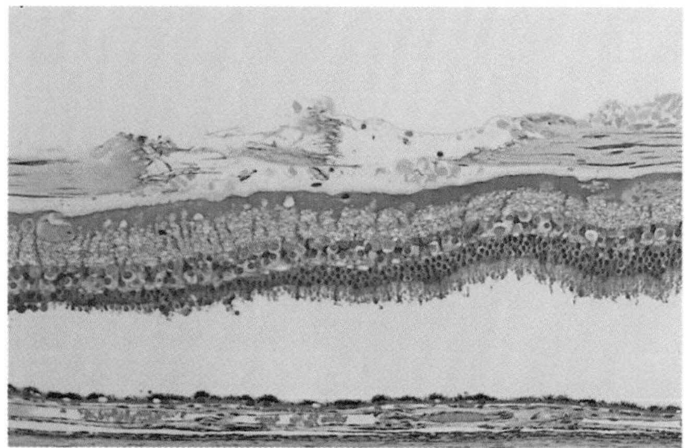

FIGURE 51–5. Photomicrograph displaying a broad area (300 μm) of full-thickness (50 μm) erbium:YAG laser ablation in this epiretinal membrane. The underlying retina is undamaged. Retinal detachment is an artifact. A fragment of the ablated tissue is in the center of this area separated from the retina. Surgery was performed in an aqueous-filled rabbit eye using a 75-μm tip probe with 0.5 mJ at 10 Hz (toluidine blue; original magnification ×62.5).

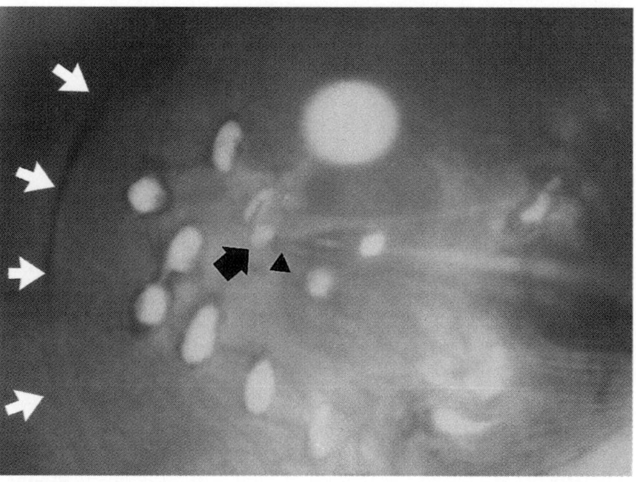

FIGURE 51–7. Erbium:YAG laser epiretinal membrane surgery in perfluoro-*N*-octane–filled rabbit eye. The perfluoro-*N*-octane bubble, which covers the epiretinal membrane, is outlined by the *white arrows*. The *black arrowhead* shows the 175-μm quartz tip in front of the membrane. The *black arrow* shows a whitish spot, indicating tissue desiccation, resulting from erbium:YAG laser delivery on the epiretinal membrane. An energy of 2 mJ was used at 5 Hz.

mote retinal injury during irradiation within the vitreous cavity, Lin and colleagues[51] used high-speed photography to explore the mechanism of Er:YAG laser–induced long-range damage in a fluid environment. In addition to tissue vaporization, they observed additional complex mechanisms of tissue interactions. Multilobed cavitation bubbles of different sizes that depend on the pulse energy (approximately 1 mm at 1 mJ) are formed during vaporization in fluid (Fig. 51–12). Loertscher and coworkers[52] measured a bubble diameter of 0.7 mm following laser delivery in water of a 5-mJ, 200-μsec pulse. Brinkmann and associates observed a bubble size of 1.5 mm after irradiation with 15 mJ in saline,[53] and Berger and colleagues[54] measured a maximum laser-generated bubble diameter of 1.2 mm after delivery of 1 mJ in saline. These cavitation bubbles in fluid appeared to influence the laser-retina interactions by three mechanisms. The first is deeper energy transmission of subsequent laser pulses through the gas bubble formed by initial pulses, permitting direct irradiation on the retina. The second mechanism is thermomechanical injury to the retina from the temperature and pressure of the traveling bubble. The third mechanism is damage by acoustic waves due to the expansion, propagation, and implosion of the bubble.[52] Berger and coworkers calculated that the Er:YAG laser tissue transection was a function of radiant exposure (in J/cm^2), but tissue injury from thermomechanical effects specifically depended on the total deposited energy. The maximum bubble was found to be a function of the cube root of the pulse energy; at constant radiant exposure, the maximum bubble diameter increases as a function of probe-tip-diameter $^2/_3$.[55] Consequently, probe tips with small diameters optimize the cutting and ablating potentials in terms of possible unintended tissue

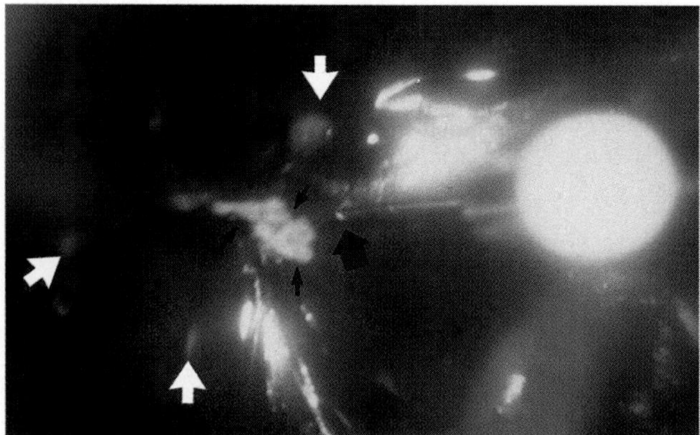

FIGURE 51–6. Erbium:YAG laser epiretinal membrane surgery in an air-filled rabbit eye. Photograph taken during laser surgery shows the 75-μm quartz delivery tip of the endoprobe *(large black arrow)* in front of an epiretinal membrane proliferating between chorioretinal scars *(white arrows)*. The surface of the membrane was completely free of fluid. Several ablation craters having a chalky appearance and a rough contour *(small black arrows)* can be visualized in the epiretinal membrane. An energy of 0.7 mJ was used at 5 Hz.

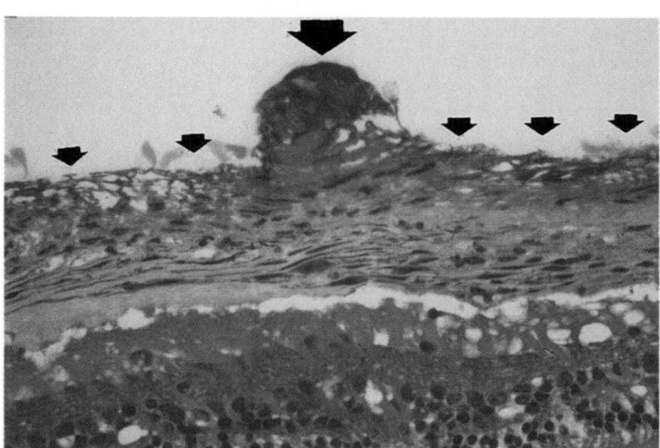

FIGURE 51–8. Photomicrograph of epiretinal membrane ablation in an air-filled rabbit eye. *Small arrows* show two adjacent ablation craters in the membrane approximately 30 μm in depth. The intervening tissue *(large arrow)* shows important coagulation. Surgery was performed with a 175-μm quartz tip endoprobe with 1 mJ at 5 Hz (toluidine blue; original magnification ×62.5).

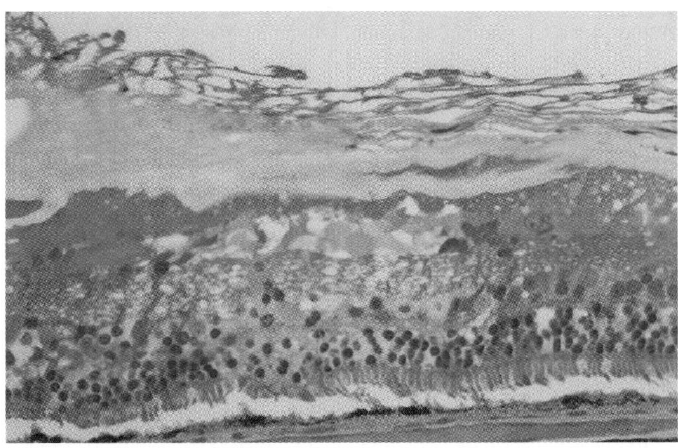

FIGURE 51–9. Photomicrograph of erbium:YAG laser epiretinal membrane ablation in perfluoro-*N*-octane–filled rabbit eye. Note the widespread vacuolization with desiccation of the treated tissue and coagulation of the underlying retina. Surgery was performed with a 175-μm tip probe with 2.5 mJ at 5Hz (toluidine blue; original magnification ×125).

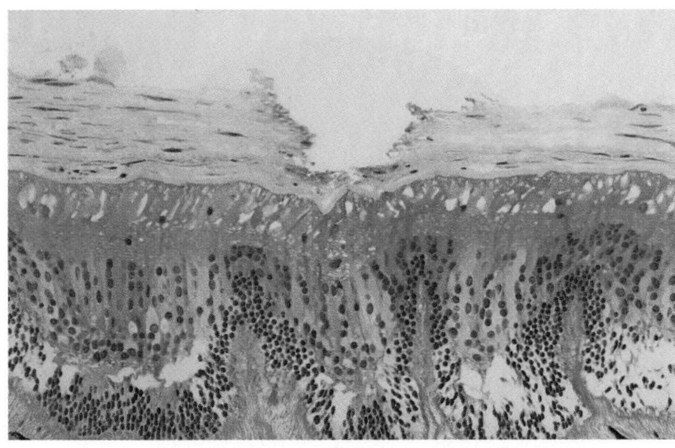

FIGURE 51–11. Photomicrograph of a serial section perpendicular to the incisions shown in Figure 51–10 reveals a nearly full-thickness cut (100 μm) without damage to the underlying retina. Collateral thermal damage is approximately 15 μm. There is a close attachment between the retina and the membrane with associated traction and alteration of the retinal architecture (toluidine blue; original magnification ×62.5).

damage; they do so by delivering low-pulse energy, resulting in higher radiant exposures.[55] These observations provide a basis for the low rate of intraoperative complications in the experimental Er:YAG laser vitreoretinal study performed by Brazitikos and coworkers,[43] in which energy was delivered to a tip diameter as low as 75 μm, yielding a higher radiant exposure at energy levels of 1 to 2 mJ that were typically used in the study. In contrast, Margolis and associates[42] noted a much higher rate of retinal injury (53%) during vitreous membrane transection that was probably a consequence of using a 200-μm tip.

CLINICAL STUDIES

D'Amico and colleagues[44] were the first to use the Er:YAG laser for clinical vitreoretinal surgery in 13 patients under a Food and Drug Administration Investigational Device Exemption for this laser system. Patients in this study underwent vitrectomy for conventional indications, including diabetic traction detachment, proliferative vitreoretinopathy, retinal detachment with posterior break, and epimacular membrane. They used a new Er:YAG laser console with a transmission system identical to that previously used for experimental surgery, with a maximum output of 5 mJ per pulse and 30 Hz. In this pioneer pilot clinical study, 48 specific intraoperative surgical maneuvers were accomplished with the Er:YAG laser, including transection of elevated membranes, incision of epiretinal membranes, drainage and relaxing retinotomy, transection of subretinal membranes, noncontact ablation of epiretinal membranes in air-filled eyes, ablation of lens remnants, posterior capsulotomy, iris surgery, and retinal vascular coagulation. Forty-five surgical maneuvers were performed in aqueous media with the probe in contact with the target tissue, and three in air-filled eyes. The Er:YAG laser showed remarkable efficacy for transection of elevated and subretinal membranes, creation of relaxing and drainage retinotomies (Fig. 51–13),

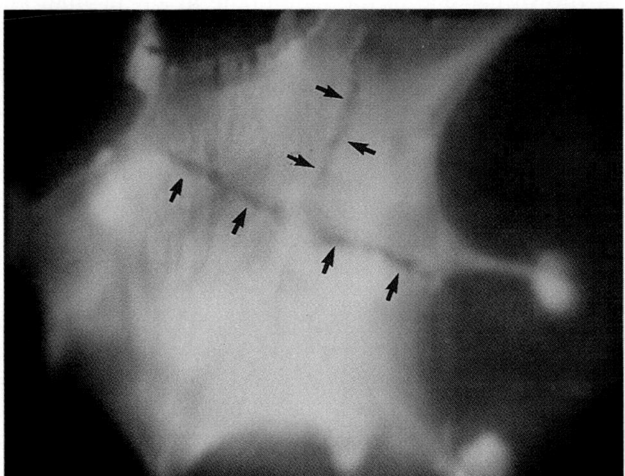

FIGURE 51–10. Postoperative photograph showing two long epiretinal membrane incisions *(arrows)* accomplished with the erbium:YAG laser using a 75-μm probe with 1 mJ at 5 Hz in an aqueous-filled rabbit eye. Endoillumination is used as a light source.

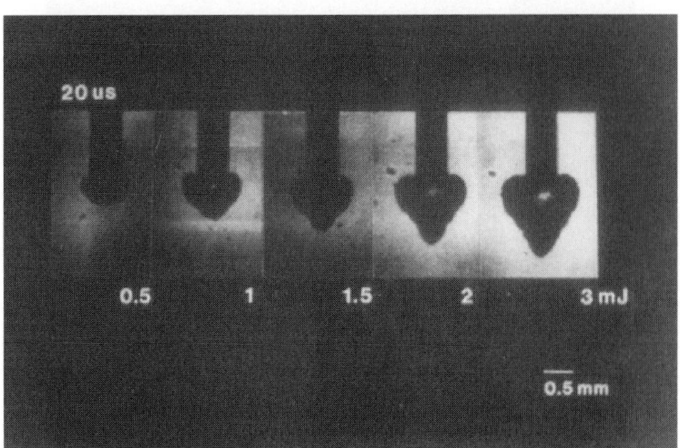

FIGURE 51–12. High-speed photographs of Er:YAG laser ablation in distilled water taken with various pulse energies at 20 μsec after the peak of the flashlamp pump pulse showing bubble formation at the tip of the probe. The diameter of the probe tip was 560 μm. (From Lin CP, Stern D, Puliafito CA: High speed photography of Er:YAG laser ablation in fluid: Implication for laser vitreous surgery. Invest Ophthalmol Vis Sci 31:2546, 1990.)

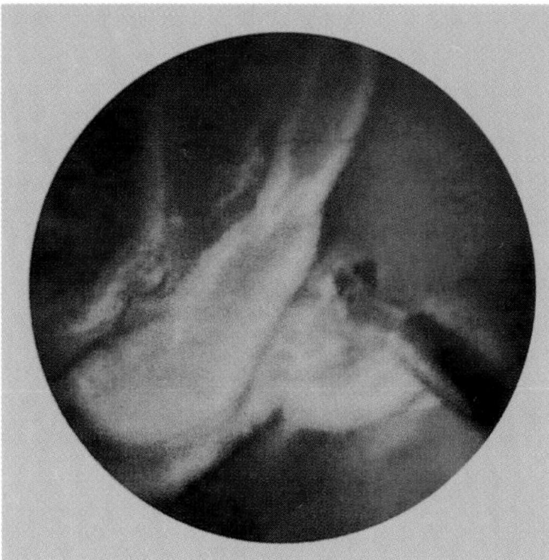

FIGURE 51–13. Retinotomy for approach to subretinal membranes with the erbium:YAG laser. Intraoperative video monitor photograph shows the 100-μm probe creating a circular opening in the detached retina. Subretinal membranes were subsequently transected with the laser through this retinotomy. (Reprinted from Am J Ophthalmol, vol 121, D'Amico DJ, Brazitikos PD, Marcellino GR, et al, Initial clinical experience with an erbium:YAG laser for vitreoretinal surgery, p 414, Copyright 1996, with permission from Elsevier Science.)

lens remnant ablation, posterior capsulotomy, and iris removal. Most incisions in epiretinal membranes were performed as part of the dissection in the posterior hyaloid in diabetic traction detachment (Figs. 51–14 and 51–15). Although these membranes were typically vascularized, the incisions proceeded without hemorrhage (see Fig. 51–15). This advantageous fine coagulation probably was due to including these fine vessels in the collateral thermal damage zone of 60 μm or less (see Fig. 51–3) along the incisions of the vascularized posterior hyaloid. However, transection of larger retinal vessels, as with relaxing retinotomy, typically caused bleeding similar to that observed with mechanical

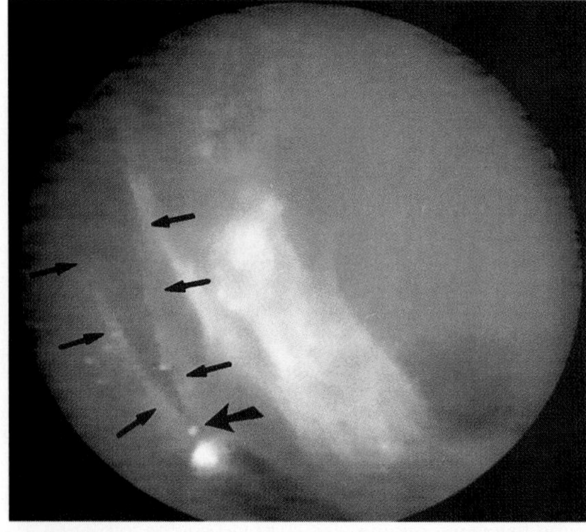

FIGURE 51–14. Intraoperative video monitor photograph during surgery for diabetic traction retinal detachment. A 100-μm tip erbium:YAG laser probe *(large arrow)* is creating an incision into the thickened posterior hyaloid *(small arrows)*.

transection of retinal vessels. In air-filled eyes, the Er:YAG laser partially or completely ablated epiretinal fibrotic tissue. Complications in this study included an extramacular retinal break (created during an epiretinal membrane incision and successfully managed with endophotocoagulation) and fine pitting of an intraocular lens during a posterior capsulotomy with a side-firing probe, which caused no symptoms.

A multicenter, prospective trial further evaluated the advantages, disadvantages, safety, complications, and applicability of the Er:YAG laser system in clinical vitreoretinal surgery.[45] The researchers enrolled 68 eyes in 66 patients with a mean follow-up of 9 months. They included data from the previously described pilot group of 13 patients. Surgical indications and the maneuvers performed in this multicenter study were identical with those of the pilot study. For a total of 174 maneuvers, surgeon's evaluation of efficacy was excellent in 55%, good in 29%, fair in 11%, and poor in 5%. Er:YAG-laser relaxing retinotomy, epiretinal and vitreous membrane surgery, capsulotomy, and transection of subretinal membrane reached high rates of excellent or good surgical efficacy. In contrast, the coagulation of blood vessels achieved only a 26% rate of good or excellent surgical efficacy. Complications included retinal injury in 5% of epiretinal membrane incisions and minor bleeding from transected retinal vessels during 29% of retinotomies.

The pilot[44] and the multicenter[45] clinical studies on the initial use of the Er:YAG laser in vitreoretinal surgery in patients confirmed the potential applicability of this technology for tractionless, noncontact or close-contact, sharp ablation, and incision of tissues within the eye. The solid-state laser was easily adapted to the operating room, and the flexible highly transmitting midinfrared fiberoptic permitted gas sterilization and subsequent use without degradation during surgery. With laser energies typically at the 1 to 2 mJ per pulse, epiretinal tissues were cut or removed without major retinal complications. For tissues away from the retina, higher energy levels were safely used. In these two studies, novel surgical approaches were introduced in clinical vitreoretinal surgery, such as direct tractionless incision of the posterior hyaloid in proliferative diabetic retinopathy, gradual removal of epiretinal tissue with the probe targeting from the vitreal side to the membrane in air- or fluid-filled eye, and creation of relaxing retinotomies displaying smooth and sharp contour. However, the major limitation of this Er:YAG laser system was the slowness of certain critical maneuvers close to the retina. This tempo resulted from the use of low pulse energies close to the retina, as well as the learning curve of surgical experience with this laser. The authors suggested that this tempo would be improved by further enhancing the laser technology, increasing the repetition rate to 100 Hz or higher, and innovation in endoprobe tip design.[44, 45] Moreover, parallel experimental studies, on measurements of bubble formation and dynamics during Er:YAG irradiation of vitreous, suggested that mechanical laser-mediated retinal injury can be minimized while efficient ablation is preserved, with pulses delivered at high repetition rates.[55]

RECENT INNOVATIONS AND FUTURE DEVELOPMENT

Current innovation in technologic development resulted in the construction of an Er:YAG laser with repetition rates

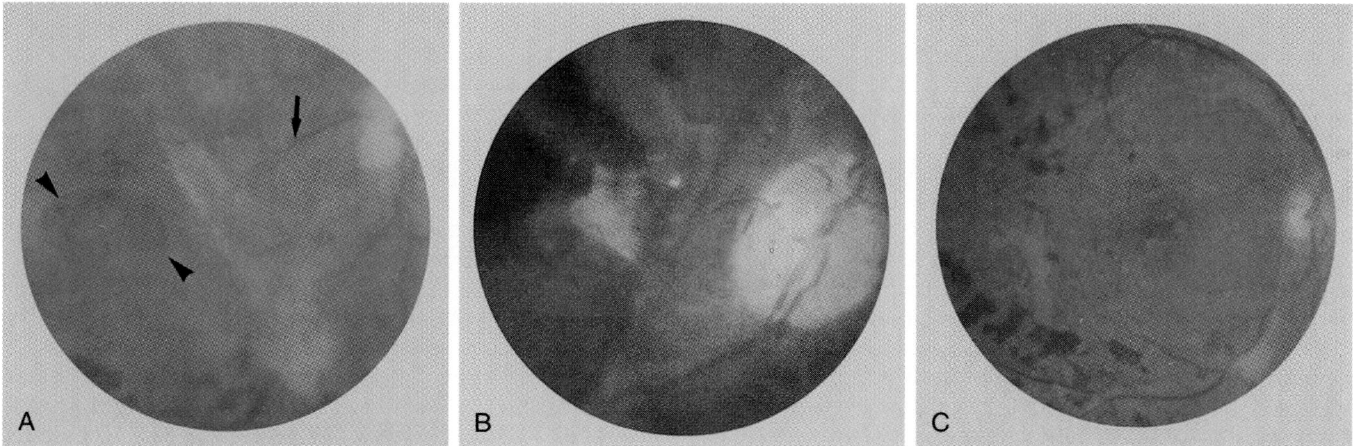

FIGURE 51–15. Erbium:YAG laser surgery for diabetic traction detachment. *A,* Preoperative fundus photograph showing the posterior hyaloid containing large new vessels *(arrow)* and a perforation above the inferior macula *(arrowheads).* The underlying fovea is detached, and visual acuity is 20/60. *B,* Intraoperative video monitor photograph of an incision in the posterior hyaloid just temporal to the optic disc taken with a 100-μm probe with the red aiming beam visible at the probe tip. The large new vessel has been transected without hemorrhage. The dissection of the posterior hyaloid was performed entirely with the laser in this eye. *C,* Fundus photograph 6 weeks after surgery. (Reprinted from Am J Ophthalmol, vol 121, D'Amico DJ, Brazitikos PD, Marcellino GR, et al, Initial clinical experience with an erbium:YAG laser for vitreoretinal surgery, p 414, Copyright 1996, with permission from Elsevier Science.)

graduated from 2 to 200 Hz.[46–49] Side-firing endoprobes were introduced, allowing new surgical approaches (Fig. 51–16). Experimental studies performed on enucleated pig eyes explored their efficacy with higher repetition rates in performing partial-thickness inner retinal ablation (see Fig. 51–16) and retinotomies.[46, 47] Compared with lower Hertz rates, high repetition rates at the level of 150 to 200 Hz resulted in better continuity and smoother contour of incisions without visible gaps in the incision despite rapid movement across the tissue; this could improve the surgical tempo. Histology revealed that when the same energy is held constant, laser penetration within the target tissue differs slightly between high and low repetition rates.[47] These findings suggested novel maneuvers, such as: (1) tractionless epiretinal membrane removal with side-firing endoprobes through energy delivery tangential to the retinal plane, (2) combined membrane and partial-thickness inner retinal ablation as an alternative to relaxing retinotomies in cases of extreme proliferative vitreoretinopathy, and (3) direct removal of the vitreous gel itself by laser energy in a process that may be called photovitrectomy.

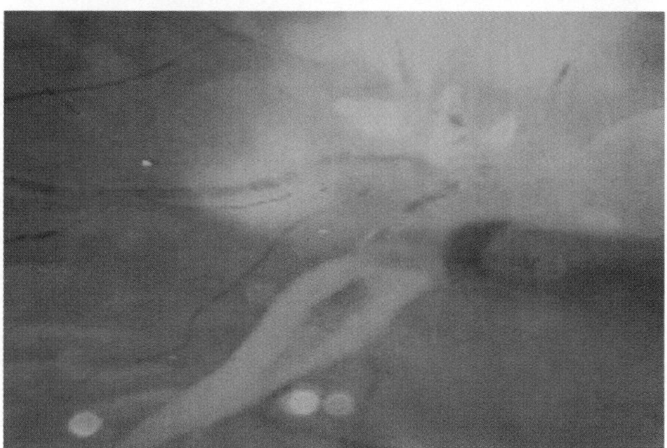

FIGURE 51–16. Intraoperative, computer-processed videotape photographs showing erbium:YAG laser retinal ablation, evident by the increased retinal transparency, performed on a retinal fold of a pig eye with a 200-μm side-firing probe (shown in the figure) using 1 mJ at 200 Hz.

Photovitrectomy is probably the most interesting future development with the Er:YAG laser, because it may allow the surgeon to perform vitreous removal and membrane microsurgery using a single surgical device. Initial investigation of the Er:YAG laser for removing vitreous used a prototype probe combining aspiration and a quartz rod of large tip diameter (600 μm). Formed animal vitreous was removed with pulse energies of 5 mJ at 30 Hz and a low combined vacuum pressure of 20 mm Hg. However, placing the tip within 2 mm of the retina caused retinal injury due to the generated mechanical acoustic waves caused by the high energy levels used in this study.[56] In a more recent study, Schmidt-Petersen and coworkers[57] used a quartz fiber tip of 500 μm and repetition rates of more than 40 Hz to ablate vitreous in enucleated pig eyes and found that the threshold for vitreous removal was 11 ± 3 mJ. A previous study already showed that continuous laser irradiation of the vitreous with 6-mJ pulses may induce a temperature rise of 20°C 500 μm away from the laser tip; it also showed that at constant laser power, the temperature profile is independent of repetition rate.[58] Future study may exploit the high Hz rates, lower energy per pulse, and side-firing endoprobes to permit the safer removal of the vitreous not only from the center of the eye but also very close to the retina.

Preliminary results with the higher (up to 200 Hz) repetition rate in clinical vitreoretinal surgery involved 32 patients who had proliferative diabetic retinopathy with traction retinal detachment and substantially thickened posterior hyaloid, advanced proliferative vitreoretinopathy, pupillary membrane, cellophane maculopathy, and retinopathy of prematurity.[48, 49] Repetition rates of 150 to 200 Hz significantly improved the tempo of epiretinal membrane surgery. As suggested in the experimental trials, it was easy to delaminate thick epiretinal fibrovascular tissue with side-firing endoprobes as opposed to the straight-firing probes used exclusively in earlier studies.[48, 49] Moreover, in some proliferative vitreoretinopathy cases, the Er:YAG laser operated in a noncontact fashion in eyes filled with perfluoro-*N*-octane (95% transmission) and gradually ablated the epiretinal membranes, resulting in progressive flattening of the detached retina.[48]

Compared with the sophisticated mechanical devices for vitreoretinal surgery, the Er:YAG laser is still in its early stages. The available experimental and clinical studies[43–49] suggest that this technology holds great promise in vitreoretinal surgery, with few laser-related intraoperative complications. Researchers noted limitations, disadvantages, and a surgical learning curve.[44, 45] Recent innovations resulting in repetition rates up to 200 Hz significantly improve the surgical speed.[46–49] Surgical experience and further technical refinement are warranted to define the role of this new technology as an adjunct to or as a replacement for conventional mechanical techniques.

Er:YAG Laser Surgery of the Lens

The maximal water absorption of the Er:YAG laser 2.94-μm wavelength resulting in a sharp containment of absorbed energy may be perfectly suited for ablation of the high water–containing crystalline lens.[24, 47, 59–62] Peyman and Katoh[24] used an Er:YAG laser to ablate the lens in rabbits; they used scanning electron and light microscopy to observe a narrow zone of coagulation damage. Gailitis and coworkers[59] studied the interaction of the 2.94-μm wavelength with human autopsy lenses. The Er:YAG laser system operated at 1 Hz in an air environment, and the energy was delivered with a beam diameter of 400 μm. The photovaporization threshold was 1.4 J/cm^2, with an ablation rate of 68 μm per pulse at 10 J/cm^2. Damage zones were 4 to 9 μm. Noecker and coworkers[60] performed ablation of human lens nuclei with a 400-μm sapphire tip in air and measured an ablation width of about 73 μm at 5 mJ (4 J/cm^2). With higher energies, lens ablation significantly increased to 130 μm at 20 mJ (16 J/cm^2). Histologic evaluation showed adjacent coagulation damage to be less than 10 μm at all energy levels tested.

Colvard and Kratz[61] performed circular openings of the anterior capsule and lens ablation using a prototype Er:YAG laser. They used a specialized probe for anterior capsulotomy, permitting redirection of the laser energy at 90 degrees to the axis of the fiber and visualization of the capsule through the clear tip. The optimal parameters in their procedure were 12 to 15 mJ of energy per pulse and a repetition rate of 10 Hz. For lens photovaporization, tips producing spot sizes of 400 to 800 μm were used, with energy levels of 20 to 60 mJ per pulse and a repetition rate of 10 to 15 Hz. They provided irrigation via a chamber maintainer infusion cannula and aspiration via a cannula inserted through a side port. In animal studies, these authors did not observe significant damage to the corneal endothelium or other intraocular structures. The FDA has granted Premarket Approval for their instrumentation for performing anterior capsulotomy as well as Investigational Device Exemption for cataract ablation. In their clinical series, the laser device was used only for ablation of the anterior and central nuclear material; the rest of the lens was removed with ultrasound. They concluded that the Er:YAG laser may help to make cataract surgery safer and reduce the learning curve associated with phacoemulsification.

Anterior capsulotomy with the Er:YAG laser was more resistant to radial tears than the can-opener method but weaker than the continuous circular capsulorrhexis technique.[62] Berger and coworkers[63] used an Er:YAG laser, directing the energy through a flexible fiberoptic to a 400-μm tip, and readily drilled hard cataractous human nucleus slabs 0.5 to 1 mm thick immersed in saline (Fig. 51–17). The ablation rate varied linearly with radiant exposure (in J/cm^2). Using an Er:YAG laser with a high repetition rate (200 Hz), Brazitikos and coworkers[47] documented the role of repetition rate in performing anterior capsulotomy and continuous high-speed nuclear ablation in enucleated pig eyes in aqueous media. With side-firing 200-μm tip probes, they effectively performed continuous circular anterior capsulotomies using 10 mJ per pulse at 30 Hz and only 2 mJ per pulse at 200 Hz (Fig. 51–18). Histology showed minimal thermal damage at the cutting edge (Fig. 51–19). With lens ablation, they observed that at low repetition rates, high-speed lens ablation was gradually reduced because of accumulation of overheated lens material at the tip of the probe, reducing subsequent energy delivery. This difficulty was overcome with repetition rates of 150 to 200 Hz and energies per pulse between 6 and 12 mJ. These parameters permitted continuous high-speed photothermal lens ablation at a good surgical tempo (see Fig. 51–18) with pulse energies significantly below those used by Colvard and Kratz.[61] Brazitikos and associates[46] concluded that high repetition rates permit continuous high-speed lens ablation with the use of lower and safer energies.

Potential advantages over the currently used phacoemulsification technique of the Er:YAG laser technology have been explored. Experiments performed in human autopsy eyes showed that even with energies as high as 16 mJ per pulse (energy levels substantially greater than those needed with high repetition rates), the Er:YAG laser is significantly safer than phacoemulsification in avoiding rupture of the posterior capsule. In addition, the type of induced capsular tear

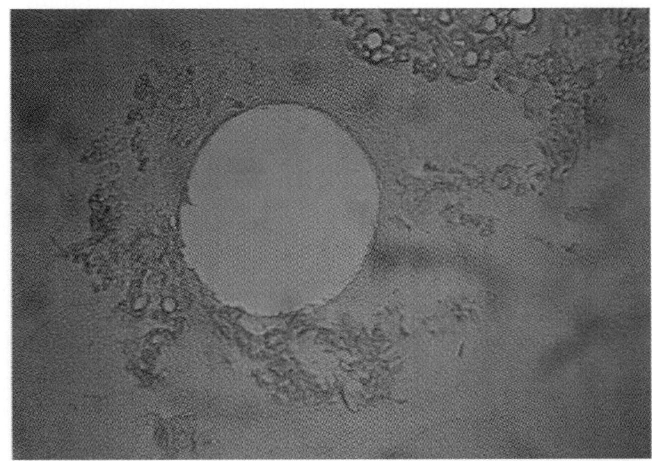

FIGURE 51–17. Photomicrograph of cataractous human lens slab drilled with the erbium:YAG laser. The laser operated in saline at a radiant exposure of 10 J/cm^2 and a repetition rate of 10 Hz, with a 400-μm probe tip diameter. Notice the minimal thermal damage along the margins of the full-thickness ablation (hematoxylin; original magnification ×20). (Courtesy of J. Talamo, M.D.)

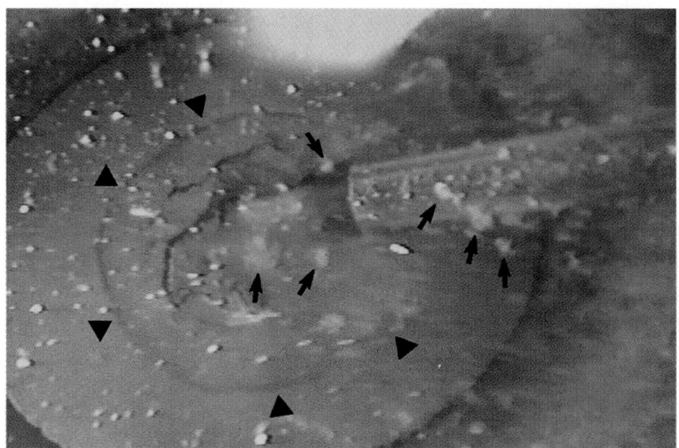

FIGURE 51–18. Computer-processed videotape photograph showing erbium:YAG laser photothermal lens ablation performed with an energy level of 10 mJ per pulse at 200 Hz with the side-firing 200-μm probe shown in the figure. *Arrowheads* outline a continuous curvilinear erbium:YAG laser photothermal capsulotomy performed with 2-mJ per pulse at 200 Hz prior to lens ablation. In this experiment, a corneal button was removed and the enucleated pig eye was submerged in balanced salt solution. The *small arrows* show some of the numerous lens debris ablated and ejected at high speed in the overlying fluid.

tended to be more localized with the Er:YAG laser and resulted less frequently in vitreous loss than phacoemulsification did.[64] The potential thermal injury to ocular structures resulting from Er:YAG laser lens ablation is surprisingly less than it is during phacoemulsification; in cadaver eyes, the temperature rise was 5 to 15 times greater after pulsed application of conventional levels of ultrasound energy than it was after Er:YAG laser irradiation of the lens. The temperature rise with the Er:YAG laser at 2 minutes was 0.5°C with irrigation and 2.5°C without irrigation. Following 2 minutes of ultrasound application, the temperature rose 2.5°C with irrigation and 35°C without irrigation.[65]

In summary, the rationale for laser technology for lens removal is to minimize surgical invasiveness with ablation of the crystalline lens through a small capsular opening. This novel technology might permit new approaches to postcataract correction, such as injection of a polymer in the capsular bag that would function as an implant with potentially preserved accommodation.[66, 67] In addition, this laser potentially is able to ablate and remove even the hardest lens nucleus, because water content and not surgical hardness is the critical factor. Finally, the Er:YAG laser's versatility in other areas of ocular surgery would be a strong advantage in multifunctional system, as opposed to ultrasound energy, which is used surgically only for lens nucleus disruption. Although this technology seems to have significant advantages over the phacoemulsification technique, further study and innovation in probe design will determine the Er:YAG laser's practical role in lens surgery.

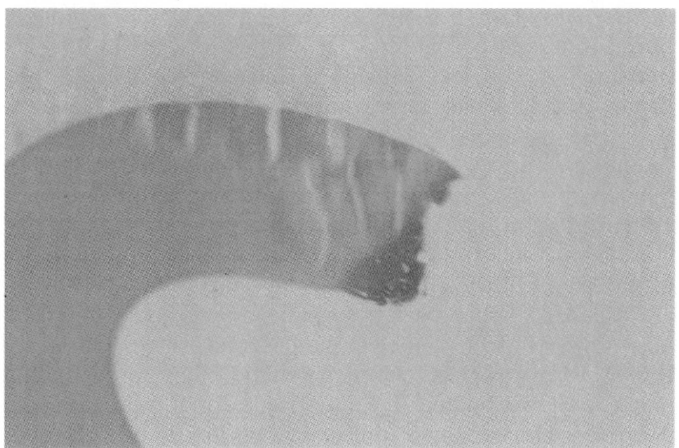

FIGURE 51–19. Photomicrograph showing the cut edge of an anterior capsule. Maximum thermal damage is approximately 25 μm. Erbium:YAG laser photothermal capsulotomy was performed in an enucleated pig eye with a 200-μm side-firing probe using 2 mJ per pulse at 200 Hz (hematoxylin; original magnification ×125).

Er:YAG Laser Surgery of the Sclera, Cornea, and Iris

SCLERAL FILTRATION SURGERY

Lasers that have been used for sclerostomy are the CO_2 (10.6-μm) laser,[68] the Er:YAG (2.94-μm) laser,[69, 70] the Er:YSGG (2.79-μm) laser,[69] the holmium:YAG (2.12-μm) laser,[70] the thulium-holmium-chromium:YAG (2.1-μm) laser,[71] the holmium:YSGC (2.1-μm) laser,[69] the continuous-wave Nd:YAG (1.06-μm) laser,[69–72] the tunable-dye (668-nm) laser,[73] and the high-power argon endolaser.[74] For infrared lasers, the thermal damage to tissue and the total laser energy required to produce sclerostomies decreases with increasing wavelength, from the 1.06-μm continuous-wave Nd:YAG, which induces 56 to 453 μm of injury, to the 2.94-μm Er:YAG laser, which produces 17 to 45 μm of thermal damage.[69] The 10.6-μm CO_2 laser typically induces a zone of thermal damage of several hundred micrometers.[22] Excimer lasers, which are the most precise for tissue incision, have been used for scleral perforation and partial trabeculectomy.[75, 76] However, as previously discussed, excimer lasers have substantial practical limitations,[34, 35] and radiation at these wavelengths may penetrate to the retina in aphakic eyes.[77]

The rationale for the Er:YAG laser in scleral surgery for filtration is to try to minimize surgical trauma with precise cutting and minimal subjacent thermal damage (Fig. 51–20). Sclerotomies performed in animal and eyebank globes confirm the low degree of thermal damage at the cutting edge.[69, 70] Arias-Puente and colleagues[78] used an Er:YAG laser for ab externo sclerostomy in human eyes with uncontrolled complicated secondary glaucomas. They operated on a total of 38 eyes and achieved intraocular pressure control without medical treatment in 55% of the eyes at 1-year follow-up. The ab interno sclerostomy technique performed with the Er:YAG laser probe en face to the trabeculum eliminates conjunctival manipulation and theoretically causes less conjunctival and episcleral trauma than current glaucoma procedures.[69, 70, 72, 79] In living rabbit eyes, however, researchers noted failed sclerostomies from fibrous tissue proliferation, occlusion by iris, and peripheral anterior synechiae.[72] Interestingly, the Er:YAG laser technology has been used to create a direct communication of the anterior chamber with Schlemm's canal through ablation of the trabecular meshwork in enucleated rabbit[80] and human autopsy eyes[80, 81] in a contact fashion with sapphire or quartz probes of 300 to

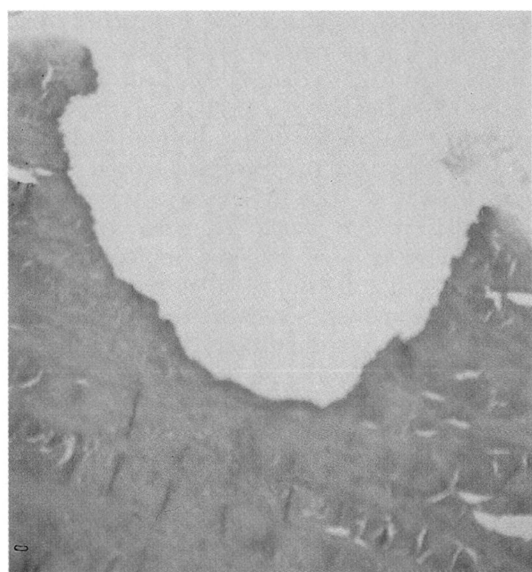

FIGURE 51–20. Photomicrograph showing erbium:YAG laser ablation crater in the sclera of an enucleated pig eye performed with a 100-μm tip probe with 12 mJ at 30 Hz in fluid. Thermal damage at the margins of the crater ranges from 15 to 50 μm (hematoxylin; original magnification ×100).

350 μm in tip diameter. Histologic study showed that an energy level of 15 mJ was optimal for efficient ablation of trabecular meshwork to Schlemm's canal, inducing minimal thermal damage.[81]

CORNEAL SURGERY

Although the 193-nm excimer laser is currently used for photorefractive keratectomy, alternatives to this technology are desirable because of the high acquisition and maintenance costs,[36] toxic gases, and possible ultraviolet mutagenesis of the excimer laser.[37–40] Midinfrared irradiation of 2.85 to 3 μm, which corresponds to the absorption peak of water (the major constituent of cornea), seems to be the most promising alternative. Laser systems generating pulses in this spectral region are the hydrogen-fluoride laser, which emits radiation at lines between 2.74 and 3 μm; the Raman-shifted Nd:YAG laser, which shifts the 1.064-μm radiation from a Q-switched Nd:YAG to 2.8 μm with methane and to 2.94 μm with deuterium as Raman-shifting media; and finally the 2.94-μm Er:YAG laser. Seiler and coworkers[82] used a hydrogen fluoride laser emitting 50-nsec pulses for corneal ablation and observed 5- to 20-μm zones of damage at the cutting edge. Loertscher and associates[83] performed corneal ablation with a multiline hydrogen-fluoride laser and observed a damage zone of 10 to 15 μm at the top of the corneal incisions. Stern and colleagues[84] made linear corneal incisions using a Raman-shifted Nd:YAG laser with a 1.5- to 10-μm collateral thermal damage zone.

The Er:YAG laser is more compact, more stable, and easier to operate than the hydrogen-fluoride and the Raman-shifted Nd:YAG lasers.[21] The laser head with the optics may be small enough to be mounted on a slit-lamp or operating microscope.[85] For corneal surgery, the laser beam is propagated through air and targeted on the corneal surface without fiberoptics. However, homogenicity of the beam profile is important for precise ablation.[85] Peyman and Katoh[24] used the Er:YAG laser to ablate a variety of ocular tissues, including cornea. In a later study, Peyman and coworkers[86] performed central corneal ablation in living rabbit eyes with an Er:YAG laser after either mechanical epithelial scrubbing or removal of an anterior central cap. The profile of the beam (3 mm in diameter) was not homogeneous, causing differences in the amount of tissue ablated within the irradiated surface. Immediately after the procedure, these authors observed some degree of thermal damage at the margin of the ablated area. Two months postoperatively, a faint stromal haze developed in some eyes, which progressively cleared. Light microscopy revealed thermal damage of approximately 40 μm at the margins and of 16 μm at the bottom of the crater. Scanning electron microscopy did not show endothelial damage despite the 300-μm ablation depth. Six months postoperatively, light microscopy showed epithelial thickening at the margins of the remodeled zone. The healing of the stroma progressed with slight disorganization of the lamellae and an increase in the population of the keratocytes. Photokeratoscopy revealed smoothness and some degree of flattening of the cornea.[86]

Preliminary studies have used the Er:YAG laser for refractive surgery in patients. Seiler and associates[85] performed corneal ablation in five blind human eyes using a pulsed Er:YAG laser, producing a circular beam of 5 mm in diameter with a homogeneous beam profile. They used 1 J per pulse at a repetition rate of up to 10 Hz with a corresponding ablation rate of 10 μm per pulse. Laser treatment followed removal of the epithelium. No recurrent erosions followed epithelial healing. At 1 month after surgery, the central flattening of the cornea was approximately 6 diopters as revealed by corneal topography. They also observed stromal haze similar to that seen after excimer laser keratectomy.

Thompson and colleagues[87] compared the Er:YAG laser with the 193-nm excimer laser in performing experimental corneal trephinations as a prelude to corneal transplantation. Excimer trephinations were sharper; however, the Er:YAG laser required less time to produce full-thickness penetration with 10 to 15 μm of thermal damage. Belgorod and coworkers[88] performed tangential corneal ablation with a pulsed Er:YAG laser in bovine eyes and measured a stromal collagen fragmentation zone of 200 to 500 nm. Compared with the Er:YAG laser, the 308-nm XeCl excimer laser induced more prominent collagen damage, whereas the 193-nm excimer laser caused less damage. Kahle and associates[36] performed gas chromatographic and mass spectroscopic analysis of human cadaver cornea tissue ablated with the 193-nm excimer and Er:YAG lasers. Their study identified molecules, typically alkanes, that were larger and fewer after excimer-laser irradiation than after Er:YAG ablation.

Experimental studies explored the role of pulse duration on the extent of the corneal thermal damage induced by the Er:YAG laser by comparing normal spiking mode (microsecond range) with Q-switched (nanosecond range) pulses.[19, 21] The 2.94-μm Er:YAG laser irradiation has an extinction length of approximately 1 μm and a thermal relaxation time of 1 μsec. Hence, single pulses lasting less than 1 μsec are necessary to decrease thermal diffusion and minimize the zone of thermal damage. Walsh and coworkers[19] and Ren and colleagues[21] used the same Er:YAG laser system for corneal ablation in enucleated bovine eyes and observed a smaller zone of collateral thermal damage with Q-switched pulses. Normal spiking mode, 200-μsec pulses with a beam

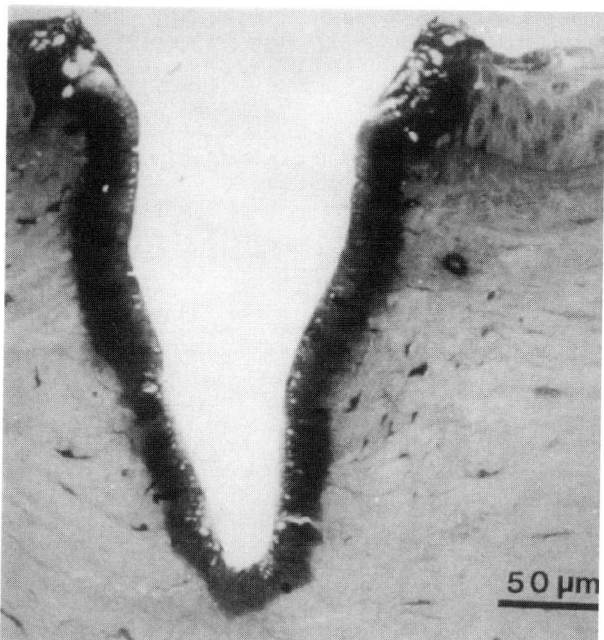

FIGURE 51–21. Typical light microscopy of calf cornea ablated by the normal spiking mode Er:YAG laser. The average width of the damage zone measured at the bottom of the cut was 16 ± 2 μm. The ablation threshold was 250 ± 20 mJ/cm². For this particular sample, the laser radiant exposure was 950 mJ/cm² (four times above threshold). (From Ren Q, Venugopalan V, Schomaker K, et al: Mid-infrared laser ablation of the cornea: A comparative study. Lasers Surg Med 12:274, 1992. Copyright © 1992 by Wiley-Liss. Reprinted by permission of Wiley-Liss, Inc., a division of John Wiley & Sons, Inc.)

diameter of 1.1 mm, induced 10 to 50 μm of collagen damage at the margin of the incisions (Fig. 51–21). Q-switched 90-nsec pulses, 420 μm in diameter at the tissue surface, caused 5 to 10 μm of damage (Fig. 51–22), indicating that Q-switched pulses may meet the criteria for precise corneal surface remodeling.[19, 21, 89]

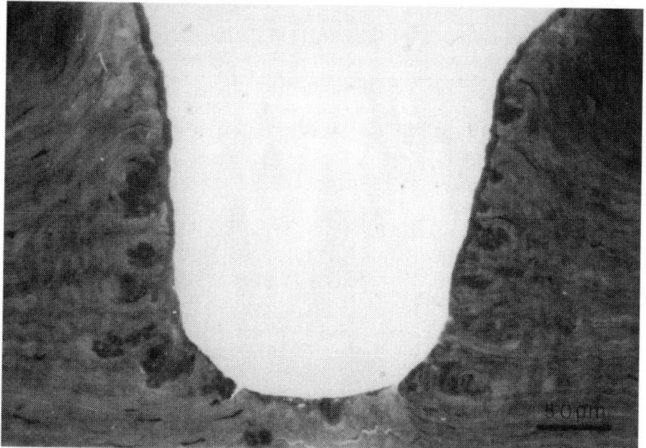

FIGURE 51–22. Typical light microscopy of calf cornea ablated by the Q-switched Er:YAG laser. The average width of damage zone measured at bottom of the cut was 4 ± 2 μm. The ablation threshold was 150 ± 10 mJ/cm². For this particular sample, the laser radiant exposure was 1.35 J/cm² (nine times above threshold). (From Ren Q, Venugopalan V, Schomaker K, et al: Mid-infrared laser ablation of the cornea: A comparative study. Lasers Surg Med 12:274, 1992. Copyright © 1992 by Wiley-Liss. Reprinted by permission of Wiley-Liss, Inc., a division of John Wiley & Sons, Inc.)

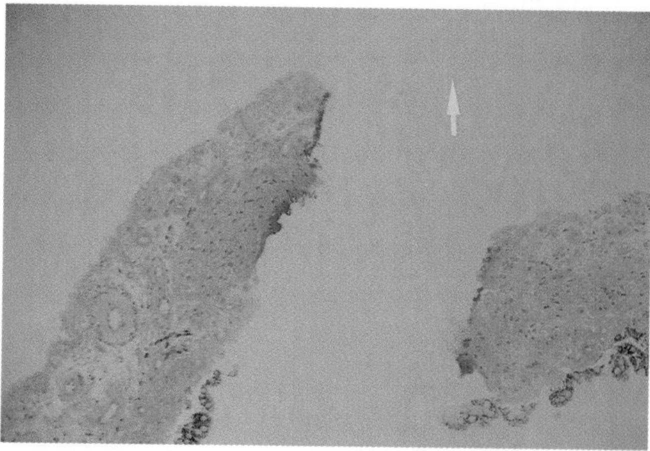

FIGURE 51–23. Photomicrograph of erbium:YAG laser iridotomy. Surgery was performed in an enucleated pig eye with a 200-μm side-firing probe with a posterior (from the epithelial side) to anterior direction, as indicated by the *white arrow*. Energy per pulse was 2.5 mJ, and the repetition rate was 200 Hz. Thermal damage at the cutting edge varies from 15 to 30 μm (hematoxylin; original magnification ×25).

IRIS SURGERY

D'Amico and coworkers[44] performed successful iris ablation at the pupil border to enlarge miotic pupils during pars plana vitrectomy in aphakic human eyes. They used hand-held quartz-tip endoprobes in a close-contact fashion in fluid media. Other researchers[47] used side-firing endoprobes to perform linear iridotomy and iridectomy in enucleated pig eyes. In this study, iris surgery was performed from the posterior epithelial iris surface with the probe operating in a up-firing fashion, as well as from the anterior surface of the iris in a down-firing fashion. Low and high repetition rates for these maneuvers yielded identical efficacy, inducing a thermal damage zone of less than 30 μm (Fig. 51–23).

REFERENCES

1. Maiman TH: Stimulated optical radiation in ruby. Nature 187:493, 1960.
2. The Diabetic Retinopathy Study Research Group: Preliminary report on effects of photocoagualtion therapy. Am J Ophthalmol 81:1, 1976.
3. The Diabetic Retinopathy Study Research Group: Photocoagulation treatment of proliferative diabetic retinopathy: The second report of diabetic retinopathy study findings. Ophthalmology 85:82, 1978.
4. Noyori KS, Campbell CJ, Rittler C, Koester CJ: The characteristics of experimental laser coagulations of the retina. Arch Ophthalmol 72:254, 1964.
5. L'Esperance FA: The ocular histopathologic effect of krypton and argon laser radiation. Am J Ophthalmol 68:263, 1969.
6. Beetham WP, Aiello LM, Balodimos MC, et al: Ruby laser photocoagulation of early diabetic neovascular retinopathy. Arch Ophthalmol 83:261, 1970.
7. Smiddy WE, Patz A, Quigley HA, Dunkelberger GR: Histopathology of the effects of tuneable dye laser on monkey retina. Ophthalmology 95:956, 1988.
8. Balles MW, Puliafito CA, D'Amico DJ, et al: Semiconductor diode laser photocoagulation in retinal vascular disease. Ophthalmology 97:1553, 1990.
9. McCullen WW, Garcia CA: Comparison of retinal photocoagulation using pulsed frequency-doubled neodymium-YAG and argon green laser. Retina 12:265, 1992.
10. Steinert RF, Puliafito CA, Trokel S: Plasma formation and shielding by three ophthalmic Nd-YAG lasers. Am J Ophthalmol 96:427, 1983.
11. Steinert RF, Puliafito CA, Kittrel C: Plasma shielding by Q-switched and mode-locked Nd-YAG lasers. Ophthalmology 90:1003, 1983.

12. Aron-Rosa D, Aron JJ, Greisemann J, Thyzel R: Use of the neodymium-YAG laser to open the posterior capsule after lens implant surgery: A preliminary report. J Am Intraocul Implant Soc 6:352, 1980.
13. Del Priore LV, Robin AL, Pollack IP: Neodymium-YAG and argon laser iridotomy: Long-term follow-up in a prospective, randomized clinical trial. Ophthalmology 95:1207, 1988.
14. Steinert RF, Wasson PJ: Neodymium:YAG anterior vitreolysis for Irvine-Gass cystoid macular edema. J Cataract Refract Surg 15:304, 1989.
15. Srinivasan R, Leigh WJ: Ablative photodecomposition on poly(ethylene terephthalate) films. J Am Chem Soc 104:6784, 1982.
16. Puliafito CA, Stern D, Kruegger RR, et al: High-speed photography of excimer laser ablation of the cornea. Arch Ophthalmol 105:1255, 1987.
17. Seiler T, Wollensak J: Myopic photorefractive keratectomy with the excimer laser: One year follow-up. Ophthalmology 98:1156, 1991.
18. Pallikaris I, Papatsanaki M, Stathi E, et al: Laser in-situ keratomileusis. Laser Surg Med 10:463, 1990.
19. Walsh JT, Flotte TJ, Deutsch TF: Er:YAG laser ablation of tissue: Effects of pulse duration and tissue type on thermal damage. Lasers Surg Med 9:314, 1989.
20. Walsh JT, Deutsch TF: Er:YAG laser ablation of tissue: Measurement of ablation rates. Lasers Surg Med 9:327, 1989.
21. Ren Q, Venugopalan V, Schomaker K, et al: Mid-infrared laser ablation of the cornea: A comparative study. Lasers Surg Med 12:274, 1992.
22. Meyers SM, Bonner RF, Rodrigues MM, Ballintine EJ: Phototransection of vitreal membranes with the carbon dioxide laser in rabbits. Ophthalmology 90:563, 1983.
23. Nelson JS, Yow L, Liaw LH, et al: Ablation of bone and methacrylate by a prototype mid-infrared erbium:YAG laser. Lasers Surg Med 8:494, 1988.
24. Peyman GA, Katoh N: Effects of an erbium:YAG laser on ocular structures. Int Ophthalmol 10:245, 1987.
25. Tsubota K: Application of erbium:YAG laser in ocular ablation. Ophthalmologica 200:117, 1990.
26. D'Amico DJ, Moulton RS, Theodossiadis PG, Yarborough JM: Erbium:YAG laser photothermal retinal ablation in enucleated rabbit eyes. Am J Ophthalmol 117:783, 1994.
27. Seiler T, Marshall J, Rothery S, Wollensak J: The potential of an infrared hydrogen fluoride (HF) laser (3.0 μm) for corneal surgery. Lasers Light Ophthalmol 1:49, 1986.
28. Borirakchanyavat S, Puliafito CA, Kliman GH, et al: Holmium-YAG laser surgery on experimental vitreous membranes. Arch Ophthalmol 109:1605, 1991.
29. McCally RL, Farrell R, Bargeron CB: Cornea epithelial damage thresholds in rabbits exposed to Tm:YAG laser radiation at 2.02 μm. Lasers Surg Med 12:598, 1992.
30. Schomacker KT, Domankevitz Y, Flotte TJ, Deutsch TF: Co:MgF$_2$ laser ablation of tissue: Effect of wavelength on ablation threshold and thermal damage. Lasers Surg Med 11:141, 1991.
31. Hale GM, Querry MR: Optical constants of water in the 200-nm to 200-μm wavelength region. Appl Optics 12:555, 1973.
32. Roberston CW, Williams D: Lambert absorption coefficients of water in infrared. J Opt Soc Am 61:1316, 1971.
33. Zolotarev MV, Mikhailov BA, Aperovich LI, Popov SI: Dispersion and absorption of liquid water in the infrared and radio regions of the spectrum. Opt Spectrosc 27:430, 1969.
34. Lewis A, Palanker D, Hemo I, et al: Microsurgery of the retina with a needle-guided 193-nm excimer laser. Invest Ophthalmol Vis Sci 33:2377, 1992.
35. Palanker D, Hemo I, Turovets I, et al: Vitreoretinal ablation with the 193-nm excimer laser in fluid media. Invest Ophthalmol Vis Sci 35:3835, 1994.
36. Kahle G, Städter H, Seiler T, Wollensak J: Gas chromatographic and mass spectroscopic analysis of excimer and erbium:yttrium aluminum garnet laser-ablated human cornea. Invest Ophthalmol Vis Sci 33:2180, 1992.
37. Marshall J, Sliney DH: Endoexcimer laser intraocular ablative photodecomposition. [Correspondence] Am J Ophthalmol 101:130, 1986.
38. Seiler T, Bende T, Winckler K, Wollensak J: Side effects in excimer corneal surgery. DNA damage as a result of 193 nm excimer laser radiation. Graefes Arch Clin Exp Ophthalmol 226:273, 1988.
39. Rasmussen RE, Hammer-Wilson M, Berns MW: Mutation and sister chromatid exchange induction in Chinese hamster ovary (Cho) cells by pulsed excimer laser radiation at 193 nm and 308 nm and continuous UV radiation at 254 nm. Photochem Photobiol 49:413, 1989.
40. Kochevar IE: Cytotoxicity and mutagenicity of excimer laser radiation. Lasers Surg Med 9:440, 1989.
41. Pitts DG, Cullen AP, Hacker PD: Ocular effects of ultraviolet radiation from 295 to 365 nm. Invest Ophthalmol Vis Sci 16:932, 1977.
42. Margolis TI, Farnarth DA, Destro M, Puliafito CA: Erbium-YAG laser surgery on experimental vitreous membranes. Arch Ophthalmol 107:424, 1989.
43. Brazitikos PD, D'Amico DJ, Bernal M-T, Walsh AW: Erbium-YAG laser surgery of the vitreous and retina. Ophthalmology 102:278, 1995.
44. D'Amico DJ, Brazitikos PD, Marcellino GR, et al: Initial clinical experience with an erbium:YAG laser for vitreoretinal surgery. Am J Ophthalmol 121:414, 1996.
45. D'Amico DJ, Blumenkranz MS, Lavin MJ, et al: Multicenter clinical experience using an erbium:YAG laser for vitreoretinal surgery. Ophthalmology 103:1575, 1996.
46. Brazitikos PD, Bochow TW, D'Amico DJ, et al: Experimental ocular surgery with a high repetition rate erbium-YAG laser. ARVO Abstracts. Invest Ophthalmol Vis Sci 37(Suppl 4):S571, 1996.
47. Brazitikos PD, D'Amico DJ, Bochow TW, et al: Experimental ocular surgery with a high repetition rate (200 Hz) erbium:YAG laser. Invest Ophthalmol Vis Sci (in press).
48. Quiroz-Mercado H, D'Amico DJ, Marcellino G: High repetition rate erbium-YAG laser for vitreoretinal surgery. Presented at the Joint XXth Meeting of the Club Jules Gonin and of the 29th Annual Scientific Session of the Retina Society, Bern, Switzerland, September 1–6, 1996.
49. Quiroz-Mercado H, Martinez JJ, D'Amico DJ, et al: High repetition rate erbium:YAG laser (200 Hz) for vitreoretinal surgery. ARVO Abstracts. Invest Ophthalmol Vis Sci 38(Suppl 4):S84, 1997.
50. Ellsworth LG, Kramer TR, Noecker RJ, et al: Retinotomy using erbium:YAG laser equipped with a contact probe on human autopsy eyes. ARVO Abstracts. Invest Ophthalmol Vis Sci 34(Suppl 4):961, 1993.
51. Lin CP, Stern D, Puliafito CA: High speed photography of Er:YAG laser ablation in fluid: Implication for laser vitreous surgery. Invest Ophthalmol Vis Sci 31:2546, 1990.
52. Loertscher H, Shi WQ, Grundfest WS: Tissue ablation through water with erbium:YAG lasers. IEEE Trans Biomed Eng 39:86, 1992.
53. Brinkmann R, Schroer F, Mohrensteder D, et al: Ablation dynamics in laser sclerostomy ab externo. ARVO Abstracts. Invest Ophthalmol Vis Sci 36(Suppl 4):S558, 1995.
54. Berger JW, Bochow TW, Kim RY, D'Amico DJ: Biophysical considerations for optimizing energy delivery during Er:YAG laser vitreoretinal surgery. Proc SPIE 2673:146, 1996.
55. Berger JW, D'Amico DJ: Modelling of Er:YAG laser-mediated explosive photovaporization: Implications for vitreoretinal surgery. Ophthalmic Surg Lasers 28:133, 1997.
56. Bochow TW, Kim R, Berger JW, D'Amico DJ: Photovitrectomy—A novel approach for vitreous removal. ARVO Abstracts. Invest Ophthalmol Vis Sci 36(Suppl 4):S834, 1995.
57. Schmidt-Petersen H, Mrochen M, Genth U, Seiler T: Erbium:YAG laser vitrectomy. ARVO Abstracts. Invest Ophthalmol Vis Sci 38(Suppl 4):S86, 1997.
58. Berger JW, Bochow TW, Talamo JH, D'Amico DJ: Measurement and modeling of thermal transients during Er:YAG laser irradiation of vitreous. Lasers Surg Med 19:388, 1996.
59. Gailitis RP, Patterson SW, Samuels MA, et al: Comparison of laser phacovaporization using the Er-YAG and the Er-YSGG laser. Arch Ophthalmol 111:697, 1993.
60. Noecker RJ, Kramer TR, Ellsworth LG, et al: Endolenticular phacolysis using erbium:YSGG and erbium:YAG lasers on human autopsy lenses: A histopathologic study. ARVO Abstracts. Invest Ophthalmol Vis Sci 34 (Suppl 4):1453, 1993.
61. Colvard DM, Kratz RP: Cataract surgery utilizing the erbium laser. *In* Fine IH (ed): Phacoemulsification: New Technology and Clinical Application. Thorofare, NJ, Slack, 1996, p 161.
62. Ryutaro O, Harigaya O, Kobayashi K: Anterior capsulotomy with a newly developed erbium:YAG laser system. Presented at the Fifth International Congress of Laser Technology in Ophthalmology, Lugano, Switzerland, June 26–29, 1996.
63. Berger JW, Kim SH, LaMarche KJ, et al: Er:YAG laser drilling of lens tissue: Predicting the ablation rate with a simple model. Proc SPIE 2393:148, 1995.
64. Snyder RW, Noecker RJ, Jones H: In vitro comparison of phacoemulsification and the erbium:YAG laser in lens capsule rupture. ARVO Abstracts. Invest Ophthalmol Vis Sci 35(Suppl 4):S798, 1994.
65. Berger JW, Talamo JH, LaMarche KJ, et al: Temperature measurements during phacoemulsification and erbium:YAG laser phacoablation in model systems. J Cataract Refract Surg 22:372, 1996.

66. Kessler J: Experiments in refilling the lens. Arch Ophthalmol 71:412, 1964.
67. Haefliger E, Parel JM, Fantes F, et al: Accomodation of an endocapsular silicone lens (phaco-ersatz) in the nonhuman primate. Ophthalmology 94:471, 1987.
68. Beckman H, Fuller TA: Carbon dioxide laser scleral dissection and filtering procedure for glaucoma. Am J Ophthalmol 88:73, 1979.
69. Özler SA, Hill RA, Andrews JJ, et al: Infrared laser sclerostomies. Invest Ophthalmol Vis Sci 32:2498, 1991.
70. Margolis TI, Farnath DA, Puliafito CA: Mid infrared laser sclerostomy. ARVO Abstracts. Invest Ophthalmol Vis Sci 29(Suppl 4):366, 1988.
71. Hoskins HD Jr, Iwach AG, Drake MV, et al: Subconjunctival THC:YAG laser limbal sclerostomy ab externo in the rabbit. Ophthalmic Surg 8:589, 1990.
72. Hill RA, Özler SA, Baerveldt G, et al: Ab-interno neodymium:YAG versus erbium:YAG laser sclerostomies in a rabbit model. Ophthalmic Surg 23:192, 1992.
73. Latina MA, March WF: Ab-interno sclerostomy using a goniolens and pulsed dye-laser in flaucoma patients. ARVO Abstracts. Invest Ophthalmol Vis Sci 32(Suppl 4):860, 1991.
74. Jaffe GJ, Williams GA, Mieler WF, Radius RL: Ab interno sclerostomy with a high-powered argon endolaser. Am J Ophthalmol 106:391, 1988.
75. Seiler T, Kriegerowski M, Bende T, et al: Partial trabeculectomy with the excimer laser (193 nm). ARVO Abstracts. Invest Ophthalmol Vis Sci 29(Suppl 4):239, 1988.
76. Berlin MS, Rajacich G, Duffy M, et al: Excimer laser photoablation in glaucoma filtering surgery. Am J Ophthalmol 103:713, 1987.
77. Keates RH, Bloom RT, Schneider RT, et al: Absorption of 308-nm excimer radiation by BSS, sodium hyaluronate and human cadaver eyes. Arch Ophthalmol 108:1611, 1991.
78. Arias-Puente A, Puy D, Garcia-Feijoo J, Garcia-Gonzalez J: Er:YAG laser sclerostomy in complicated secondary glaucomas. ARVO Abstracts. Invest Ophthalmol Vis Sci 36(Suppl 4):S557, 1995.
79. Kobayashi K, Mizota A, Takasoh M, Momiuchi M: Internal contact sclerostomy with erbium YAG laser. ARVO Abstracts. Invest Ophthalmol Vis Sci 36(Suppl 4):S557, 1995.
80. McHam ML, Schuman JS, Eisenberg DL, Wang N: Er:YAG laser sclerectomy and laser trabecular ablation with a sapphire optical fiber. ARVO Abstracts. Invest Ophthalmol Vis Sci 36(Suppl 4):S557, 1995.
81. Kramer TR, Noecker RJ, Ellsworth LG, et al: Laser trabecular ablation of human autopsy eyes with erbium:YAG laser: A histopathologic study. ARVO Abstracts. Invest Ophthalmol Vis Sci 33(Suppl 4):1141, 1993.
82. Seiler T, Marshall J, Rothery S, Wollensak J: The potential of an infrared hydrogen fluoride (HF) laser (3.0 μm) for corneal surgery. Lasers Ophthalmol 1:49, 1986.
83. Loertscher H, Mandelbaum S, Parrish RK, Parel JM: Preliminary report on corneal incisions created by a hydrogen fluoride laser. Am J Ophthalmol 102:217, 1986.
84. Stern D, Puliafito CA, Dobbi ET, Reidy WI: Infrared laser surgery of the cornea: Studies with a Raman-shifted Nd:YAG laser at 2.80 and 2.92 μm. Ophthalmology 95:1434, 1988.
85. Seiler T, Schmidt-Petersen H, Leiacker R, et al: Erbium:YAG laser photoablation of human cornea. Am J Ophthalmol 120:668, 1995.
86. Peyman GA, Badaro RM, Khoobehi B: Corneal ablation in rabbits using an infrared (2.9 mm) erbium:YAG laser. Ophthalmology 96:1160, 1989.
87. Thompson KP, Barraquer E, Parel JM, et al: Potential use of lasers for penetrating keratoplasty. J Cataract Refract Surg 15:397, 1989.
88. Belgorod BM, Ediger MN, Weiblinger RP, Erlandson RA: Tangential corneal surface ablation with 193- and 308-nm excimer and 2396-nm erbium-YAG laser irradiation. Arch Ophthalmol 110:533, 1992.
89. Seiler T, Wollensak J: Fundamental mode photoablation of the cornea for myopic correction. 1: Theoretical background. Lasers Light Ophthalmol 5:199, 1993.

CHAPTER 52

Photodynamic Therapy

Deeba Husain, Evangelos S. Gragoudas, and Joan W. Miller

Photodynamic therapy (PDT) involves the use of photoactivatable compounds (photosensitizers) that accumulate in and are retained by proliferating tissues. Activation of these molecules by light at the appropriate wavelength generates active forms of oxygen and free radicals, which result in photochemical damage to cells that contain the photosensitizer. Thus, PDT can be used to treat diseased areas selectively while sparing the normal tissue. PDT has been extensively studied in the treatment of neoplasia and more recently for neovascularization. In ophthalmology, it is being investigated as a treatment modality for choroidal neovascularization (CNV) in age-related macular degeneration and choroidal melanoma.

Historical Background

The earliest report on the action of light-activated chemicals on biologic systems was published in 1900 by Raab, who described the lethal effect of light on paramecia treated with acridine dye.[1] Raab noted that paramecia in a flask died on exposure to light after incubation with acridine dye, whereas dye alone, light alone, or dye after exposure to light did not cause cell death. In 1904, Von Tappeiner and Jodlbauer demonstrated the oxygen dependence of this photosensitization reaction and coined the term *photodynamic action*.[2]

Meyer-Betz demonstrated the photosensitizing properties of hematoporphyrin derivative (HPD) in 1913.[3] Policard reported fluorescence in experimental rat sarcomas under the Wood light due to excitation of endogenous porphyrins.[4] In 1942, Aueler and Banzer first used HPD for photodynamic destruction of tumors in animals.[5] In 1961, Lipson and colleagues reported on the use of HPD for fluorescence detection of neoplastic tissue and subsequent treatment in patients with breast cancer.[6] In 1972, Diamond and coworkers showed destruction of glioma cells in culture and subsequently treated transplanted gliomas in rats with HPD and light.[7] Dougherty and associates used the term *photoradiation therapy* to describe the treatment of tumors in animals using filtered visible light and HPD.[8]

In 1978, Dougherty and colleagues reported the first large series of patients with cutaneous malignancies that exhibited partial or complete response to photoradiation therapy using HPD and light.[9] The active components of HPD were identified to be dihematoporphyrin ethers and esters (DHE), and the commercial preparation of DHE is known as porfimer sodium, or Photofrin. Phase III clinical trials were initiated with porfimer sodium in the 1980s for the treatment of bladder carcinoma, endobronchial carcinoma, and obstructive esophageal carcinoma.[10] Porfimer sodium has been used extensively in clinical trials. It is approved for the treatment of superficial bladder cancer in Canada. In Japan, early cancers of the lung, esophagus, stomach, and cervix have been treated with porfimer sodium.[11] In North America and Europe, phase III clinical trials with porfimer sodium have shown its beneficial effect in the palliative treatment of lung and esophageal cancers and in the prophylactic treatment of papillary bladder cancer.[12] Preliminary trials in the treatment of basal cell carcinoma, metastatic skin lesions, and the elimination of leukemia progenitor cells in the marrow of patients with chronic myelogenous leukemia have shown the benefit of PDT with benzoporphyrin derivative.[12] Nononcologic conditions outside the eye that are well suited to treatment with PDT include psoriasis, atherosclerotic plaque and restenosis, bone marrow purging for the treatment of leukemias with autologous bone marrow transplant, inactivation of viruses in blood or blood products, and several autoimmune conditions including rheumatoid arthritis.[13] Porfimer sodium has been approved for human use in the Netherlands for early and late esophageal and lung cancer. Japan has approved the use of porfimer sodium for PDT of early stomach, esophageal, lung, and cervical cancer and cervical dysplasia.[14]

Mechanism of Action

PDT requires the administration of a photosensitizer dye that accumulates in neoplastic and neovascular tissues. The targeted tissue is then irradiated using light of a wavelength at an absorption peak of the dye. A photochemical reaction is initiated with the absorption of light by the photosensitizer molecule in the ground state (S), which is excited to enter a higher-energy triplet state (^3S). The ^3S molecules are short-lived reactive species that transfer their energy via two pathways that can cause cytotoxicity. Energy can be transferred from the ^3S photosensitizer to molecular oxygen, converting it to singlet oxygen ($^1O_2$) while returning to their ground state (type II reaction).[15] The ^3S molecules may also directly transfer energy through a free radical mechanism to form cytotoxic intermediates (type I reaction) (Fig. 52–1). The type II–mediated pathway accounts for the majority of tissue destruction and is responsible for the oxygen dependence of PDT. The extent of oxygen dependence varies somewhat among photosensitizers; under anoxic conditions, PDT effects are abolished for porfimer sodium.[16]

PDT offers some degree of selectivity in the destruction of tumor and neovascular tissue, with minimal local and systemic side effects. This is due to two factors: a preferential

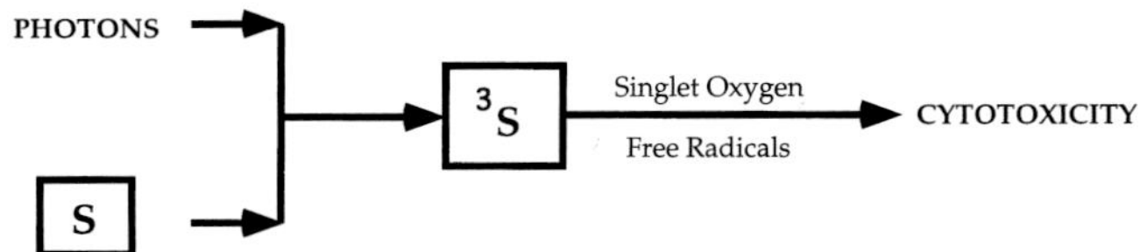

FIGURE 52–1. Schematic representation of photodynamic action. Photons are absorbed by photosensitizer molecules in ground state (S). This causes them to enter a higher energy excited triplet state (^3S). The short-lived reactive triplet state photosensitizer molecule leads to transfer of energy causing the formation of singlet oxygen and free radicals that cause cytotoxicity.

localization of the photosensitizer in these tissues and precise laser light irradiation of the targeted tissue.[17] The mechanism of accumulation of the photosensitizer in the neovascular and neoplastic tissue is not known, but several theories have been proposed. Photosensitizers are taken up by most tissues of the body but are retained longer in neoplastic tissue, as well as in normal liver, spleen, kidney, and wound healing tissue. Henderson and Dougherty have suggested that pooling and retention of photosensitizers in tumors could be due to a larger interstitial space and poor lymphatic network.[18] The cells with high mitotic activity, such as tumor and neovascular endothelial cells, have a high expression of low density lipoprotein (LDL) receptors (e.g., the apo B/E receptor),[19] which might cause more efficient uptake of LDL-bound molecules by receptor-mediated endocytosis.[20] Therefore, various methods to enhance the LDL-mediated mechanism have been investigated, including formulation of photosensitizer in liposomes and lipid emulsions, as well as preincorporation with LDL. Selective localization of photosensitizers in tumors has also been improved by binding the dye to targeting molecules such as monoclonal antibodies that recognize specific antigens on tumor cells.[21]

The mechanisms of PDT-mediated tissue destruction include cellular, vascular, and immunologic damage. Direct cellular destruction is due to the damage of cellular membranes through lipid peroxidation and protein damage by $^1O_2$ and free radical intermediates,[10] leading to structural and functional damage to cellular membranes. Direct damage to nuclear components and apoptotic mechanisms has also been reported.[22] Vascular damage is an important mechanism of tissue destruction in PDT with certain photosensitizers and probably is secondary to endothelial damage and subsequent platelet aggregation, as well as vessel thrombosis. Eicosanoids are released after PDT, including thromboxane, histamine, and tumor necrosis factor-α, and may contribute to vascular occlusion.[23] Finally, immunomodulation may play a role in PDT-induced tissue destruction. Treatment of various tumors with PDT has demonstrated increased tissue levels of cytokines,[24] enhanced killing activity of specific cytotoxic T lymphocytes,[25] increased natural killer cell activity,[26] and tumor-associated macrophage accumulation in tissue[27] with release of tumor necrosis factor-α and macrophage-mediated cytotoxicity. Researchers are investigating immunomodulation after PDT for application in organ transplantation and the treatment of autoimmune diseases.

Clinically Approved Photosensitizers

The effective penetration depth of PDT depends on the wavelength of the light and optical properties, such as absorption and scatter of the targeted tissue. Typically, the effective penetration depth is 2 to 3 mm at 630 nm and increases to 5 to 6 mm at longer wavelengths (700 to 800 nm).[28] These values can be altered by changing the biologic and physical characteristics of the photosensitizer. In general, photosensitizers with longer wavelengths and higher molar absorption at these wavelengths are more efficient photodynamic agents[14] (Fig. 52–2).

Most clinical experience comes from the porphyrin family of photosensitizers, including HPD and DHE. DHE is a complex mixture of oligomeric esters and ethers of HPD with inherent variability[29] (Fig. 52–3). The commercial preparation of DHE is porfimer sodium (see Fig. 52–3*A*). Porfimer sodium has been extensively studied in clinical trials for superficial bladder cancer, obstructive tumors of the lung and esophagus, and early cancers of the lung, stomach, and cervix. It causes effective photodynamic tumor damage but leads to prolonged skin photosensitivity requiring about 48 hours of hospitalization after treatment. It also is poorly characterized chemically and has relatively low absorption in the wavelength region of therapeutic interest (600 to 1100 nm).[14] This has provided an incentive to develop second-generation photosensitizers.

BPD, a second-generation photosensitizer, is formally a chlorin because it has a reduced pyrrole ring as well as a fused six-membered isocyclic ring[30] (see Fig. 52–3*B*). The light absorption maximums of BPD at 354, 418, 574, 626, and 688 nm. allow deeper tissue penetration and effective treatment. BPD has a rapid rate of clearance, with no significant photosensitivity after 24 hours, and is metabolized to inactive forms prior to excretion through feces.[31] Phase III clinical trials are in progress for the treatment of exudative age-related macular degeneration with BPD, and a small pilot trial is investigating PDT using BPD for psoriatic arthritis.

Other second-generation photosensitizers undergoing clinical trials include monoaspartyl chlorin e6 (NPe6) (see Fig. 52–3*C*) with a light absorption maximum at 660 to 665 nm; mesotetra hydroxyphenyl chlorin (mTHPC) (see Fig. 52–3*D*) with a light absorption maximum at 650 nm; tin etiopurpurin (SnEt2) (see Fig. 52–3*E*) with a light absorption maximum at 660 to 665 nm; and 5-amino-levulinic acid (ALA) (see Fig. 52–3*F*), a precursor of protoporphyrin IX in heme biosynthesis, with a light absorption maximum of 630 nm[17] (see Fig. 52–3).

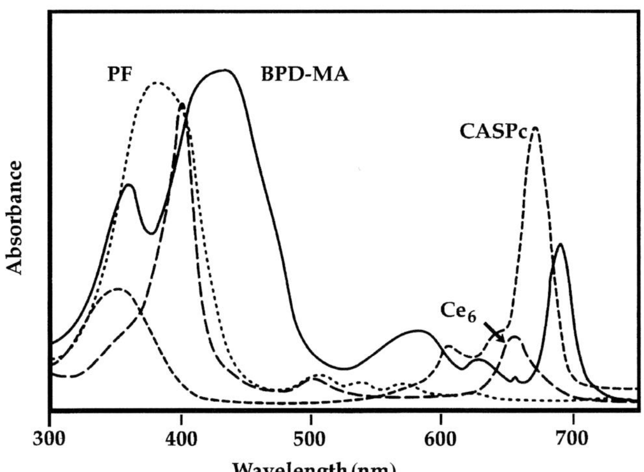

FIGURE 52–2. Absorption spectra of selected photosensitizers that have been used in photodynamic therapy. PF, photoferin; BPD-MA, benzoporphyrin derivative monoacid; Ce6, chlorin 6; CASPc, chloroaluminum sulfonated phthalocyanine. (From Lui H, Anderson RR: Photodynamic therapy in dermatology: Recent developments. Dermatol Clin 11:1–13, 1993.)

Photosensitizers in Ophthalmology (Table 52–1)

RETINOBLASTOMA

PDT of experimental retinoblastoma-like tumor in animals has shown effective regression. Winther suggested that PDT using porfimer sodium leads to early destruction of cells due to direct damage to the neoplastic cells and delayed effect due to damage of the vascular supply of the tumor.[32] The side effects of the treatment include leukocytic infiltration of the cornea and conjunctiva and edema of the retina with severe disorganization and damage to photoreceptors.[33] PDT using DHE caused complete remission in 15 to 25% of fast-growing rat retinoblastoma-like tumor, although some of the treated eyes had intraocular hemorrhage and reversible corneal clouding.[34]

There are few clinical reports of PDT for treatment of retinoblastoma. Ohnishi and coworkers treated five patients with retinoblastoma with PDT using HPD (dye dose 2.5 to 5 mg/kg and light absorption at 488 to 514.5 nm), four of whom had undergone previous irradiation. PDT resulted in thrombus formation, angionecrosis, and tumor cell death up to a depth of 6 mm in the tumor.[35] Murphee successfully treated two patients with recurrent retinoblastoma with PDT using HPD and continuous-wave argon green laser.[36] The role of PDT in the treatment of retinoblastoma is not well established, and further studies are needed.

OCULAR MELANOMA

Various investigators have studied the effect of PDT on experimental choroidal melanoma. PDT with HPD for the treatment of Greene hamster melanoma in rabbits caused complete tumor destruction in some tumors, but superficial necrosis occurred.[37] Second-generation photosensitizers such as chloroaluminum sulfonated phthalocyanine (CASPc)[38, 39] and BPD[40] have yielded favorable results in the treatment of amelanotic Greene hamster melanoma in the rabbit eye. Pigmented murine melanoma in a rabbit model has been treated with CASPc and argon dye laser at 25 to 70 J/cm^2; tumor regression was noted in 12 of the 20 animals treated.[41] PDT using BPD was performed in 18 rabbit eyes with pigmented melanoma, and regression occurred in all tumors treated with 60 J/cm^2 (Fig. 52–4*A* and *B*).[42] Histologic examination showed acute vascular damage to the full thickness of the tumor (up to 4.6 mm),[42] and necrosis with mononuclear and macrophage infiltration was prominent at 1 month of follow-up.[43]

Hu and colleagues studied photoimmunotherapy of human uveal melanoma cells (RPMI1846) in vitro.[44] The photosensitizer chlorin e6 monoethylenediamine monoamide (CMA) was conjugated with melanoma reactive monoclonal antibody IG12. Target cells preincubated with CMA were irradiated with 5 to 40 J/cm^2 light and compared with control

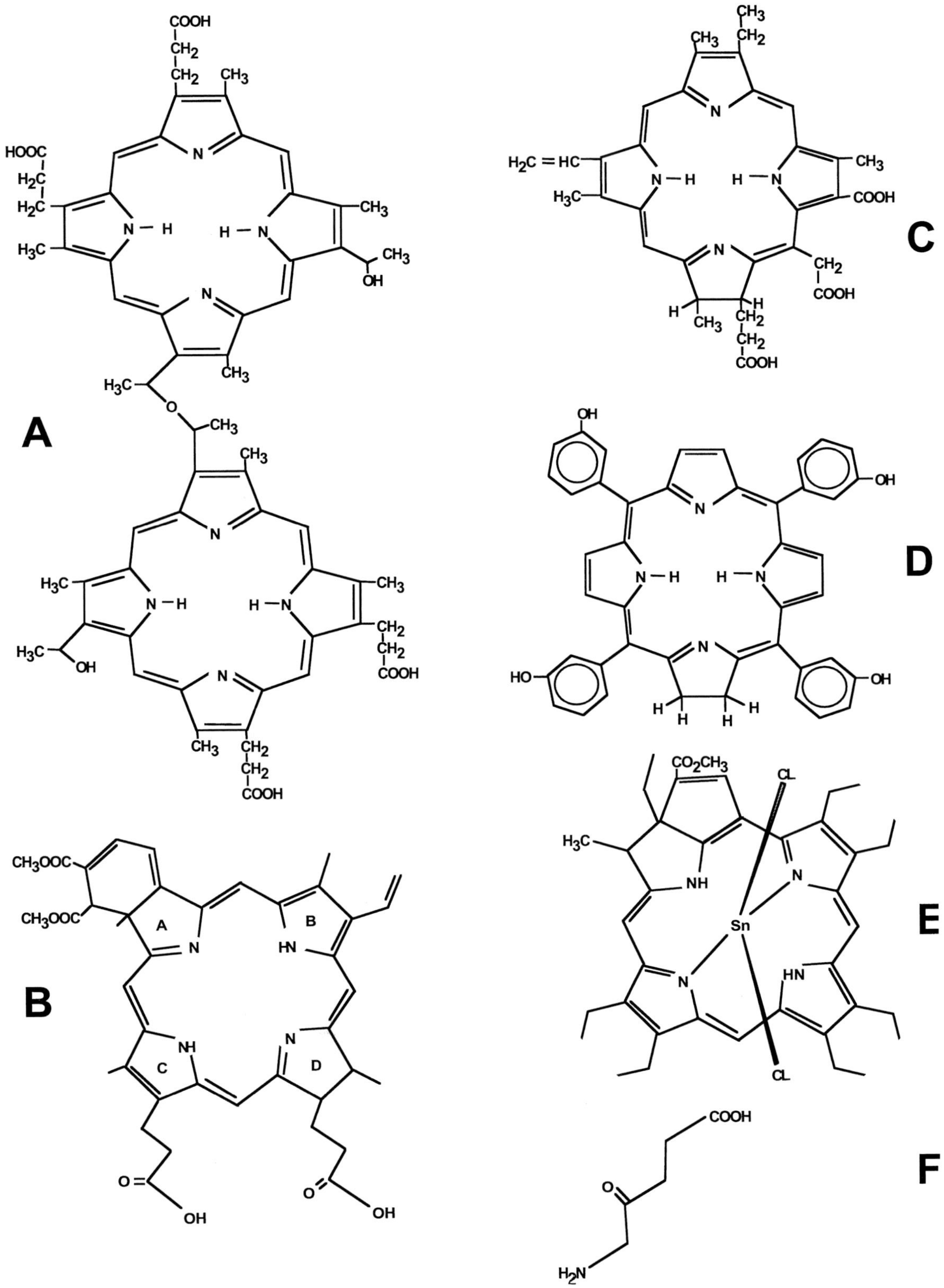

FIGURE 52–3. Chemical structures of: *(A)* Dihematoporphyrin ether, DHE; *(B)* Benzoporphyrin derivative monoacid, BPD-MA; *(C)* Mono-aspertyl chlorin e6, NP e6; *(D)* Meta-tetra (hydroxyphenyl) chlorin, mTHPC; *(E)* Tin-etio-purpurin, SnET2; *(F)* 5-amino-levulinic acid, ALA.

TABLE 52–1. **Photosensitizers in Ophthalmology**

Xanthene derivatives
Rose bengal
Tetrapyrrole derivatives
Hematoporphyrin derivative
Photofrin (dihematoporphyrin ether)
Benzoporphyrin derivative
Chlorins and Bacteriochlorins
Mono-aspartyl chlorin e6
Bacteriochlorin a
Tin etiopurpurin
Phthalocyanines
Chloroaluminum sulfonated phthalocyanine
Zinc phthalocyanine

cells that were treated with CMA alone or light alone. The authors found that the immunoconjugate was effective in photodestruction of human uveal cells in vitro and that phototoxicity was selective and more potent than free CMA.

Ocular melanoma appears to be a suitable candidate for PDT. The presence of leaky tumor vasculature and an intact blood-retinal barrier in adjacent tissues may result in enhanced localization of photosensitizer within tumor. Tse and associates treated three patients with HPD and light at 630 nm; only one treated at a higher light dose of 2160 J/cm^2 showed response in the form of limited tumor necrosis.[45] Bruce treated 24 patients with choroidal melanoma using HPD and light.[46] Complete regression occurred in 8 of the 11 patients with small tumors; the larger tumors remained stable. Common side effects included skin sensitivity, chemosis, and iritis. Less common side effects were cataract, vitritis, choroidal detachment, exudative retinal detachment, and delayed chorioretinal scarring. Sery and colleagues treated five patients with PDT using HPD when the tumor failed to respond to conventional treatment.[47] The tumors showed superficial regression, but the results were disappointing because surgical intervention became necessary in all cases. Favilla and coworkers treated 19 patients with choroidal melanomas that were 7 to 10 mm in height.[48] Six of these treated patients showed complete regression, and 8 showed no regression. These clinical reports are inconclusive in determining the role of PDT in the treatment of patients with ocular melanoma. However, patient selection in these early reports was for large tumors, with a resultant high complication rate. Clinical investigation with newer photosensitizers and smaller tumors is warranted.

IRIS MELANOMA

Different photosensitizers have been tested in the experimental Greene hamster model of iris and ciliary body melanoma in the rabbit eye. Small tumors of up to 4 mm in height have shown complete necrosis when treated with PDT using HPD at a dose of 2.5 mg/kg and light at 102 J/cm^2. PDT with higher doses of light ($>$ 180 J/cm^2) or dye (7.5 to 10 mg/kg) led to side effects such as corneal and conjunctival edema, intraocular hemorrhage, and intraocular inflammation.[49] PDT of iris melanoma model with CASPc and light at 20 J/cm^2 demonstrated tumor growth arrest. Treatment at light doses higher than 60 J/cm^2 led to permanent tumor growth arrest but also caused side effects similar to those occurring with PDT using HPD at higher doses.[37] PDT of this model using lipoprotein-bound BPD-MA and light at 692 nm and 100 J/cm^2 demonstrated necrosis of iris tumor and formation of an avascular fibrotic scar. Histologically, destruction of the neovascular endothelial cells and intracellular tumor cell damage occurred.[50]

Tse and associates studied the effect of PDT on iris melanoma in two patients using HPD and light at 630 nm. Both eyes showed complete tumor regression; 1 year later, histopathology revealed few tumor cells at the peripheral iris.[45] One patient with multinodular iris melanoma treated with HPD (2.5 mg/kg) and light at 630 nm showed no response to PDT.[47] In 1992, Davidorf and Davidorf treated four patients with iris melanoma using HPD (2.5 mg/kg) and red light at 1.72 $\times$ 10^6 J/cm^2.[51] The eye of the first patient was enucleated and showed tumor necrosis. The three subsequent patients showed complete tumor ablation with no evidence of regrowth. The side effects listed in the clinical reports were similar to those in the experimental data and were related to higher light and dye doses. The efficacy of PDT in the treatment of iris melanoma has been demonstrated, but further investigations are required to determine optimal treatment parameters and long-term effects.

CORNEAL NEOVASCULARIZATION

Epstein and colleagues performed PDT of experimental corneal neovascularization (created by intrastromal interleukin-2 injection).[52] PDT was performed using intravenous

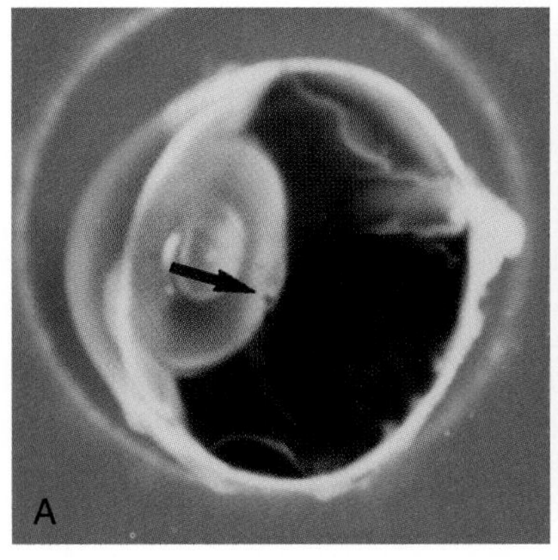

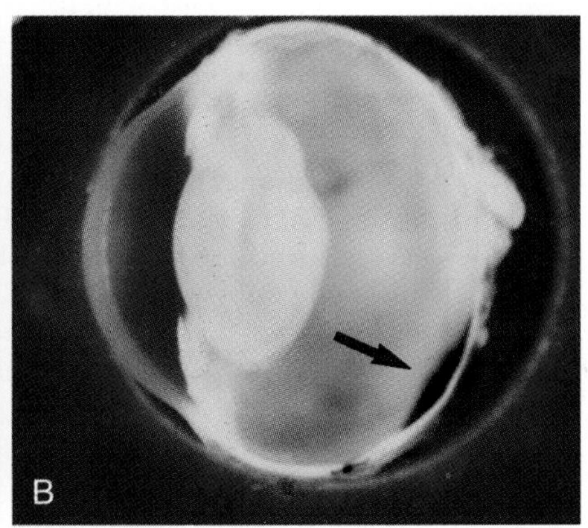

FIGURE 52–4. Cross section of tumor-bearing eyes. *A,* One month after treatment with benzoporphyrin derivative monoacid and light at 150 J/cm^2. *B,* Two weeks after treatment with light only (150 J/cm^2). A small pigmented choroidal nodule *(black arrow)* is seen at the tumor site in the eye treated with benzoporphyrin derivative and light contrasted with the large pigmented mass abutting the posterior surface of the lens in the control eye. (From Young LHY, Howard MA, Hu LK, et al: Photodynamic therapy of pigmented choroidal melanoma using a liposomal preparation of benzoporphytin derivative. Arch Ophthalmol 114:186–192, 1996.)

DHE and irradiation at 72 hours with light at 514 nm. PDT caused significant reduction in the corneal neovascularization. The side effects included blepharitis (9%) and iris damage (18%), but no side effects occurred with the posterior segment. PDT with light at 514 nm thus was shown to be efficacious for the treatment of corneal neovascularization in this model. The literature contains no clinical reports of PDT for corneal neovascularization.

IRIS NEOVASCULARIZATION

PDT has been efficacious in the treatment of iris neovascularization in experimental models in the primate eye. Iris neovascularization was created by laser occlusion of the branch retinal veins. PDT using HPD (3 mg/kg) and light at 675 nm caused iris neovascular occlusion at 24 hours after treatment but was accompanied by anterior chamber inflammation and recurrence of neovascularization.[53] Miller and coworkers used CASPc (0.5 to 1 mg/kg) and light at 675 nm to treat rubeosis iridis in this model.[54] They found thrombotic occlusion at 1 hour after treatment and a transient rise of intraocular pressure, but they noted minimal anterior chamber reaction. New vessels recurred on the iris surface after 7 days of follow-up. Recent work using liposomal BPD[55] (0.75 mg/kg) and light at 689 nm (150 J/cm^2) has demonstrated effective occlusion of experimental iris neovascularization at 24 hours after PDT, with no significant intraocular inflammation or rise of intraocular pressure. Iris neovascularization recurred at 7 to 9 days of follow-up. This may be new neovascularization due to continued ishemic stimulus from the laser vein occlusion for creation of the model or due to recanalization of the treated neovascularization. The currently established treatment of rubeosis iridis and neovascular glaucoma is retinal ablation by panretinal photocoagulation. Normally, this treatment requires 4 to 6 weeks to take effect, during which time angle closure and glaucomatous damage may continue. The findings from the experimental work on iris neovascularization demonstrate that PDT leads to effective acute vascular occlusion and may offer an adjunctive therapy to panretinal photocoagulation for rubeosis iridis and neovascular glaucoma.

CHOROIDAL NEOVASCULARIZATION

PDT is a potentially selective treatment modality for neovascularization. It may offer a treatment for CNV when the neovascularization can be occluded and the overlying neurosensory retina is spared. This may prevent the sudden decrease of vision that complicates thermal photocoagulation of subfoveal CNV. Several investigators have studied the efficacy of various photosensitizers for PDT of experimental CNV. Experimental CNV was created in a monkey model by inducing argon laser injury to the macula, which led to development of CNV in 2 to 4 weeks[56] (Fig. 52–5*A–C*).

In 1987, Thomas and Langhofer used DHE and achieved successful thrombosis of experimental CNV without occlusion of the choriocapillaris in the monkey model.[57] The treatment parameters included 8 mg/kg of DHE given intravenously with irradiation performed 12 hours after dye injection. The light source used was argon green laser, with a single spot size of 200 μm at a fluence of 1.6 J/cm^2 and a power of 100 mW delivered over 0.1 second. The light parameters used imply a thermal component to injury rather than a photochemical one, because the irradiance was 318 W/cm^2. Also, as mentioned earlier, hematoporphyrins have negative attributes of chemical variability and prolonged skin photosensitivity lasting a month or longer.

Kliman and associates studied PDT of experimental CNV using CASPc.[58] A dye dose of 0.5 mg/kg was injected intravenously, followed by light irradiation at 675 nm generated from an argon pumped dye laser. Effective CNV occlusion occurred acutely when irradiation was performed 5 to 30 minutes after dye injection at powers of 5 to 10 mW for 15 seconds to 5 minutes using a spot size of 1500 μm. These parameters correspond to an irradiance of 282 to 565 mW/cm^2 and a fluence of 4.24 to 170 J/cm^2. These preliminary studies suggest that closure of experimental CNV can be accomplished over a wide range of treatment parameters, but the selectivity of effect and the damage to retinal structures were not investigated. The drawback of this photosensitizer is that its safety for human use has not been studied.

Miller and Miller studied the efficacy of rose bengal, a xanthene derivative, to treat experimental CNV.[59] The illumination source used was a CSO SL-300 slit lamp fitted with filters to deliver light at 510 to 750 nm. Rose bengal was used at a dose of 40 mg/kg; irradiation was 20 to 70 minutes after dye injection using 12.7 mW/cm^2. PDT with rose bengal led to disruption of CNV but did not destroy the new vessels completely, and the required dye dose was 27 times higher than the dose that has been demonstrated to be safe clinically.

Preliminary work has been carried out with tin-etiopurpurins.[60] The treatment parameters include a dye dose of 1 mg/kg with light at 665 nm, irradiance of 600 mW/cm^2, and fluence of 35 to 70 J/cm^2. A spot size of 1200 μm was used, and light exposure lasted 60 to 120 seconds. This treatment is effective in closure of experimental CNV. Again, selectivity and effects on normal retinal structures were not studied.

Newer photosensitizers have been used to occlude normal choroidal vasculature; the potential use of these dyes to treat CNV has been extrapolated. Mori and coworkers have demonstrated effective and selective occlusion of choroidal vessels in Japanese monkey eyes using 2 to 10 mg/kg of mono-l-aspertyl chlorin e6 (NP e6) and light at 664 nm (0.4 to 7.5 J/cm^2).[61] Obana and colleagues performed PDT in pigmented rabbits and Long Evan's rats retina and choroid using ATX-S10, a new chlorin derivative (2 to 12 mg/kg) and light at 672 nm (3.5 J/cm^2).[62] Histopathology of these eyes demonstrated photothrombosis of choriocapillaris and choroidal vessels with no obvious damage to the neurosensory retina.

Our laboratory has used a tetrapyrrole derivative monoacid (BPD). This photosensitizer has a long absorption wavelength at 690 nm,[63] thus allowing deeper tissue penetration for effective treatment through blood, fluid, and fibrosis, which is important in the treatment of CNV. When injected intravenously, BPD has a serum half-life of 30 minutes. The highest tissue levels are reached in 3 hours, declining rapidly and cleared in the first 24 hours, thus reducing the risk of the systemic photosensitivity.[64] BPD is safe for human use and was first studied in clinical trials in dermatology for malignant skin tumors.[65]

Initial studies in experimental CNV used a lipoprotein-associated preparation of BPD at doses of 1 to 2 mg/kg and

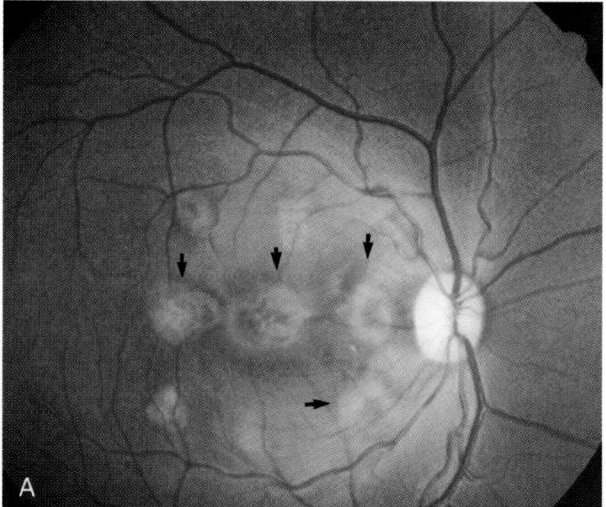

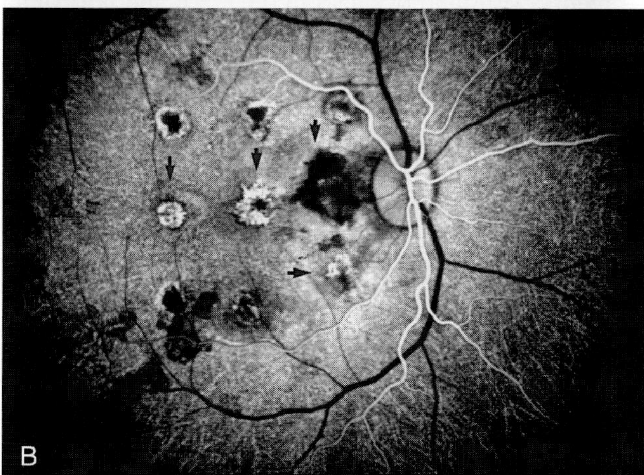

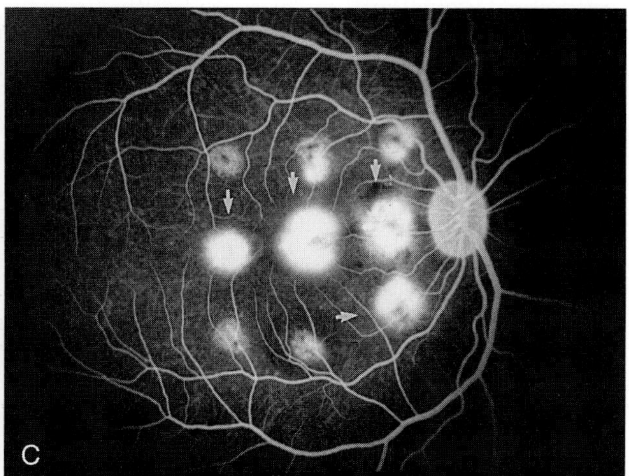

FIGURE 52–5. *A,* Fundus photograph showing elevated yellow-gray areas *(arrows)* of choroidal neovascularization in the experimental model of choroidal neovascularization in the monkey eye. *B,* Early phase fluorescein angiogram of the eye in *A* showing the typical lacy pattern of hyperfluorescence in areas of experimental CNV *(arrows). C,* Late-phase angiogram of the eye in *B* showing increasing hyperfluorescence and fluorescein leakage by the CNV *(arrows).* (*A–C,* From Husain D, Miller JW, Michaud N, et al: Intravenous infusion of liposomal benzoporhyrin derivative verteporfin for photodynamic therapy of experimental choroidal neovascularization. Arch Ophthalmol 114[8]:978–985, 1996.)

light at 692 nm generated from an argon/dye laser that was delivered via a slit-lamp delivery system with a spot size of 1250 μm. Effective vascular occlusion occurred when irradiation was performed 1 to 80 minutes after the dye injection, with a fluence of 50 to 150 J/cm^2 and irradiance of 150 to 600 mW/cm^2.[66] No thermal damage occurred at irradiances as high as 1800 mW/cm^2.[67]

The liposomal preparation of BPD was used to further refine dosimetry.[68] The liposomal preparation is not a delivery system, but it provides a safe method for solubilizing BPD for intravenous administration. The mechanism of photosensitizer uptake by the neovascular tissue is not known, but it has been observed that neovascular and neoplastic tissue increase lipoprotein receptors, which may enhance preferential uptake of the photosensitizer.[69] BPD fundus angiography has also demonstrated that liposomal BPD accumulates in CNV.[70]

The effect of PDT using liposomal BPD was recorded by fundus photography and fluorescein angiography and was confirmed by histopathology.[68] Dye doses of 0.25 to 1 mg/kg of liposomal BPD were studied; a minimal dose of 0.375 mg/kg caused effective closure of CNV. Irradiation was performed 5 to 120 minutes after the dye injection, but irradiation at 5 minutes after dye injection caused occlusion of choroidal vessels in the normal eye, whereas irradiation after 50 minutes caused occlusion in only 41% of the CNV. The optimal time for irradiation appeared to be 20 to 50 minutes after a bolus intravenous injection of dye with a spot size of 1250 μm at an irradiance of 600 mW/cm^2 and a fluence of 150 J/cm^2.[68]

Because damage to normal retina and choroidal structures was difficult to assess in experimental CNV models, the selectivity of PDT was assessed in normal retina and choroid using the same parameters as for CNV.[68] Fluorescein angiography demonstrated early hypofluorescence in the treated areas, followed by hyperfluorescence starting at the periphery of the lesion in the later frames of the angiogram. A grading system for assessing damage to retina and choroid was devised. Damage to retinal pigment epithelium and choriocapillaris occurred in all irradiated eyes; the grading scheme was based on the damage to the neurosensory retina and medium to large choroidal vessels. Grade I damage denotes occasional pyknosis in the outer nuclear layer (ONL), grade II denotes less than 20% pyknosis in the ONL, grade III denotes less than 50% pyknosis in the ONL, grade IV denotes greater than 50% pyknosis in the ONL, and grade V denotes greater than 50% damage in the ONL, damage to the larger choroidal or any retinal vessel, or both. Some damage to the photoreceptors occurred throughout all grades, typically mild vacuolization and disorientation of the inner and outer segments of the photoreceptors. PDT with 1 mg/kg liposomal BPD led to grade V damage to the retina and choroid. When PDT was performed with liposomal BPD doses of 0.25, 0.375, or 0.5 mg/kg, at 20 to 50 minutes after dye injection, the retinal structure was well preserved and PDT was sufficiently selective.

Dosimetry experiments were performed using a bolus intravenous injection of liposomal BPD-MA, but liposomal drugs are typically used clinically as an intravenous infusion, and clinical trials in dermatology using liposomal BPD reported successful administration of the dye by infusion. Further studies were designed to evaluate the efficacy and parameters for PDT of experimental CNV using an intravenous infusion of liposomal BPD.[71] A slow infusion of BPD (over 45 minutes) showed effective closure when PDT was performed within 30 to 45 minutes of the start of dye infusion. These results are similar to those found with the bolus dye delivery, but the time window for irradiation from the end of dye infusion is smaller. Therefore, a faster infusion was tested (10 minutes), and closure was effective when irradiation was performed 20 to 30 minutes from the start of infusion using light at 689 nm with a spot size of 1250 to 3000 μm at 600 mW/cm² and 150 J/cm². Fluorescein angiography (Fig. 52–6*A–C*) showed closure of experimental CNV, which was confirmed by histopathology. Light microscopy showed occluded vessels in the area of CNV and closure of the underlying choriocapillaris; the overlying retina was essentially normal. Electron microscopy of the vessels in the CNV showed occlusion of the lumen with red blood cells, white blood cells, and platelets; damaged endothelial cells showed swelling and vacuolation of the cytoplasm with breaks in the nuclear membrane.[71]

Light irradiation of normal monkey retina and choroid with the same parameters was used to study the selectivity of PDT using liposomal BPD. Fundus photography taken at 24 hours after PDT demonstrated mild graying of the retina at the treated areas (Fig. 52–7*A*). Fluorescein angiography of these areas showed early hypofluorescence (see Fig. 52–7*B*) with late staining starting from the edges of the lesion (see Fig. 52–7*C*). Light and electron microscopy of the lesions showed occlusion of the choriocapillaris and damage to the retinal pigment epithelium in all cases. Most eyes showed preservation of the medium and larger choroidal vessels and some disarray and vacuolation of the outer segments, with mild pyknosis in the ONL and normal inner retina.

The long-term effect of BPD on treated CNV has been studied.[72] Monkey eyes were followed up for 4 weeks after PDT. Persistent closure of CNV occurred in most eyes that had been treated with optimal parameters, with histopathology showing a fibrous scar enclosed by proliferating retinal pigment epithelium cells with few open capillaries. In nor-

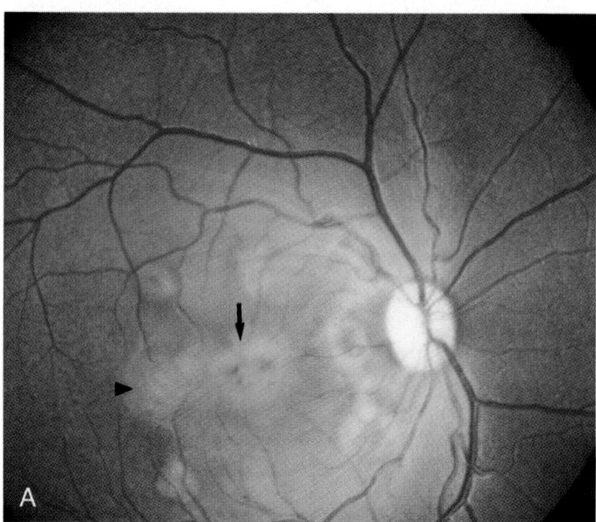

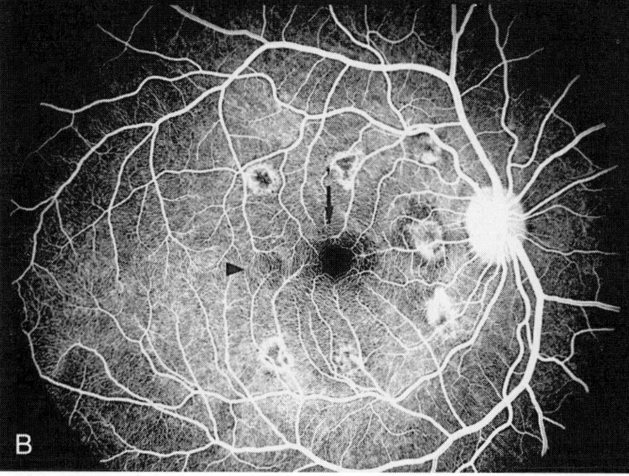

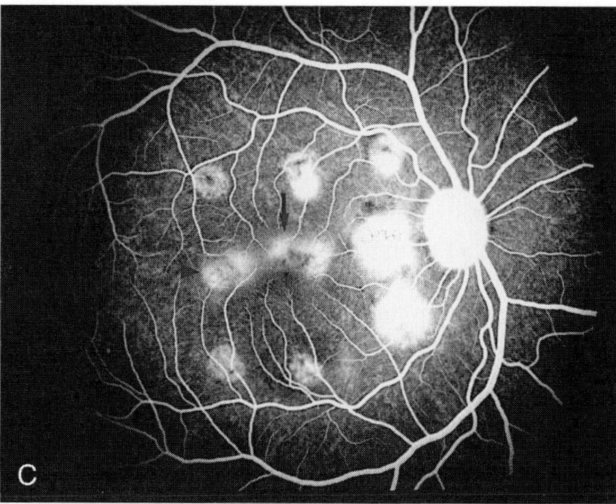

FIGURE 52–6. *A,* Fundus photograph 24 hours after photodynamic therapy with irradiation performed at the end of slow dye infusion to the foveal choroidal neovascularization *(arrow)* and at the end of flush infusion to the choroidal neovascularization temporal to the fovea *(arrowhead),* showing mild graying of the two treated areas. *B,* Early-phase fluorescein angiogram 24 hours after PDT using liposomal benzoporphyrin derivative at the end of slow dye infusion *(arrow)* and at the end of flush *(arrowhead),* illustrates hypofluorescence (occlusion of CNV) in both areas with perfusion of the overlying normal retinal capillaries confirming occlusion of CNV. *C,* Late-phase angiogram of eye in Figure 52–4, showing staining at the edge of the irradiated area. This most likely represents leakage from perfused choriocapillaris through damaged RPE. (*A–C,* From Husain D, Miller JW, Michaud N, et al: Intravenous infusion of liposomal benzoporphyrin derivative verteporfin for photodynamic therapy of experimental choroidal neovascularization. Arch Ophthalmol 114[8]:978–985, 1996.)

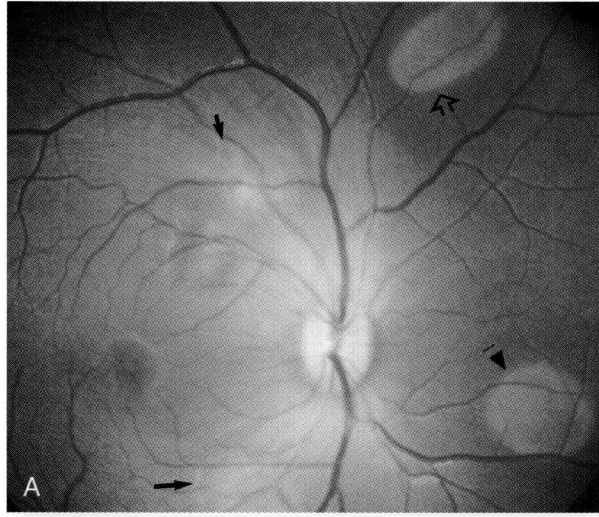

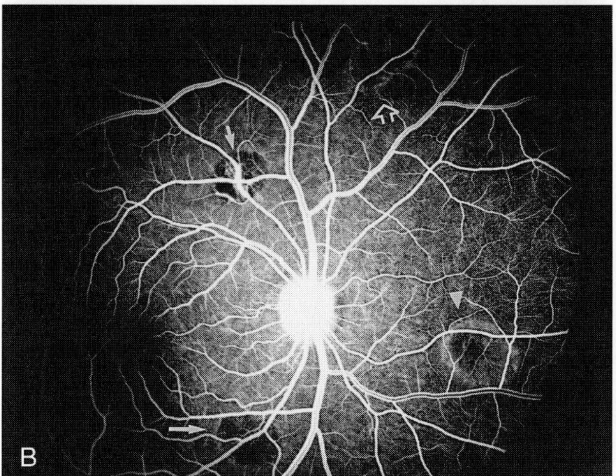

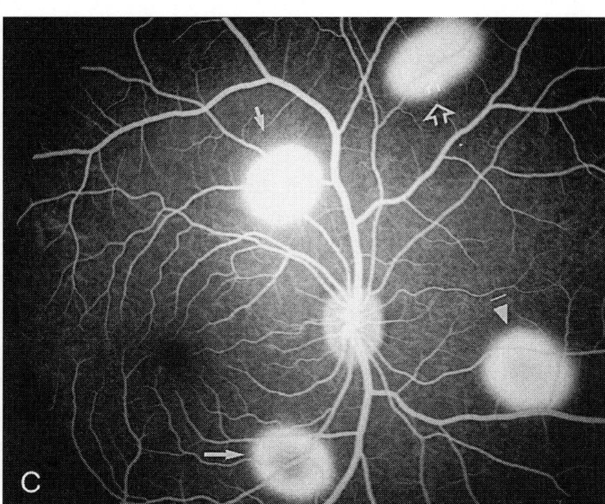

FIGURE 52–7. *A,* Fundus photograph 24 hours after photodynamic therapy of a normal retina and choroid, showing mild graying of the areas irradiated at the end of dye infusion *(small arrow),* at the end of a flush *(long arrow),* 10 minutes after the end of a flush infusion *(hollow arrow),* and 20 minutes after the end of a flush *(arrowhead). B,* Early-phase fluorescein angiogram of the eye in *A,* taken 24 hours after photodynamic therapy of the normal retina and choroid, showing hypofluorescence of the irradiated areas. *C,* Late-phase angiogram of the eye in *B,* showing staining of the irradiated area starting from the periphery of the lesion. This staining is most likely occurring as described in Figure 52–5. (*A–C,* From Husain D, Miller JW, Michaud N, et al: Intravenous infusion of liposomal benzoporphyrin derivative verteporfin for photodynamic therapy of experimental choroidal neovascularization. Arch Ophthalmol 114[8]:978–985, 1996.)

mal eyes treated with CNV, the choriocapillaris was reperfused at 4 weeks. The retinal pigment epithelium showed irregular pigmentation with liposomes, phagosomes, and melanosomes, indicating some recovery of function. A layer of pigmented macrophages was seen over the RPE. The photoreceptors were mildly disorganized. The rest of the neurosensory retina appeared to be normal. Thus, the damage to normal retina and retinal pigment epithelium caused by PDT at 24 hours showed histologic recovery at 4 weeks.

Long-term recurrence or persistence of CNV after PDT may necessitate repeat treatments, so the effect of repeat treatments on normal monkey retina and choroid was evaluated.[73] Three consecutive treatments were placed in the monkey eye, using different doses of liposomal BPD doses (6, 12, and 18 mg/m^2) but constant light dose (689 nm; 600 mW/cm^2; 100 J/cm^2). Treatments were separated by 2 weeks, with histopathologic examination at 2 and 6 weeks after the third treatment. Damage to the retina, choroid, and optic nerve was minimal in animals treated at 6 mg/m^2. Higher dye doses led to significant cumulative damage to the normal retina, choroid, and optic nerve.

The studies of PDT using liposomal BPD in monkeys suggested that selective closure of CNV could be achieved. A clinical trial of PDT for CNV was sponsored by QLT Phototherapeutics and CIBA Vision Ophthalmics. Eligibility criteria for the study included subfoveal choroidal neovascularization with a classic component secondary to age-related macular degeneration (AMD) or other etiologies. CNV lesions had to be less than or equal to 9 macular photocoagulation study (MPS) disc areas, and refracted vision (by protocol) had to be 20/40 or worse. Patients were treated under a clinical protocol with IRB approval. The treatment protocol included intravenous administration of liposomal BPD followed by timed irradiation using light at 689 nm from a Coherent Ocular Photoactivation Diode and laser delivery system. Regimens of dye dose, light dose, and timing of irradiation varied. Follow-up was carried out for 3 months with refracted visual acuity, ophthalmic examination, fundus photography, and angiography.

A dose escalation protocol reported on 61 patients.[74, 75] Dye doses were 6 or 12 mg/m^2 of liposomal BPD with light at 689 nm with a fluence of 50 to 150 J/cm^2 and an irradiance of 600 mW/cm^2. Most cases demonstrated absence of leakage from classic CNV in the early phase of the angiogram at 1 week of follow-up, suggesting occlusion of the classic CNV. At 4 weeks after treatment, most patients showed reperfusion of a portion of CNV. At 12 weeks of follow-up, some cases had recurred, defined as extension of the CNV beyond the original borders. Adverse ocular side effects were noted only at the highest light doses with a significant loss of vision in three patients. Side effects attributed to PDT included retinal arteriolar, venular, and capillary occlusion. Side effects that could be attributed to the disease process itself or to PDT included vitreous hemorrhage.

A phase III clinical trial was initiated in December 1996, as a randomized, placebo-controlled, double-masked, multicenter study designed to determine the effect of PDT on vision in patients with subfoveal CNV secondary to AMD. Eligibility criteria include subfoveal new or recurrent CNV secondary to AMD with a classic component. Patients undergo retreatment with PDT if angiographic leakage is apparent on follow-up. The study is being carried out at approximately 19 centers in North America and Europe.

PDT using liposomal BPD has shown early angiographic occlusion of CNV in patients; nonselective side effects occur only at higher light doses. In the experimental models, PDT has also been efficacious in the treatment of iris and corneal neovascularization, and it offers an adjunctive therapy to the existing modalities for these conditions. Clinical reports have shown that PDT's effect on ocular tumors varies. PDT of the experimental tumors, both melanoma and retinoblastoma, has been promising, and PDT of small tumors may be a useful treatment that might preserve vision. Further research is required to determine the suitable photosensitizer and the optimal treatment parameters for the ocular applications of PDT. New photosensitizers that may have improved characteristics for PDT of ocular structures continue to be developed. Future strategies may address improved selectivity by complexing photosensitizers to agents that target tumors and neovasculature. Finally, PDT may be used in a multifaceted approach, perhaps combining photodynamic, antiangiogenic, and immunogenic modalities.

REFERENCES

1. Raab O: Ueber die Wirkung Fluorescierenden Stoffe Auf Infusorien. Z Biol 39:524–546, 1900.
2. Von Tappeiner H, Jodlbauer A: Ueber wirking der photodynamischen (fluorescierenden) Stoffe auf Protozoan und Enzyme. Dtsch Arch Klin Med 80:427–487, 1904.
3. Meyer-Betz F: Untersuchungen uber die Biologische (photodynamische) Wirkung des hamatoporphyrins und anderer Derivative des Blut-und-Gallenfarb-stoffs. Dtsch Arch Klin Med 112:476–503, 1913.
4. Policard A: Etude sur les aspects offerts par des tumeurs experimentales examinees a la lumiere de Wood. C R Soc Biol 91:1423–1428, 1924.
5. Aueler H, Banzer G: Untersuchungen uber die rolle der Porphyrine bei geschwulstkranken Menschen und Tieren. Z Krebsforsch 53:65–68, 1942.
6. Lipson RL, Baldes EJ, Olsen EM: Hematoporphyrin derivative for detection and management of cancer. Proceedings of the IXth International Cancer Congress, 1966, p 393.
7. Diamond I, Granelli SG, McDonough AF, et al: Photodynamic therapy of malignant tumors. Lancet 2:1175, 1972.
8. Dougherty TJ, Grindley GB, Fiel R, et al: Photoradiation therapy II. Cure of animal tumors with hematoporphyrin and light. J Natl Cancer Inst 55:115–121, 1975.
9. Dougherty TJ, Kaufman JE, Goldfarb A, et al: Photoradiation therapy for the treatment of malignant tumours. Cancer Res 38:2628–2635, 1978.
10. Lui H, Anderson RR: Photodynamic therapy in dermatology: Recent developments. Dermatol Clin 31:1–13, 1993.
11. Kato H, Horai T, Fruruse K, et al: Photodynamic therapy of cancers: A clinical trial of porfimer sodium in Japan. Jpn J Cancer Res 84:1209–1214, 1993.
12. Levy JG: Photosensitizers in photodynamic therapy. Semin Oncol 21(6 Suppl 15):4–10, 1994.
13. Richter AM, Chowdhary R, Ratkay L, et al: Non-oncologic potentials for the photodynamic therapy. Proc Soc Photo-Optical Instr Eng 2078:293–304, 1994.
14. Hasan T, Parish JA: Photodynamic therapy of cancer. *In* Holland JF, Frei E, et al (eds): Cancer Medicine, 4th ed, vol I. Baltimore, Williams & Wilkins, 1996, pp 739–751.
15. Foote CS: Photosensitized autooxidation and singlet oxygen: Consequences in biological systems. *In* Proyer WA (ed): Free Radicals in Biology, vol 2. New York, Academic, 1976, p 85.
16. Henderson BW: Probing the effects of photodynamic therapy through in vivo-in vitro methods. *In* Kessel D (ed): Photodynamic Therapy of Neoplastic Disease, vol I. Boca Raton, FL, CRC, 1990, pp 169–188.
17. Fisher AMR, Murphree AL, Gomer CJ: Clinical and preclinical photodynamic therapy. Lasers Surg Med 17:2–31, 1995.
18. Henderson BW, Dougherty TJ: How does photodynamic therapy work? Photochem Photobiol 55:931–948, 1992.
19. Jori G: Low density lipoproteins-liposome delivery system for tumor photosensitizers in vivo. *In* Handerson BW, Dougherty TJ (eds): Photodynamic Therapy, Basic Principles and Clinical Applications. New York, BC Dekker, 1992, pp 173–186.
20. Kessel D: Porphyrin-lipoprotein association as a factor in porphyrin localization. Cancer Lett 33:183–188, 1986.
21. Jiang FN, Allison B, Lui D, et al: Enhanced photodynamic killing of target cells by either monoclonal antibody or low density lipoprotein mediated delivery systems. J Controlled Release 19:41–58, 1992.
22. Agarwal ML, Larkin HE, Zaidi SIA, et al: Phospholipase activation triggers apoptosis in photosensititzed mouse lymphoma cells. Cancer Res 53:5897–5902, 1993.
23. Fingar VH, Weiman TJ: Studies on the mechanism of photodynamic therapy induced tumor destruction. Proceedings of the SPIC Conference, "Photodynamic Therapy Mechanisms II." 1990, pp 168–177.
24. Nseyo UO, Whalen RK, Duncan MR, et al: Urinary cytokines following photodynamic therapy for bladder cancer: Preliminary report. Urology 36:167–171, 1990.
25. Steele JK, Lui D, Stammers AT, et al: Suppressor deletion therapy: Selective elimination of T-suppressor cells in vivo using Hp conjugate to a monoclonal antibody permits animal to reject synergic tumor cells. Cancer Immunol Immunother 26:125–131, 1988.
26. Gomer CJ, Ferrario A, Hayashi N, et al: Molecular and tissue response following photodynamic therapy. Lasers Surg Med 8:450–463, 1988.
27. Evans S, Matthews W, Perry R, et al: Effect of photodynamic therapy on tumor necrosis factor production by murine macrophages. J Natl Cancer Inst 82:34–39, 1990.
28. Svaasand LO, Ellingson R: Optical properties of human brain. Photochem Photobiol 38:283–299, 1983.
29. Dougherty TJ, Potter WR, Weishaupt KR: The structure of active component of hematoporphyrin derivative. *In* Doirin DR, Gomer CJ (eds): Porphyrin Localization and Treatment of Tumors. New York, Alan R. Liss, 1984, pp 304–314.
30. Richter AM, Waterfield E, Jain AK, et al: In vitro and phototoxic properties of four structurally related benzoporphyrin derivatives. Photochem Photobiol 52:495–500, 1990.
31. Richter AM, Jain AK, Canaan AJ, et al: Photosensitizing efficiency of two regioisomers of the benzoporphyrin derivative monoacid ring A. Biochem Pharmacol 43:2349–2358, 1992.
32. Winther J: Photodynamic therapy effect in an intraocular retinoblastoma-like tumor assessed by an in vivo to in vitro colony forming assay. Br J Cancer 59(6):869–872, 1989.
33. Winther J, Ehlers N: Histopathological changes in an intraocular retinoblastoma-like tumor following photodynamic therapy. Acta Ophthalmol 66(1):69–78, 1988.
34. Winther J: Porphyrin photodynamic therapy in an experimental retinoblastoma model. Ophthalmic Paediatr Genet 8(1):49–52, 1987.
35. Ohnishi Y, Yamana Y, Minei M: Photoradiation therapy using argon laser and a hematoporphyrin derivative for retinoblastoma: A preliminary report. Jpn J Ophthalmol 30:409–419, 1986.
36. Murphee AL: Retinoblastoma. *In* Ryan SJ, Ogden TE (eds): Retina, vol 1. St. Louis, CV Mosby, 1989.
37. Lui LHS, Chuo N: Hematoporphyrin phototherapy for experimental intraocular malignant melanoma. Arch Ophthalmol 101:901–903, 1983.
38. Panagopoulos JA, Svitra PP, Puliafito CA, et al: Photodynamic therapy for experimental melanoma using chloraluminum sulfonated phthalocyanine. Arch Ophthalmol 107:886–890, 1989.
39. Ozler SA, Nelson SJ, Liggett PE, et al: Photodynamic therapy of experimental subchoroidal melanoma using chloroaluminum sulfonated phthalocyanine. Arch Ophthalmol 110:555–561, 1992.

40. Schmidt U, Birngruber R, Gragoudas E, et al: Photodynamic therapy of experimental choroidal melanoma using a lipoprotein-delivered benzoporphyrin. Ophthalmology 104:89–99, 1994.
41. Gonzalez VH, Hu LK, Theodossiadis PG, et al: Photodynamic therapy of pigmented choroidal melanomas. Invest Ophthalmol Vis Sci 36(5):871–878, 1995.
42. Kim RY, Hu LK, Foster SB, et al: Photodynamic therapy of pigmented choroidal melanomas of greater than 3-mm thickness. Ophthalmology 103(12):2029–2036, 1996.
43. Young LHY, Howard MA, Hu LK, et al: Photodynamic therapy of pigmented choroidal melanoma using a liposomal preparation of benzoporphyrin derivative. Arch Ophthalmol 114:186–192, 1996.
44. Hu LK, Hasan T, Gragoudas ES, et al: Photoimmunotherapy of human uveal melanoma cells. Exp Eye Res 61:385–391, 1995.
45. Tse DT, Dutton JJ, Weingeist TA, et al: Hematoporphyrin photoradiation therapy for intraocular and orbital malignant melanoma. Arch Ophthalmol 102:833–838, 1984.
46. Bruce RA Jr: Evaluation of hematoporphyrin photoradiation therapy to treat choroidal melanoma. Lasers Surg Med 4:59–64, 1984.
47. Sery TW, Sheilds JA, Ausberger JJ, et al: Photodynamic therapy of human ocular cancer. Ophthalmic Surg 18:413–418, 1987.
48. Favilla I, Cote M, Gomer CJ, et al: Photodynamic therapy of posterior melanomas. Br J Ophthalmol 75:718–721, 1991.
49. Sery TW, Dougherty TJ: Photoradiation of rabbit ocular malignant melanoma sensitized with hematoporphyrin derivative. Curr Eye Res 45:3718–3725, 1984.
50. Schmidt-Erfurth U, Hasan T, Flotte T, et al: Photodynamic therapy of experimental, intraocular tumors with benzoporphyrin-lipoprotein. Ophthalmologe 91(3):348–356, 1994.
51. Davidorf J, Davidorf F: Treatment of iris melanoma with photodynamic therapy. Ophthalmic Surg 23:522–527, 1992.
52. Epstein RJ, Hendricks RL, Harris DM: Photodynamic therapy of corneal neovascularization. Cornea 10(5):424–432, 1991.
53. Packer AJ, Tse DT, Gu X-Q, et al: Hematoporphyrin photoradiation for iris neovascularization. Arch Ophthalmol 102:1193–1197, 1984.
54. Miller JW, Stinson WG, Gregory WA: Phthalocyanine photodynamic therapy of experimental iris neovascularization. Ophthalmology 98:1711–1719, 1991.
55. Husain D, Miller JW, Kenney AC, et al: Photodyanmic therapy and digital angiography of experimental iris neovascularization using liposomal benzoporphyrin derivative. Ophthalmology 104(8):1242–1250, 1997.
56. Ohkuma H, Ryan SJ: Experimental subretinal neovascularization in the monkey. Arch Ophthalmol 101:1102–1110, 1982.
57. Thomas EL, Langhofer M: Closure of experimental subretinal neovascular vessels with dihematoporphyrin ether augmented argon green laser photocoagulation. Photochem Photobiol 46:5881–5886, 1987.
58. Kliman, Puliafito CA, Stern D, et al: Phthalocyanine photodynamic—The new strategy for closure of choroidal neovascularization. Laser Surg Med 15(1):2–10, 1994.
59. Miller H, Miller B: Photodynamic therapy of subretinal neovascularization in the monkey eye. Arch Ophthalmol 111:855–860, 1993.
60. Baumal CR, Puliafito CA, Pieroth L, et al: Photodynamic therapy (PDT) of experimental choroidal neovascularization with tin ethyl etiopurpurin. [Abstract] Invest Ophthalmol Vis Sci 37(3):S122, 1996.
61. Mori K, Ohta M, Katagiri T, et al: Photodynamic therapy (PDT) with combination of a new sensitizer: NPe6 and a diode laser emitting at 664 nm. [Abstract] Invest Ophthalmol Vis Sci 37(3):S3177, 1996.
62. Obana A, Gohto Y, Miki T, et al: Photodynamic therapy of choroidal vessels using a newly developed chlorin derivative (ATX-S10). [Abstract] Invest Ophthalmol Vis Sci 37(3):S549, 1996.
63. Richter A, Waterfield E, Jain A, et al: Photosensitizing potency of structural analogs of benzoporphyrin derivative (BPD-MA) in a mouse model. Br J Cancer 63:87–93, 1991.
64. Richter AM, Cerruti-Sola S, Sternberg ED, et al: Biodistribution of tritiated benzoporphyrin derivative (3H-BPD-MA), a new photosensitizer, in normal and tumor-bearing mice. J Photochem Photobiol 5:231–244, 1990.
65. Lui J, Hruza L, Kollias N, et al: Photodynamic therapy of malignant skin tumors with benzoporphyrin derivative-monoacid ring A (BPD-MA): Preliminary investigations. *In* Anderson RR, et al (eds): Proceedings of Lasers in Otolaryngology, Dermatology, and Tissue Welding, January 16–18, 1993. Progress in Biomedical Optics, Proceedings of SPEI v. 1876. Los Angeles, Bellingham WA, SPEI, 147–151, 1993.
66. Miller JW, Walsh AW, Kramer M, et al: Photodynamic therapy of experimental choroidal neovascularization using lipoprotein delivered benzoporphyrin. Arch Ophthalmol 113:810–818, 1995.
67. Moulton RS, Walsh AW, Miller JW, et al: Response of retinal and choroidal vessels to photodynamic therapy using benzoporphyrin derivative. [Abstract] Invest Ophthalmol 34(3):S2294, 1993.
68. Kramer M, Miller JW, Michaud N, et al: Liposomal benzoporphyrin derivative verteporfin photodynamic therapy: Selective treatment of choroidal neovascularization in monkeys. Ophthalmology 103(3):427–438, 1996.
69. Allison BA, Pritchard PH, Levy JG: Evidence of low-density lipoprotein receptor mediated uptake of BPD. Br J Cancer 69(5):833–839, 1994.
70. Kramer M, Kenney AG, Delori F, et al: Imaging of experimental choroidal neovascularization (CNV) using liposomal benzoporphyrin derivative mono-acid (BPD-MA) angiography. [Abstract] Invest Ophthalmol Vis Sci 36(4):S236, 1995.
71. Husain D, Miller JW, Michaud N, et al: Intravenous infusion of liposomal benzoporphyrin derivative verteporfin for photodynamic therapy of experimental choroidal neovascularization. Arch Ophthalmol 114(8):978–985, 1996.
72. Husain D, Miller JW, Michaud N, et al: Long term effects of photodynamic therapy (PDT) using liposomal benzoporphyrin derivative (BPD) on experimental choroidal neovascularization (CNV) and normal retina choroid. [Abstract] Invest Ophthalmol Vis Sci 37(3):1013, 1996.
73. Reinke MH, Canakis C, Husain D, et al: Photodynamic therapy retreatment of normal retina and choroid in the primate. [Abstract] Invest Ophthalmol Vis Sci 38(4):75, 1997.
74. Schmidt-Erfurth U, Miller JW, Sickenberg M, et al: Photodynamic therapy of subfoveal choroidal neovascularization using benzoporphyrin derivative: First results of multicenter trial. [Abstract] Invest Ophthalmol Vis Sci 37(3):B492, 1996.
75. Miller JW, Schmidt-Erfurth U, Sickenberg M, et al: Selected angiographic findings following photodynamic therapy of subfoveal choroidal neovascularization using BPD. [Abstract] Invest Ophthalmol Vis Sci 37(3):1014, 1996.

CHAPTER 53

Excimer Laser Physics and Biology

Elizabeth A. Davis, Juan-Carlos Abad, and Dimitri T. Azar

Excimer laser surgery has become the most commonly performed refractive surgical procedure in many regions of the world. As with other refractive procedures, it is desired by patients for a variety of reasons. Certain jobs require better uncorrected visual acuity than may be attainable with glasses. Some patients have ocular or medical conditions that prohibit contact lens wear. In other cases, patients with anisometropia may have spectacle-related anisophoria that results in intolerable asthenopia. Still other patients opt to be free of glasses or contact lenses for reasons of convenience or cosmesis.

Although many physicians had been skeptical about performing refractive surgery on ametropic eyes that are otherwise healthy, growing experience and improved outcomes have increased the acceptance of this new field of ophthalmology. Nevertheless, we must continue to monitor the safety, reliability, predictability, reproducibility, and stability of refractive techniques through ongoing controlled multicenter trials.

OPHTHALMIC LASERS

Lasers are used extensively to treat ophthalmic disease. The application of laser surgery to the cornea for refractive purposes results from the fact that the cornea accounts for two-thirds of the optical power of the eye. Thus, variations in corneal curvature can affect the ability of the eye to focus incoming light onto the retina. Surgical alteration of the cornea has been employed for decades in various modalities using incisional techniques or lamellar procedures and, more recently, lasers to achieve the same goal. Figure 53–1 shows the various laser modalities currently available that may alter corneal tissue using photothermal, photochemical, and photodisruptive mechanisms.

Photocoagulation is routinely employed to treat macular degeneration, macular edema, and diabetic retinopathy. Both laser trabeculoplasty and laser iridotomy have been useful in glaucoma management. The development of the infrared neodymium:yttrium-aluminum-garnet (Nd:YAG) laser has permitted noninvasive treatment of posterior capsule opacities after cataract surgery as well as the lysing of vitreous bands. Each of these procedures employs laser energy to remove tissue by local heating. The high power of the laser, together with the ability to focus the radiation on a very small, precise area, results in vaporization of the water within the tissue. Despite the ability to focus the laser beam to spot sizes on the order of micrometers, diffusion of heat and deep penetration of the radiation into tissue can result in regions of thermal damage significantly larger than the size of the focal spot.[1] This effect may be desirable when photocoagulation for hemostasis is needed but counterproductive when the destruction of precise areas of tissue is required. With the development of high-powered pulsed lasers emitting in the ultraviolet (UV) region of the spectrum, the ability to remove tissue in discrete regions became possible.

PHOTOREFRACTIVE KERATECTOMY AND LASER IN SITU KERATOMILEUSIS

The excimer laser was first developed in 1975 and initially used in industry for the etching of various materials. The first description of the corneal epithelial damage induced by an excimer laser was in 1981.[2] In 1983, it was reported that controlled ablation of corneal tissue could be performed using 193-nm-wavelength UV with minimal damage to surrounding structures.[3–5]

Before the introduction of the excimer laser, interest in reshaping the corneal curvature to change its refractive power was growing in ophthalmology. Lamellar and incisional techniques using diamond blades were already being performed. However, it soon became apparent that the excimer laser was a much more precise method of incising the corneal surface.[6] Additionally, the unique characteristics of the excimer laser–cornea interaction made it possible to actually reprofile the anterior surface of the cornea.[7–10] This technique of *photorefractive keratectomy* (PRK) is now used to treat refractive errors.

Another method of altering the anterior corneal curvature is *laser in situ keratomileusis* (LASIK). It involves elevating a hinged flap of epithelium and anterior stroma with a microkeratome. The laser beam is then applied directly to the exposed stromal bed.[11–13] After laser treatment, the flap is repositioned in its bed. In most cases, sutures are not necessary because the action of the endothelial pump keeps the flap in place.

Excimer Laser

LASER BIOPHYSICS

Laser Composition and Energy

Excimers, or *excited dimers*, are molecules of two identical components in an energized state. Radiation is emitted as

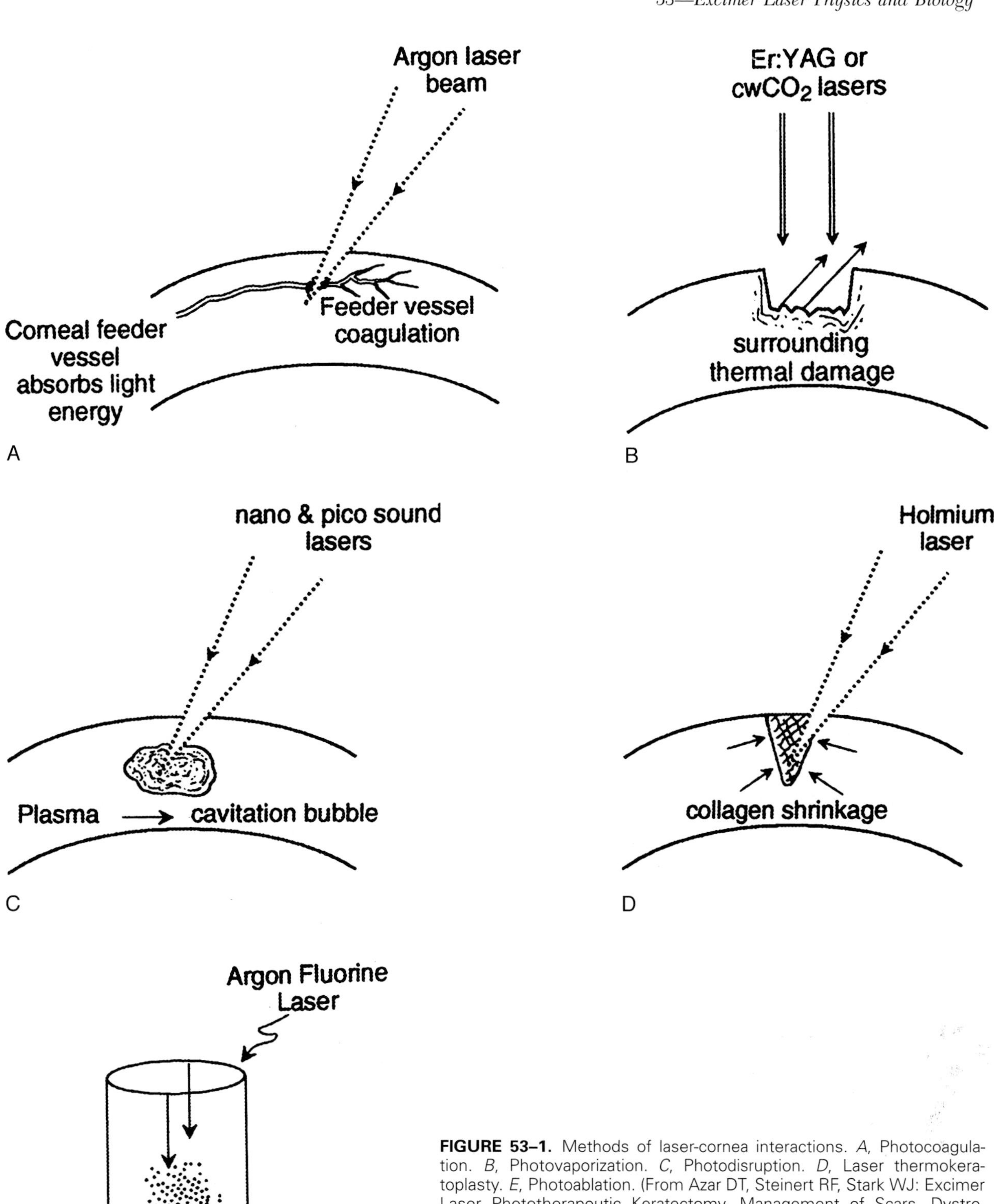

FIGURE 53–1. Methods of laser-cornea interactions. *A*, Photocoagulation. *B*, Photovaporization. *C*, Photodisruption. *D*, Laser thermokeratoplasty. *E*, Photoablation. (From Azar DT, Steinert RF, Stark WJ: Excimer Laser Phototherapeutic Keratectomy. Management of Scars, Dystrophies, and PRK Complications. Baltimore, Williams & Wilkins, 1997.)

decay occurs from the excited state to the ground state. Various combinations of a rare gas (such as argon, xenon, or krypton) and a halogen (e.g., fluorine, bromine, or chlorine) can be used as the active laser medium. Emission of UV light occurs when a high-voltage current is applied to the gas mixture after it has been ionized by a set of electrodes. The wavelength of light emitted depends on the composition of the medium (argon fluoride: 193 nm; krypton chloride: 222 nm; krypton fluoride: 248 nm; xenon chloride: 308 nm; xenon fluoride: 351 nm).

Corneal Ablation

Excimer lasers are able to break intermolecular bonds because the photons they emit have an energy that exceeds that of a typical peptide bond. When the concentration of photons or energy density of laser light exceeds a critical value, the broken bonds are unable to recombine, and the material decomposes ablatively, hence the name *ablative photodecomposition* or *photoablation*.[14–16] Molecular fragments are ejected into the atmosphere because of the rapid expansion in the volume of the decomposed tissue and the acquisition of kinetic energy from the excess energy of the photons (Fig. 53–2). Only those molecules that absorb the UV light are affected, and the surrounding tissue shows no conductive effects. Furthermore, it is thought that bond breaking minimizes heating of the tissue and thermal damage to adjacent areas.

Laser Variables

Wavelength. Krueger and colleagues[17] compared the tissue effects of the four major wavelengths produced by the excimer laser (ArF, KF, XeCl, XeF). The 193-nm wavelength of the ArF gas mixture demonstrated much smoother and more precise corneal tissue ablation compared with the other wavelengths, which were associated with greater amounts of thermal damage to adjacent tissue. As a result of these findings, ArF is the most commonly used gas mixture in clinical excimer lasers today.

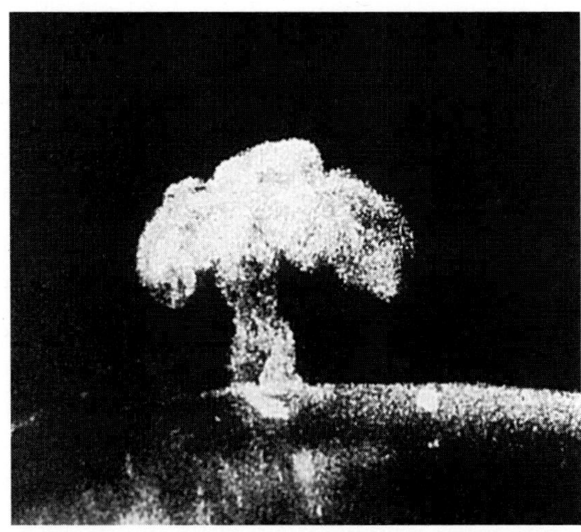

FIGURE 53–2. Photograph of ejection plume during excimer laser ablation of the cornea. (From Puliafito CA, Stern D, Kreuger RR, Mandel ER: High-speed photography of excimer laser ablation of the cornea. Arch Ophthalmol 105:1255–1259, 1987.)

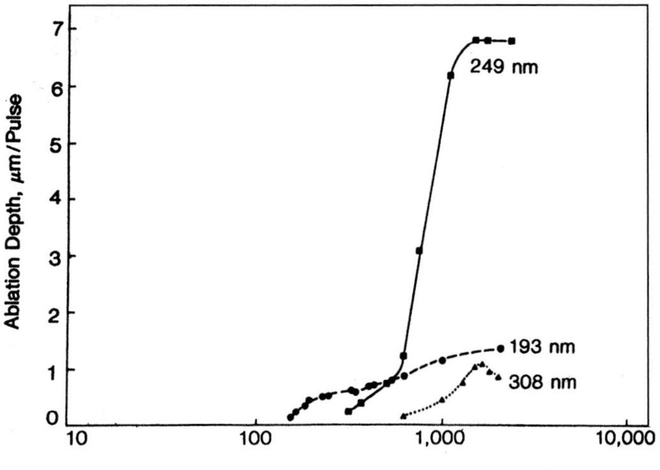

FIGURE 53–3. Corneal ablation depth as a function of pulse radiance for three wavelengths produced by the excimer laser. Note the flatness of the 193-nm curve compared with the others, allowing a more controlled ablation of the tissue. (From Krueger RR, Trokel SL, Schubert HD: Interaction of ultraviolet laser light with the cornea. Invest Ophthalmol Vis Sci 26:1455–1464, 1985 © Association for Research in Vision and Ophthalmology; Krueger RR, Trokel SL: Quantitation of corneal ablation by ultraviolet laser light. Arch Ophthalmol 103:1741–1742, 1985.)

Ablation Threshold. The *irradiance* of a laser is the quantity of laser light per unit area incident on the tissue surface measured in watts per square meter. It is thus a measure of energy density. Irradiance is a function of both the output energy of the laser and the beam diameter. In contrast, *fluence* is laser energy per unit *volume*.

There appears to be a threshold level of irradiance below which no ablation occurs and the cornea appears grossly unaffected. With low levels of irradiance, a slight surface clouding of the epithelium occurs. Progressively increasing levels of irradiance result in ablation. Krueger and colleagues[17] showed that the threshold for corneal ablation increases at lower pulse rates, except for 193-nm radiation, for which the threshold remains constant (50 mJ/cm^2), suggesting that a build-up of energy does not contribute to tissue removal. For longer UV wavelengths, the ablation threshold increases logarithmically (Fig. 53–3).

Ablation Depth (Ablation Rate). Above threshold, for a given irradiance each laser pulse removes a constant amount of tissue. Increasing irradiance results in a greater ablation depth and is a function of wavelength. The relationship between irradiance and ablation depth has a shallower slope for the 193-nm wavelength compared with other wavelengths, thus allowing a more controlled ablation of tissue.[18]

Efficiency of tissue ablation is desirable when removing corneal tissue. The minimal laser energy that achieves the necessary amount of tissue removal should be used in order to avoid unwanted heat, shock waves, or photochemical effects both locally and at distant sites from the excess unused energy. Several experimental studies on animal corneas have demonstrated different values for the most efficient ablation energy density.[18–21] Clinical studies in humans have estimated the ablation depth while compensating for the healing response. Using 160 to 180 mJ/cm^2, an ablation rate between 0.21 and 0.27 μm per pulse (VISX laser, Santa

Clara, CA) and 0.26 μm per pulse (Summit laser, Waltham, MA) was estimated when human trials began and later confirmed with Scheimpflug's photography of the cornea before and after PRK.[22] In cases of corneal scars, the ablation rate can differ significantly from that of the surrounding normal stroma. This must be taken into account when performing phototherapeutic keratectomy.

Ablation Frequency (Hertz). Most excimers ablate tissue with pulses of laser at a frequency of 5 to 10 Hz (pulses per second). Higher frequencies result in shorter procedures and a better ease of patient fixation as well as less stromal dehydration. However, if the laser frequency is faster than the thermal relaxation time of the adjacent tissues, thermal damage occurs. In experimental studies in rabbit eyes, it was determined that for an irradiance of 300 mJ/cm^2, the repetition rate should not exceed 63 Hz.[23] If the irradiance is 150 mJ/cm^2, the upper limit increases to 82 Hz. In addition, the limited rate of clearance of the plume of ablated tissue may further limit the predictability of surgical outcomes as the ablation frequency is increased.

Tissue Variables

Surface Regularity. Excimer laser application to the cornea results in a precise, smooth area of ablation. Homogeneity in the energy of the laser beam is critical for achieving such smoothness and uniformity. If there are parts of the beam of higher energy, or "hot spots," irregular ablation may result. There are several methods of beam reshaping in order to achieve beam homogeneity. These include a rotating dove prism,[8, 24] a rotating slit beam,[25] a prismatic integrator with telescopic zoom,[26] and an absorbing cell system.[27]

Stromal Hydration. Uniformity of ablation also depends on the hydration of the tissue. Once the corneal epithelium is removed, the corneal stroma can swell. Dehydration of the superficial stroma may be promoted by the light of the operating microscope. This is of importance because deeper ablations occur when the tissue is dehydrated.[28, 29]

In some of the early clinical studies a nitrogen gas blower was employed. This resulted in even tissue dehydration and predictable ablation. However, corneas treated in this manner developed increased reticular haze. Thus, the clinical use of the nitrogen gas blower was abandoned.

To minimize changes in stromal hydration, photoablation should be performed soon after the epithelium is removed. Furthermore, no additional fluid should be applied to the cornea whenever possible. In some cases, fluid may accumulate centrally, resulting in nonuniform ablation and the development of a central island. Further discussion of this topic is found later.

Surface Phenomena

Shock Waves. When the excimer laser strikes the corneal surface, a shock wave is produced that propagates in the air above the eye. The velocity of the shock wave is on the order of 1 km/sec but varies with the laser wavelength and the energy of ablation. Because the shock wave consists of an expanding high-temperature and high-pressure gas cloud, corneal tissue injury may occur. Thermal denaturation of surface collagen may result in pseudomembrane formation.[6] Stromal vacuoles and an increased number of keratocytes have also been observed in the later stages of wound healing.[7] Furthermore, a pressure of up to 100 atmospheres may be generated, resulting in mechanical stress to the cornea and structural changes beneath the ablation surface.

Gaseous and Particulate Ejection. When excimer laser energy is applied to the cornea, an ablation plume of particulate matter is ejected from the surface in a mushroom cloud at supersonic velocity (see Fig. 53–2).[30] Some particles are below optical resolution but have been shown by mass spectrometry to be primarily H_2O radicals, simple carbons, hydrocarbons, and some alkanes.[31, 32] With recoil of the ejection plume, a surface wave is produced that propagates across the corneal surface at several meters per second.[33] It is possible that the displacement of corneal tissue by the surface wave could cause structural injury, although this has not been observed histopathologically.

Surface fluid from within the cornea may be produced by both the shock wave and the surface wave. This could potentially lead to attenuation of ablation and topographic steep central islands.

Surface Heating. Excimer laser photoablation is primarily a nonthermal process. Nevertheless, as energy is released during molecular bond breakage, heat is generated. In general, the average corneal temperature increase is 20°C.[34] These temperature spikes could lead to keratocyte injury at the cellular level and impairment of wound healing. Methods of cooling the corneal surface or reducing this temperature increase might avoid these potential adverse effects.

Pseudomembrane Formation. When corneal tissue is subjected to excimer laser photoablation, light microscopic examination of the epithelial aspect of the ablated areas shows that it appears to have clean edges with no detectable cellular injury other than pale-staining cytoplasms of the cells bordering the incision. Electron microscopy has revealed that these cells have no cell membrane adjacent to the ablated area but are bordered by an electron-dense condensation.[35] This condensation has been termed a *pseudomembrane*. Pseudomembranes are not observed in some corneas. Furthermore, greater energy densities result in thicker pseudomembranes. The cause of this pseudomembrane is unknown, but it has been postulated to be due to a thermal effect or the result of the uncoupling of organic double bonds formed during photoablation.[9]

The presence of a pseudomembrane is thought to have a beneficial effect for clinical excimer laser applications. It may serve as a scaffold for wound reepithelialization, and it may provide a barrier to the passage of water, thus preventing significant corneal edema. It is likely that the role of the pseudomembrane may be insignificant in comparison with that of other biochemical mediators and peptides that have been clearly shown to affect corneal wound healing.[36–55]

Biologic Effects: Corneal Abnormality After Laser Surgery

EPITHELIAL EFFECT

The earliest cellular response to excimer laser photoablation of the cornea is reepithelialization.[36] Initially, the epithelium migrates from the wound periphery centrally to cover the defect; peripheral cells undergo mitosis and provide the cells to form an initial covering of three to five cell layers.

Subsequently, hyperplasia occurs, with the greatest amount of thickening developing in the deepest part of the ablation.[10, 37, 38] Studies have shown that surface reepithelialization begins immediately after surgery and is complete within 3 to 5 days of 6-mm diameter treatments.[39–41]

Although immunolocalization studies indicate the presence of normal epithelial adhesion structures (hemidesmosomes, anchoring fibril components),[42] recent electron microscopic studies of human specimens have shown significant delays in normalization of components of the epithelial basement membrane and anchoring fibrils.[42, 43] These abnormalities were present up to 6 months postoperatively and did not normalize until 1 year (Fig. 53–4).[42] Despite this abnormality, the incidence of recurrent epithelial erosions after laser corneal photoablation is infrequent. In fact, the excimer laser has been successfully used for treatment of recurrent epithelial erosions.[44, 45]

BOWMAN'S MEMBRANE EFFECT

Excimer laser treatment of the cornea results in the removal of Bowman's membrane, which is the acellular anterior zone of the stroma. Unlike the overlying epithelium, Bowman's layer does not regenerate. Although other mechanisms that destroy Bowman's membrane can result in scarring, photoablation does not appear to be associated with this effect.[46, 47]

STROMAL EFFECT

In the first 24 hours after photoablation, there is an influx of polymorphonuclear leukocytes into the stroma[48, 49] and an increase in tear plasmin levels that contribute to the removal and repair of collagen and extracellular matrix.[50] There is an initial decrease in the most superficial keratocytes. However, over the ensuing 2 weeks, these cells not only repopulate the area but increase in density up to three times their original number.[38, 49] New collagen and proteoglycan matrix is produced by these cells and can result in corneal haze. This haze can be seen as early as 1 week after treatment, and it peaks at 3 to 6 months.[47] Malley and coworkers[39] postulated that subepithelial haze is due to the production of disorganized layers of type III collagen and the absence of normal keratan sulfate in the subepithelial space. Haze tends to disappear by 12 to 18 months in most cases[51] and correlates with remodeling of the subepithelial zone, the disappearance of fibroblasts and type III collagen, and the emergence of a normal lamellar structure populated by keratocytes. In some cases, however, the extracellular matrix organizes into an irregularly arranged fibrous tissue that appears as a scar clinically.

The stromal changes after LASIK have been less extensively studied. There appears to be less collagen deposition after a lamellar keratectomy compared to a superficial keratectomy (excimer or mechanical).[6, 36] Additionally, one study revealed decreased metalloproteinase (a collagenase involved in wound repair) levels after LASIK compared with PRK.[52] Clinical experience supports these results as well. In human studies, the incidence of stromal haze is significantly lower after LASIK than after PRK.[53–55]

DESCEMET'S MEMBRANE EFFECT

Rabbit studies have shown an amorphous fibrogranular material in the middle and anterior part of Descemet's membrane beneath the 6-mm ablation zone,[49] but this effect has been observed in only a single human specimen.[38] The cause and clinical implications of this finding are uncertain.

ENDOTHELIAL EFFECT

The incidence of significant endothelial cell injury and loss is low after excimer laser therapy and tends to correlate with the depth and energy density of ablation.[56] Clinical studies have reported zero to 13% overall cell loss up to 1 year after PRK.[57–59] Although the excimer laser is absorbed within a few micrometers of corneal tissue, endothelial damage might occur from secondary shock waves, fluorescence, secondary irradiation, or posterior migration of toxic byproducts.[6, 49, 56, 60]

Clinical Effect of Laser Surgery

Numerous human clinical trials have been performed to determine the results of excimer laser treatment of myopia.

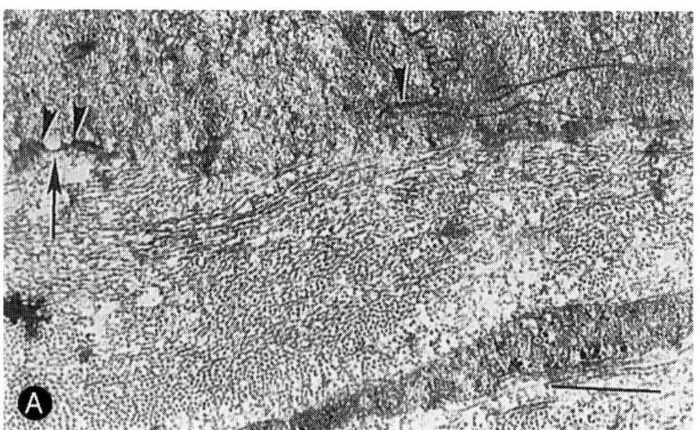

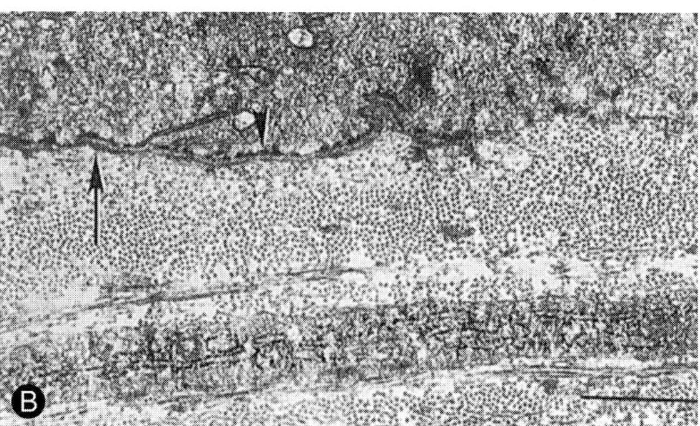

FIGURE 53–4. Basement membrane zone of a 33-year-old patient 6 months after excimer physiotherapeutic keratectomy. Bars indicate 1 micrometer. *A*, Areas of absent and discontinuous basement membrane *(arrow)* are noted. Hemidesmosomes *(arrowheads)* are present in areas that correspond to the basement membrane segments. Anchoring fibrils are absent. *B*, Electron microscopic appearance of another treated region showing greater basement membrane *(arrow)* and hemidesmosome *(arrowhead)* re-formation. Stromal keratocytes are noted in proximity to the epithelial basement membrane. (From Fountain TR, de la Cruz Z, Green WR, et al: Reassembly of corneal epithelial adhesion structures after excimer laser keratectomy in humans. Arch Ophthalmol 112:967–972, 1994.)

PRK results have been most extensively studied. Many of these studies have arbitrarily been divided into three categories: low-myopia studies (≤ 6 D; Table 53–1), high-myopia studies (>6 D; Table 53–2), and combined low- and high-myopia studies (1 to 25 D; Table 53–3). It is beyond the scope of this chapter to go into detail about each study, but several generalizations can be made from the data. For patients undergoing PRK with low myopia, uncorrected visual acuity outcomes were better and a higher percentage of patients were within 1 D of emmetropia. Patients with high myopia had a higher incidence of postoperative haze formation.

HAZE

A certain degree of haze occurs in all corneas after excimer laser treatment as a result of new collagen and proteoglycan matrix formation. Haze may be mild or intense, and it may or may not disappear. Haze is typically associated with refractive regression.

It is known that topical corticosteroids inhibit fibroblast proliferation[61] and hence new collagen formation. Indeed, experimental studies have shown that topical steroids prevent haze after photoablation[62]. However, a prospective randomized double-blind study revealed no significant difference in the development of anterior stromal haze in eyes treated with topical steroids compared with placebo controls.[63, 64] Hence, topical steroid use is not advocated after uncomplicated excimer laser treatment, particularly in view of its potential side effects. It has been found to be useful to treat haze once it occurs and to reverse the associated refractive regression.

A wide variety of nonsteroidal agents has been investigated as potential modulators of stromal healing. These include antifibrotic agents (mitomycin,[62] interferon alfa-2b,[65] pirenzepine[66]), protease inhibitors (aprotinin[50, 67]), antibodies to tissue growth factor-β and sodium hyaluronate,[68] nonsteroidal antiinflammatory agents,[69] and pentoxifylline.[70] Cooling the cornea during photoablation to reduce the production of heat-shock proteins has also been investigated.[71] Whether any of these agents or methods will be clinically useful is unknown.

OCULAR HYPERTENSION

Ocular hypertension can occur after PRK and is related to the use of topical steroids. The incidence ranged from 0.27 to 25.3% in the study by Brancato and associates.[72] The increase in pressure is usually transient and responds well to either discontinuing the steroid or treating with topical antihypertensives. However, rare cases of progressive visual field loss and optic nerve cupping have been reported.[73]

GLARE AND HALOES

Glare and haloes are visual phenomena experienced by some patients when incoming light is scattered by either corneal opacities or corneal irregularities. The symptoms are more apparent at night when the pupil enlarges and allows more light to enter the eye. The reported incidence of these symptoms ranges from 5 to 78%.[74–76]

When the cornea is clear, the visual phenomena seem to result from the spherical aberration induced in the centrally flattened cornea.[77, 78] A study by O'Brart and associates[79] examined 43 patients who underwent bilateral PRK. The first eye was treated with a 4-mm ablation zone and the second eye with a 5-mm ablation zone. Their results showed that larger ablation zones correlated with decreased halos and better night vision.

The management of halos following PRK depends on the cause. If the cause is corneal haze, reinstituting topical steroid therapy can be tried. If there is also residual myopia, re-treatment may be considered. If the initial ablation zone was small, this may be increased on re-treatment. A blended peripheral transition zone can be subsequently employed to minimize the depth of laser ablation.[79] If the eye is emmetropic or hyperopic, a trial of minus lens overcorrection or weak miotics at bedtime may be of use.[79]

DECENTRATION

Incorrect centration of the ablation zone can occur during PRK. This may result from patients moving their eyes during the procedure or inaccurate marking of the optical center of the cornea by the surgeon. Most surgeons now routinely center the optical zone of the excimer treatment around the center of the pupil rather than around the visual axis of the eye.[80, 81] Decentered ablations can result in irregular astigmatism and loss of uncorrected visual acuity or sometimes best-corrected visual acuity.[82–86]

Small decentrations are usually of no visual significance and can be left alone. Large (≥ 1 mm) decentrations, however, need addressing. If undercorrection is also present, re-treatment with a larger ablation zone that encompasses the decentered area may be attempted.[87] If not, a rigid gas-permeable contact lens may neutralize irregular astigmatism.

CENTRAL ISLANDS

Central islands are areas of corneal steepening within the ablation zone. These islands typically measure 1 to 3 mm in diameter and are 1 to 3 D in height. They may result in irregular astigmatism, monocular diplopia, haloes, and glare.[87] One of the causes of central islands is thought to be nonuniform corneal hydration. If an area of the cornea within the ablation zone is better hydrated than the surrounding areas, relatively less ablation occurs in that region. Another cause for central islands is plume generation. In the past, nitrogen blowers eliminated this problem. Scanning lasers also do not create central islands since the beam moves away from the plume as ablation occurs.

The reported incidence of central islands varies depending on the author, the laser treatment center, and the time after PRK when corneal topography is performed. In a study by Lin[88] of 502 eyes undergoing PRK using the VISX excimer laser, the incidence of central islands at 1 month was 26%. This decreased to 18% at 3 months, 8% at 6 months, and 2% at 12 months, possibly as the result of corneal remodeling.

VISX has subsequently revised its algorithm with new software that applies additional laser pulses to the central 2.5 mm to minimize the problem of central islands.

ASTIGMATISM

Both regular and irregular astigmatism can occur after PRK. Irregular astigmatism may result from nonuniform epithelial

Text continued on page 598

TABLE 53–1. **Low-Myopia Studies**

Author/Laser/Year	Low Myopes (No. of Eyes in Main Study)	Mean Follow-Up (Mo)	Attempted Correction (D)	Single or Multi-Zone (mm)	OZ (mm)	UCVA 20/40 (%)	UCVA 20/20 (%)
McDonald (USA)/ VISX/1991	7 (18)	12	−2.25 to −5.00	Single	5.00	86	
Gartry (UK)/ Summit/1992	120 (120)	18	−2.00 to −7.00	Single	4.00	See below	See below
	20		−2.00			90	55
	20		−3.00			78	56
	20		−4.00			59	47
	20		−5.00			63	50
	20		−6.00			63	25
Brancato (Italy)/ Summit/1993	146 (330)	12	−0.8 to −6.00	Single	3.50–5.00	Mean UCVA 20/32 at 12 mo	Mean UCVA 20/32 at 12 mo
Kim (Korea)/ Summit/1993	135 (202) Preop Myopia: −2.00 to −7.00 D (group 1)	12	−2.00 to −6.00	Single	5.00	98.5	
	67 (202) Preop myopia: −7.25 to −13.50 D (group 2)	12	−6.00	Single	5.00	62.7	
Maguen (USA)/ VISX/1994	122 (122)	12	−1.00 to −6.00	Single	? 6.00	89	37
	48 (48)	24				92	48
	9 (9)	36				90	80
Hamberg-Nystrom (Sweden)/ Summit/1994	20 (20)	12	−2.00 to −5.00	Single	5.00	100	80
Hamberg-Nystrom (Sweden)/VISX/ 1994	20 (20)	12	−2.00 to −5.00	Single	5.00	85	35
O'Brart (UK)/ Summit/1994	33 (33) first eyes	24	−2.00 to −6.00	Single	4.00	Not studied	Not studied
	33 (33) second eyes	12	−2.00 to −6.00	Single	5.00	Not studied	Not studied

±1 D (%)	Corneal Haze	Topical Steroids	Increased IOP (%)	Loss BCVA 2 Lines (%)	Loss BCVA >2 Lines (%)	Remarks or Comments
57	0% > grade 1 + haze	Yes	0	0	0	
See below 95 70 40 50 40	Maximal	Yes	12 (overall study)	3	0	Halo effect in 78%, major halo problem in 10%. Significant decentration in 1% due to patient movement. In −2 to −5 D groups, refraction stable after 3 mo. In −7 D group, 2 D of regression from 3 to 6 mo.
71.2	Haze level proportional to attempted correction	Yes	25.3	2.4	0	9.4% had late epithelial healing (>4 days); 10.6% had decentration of ablation zone >1 mm. Overall, glare or halos seen in 10%. Myopic regression seen in 4% of overall study group.
91.4	0% with grade 2 haze or worse	Yes	14.1	8.1 (2 lines or more)		
51.7	3% with grade 2 haze or worse	Yes	23.9	17.9 (2 lines or more)		Same as above.
79 (12 mo) 86 (24 mo) 90 (36 mo)	Haze maximal from 1–6 mo; most common grading 1.5	Yes	10.8 (at any time)	4 (12 mo)	0 (12 mo)	One-third of eyes received N_2 flow and two-thirds did not. 5% of all eyes developed central islands; all such eyes did not receive N_2 flow. In 1.25% of eyes, islands persisted beyond 6 mo. Two eyes developed myopic regression, and 1 eye was retreated.
Not studied	Not studied	Yes	Maximum 18 mm Hg	Not studied	Not studied	Median spherical equivalent at 12 mo was 0.00 D. This result was statistically different from that of VISX laser (−0.5 D). No statistical difference in IOPs, contrast sensitivity, or centration.
Not studied	Not studied	Yes	Maximum 21 mm Hg	Not studied	Not studied	Median spherical equivalent at 12 mo was −0.50 D. Difference from that of Summit laser (0.00 D) statistically significant.
0 > +1.00 D	Maximal at 3 mo	Yes (19 eyes) No (14 eyes)	Not reported	0	0	Magnitude of halos, as measured with a computer program, statistically less in eyes treated with 5.00-mm ablation zone. Mean postoperative refractive change significantly greater for 5-mm ablation zone ($P < .01$). No significant difference between two groups in terms of anterior stromal haze.
15 > +1.00 D	Maximal at 3 mo	Yes (19 eyes) No (14 eyes)	Not reported	0	0	

From Chan TK, Ashraf MF, Azar DT: Photorefractive keratectomy (PRK) outcomes and complications. *In* Azar DT, Steinert RF, Stark WJ (eds): Excimer Laser Phototherapeutic Keratectomy. Baltimore, Williams & Wilkins, 1997, pp 160–161.

Abbreviations: OZ, optical zone; UCVA, uncorrected visual acuity; IOP, intraocular pressure; BCVA, best corrected visual acuity.

TABLE 53–2. **High-Myopia Studies**

Author/Laser/ Year	Low Myopes (No. of Eyes in Main Study)	Mean Follow-Up (Mo)	Attempted Correction (D)	Single or Multi-Zone (mm)	OZ (mm)	UCVA 20/40 (%)	UCVA 20/20 (%)
McDonald (USA)/ VISX/1991	11 (18)	12	−5.01 to −8.00	Single	5.00 (≤6 D) 4.50 (−6.01 to −7.00) 4.25 (−7.01 to −8.00)	18	
Brancato (Italy)/ Summit/1993	145 (330)	12	−6.10 to −9.90	Single	3.50–5.00	Mean UCVA 20/63 at 12 mo	Mean UCVA 20/63 at 12 mo
	39 (330)	12	−10.00 to −25.00	Double	First zone 3.50–4.80 Second zone 3.80–5.00	Mean UCVA 20/63 at 12 mo	Mean UCVA 20/63 at 12 mo
Heitzman (USA)/ VISX/1993	23 (23)	7.5	−8.00 to −19.50	Multi	4.00, 5.00, 6.00	52	
Buratto (Italy)/ Summit/1993	40 (40)	24	−6.00 to −10.00	Single	4.30 or 4.50	Not reported	Not reported
Sher (USA)/VISX/ 1994	47 (47)	6–12	−8.00 to −15.25 (mean −11.2)	Single	5.50–6.20	60	Not reported
Talamo (USA)/ VISX/1995	46	6	−6.00 to −8.00 (mean −6.98)	Single (67%) Double (33%)	6.00: single 6.00 and 5.00: double	74	17

TABLE 53–3. **Combined Low- and High-Myopia Studies**

Author/Laser/Year	Low Myopes (No. of Eyes in Main Study)	Mean Follow-Up (Mo)	Attempted Correction (D)	Single or Multi-Zone (mm)	OZ (mm)	UCVA 20/40 (%)	UCVA 20/20 (%)
Seiler (Germany)/ Summit/1991	26	12	−1.4 to −9.25 (mean −4.5)	Single	3.5	96 (except 3 eyes intentionally undercorrected)	47.8 (except 3 eyes intentionally undercorrected)
Tengroth (Sweden)/ Summit/1993	420	12	−1.25 to −7.50 (mean −4.5)	Single	4.50 (<−5.5) 4.30 (≥−5.5)	91	Not reported
Ficker (UK)/ Summit/1993	61	12	−1 to −10	Single	5.00 (≤−8.0) 4.50 (>−8.0)	81	Not reported
Epstein (Sweden)/ Summit/1994	495	24	−1.25 to −7.50 (mean 4.05)	Single	4.50 (<5.50) 4.30 (5.50–7.50)	91	Not reported

±1 D (%)	Corneal Haze	Topical Steroids	Increased IOP (%)	Loss BCVA 2 Lines (%)	Loss BCVA >2 Lines (%)	Remarks or Comments
18	5.8% had > grade 1 + haze	Yes	0	0	0	One eye lost 3 lines BCVA due to irregular astigmatism; 2 lines regained by hard contact lens refraction. Another eye lost 2 lines of BCVA due to irregular astigmatism from decentered ablation; both lines regained with hard contact lens refraction.
34.5 28.2	Positive correlation between corneal haze and attempted correction	Yes	25.3 (overall study)	2.4 (overall study)	0	In overall study, 9.4% had late reepithelialization (>4 days) and 10.6% had decentration of ablation zone >1 mm.
39	Peak at 3 mo. 8.7% grade 2+ haze	Yes	0	15	0	Loss of BCVA due to irregular astigmatism and corneal haze. One eye had decentration of ablation zone of 2.4 mm. 12% developed central islands. Two eyes had myopic regression and were retreated. One eye underwent radial keratotomy for regression.
35	Grade 1+ in 77.5% Grade 2+ in 7.5%	Yes	7.5	40		Mean SE was −8.12 D preoperatively and −2.31 D at 24 mo. Halos in 5%, glare in 10%, irregular astigmatism in 2.5%. 65% had myopic regression exceeding −1 D. UCVA was 20/100 in 60%.
58 (excluding retreatments) 47 (all cases)	Peak at 3 mo. 8.7% grade 2+	Yes	0	15	0	Irregular astigmatism and corneal haze were causes of loss of BCVA. One eye had decentration of ablation zone of 2.4 mm. 12% developed central islands.
67	11% grade 1+ or more	Yes	0	2 (irregular astigmatism)		Single-zone ablations had better refractive and visual acuity outcomes than double-zone ablations. Mean UCVA was 20/30 and 20/50 for single-zone and double-zone ablations, respectively. Also 76% and 36% were within 1 D of emmetropia, respectively.

From Chan TK, Ashraf MF, Azar DT: Photoreactive keratectomy (PRK) outcomes and complications. *In* Azar DT, Steinert RF, Stark WJ (eds): Excimer Laser Phototherapeutic Keratectomy. Baltimore, Williams & Wilkins, 1997, pp 162–163.

Abbreviations: OZ, optical zone; UCVA, uncorrected visual acuity; IOP, intraocular pressure; BCVA, best corrected visual acuity; SE, spherical equivalent.

±1 D (%)	Corneal Haze	Topical Steroids	Increased IOP (%)	Loss BCVA 2 Lines (%)	Loss BCVA >2 Lines (%)	Remarks or Comments
92	All eyes except one had grade 1+ or less haze	Yes	3.1	0	0	One eye developed myopic regression with grade 1+ haze and was retreated. Six patients had persistent halos.
86	Mean haze at 12 mo was 0.77+. 3 or 4+ haze always correlated to regression. Haze reversed with topical steroids.	In substudy: group 1: treated for 3 mo group 2: treated for 5 weeks	13	Not reported	Not reported	Group 1 eyes regressed significantly less than group 2 eyes (*P* < .01). Glare and halos not significant problem.
81 87.5	Mean grading at 12 mo): 1+ Grade 2+: 3% Grade 3+: 1%	Yes Yes	Not reported 13	0 0	0 0	Regression to myopia more common in eyes treated for more than −4.00 D. Glare not significant problem. Subgroup analysis showed that eyes with low myopia (less than −3.9 D) had significantly better refractive outcomes than eyes with higher myopia.

From Chan TK, Ashraf MF, Azar DT: Photoreactive keratectomy (PRK) outcomes and complications. *In* Azar DT, Steinert RF, Stark WJ (eds): Excimer Laser Phototherapeutic Keratectomy. Baltimore, Williams & Wilkins, 1997, pp 164–165.

Abbreviations: OZ, optical zone; UCVA, uncorrected visual acuity; IOP, intraocular pressure; BCVA, best corrected visual acuity.

healing. This tends to resolve once the epithelium has completely healed. Other causes of irregular astigmatism, such as decentration and central islands, have already been discussed.

Increases in regular astigmatism after PRK are infrequent. Nevertheless, changes in cylindrical power or axis have been reported and may be the result of improper laser alignment or corneal wound healing and remodeling.

REGRESSION OF EFFECT

Both epithelial hyperplasia and the stromal response to excimer laser photoablation can lead to a regression of the refractive effect. Modulation of this response with topical corticosteroids was examined in a prospective double-blind randomized study comparing 0.1% dexamethasone to placebo in −3-D or −6-D procedures.[63, 64] Although 6-week outcomes showed a significantly greater change in mean refraction in the corticosteroid-treated group, this difference became statistically insignificant after corticosteroids were discontinued at 3 months. Because of the regression effect, most excimer lasers have been designed to overcorrect patients initially and allow the healing response to bring the patient's refraction back toward the target power.

PAIN

As with corneal abrasions, the epithelial defect produced by excimer PRK can be associated with significant postoperative pain. The neural response to excimer PRK seems to be exaggerated compared with that of manual deepithelialization, as demonstrated in rabbit eyes.[89] Another animal study showed a marked rise in prostaglandin E_2 levels after PRK that was blunted more dramatically by diclofenac sodium than fluorometholone.[90] This finding prompted a clinical study comparing the degree of pain and discomfort in patients undergoing bilateral PRK with one eye treated with a contact lens, cycloplegic, and 0.1% fluorometholone and the other eye treated with the same regimen plus 0.1% diclofenac sodium.[91, 92] Patients in the diclofenac sodium group experienced significantly less pain.

Use of topical nonsteroidal agents alone without concomitant use of a topical corticosteroid may be associated with sterile stromal infiltrates. Hence, it is advocated that the use of topical nonsteroidals be accompanied by the use of a topical corticosteroid to prevent this effect.

The use of a topical anesthetic (1% tetracaine) for 24 hours to control pain after PRK was evaluated in a prospective randomized double-blind trial.[93] Significant reduction of pain occurred in the anesthetic-treated group compared with the controls without impairment of wound healing or visual performance.

After LASIK, mild pain is associated with the shock wave and surgical incision, but the absence of an epithelial defect seems to speed recovery from the procedure.

PRK is associated with a transient decrease in corneal sensation for approximately 3 months[94] as a result of the ablation of the subepithelial nerve plexus. However, this does not seem to impair reepithelialization. LASIK, on the other hand, results in less corneal anesthesia.

REFERENCES

1. Cummins L, Nauenberg M: Thermal effects of laser radiation in biological tissue. Biophys J 42:99–102, 1983.
2. Taboada JM, Kessel GW, Reed RD: Response of the corneal epithelium to KrF excimer laser pulses. Health Phys 40:677, 1981.
3. Trokel SL, Srinivasan R, Braren B: Excimer laser surgery of the cornea. Am J Ophthalmol 96:710, 1983.
4. Seiler T, Wollensak J: In vivo experiments with the excimer laser—Technical parameters and healing processes. Ophthalmologica 192:65–70, 1986.
5. Srinivasan R, Sutcliffe E: Dynamics of the ultraviolet laser ablation of corneal tissue. Am J Ophthalmol 103:470–471, 1987.
6. Marshall J, Trokel S, Rothery S, Schubert H: An ultrastructural study of corneal incisions induced by an excimer laser at 193 nm. Ophthalmology 92:749–758, 1985.
7. Marshall J, Trokel S, Rothery S, et al: Photoablative reprofiling of the cornea using an excimer laser: Photorefractive keratectomy. Lasers Ophthalmol 1:21, 1986.
8. Munnerly CR, Koons SJ, Marshall J: Photorefractive keratectomy: A technique for laser refractive surgery. J Cataract Refract Surg 14:46–52, 1988.
9. Trokel S: Evolution of excimer laser corneal surgery. J Cataract Refract Surg 15:373–383, 1989.
10. Taylor DM, L'Esperance F Jr, Del Pero R, et al: Human excimer laser lamellar keratectomy: A clinical study. Ophthalmology 96:654–664, 1989.
11. Barraquer JI: Queratoplastia refractiva. Estudios Inform Oftal Inst Barraquer 10:2–10, 1949.
12. Ruiz LA, Rowsey JJ: Invest Ophthalmol Vis Sci 29(Suppl):392, 1988.
13. Pallikaris IG, Papatzanaki ME, Stathi EZ, et al: Laser in situ keratomileusis. Lasers Surg Med 10:463–468, 1990.
14. Srinivasan R: Kinetics of the ablative photodecomposition of organic polymers in the far ultraviolet (193 nm). J Vac Sci Technol B 1:923–926, 1983.
15. Keyes T, Clarke RH, Isner JM: Theory of photoablation and its implications for laser phototherapy. J Phys Chem 89:4194–4196, 1985.
16. Krauss JM, Puliafito CA, Steinert RF: Laser interactions with the cornea. Surv Ophthalmol 31:37–53, 1986.
17. Krueger RR, Trokel SL, Schubert HD: Interaction of ultraviolet laser light with the cornea. Invest Ophthalmol Vis Sci 26:1455–1464, 1985.
18. Krueger RR, Trokel SL: Quantitation of corneal ablation by ultraviolet laser light. Arch Ophthalmol 103:1741–1742, 1985.
19. Puliafito CA, Wong K, Steinert RF: Quantitative and ultrastructural studies of excimer laser ablation of the cornea at 193 and 248 nanometers. Lasers Surg Med 7:155–159, 1987.
20. Van Saarloos PP, Constable IJ: Bovine corneal ablation by ultraviolet laser light. Arch Ophthalmol 103:1741–1742, 1985.
21. Seiler T, Kriegerowski M, Schnoy N, Bende T: Ablation rate of human corneal epithelium and Bowman's layer with the excimer laser (193 nm). Refract Corneal Surg 6:99–102, 1990.
22. Huebscher HJ, Genth U, Seiler T: Determination of excimer laser ablation rate of the human cornea using Scheimpflug videography. Invest Ophthalmol Vis Sci 37:42–46, 1996.
23. Bende T, Seiler T, Wollensak J: Side effects in excimer corneal surgery: Corneal thermal gradients. Graefes Arch Exp Ophthalmol 226:277, 1988.
24. Mandel ER, Krueger RR, Puliafito CA, et al: Excimer laser large area ablation of the cornea. Invest Ophthalmol Vis Sci 28(Suppl.):275, 1987.
25. Hanna K, Chastang JC, Pouliquen Y, et al: A rotating slit delivery system for excimer laser refractive keratoplasty. Am J Ophthalmol 103:474, 1987.
26. Forster W, Beck R, Busse H: Design and development of a new 193-nanometer excimer laser surgical system. Refract Corneal Surg 9:293–299, 1993.
27. Fyodorov SN, Semyonav AD, Magaramov JA, et al: PRK using an absorbing cell delivery system for correction of myopia from 4 to 26 D in 3251 eyes. Refract Corneal Surg 9 (Suppl):123–124, 1993.
28. Dougherty PJ, Wellish KL, Maloney RK: Excimer laser ablation rate and corneal hydration. Am J Ophthalmol 118:169–176, 1994.
29. Filatov V, Kim SH, Kenyon KR, Talamo JH: The effect of tissue hydration on the corneal surface smoothness following excimer photorefractive keratectomy in rabbits. Invest Ophthalmol Vis Sci 36 (Suppl):S707, 1995.
30. Puliafito CA, Stern D, Krueger RR, Mandel ER: High-speed photogra-

phy of excimer laser ablation of the cornea. Arch Ophthalmol 105:1255–1259, 1987.
31. Kermani O, Koort HJ, Roth E, et al: Mass spectroscopic analysis of excimer laser ablated material from human corneal tissue. J Cataract Refract Surg 14:638–641, 1988.
32. Kahle G, Stadter H, Seiler L, et al: Gas chromatographic and mass spectroscopic analysis of excimer and erbium:yttrium aluminum garnet laser–ablated human cornea. Invest Ophthalmol Vis Sci 33:2180–2184, 1992.
33. Bor Z, Hopp B, Racz B, et al: Plume emission, shock wave, and surface wave formation during excimer laser ablation of the cornea. Refract Corneal Surg 9 (Suppl):S111–S114, 1993.
34. Berns MW, Liaw LH, Olivia A, et al: An acute light and electron microscopic study of ultraviolet 193-nm excimer laser corneal incisions. Ophthalmology 95:1422–1433, 1988.
35. Marshall J, Trokel S, Rothery S, Krueger RR: A comparative study of corneal incisions induced by diamond and steel knives and two ultraviolet radiations from an excimer laser. Br J Ophthalmol 70:482–501, 1986.
36. Tuft SJ, Zabel RW, Marshall J: Corneal repair following keratectomy: A comparison between conventional surgery and laser photoablation. Invest Ophthalmol Vis Sci 30:1769–1777, 1989.
37. Campos M, Cuevas K, Shieh E, et al: Corneal wound healing after excimer laser ablation in rabbits: Expanding versus contracting apertures. Refract Corneal Surg 8:378–381, 1992.
38. Wu WCS, Stark WJ, Green WR: Corneal wound healing after 193-nm excimer laser keratectomy. Arch Ophthalmol 109:1426–1432, 1991.
39. Malley DS, Steinert RF, Puliafito CA, et al: Immunofluorescence study of corneal wound healing after excimer laser anterior keratectomy in the monkey eye. Arch Ophthalmol 108:1316–1322, 1990.
40. Kornmehl EW, Steinert RF, Puliafito CA, Reidy W: Morphology of an irregular corneal surface following 193 nm ArF excimer laser large area ablation with 0.3% hydroxypropyl methylcellulose 2910 and 0.1% dextran70, 1% carboxymethyl cellulose sodium or 0.9% saline. Invest Ophthalmol Vis Sci 31:245, 1990.
41. DelPero RA, Gistad JE, Roberts AD, et al: A refractive and histopathologic study of excimer laser keratectomy in primates. Am J Ophthalmol 109:419–429, 1990.
42. Fountain TR, De La Cruz Z, Green WR, et al: Reassembly of corneal epithelial adhesion structures following human excimer laser keratectomy. Arch Ophthalmol 112:967–972, 1994.
43. Ahmad OF, Green WR, Stark WJ, et al: Excimer laser keratectomy: Morphometric analysis of epithelial basement membrane and hemidesmosome reformation. Invest Ophthalmol Vis Sci 34 (Suppl):703, 1993.
44. Vrabec MP, McDonald DS, Chase DS, et al: Traumatic corneal abrasions after excimer laser keratectomy. Am J Ophthalmol 116:101–102, 1993.
45. Hahn T, Woo J, Kim J: Phototherapeutic keratectomy in nine eyes with superficial corneal diseases. Refract Corneal Surg 9 (Suppl):S115–S118, 1993.
46. Kerr-Muir MG, Trokel S, Marshall J: Ultrastructural comparison of conventional surgical and argon fluoride excimer laser keratectomy. Am J Ophthalmol 103:448–453, 1987.
47. Binder PS: What we have learned about corneal wound healing from refractive surgery. J Refract Corneal Surg 5:98–120, 1989.
48. Aron-Rosa DS, Boerner CF, Bath P, et al: Corneal wound healing after excimer laser keratotomy in a human eye. Am J Ophthalmol 103:454–464, 1987.
49. Hanna KD, Pouliquen Y, Waring GO, et al: Corneal stromal wound healing in rabbits after 193-nm excimer laser surface ablation. Arch Ophthalmol 107:895, 1989.
50. Lohmann CP, Marshall J: Plasmin- and plasminogen-activator inhibitors after excimer laser photorefractive keratectomy: New concept in prevention of postoperative myopic regression and haze. Refract Corneal Surg 9:300–302, 1993.
51. Lohmann CP, Gartry DS, Muir MK, et al: Corneal haze after excimer laser refractive surgery: Objective measurement and functional implications. Eur J Ophthalmol 1(4):173–180, 1991.
52. Pluznik DT, Azar DT, Jain S, et al: Matrix metalloproteinase expression and corneal haze measurement after excimer keratomileusis in situ. Invest Ophthalmol Vis Sci 36(Suppl):S29, 1995.
53. Buratto L, Ferrari M, Rama P: Excimer laser intrastromal keratomileusis. Am J Ophthalmol 113:291–295, 1992.
54. Pallikaris IG, Siganos DS: Excimer laser in situ keratomileusis and photorefractive keratectomy for correction of high myopia. J Refract Surg 11 (Suppl):498–510, 1995.
55. Kremer FB, Dufek M: Excimer laser in situ keratomileusis. J Refract Surg 11 (Suppl):244–247, 1995.
56. Zabel R, Tuft S, Marshall J: Excimer laser photorefractive keratectomy: Endothelial morphology following area ablation of the cornea. Invest Ophthalmol Vis Sci 29 (Suppl):804, 1993.
57. Carones F, Brancato R, Venturi E, et al: The corneal endothelium after myopic excimer laser photorefractive keratectomy. Invest Ophthalmol Vis Sci 34 (Suppl):390, 1988.
58. Beldavs R, Thompson K, Waring GO III, et al: Quantitative specular microscopy after PRK. Ophthalmology 99:125, 1992.
59. Amano S, Shimuzu K: Corneal endothelial changes after excimer laser photorefractive keratectomy. Am J Ophthalmol 116:692–694, 1993.
60. Dehm EJ, Puliafito CA, Adler CM, Steinert RF: Corneal endothelial injury in rabbits following excimer laser ablation at 193 and 248 nm. Arch Ophthalmol 104:1364–1368, 1986.
61. Aquavella J, Gassett A, Dohlman C: Corticosteroids in corneal wound healing. Am J Ophthalmol 58:621–626, 1964.
62. Talamo JH, Gollamudi S, Green WR, et al: Modulation of corneal wound healing after excimer laser keratomileusis using topical mitomycin C and steroids. Arch Ophthalmol 109:1141–1146, 1991.
63. Gartry D, Muir MG, Lohmann CP, et al: The effect of topical corticosteroids on refractive outcome and corneal haze after photorefractive keratectomy. Arch Ophthalmol 110:944–952, 1992.
64. Gartry DS, Kerr-Muir MG, Marshall J: The effect of topical corticosteroids on refraction and corneal haze following excimer laser treatment of myopia: An update. A prospective, randomized, double-masked study. Eye 7:584–590, 1993.
65. Morlet N, Gillies MC, Crouch R, Maloof A: Effect of topical interferon-alpha 2b on corneal haze after excimer laser photorefractive keratectomy in rabbits. Refract Corneal Surg 9:443–451, 1993.
66. Lam DSC, Chew SJ, McDonald MB, Beuerman RW, et al: Modulation of corneal wound healing after excimer laser keratoplasty with muscarinic and histamine receptor antagonists. Invest Ophthalmol Vis Sci 34 (Suppl):S705, 1993.
67. O'Brart D, Lohmann CP, Klonos G, et al: The effects of topical corticosteroids and plasmin inhibitors on refractive outcome, haze and visual performance after photorefractive keratectomy. Ophthalmology 101:1565–1574, 1994.
68. Algawi K, Agrell B, Goggin M, O'Keefe M: Randomized clinical trial of topical sodium hyaluronate after excimer laser photorefractive keratectomy. J Refract Surg 11:42, 1995.
69. Nassaralla BA, Szerenyi K, Wang XW, et al: Effect of diclofenac on corneal haze after photorefractive keratectomy in rabbits. Ophthalmology 102:469–474, 1995.
70. Abad JC, Liw JE, Pepiu A, et al: Evaluation of pentoxifylline in the prevention of haze after photorefractive keratectomy (PRK) in the rabbit. Invest Ophthalmol Vis Sci 37 (Suppl):S58, 1996.
71. Tsubota K, Toda I, Itoh S: Reduction of subepithelial haze after photorefractive keratectomy by cooling the cornea. Am J Ophthalmol 115:820–821, 1993.
72. Brancato R, Tavola A, Carones F, et al: Excimer laser photorefractive keratectomy for myopia: Results in 1165 eyes. Refract Corneal Surg 9:95–104, 1993.
73. Kim JH, Sah WJ, Hahn TW, et al: Some problems after photorefractive keratectomy. J Refract Corneal Surg 10 (Suppl):S226–S230, 1994.
74. Gartry DS, Kerr-Muir MJ, Marshall J: Excimer laser photorefractive keratectomy: 18 month follow up. Ophthalmology 99:1209–1219, 1992.
75. Kim JH, Hahn TW, Lee YC, Joo CK, Sah WJ: Photorefractive keratectomy in 202 eyes: One year results. Refract Corneal Surg 9 (Suppl 2): S11–S16, 1993.
76. Buratto L, Ferrari M: Photorefractive keratectomy for myopia from 6.00 to 10.00 D. Refract Corneal Surg 9 (Suppl):S34–S36, 1993.
77. Seiler T, Schmidt-Petersen H, Wollensak J: Complications after myopic photorefractive keratectomy, primarily with the Summit excimer laser. *In* Salz JJ (ed): Corneal Laser Surgery. St. Louis, CV Mosby, 1995, pp 131–142.
78. Seiler T, Reckmann W, Maloney RK: Effective spherical aberration of the cornea as a quantitative descriptor in corneal topography. J Cataract Refract Surg 19 (Suppl):155–165, 1993.
79. O'Brart DPS, Lohmann CP, Fitzke FW, et al: Night vision after excimer laser photorefractive keratectomy: Haze and haloes. Eur J Ophthalmol 4:43–51, 1994.
80. Uozato H, Guyton DL: Centering corneal surgical procedures. Am J Ophthalmol 103:264–275, 1987.
81. Maloney RK: Corneal topography and optical zone location in photorefractive keratectomy. Refract Corneal Surg 6:363–371, 1990.

82. Heitzmann J, Binder PS, Kassar BS, Nordan LT: The correction of high myopia using the excimer laser. Arch Ophthalmol 111:1627–1634, 1993.
83. Maguire LJ, Zabel RW, Parker P, et al: Topography and ray tracing analysis of patients with excellent visual acuity 3 months after excimer laser photorefractive keratectomy for myopia. Refract Corneal Surg 7:122–128, 1991.
84. Gimbel HV, Van Westenbrugge JA, Johnson WH, et al: Visual, refractive and patient satisfaction results following bilateral photorefractive keratectomy. Refract Corneal Surg 9 (Suppl 2):S5–S10, 1993.
85. Taylor HR, Guest CS, Kelly P, et al: Comparison of excimer laser treatment of astigmatism and myopia. Arch Ophthalmol 111:1621–1626, 1993.
86. Cavanaugh TB, Durrie DS, Riedel SM, et al: Topographical analysis of the centration of excimer laser photorefractive keratectomy. J Cataract Refract Surg 19 (Suppl):136–143, 1993.
87. Maguen E, Machat JJ: Complications of photorefractive keratectomy, primarily with the VISX excimer laser. *In* Salz JJ (ed): Corneal Laser Surgery. St. Louis, CV Mosby, 1995, pp 143–158.
88. Lin DTC: Corneal topographic analysis after excimer laser photorefractive keratectomy. Ophthalmology 101:1432–1439, 1994.
89. Beuerman RW, McDonald MB, Varnell RJ, Thompson HW, et al: Neurophysiological evaluation of corneal nerves in rabbits following excimer photorefractive keratectomy. Invest Ophthalmol Vis Sci 34: 704, 1993.
90. Phillips AF, Szerenyi K, Campos M, et al: Arachidonic acid metabolites after excimer laser corneal surgery. Arch Ophthalmol 111:1273–1278, 1993.
91. Eiferman RA, Hoffman RS, Sher NA: Topical diclofenac reduces pain after photorefractive keratectomy. Arch Ophthalmol 111:1022, 1993.
92. Sher NA, Frantz JM, Talley A: Topical diclofenac in the treatment of ocular pain after excimer photorefractive keratectomy. Refract Corneal Surg 9:425, 1993.
93. Verma S, Corbett MC, Marshall J: A prospective, randomized, double-masked trial to evaluate the role of topical anesthetics in controlling pain after photorefractive keratectomy. Ophthalmology 102:1918–1924, 1995.
94. Campos M, Garbus J, McDonnell PJ: Corneal sensitivity after photorefractive keratectomy. Am J Ophthalmol 114:51–54, 1992.

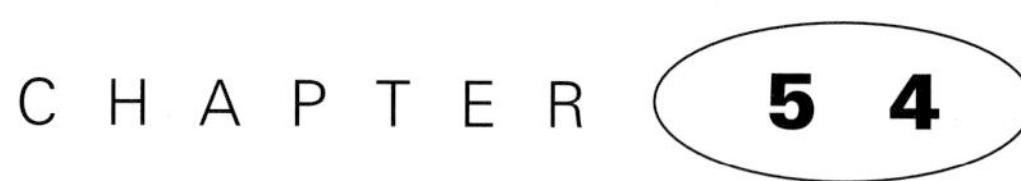

New Lasers for Glaucoma Surgery

Mark A. Latina, Santiago Antonio B. Sibayan, and Michael S. Berlin

Lasers have revolutionized our approach to the treatment of glaucoma. The development of various innovative laser surgical techniques has provided us with a whole new means of treating this sight-threatening disease.

The most widely available and commonly performed techniques in glaucoma laser surgery (iridotomy, argon laser trabeculoplasty, gonioplasty, and trabeculectomy flap suture lysis) have been extensively documented and have changed little since the late 1980s. In recent years, however, a large number of new glaucoma laser procedures have been proposed. These include selective laser trabeculoplasty, trabecular ablation, laser goniotomy, laser sclerostomy, laser sinusotomy, cyclophotocoagulation, and laser bleb revision. This review addresses the current status of these procedures that have been proposed or are under development.

Trabecular Meshwork Procedures

CONTINUOUS-WAVE LASER TRABECULOPLASTY

In primary open-angle glaucoma (OAG), the trabecular meshwork is the main source of outflow resistance. Laser trabeculoplasty has been proved to be effective in increasing fluid outflow through the trabecular meshwork. The mechanism by which it works, however, remains poorly understood. One proposed mechanism of action is heat-induced modification of collagen in the trabecular meshwork, leading to widening of intertrabecular spaces.[1] Another proposed mechanism of action is the stimulation of trabecular meshwork cell division and repopulation and rejuvenation of trabecular structure, resulting in enhancement of aqueous outflow.[2]

Various types of continuous-wave (CW) lasers have been used to perform trabeculoplasty. The use of the argon laser ($\lambda =$ 488 or 514.5 nm), as first described by Wise and Witter in 1979,[1] is currently the most commonly performed method of laser trabeculoplasty. With this technique, long-term intraocular pressure (IOP) drops of up to 10 mm Hg have been reported.[1, 3] More recently, the diode laser ($\lambda = 810$ nm) has been used to perform trabeculoplasty. In a prospective study comparing diode laser trabeculoplasty with argon laser trabeculoplasty, Brancato and coworkers[4] have demonstrated that both lasers are equally effective in lowering the IOP. In contrast, Englert and associates[5] have found argon laser trabeculoplasty to be more effective than diode laser trabeculoplasty. Further studies are necessary to determine the comparative efficacy of these lasers.

The use of the CW frequency-doubled Nd:yttrium-aluminum-garnet (YAG) laser ($\lambda = 532$ nm) is under investigation.[6] Histologic studies have shown thermal and coagulative changes in the trabecular meshwork that are comparable to those seen after treatment with the argon laser. Clinical studies using this laser are pending.

SELECTIVE LASER TRABECULOPLASTY

Selective laser trabeculoplasty is a new approach to the treatment of OAG. This procedure selectively targets pigmented trabecular meshwork cells without causing collateral thermal and coagulative damage to surrounding cells or structures.

Unlike conventional argon or diode laser trabeculoplasty, which is accomplished with the use of CW lasers, selective laser trabeculoplasty is performed with a Q-switched frequency-doubled Nd:YAG laser (λ = 532 nm) with a pulse duration of 3 nsec. Using such a laser, Latina and Park[7] demonstrated that selective targeting of pigmented trabecular meshwork cells can be achieved in cell culture. In studies performed in owl monkeys, Latina and Sibayan have demonstrated that selective targeting of pigmented cells can also be achieved in vivo without thermal damage to the trabecular meshwork (Fig. 54–1).[8]

A preliminary clinical trial has been performed to study the safety and efficacy of this procedure in lowering the IOP in patients with glaucoma. Latina and colleagues[9] treated 53 eyes with OAG that were on maximum tolerated medical therapy. Patients were divided into two treatment groups. The first group consisted of patients who had not undergone previous argon laser trabeculoplasty, and the second group was composed of individuals who had previously undergone argon laser trabeculoplasty. In this study, there were 25 females and 28 males. Racial composition was as follows: 30 whites, 18 African Americans, and 5 Hispanics. Patients were treated by applying 50 laser spots over 180 degrees of the nasal trabecular meshwork using the Coherent Selecta 7000 (Coherent Laser, Palo Alto, CA). Follow-up was for up to 26 weeks.

The average preoperative IOP was 24.6 mm Hg. There was an average IOP drop of 30.2% at 1 day (7.5 mm Hg IOP reduction), 22.3% at 8 weeks (5.6 mm Hg IOP reduction), and 18.7% at 26 weeks (4.6 mm Hg IOP reduction).

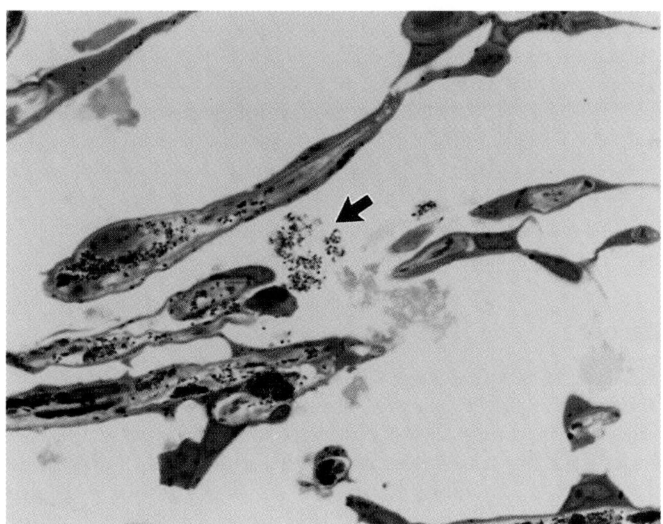

FIGURE 54–1. Histologic section of owl monkey trabecular meshwork 24 hours after treatment with selective laser trabeculoplasty. Disrupted pigmented cell and cellular remnants are present *(arrow)*. Trabecular beams and overall trabecular meshwork structure remain intact. There is no evidence of thermal damage.

There were no serious adverse effects. IOP elevations of 8 mm Hg or greater occurred in 9% of eyes within 2 hours after treatment. These pressure spikes responded to medical therapy that resulted in IOP reduction within 24 hours.

Seventy percent of eyes responded to treatment, with an IOP reduction of 3 mm Hg or more. Responders in both treatment groups had comparable IOP drops (23.5% IOP reduction for the OAG with no prior argon laser trabeculoplasty group versus 24.2% IOP reduction for the OAG with prior argon laser trabeculoplasty group). Both groups showed a statistically significant drop in IOP compared with baseline (P<.001).

This preliminary clinical trial suggests that selective laser trabeculoplasty is a clinically safe and effective method of reducing the IOP in patients with OAG. The data also suggest that this procedure is effective in treating patients with prior argon laser trabeculoplasty and that a similar IOP drop may be achieved in this subgroup of patients. Treatment of this subgroup may be important because many of these patients may be able to avoid filtration surgery if treated with selective laser trabeculoplasty. Because the technique is less destructive to the trabecular meshwork than argon laser trabeculoplasty (there is no collateral thermal damage or scarring of the trabecular meshwork), this procedure could potentially be repeated many times. Further clinical trials are in progress and should lead to more information on the efficacy of this procedure.

TRABECULAR ABLATION

Trabecular ablation is a technique that aims to create direct communication between the anterior chamber and the canal of Schlemm. Outflow facility is improved by eliminating the trabecular meshwork, which has been estimated to account for 75% of outflow resistance.[10] This procedure is a relatively new technique that is currently being investigated by several groups using various types of lasers.

Vogel and coworkers[11] claim that the excimer laser is ideal for this procedure since tissue can be ablated with minimal thermal effects and necrosis (Fig. 54–2). Using a 308-nm excimer laser delivered through a goniolens, they performed trabecular ablation in 42 eyes that were candidates for trabeculectomy (34 with primary OAG and 8 with low-tension glaucoma). Three to five pores were ablated within the trabecular meshwork. In primary OAG patients, the average IOP drop was 4.7 mm Hg over a follow-up period of 5.7 months. Low-tension glaucoma patients had comparable results, with an average IOP decrease of 4.5 mm Hg over a follow-up period of 6.1 months.[12]

Vivar and colleagues[13] have performed a similar technique with the use of a Ti-sapphire laser (λ = 790 nm) delivered gonioscopically over 3 clock hours of the trabecular meshwork. They claim a high success rate, with good IOP control and minimal complications.

Some lasers, however, appear to be less promising. Using an Er:YAG laser (λ = 2.94 μm) delivered gonioscopically, Dietlein and associates[14] performed ab interno photoablation of the trabecular meshwork of 15 rabbits. They reported substantial collateral thermal damage, progressive fibroblastic and endothelial proliferation, and dense scar tissue formation.

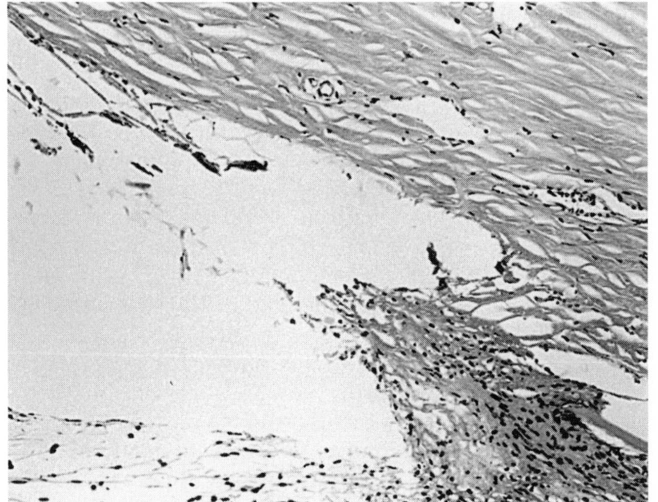

FIGURE 54–2. Photomicrograph of the trabecular meshwork of a human eye after excimer laser ablation. The trabecular meshwork and the inner wall of the canal of Schlemm are completely removed. Thermal reaction, as indicated by dark staining, is minimal. (From Vogel M, Lauritzen K, Quentin C-D: Punktuelle Ablation des Trabekelwerks mit dem Exzimer laser beim primaeren Offenwinkelglaukom. Ophthalmologe 93:565–568, 1996. Copyright Springer-Verlag.)

LASER GONIOTOMY

Primary infantile glaucoma (congenital glaucoma) is caused by a developmental defect of the trabecular meshwork. In this condition, trabecular pillars cause traction on the iris root and result in compaction of the trabecular meshwork. Goniotomy, the current treatment of choice for congenital glaucoma, severs trabecular beams bridging the anterior chamber angle, resulting in decreased resistance to aqueous humor outflow. It is usually performed with the use of a Barkan blade or an irrigating needle and is associated with such complications as cyclodialysis, hemorrhage from the iris root, and trauma to the external wall of the canal of Schlemm. Since laser techniques are generally safer and more reproducible than conventional surgery, they may be able to reduce the complications associated with surgical goniotomy.

Goniotomy requires a cornea that is clear enough to allow visualization of the anterior chamber by direct gonioscopy. Unfortunately, since primary infantile glaucoma is commonly associated with cloudy corneas, the view of the angle is often obscured. Endoscopic techniques allow visualization of the angle, even in the presence of cloudy corneas.

Jacobi and coworkers[15] successfully performed laser goniotomy under endoscopic guidance in porcine cadaver eyes. This was achieved using an Er:YAG endoprobe and a microendoscope inserted through separate limbal paracenteses. Laser ablation of the pectinate ligaments was achieved without tissue damage to adjacent structures. Shetlar and associates[16] have also achieved good results in porcine cadaver eyes using a free-electron laser tuned to a wavelength of 4 μm.

Laser Filtration Procedures

LASER SCLEROSTOMY

Laser sclerostomy is the creation of a fistula between the anterior chamber and the subconjunctival space. This procedure enables aqueous humor to bypass the trabecular meshwork, resulting in reduction of the IOP. It has been performed with the use of various lasers, such as the CW Nd:YAG,[17, 18] THC:YAG (thallium, holmium, chromium: YAG; also known as holmium:YAG),[19, 20] Er:YAG,[21, 22] Q-switched Nd:YAG,[23] flashlamp pulsed-dye,[24] excimer,[25] and diode.[26] Currently, only the CW Nd:YAG and THC:YAG lasers are approved by the Food and Drug Administration for laser sclerostomy.

Laser sclerostomy has been presented as a less invasive alternative to conventional glaucoma filtration surgery. It can be performed relatively rapidly and easily on an outpatient basis. It involves minimal surgical manipulation of ocular tissues, thus the stimuli for conjunctival scarring are reduced. Since conjunctival incisions are small or absent, the risk of wound leaks may be decreased. Laser sclerostomy therefore has the potential advantage of improving the success rate of filtration surgery.

One major disadvantage of laser sclerostomy is that most techniques result in full-thickness filters and can be associated with such complications as overfiltration, hypotony, and choroidal effusion. This problem persists and is one of the main reasons why this technique has not yet achieved widespread acceptance.

Delivery

Laser sclerostomy techniques fall into two main categories: ab externo and ab interno. In the ab externo approach, laser energy is delivered using a fiberoptic probe inserted through a subconjunctival flap or partial-thickness corneal flap. In the ab interno technique, sclerostomies can be performed either invasively with the use of a fiberoptic probe inserted though a paracentesis, or noninvasively with the use of a goniolens.

Various types of fiberoptic probes have been devised. A sharp sapphire tip scalpel coupled to a fiberoptic delivery system has been used for the delivery of CW Nd:YAG lasers.[17, 18] The Er:YAG laser[21] and the 308-nm ultraviolet excimer laser[25] utilize blunt fiberoptic probes that are applied perpendicular to the limbus and are advanced while in direct contact with the tissue. Side-firing laser probes that are applied tangential to the limbus have been used for delivery of the THC:YAG laser.[19, 20]

Gonioscopic laser sclerostomy usually requires lenses with special characteristics. One such example is the Lasag CGF goniolens, which features a flange adapted to allow a bleb to form while the lens is in place on the eye.

Lasers

Most laser sclerostomy research has elucidated the efficacy of various laser types and analyzed their histologic effects. Direct experimental and clinical comparison between lasers is difficult, however, because of differing treatment parameters for the wavelength, power, pulse duration, pulse frequency, beam diameter, patient composition, and criteria for success.

THC:YAG, CW Nd:YAG, and diode lasers create thermal damage to tissue.[27, 28] In contrast, the Er:YAG laser has a minimal thermal effect and produces the least thermal damage of all nonexcimer lasers. This theoretically makes it well suited for sclerostomy procedures. By delivering laser energy at a wavelength of 2.94 μm, which is very close to the absorption peak of water in the infrared region, the Er:YAG laser is highly absorbed by all water-containing tissues. This results in reduced penetration depth and thermal damage radius.[21] However, the Er:YAG applicator probe tip should be placed in direct contact with the sclera, otherwise laser energy will be absorbed by water between the tip and the target tissue. This results in conversion of most of the laser energy into heat, consequently increasing thermal damage.

Clinical application of the Er:YAG laser has been limited because of the lack of an acceptable fiberoptic delivery system. However, McHam and coworkers[21] have demonstrated that a single crystal sapphire fiberoptic is a reliable and efficient means of delivering the Er:YAG wavelength to create laser sclerostomies with minimal thermal damage in rabbits.

Ab Externo Laser Sclerostomy

The THC:YAG and the Er:YAG are the two lasers that have been most extensively studied to perform ab externo laser sclerostomies. These techniques involve the use of a fiberoptic delivery system attached into a handpiece. To perform the procedure, retrobulbar anesthesia is administered, and a 1- to 2-mm conjunctival stab incision is made 5 to 15 mm away from the intended sclerostomy site. The laser probe is advanced subconjunctivally and placed in contact with the sclera just posterior to the limbus. The laser is then fired until an adequate opening between the anterior chamber and the subconjunctival space is formed.

Iwach and associates[20] reported their 4-year experience with the THC:YAG laser sclerostomy. Success was defined as an IOP of 22 mm Hg or less, or a drop of at least 30% in patients with preoperative IOPs of 22 mm Hg or less. In a total of 103 procedures performed in 87 eyes, the estimated success rate in eyes in which only one sclerostomy was performed was 39% at 2 years and 26% at 4 years. In comparison, eyes that underwent up to two sclerostomies had higher success rates (44 and 36% at 2 and 4 years, respectively).

Schuman and colleagues[19] reported results of THC:YAG laser sclersostomy in 49 eyes with a mean follow-up of 1 year. With this procedure, they were able to achieve an average IOP reduction of 7.2 mm Hg (The mean preoperative IOP was 26.9 mm Hg; the mean postoperative IOP was 19.7). Thirty patients (61%) achieved final IOPs that ranged from 5 to 22 mm Hg. Complications encountered included suprachoroidal hemorrhage and hypotony.

Er:YAG laser sclerostomy was performed by Jacobi and coworkers[22] in 26 patients. Transient postoperative hypotony associated with overfiltration was a common complication. Later in the course, occlusion of the fistula occurred, leading to filter failure. The half-lives of functional filtering blebs were estimated to be as short as 36 days. These findings led the investigators to conclude that this procedure is unsuitable for long-term pressure control.

Schmidt-Erfurth and colleagues[29] have reported the use of adjunctive mitomycin C in THC:YAG or Er:YAG laser sclerostomy. Immediately before the sclerostomy was performed, mitomycin C (0.5 mg/mL) was applied with a soaked sponge over the prospective filter bleb site for 3 to 5 minutes. Their results demonstrated a success rate of 65% in the mitomycin C–treated group versus 41% in the sclerostomy-alone group (success was defined as a reduction of IOP to a level of 22 mm Hg or less and the presence of a prominent bleb). However, hypotony was more frequent and more pronounced in the group that was treated with mitomycin C. The incidence of iris incarceration was also higher in the mitomycin C–treated group (69%) compared with the sclerostomy-alone group (45%). Whether adjunctive administration of antimetabolites during laser sclerostomy would be of significant benefit in enhancing the success of this procedure requires further investigation.

Invasive ab Interno Sclerostomy

Ab interno laser sclerostomies have been performed with a CW Nd:YAG laser delivered through a synthetic sapphire tip laser scalpel. To perform this procedure, one creates a beveled corneal incision at the limbus and deepens the anterior chamber with sodium hyaluronate. A 200-μm sapphire laser tip is introduced across the anterior chamber to the opposite side, keeping the tip parallel to the iris. The tip is then positioned at the level of the trabecular meshwork and the laser is fired. To aid the procedure, one can indent the eye with a muscle hook just beneath the site of the intended sclerostomy. The end-point is visualization of the tip in the subconjunctival space and ballooning of the conjunctiva.

Wilson and Javitt[18] performed this procedure in five aphakic patients with an average follow-up time of 25 months. They reported three successes with an average postoperative IOP of 15 mm Hg. No intraoperative complications were noted. However, choroidal detachment was observed in all patients and required drainage in one. In another study, Lui and Higginbotham performed a similar procedure in nine eyes.[30] They reported that only four of nine procedures performed were successful. Hyphema was a common postoperative complication.

The excimer laser[25] and the diode laser[26] have been used to perform ab interno sclerostomies in rabbits. Although the experimental results appear promising, studies using these lasers in humans have not yet been performed.

Noninvasive ab Interno Sclerostomy

The ideal laser filtration procedure is one that can be performed in the office setting without violating ocular tissue with surgical instruments, using only laser energy and appropriate lenses to conduct the procedure. The goal would be to replace conventional filtration surgery with a completely outpatient procedure, just as laser iridotomy has replaced surgical iridectomy. Such has been the impetus behind the development of noninvasive ab interno sclerostomy.

The Q-switched Nd:YAG laser was used in one of the first successful noninvasive ab interno approaches to laser sclerostomy. This technique was pioneered by March and coworkers.[23] With the use of a special goniolens, this procedure could be performed in the office with minimal manipulation of ocular tissues. One major drawback was that it was necessary to use a significant amount of energy (as much as 27 J), which often resulted in damage to surrounding tissues.

Latina and coworkers[24] developed an alternative gonio-

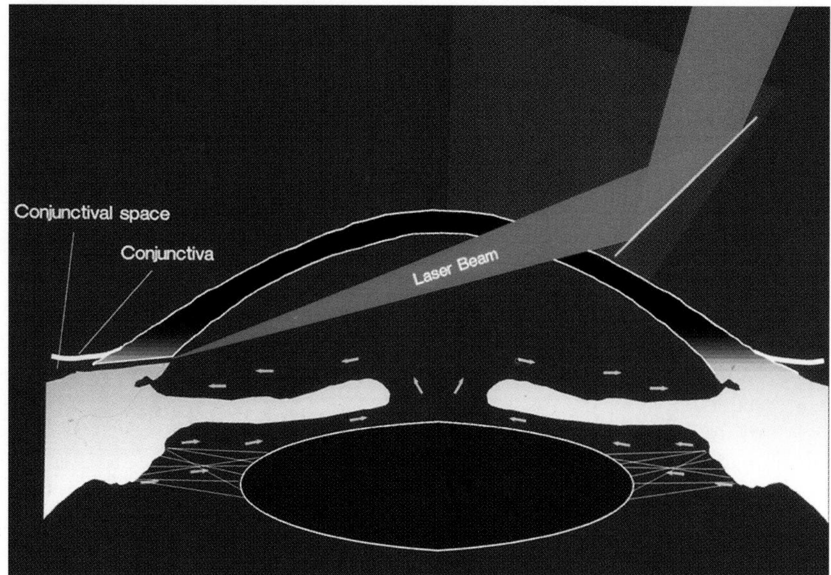

FIGURE 54–3. Schematic representation of gonioscopic ab interno sclerostomy. A laser beam is directed through a goniolens onto the region of dyed sclera to create a fistula. (From Latina MA, Dobrogowski M, March WF, Birngruber R: Laser sclerostomy by pulsed-dye laser and goniolens. Arch Ophthalmol 108:1745–1750, 1990. Copyright 1990, American Medical Association.)

scopic ab interno sclerostomy using a technique termed *dye-enhanced sclerostomy*. In this procedure, laser energy was transmitted across the cornea and anterior chamber and absorbed by the sclera (Fig. 54–3). The optical absorption of sclera was enhanced by noninvasive iontophoretic administration of methylene blue (Fig. 54–4). The emission wavelength of a flashlamp pulsed-dye laser was matched to the absorption peak of methylene blue. Thermal damage to the surrounding tissue was minimized by using a short pulse duration (7 μsec). In their pilot clinical study, complete fistula formation was achieved in only 55% of eyes. With success defined as an IOP of 22 mm Hg or lower, only 53% were successful at 9 months. The sclerostomy formed was conical with a small external aperture, which probably contributed to the failure of filtration. Although postoperative complications were minimal, the authors concluded that the long-term IOP control was unacceptable.

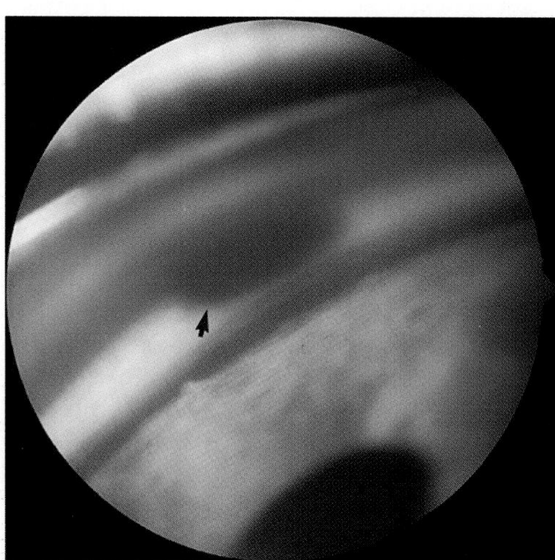

FIGURE 54–4. Gonioscopic view of dyed sclera *(arrow)* before treatment with gonioscopic ab interno sclerostomy. (From Latina MA, Dobrogowski M, March WP, Birngruber R: Laser sclerostomy by pulsed-dye laser and goniolens. Arch Ophthalmol 108:1745–1750, 1990. Copyright 1990, American Medical Association.)

Chuck and associates[31] attempted to refine the ab interno laser sclerostomy procedure testing other dyes such as fluorescein, rose bengal, and indocyanine green. Their results suggest that rose bengal and indocyanine green localize in the sclera better than methylene blue and that the use of these agents in conjunction with appropriate laser sources may lead to better procedure efficiency. Arya and colleagues[32] utilized a microsecond pulsed-diode laser to create a full-thickness fistula in cadaver sclera dyed with indocyanine green. Clinical trials are needed to evaluate the efficacy of these approaches.

Comment

Although laser sclerostomy has many theoretical advantages over conventional filtration surgery, several risks and complications remain. Many of the procedures reported still require an operating room environment with monitored anesthesia. Although laser sclerostomy is simpler and more rapidly performed than conventional filtration surgery, it is still associated with such complications as flat chambers, iris incarceration into the fistula, suprachoroidal hemorrhage, hyphema, misdirected fistulas, conjunctival buttonholes, and endophthalmitis. It is unlikely that laser sclersotomy will gain widespread clinical acceptance until the success rate of the procedure is improved and the complication rate is reduced compared with those of conventional filtration surgery. The authors do not find any compelling indications to perform laser sclerostomy procedures instead of other glaucoma surgical procedures currently available.

LASER SINUSOTOMY

Krasnov[33] originally described the technique of sinusotomy, the procedure of unroofing the canal of Schlemm, allowing aqueous humor to percolate into the subconjunctival space. This technique may be of particular benefit to patients who have glaucoma secondary to elevated episcleral venous pressure (e.g., Sturge-Weber syndrome, dural shunt syndrome). Seiler and coworkers[34] and Kuwayama and colleagues[35] described the use of the 193-nm excimer laser to create a sinusotomy and referred to this technique as *partial external trabeculectomy.* This was performed by dissecting the conjunctiva to allow exposure of the limbus, followed by excimer laser ablation of tissue within this region. The end-point was to expose the juxtacanalicular meshwork, leaving a thin layer of trabecular meshwork behind. Since aqueous humor does not allow transmission of ultraviolet light, ablation stops automatically once resistance to aqueous flow is eliminated.[35] Histologic studies using cadaver eyes show that this procedure does not result in a full-thickness opening into the anterior chamber and that the remaining trabecular tissue may act as a microporous passive filter.[36]

Campos and coworkers[37] described a method of performing sinusotomy without conjunctival dissection. This was performed in rabbits and human eye bank eyes using a 193-nm ArF excimer laser. In the rabbit experiments, the conjunctiva was pulled over the corneoscleral limbus, and a slit-shaped excimer beam was used to ablate through conjunctiva and sclera until the outer wall of the canal of Schlemm was perforated (Figs. 54–5 and 54–6). On completion of the procedure, the conjunctiva was allowed to retract, and a bleb immediately formed. The small slit created in the conjunctiva was sutured. The IOP in rabbits decreased from a preoperative level of 10 mm Hg to 4.9 mm Hg postoperatively. Brooks and associates[38] have also described a similar technique. This procedure has the advantage of minimizing trauma to the conjunctiva, thus potentially increasing the chances for developing a successful filter.

Allan and coworkers[39–41] have also used a transconjunctival technique to create laser sclerostomies. Their technique is similar to those that have been employed by Campos and Brooks for creating sinusotomies. However, instead of creating partial-thickness ablations, they achieved full-thickness openings between the anterior chamber and the subconjunctival space. A 6-month follow-up study demonstrated good IOP control (≤16 mm Hg) in eight of nine eyes treated with this procedure. This procedure, however, has been associated with hyphema, early postoperative hypotony, temporary fibrinous occlusion of the sclerostomy, and suprachoroidal hemorrhage.

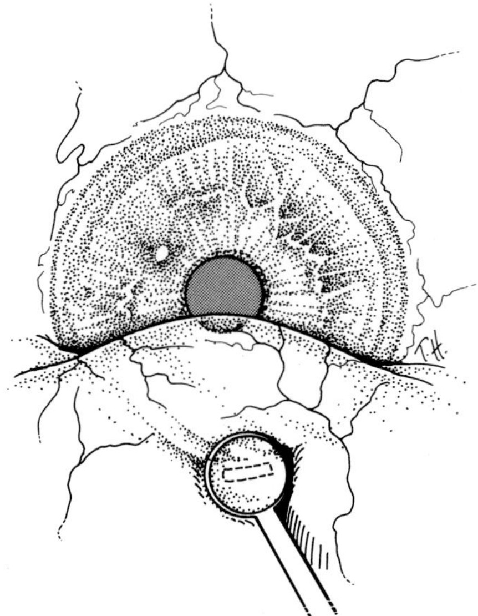

FIGURE 54–5. Illustration of the technique of transconjunctival sinusotomy. The conjunctiva is advanced over the cornea, and a ring is placed over the conjunctiva at the location of the canal of Schlemm. An excimer laser is focused over this area and is used to perform transconjunctival ablation of the outer wall of the canal of Schlemm. (From Campos, M, Lee PP, Trokel SL, et al: Transconjunctival sinusotomy using the 193-nm excimer laser. Acta Ophthalmol 72:707–711, 1994.)

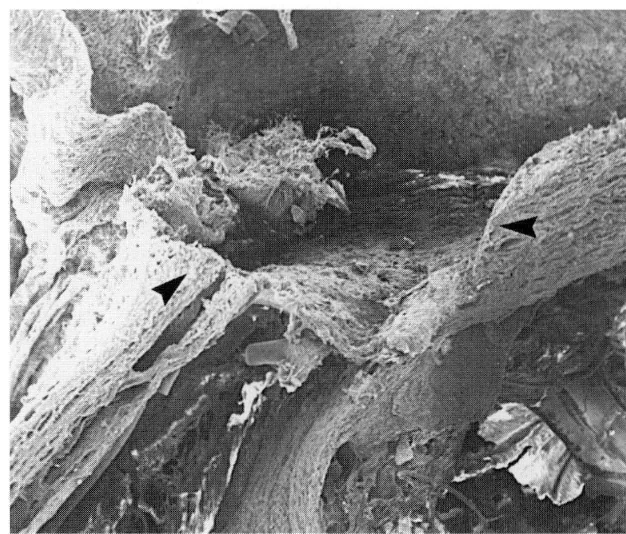

FIGURE 54–6. Scanning electron micrograph of rabbit eye after transconjunctival laser sclerostomy. Partial-thickness ablation of the eye wall at the corneoscleral limbus and removal of the outer wall of the canal of Schlemm are revealed *(arrows).* Thermal damage to adjacent tissue is minimal. (From Campos M, Lee PP, Trokel SL, et al: Transconjunctival sinusotomy using the 193-nm excimer laser. Acta Ophthalmol 72:702–711, 1994.)

Zimmerman is investigating *laser trabeculodissection*, a modification of laser sinusotomy. In this technique, a partial-thickness scleral flap is surgically dissected and the excimer laser is used to dissect tissue to the level of the trabecular meshwork, leaving a thin membrane behind. Unlike laser sinusotomy, this is a true guarded procedure (Zimmerman T, personal communication, 1996).

Laser Cyclophotocoagulation

In contrast to glaucoma filtration procedures, which lower the IOP by increasing aqueous humor outflow, cyclodestructive procedures reduce the IOP by decreasing aqueous humor production. In the latter group of procedures, the secretion of aqueous humor is reduced by partial destruction of the ciliary epithelium, stroma, and ciliary body vascular supply. Cyclodestructive procedures are particularly useful for the treatment of glaucoma that is refractory to other therapies.

Various modalities have been used to perform cyclodestructive procedures. These include diathermy,[42] cyclocryotherapy,[43] and xenon arc cyclophotocoagulation (CPC).[44] Laser energy as a means of cyclodestruction was first employed by Beckman and colleagues[45] in 1972 when they applied a ruby laser via a transscleral approach. Other lasers that have been used for CPC include the Nd:YAG,[46, 47] argon,[48, 49] and 780 to 830 nm infrared diode lasers.[50]

Lasers can be delivered transsclerally by a noncontact method (through a slit-lamp system)[45, 46, 50] or a contact method (through a fiberoptic probe applied on the sclera).[47, 51] Lasers may also be delivered directly to the ciliary body.[48, 49]

Despite the advances in cyclodestructive procedures, they are still associated with postoperative problems such as inflammation, postoperative pressure spikes, long-term hypotony, cystoid macular edema, and phthisis bulbi. As a result, these techniques are still often considered a last resort. The current challenge in cyclodestructive procedure research is to develop a technique that is associated with fewer complications. The following discussion focuses on the latest products of such research.

PHOTODYNAMIC THERAPY OF THE CILIARY BODY

Photodynamic therapy utilizes the biologic effects that result from the interaction of photosensitizers with light. Excitation of a photosensitizing dye by an appropriate wavelength induces the production of reactive oxygen species and singlet oxygen. These highly reactive products interact with various biologic molecules, resulting in cell death. Although photodynamic therapy has been used mainly for oncologic applications, it has recently been applied to other nononcologic uses.[52]

Tsilimbaris and coworkers[53] used photodynamic therapy to perform CPC in albino rabbits. Phthalocyanine, a photosensitizer, was administered intravenously and the ciliary body was irradiated transsclerally with a 670-nm diode laser. This resulted in IOP reduction that lasted for approximately 2 weeks. Histologic analysis of the treated ciliary body revealed vascular thrombosis and endothelial cell damage, as well as disruption of the ciliary epithelium. They have postulated that the decreased secretory function of the ciliary body may be due to vascular compromise alone or in combination with a direct photodynamic effect on the endothelium.

Further studies are necessary to determine whether photodynamic therapy of the ciliary body can provide a safe and effective means of lowering the IOP.

KRYPTON RED AND 670-NM DIODE LASER CYCLOPHOTOCOAGULATION

The success of CPC is highly dependent on the degree of absorption of laser energy by the ciliary body. Theoretically, krypton red (λ = 647 nm) and 670-nm diode lasers would be ideal for the direct treatment of the ciliary body since these wavelengths are close to the absorption peak of the ciliary body.[54, 55] However, for transscleral approaches, the light transmission characteristics of sclera must be taken into consideration. Transscleral penetrance increases with an increase in wavelength and is poorer at 647 nm and 670 nm when compared with the longer wavelengths that are currently in common use for CPC (Nd:YAG λ = 1064 nm; infrared diode λ = 810 nm).[55, 56]

It has been shown that compression of the sclera by the laser delivery probe during contact application increases the scleral transmission of light, especially for short wavelengths.[56] Moreover, because the ciliary body absorbs red wavelengths (i.e., 647 and 670 nm) better than infrared wavelengths (i.e., 810 and 1064 nm), less energy is required to cross the sclera to produce adequate cyclophotocoagulative effects.[57] Krypton red and 670-nm diode lasers may therefore provide an effective means of conducting CPC.

Immonen and associates[54] performed krypton red laser CPC in 62 eyes. They reported an average IOP drop of 13.9 mm Hg 6 months after the procedure. A relatively low incidence of complications was reported. Only a mild to moderate degree of inflammation was noted postoperatively. Just 2 of 55 eyes were hypotonous at the 6-month follow-up period. They did not observe any cyclodestruction-related decreases in visual acuity. Although these findings appear promising, more studies are needed to prove the safety and efficacy of this procedure.

ENDOSCOPIC CYCLOPHOTOCOAGULATION

Transscleral cyclodestructive procedures have the disadvantage of being performed without direct visualization of the ciliary processes. Therefore, it is not possible to precisely apply treatment and quantitate the amount of ciliary destruction. Furthermore, transscleral procedures result in damage adjacent to the target tissue. Direct treatment of ciliary processes would eliminate such problems.

In order to avoid such problems, methods such as transpupillary argon laser CPC[48] and ciliary body endophotocoagulation with transpupillary visualization during pars plana vitrectomy[49] have been devised. These procedures have not achieved widespread use because of the difficulty of visualizing ciliary processes in vivo. The iris obstructs the view of the ciliary processes and must be well dilated or surgically removed in order to allow proper visualization. Furthermore, scleral depression is necessary to permit an adequate view of these structures.

Uram[58] has coupled the technique of endoscopic visualization of ciliary processes with delivery of a diode laser. The combination endoscope–laser probe used for this procedure is a 20-gauge instrument that is inserted through the pars plana. With this method, he has been able to visualize ciliary processes clearly and to deliver laser energy directly to these structures with accuracy. He performed this procedure in 10 patients with neovascular glaucoma. Ninety to 180 degrees of the ciliary processes were treated. Over a mean follow-up period of 8.8 months, he achieved an average decrease in IOP of 28.3 mm Hg (mean preoperative IOP was 43.6 mm Hg; mean postoperative IOP was 15.3 mm Hg). No intraoperative complications were noted, and postoperative inflammation was not prominent.

Laser Bleb Revision and Remodeling

TREATMENT OF HYPOFUNCTIONING BLEBS

After filtration surgery, aqueous flow into the subconjunctival space must be established in the immediate postoperative period and maintained thereafter for adequate bleb development to occur and for continued bleb function. Inadequate aqueous flow can occur at any time after surgery and can lead to subsequent filter failure. This may be due to a variety of factors that result in occlusion of the sclerostomy, the formation of episcleral membranes, or the development of subconjunctival fibrosis.[59]

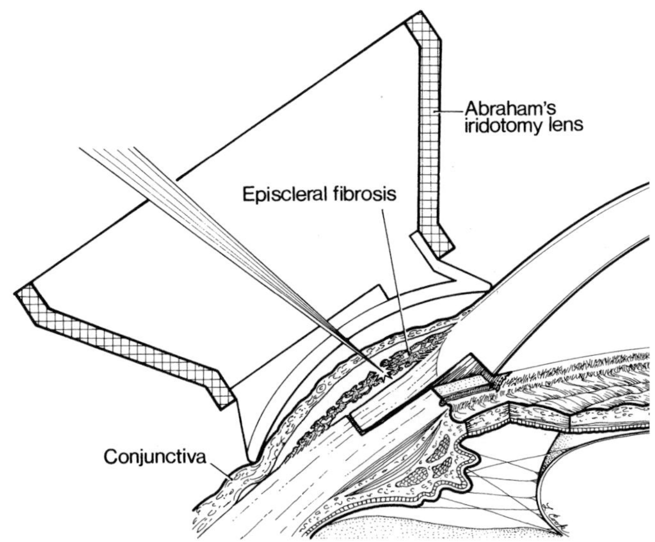

FIGURE 54–7. Sagittal section illustrating disruption of episcleral fibrotic tissue using the neodymium:yttrium-aluminum-garnet laser delivered transconjunctivally through an Abraham iridotomy lens. (From Latina MA, Rankin GA: Internal and transconjunctival Nd:YAG laser revision of late failing filters. Ophthalmology 98:215–221, 1991.)

The use of lasers to revise failed filtration sites provides the advantage of avoiding surgical entry into the eye. Revision of failed filters has been performed using argon and Q-switched Nd:YAG lasers delivered with the use of a slit lamp via ab interno and ab externo approaches. Q-switched Nd:YAG lasers are more versatile than argon lasers because they cut tissue by photodisruption and do not require chromophores for the absorption of laser energy.[59]

Latina and Rankin[60] have successfully utilized the Q-switched Nd:YAG laser for transconjunctival revision of filters that had failed owing to episcleral membrane formation or subconjunctival fibrosis. This technique is indicated if there is no internal obstruction, or if internal revision fails to reestablish adequate filtration. To conduct the procedure, one places an Abraham iridotomy lens over the bleb and focuses the laser on the obstruction to be disrupted (Fig. 54–7). A relatively transparent portion of the bleb is necessary to allow the laser to focus on the target subconjunctival tissues in the bleb. Using such a technique, the investigators reported lowering of IOP in all seven cases that they presented.

TREATMENT OF LARGE, OVERFUNCTIONING, LEAKING BLEBS

Functional filtering blebs are a desired result in glaucoma filtering surgery. However, if the blebs become extremely large, a variety of problems may arise. Relatively minor problems include foreign body sensation, dry eye, and difficulty with blinking. More serious complications, such as hypotony, dellen formation, bleb leak or rupture, and endophthalmitis may also develop, particularly if the bleb is thin-walled. Such blebs can be revised with the use of lasers.

Fink and coworkers[61] reported the use of the argon laser for the treatment of large filtering blebs in four patients. Methylene blue or rose bengal was applied over the surface of the bleb to act as a chromophore. The argon laser was then used to burn the surface until visible shrinkage was appreciated. All four patients developed a significant amount of bleb shrinkage accompanied by a rise in IOP. However, transient bleb leaks developed in two patients. This was attributed to overtreatment of thin areas of conjunctiva.

Lynch and associates[62] performed a clinical bleb-remodeling trial by using a CW Nd:YAG laser. Grid patterns of 30 to 40 spots were applied over large, overfiltering and leaking blebs. After laser treatment, most blebs became lower and thicker. An increase in IOP was also observed.

Conclusion

The tremendous advances in ophthalmic laser therapeutics are expected to continue, even if only a fraction of the techniques developed become feasible. Although these techniques may not totally supplant conventional surgical methods, they will definitely be welcome additions to our currently available surgical armamentarium.

REFERENCES

1. Wise JB, Witter SL: Argon laser therapy for open-angle glaucoma: A pilot study. Arch Ophthalmol 97:319–322, 1979.
2. Van Buskirk EM, Pond V, Rosenquist RC, Acott TS: Argon laser trabeculoplasty. Studies of mechanism of action. Ophthalmology 91:1005–1010, 1984.
3. Shingleton BJ, Richter CU, Bellows AK, et al: Long-term efficacy of argon laser trabeculoplasty. Ophthalmology 94:1513–1518, 1987.
4. Brancato R, Carassa R, Trabucci G: Diode laser compared with argon laser for trabeculoplasty. Am J Ophthalmol 112:50–55, 1991.
5. Englert JA, Cox TA, Allingham RR, Shields MB: Argon versus diode laser trabeculoplasty. Invest Ophthalmol Vis Sci 38 (Suppl):168, 1997.
6. Abreu MM, Massilon LJ, Sierra RA, Netland PA: Trabeculoplasty with frequency-doubled Nd:YAG laser versus argon laser in animal eyes. Invest Ophthalmol Vis Sci 38 (Suppl):168, 1997.
7. Latina MA, Park C: Selective targeting of trabecular meshwork cells: In vitro studies of pulsed and CW laser interactions. Exp Eye Res 60:359–371, 1995.
8. Latina, MA, Sibayan SA: In vivo selective targeting of trabecular meshwork cells by laser irradiation — A potential treatment for glaucoma. Invest Ophthalmol Vis Sci 37 (Suppl):408, 1996.
9. Latina MA, Sibayan SA, Shin DH, et al: Q-switched 532-nm Nd:YAG laser trabeculoplasty ("selective laser trabeculoplasty"): A multicenter clinical trial. Ophthalmology 105(11):2082–2090, 1998.
10. Grant WM: Further studies on facility of flow through the trabecular meshwork. Arch Ophthalmol 60:523–533, 1958.
11. Vogel M, Lauritzen K, Quentin C-D: Punktuelle Ablation des Trabekelwerks mit dem Exzimerlaser beim primären Offenwinkelglaukom (Targeted ablation of the trabecular meshwork with the excimer laser in primary open-angle glaucoma). Ophthalmologe 93:565–568, 1996.
12. Lauritzen K, Vogel M: Trabecular meshwork ablation with excimer laser — a new concept of therapy for glaucoma patients. Invest Ophthalmol Vis Sci 38 (Suppl):167, 1997.
13. Vivar A, Lowery J, Rostrepo OL, Simon G: A one-year follow-up clinical results following gonioscopic laser trabecular ablation (GLTA) with a Ti-sapphire laser for the treatment of glaucoma. Invest Ophthalmol Vis Sci 37 (Suppl):263, 1996.
14. Dietlein TS, Jacobi PC, Krieglstein GK: Experimental erbium:YAG laser photoablation on trabecular meshwork in rabbits. Invest Ophthalmol Vis Sci 37 (Suppl):260, 1996.
15. Jacobi PC, Dietlein TS, Krieglstein GK: Experimental microendoscopic photoablative laser goniotomy as a surgical model for the treatment of dysgenetic glaucoma. Graefes Arch Clin Exp Ophthalmol 234:670–676, 1996.
16. Shetlar DJ, Joos KM, Shen JH, Robinson RD: Endoscopic goniotomy with the free electron laser. Invest Ophthalmol Vis Sci 38 (Suppl):169, 1997.
17. Javitt JC, O'Connor SS, Wilson RP, Federman IL: Laser sclerostomy

ab interno using a continuous wave Nd:YAG laser. Ophthalmic Surg 20:552–556, 1989.
18. Wilson RP, Javitt JC: Ab interno laser sclerostomy in aphakic patients with glaucoma and chronic inflammation. Am J Ophthalmol 110:178–184, 1990.
19. Schuman JS, Stinson WG, Hutchinson T, et al: Holmium laser sclerectomy: Success and complications. Ophthalmology 100:1060–1065, 1993.
20. Iwach AG, Hoskins HD, Mora JS, et al: Update on the subconjunctival THC:YAG (holmium) laser sclerostomy ab externo clinical trial: A four-year report. Ophthalmic Surg Lasers 27:823–831, 1996.
21. McHam ML, Eisenberg DL, Schuman JS, Wang N: Erbium:YAG laser sclerectomy with a sapphire optical fiber. Ophthalmic Surg Lasers 28:55–58, 1997.
22. Jacobi PC, Dietlein TS, Krieglstein GK: Prospective study of ab externo erbium:YAG laser sclerostomy in humans. Am J Ophthalmol 123:478–486, 1997.
23. March WF, Gherezghiher T, Koss MC, Nordquist RE: Experimental YAG laser sclerostomy. Arch Ophthalmol 102:1834–1836, 1984.
24. Latina MA, Melamed S, March WF, et al: Gonioscopic ab-interno laser sclerostomy: A pilot study in glaucoma patients. Ophthalmology 99:1736–1744, 1992.
25. Berlin MS, Rajacich G, Duffy M, et al: Excimer laser photoablation in glaucoma filtering surgery. Am J Ophthalmol 103:713–714, 1987.
26. Karp CL, Higginbotham EJ, Edward DP, Musch DC: Diode laser surgery: Ab interno and ab externo versus conventional surgery in rabbits. Ophthalmology 100:1567–1573, 1993.
27. Van der Zypen E, England C, Frankhauser F, Kwasniewska S: Sklerostomie mit Hilfe verschiedener Lasermodalitäten. Klin Monatsbl Augenheilkd 204:427–429, 1994.
28. Van der Zypen E, England C, Frankhauser F, Kwasniewska S: Sclerostomy ab interno using long-wave laser modalities: Acute morphological effects. Ger J Ophthalmol 4:7–10, 1995.
29. Schmidt-Erfurth U, Wetzel W, Dröge G, Birngruber R: Mitomycin-C in laser sclerostomy: Benefit and complications. Ophthalmic Surg Lasers 28:14–20, 1997.
30. Pappas RM, Higginbotham EJ, Choe HS: Advances in laser sclerostomy: How far have we come? Ophthalmic Surg Lasers 28:751–757, 1997.
31. Chuck RS, Fischer H, Po S, et al: Optimization of dye-enhanced ab interno laser sclerostomy. Invest Ophthalmol Vis Sci 37 (Suppl):262, 1996.
32. Arya AV, Schuman JS, Scott W, et al: Indocyanine green enhanced pulsed diode laser sclerectomy. Invest Ophthalmol Vis Sci 37 (Suppl):260, 1996.
33. Krasnov MM: Externalization of Schlemm's canal (sinusotomy) in glaucoma. Br J Ophthalmol 52:157–161, 1968.
34. Seiler T, Kriegerowski M, Bende T, Wollensak J: Partielle externe Trabekulektomie. Klin Monatsbl Augenheilkd 195:216–220, 1989.
35. Kuwayama Y, Takagi T, Tanaka M, Takeuchi R: 193 nm excimer laser partial external trabeculectomy. Invest Ophthalmol Vis Sci 33 (Suppl):1017, 1992.
36. Bertagno R, Giordano G, Murialdo U, et al: Excimer laser photoablative filtration surgery: Histology and ultrastructure in 4 human cadaver eyes. Int Ophthalmol 18:159–161, 1994.
37. Campos M, Lee PP, Trokel SL, et al: Transconjunctival sinusotomy using the 193-nm excimer laser. Acta Ophthalmol 72:707–711, 1994.
38. Brooks AMV, Samuel M, Carroll N, et al: Excimer laser filtration surgery. Am J Ophthalmol 119:40–47, 1995.
39. Allan BDS, van Saarloos PP, Russo AV, et al: Excimer laser sclerostomy: The in vitro development of a modified open mask delivery system. Eye 7:47–52, 1993.
40. Allan BDS, van Saarloos PP, Cooper RL, et al: 193-nm Excimer laser sclerostomy using a modified open mask delivery system in rhesus monkeys with experimental glaucoma. Graefes Arch Clin Exp Ophthalmol 231:662–666, 1993.
41. Allan BDS, van Saarloos PP, Cooper RL, Constable IJ: 193 nm Excimer laser sclerostomy in pseudophakic patients with advanced open angle glaucoma. Br J Ophthalmol 78:199–205, 1994.
42. Weve H: Die Zyklodiathermie das Corpus ciliare bei Glaukom. Zentralbl Ophthalmol 29:562–569, 1933.
43. Bietti G: Surgical intervention on the ciliary body: New trends for the relief of glaucoma. JAMA 142:889–897, 1950.
44. Weekers R, Lavergne G, Watillion M, et al: Effects of photocoagulation of ciliary body upon ocular tension. Am J Ophthalmol 52:156–163, 1961.
45. Beckman H, Kinoshita A, Rota AN, Sugar HS: Transscleral ruby laser irradiation of the ciliary body in the treatment of intractable glaucoma. Trans Am Acad Ophthalmol Otolaryngol 76:423–436, 1972.
46. Beckman H, Sugar HS: Neodymium laser cyclocoagulation. Arch Ophthalmol 90:27–28, 1973.
47. Schuman JS, Bellows AR, Shingleton BJ, et al: Contact transscleral Nd:YAG laser cyclophotocoagulation: Midterm results. Ophthalmology 99:1089–1095, 1992.
48. Lee P-F, Pomerantzeff O: Transpupillary cyclophotocoagulation of rabbit eyes: An experimental approach to glaucoma surgery. Am J Ophthalmol 71:911–920, 1971.
49. Shields MB: Cyclodestructive surgery for glaucoma: Past, present and future. Trans Am Ophthalmol Soc 83:285–303, 1985.
50. Hennis HL, Stewart WC: Semiconductor diode laser transscleral cyclophotocoagulation in patients with glaucoma. Am J Ophthalmol 113:81–85, 1992.
51. Gaasterland DE, Pollack IP: Initial experience with a new method of laser transscleral cyclophotocoagulation for ciliary ablation in severe glaucoma. Trans Am Ophthalmol Soc 90:225–246, 1992.
52. Fisher AMR, Murphree AL, Gomer CJ: Clinical and preclinical photodynamic therapy. Lasers Surg Med 17:2–31, 1995.
53. Tsilimbaris MK, Naoumidi II, Naoumidis LP, et al: Transscleral ciliary body photodynamic therapy using phthalocyanine and a diode laser: Functional and morphologic implications in albino rabbits. Ophthalmic Surg Lasers 28:483–494, 1997.
54. Immonen IJR, Puska P, Raitta C: Transscleral contact krypton laser cyclophotocoagulation for treatment of glaucoma. Ophthalmology 101:876–882, 1994.
55. Immonen I, Viherkoski E, Peyman GA: Experimental retinal and ciliary body photocoagulation using a new 670-nm diode laser. Am J Ophthalmol 122:870–874, 1996.
56. Vogel A, Dlugos C, Nuffer R, Birngruber R: Optical properties of human sclera, and their consequences for transscleral laser applications. Lasers Surg Med 11:331–340, 1991.
57. Immonen I, Suomalainen V-P, Kivelä T, Viherkoski E: Energy levels needed for cyclophotocoagulation: A comparison of transscleral contact CW-YAG and krypton lasers in the rabbit eye. Ophthalmic Surg 24:530–533, 1993.
58. Uram M: Ophthalmic laser microendoscope ciliary process ablation in the management of neovascular glaucoma. Ophthalmology 99:1823–1828, 1992.
59. Latina MA, Shields SR: Laser revision of failing filters. Ophthalmol Clin North Am 6:437–447, 1993.
60. Latina MA, Rankin GA: Internal and transconjunctival neodymium:YAG laser revision of late failing filters. Ophthalmology 98:215–221, 1991.
61. Fink AJ, Boys-Smith JW, Brear R: Management of large filtering blebs with the argon laser. Am J Ophthalmol 101:695–699, 1986.
62. Lynch MG, Roesch M, Brown RH: Remodeling filtering blebs with the neodymium-YAG laser. Ophthalmology 103:1700–1705, 1996.

INDEX

Note: Page numbers in *italics* refer to illustrations; page numbers followed by t refer to tables.

C

D

E

G

L

M

N

O

Q

S

T

V

W

X